Essentials of Modern Neuroscience

Essentials of Modern Neuroscience

Editors

Franklin R. Amthor, PhD
Professor of Psychology
University of Alabama at Birmingham
Birmingham, Alabama

Anne B. Theibert, PhD
Professor of Neurobiology
University of Alabama at Birmingham
Birmingham, Alabama

David G. Standaert, MD, PhD
John N. Whitaker Professor and Chair
Department of Neurology
University of Alabama at Birmingham
Birmingham, Alabama

Erik D. Roberson, MD, PhD
Rebecca Gale Endowed Professor
Department of Neurology
University of Alabama at Birmingham
Birmingham, Alabama

New York   Chicago   San Francisco   Athens   London   Madrid   Mexico City
Milan   New Delhi   Singapore   Sydney   Toronto

Essentials of Modern Neuroscience

Copyright © 2020 by McGraw Hill. All rights reserved. Printed in China. Except as permitted under the United States Copyright Act of 1976, no part of this publication may be reproduced or distributed in any form or by any means, or stored in a data base or retrieval system, without the prior written permission of the publisher.

1 2 3 4 5 6 7 8 9   DSS   25 24 23 22 21 20

ISBN 978-0-07-184905-0
MHID 0-07-184905-X

This book was set in Minion Pro by Cenveo® Publisher Services.
The editors were Michael Weitz and Peter Boyle.
The production supervisor was Richard Ruzycka.
Project management was provided by Anupriya Tyagi, Cenveo Publisher Services.

This book is printed on acid-free paper.

Cataloging-in-publication data for this book is on file at the Library of Congress.

McGraw Hill books are available at special quantity discounts to use as premiums and sales promotions, or for use in corporate training programs. To contact a representative, please visit the Contact Us pages at www.mhprofessional.com.

Contents

About the Authors

Franklin R. Amthor, PhD, is a professor of Psychology at the University of Alabama at Birmingham (UAB). Dr. Amthor's research interests evolved from his undergraduate electrical engineering background at Cornell University into artificial intelligence simulations involving Perceptrons, and then visual neuroscience. His Ph.D. work was done at Duke University in Biomedical Engineering on quantitative analysis of retinal ganglion cell responses. He did a postdoctoral fellowship at the School of Optometry at UAB, and then was an NEI R01 funded principal investigator who led a team determining the relationship between mammalian ganglion cell physiology, morphology, and central projections. More recently, he has worked on retinal circuitry underlying the responses of different retinal ganglion cell classes, and on assistive devices for the blind.

Anne B. Theibert, PhD, is a professor of Neurobiology at the University of Alabama at Birmingham (UAB). Dr. Theibert is a researcher, teacher, and course director in both the UAB College of Arts and Sciences and School of Medicine (SoM). She received her B.A. in Chemistry from Goucher College, and Ph.D. in Biological Chemistry from Johns Hopkins University. Following a postdoctoral fellowship in the Neuroscience Department at Johns Hopkins, she was recruited to the SoM faculty at UAB in 1991, and directed an NIH-funded basic research program for 17 years, concentrating on cell signaling during neuronal development, with a focus on understanding pathways disrupted in neurodevelopmental disorders. In 2008, Dr. Theibert cofounded the UAB Undergraduate Neuroscience Program (UNP) and served as Director of the UNP during its first decade. She currently teaches neuroscience and nervous system development to UAB professional and graduate students, and directs and teaches undergraduate courses in cellular, molecular, systems and cognitive neuroscience.

David G. Standaert, MD, PhD, is a professor and chair of the Department of Neurology at the University of Alabama at Birmingham (UAB), where he holds the John N. Whitaker Endowed Chair in Neurology. He is a physician-scientist with interests in Parkinson disease and other disorders of movement. He received his A.B. with high honors from Harvard College, and M.D. and Ph.D. degrees from Washington University in St. Louis. He was a resident in neurology at the Hospital of the University of Pennsylvania, and a fellow in movement disorders at Massachusetts General Hospital. He joined the faculty of Harvard Medical School in 1995, and relocated to UAB in 2006. Currently he directs the NIH-funded Alabama Morris K. Udall Center of Excellence in Parkinson's Disease Research. He is Chairman of the Scientific Advisory Board of the American Parkinson Disease Association, Deputy Editor of the journal *Movement Disorders*, a Fellow of both the American Neurological Association and the American Academy of Neurology, a Councilor of the Association of University Professors of Neurology, and a member of the NIH/NINDS Board of Scientific Counselors. His lab has a long-standing interest in the basic mechanisms underlying Parkinson disease as well as the complications of therapy.

Erik D. Roberson, MD, PhD, is the Rebecca Gale endowed professor of Neurology and Neurobiology at the University of Alabama at Birmingham (UAB). Dr. Roberson is a physician-scientist whose research is dedicated to reducing the impact of age-related cognitive disorders. He received his A.B. with highest honors from Princeton University and then earned his M.D. and Ph.D. in neuroscience at Baylor College of Medicine. He was a resident and chief resident in neurology at the University of California San Francisco, where he also completed a clinical fellowship in behavioral neurology. In addition to his laboratory focused on understanding mechanisms and identifying new treatments for dementia, Dr. Roberson directs the Alzheimer's Disease Center and the Center for Neurodegeneration and Experimental Therapeutics at UAB. He also cares for patients in the UAB Memory Disorders Clinic and leads clinical trials testing new dementia treatments.

Contributors

Shruti P. Agnihotri, MD
Assistant Professor of Neurology
University of Alabama at Birmingham
Birmingham, Alabama
Chapter 32

Rachel C. Besing, PhD
Assistant Professor of Psychology
Brescia University
Owensboro, Kentucky
Chapter 23

Stephen Brackett, MD
Clinical Assistant Professor of Psychiatry
University of Alabama at Birmingham
Birmingham, Alabama
Chapter 43

Yoon-Hee Cha, MD
Associate Professor of Neurology
University of Minnesota
Minneapolis, Minnesota
Chapter 36

Christopher M. Ciarleglio, PhD
Chair of Science and Director of the Advanced
    Science Academy
Morris Catholic High School
Denville, New Jersey
Chapter 23

Karen Cropsey, PsyD
Professor of Psychiatry
University of Alabama at Birmingham
Birmingham, Alabama
Chapter 43

Joseph T. Daley, MD
Associate Professor of Neurology
University of Alabama at Birmingham
Birmingham, Alabama
Chapter 34

Lindsey Elliott, PhD
Graduate Student
University of Alabama at Birmingham
Birmingham, Alabama
Chapter 41

Aaron D. Fobian, PhD
Assistant Professor of Psychiatry
University of Alabama at Birmingham
Birmingham, Alabama
Chapter 41

Karen L. Gamble, PhD
Associate Professor of Psychiatry
University of Alabama at Birmingham
Birmingham, Alabama
Chapter 23

Cristin F. Gavin, PhD
Assistant Professor of Neurobiology
University of Alabama at Birmingham
Birmingham, Alabama
Chapters 10 & 20

Merida Grant, PhD
Associate Professor of Psychiatry
University of Alabama at Birmingham
Birmingham, Alabama
Chapter 42

Rabia Jamy, MD
Neurology Resident
University of Alabama at Birmingham
Birmingham, Alabama
Chapter 29

Mohamed Kazamel, MD
Assistant Professor of Neurology
University of Alabama at Birmingham
Birmingham, Alabama
Chapter 31

Nina Kraguljac, MD
Assistant Professor of Psychiatry
University of Alabama at Birmingham
Birmingham, Alabama
Chapter 38

Robin A.J. Lester, PhD
Professor of Neurobiology
University of Alabama at Birmingham
Birmingham, Alabama
Chapter 5

Li Li, MD, PhD
Associate Professor of Psychiatry
University of Alabama at Birmingham
Birmingham, Alabama
Chapter 39

Michael Lyerly, MD
Associate Professor of Neurology
University of Alabama at Birmingham
Birmingham, Alabama
Chapter 24

Lydia Marcus, MD
Assistant Professor of Pediatrics
University of Alabama at Birmingham
Birmingham, Alabama
Chapter 35

Jesse Tobias C. Martinez, Jr., MD
Assistant Professor of Psychiatry
University of Alabama at Birmingham
Birmingham, Alabama
Chapter 40

William Meador, MD
Associate Professor of Neurology
University of Alabama at Birmingham
Birmingham, Alabama
Chapter 30

Daniel Mirman, PhD
Senior Lecturer
The University of Edinburgh
Edinburgh, United Kingdom
Chapter 21

Marissa C. Natelson Love, MD
Assistant Professor of Neurology
University of Alabama at Birmingham
Birmingham, Alabama
Chapter 29

Lucas Pozzo-Miller, PhD
Professor of Neurobiology
University of Alabama at Birmingham
Birmingham, Alabama
Chapter 2

Brian Samuels, MD, PhD
Associate Professor of Ophthalmology
University of Alabama at Birmingham
Birmingham, Alabama
Chapter 37

Samantha Schiavon, MA
Graduate Student
University of Alabama at Birmingham
Birmingham, Alabama
Chapter 43

Angela Hays Shapshak, MD
Associate Professor of Neurology
University of Alabama at Birmingham
Birmingham, Alabama
Chapter 33

Michelle Sisson, MA
Graduate Student
University of Alabama at Birmingham
Birmingham, Alabama
Chapter 43

Robert E. Sorge, PhD
Associate Professor of Psychology
School of Medicine
University of Alabama at Birmingham
Birmingham, Alabama
Chapter 15

Victor W. Sung, MD
Associate Professor of Neurology
University of Alabama at Birmingham
Birmingham, Alabama
Chapter 28

Ashley Thomas, MD
Associate Professor of Neurology
University of Alabama at Birmingham
Birmingham, Alabama
Chapter 27

Stacie K. Totsch, PhD
Division of Pediatric Hematology and Oncology
Department of Pediatrics
University of Alabama at Birmingham
Birmingham, Alabama
Chapter 15

Paula Warren, MD
Neurooncologist
Hattiesburg Clinic
Hattiesburg, Mississippi
Chapter 25

Cristina Wohlgehagen, MD
Headache Specialist and Founder
International Headache Center
Dallas, Texas
Chapter 26

Yesie Yoon, MD
Assistant Professor of Psychiatry
University of Alabama at Birmingham
Birmingham, Alabama
Chapter 44

Preface

Why does the world need another neuroscience text? Students study neuroscience for a variety of purposes that range from molecular basic science, to systems, to clinical. Although there are many neuroscience texts that cover some of these areas well, few attempt to cover the entire range. Moreover, texts that attempt to cover such a broad range of neuroscience content are often too large to be tractable, or differentiate poorly between basic science and clinical sections.

Essentials of Modern Neuroscience has been written for students in the medical and other health professions with the goal of being accessible, coherently organized, and universal in its coverage of basic science and clinical neuroscience. It is thus divided into two main parts, the first being a thorough treatment of the basic science of the anatomy and function of the nervous system, and the second comprising an extended treatment of nervous system disorders and therapeutics.

Part I, Anatomy & Function of the Nervous System, was written with two goals: (1) It stands alone as a concise introductory text for neuroscience, and could be used as such, and (2) its organization allows it to be used as a good reference for the clinical sections when basic science background is needed. Section I gives a systematic explanation of the layout of the central and peripheral nervous systems, concentrating on their role in nervous system function. Section II then covers modern molecular neuroscience, starting with a complete treatment of the cellular biophysics underlying the resting and action potentials, then covering synaptic transmission, neurotransmitter systems, and synaptic plasticity. Section III, Systems Neuroscience: Sensory & Motor Systems, considers all the sensory systems from transduction to central processing.

It then moves to motor systems, covering the pyramidal and extrapyramidal cortical-spinal pathways, and then the autonomic and enteric nervous systems. Section IV is Cognitive Neuroscience, investigating the neural basis of consciousness, learning and memory, language, emotion, and circadian rhythms.

Part II, Nervous System Disorders & Therapeutics, introduces students to the major disorders of the nervous system and commonly used therapeutics, building on the foundation laid down in Part I, and is organized by clinical specialty. Section V is comprised of 12 chapters surveying disorders treated by neurologists and neurosurgeons. Section VI covers otological, vestibular, and ophthalmological disorders. Finally, Section VII covers the world of psychiatric disorders with seven chapters ranging from thought and mood disorders to addiction and functional disorders. Written by clinicians, the chapters of Part II are intended to prepare students for initial clinical encounters in each of these specialty areas. Each chapter begins with a description of disease prevalence and burden to help students understand which disorders they are most likely to encounter and which have the biggest impact. Discussions of the diagnosis, key features, and treatment of these disorders are aimed at preparing students for board-type examinations. Case studies help consolidate the presentation of classic diseases.

Acknowledgment

F.R.A. would like to thank Prof. Karlene Ball, chair of the UAB Psychology Dept. while the book was being written, who supported F.R.A.'s academic efforts.

PART I
ANATOMY & FUNCTION OF THE NERVOUS SYSTEM

SECTION I

Organization & Structure of the Nervous System

Organization & Cells of the Nervous System

Anne B. Theibert

OBJECTIVES

After studying this chapter, the student should be able to:

- Outline the major anatomic components of the central nervous system (CNS) and peripheral nervous system (PNS).
- Diagram the functional areas of the brain and spinal cord.
- Describe the types of nerves and ganglia in the PNS and their structure.
- Distinguish the different categories of neurons.
- Identify the neuronal organelles and their biochemical functions.
- Diagram the specialized neuronal processes and their functions.
- Describe the main CNS and PNS glial cells and their functions.

OVERVIEW: THE NERVOUS SYSTEM

The nervous system mediates a wide range of functions, from detection of environmental stimuli, to control of muscle contraction, to problem solving, language, and memory. The nervous system is divided into 2 main parts, the central nervous system (CNS) and the peripheral nervous system (PNS) (Figures 1–1 and 1–2). Anatomically, the CNS is divided into the brain and spinal cord, whereas the PNS is composed of ganglia and nerves, including cranial and spinal nerves and their branches. Functionally, the PNS can be divided into the somatic, autonomic (visceral), and enteric nervous systems. In the overall flow of information, the PNS detects and relays sensory information about the external and internal environments to the CNS. The CNS receives, integrates, and stores information and controls the output to the PNS to generate responses and behavior.

At the cellular level, the nervous system is composed of neurons and glial cells (Figure 1–3). Neurons (also called nerve cells or neuronal cells) are the main signaling cells that communicate with other neurons, muscles, or glands. Neurons can be categorized by their function as sensory neurons, motor neurons, or interneurons or by their morphology or neurotransmitter. Glial cells (also called neuroglia or glia) are the support cells in the nervous system. Astrocytes and satellite cells provide structural and metabolic support, oligodendrocytes and Schwann cells furnish myelination of axons,

pericytes regulate capillaries, ependymal cells synthesize cerebrospinal fluid (CSF), microglia are immune cells, and enteric glia are part of the gastrointestinal (GI) tract. Neurons have a cell body where the nucleus and majority of cellular organelles are located and many biochemical activities occur. Neurons also contain specialized processes and regions that allow them to send and receive signals rapidly and precisely. The axon is a process by which electrical signals are conducted and where signals are sent to other neurons or target cells. The dendrites are branched processes that receive signals from other neurons. The synapse is a structure where signals are transmitted, via synaptic transmission, from the axon to its target. Neurons can receive thousands of synaptic inputs, can form neural circuits, and function in networks that underlie sensations, cognitive functions, and the generation of responses and behavior.

CNS COMPONENTS, COVERINGS, & VASCULATURE

The brain and spinal cord compose the CNS. The brain is enclosed within the cranial cavity and is protected by the cranium (skull) and meninges (Figure 1–4). The meninges are a 3-membrane system that covers, protects, and nourishes the brain and spinal cord. The outer dura mater is a thick tough membrane that is connected to the cranium and protects the brain. The middle membrane, called the arachnoid mater,

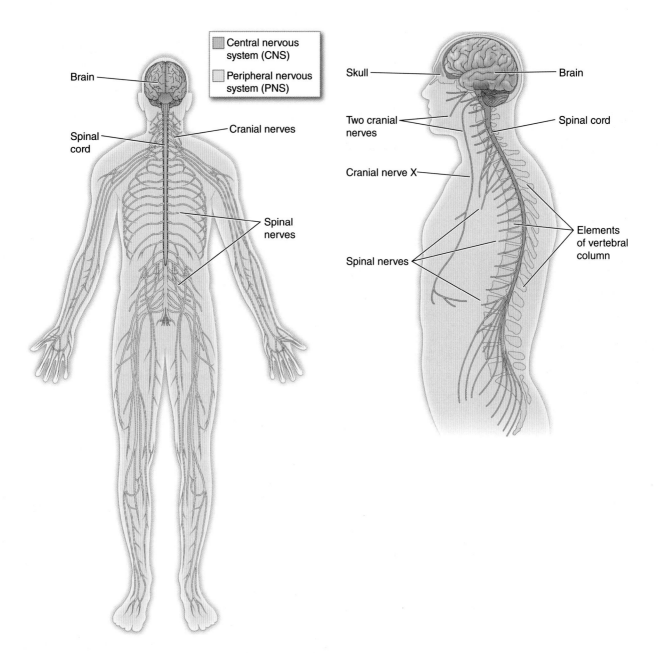

FIGURE 1-1 Anatomic divisions of the nervous system and their structures: CNS and PNS. Forming the CNS, the brain (encased in the skull) is continuous with the spinal cord (encased in the spinal column). Forming the PNS, cranial nerves emerge from the brainstem, while spinal nerves emerge from the spinal cord. In the PNS, nerves are associated with spinal, cranial or autonomic ganglia, which are not shown.

cushions the brain. Below the arachnoid is the subarachnoid space, which contains CSF and where specialized regions called arachnoid granulations resorb CSF. The innermost layer, the pia mater, is a thin layer that adheres to the surface of the brain and follows its contours, forming a barrier but with many capillaries that nourish the brain and spinal cord.

The brain has 3 main regions: the forebrain, brainstem, and cerebellum. The inner spaces of these regions form the ventricles, which produce and circulate CSF and are connected to form the ventricular system (Figure 1–5). Both the meninges and brain are highly vascularized. Two main pairs of arteries supply blood to the brain (Figure 1–6). The internal

carotid arteries, which are branches from the common carotid artery, supply the anterior brain, whereas the vertebral arteries, which are branches from the subclavian artery, supply the posterior brain and brainstem. The main venous blood outflow from the brain is via the jugular veins.

CNS capillaries are specialized in that their vascular endothelial cells form tight junctions and are enveloped in glial cells, together producing the blood–brain barrier (BBB). The BBB is a selective permeability barrier that prevents the direct movement of unwanted molecules, immune cells, and pathogens into the brain. The BBB allows the passage of water, oxygen, carbon dioxide, and lipid-soluble molecules, including

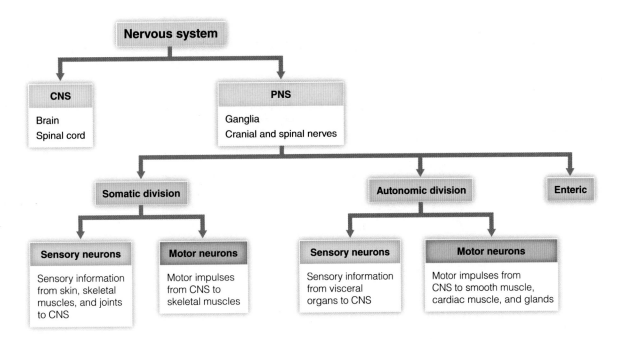

FIGURE 1-2 Functional divisions of the nervous system: CNS and PNS.

steroid hormones, by passive diffusion. Astrocytes selectively transport ions and molecules such as glucose and amino acids and release them into the extracellular fluid to supply neurons and other glia with essential nutrients.

BASIC BRAIN ANATOMY

The forebrain is the largest part of the brain and contains the cerebrum and diencephalon (Figure 1–7). The cerebrum is formed by the large left and right cerebral hemispheres, which are separated by the medial longitudinal fissure, and contains the outer cerebral cortex, inner cerebral white matter, and subcortical nuclei. The cerebrum encloses the lateral ventricles and overlies the diencephalon, a structure that contains the thalamus and hypothalamus and that surrounds the third ventricle. Functionally, the forebrain is involved in receiving sensory information from the PNS and generating outgoing motor information, and is where executive and cognitive functions are generated. The oldest part of the brain, the brainstem, is composed of the midbrain, pons, and medulla and serves to relay information from the spinal cord and cerebellum to the forebrain and vice versa. In addition, the brainstem regulates vital functions, such as breathing, consciousness, and control of body temperature. The cerebral aqueduct and fourth ventricle lie inside the brainstem. Connected to the pons, the cerebellum forms the posterior-most region of the brain and is involved in control and coordination of movement and some cognitive tasks.

Examination of postmortem fixed brain tissue reveals that each of these brain regions contains gray and white matter areas (Figure 1–8). In living tissue, gray matter appears pinkish light brown. Gray matter contains mainly neuronal cell bodies, their dendrites, and associated glial cells. In the brain, 2 types of gray matter are present. Cortical gray matter forms the outer regions of the cerebrum and cerebellum and is distinguished by its layered organization of neurons. The other type of gray matter is called a nucleus, an aggregate of cell bodies with similar morphology and function found below the cortex (subcortical nuclei) and in the brainstem and cerebellum. White matter contains predominantly myelinated axons (which, because of their fatty rich myelin membrane, produce the white appearance) and white matter glial cells. White matter contains bundles of myelinated axons that are referred to as tracts in the CNS. In the brain, the white matter tracts include projection tracts that connect neurons in the forebrain to neurons in the brainstem or spinal cord, association tracts that connect one cortical region to another, and commissural tracts, which connect areas from one side of the brain to the other.

The exterior surface of the cerebrum is distinguished by many gyri (singular: gyrus) and sulci (singular: sulcus) that produce the characteristic folded appearance of the human and many mammalian brains. A sulcus is a groove or furrow in the cerebral cortex, whereas a gyrus is a crest or ridge. The folding created by gyri and sulci facilitates a larger surface area of cerebral cortex to fit inside the skull. Deep sulci separate the cortex into 4 cortical lobes on each side, called the frontal, parietal, temporal, and occipital lobes, named for the cranial bones that overlie each (Figure 1–9). The central sulcus forms the division between the frontal and parietal lobe. The lateral sulcus (also called the Sylvian fissure) separates the temporal lobe from the frontal and parietal lobes. The parieto-occipital sulcus forms the boundary between the parietal and occipital lobes. Many additional sulci and gyri are present in the

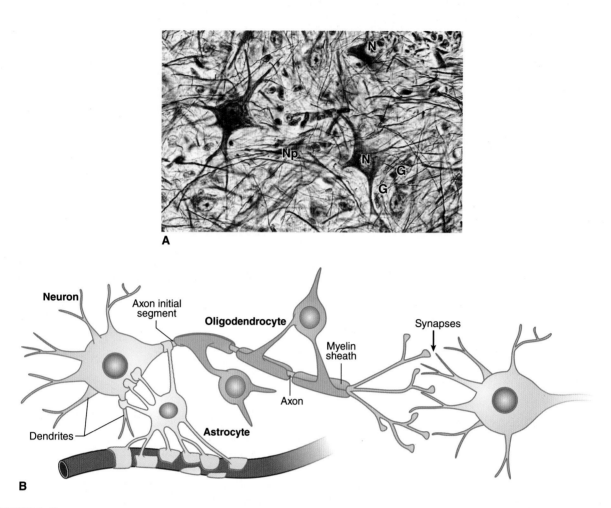

FIGURE 1–3 Cellular components of the nervous system. **A.** Micrograph showing neuronal cell bodies (N) and smaller glial (G) cells that surround them in the CNS. Use of a hematoxylin stain with gold chloride shows the neuropil (Np), which is the dense network of axons and dendrites. **B.** Neurons and glia in the CNS. A typical projection/principal interneuron has a cell body (or soma), multiple dendrites, which receive synaptic responses, and an axon, which sends electrical signals and is insulated by a myelin sheath derived from specialized membrane processes of oligodendrocytes. Astrocytes perform supportive roles in the CNS, and their processes are closely associated with neuronal synapses and capillaries. (Part A, reproduced with permission from Young B, Heath JW: *Wheater's Functional Histology: A Text and Colour Atlas*. Edinburgh: Churchill Livingstone; 2000; part B, reproduced with permission from Katzung BG: *Basic & Clinical Pharmacology*, 14th ed. New York, NY: McGraw Hill; 2018.)

cerebral cortex, with all cortical gyri and sulci containing an outer layer of cortical gray matter and a thin layer of underlying white matter. Each of the 4 main lobes contains distinct anatomic and functional areas.

BASIC SPINAL CORD ANATOMY

The spinal cord emerges caudally from the brainstem, within the spinal canal, and is protected by the vertebral column (also called the spine) and meninges (Figure 1–10). Along their length, the vertebral column and spinal cord inside are separated into 5 regions, called cervical, thoracic, lumbar, sacral, and coccygeal segments. Similar to the brain, the spinal cord is composed of gray and white matter regions but with an opposite organization. Spinal gray matter, composed of neuronal cell bodies, dendrites, and glia, is located medially and is surrounded by spinal white matter, which contains tracts and glia, located in the lateral areas of the spinal cord. The gray matter surrounds the inner central

canal, which provides CSF to the spinal cord. Spinal gray matter is separated anatomically and functionally into dorsal (posterior) and ventral (anterior) horns on each side. Sensory information is carried by afferent axons of spinal nerves, which enter the cord via the dorsal roots. These sensory axons branch, and one branch can synapse on interneurons in the dorsal horn, whereas the other branch can ascend to the brain. These axons form the ascending tracts in the spinal cord. Descending tracts in the white matter provide outgoing motor information from the cerebrum or brainstem. The axons in the descending tracts synapse on motor neuron cell bodies in the ventral/anterior horns. The ventral horn motor neurons extend their axons out of the cord via the ventral root, and their axons form the motor components of the spinal nerves. Because the lower motor neurons cell bodies lie in the spinal cord, while their axons form the motor components of the spinal nerves, they are considered part of both the CNS and PNS. The anatomy of the brain and spinal cord is described in greater detail in Chapter 3.

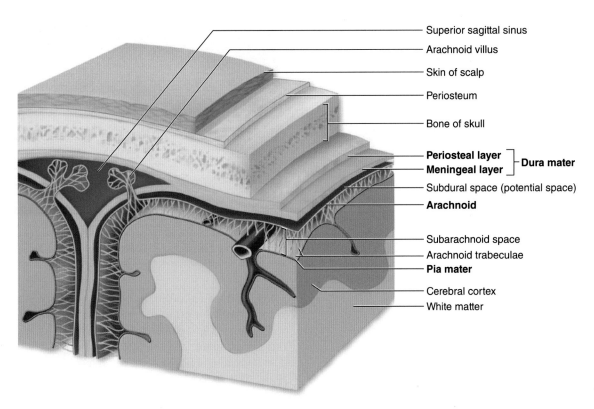

Superior sagittal sinus
Arachnoid villus
Skin of scalp
Periosteum
Bone of skull
Periosteal layer ⎤
Meningeal layer ⎦ **Dura mater**
Subdural space (potential space)
Arachnoid
Subarachnoid space
Arachnoid trabeculae
Pia mater
Cerebral cortex
White matter

FIGURE 1-4 Meninges around the brain. Composed of the dura mater, arachnoid mater, and pia mater, the meninges form a membrane system that surrounds the brain and the spinal cord. The diagram also show the subarachnoid space filled with cerebrospinal fluid (CSF), and arachnoid villi, which function to resorb CSF and transfer it into the blood. (Reproduced with permission from McKinley MP, O'Loughlin VD, Bidle TS. *Anatomy and Physiology: An Integrative Approach.* New York, NY: McGraw Hill; 2013.)

PNS: FUNCTIONAL DIVISIONS

The PNS has 3 functional divisions: the somatic, autonomic (also called visceral), and enteric nervous systems. The somatic nervous system mediates conscious/voluntary movement via regulation of skeletal muscle contraction and provides sensory information from the skin, muscles, and joints. The autonomic nervous system involves unconscious/involuntary control of cardiac muscle, smooth muscle, and glands. Its sensory

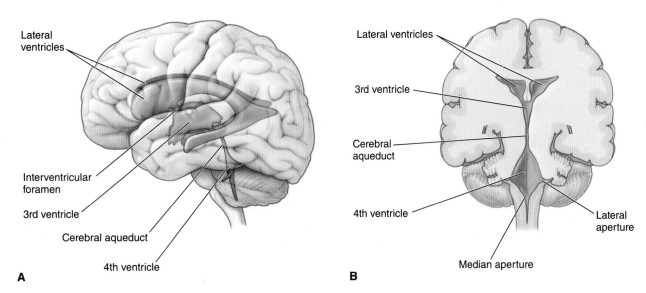

Lateral ventricles
Interventricular foramen
3rd ventricle
Cerebral aqueduct
4th ventricle

A

Lateral ventricles
3rd ventricle
Cerebral aqueduct
4th ventricle
Median aperture
Lateral aperture

B

FIGURE 1-5 The ventricular system. **A.** Three-dimensional lateral view of the ventricles of the brain. **B.** Coronal section of the brain showing the ventricles. The ventricles are lined with ependymal cells, and contain the choroid plexus, which synthesize cerebrospinal fluid (CSF). The two lateral ventricles lie within the left and right cerebrum, the third ventricle (between the halves of the diencephalon), the cerebral aqueduct, and the fourth ventricle within the brainstem. (Reproduced with permission from Morton DA, Foreman KB, Albertine KH. *The Big Picture: Gross Anatomy,* 2nd ed. New York, NY: McGraw Hill; 2019.)

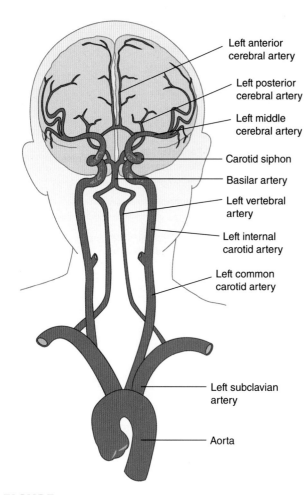

FIGURE 1–6 Blood supply to the brain and the major cerebral arteries. Arterial blood for the brain enters the cranial cavity by way of two pairs of large vessels. The pair of internal carotid arteries supplies arterial blood to most of the forebrain while the pair of vertebral arteries supplies the brainstem, cerebellum, occipital lobe, and parts of the thalamus. (Reproduced with permission from Waxman SG. *Clinical Neuroanatomy,* 28th ed. New York, NY: McGraw Hill; 2017.)

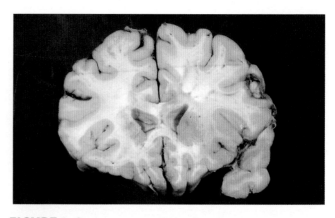

FIGURE 1–8 Brain gray and white matter areas. Coronal section from postmortem human brain. (Reproduced with permission from Kemp WL, Burns DK, Travis Brown TG. *Pathology: The Big Picture.* New York, NY: McGraw Hill; 2008.)

component, often called the visceral sensory system, provides information from the viscera, the internal organs, and vasculature. The autonomic motor system is divided into the sympathetic and parasympathetic nervous systems. The sympathetic nervous system, referred to as the "fight or flight" system, is activated under conditions requiring mobilization of energy. The parasympathetic nervous system, referred to as the "rest and digest" or "feed and breed" system, is activated when organisms are in a relaxed state. The enteric nervous system, which is also under involuntary control, governs the GI system. Although it receives considerable input from the autonomic nervous system, the enteric nervous system can function independently and is considered a separate system in the PNS.

PNS: ANATOMIC COMPONENTS

Anatomically, the PNS is composed of ganglia and nerves. Ganglia are clusters of functionally related neuronal cell bodies and their accompanying glial cells in the PNS.

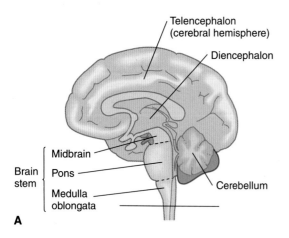

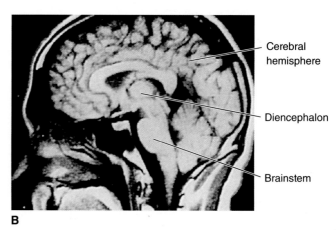

FIGURE 1–7 Major anatomic divisions of the brain. **A.** Illustration of the midsagittal plane. **B.** Magnetic resonance image of a midsagittal section through the head. (Reproduced with permission from Waxman SG. *Clinical Neuroanatomy,* 28th ed. New York, NY: McGraw Hill; 2017.)

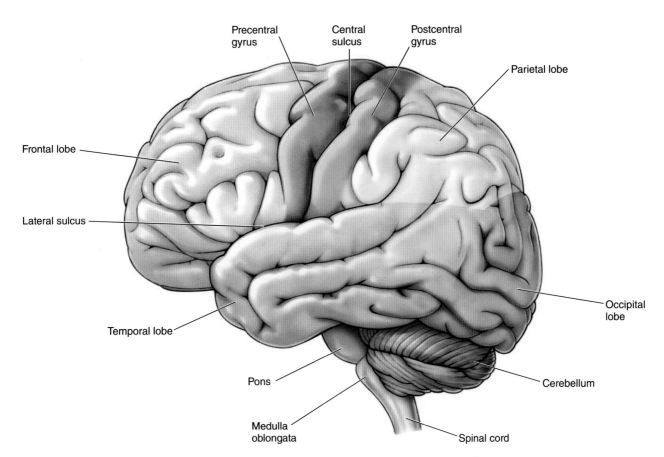

FIGURE 1–9 Lateral view of the brain. This view illustrates the left cerebral hemisphere with its major sulci and gyri, cortical areas, and several subcortical structures. (Reproduced with permission from Morton DA, Foreman KB, Albertine KH. *The Big Picture: Gross Anatomy,* 2nd ed. New York, NY: McGraw Hill; 2019.)

Cell bodies of somatic sensory neurons form the dorsal root ganglia, whereas cell bodies of autonomic neurons form the sympathetic and parasympathetic ganglia. The sympathetic ganglia lie outside of but close to the spinal cord and communicate to form the sympathetic chain. The parasympathetic ganglia in the body lie close to the organ they innervate. The cranial ganglia contain parasympathetic or sensory cell bodies.

Nerves are bundles of axons ensheathed in connective tissue that innervate all parts of the body, sending messages to and receiving messages from the CNS (Figure 1–11). The neuronal cell bodies that give rise to nerves do not lie within the nerves themselves. Rather, their cell bodies reside within the brain, spinal cord, or ganglia. Nerves can contain both efferent and afferent axons. Efferent axons transmit motor signals from the CNS to the PNS and can be somatic or autonomic. Afferent axons transmit sensory signals from the PNS to the CNS; afferents can be somatic or visceral. Afferent and efferent axons are protected by several layers of connective tissue, which together with glia and blood vessels form nerves.

Spinal and cranial nerves supply input to and output from the CNS. There are 31 pairs of spinal nerves, which emerge from and travel to the spinal cord and which are named for the spinal cord segment to which they connect (Figure 1–11).

Spinal nerves are mixed nerves, containing both motor efferents and sensory afferents and containing both somatic and autonomic components. As they leave or enter the spinal cord, the afferents from the dorsal root and efferents from the ventral root bundle together, but then branch to form the rami (singular: ramus). The gray and white rami contain autonomic components, whereas the dorsal/posterior and ventral/anterior rami contain both somatic and autonomic components. Some rami form a nerve plexus, a network of interconnecting nerves. In the somatic motor system, axons emerge from lower motor neurons in the spinal cord, travel in the spinal nerves, and directly innervate skeletal muscles. In the autonomic nervous system, motor neurons in the spinal cord (called preganglionic neurons) send their axons to synapse onto a postganglionic neuron (whose cell bodies lie in the autonomic ganglia), which then send axons to innervate the target organ. Some nerve components form large distinctive bundles or branches and are referred to by their specific names, such as the splanchnic nerves or sciatic nerve.

Sensory and motor information for the head and neck (and several other parts of the body) is supplied by the 12 pairs of cranial nerves. The majority (10 of 12) of the cranial nerves are part of the PNS, with their cranial nerve nuclei located in the brainstem and nerves traveling outside the CNS.

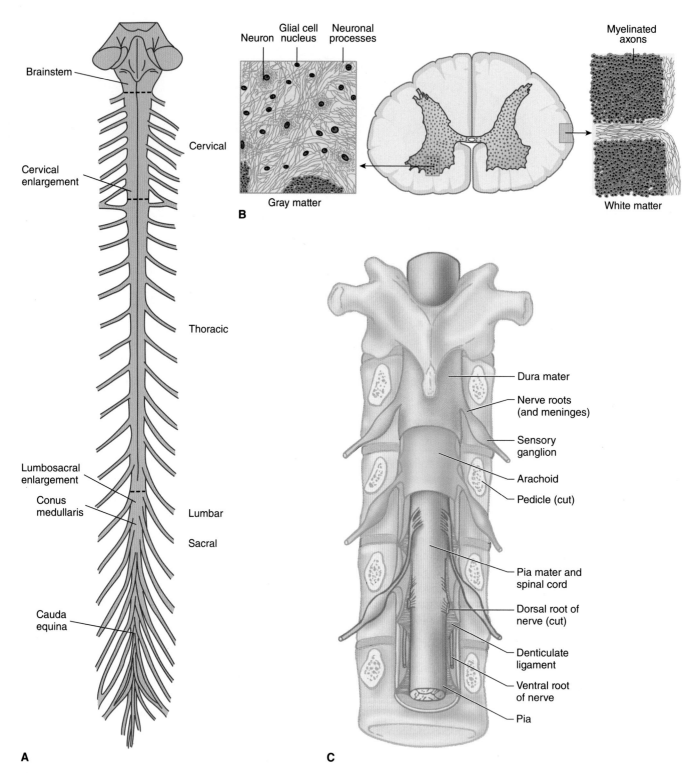

FIGURE 1–10 Spinal cord anatomy. **A.** Schematic dorsal view of an isolated spinal cord and proximal regions of spinal nerves, indicating the major anatomic regions along the cord. **B.** Cross section through the spinal cord, showing gray matter (which contains neuronal and glial cell bodies, axons, dendrites, and synapses) and white matter (which contains myelinated axons and associated glial cells). Spinal gray matter is called the dorsal and ventral horns. Spinal cord white matter contains ascending and descending tracts. **C.** Dorsal view of the spinal cord showing the three meninges membranes and part of the vertebrae. The spinal nerves emerge from the ventral roots and enter via the dorsal roots. The spinal (dorsal root) ganglia that contain the sensory neuron cell bodies are shown. (Part A, reproduced with permission from Waxman SG. *Clinical Neuroanatomy,* 28th ed. New York, NY: McGraw Hill; 2017; part B, reproduced with permission from Junqueira LC, Carneiro J, Kelley RO: *Basic Histology: Text & Atlas.* 11th ed. McGraw Hill, 2005; part C, reproduced with permission from Butterworth JF, Mackey DC, Wasnick JD. *Morgan and Mikhail's Clinical Anesthesiology,* 5th ed. New York, NY: McGraw Hill; 2013.)

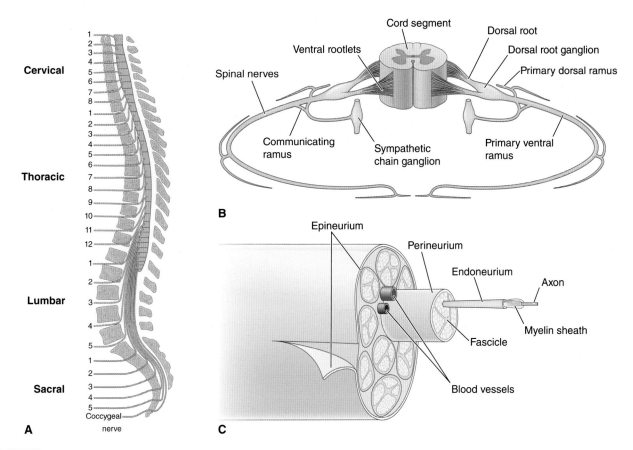

FIGURE 1–11 Spinal cord, vertebral column, and spinal nerve organization. **A.** Schematic view of the spinal cord, vertebral column, and spinal nerves along the anterior-posterior axis. **B.** Spinal nerves emerge from and enter into the spinal cord. Motor axons (from both somatic and autonomic motor neurons) emerge via the ventral roots while sensory axons (from both somatic and visceral sensory neurons) enter into the cord via the dorsal roots. After a spinal nerve forms from the dorsal and ventral roots, it branches into the dorsal ramus and ventral ramus. The spinal (dorsal root) ganglia contain cell bodies of somatic sensory neurons, and lie adjacent to the cord. Autonomic ganglia are not shown. **C.** Nerves contain myelinated axons, unmyelinated axons, the myelinating Schwann cells (not shown), and blood vessels. Nerve components are ensheathed in layers of connective tissue called the endoneurium, perineurium, and epineurium.

Two cranial nerves, the olfactory nerve (CN I) and the optic nerve (CN II), are CNS nerves because they emerge from the cranium and travel within the CNS. Many of the cranial nerves are mixed, with both somatic and autonomic efferents and afferents, but a few are dedicated to either motor or sensory functions. Cranial nerves with sensory or parasympathetic components have associated ganglia, which lie just outside of the brainstem. Furthermore, sensory afferents can mediate both general, somatic sensations, such as touch, pain, and temperature, and special sensations, such as taste, hearing, vision, and smell.

FUNCTIONAL CATEGORIES OF NEURONS

The 2 main cellular components of the nervous system are neurons and glial cells. In addition, the CNS and PNS are highly vascularized and contain numerous blood vessel cells. However, because vascular endothelial and smooth muscle cells derive from mesoderm and are also found outside the nervous system, they are not considered cells of the nervous system. The brain is estimated to contain approximately 86 billion neurons and about the same number of or more glial cells.

Neurons are signaling cells that transmit electrical and chemical signals. The vast majority of neurons are electrically excitable, meaning they can produce and conduct action potentials (Figure 1–12). Most neurons function as part of neuronal circuits. Neurons are distinguished from other cells by a variety of features. Morphologically, they extend specialized membrane processes including axons (for sending information), dendrites and small protrusions called dendritic spines (for receiving information), and membrane subdomains called synapses (where information is transformed and transferred from the axon to the receiving cell). Biochemically, neurons synthesize, package, and release neurotransmitters. Physiologically, they produce and conduct action potentials along the axon and graded potentials along the dendrites and cell bodies, and their receptors can detect different forms of energy, such as light and sound waves, and convert those into electrical or chemical signals. Each of these specialized functions ensures that neurons communicate specifically and rapidly with their targets.

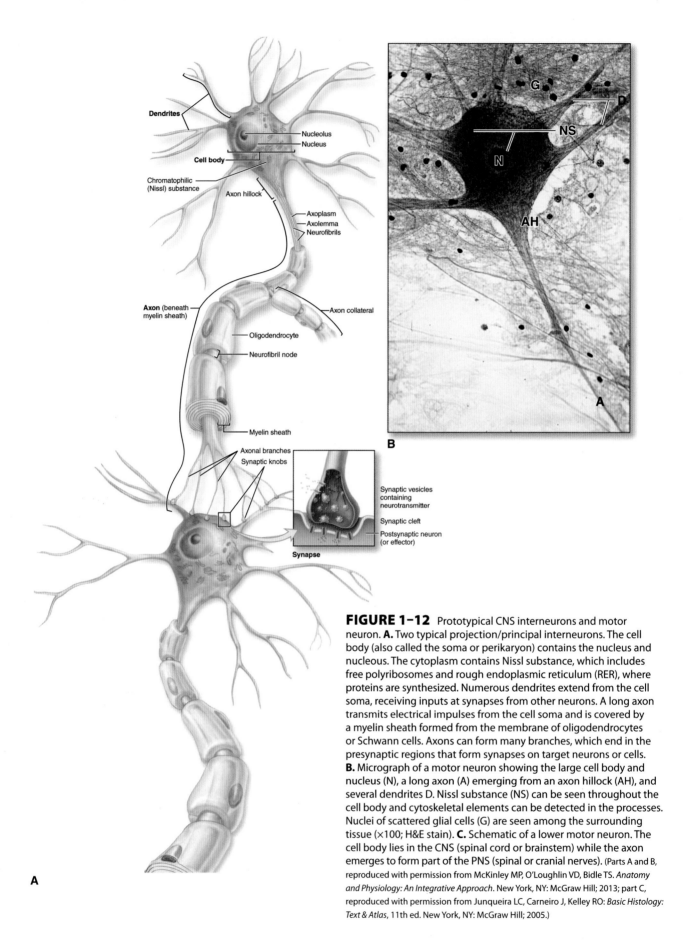

Dendrites

Nucleolus
Nucleus

Cell body

Chromatophilic
(Nissl) substance

Axon hillock

Axoplasm
Axolemma
Neurofibrils

Axon (beneath
myelin sheath)

Axon collateral

Oligodendrocyte

Neurofibril node

Myelin sheath

Axonal branches
Synaptic knobs

Synaptic vesicles
containing
neurotransmitter
Synaptic cleft
Postsynaptic neuron
(or effector)

Synapse

A

B

G

D

NS

N

AH

A

FIGURE 1–12 Prototypical CNS interneurons and motor neuron. **A.** Two typical projection/principal interneurons. The cell body (also called the soma or perikaryon) contains the nucleus and nucleous. The cytoplasm contains Nissl substance, which includes free polyribosomes and rough endoplasmic reticulum (RER), where proteins are synthesized. Numerous dendrites extend from the cell soma, receiving inputs at synapses from other neurons. A long axon transmits electrical impulses from the cell soma and is covered by a myelin sheath formed from the membrane of oligodendrocytes or Schwann cells. Axons can form many branches, which end in the presynaptic regions that form synapses on target neurons or cells. **B.** Micrograph of a motor neuron showing the large cell body and nucleus (N), a long axon (A) emerging from an axon hillock (AH), and several dendrites D. Nissl substance (NS) can be seen throughout the cell body and cytoskeletal elements can be detected in the processes. Nuclei of scattered glial cells (G) are seen among the surrounding tissue (×100; H&E stain). **C.** Schematic of a lower motor neuron. The cell body lies in the CNS (spinal cord or brainstem) while the axon emerges to form part of the PNS (spinal or cranial nerves). (Parts A and B, reproduced with permission from McKinley MP, O'Loughlin VD, Bidle TS. *Anatomy and Physiology: An Integrative Approach.* New York, NY: McGraw Hill; 2013; part C, reproduced with permission from Junqueira LC, Carneiro J, Kelley RO: *Basic Histology: Text & Atlas,* 11th ed. New York, NY: McGraw Hill; 2005.)

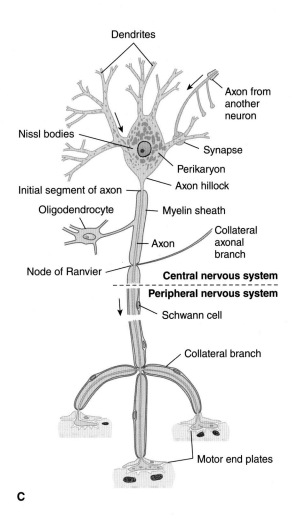

FIGURE 1–12 *(Continued)*

Hundreds of different types of neurons have been identified in the human nervous system. One way neurons can be categorized is by their general function, as sensory neurons, motor neurons, or interneurons. There are 3 types of sensory neurons (also called afferent neurons) that detect and convey signals from the external and internal environments. Special sense neurons are located in special sense organs of the CNS (eg, photoreceptor cells) or the PNS (eg, hair cells). Somatosensory and visceral sensory neuron cell bodies are found in the PNS, although their axons enter the CNS and branches form components of ascending sensory tracts in the CNS. Four types of motor neuros (also called efferent neurons) are involved in control of the somatic and autonomic motor systems. Upper motor neuron cell bodies are located in either the motor cortex or brainstem, and their axons project to lower motor neurons, and those lie entirely in the CNS. Somatic and autonomic (preganglionic) lower motor neuron cell bodies are found in the spinal cord or brainstem, with their axons emerging from those regions to form the motor efferents of the spinal and cranial nerves. Thus, lower motor neurons are considered part of both the CNS and PNS. Both the cell bodies (in sympathetic or parasympathetic ganglia) and axons of postganglionic autonomic motor neurons lie entirely in the PNS.

All of the other neurons in the CNS are called interneurons (or in some cases, just neurons). There are 2 types of interneurons, which are distinguished by whether they function locally or send their axons to other parts of the CNS. Local interneurons (also called local circuit neurons) work within the same brain region, usually have short unmyelinated axons, and form circuits with nearby neurons. Projection neurons (also called principal or relay neurons) extend their axons, which are usually long and myelinated, to another brain or spinal cord region. Interneurons are also named by their morphology, neurotransmitter they release, type of response they produce in their target cells, electrophysiology properties, and/or by the person who first discovered them.

CLASSIFICATION OF NEURONS BY MORPHOLOGY

Morphologically, neurons vary widely with respect to their size and level of dendritic branching (Figure 1–13). Most interneurons and motor neurons have a single axon and multiple dendrites and are called multipolar neurons. A few populations of interneurons called bipolar neurons contain a single axon and

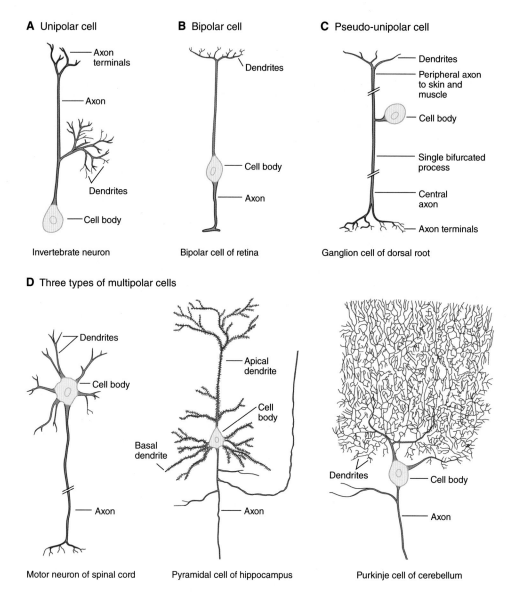

A Unipolar cell

Axon terminals
Axon
Dendrites
Cell body

Invertebrate neuron

B Bipolar cell

Dendrites
Cell body
Axon

Bipolar cell of retina

C Pseudo-unipolar cell

Dendrites
Peripheral axon to skin and muscle
Cell body
Single bifurcated process
Central axon
Axon terminals

Ganglion cell of dorsal root

D Three types of multipolar cells

Dendrites
Cell body
Axon

Motor neuron of spinal cord

Apical dendrite
Cell body
Basal dendrite
Axon

Pyramidal cell of hippocampus

Dendrites
Cell body
Axon

Purkinje cell of cerebellum

FIGURE 1–13 Morphologic categories of neurons as unipolar, bipolar, or multipolar based on the number of processes that originate from the cell soma. **A.** Unipolar cells have a single process emanating from the cell soma and are characteristic of the invertebrate nervous system. **B.** Bipolar cells have a single dendrite that receives electrical signals and an axon that transmits signals to other cells. **C.** Pseudo-unipolar cells transmit somatosensory information. They contain one axon branch that extends to the skin or muscle, and another axon branch extends to the spinal cord. **D.** Multipolar cells have a single axon and many dendrites. The most common type of neuron in the mammalian nervous system, three examples are shown. Spinal motor neurons innervate skeletal muscle fibers. Pyramidal cells are found in the cerebral cortex, and have a roughly triangular cell body; apical dendrites emerge from the apex and the basal dendrites from the base. Purkinje cells of the cerebellum are characterized by an extensive dendritic tree that accommodates enormous synaptic inputs. (Parts A and B, reproduced with permission from Kandel ER, Schwartz JH, Jessell TM, et al: *Principles of Neural Science*, 5th ed. New York, NY: McGraw Hill; 2013; parts C and D, adapted with permission from Ramón y, Cajal S: *Histology*, 10th ed. Baltimore, MD: Wood; 1933.)

only a single dendrite. Unipolar neurons, which contain only 1 process, are common in insects but are found in only a few brain regions in mammals. Sensory neurons do not have typical dendrites because they do not receive information from synapses, but rather have specialized sensory receptor regions to detect signals from the environment. Some sensory neurons (eg, photoreceptor, taste, and hair cells) also do not have axons but synapse onto another neuron that relays its sensory information. In other sensory neurons (eg, somatosensory neurons), the receptive region is connected to an axon, which transmits the sensory

signal past the cell body and via its other axon branch into the CNS. These are called pseudounipolar neurons.

Some neurons (also called cells) are named based on their morphology (Figure 1–14). Pyramidal neurons are located in the cerebral cortex, hippocampus, and amygdala and have triangle-shaped cell bodies, with 1 large apical dendrite and several basal dendrites. Their dendrites contain many dendritic spines. Located in layers 3 to 6 of the cerebral cortex, many pyramidal neurons are projection neurons that send their axons out of the cerebral cortex. Spindle neurons are a subtype of pyramidal cell

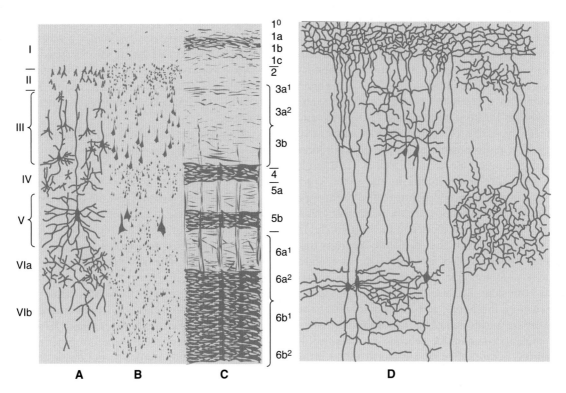

FIGURE 1–14 Neuronal organization of the cerebral cortex. **A.** Golgi neuronal stain. **B.** Nissl cellular stain. **C.** Weigert myelin stain. **D.** Neuronal connections. Roman and Arabic numerals indicate the layers of the neocortex; 4, external line of Baillarger (line of Gennari in the occipital lobe); 5b, internal line of Baillarger. (Parts A-C, reproduced with permission from Ranson SW, Clark SL: *The Anatomy of the Nervous System,* 10th ed. Philadelphia, PA: Saunders; 1959; part D, reproduced with permission from Ganong WF: *Review of Medical Physiology,* 22nd ed. New York, NY: Appleton & Lange; 2005.)

with an elongated cell body and only a single apical dendrite and are found in only 3 regions in the cerebral cortex. Stellate cells/ neurons have a star shape with multiple dendrites that radiate from the cell's body. Found in many brain regions, including the cerebral cortex, cerebellum, and striatum, stellate cell dendrites can either contain (spiny) or lack (aspiny) dendritic spines. Many stellate cells are local circuit neurons. Granule cells are also found in a variety of brain regions, including the cerebellum, hippocampus, cerebral cortex, and olfactory bulb, and are characterized by having a very small cell body. Many granule cells are local interneurons. Basket cells are another type of local interneuron, also found in the cerebellum, cerebral cortex, and hippocampus. Their name derives from the basket-like nest that their axons form around their target cells.

CLASSIFICATION OF NEURONS BY NAMES & NEUROTRANSMITTER

Neurons have also been named by the researchers who first identified them. Purkinje neurons, discovered by Jan Purkinje, are very large projection neurons that send the sole output from the cerebellar cortex. Underneath the cerebellar Purkinje neurons are a population of neurons called Lugaro cells, identified by Ernesto Lugaro. These spindle-shaped neurons have 2 dendrites that emerge from opposite poles of the cell body and provide information to many cells in the cerebellum. Also located in the cerebellum are the Golgi cells, discovered by

Camillo Golgi, which are located in the granule cell layer and provide inputs to the granule cells. First described by Vladimir Betz, Betz cells are very large pyramidal neurons, a type of projection neuron, with the upper motor neurons located in layer 5 of the primary motor cortex. Discovered by Birdsey Renshaw, Renshaw cells are interneurons found in the spinal cord gray matter that provide and receive inputs to and from lower motor neurons. Constantin von Economo first identified and named the spindle neurons described earlier, which are found in only hominids, whales, dolphins, and elephants.

Other criteria by which neurons can be classified are by their neurotransmitter and the response they produce in their targets, which can be excitatory, inhibitory, or modulatory. Approximately 90% of brain neurons use either glutamate or γ-aminobutyric acid (GABA) as their neurotransmitter, with the other 10% of neurons using acetylcholine or one of the biogenic amines (ie, norepinephrine, epinephrine, dopamine, or serotonin). Neurons that release glutamate are called glutamatergic neurons. Glutamatergic neurons are found throughout the brain and spinal cord. Although glutamate can act on several types of postsynaptic receptors, the majority (in terms of numbers) of glutamate receptors are ionotropic receptors that produce an excitatory response. Therefore, glutamatergic neurons are also referred to as excitatory neurons. An important class of glutamatergic neurons are the pyramidal neurons in the hippocampus and cerebral cortex, many of which are projection/principal neurons.

Neurons that release GABA as their neurotransmitter are GABAergic neurons. The most prevalent effect of GABA is an inhibitory response, and accordingly, GABAergic neurons are categorized as inhibitory interneurons. Inhibitory interneurons are found throughout most regions of the brain and are abundant in the cerebral cortex, cerebellum, and striatum. Cerebellar Purkinje neurons are GABAergic and are one of the few types of projection/principal neurons that are inhibitory. The neurotransmitter glycine also produces inhibition, and glycinergic neurons, as well as GABAergic neurons, are inhibitory interneurons in the spinal cord. Other brain neurons release acetylcholine (called cholinergic neurons) or one of the monoamines. In the brain, many cholinergic neuron cells bodies are located in the basal forebrain and project to many areas of the cerebrum. Neurons that release biogenic amines, called noradrenergic, adrenergic, dopaminergic, or serotonergic neurons, have cell bodies located in the brainstem. Because these neurons produce a variety of excitatory, inhibitory, and modulatory effects on their targets, they are usually named for their neurotransmitter. In the PNS, somatic lower motor neurons are classified as excitatory neurons because they release acetylcholine at the neuromuscular junction, which always produces an excitatory response in the muscle cell.

NEURONAL ORGANELLES & GENE EXPRESSION

Similar to other cells, neurons possess a plasma membrane that functions as a selective permeability barrier to the extracellular fluid and that encloses the cytoplasm containing the nucleus, cytosol, and typical complement of cellular organelles and biochemical activities (Figure 1–15). The cell body of the neuron, also called the cell soma, can vary in diameter from approximately 100 μm to approximately 10 μm. The organelles include the nucleus, smooth and rough endoplasmic reticulum (ER), Golgi apparatus, lysosomes, proteasomes, and mitochondria, several of which are also localized in the axon and dendrites. Neurons contain a robust cytoskeleton with typical filaments and cytoskeletal motor proteins, which are important in the development, structure, and function of axons and dendrites.

After neurons undergo their final division during embryonic development, they become postmitotic, and the vast majority of neurons do not proliferate in the postnatal and adult brain. However, in the mammalian dentate gyrus of the hippocampus and striatum and the olfactory bulb in rodents, adult neurogenesis can lead to the generation of new neurons. The precursors for adult neurogenesis in the hippocampus have been identified as neural precursor cells that lie in the subgranular zone. The newly produced neurons migrate, differentiate into mature neurons, and form connections with existing neurons. Shown to be stimulated by exercise and activity, adult neurogenesis has been implicated in learning and memory, and errors in neurogenesis have been proposed to contribute to depression and schizophrenia.

Because mature neurons do not divide, the main activities that occur in the nucleus are transcription, the synthesis of RNA from the DNA, assembly of ribosome subunits, and the modification of DNA and DNA-binding proteins in what are referred to as epigenetic changes. Ribosomal RNA combines with proteins to form the ribosome subunits in the nucleolus. mRNA and tRNA are transcribed and transported through the nuclear pores to the cytoplasm, where they control translation, which is the synthesis of proteins by the ribosomes. In the nucleus, mRNAs are transcribed as precursors that undergo modifications and splicing to form mature mRNAs that are then transported out of the nucleus and translated using the genetic code (Figure 1–16).

Translation is the process by which ribosomes synthesize proteins, with the sequence of amino acids determined by the codons in the mRNA and its parent gene. Translation occurs in the cytoplasm on either free or ER-bound ribosomes. Proteins that are entirely water soluble, called cytoplasmic or cytosolic proteins, are synthesized on free ribosomes that, as they translate the mRNA, form polysomes. Proteins that have hydrophobic stretches of amino acids, called transmembrane spanning domains, that cause them to integrate into the membrane are synthesized on ribosomes that associate with the ER, called rough ER. Transmembrane proteins are also called integral membrane proteins. Once a transmembrane protein has been synthesized, it must traffic to its location in the plasma membrane or intracellular membrane compartment. The rough ER also synthesizes proteins and peptides destined to be secreted from neurons.

It is estimated that the human genome contains approximately 20,000 protein-coding genes. Through the process of alternative splicing, different protein variants of many genes can be produced. The control of the types and amounts of proteins that a cell expresses is referred to as gene expression (Figure 1–16). The regulation of gene expression can occur at many points along the path from DNA to protein, including at the transcriptional level by control of transcription factors and epigenetic modifications,

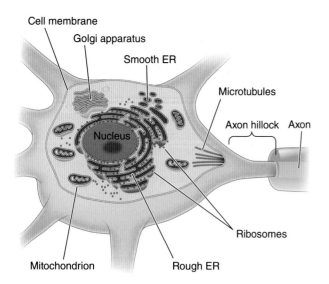

FIGURE 1–15 Neuronal organelles located in the cell body. ER, endoplasmic reticulum.

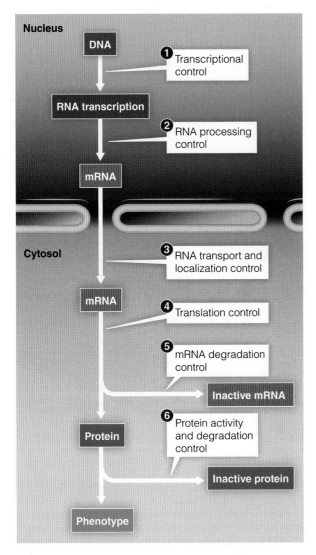

FIGURE 1–16 Regulation of gene expression in neurons.

mRNA processing, export and turnover, and in the processes of translation and protein degradation. Gene expression and control of protein expression determine the morphologic and functional phenotype of a cell. Neurons express approximately 14,000 protein-coding genes, with approximately 8000 of these expressed in other cells and involved in fundamental cellular processes and metabolism. Approximately 6000 protein-coding genes are neuronal specific genes that are only expressed in neurons and include types of transporters, channels, neurotransmitter synthetic enzymes, cytoskeletal associated proteins, scaffolding proteins, and receptors.

NEURONAL MEMBRANES & TRAFFICKING

The neuronal plasma membrane and other membrane-enclosed organelles are formed from a phospholipid bilayer and transmembrane proteins (Figure 1–17). Membranes also contain cholesterol and sphingolipids. In neurons, lipids are synthesized in the smooth ER or, in the case of cholesterol, obtained from the diet or liver. Transmembrane proteins become incorporated into the ER membrane during translation. Following translation in the rough ER, transmembrane and secreted proteins and peptides are transported via small vesicles to the Golgi, where they are further modified and then sorted and packaged into vesicles, called secretory vesicles, at the trans-Golgi network to be transported to their final destination. Called the biosynthetic or secretory pathway, it is involved in the synthesis and delivery of lipids and transmembrane proteins to the plasma membrane; the secretion of proteins and peptides outside the neuron; formation of organelles in the endosomal pathway, including the early endosome and lysosome; and production of the precursors needed to form synaptic vesicles. Proteins and lipids move between membrane compartments by a process called membrane trafficking.

Proteins and lipids are also retrieved from the plasma membrane through trafficking in the endosomal pathway. Plasma membrane lipids and transmembrane proteins undergo endocytosis, where a small patch of the membrane folds inward into the cytoplasm and pinches off to form a small endocytic vesicle. This vesicle then traffics to and fuses with the early endosome, where the proteins are sorted into small vesicles that bud off and are trafficked to different compartments. Transmembrane proteins can travel by recycling vesicles back to the plasma membrane. A specific type of endocytosis, called receptor-mediated endocytosis, is used to bring key nutrients such as cholesterol and iron into the cell. In this process, the receptors bind and deliver their nutrients to endosomal compartments and can recycle back to the plasma membrane. Transmembrane proteins that have been damaged will traffic to the late endosome and then fuse with the lysosome. A lysosome is a membrane-bound compartment with an acidic pH that contains a variety of degradative enzymes inside, which can degrade proteins, nucleic acids, and lipids. Lysosomes can also function to degrade cytoplasmic proteins or damaged organelles, such as mitochondria, by fusing with compartments in the autophagy pathway. Another intracellular compartment, called the proteasome, is involved in degrading mainly cytoplasmic proteins. Located in the cytoplasm or nucleus, proteasomes are large complexes of proteins that lack membranes. Proteasomes bind damaged proteins, unravel them, and then cleave them with proteases to produce small peptides that can be further degraded to amino acids.

NEURONAL ENERGETICS

It has been estimated that the brain consumes approximately 20% of the energy and oxygen in the body, although it only composes approximately 2% of the body's mass. In order to meet its energy demands, neurons require energy substrates, oxygen, and mitochondria located in the cell soma, axons, and dendrites. The main energy currency in the cell

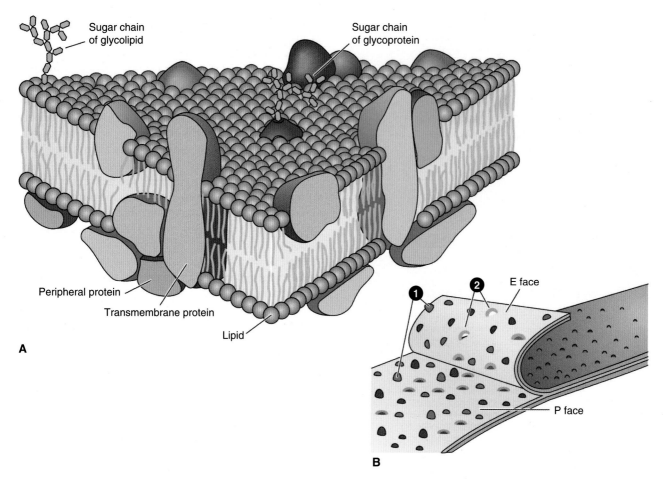

FIGURE 1-17 The neuronal plasma membrane is composed of the lipid bilayer and transmembrane proteins. **A.** The fluid mosaic model of membrane structure emphasizes that the phospholipid bilayer of a membrane contains proteins inserted in it or associated with its surface (peripheral proteins) and that many of these proteins move within the fluid lipid phase. Integral proteins embedded in the lipid layers are called transmembrane proteins. **B.** When cells are frozen and fractured (cryofracture), the lipid bilayer of membranes is often cleaved along the hydrophobic center. Electron microscopy of cryofracture preparation replicas provides a useful method for studying membrane structures. Most of the protruding membrane particles seen (1) are proteins or aggregates of proteins that remain attached to the half of the membrane adjacent to the cytoplasm (P or protoplasmic face). Fewer particles are found attached to the outer half of the membrane (E or extracellular face). Each protein bulging on one surface has a corresponding depression (2) on the opposite surface. (Reproduced with permission from Mescher AL. *Junqueira's Basic Histology: Text & Atlas,* 15th ed. New York, NY: McGraw Hill; 2018.)

is adenosine triphosphate (ATP). ATP can be generated by glycolysis, an anaerobic process that takes place in the cytoplasm, converting glucose into pyruvate, reduced nicotinamide adenine dinucleotide (NADH), and ATP. Pyruvate can be converted to lactate or shuttled with NADH into mitochondria, which synthesize ATP via the enzymes in the Krebs cycle and oxidative phosphorylation, with a yield of approximately 16 ATP molecules per pyruvate/NADH. Neurons do not contain large stores of glucose in glycogen, and therefore, they depend on nearby astrocytes to take up glucose from capillaries and release glucose and its glycolytic product lactate into the extracellular space. Neurons convert lactate back into pyruvate via lactate dehydrogenase and shuttle the pyruvate into mitochondria. Neurons are highly dependent on mitochondria for the synthesis of ATP, and conditions that lead to anoxia can rapidly lead to neuronal damage and cell death.

THE AXON

The axon is a structure that is unique to neurons (Figure 1–18). It is a process that is specialized for the generation and conduction of electrical signals called action potentials, which are sent along the axon, in some cases over long distances, to the end of the axon called the presynaptic terminus. At the terminus, the action potential electrical signal is converted into a chemical signal in the form of neurotransmitter release. Axons can be small or large in diameter, ranging from less than 1 to 10 μm. Axons can be long or short and unmyelinated or myelinated. Projection neurons and sensory neurons extend the longest axons, which are usually myelinated and can be centimeters to a meter in length. Local circuit neurons are usually unmyelinated and only a few millimeters in length. Axons can be unbranched with 1 main output or be highly branched, with the branches called collaterals, each of which can form a separate output.

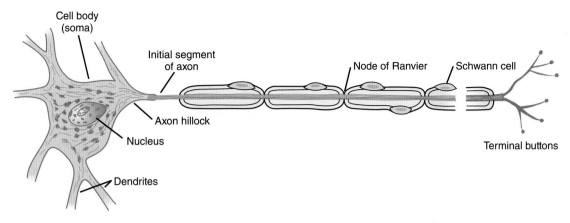

FIGURE 1–18 Neuron with a myelinated axon. A neuron is composed of a cell body (soma) with a nucleus, several processes called dendrites, and an axon that originates from the axon hillock. The first portion of the axon is called the initial segment. When myelinated as shown, a myelin sheath forms from an oligodendrocyte (CNS) or Schwann cell (PNS) and surrounds the axon, except at its ending and at the nodes of Ranvier. Terminal buttons (boutons) are located at the terminal endings. (Reproduced with permission from Barrett KE, Barman SM, Brooks HL et al: *Ganong's Review of Medical Physiology,* 26th ed. New York, NY: McGraw Hill; 2019.)

All axons have several common features. The axon emerges from the neuronal cell body at a region called the axon hillock, which tapers to form the initial segment. The axon hillock helps provide a barrier to the random diffusion of organelles, and many organelles require axonal transport to move from the cell body to the axon. The axon hillock also blocks diffusion of plasma membrane proteins from the cell body membrane to the axonal membrane. The initial segment is adjacent to the axon hillock and is the region where the action potential is generated. Even in myelinated axons, the initial segment is unmyelinated and is the regions where voltage-gated sodium channels are highly concentrated. The end of the axon is called the axon terminal, presynaptic terminus, or synaptic bouton. If the axon is myelinated, the myelin membrane does not cover the presynaptic terminus.

Axons contain cytoskeletal proteins that provide structure and important functions. The largest filaments, called microtubules (MTs), give the axon stability and provide tracks to move organelles and large protein complexes up and down the axon. MTs are formed by polymerization of tubulin subunits with microtubule-associated proteins (MAPs) that associate and regulate polymerization and bundling of MTs. In addition, MT-based motors bind MTs and use the energy released by ATP hydrolysis to move cargoes along MT filaments in fast axonal transport, a type of axoplasmic transport (Figure 1–19). The kinesin family of MT-based motors moves cargoes from the cell body in the anterograde direction to the axon terminus, whereas the dynein family of MT-based motors moves cargoes in the retrograde direction, from the axon terminus to the cell body. Important cargoes moved in fast axonal transport include mitochondria, lysosomes, mRNA, ribosomes, and vesicles. Vesicles provide lipids and transmembrane proteins destined for the axonal plasma membrane, synaptic vesicle components, and peptides destined for secretion by the presynaptic terminus. Many soluble proteins and cytoskeletal components use slow axonal transport to travel along the axon.

Two other cytoskeletal filaments, an intermediate filament called neurofilament and the microfilaments composed of actin, are expressed in neurons. Mechanically strong, neurofilaments serve a mainly structural role and ensure the diameter of the axon does not diminish along its length. Actin microfilaments are found associated with the plasma membrane, along with dozens of actin-binding proteins that regulate the assembly, disassembly, and bundling of the actin filaments and binding to the plasma membrane. During development, actin filaments and the actin-based motor, called myosin, are used to provide the mechanical forces that drive the motility of the growing axon. In mature axons, actin is localized in a mesh that underlies the axonal plasma membrane and at the presynaptic terminus. Because MTs do not extend into the axon terminus, actin and myosin are involved in transporting cargoes in the axon terminal and providing scaffolds that tether transmembrane proteins at specific regions of the axonal or presynaptic membrane.

DENDRITES & SYNAPSES

Dendrites are branched processes that are specialized for receiving information (Figure 1–20). Presynaptic axon terminals form synapses on dendrites, which then produce postsynaptic signals that are passively transmitted to the cell body. Dendrites can be highly branched and referred to as the dendritic tree or arbor. The number of inputs that a neuron receives is proportional to its dendritic area. Dendrites can be distinguished from axons by their appearance. Unlike axons, which have a constant diameter, dendrites taper as they extend from the cell body. Dendrites are usually shorter than axons and may be studded with dendritic spines. Similar to the axon, dendrites contain mitochondria, secretory and endocytic vesicles, early endosomes, and an organized cytoskeleton, including MTs, microfilaments, and their regulatory proteins and motors. In addition, axons and dendrites

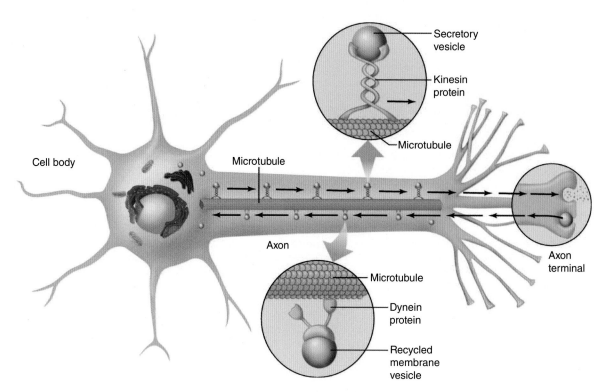

FIGURE 1–19 The axonal cytoskeleton and fast axonal transport (FAT). FAT occurs at a rate of about 400 involves the transport of vesicles and organelles along microtubules (MT) and involves MT based motor proteins dynein and kinesin. Anterograde (orthograde) transport occurs along microtubules from the cell body to the presynaptic region, while retrograde transport occurs from the presynaptic terminus to the cell body. (Reproduced with permission from Widmaier EP, Raff H, Strang KT. *Vander's Human Physiology.* New York, NY: McGraw Hill; 2008.)

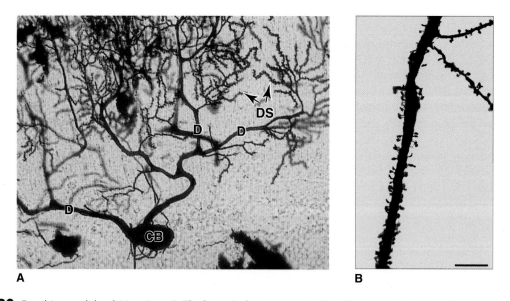

FIGURE 1–20 Dendrites and dendritic spines. **A.** The large Purkinje neuron in this silver-stained section of cerebellum has many dendrites (D) emerging from its cell body (CB) and forming branches. Each of the small dendritic branches has many tiny projecting dendritic spines (DS) spaced closely along their length, each of which is a site of a synapse with another neuron. Dendritic spines are highly dynamic, the number and morphology of synapses can change (×650; Silver stain). **B.** Dendrite from a pyramidal neuron in the motor cortex. Note the spines on the main dendrite and on its smaller branches, and note that spines have different lengths and shapes. Scale = 10 μm. (Part A, reproduced with permission from Berman I. *Color Atlas of Basic Histology,* 3rd ed. New York, NY: McGraw Hill; 2003; part B, used with permission from Dr. Andrew Tan, Yale University.)

contain ribosomes and mRNA that mediate local protein synthesis within these processes. The dendrites of some neurons contain dendritic spines along their length. Dendritic spines are actin-rich small protrusions that can have a bulbous head and are the regions where the majority of excitatory glutamate synapses occur on the dendrite. Spines are dynamic structures that can undergo changes in shape, size, and number, and this morphologic spine plasticity (and the functional plasticity of the synapses they contain) has been implicated in learning and memory.

The synapse is the structure where synaptic transmission occurs (Figure 1–21). The axon terminal is the part of the axon that forms a synapse with another neuron, muscle, or gland. When a neuron makes a synaptic connection with another cell, it is said to innervate that cell. The connections between an axon and a muscle or gland are also referred to as junctions. In neurons, synapses occur between an axon and a dendrite (axodendritic synapses), an axon and the cell body (axosomatic synapses), or an axon and another axon (axoaxonic synapses). If the axons form short branches at their ends and synapse on dendrites or cell bodies, these branches are called the terminal arbor. Some axons form bulbous presynaptic swellings and synapse on a dendrite without terminating there, but continue on to form additional synapses. These are called the en passant synapses.

Two different types of synapses, named electrical and chemical synapses, mediate transmission. Although fairly rare in the human CNS, electrical synapses allow for the direct flow of ions (current) through gap junctions between the pre- and postsynaptic neuron. The vast majority of synapses in the human brain are chemical synapses, which involve the release of neurotransmitter from the presynaptic terminus and production of electrical and other signaling responses in the postsynaptic neuron (Figure 1–22). In chemical synapses, the presynaptic terminus is distinguished by the presence of synaptic vesicles and specializations called active zones. The synaptic cleft (20 to 40 nm wide) separates the pre- and postsynaptic membrane, although synaptic adhesion molecules from the presynaptic and postsynaptic membrane bind across the synaptic cleft to help produce the stability and specificity of the synapse. The postsynaptic membrane contains neurotransmitter receptors that are tethered at the synapse by scaffolding and cytoskeletal proteins, forming a region called the postsynaptic density in excitatory/glutamatergic synapses.

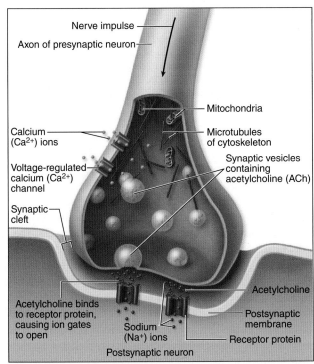

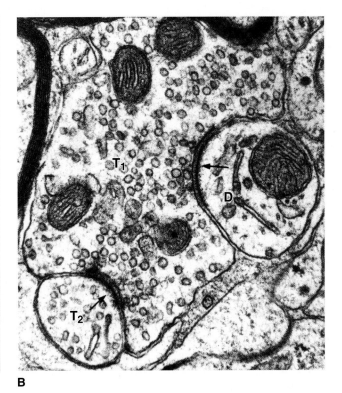

A

B

FIGURE 1–21 Synapse structure: major components of the synapse. **A.** Diagram showing a synapse releasing neurotransmitter (NT) by exocytosis from the terminal bouton. Presynaptic terminals always contain a large number of synaptic vesicles containing NT, numerous mitochondria, and endoplasmic reticulum ER. **B.** Electron micrograph showing a large presynaptic terminal (T_1) filled with synaptic vesicles and asymmetric electron-dense regions around 20- to 30-nm-wide synaptic clefts (arrows). The postsynaptic membrane contains NT receptors. The postsynaptic membrane on the right is part of a dendrite (**D**), associated with fewer vesicles of any kind, showing this to be an axodendritic synapse. On the left is another presynaptic terminal (T_2), suggesting an axoaxonic synapse with a role in modulating activity of the other terminal (×35,000). (Part A, reproduced with permission from McKinley MP, O'Loughlin VD. *Human Anatomy*, 3rd ed. New York, NY: McGraw Hill; 2012; part B, reproduced with permission from Mescher AL. *Junqueira's Basic Histology: Text & Atlas*, 15th ed. New York, NY: McGraw Hill; 2018.)

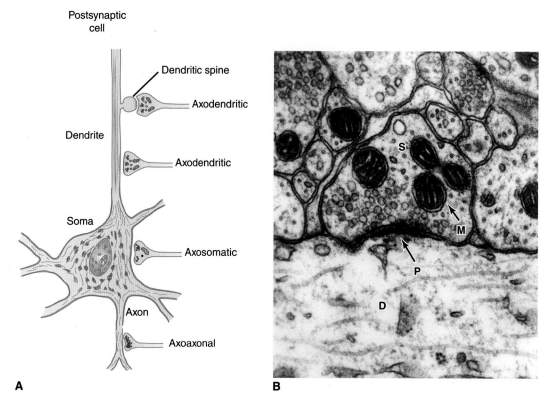

A   **B**

FIGURE 1–22 Synapse structure: morphologic types of synapses. **A.** Diagram showing the three common morphologic types of synapses. Presynaptic axons synapse on either the dendritic shaft or dendritic spine forming axodendritic synapses, and tend to be excitatory synapses. Axosomatic sysnapses occur on the cell body/soma and tend to be inhibitory synapses. Less numerous axoaxonic synapses occur between a presynaptic axon and a postsynaptic axon and tend to modulate the release of neurotransmitter. **B.** Electron micrograph of a synapse showing the presynaptic knob (S) ending on the shaft of a dendrite (D) in the central nervous system. M, mitochondrion; P, postsynaptic density (×56,000). (Reproduced with permission from Barrett KE, Barman SM, Brooks HL et al: *Ganong's Review of Medical Physiology,* 26th ed. New York, NY: McGraw Hill; 2019.)

GLIAL CELLS & THEIR FUNCTIONS

Neurons, axons, and synapses are surrounded by glial cells that provide structural, metabolic, and functional support in the CNS and PNS (Figures 1–23 and 1–24). Glial cells can be categorized as macroglia and microglia. Similar to neurons, macroglia are derived from the ectoderm, either the neural tube (CNS glia) or the neural crest cells (PNS glia), and include astrocytes, satellite cells, pericytes, oligodendrocytes, Schwann cells, ependymal cells, and enteric glia. There is only 1 type of microglia cell, constituting approximately 15% to 20% of total cells in the brain and functioning as the resident immune cells in the CNS. Originally thought to develop from mesoderm, microglia are likely derived from the embryonic yolk sac and are distinguished by their small cell bodies and short processes. Microglia exhibit both phagocytic and antigen-presenting functions that defend the CNS from infection by bacteria, viruses, and fungi. In addition, microglia are involved in maintaining overall brain health as they constantly scavenge the CNS for extracellular protein aggregates called plaques and damaged neurons and synapses. As phagocytic cells, microglia have also been implicated in dendritic spine removal underlying spine plasticity.

Astrocytes in the CNS and satellite cells in the PNS provide structural and metabolic support in the nervous system. Deriving their name from their star-like appearance, astrocytes (also called astroglia) are the most abundant glia in the CNS. Gray matter, type I protoplasmic astrocytes support neuronal cell bodies and dendrites, whereas white matter, type II fibrous astrocytes support axons and their myelinating cells, the oligodendrocytes. Astrocytes form structures called end feet on capillaries, a component of the BBB. Transporter proteins on the end feet allow astrocytes to take up important molecules such as glucose, lactate, amino acids, and other metabolites from the blood and release them into the extracellular fluid around neurons. Through this mechanism, astrocytes provide key nutrients to nearby neurons, axons, and oligodendrocytes. Astrocytes also express ion channels and ion transporters, which enable them to regulate the ionic concentration of the extracellular fluid.

As a result of their proximity to synapses and expression of neurotransmitter transporters, astrocytes can function in the modulation of synaptic transmission, forming the tripartite synapse (Figure 1–25). In addition, astrocytes express neurotransmitter receptors and release gliotransmitters such as ATP, which allow communication with neurons and among astrocytes. Following injury to the CNS, astrocytes respond by

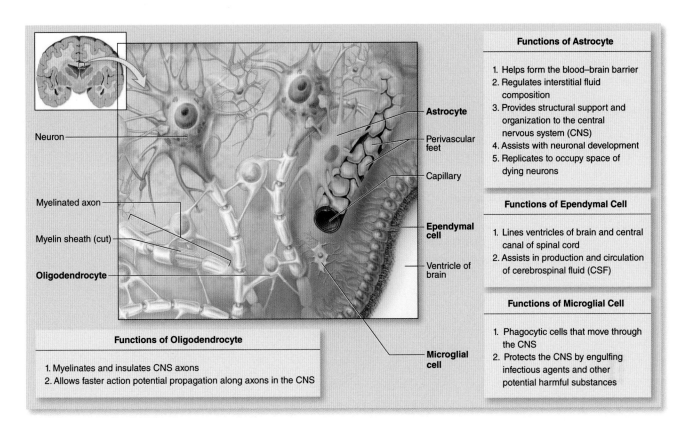

Functions of Astrocyte

1. Helps form the blood–brain barrier
2. Regulates interstitial fluid composition
3. Provides structural support and organization to the central nervous system (CNS)
4. Assists with neuronal development
5. Replicates to occupy space of dying neurons

Functions of Ependymal Cell

1. Lines ventricles of brain and central canal of spinal cord
2. Assists in production and circulation of cerebrospinal fluid (CSF)

Functions of Microglial Cell

1. Phagocytic cells that move through the CNS
2. Protects the CNS by engulfing infectious agents and other potential harmful substances

Functions of Oligodendrocyte

1. Myelinates and insulates CNS axons
2. Allows faster action potential propagation along axons in the CNS

FIGURE 1–23 Glial cells of the central nervous system (CNS). There are five major types of glial cells located in the CNS: oligodendrocytes, astrocytes, ependymal cells, microglial cells, and pericytes. CNS glia are located in both the brain and spinal cord. The interrelationships and major functions of these cells are shown diagrammatically here. Pericytes (which are not shown) are involved in regulating the blood-brain barrier. (Reproduced with permission from McKinley MP, O'Loughlin VD, Bidle TS. *Anatomy and Physiology: An Integrative Approach.* New York, NY: McGraw Hill; 2012.)

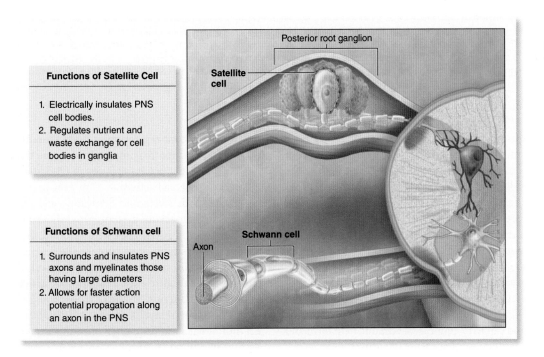

Functions of Satellite Cell

1. Electrically insulates PNS cell bodies.
2. Regulates nutrient and waste exchange for cell bodies in ganglia

Functions of Schwann cell

1. Surrounds and insulates PNS axons and myelinates those having large diameters
2. Allows for faster action potential propagation along an axon in the PNS

FIGURE 1–24 Glial cells of the peripheral nervous system (PNS). Two types of glial cells are located in the PNS: Schwann cells (alternatively called neurolemmocytes), which are located within and surround axons in nerves, and satellite cells, which surround the nerve cell bodies and are thus found only in ganglia. Major functions of these cells are indicated. (Reproduced with permission from McKinley MP, O'Loughlin VD, Bidle TS. *Anatomy and Physiology: An Integrative Approach.* New York, NY: McGraw Hill; 2012.)

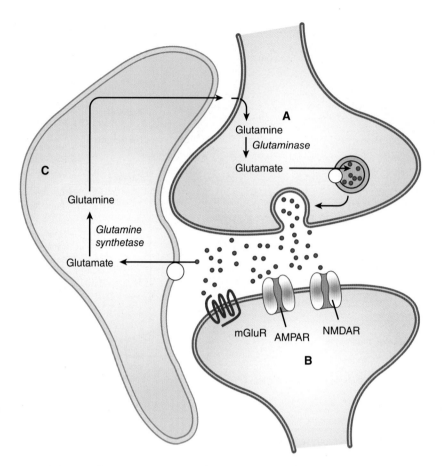

FIGURE 1–25 Astrocytes contribute to the tripartite synapse. Schematic diagram of a glutamate synapse. Astrocytes can regulate synaptic glutamate levels at glutamateric synapses. Glutamine is imported into the presynaptic glutamatergic neuron (**A**) and converted into glutamate by glutaminase. The glutamate is then transported in vesicles by the vesicular glutamate transporter. Upon release into the synapse, glutamate can bind to and activate AMPA and NMDA types of ionotropic glutamate receptors (AMPAR, NMDAR) and with metabotropic receptors (mGluR) on the postsynaptic neuron (**B**). Synaptic transmission is terminated by transport of the synaptic glutamate into a neighboring astrocyte (**C**) (or into the presynaptic and postsynaptic neurons, which is not shown) by a glutamate transporter. It is converted into glutamine by glutamine synthetase and transported back into the extracellular fluid where it can be taken up by the presynaptic axon. By regulating the levels of glutamate, the magnitude and duration of the postsynaptic responses can be modulated. It has also been proposed that astrocytes may release gliotransmitters into the synapse that can also modulate synaptic transmission (not shown). (Reproduced with permission from Katzung BG: *Basic & Clinical Pharmacology*, 14th ed. New York, NY: McGraw Hill; 2018.)

transforming into reactive glia, releasing immune modulatory factors, and forming glial scars, which can replace regions of lost neurons but impede the regeneration of axons. In the PNS, satellite cells are located in ganglia where they surround sensory and autonomic neuronal cells bodies and perform similar metabolic support functions.

Although the exact mechanism(s) have not been determined, in response to neuronal activity, neurons and astrocytes release vasodilators and vasoconstrictors that affect capillary blood flow. By releasing vasomodulators, neurons and astrocytes may regulate vascular endothelial cells directly and/or through another type of glial cell, the pericytes. Pericytes are contractile cells that surround capillary endothelial cells and help form and maintain the tight junctions that ensure the BBB (**Figure 1–26**). In addition, as contractile cells, pericytes can regulate contraction and relaxation that control capillary blood flow. Arterioles, which are larger blood vessels lined with vascular smooth muscle, have also been implicated as cells that respond to neuronal

activity–dependent regulation of brain blood flow. Functional magnetic resonance imaging (fMRI) is a functional neuroimaging technique that detects changes in blood flow as an indirect measure of neuronal activity.

Oligodendrocytes and Schwann cells are the myelinating cells in the nervous system, providing specialized plasma membrane projections that wrap around the axon multiple times. With its high lipid content (80% lipid and 20% protein), the myelin membranes form an insulating sheath that ensures fast and efficient conduction of action potentials by salutatory conduction. In the CNS, each oligodendrocyte can form 1 segment of myelin for many (up to 50) adjacent axons. An individual axon (especially the longer ones) is myelinated by multiple oligodendrocytes along its length. In the CNS, axons larger than 1 μm are usually myelinated. Along the axon, myelinated segments are separated by small unmyelinated regions called nodes of Ranvier. The axon at the nodes has access to the extracellular fluid and is the region where

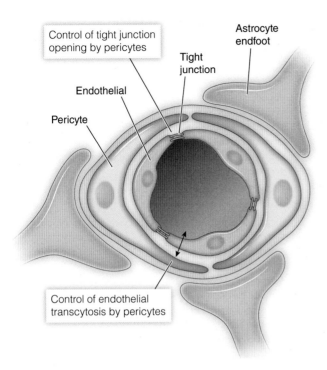

FIGURE 1–26 Glia and the blood-brain barrier. Diagram shows the cellular components of CNS capillaries. The blood-brain barrier is formed by specialized vascular endothelial cells (pink) in CNS capillaries, which form tight junctions that prevent the diffusion of water-soluble molecules, and movement of immune and pathogenic cells from the blood into the CNS. The endothelial cells are covered by pericytes (blue), a type of contractile glial cell, which help regulate the tight junctions and also control the diameter of the capillary and modulate blood flow. Surrounding the pericytes are astrocytic end feet (green) that function to transport essential nutrients from the blood into CNS tissue and release factors that affect contraction of pericytes.

the action potential is regenerated. Oligodendrocytes also provide trophic support to axons at the nodes. Similar to reactive glia, oligodendrocytes form barriers to axon regeneration in the CNS. If oligodendrocytes become damaged or die, oligodendrocyte precursor cells in the subventricular zone can differentiate and replace oligodendrocytes to remyelinate axons.

In the PNS, sensory and motor axons are myelinated by Schwann cells residing within the nerve. An individual Schwann cell is associated with only 1 axon, covering approximately 100 μm of the axon segment. Therefore, an axon may require many hundreds to thousands of Schwann cells to myelinate it along its length. Schwann cells also associate with unmyelinated axons in nerves, providing trophic support to their associated axons. In contrast to the CNS, following injury in the PNS, axons regenerate, an activity promoted by Schwann cells. Additional roles for Schwann cells include modulation of neuromuscular synaptic activity and presentation of antigens to immune cells. Nerves also contain capillaries with associated pericytes. The presence of the pericytes and several layers of connective tissue around the axons isolates the axons from the capillaries and establishes the blood–nerve barrier.

Ependymal cells are glia cells found in the CNS where they line the ventricles and central canal and form the choroid plexus. Forming an epithelial layer, ependymal cells produce and circulate CSF for the brain and spinal cord. Within the 4 brain ventricles (2 lateral ventricles and third and fourth ventricles), a population of specialized ependymal cells and capillaries together form a structure called the choroid plexus, which produces the majority of CSF. CSF is formed as plasma is filtered from the blood through the ependymal cells. Choroid plexus ependymal cells actively transport sodium, chloride, and bicarbonate ions, with the accompanying water, into the ventricles. Tight junctions formed between ependymal cells establish the blood–CSF barrier, and cilia on their apical surface facilitate the circulation of CSF. The other part of the blood–CSF barrier is formed by the tight junctions between the cells in the arachnoid membrane.

Other types of glia found in the PNS include cells that surround several types of sensory neuron receptors and enteric glia. Two major populations of enteric glia are found in the enteric nervous system and the epithelium throughout the intestinal mucosa. Enteric glia may communicate with a variety of cells in the GI system, including enteric neurons, enteric endocrine cells, immune cells, and epithelial cells. Proposed functions for enteric glia include regulation of fluid secretion, intestinal motility, enteric neurotransmission, neurogenesis, and immune signaling.

SUMMARY

- The nervous system has 2 major divisions: the CNS and the PNS.
- The PNS detects information about the environment and sends sensory information to the CNS. The CNS receives, integrates, and stores information and sends signals to the PNS, generating responses and behavior.
- The 2 major cell types in the nervous system are neurons, which are the signaling cells, and glial cells, which are the support cells.
- The CNS includes the brain and spinal cord. Both are protected by bones and the meninges and are highly vascularized. The brain surrounds the ventricles, which produce and circulate CSF.
- The blood–brain barrier is formed by special vascular endothelial cells and glial cells that prevent the entry of unwanted molecules and cells into the CNS.
- The brain is composed of 3 major regions: the forebrain, brainstem, and cerebellum.
- In the CNS, gray matter regions contain neuronal cells bodies, dendrites, and glia. White matter regions are enriched in myelinated axons and glia.
- Ridges (gyri) and furrows (sulci) create the folded surface of the brain. Deep sulci divide the cerebral cortex into the frontal, parietal, temporal, and occipital lobes.

- In the PNS, the somatic division controls skeletal muscle contraction and receives sensory information from skin, muscles, and joints. The autonomic division controls smooth and cardiac muscles and glands and receives sensory information from the viscera.

- The spinal cord is organized into the cervical, thoracic, lumbar, sacral, and coccygeal segments. Dorsal gray matter receives input from sensory afferents. Ventral gray matter sends output via motor efferents.

- The PNS is organized into ganglia and nerves (spinal and cranial), which enclose axons of sensory and motor neurons.

- The neuronal plasma membrane encloses the cytoplasm and nucleus; typical cellular organelles perform transcription, translation, membrane trafficking, protein turnover, and energy production.

- Axons generate and conduct action potentials, the output signals from the neuron. Cytoskeletal proteins in the axon are involved in structural support and fast and slow axonal transport. The end of the axon forms the presynaptic terminus.

- Dendrites receive inputs from axons via synapses. Some dendrites contain dendritic spines, small protrusions where synapses form. Synapses are also located on the cell body and other axons.

- Glial cells are support cells in the CNS and PNS. Astrocytes and satellite cells provide metabolic support; oligodendrocytes and Schwann cells furnish myelination; pericytes regulate capillaries; ependymal cells synthesize CSF; microglia are immune cells; and enteric glia function in the GI tract.

SELF-ASSESSMENT QUESTIONS

1. Following an injury in the workplace that affected a patient's right arm, causing loss of movement of that limb, it was determined that the injury had disrupted axoplasmic transport in the sensory and motor nerves of that limb. Which of the following statements accurately reflects a fundamental property of axonal transport?

   A. Large membranous organelles are transported by slow axonal transport.
   B. Cytosolic proteins are transported by fast axonal transport.
   C. Retrograde transport is generally limited to a fixed rate of movement of particles.
   D. Anterograde transport is dependent on microtubules.
   E. The motor protein kinesin specifically governs slow axonal transport.

2. Which of the following best describes the characteristic of white matter?

   A. White matter contains neuronal cell bodies, dendrites, and synapses.
   B. White matter contains myelinated axons, astrocytes, and oligodendrocytes.
   C. White matter contains pericytes and ependymal cells.
   D. White matter contains all neurons and glia in the central nervous system (CNS).
   E. White matter includes all tracts and nerves in the CNS and peripheral nervous system (PNS).

3. Which of the following best describes the functions of astrocytes?

   A. Astrocytes form cerebral blood vessels and the blood–brain barrier.
   B. Astrocytes line the brain ventricles and form the brain capillaries.
   C. Astrocytes provide energy substrates for neurons and can regulate blood flow.
   D. Astrocytes are the major immune cells of the CNS and become "reactive glia" following injury.
   E. Astrocytes form the postsynaptic component of the tripartite synapse.

4. Which of the following best describes neurons and their processes?

   A. All neurons are signaling cells that communicate via electrical and/or chemical information with other neurons or target cells.
   B. All neurons are multipolar cells, with 1 large axon and multiple branched dendrites.
   C. All neuronal cell bodies are located in the CNS, but their axons can extend into the PNS.
   D. All axons are myelinated and highly branched at their termini.
   E. All dendrites contain small protrusions called dendritic spines, which increase the surface area of the dendrite.

5. Which of the following best characterizes the blood–brain barrier (BBB)?

   A. The presence of the BBB prevents hydrophobic molecules such as steroids and gases from entering into the neural tissue of the brain.
   B. The BBB prevents entry of most pathogenic cells but allows the majority of immune cells into the brain to prevent infection.
   C. The majority of CNS neurons and astrocytes come in direct contact with brain capillaries to ensure access to energy substrates and oxygen.
   D. The BBB forms during neurulation to prevent migration of PNS neurons into the CNS.
   E. The BBB is formed by vascular endothelial cells and pericytes, with astrocytic end feet surrounding them.

Development of the Nervous System

Lucas Pozzo-Miller & Anne B. Theibert

OBJECTIVES

After studying this chapter, the student should be able to:

- Outline the major stages, structures, and processes underlying the development of the human nervous system.
- Diagram the 5 major brain vesicles and what regions they form in the brain.
- Describe the general time course for each of the major stages of CNS development.
- Explain the identified cellular mechanisms underlying neurulation, neurogenesis, neuronal migration, gliogenesis, neural apoptosis, axonal and dendritic outgrowth, synaptogenesis, synaptic refinement, and myelination.
- Identify which processes depend on hardwired genetic programs and which ones are modified by experience-driven neuronal activity.
- Describe the underlying basis of congenital birth defects that affect the brain.

CENTRAL NERVOUS SYSTEM DEVELOPMENT: OVERVIEW & TIMELINE

Development of the human nervous system involves the generation of the central nervous system (CNS) and peripheral nervous system (PNS) and occurs during embryonic, fetal, and postnatal periods. The study of nervous system development allows a better understanding of the structural organization of the adult nervous system and helps in comprehending the basis of congenital disorders that affect brain function and cause cognitive disorders. Key prenatal stages in neural development include gastrulation, neural induction (NI), neurulation, neurogenesis, gliogenesis, neural migration, and synaptogenesis. Through these prenatal stages, the gross structures of the brain, spinal cord, and nerves are formed; most neuronal and some glial populations are generated; some synapses are formed; and development is governed predominantly by hardwired intrinsic genetic programs that control gene expression and cell–cell interactions. At birth, the mass of the human brain is approximately 350 to 400 g. Postnatally, additional glial cell populations develop, myelination rapidly takes place, dendrites become highly branched, and many more synapses are established. From birth through adolescence, synapses are stabilized and pruned by activity-dependent processes for the construction of neural circuits. This enables experience-driven neuronal activity to influence the wiring of the brain. Postnatally, the human brain nearly quadruples its mass to approximately 1300 to 1400 g in adults.

Errors in development of the nervous system can result from exposure to teratogens or genetic anomalies or mutations, which can produce sensory, motor, behavioral, or cognitive deficits and also make the brain susceptible to disorders that develop in late adolescence or adulthood. A teratogen is defined as a chemical, infectious agent, physical condition, or deficiency that, upon exposure, may cause birth defects or impair future intellectual, behavioral, or emotional functioning via a toxic effect on the developing embryo, fetus, or child. Teratogens include chemical agents such as alcohol, tobacco, environmental toxins, heavy metals, therapeutic drugs and drugs of abuse, infectious agents such as bacteria and viruses, physical injury and emotional stressors, and deficiencies such as malnutrition or hypoxia. The effects of teratogens are determined by the dose or level, timing and duration of exposure, and interactions with genetic factors. The developmental time when a particular organ is most susceptible to teratogenic damage is during the prenatal critical period, usually when morphogenesis, cell proliferation, and cellular differentiation are occurring in that organ (Figure 2–1). The prenatal critical period for brain development is from approximately 2 to 18 weeks (Figure 2–2).

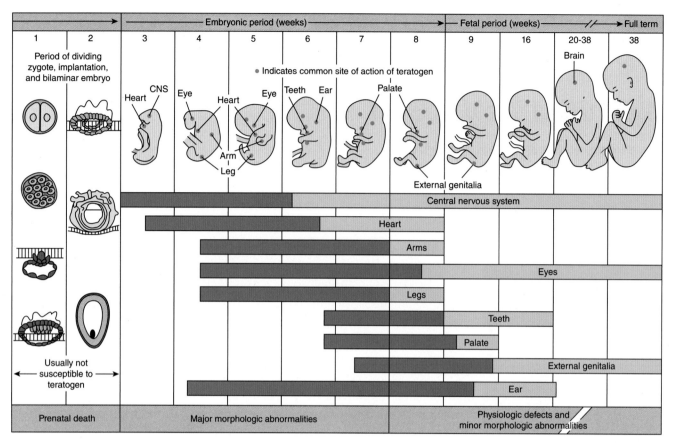

FIGURE 2-1 Illustration of the critical or sensitive periods of human prenatal development. During the first 2 weeks of development, the embryo is typically not susceptible to teratogens. During these pre-differentiation stages, a substance either damages all or most of the cells of the embryo, resulting in its death, or it damages only a few cells, allowing the embryo to recover without developing defects. Dark blue denote highly sensitive stages; light blue denote stages that are less sensitive to teratogens. (Reproduced with permission from Moore KL. *The Developing Human: Clinically Oriented Embryology.* 4th ed. Philadelphia, PA: Saunders/Elsevier; 1988.)

However, because the brain continues to develop throughout gestation, postnatally and through young adulthood, exposure to teratogens after the prenatal critical period can also lead to intellectual, emotional, and behavioral disabilities.

EARLY DEVELOPMENT: THE EPIBLAST & GASTRULATION

Human development begins with fertilization of the egg cell (ovum) by a sperm cell and is followed by the embryonic period (up to 8 weeks after fertilization) and the fetal period (8 weeks to birth at approximately 38 weeks; Figure 2–3). All developmental times here refer to after fertilization in humans.

The fertilized egg, called the zygote, undergoes a series of cell divisions to produce the blastocyst, a fluid-filled cavity containing the inner cell mass (ICM) and lined by trophoblasts. Following implantation (between 8 and 10 days), the ICM of the blastocyst reorganizes to form the bilaminar embryonic disc, composed of the epiblast and underlying hypoblast. The epiblast is a flat disc of cells that gives rise to the entire embryo. The hypoblast forms the yolk sac, while the trophoblasts form the trophectoderm, which gives rise to the placenta. At about

day 16, the embryonic disc undergoes the process of gastrulation (Figure 2–4). First, cells in the midline of the epiblast disc form a surface indentation called the primitive pit, which elongates to generate the primitive streak, a morphologic groove in the epiblast along the anterior-posterior axis of the embryo. During gastrulation, epiblast cells proliferate and migrate, with migrating cells moving first medially toward the primitive streak, and then ventrally, underneath the streak, and finally moving away from the midline in a process called ingression. Cells ingress in successive waves. Cells that migrate first push the hypoblast cells aside and form the inner layer, the endoderm, which gives rise to the lining of organs of the digestive and respiratory systems and several glands. Cells ingressing next will come to lie on top of the endoderm and form the middle layer, the mesoderm, which gives rise to the muscles, bones, cardiovascular system, and blood cells. Cells that do not ingress remain on the surface and become the outer layer, the ectoderm, which gives rise to the entire nervous system, epidermis (skin), some connective tissues, and related structures. Following gastrulation, the embryonic disc is transformed into the 3 primary germ layers (the trilaminar gastrula), and all 3 axes of the embryo are established: anterior-posterior (rostral-caudal), dorsal-ventral, and medial-lateral axes.

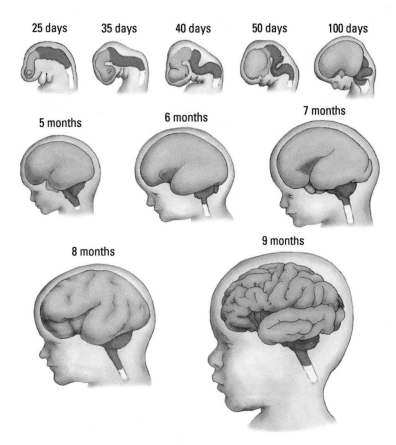

FIGURE 2–2 Prenatal growth and development of the human brain showing a series of embryonic and fetal stages. The numbers below each image refers to the gestational week used in human obstetrics, which is the time after fertilization plus two weeks. (Reproduced with permission from Balter L: *Parenthood in America: An encyclopedia.* Santa Barbara, CA: ABC-CLIO; 1999.)

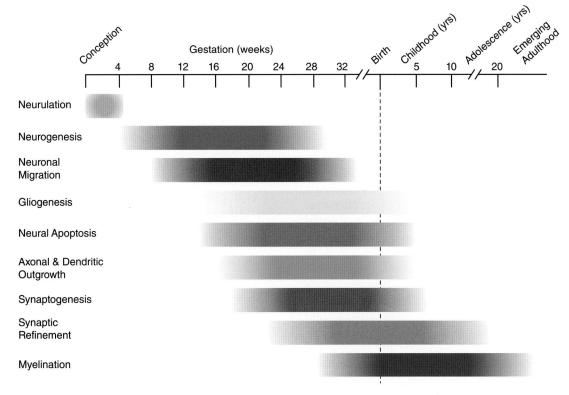

FIGURE 2–3 Timeline of processes in human brain development indicating general developmental events.

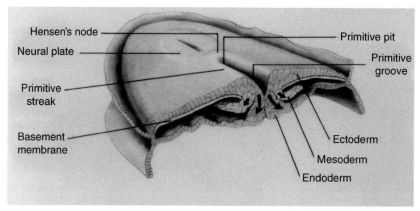

A

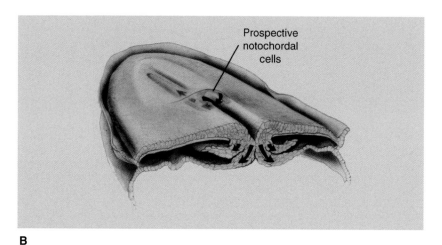

B

FIGURE 2–4 Gastrulation in vertebrates. The organizer for gastrulation in the vertebrate embryo is the "primitive node," which is called Hensen's node in avian development. **A.** Prospective endodermal and mesodermal cells of the epiblast migrate toward the primitive streak and ingress (*arrows*) through the primitive groove to become the definitive endoderm and mesoderm. The cells that do not migrate will remain on the outer layer and form the ectoderm **B.** Prospective notochordal cells in the cranial margin of Hensen's node will ingress through the primitive pit (*arrows*) during primitive streak regression to become the notochordal process. (Reproduced with permission from Dias MS, Walker ML: The embryogenesis of complex dysraphic malformations: a disorder of gastrulation? *Pediatr Neurosurg.* 1992;18(5-6):229-253.)

NEURAL INDUCTION & FORMATION OF THE NEURAL PLATE

The next important stage, beginning at approximately 17 days after fertilization, is the process of neural induction (Figure 2–5), which leads to the specification of neural and nonneural ectoderm. The formation of the notochord, a distinct cylinder of mesodermal cells at the midline of the gastrula, is a key step in NI. The notochord, together with the adjacent paraxial mesoderm, releases diffusible factors called morphogens. Morphogens are signaling molecules that form gradients and trigger highly orchestrated cascades of gene expression that control the levels and types of proteins expressed in the cell and underlie the specification toward a particular cell fate, as well as morphogenetic movements. Approximately half of the ectodermal cells, located closer to the midline, receive higher concentrations of

neural-inducing morphogens and thus become specified as the neural ectoderm (neuroectoderm), change their shape, and form the neural plate. The lateral ectoderm located further away from the midline becomes the epidermal (nonneural) ectoderm.

Well studied in amphibians, NI involves morphogens released by the notochord, which inhibit signaling of bone morphogenetic proteins (BMPs) in the overlying ectoderm. Expressed throughout the developing embryo, BMPs are growth factors members of the transforming growth factor-β superfamily that regulates a family of transcription factors. Inhibition of BMP signaling allows neural commitment genes to be expressed, including transcription factors, which then alter gene expression in the developing neural plate cells, furthering the cells along the path of neural commitment. Ectoderm cells in which BMP signaling is inhibited become neural cells, whereas cells that do not receive sufficient levels of morphogens become epidermis. In mammals, other growth

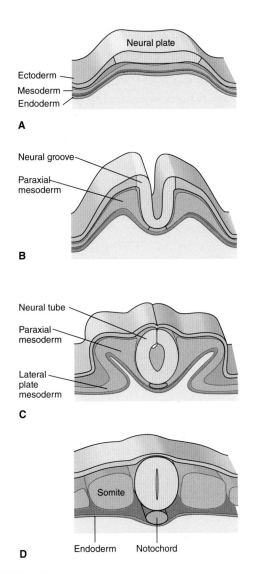

A

B

C

D

FIGURE 2–5 The neural plate folds during neurulation to form the neural tube and neural crest. **A.** Early in embryogenesis three germ cell layers—the ectoderm, mesoderm, and endoderm—lie close together. A group of mesoderm cells at the midline form the notochord. The ectoderm gives rise to the neural plate, the precursor of the central and peripheral nervous systems. **B.** The neural plate buckles at its midline to form the neural groove and elevates the neural folds. **C.** Closure of the dorsal neural folds forms the neural tube, which gives rise to the CNS. The group of cells that lies above the developing neural tube and below the non-neural ectoderm form the neural crest cells, which give rise to the PNS. **D.** The neural tube lies over the notochord and is flanked by somites, an ovoid group of mesodermal cells that give rise to muscle and cartilage. (Reproduced with permission from Kandel ER, Schwartz JH, Jessell TM, et al: *Principles of Neural Science,* 5th ed. New York, NY: McGraw Hill; 2013.)

factors, such as fibroblast growth factor (FGF), are implicated in NI. The neural plate starts to differentiate from the surrounding nonneural plate as neural plate cells become tall columnar epithelial cells. The neural plate is wider in its rostral region, which will develop into the brain, and narrower at the caudal end, which will form the spinal cord.

NEURULATION: FORMATION OF THE NEURAL TUBE & NEURAL CREST

The next critical stage is neurulation, which occurs during the third and fourth weeks after fertilization, and leads to the transformation of the neural plate into the neural tube (Figure 2–5). Concomitant with neurulation is the formation of neural crest cells and placodes. Neural tube cells give rise to neurons and glia in the CNS, whereas neural crest cells give rise to neurons and glia of the PNS; placodes give rise to special sensory neurons and ganglia of several cranial nerves. Neurulation involves large morphologic changes as the neural plate cells bend, fold, and fuse to transform the neural plate into a tube of cells, with the overlying neural crest cells. Primary neurulation forms the brain and the majority of the spinal cord, whereas secondary neurulation forms the sacral region of the spinal cord.

Primary neurulation begins at approximately day 18, when the neural plate begins to fold inward, forming the neural groove along the midline of the neural plate running rostral to caudal. Cells in the neural groove become attached to the notochord and change shape, which induces the folding of the neural plate. As the neural groove deepens, this folding causes cells at the margins of the neural plate, called the neural folds, to become elevated and approach each other in the dorsal midline. Cells within the neural folds come in close apposition to each other and adhere via specific cell adhesion molecules such N-cadherin, which then promote the closure of the neural tube. Neural plate cells located in the lateral edges of the neural folds are excluded from the tube and, as the tube closes, aggregate just above (dorsal to) the neural tube and become neural crest cells. Neural crest cells are a transient population of progenitor cells that migrate to form the sensory and postganglionic autonomic neurons in the PNS and glial cells of the PNS and contribute to some glands and tissues (see later discussion). The closure of the neural tube separates it from the neural crest cells and the overlying nonneural (epidermal) ectoderm. During this period, cranial placodes develop within the medial epidermal ectoderm, which give rise to sensory neurons in the nose and ear and several cranial ganglia.

During primary neurulation, the closure of the neural tube begins on day 20 at the level of the fourth somite, where the future cervical spinal cord will be located. The closure is asynchronous, proceeding rostrally and caudally such that the ends of the neural tube close at different times. The anterior neuropore closes at approximately day 24, whereas the posterior neuropore closes at about day 26. After the posterior neuropore closes, the process of secondary neurulation forms the most rostral region of the spinal cord. During secondary neurulation, the neural ectoderm and some cells from the endoderm form the medullary cord, which condenses, separates, and then forms cavities that merge with the rostral cord to form a single tube. Failure of the neural tube to close normally produces neural tube defects, including spina bifida, the most common congenital birth defect affecting the nervous system (discussed in Chapter 35).

REGIONALIZATION & PATTERNING IN THE CNS

The anterior/rostral neural tube gives rise to the brain, while the posterior/caudal neural tube forms the spinal cord. As the neural tube is closing, between 3 and 4 weeks after fertilization, key morphologic changes occur along the anterior-posterior axis, when transient morphologic segments of the developing neural tube, called neuromeres, establish regions of the embryonic brain and spinal cord. Through a transient blockage, the pressure of the fluid inside the rostral/anterior tube increases. Differential cell adhesion leads to the ballooning of the rostral/anterior (also called cranial) tube in 3 regions, forming the 3 primary vesicles. These large macroscopic vesicles divide the neural tube into the prosencephalon (forebrain), mesencephalon (midbrain), and rhombencephalon (hindbrain) (Figure 2–6 and Figure 2–7). The entire brain is formed from these 3 primary vesicles, whereas the ventricular system is formed from the lumen of the neural tube.

By 5 weeks, 2 of the primary vesicles enlarge and undergo an additional division to yield a total of 5 vesicles. The prosencephalon, also called the cerebrum, divides to form the telencephalon and diencephalon. As the telencephalon develops, it is tethered at the rostral midline, so it bulges to form the right and left cerebral hemispheres. As it develops, the telencephalon expands to surround the diencephalon and forms 2 gray matter regions: the dorsal telencephalon (pallium), which forms the cerebral cortex and hippocampus, and the

ventral telencephalon (subpallium), which gives rise to the basal ganglia and olfactory bulbs. Regions from both the pallium and subpallium form the amygdala. The diencephalon develops into the thalamus, hypothalamus, and optic vesicles, which give rise to the optic nerve and retina. The mesencephalon, which does not undergo a secondary division, forms the midbrain, with the dorsal mesencephalon forming the tectum (containing the superior and inferior colliculi) and the ventral regions forming the midbrain tegmentum. The rhombencephalon divides to form the metencephalon (future pons and cerebellum) and myelincephalon (future medulla oblongata). Together, the midbrain, pons, and medulla form the brainstem. The myelincephalon connects with the caudal neural tube, which develops into the spinal cord.

Concomitant with the formation of the vesicles, the neural tube bends along its anterior-posterior axis at 3 flexures that give an appearance of a cane at this stage. The first flexure is the cephalic flexure, occurring between the end of the third week and the beginning of the fourth week, and is located at the region of the midbrain; this flexure results in the forebrain bending ventrally to form a crook that resembles the cane handle. The cervical flexure occurs next, at approximately 5 weeks, and is located at the junction between the hindbrain and the spinal cord. The third flexure, the pontine flexure, occurs at the seventh week, and is located between the metencephalon and myelincephalon. Although this flexure does not persist as a bend in the axis of the hindbrain, it affects the future development of the rhombencephalon.

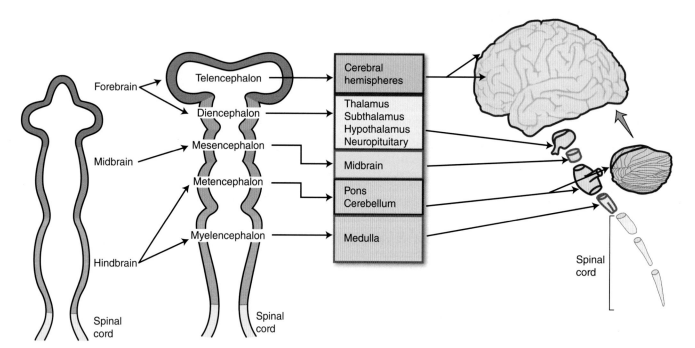

FIGURE 2–6 Illustration of regionalization that underlies the formation of major anatomic parts of the central nervous system. Early development of the neural tube produces the three primary vesicles called the forebrain (prosencephalon), midbrain (metencephalon), and hindbrain (rhombencephalon) shown on the left. Next the forebrain divides to form the telencephalon and diencephalon, the midbrain does not divide, while the hindbrain divides into the metencephalon and myelincephalon, shown in the center of the figure. Differentiation of each of the five vesicles produces the major brain structures indicated in the image on the right side of the figure. (Reproduced with permission from Kibble JD, Halsey CR. *Medical Physiology: The Big Picture.* New York, NY: McGraw Hill; 2009.)

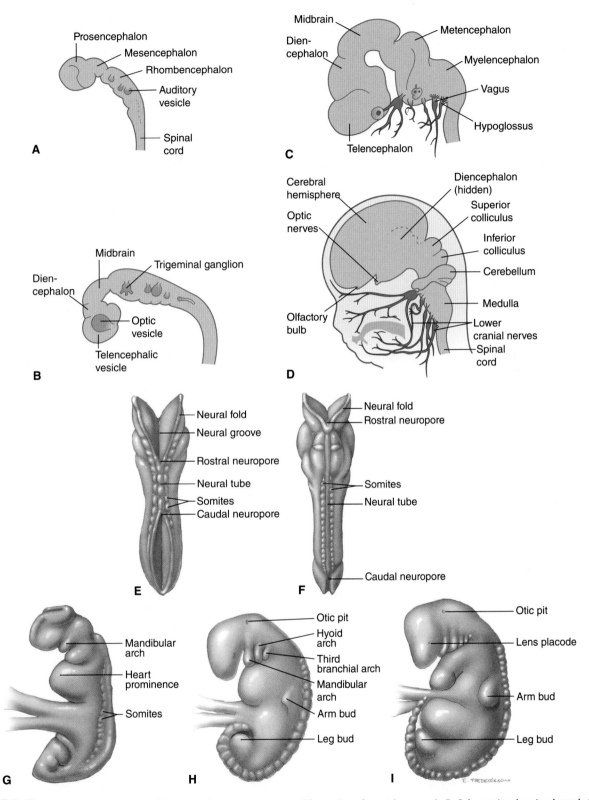

FIGURE 2–7 Stages in development of the central nervous system and formation of cranial nerves. **A–D.** Schematics showing lateral views of regionalization and flexure of the neural tube during development from 3 to 5 embryonic vesicles, and formation of several cranial nerves. Four stages in early development are illustrated (times are approximate.) A: 3 ½ weeks. B: 4 ½ weeks. C: 7 weeks. D: 11 weeks. **E–I.** Illustrations depicting closure of the neural tube and regionalization in 3- to 4-week-old embryos. E, F. Dorsal views of embryos during 22 to 23 days of development showing 8 and 12 somites, respectively, before closure of the neural tube with the rostal and caudal neuropores. G-I. Lateral views of embryos during 24 to 28 days, showing 16, 27, and 33 somites, respectively. All times reflect days or weeks post-fertilization. (Parts A–D reproduced with permission from Waxman SG. *Clinical Neuroanatomy*, 28th ed. New York, NY: McGraw Hill; 2017.)

The lumen of the neural tube becomes the ventricular system and the central canal, which generate and contain the cerebrospinal fluid (CSF). The lumen of the telencephalon becomes the lateral (first and second) ventricles in the right and left cerebral cortex. The lumen of the diencephalon forms the third ventricle. The cerebral aqueduct is formed in the lumen of the mesencephalon (midbrain). The fourth ventricle is formed from the rhombencephalon (metencephalon and myelincephalon), and the central canal is formed from the lumen of the spinal cord. Glial cells called ependymal cells line the ventricles, form part of the choroid plexus, and produce the CSF that fills the ventricular system and the central canal.

The CNS is patterned along its anterior-posterior axis, which is best characterized in the hindbrain. The hindbrain divides into segments that are slightly constricted swellings called rhombomeres. These rhombomeres form the rhombencephalon, which in turn forms the hindbrain. Each rhombomere segment develops its own set of ganglia and nerves that are later responsible for rhythmic behaviors, such as respiration, mastication, and walking. The morphogens FGF and retinoic acid regulate rhombomere development. Each rhombomere expresses its own unique set of genes, a process governed by the expression of specific transcription factors of the homeobox domain (Hox) gene family.

The CNS is also patterned along its dorsal-ventral axis. Neural tube cells at the ventral midline form the floor plate, whereas cells at the dorsal region become the roof plate. Exposure of these regions of the neural tube to different gradients of morphogens from the underlying notochord and the overlying dorsal ectoderm leads to differential gene expression that impacts the differentiation of neurons in the dorsal and ventral tube. An important morphogen released from the notochord and its overlying floor plate is sonic hedgehog (SHH). Morphogens released from the roof plate include BMPs. These morphogen gradients lead to the formation of a longitudinal groove, called the sulcus limitans, during the fourth week, which appears in the lateral wall of the neural tube throughout the future spinal cord and brainstem. The sulcus limitans separates the neural tube into the dorsal alar plate and the ventral basal plate. This division is functionally important because neurons derived from the alar plate of the spinal cord form the dorsal gray matter (posterior horns), which differentiates into sensory relay neurons, whereas neurons derived from the basal plate form the ventral gray matter (anterior horns), which differentiates into motor neurons.

Similar distinctions are present in the brainstem, but with a medial-lateral arrangement. With the formation of the pontine flexure and the fourth ventricle, the rhombencephalon undergoes a shape change that pushes the dorsal alar plate laterally and shifts the ventral basal plate medially. Although the sulcus limitans does not extend beyond the brainstem, the dorsal and ventral regions of the prosencephalon and mesencephalon are exposed to similar gradients of morphogens that influence their development into morphologically and functionally distinct brain regions. Indeed, mutations in *SHH*

cause a severe congenital malformation called holoprosencephaly (type 3), in which there is a loss of the central midline in the developing brain (see Chapter 35).

NEUROGENESIS & GLIOGENESIS

Once the neural tube closes and undergoes the morphologic changes described earlier, neurons and glia are generated from the neural tube through proliferation and differentiation, called neurogenesis (**Figure 2–8**) and gliogenesis. As newly born neurons and glia are generated, they also undergo migration to their final location in the brain. The majority of neurogenesis occurs during prenatal development, although a few neuronal populations are generated postnatally. Gliogenesis involves the formation of astrocytes, oligodendrocytes, and ependymal cells during the late prenatal and early postnatal periods. Different populations of neural cells develop at different times in different regions of the nervous system. Beginning after the closure of the neural tube at 4 weeks after fertilization and continuing through the early postnatal period, the peak in neurogenesis occurs between the fifth week and fifth month of gestation. It has been estimated that during its peak, approximately 250,000 neurons are produced per minute. Because the brain contains approximately 86 billion neurons, this is a period of robust neuronal proliferation and differentiation. Glia outnumber neurons in most brain regions, usually developing after neurons in a given region. Glia are continuously replaced in the adult nervous system from glial progenitors, while new neurons are generated at a very low rate only in a few specific brain regions in the adult brain, in a process called adult neurogenesis.

After the neural tube closes, it is composed of a single layer of cells called the germinal neuroepithelium (NE). NE cells develop into neural stem cells (NSCs) and neural progenitor cells (NPCs), which are populations of self-renewing cells that generate all the neurons and glial cells of the CNS. NSCs have the capacity for unlimited self-renewal and multipotency. As NSCs proliferate, they give rise to NPCs, cells that have more limited capacity for self-renewal and more restricted potency. NPCs give rise to lineage-restricted cells that migrate and differentiate into different types of neurons and glial cells.

An important type of NSC are the radial glial cells (RGC). RGCs, so named because they initially express a glial-specific protein and guide the radial migration of neurons, actually give rise to the majority of principal neurons of the cerebral cortex that use the excitatory neurotransmitter glutamate. Initially, NE cells proliferate and generate RGCs, both of which proliferate in the area next to the lumen of the neural tube (the future ventricle), forming the ventricular zone (VZ). The NE cells and RGCs are also referred to as apical progenitors. In the VZ, dividing RGCs undergo either symmetric divisions that lead to self-renewal or asymmetric cell divisions that produce 1 self-renewing daughter cell and another daughter cell that is either a postmitotic neuron or a specific type of NPC.

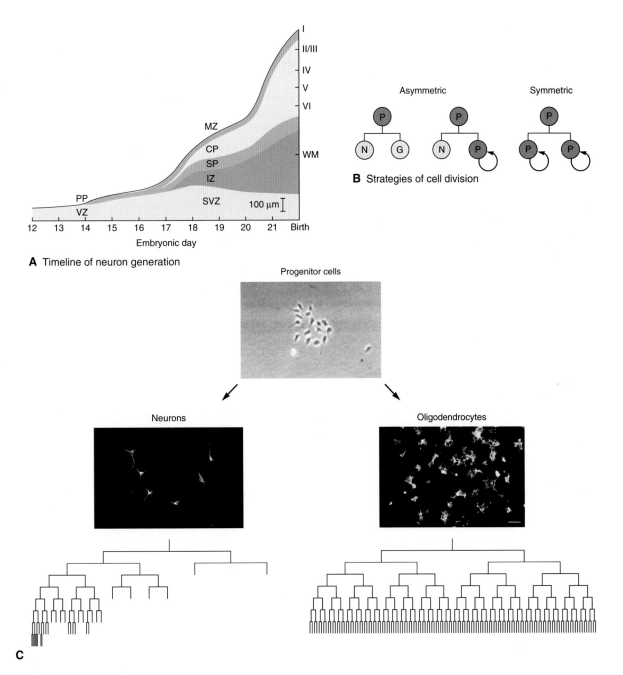

FIGURE 2–8 Neurogenesis and gliogenesis in the cerebral cortex. **A.** Temporal sequence of neurogenesis in the mouse cerebral cortex. Neurons begin to accumulate in the cortical plate (CP) during the last 5 days of embryonic development. Within the CP, neurons populate the deep layers before the superficial layers. (IZ, intermediate zone; MZ, marginal zone; PP, preplate; SP, subplate; SVZ, subventricular zone; VZ, ventricular zone; WM, white matter.) **B.** Neural progenitor cells have two different modes of division. A progenitor cell (P) undergoes asymmetric division to generate a neuron (N) and a glial cell (G) (left). Or a progenitor cell can undergo asymmetric division to give rise to another progenitor cell and a neuron (middle). Asymmetric divisions contribute to the generation of neurons at early stages of development, and of glial cells at later stages. A progenitor cell undergoes symmetric division to generate two additional progenitor cells (right). **C.** Time-lapse microscopy illustrates the divisions and differentiation of isolated rodent cortical progenitor cells. Lineage analysis illustrates cells that undergo predominantly asymmetric division, giving rise to neurons (left), or symmetric division that gives rise to oligodendrocytes (right). (Parts A and B, reproduced with permission from Kandel ER, Schwartz JH, Jessell TM, et al: *Principles of Neural Science,* 5th ed. New York, NY: McGraw Hill; 2013; part C, reproduced with permission from Qian X, Goderie SK, Shen Q, et al: Intrinsic programs of patterned cell lineages in isolated vertebrate CNS ventricular zone cells, *Development.* 1998 Aug;125(16):3143-3152.)

RGCs generate 2 main types of progenitors. One type, called short neural precursors, remains in the VZ and constitutes a third category of apical progenitors. The other RGC progeny is the intermediate progenitor cell (IPC), also called basal progenitor or bRGC, the majority of which migrate to an adjacent region called the subventricular zone (SVZ), where further neurogenesis takes place. Subsequent symmetrical divisions of these progenitor cells produce self-renewing daughter cells, whereas asymmetric divisions produce daughter cells with more restricted lineage. There is a distinct progression of lineage differentiation whereby RGCs first give rise to neurons and later to astrocytes and oligodendrocytes.

MIGRATION & DIFFERENTIATION IN THE CNS

Concomitant with neurogenesis is the process of neuronal migration, during which differentiating neurons travel from their origin or birthplace to their final position in the brain. The formation of the cerebral cortex (corticogenesis) is an excellent model for the characterization of neuronal migration. Neurons formed in the VZ or SVZ migrate to their final locations in the neocortex, occurring between gestational weeks 7 and 18 in humans. A key event is the formation of the cortical plate, which includes the cortical layers 2 to 6. Corticogenesis begins with the formation of a region called the preplate (a layer that forms between the outer pial surface and the VZ/SVZ). The first-born postmitotic neurons, Cajal-Retzius cells and subplate neurons, leave the stem cell niche in the VZ/SVZ and migrate outward along the scaffolding fibers provided by RGCs to form the preplate. The preplate then separates into 2 components, as Cajal-Retzius cells migrate outward to form the marginal zone (above the cortical plate and containing layer 1) and the subplate neurons form the deeper subplate region that will become the intermediate zone.

Subsequent waves of postmitotic cells migrate along RGCs, and these new neurons form the cortical plate, which separates the superficial marginal zone and the intermediate zone (Figure 2–9). This phase involves the appearance of well-defined cell layers in the cortical plate (cortical layers 2 to 6), as each wave of newly generated neurons migrates past their predecessors to progressively more peripheral zones, while the earlier generated neurons are differentiating. In this way, the cortex is said to develop in an inside-out manner. The intermediate zone becomes the white matter region just below the cortical gray matter. The transition from preplate to cortical plate is a period during which cortical malformations are thought to occur (see Chapter 35). The extracellular matrix protein reelin (encoded by the *RELN* gene) and its plasma membrane receptors are implicated in neuronal migration during corticogenesis because mutations in those genes cause cortical malformations.

The majority of excitatory neurons in the neocortex (approximately 75% of the total cortical neurons) are generated from RGC precursors in the VZ or SVZ immediately below their adult location, where they arrive by radial migration as described earlier. In contrast, the majority of inhibitory interneurons (approximately 25% of cortical neurons) migrate tangentially (parallel to the ventricular surface) to reach their appropriate location in the cortex, in a process that is independent of radial glial fibers. An important structure in tangential migration is the ganglionic eminence, a transitory structure located in the ventral VZ of the telencephalon that helps guide cortical inhibitory interneurons to their destination in the cortex. A third type of migration is axophilic migration, which uses existing axon tracts to guide the migration of developing neurons.

As development proceeds, mitotically active neural progenitor cells give rise to postmitotic cells that, via different patterns of gene expression, differentiate into specific types of neurons and glial cells. Cellular differentiation during development is the result of the orchestrated activity of gene regulatory networks. One well-documented way that gene expression is controlled is via transcription, which is controlled by transcription factors and epigenetics. Control of gene expression depends on both intrinsic factors (proteins and mRNAs inherited from the mother cell after cell division) and extrinsic cues, including molecules found in the environment that function through receptor signaling pathways to control gene regulatory proteins. Gene expression controls the levels of protein expression, which influences specific biochemical, functional, and structural characteristics of different classes of neurons and glial cells.

Much research in the past 3 decades has focused on identifying the extracellular factors, receptors, and gene regulatory networks involved in controlling neuronal and glial cell differentiation, prompted in part by the potential for cell replacement therapy to treat neurodegenerative and other neurologic disorders, as well as brain and spinal cord injury. These studies have led to the identification of many genes that contribute to the neuron–glia fate decision, including many of the morphogens mentioned earlier, as well the proneural, neurogenic, and Hes genes in the basic helix-loop-helix (bHLH) transcription factor families, the Sox and Pax families of transcriptional regulators, and signaling pathways involving Notch.

An important structural feature of the human brain is the presence of several convolutions in the surface of the cerebral cortex. The grooves or depressions in the surface of the cerebral cortex are called sulci (singular: sulcus), and the bumps or ridges are called gyri (singular: gyrus), which are formed through the process of gyrification. The thickness of the 6-layered cerebral cortex (2 to 4 mm) is similar across all mammals. Because the brain is confined within the skull, brain size is limited, and the adult human cortex must fold and wrinkle to allow an expansion of cortical surface area during human fetal development. Beginning at approximately 10 weeks after fertilization, the primary cortical gyri form first, followed later by the development of secondary and tertiary gyri. Differential proliferation and differentiation in the VZ and SVZ progenitor zones may underlie differences in cortical size and gyrification among mammals. Errors that produce changes in the structure of gyri and sulci in the cerebral cortex are associated with various disorders, including lissencephaly (smooth brain), pachygyria, and polymicrogyria. These disorders reflect atypical neurogenesis and/or corticogenesis and cause various neurologic symptoms, such as epilepsy, muscle weakness, and intellectual disability (see Chapter 35).

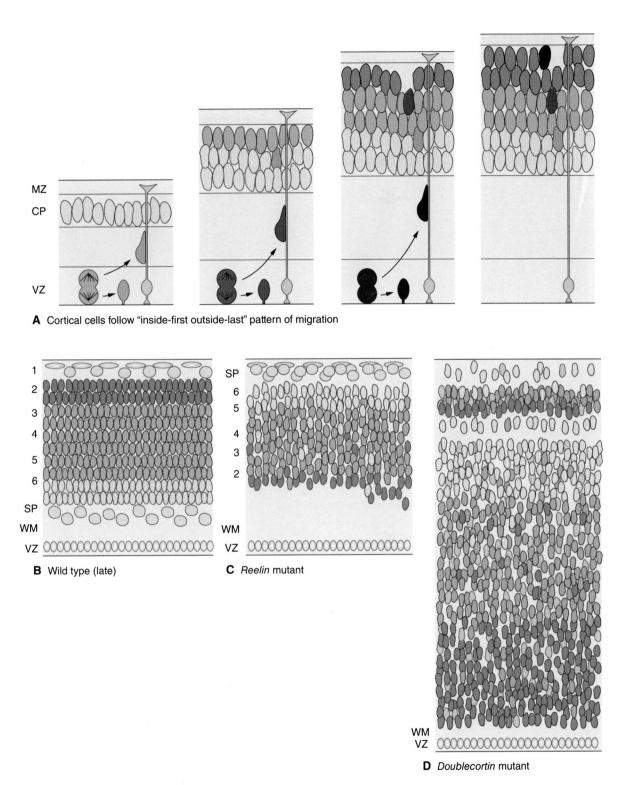

A Cortical cells follow "inside-first outside-last" pattern of migration

B Wild type (late)

C *Reelin* mutant

D *Doublecortin* mutant

FIGURE 2–9 Migration of neurons during cortical development produces the layered organization of the cerebral cortex. **A.** During typical cerebral cortical development mouse neurons use radial glial cells as migratory scaffolds as they enter the cortical plate. As they approach the pial surface, neurons stop migrating and detach from radial glial cells. (CP, cortical plate; MZ, marginal zone; VZ, ventricular zone.) **B.** An orderly inside-out pattern of neuronal migration results in the formation of six neuronal layers in the mature cerebral cortex, arranged between the white matter (WM) and subplate (SP). **C.** In the mouse mutant *reeler*, which lacks functional reelin protein, the layering of neurons in the cortical plate is severely disrupted and partially inverted. In addition, the entire cortical plate develops beneath the subplate. **D.** In *doublecortin* (*dcx*) mutants the cortex is thickened, neurons lose their characteristic layered identity, and some layers contain fewer neurons. A similar disruption is observed in *Lis1* mutants, which underlies certain forms of human lissencephaly. (Adapted with permission from Olson EC, Walsh CA: Smooth, rough and upside-down neocortical development, *Curr Opin Genet Dev.* 2002 Jun;12(3):320-327.)

AXONAL OUTGROWTH & PATHFINDING

As neurons migrate and differentiate, they begin to extend their axon first, followed by several dendrites, sometimes after they have arrived at their final location (**Figure 2–10**). Axons are guided toward their targets by a specialized structure at the tip of the growing process called the growth cone. A growth cone is a highly dynamic structure that senses guidance cues through specific membrane receptors and ion channels and translates extracellular signals into changes in the cytoskeleton that result in a tropic (movement) behavior. Axons are guided

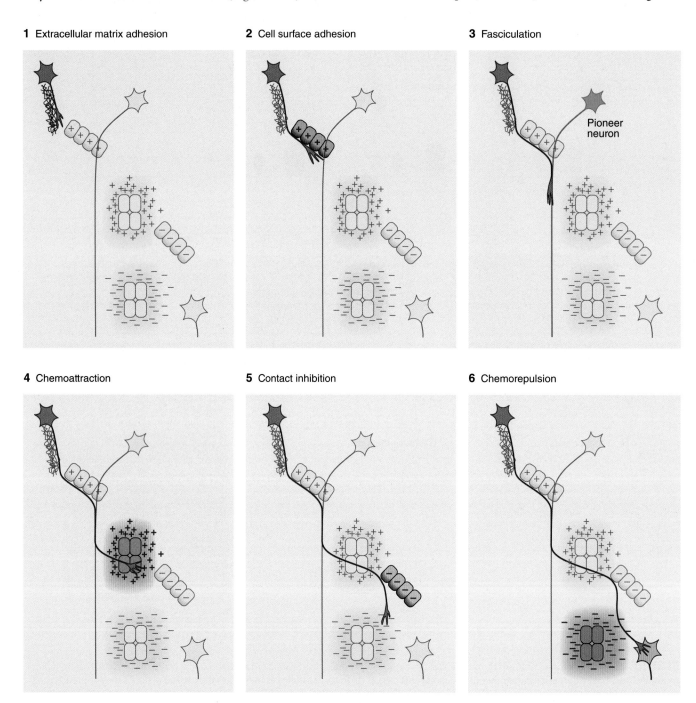

FIGURE 2–10 Axonal outgrowth and guidance is directed by a variety of mechanisms, involving both short and long range cues that can act as attractants or repellents. In many cases it is the axonal tip or growth cone that mediates the interaction. 1. Interactions with molecules in the extracellular matrix can promote growth. 2. The axon can interact with adhesive cell-surface molecules on neural cells. 3. The growing axon can adhere to another axon from a "pioneer" neuron and track along it, a process termed *fasciculation*. 4. The growing axon can be attracted by soluble chemical signals. 5. Cell-surface repellent cues expressed on intermediate targets can cause the axon to turn away. 6. The growing axon can be repelled by soluble chemical signals. (Reproduced with permission from Kandel ER, Schwartz JH, Jessell TM, et al: *Principles of Neural Science*, 5th ed. New York, NY: McGraw Hill; 2013.)

to their target by environmental cues that include soluble, cell-associated or matrix-attached molecules that act as either repellents or attractants.

In many brain regions, there are 2 main types of neurons: projection neurons, whose axons project outside of that region, and local circuit neurons, which project only to neighboring neurons within the same region. For axons that travel long distances, the axon is guided toward its postsynaptic partner by a series of intermediate targets and gradients of diffusible and tethered cues. A number of diffusible guidance cues and their receptors have been identified and include secreted proteins (and their cognate receptors) called netrins (DCC and Unc5), Slit (Robo), ephrins (Eph receptors), and semaphorins (plexins and neuropilins). Developmental morphogens such as BMPs, FGF, and Wnts also contribute to growth cone navigation. Cell adhesion molecules, such as immunoglobulin superfamily cell adhesion molecules and cadherin, and extracellular matrix proteins provide cell-attached and nondiffusible, tethered cues. Although less well characterized and usually much shorter in length, developing dendrites also project growth cones, with dendritic outgrowth likely governed by similar types of mechanisms used by the growing axon.

NEURONAL SURVIVAL & APOPTOSIS

During nervous system development, neurogenesis and gliogenesis produce more neurons and glial cells than are needed in the adult nervous system. Physiologic neural cell loss through apoptosis (programmed cell death) removes approximately one-third to one-half of all developing neural cells, including neural progenitors, postmitotic neurons, and glial cells. Apoptosis is critical to adjust the size of the input population to match the size of the target population, thus preventing erroneous or unnecessary connections.

Neurons depend on both survival factors in the environment and functional synaptic connections for their survival. Best characterized for neurons of the PNS, it was hypothesized that growing axons compete for limiting amounts of target-derived trophic factors and that axons that fail to receive sufficient trophic support do not survive (Figure 2–11). Classical studies on target-derived factors that support sympathetic neuron survival led to the discovery of nerve growth factor (NGF). Subsequently, the related neurotrophins, neurotrophin (NT)-3, NT-4, and brain-derived neurotrophic factor (BDNF), were identified. In both the CNS and PNS, neurotrophins and

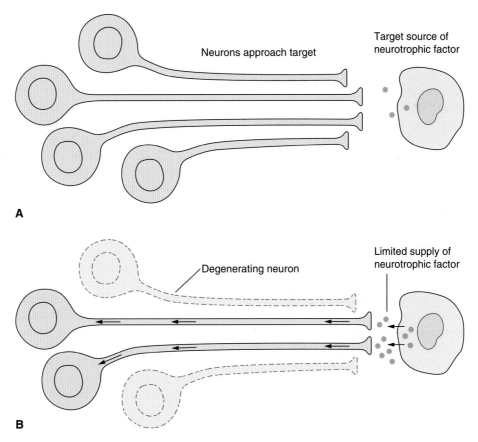

FIGURE 2–11 The neurotrophic factor hypothesis. **A.** Neurons extend their axons to target cells, which secrete low levels of neurotrophic factors. (For simplicity only one target cell is shown.) The neurotrophic factor binds to specific receptors, which leads to the promotion of neuronal survival. **B.** Neurons that fail to receive adequate amounts of neurotrophic factor stimulation die through a program of cell death termed apoptosis.

a variety of other trophic factors produced during different stages of development contribute to the survival of specific neuronal classes. Other trophic factors include BMPs, glial cell line–derived neurotrophic factor, ciliary neurotrophic factor, insulin-like growth factor, cytokines, and even classical neurotransmitters such as glutamate, which can support neuronal survival. Once functional synaptic connections have been established, activity also contributes to neuronal survival. Interestingly, some trophic factors such as BDNF play important roles not only in survival, but also neurogenesis and synaptic plasticity in the adult brain. Because adult neurons die by apoptosis in neurodegenerative disorders, identification of the molecular mechanisms underlying neuronal apoptosis is an intensely studied topic with the goal of identifying novel treatments and strategies to prevent apoptosis in the adult brain.

SYNAPTOGENESIS & SYNAPTIC REFINEMENT

Once neurons have reached their final destinations and extended their axon and dendrites and the axonal growth cone has contacted its postsynaptic target, a synapse is ready to be formed. Formation of a synapse between a neuron and its target cell is termed *synaptogenesis* and occurs prenatally, throughout postnatal development and adolescence, as well as into adulthood. Neurons form synapses in order to communicate with other neurons in the CNS or with target muscles or glands in the PNS, for the establishment of functional neural circuits that mediate sensory and motor processing, and underlie behavior and memory. Chemical synapses use neurotransmitters that diffuse across the extracellular space between presynaptic and postsynaptic neurons and bind to selective membrane receptors, whereas electrical synapses formed by gap junction channels allow direct electrical communication between neurons. Many different morphologic and functional types of chemical synapses exist in the CNS. Chemical synapses are formed between the specialization of a presynaptic axon, called a presynaptic terminal or bouton, and a dendrite, cell body, or presynaptic terminal of the postsynaptic neuron. Synapses on dendrites can be formed on the shaft of the dendrite or on small protrusions called dendritic spines. Dendrites undergo extensive branching during postnatal development, which increases the area and number of synapses that can form on the dendrites.

During CNS synaptogenesis, the presynaptic growth cone contacts the postsynaptic neuron, which sends retrograde signals that transform the growth cone into a presynaptic terminal. If the target is a dendrite, a dynamic protrusion called a filopodium attracts the presynaptic growth cone and helps initiate synapse formation. Once contacted, the presynaptic and postsynaptic compartments become highly specialized with the clustering of multiple proteins in and near the plasma membranes of both regions. Many of the presynaptic and postsynaptic proteins, including the synaptic vesicle release machinery, ion channels, receptors, and scaffolds,

are delivered to the developing synapses in preassembled membrane-bound packets. Contact between the 2 neurons involves the binding of cell adhesion molecules, such as neuroligin and neurexin, synCAMs, cadherins, ephrins, and Eph receptors, across the synaptic cleft, which adheres the synaptic partners to each other. Some synapses have been shown to be active within minutes after initial contact, but it usually takes much longer (hours to days) for mature synapses to become functional.

The development of proper brain function involves a careful balance between the production and elimination of cells and synapses. Neurons often extend axonal branches and form synapses with both appropriate and inappropriate targets, and the inappropriate connections are eventually pruned away. During development and throughout life, synapses are reconfigured both morphologically and functionally, through a process called synaptic refinement, a type of synaptic plasticity that involves the formation of new synapses, elimination of unwanted or unused synapses, and changes in synaptic morphology and synaptic transmission, called synaptic strength (Figure 2–12). Although initial synapse formation does not depend on neuronal activity, elimination of supernumerary and inappropriate synapses and the ongoing modification of existing synapses depend on neuronal activity. Activity-dependent mechanisms driven by sensory inputs and behavioral experiences modulate the development of neural circuits and their connectivity maps.

Many synapses that form during prenatal and early postnatal periods are eliminated between early childhood and the onset of puberty. Synaptic refinement and circuit formation occur and peak at different developmental times, called sensitive and critical periods, in different brain systems. Developmental sensitive and critical periods are time windows when experiences have a greater impact on certain areas and functions of brain development and when the brain is most likely to strengthen important connections and eliminate unneeded ones in specific brain regions. A postnatal critical period is a somewhat narrower window during the sensitive period, during which the nervous system is especially impacted by environmental stimuli (Figure 2–13); if the organism does not receive the appropriate stimulus during the critical period for a given skill or function, it may be difficult, or even impossible, to develop that function later in life. Critical periods for development of the visual and auditory systems occur in the first 6 to 9 months, whereas language peaks around 6 to 12 months and higher cognitive functions peak in childhood. Lifelong changes in the strength of synapses, so called synaptic plasticity, is considered a key mechanism that underlies learning and memory and is discussed in detail in Chapter 10.

MYELINATION

Myelination, the formation of the insulating myelin sheath around axons, begins in late embryonic stages and continues through early postnatal stages and adolescence (Figure 2–14).

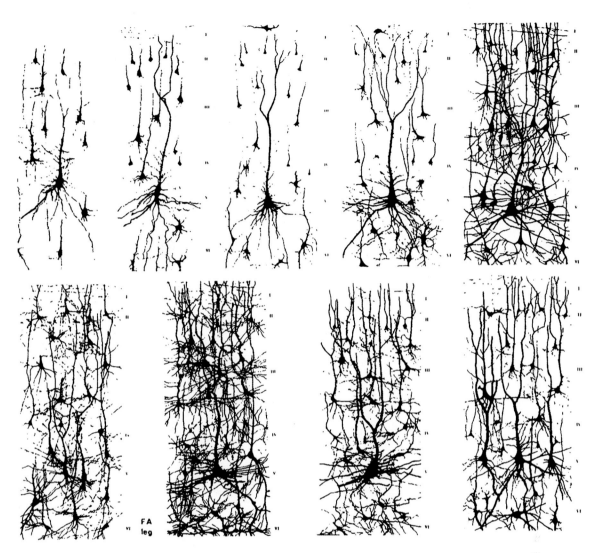

FIGURE 2–12 Dendritic arborization, synaptogenesis, and synapse refinement in the postnatal development of the cerebral cortex. Cox-Golgi preparations of the leg area of the motor cortex (area 4). *Upper row, left to right:* 1 month premature (8 months gestation); newborn at term; 1 month; 3 months; and 6 months. *Lower row, left to right:* 15 months; 2 years; 4 years; 6 years. Apical dendrites of Betz cells have been shortened, all to the same degree, for the purposes of display. (Used with permission from T. Rabinowicz, University of Lausanne.)

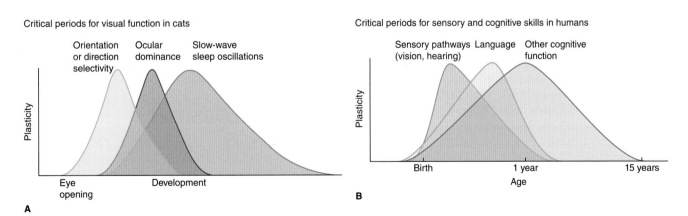

FIGURE 2–13 The timing of critical periods varies with brain function. **A.** In cats the critical periods for development of orientation or direction selectivity in visual neurons occur earlier than those for establishment of ocular dominance and slow-wave sleep oscillation. **B.** In humans the timing of periods for development of sensory processing, language, and cognitive functions varies. (Part A, reproduced with permission from Hensch TK: Critical period plasticity in local cortical circuits. *Nat Rev Neurosci.* 2005 Nov;6(11):877-888; part B, adapted with permission from Nelson CA, Zeanah CH, Fox NA: How Early Experience Shapes Human Development: The Case of Psychosocial Deprivation, *Neural Plast.* 2019 Jan 14;2019:1676285.)

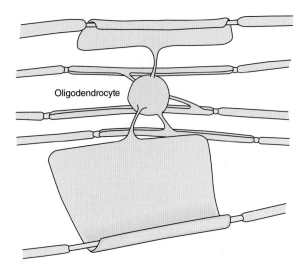

A Myelination in the central nervous system

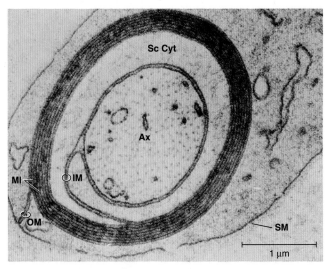

B Myelination in the peripheral nervous system

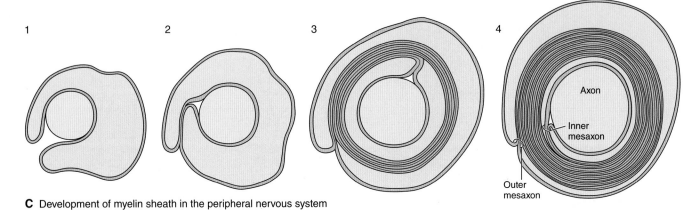

C Development of myelin sheath in the peripheral nervous system

FIGURE 2–14   Myelination of axons in the central and peripheral nervous systems. **A.** Illustration showing axons in the central nervous system are wrapped in several layers of myelin produced by oligodendrocytes. Each oligodendrocyte can myelinate multiple axons. **B.** Electron micrograph of a transverse section through an axon (Ax) in the mouse sciatic nerve shows the origin of a sheet of myelin (MI) at the inner mesaxon (IM), which arises from the surface membrane (SM) of a Schwann cell, and is continuous with the outer mesaxon (OM). The Schwann cell cytoplasm (Sc Cyt) is squeezed out as the myelin layers become compact. **C.** A peripheral nerve fiber is myelinated by a Schwann cell in sequential stages. In stage 1 the Schwann cell surrounds the axon. By stage 4 a mature myelin sheath has formed. (Part C, reproduced with permission from Williams PL, Warwick R, Dyson M, et al: *Gray's Anatomy.* 37th ed. Edinburgh, United Kingdom: Churchill Livingstone; 1989.)

The myelinating cells of the CNS, oligodendrocytes, develop from precursors called oligodendrocyte precursor cells and, in general, myelinate axons that are larger than 1 μm in diameter. Oligodendrocytes are numerous in white matter (where 1 oligodendrocyte can myelinate up to 50 axons), whereas satellite oligodendrocytes are located in gray matter. The myelin sheath provides electrical insulation for axons that ensures efficient and fast conduction of action potentials, in addition to providing trophic and metabolic support for the axons. Myelination is especially important for long axons that travel long distances to their targets, such as fibers from projection neurons. Once myelinated, axons from similar regions bundle together to form the major white matter systems in the brain: the cortical white matter, the corpus callosum, and the internal capsule, as well as the major tracts in the spinal cord. Impairments in the function of oligodendrocytes cause myelination defects that lead to demyelinating disorders and hypomyelinating leukodystrophies (described in Chapter 35).

PNS DEVELOPMENT

The vast majority of neurons and glia of the PNS are generated from neural crest cells (Figure 2–15). Formed from the margins of the developing neural plate (the neural folds), neural crest cells are ectoderm derivatives that first aggregate above the roof of the neural tube, but then migrate away to give rise to peripheral neurons and glial cells, as well as pigmented skin cells and parts of glands and facial structures.

Cells from the cranial neural crest migrate dorsolaterally, forming the craniofacial mesenchyme that differentiates

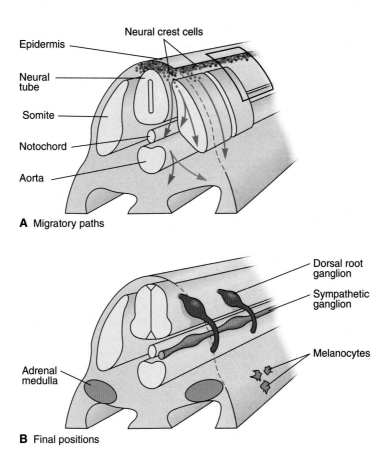

A Migratory paths

B Final positions

FIGURE 2–15 Neural crest cell migration and differentiation forms the peripheral nervous system. **A.** Cross section through the middle part of the trunk of a chick embryo shows the main pathways of neural crest cells. Some migratory cells migrate along a superficial pathway, just beneath the ectoderm, and differentiate into pigment cells of the skin. Others migrate along a deeper pathway that takes them through the somites, where they coalesce to form dorsal root sensory ganglia. Still others migrate between the neural tube and somites, past the dorsal aorta. These cells differentiate into sympathetic ganglia and adrenal medulla. **B.** The final settling positions of neural crest cells, after they have completed their migration and undergone differentiation. (Reproduced with permission from Kandel ER, Schwartz JH, Jessell TM, et al: *Principles of Neural Science*, 5th ed. New York, NY: McGraw Hill; 2013.)

into the sensory components of cranial nerves, various cranial ganglia, PNS glia, and craniofacial cartilage and bone. Entering the pharyngeal pouches and arches, some cells contribute to the thymus, odontoblasts of the tooth primordia, and bones of the jaw and middle ear. The trunk neural crest produces cells that form 1 of 2 pathways. Cells that migrate dorsolaterally into the ectoderm and toward the ventral midline become pigment-synthesizing melanocytes. Cells that migrate ventrolaterally through the anterior portion of each sclerotome and remain there form the sensory neurons of the dorsal root ganglia, whereas those that continue to migrate ventrally form the sympathetic ganglia, adrenal medulla, Schwann cells, and the aortic nerve clusters. Cells from the vagal and sacral neural crest give rise to the ganglia of the enteric nervous system and the parasympathetic ganglia. Cells from the cardiac neural crest develop into cartilage, connective tissue, and neurons of some pharyngeal arches, in addition to musculo-connective tissue of the large arteries in the heart and regions of the heart septum and semilunar valves, as well as melanocytes. Finally, some PNS neurons

are derived from the neural placodes, small islands of neural ectoderm located in the medial regions of epidermal ectoderm after the neural tube closes. Neural placodes give rise to olfactory and auditory sensory neurons and contribute to several ganglia in cranial nerves.

SUMMARY

- Nervous system development begins in the embryonic period and continues through fetal stages and during postnatal life.

- Prenatal development is governed mainly by intrinsic hardwired genetic programs that involve gene expression and cell–cell interactions.

- The entire nervous system develops from the ectoderm layer.

- Neural induction involves the release of morphogens from the notochord, which control differentiation of overlying ectoderm cells that generate the neural plate.

- Neurulation leads to the formation of the neural tube, which gives rise to neurons and glial cells of the CNS.
- During neurulation. the neural crest forms above (dorsal to) the neural tube, and neural crest cells migrate to form the PNS.
- Neurogenesis and gliogenesis involve the proliferation and differentiation of neural stem cells and neural progenitor cells.
- Newly generated neurons and glia migrate to their final position in the brain.
- The formation of gyri and sulci through gyrification significantly increases the surface area of the cerebral cortex.
- Outgrowth of axons and dendrites involves guidance from environmental cues.
- Final neuron numbers are determined by neurogenesis, neuronal survival, and cell death (apoptosis) modulated by neurotrophins.
- Synapse formation (synaptogenesis) occurs in prenatal and postnatal periods, followed by activity-dependent pruning during postnatal sensitive and critical periods.
- Postnatal development is controlled mainly by extrinsic, activity-dependent mechanisms that impact neuronal survival, synapses, and neural circuits.
- Synapse number and strength are dynamic and modified throughout life by experience-driven neuronal activity.
- Myelination of CNS axons by oligodendrocytes during early postnatal development produces white matter in the CNS.
- Neural crest cells migrate and differentiate into neurons and glial cells in the PNS and several types of nonneural cells.

SELF-ASSESSMENT QUESTIONS

1. Which of the following best describes the process of neural induction (NI)?
   A. NI involves the release of morphogens by the notochord that inhibit bone morphogenetic proteins (BMP) signaling in the overlying ectoderm.
   B. NI involves morphogens released by the neural plate to the underlying notochord.
   C. In NI. morphogens stimulate the developing gastrula to form the 3 primary germ layers.
   D. NI occurs following neurulation, during segmentation and flexure.
   E. NI involves induction of the mesoderm to form neural mesoderm.

2. Which of the following best characterizes development of the neural tube?
   A. Errors in neuronal and glial migration produce microcephaly.
   B. Errors in proliferation and expansion of the neural tube produce neural tube defects.
   C. It forms from the neural plate in the process of "neural flexure" following gastrulation.
   D. It gives rise to the vast majority of neurons and glia of the central nervous system (CNS).
   E. The lumen of the neural tube forms the meninges and blood supply of the brain and spinal cord.

3. Which of the following best describes regionalization of the neural tube during development?
   A. The myelencephalon gives rise to the cerebellum.
   B. The mesencephalon gives rise to the midbrain.
   C. The telencephalon gives rise to the thalamus and hypothalamus.
   D. The diencephalon gives rise to the forebrain.
   E. The metencephalon gives rise to the pons and medulla oblongata.

4. Which of the following best characterizes neurogenesis and gliogenesis?
   A. For most regions of the cerebral cortex, glial cells are generated and differentiate before neurons.
   B. The majority of neurons are produced from the neural tube, whereas the majority of glia are produced from neural crest cells.
   C. Both neurons and glia develop from neural stem cells and neural progenitor cells.
   D. Both neurogenesis and gliogenesis occur predominantly postnatally.
   E. Neurogenesis and gliogenesis begin before neurulation and closure of the neural tube.

5. Synaptogenesis involves the formation of synapses, which are:
   A. formed only between neuronal axons and dendrites.
   B. eliminated by apoptosis during the prenatal critical period.
   C. stable structures that are formed predominantly during prenatal development.
   D. important for neuronal migration along radial glial cells.
   E. dynamic structures that can undergo synaptic refinement and be modified by experience.

Functional Anatomy of the Nervous System I: Cerebrum & Subcortical Structures

Anne B. Theibert

OBJECTIVES

After studying this chapter, the student should be able to:

- Outline the 5 embryonic vesicles and explain what they give rise to in the human brain.
- Identify and define the major anatomic components of the forebrain derived from the telencephalon and diencephalon: the cerebral hemispheres, cerebral cortices, cerebral white matter, and subcortical structures.
- Identify the major sulci and gyri, gray and white matter regions, organization of the cerebral cortex, and types of white matter tracts.
- Describe the anatomy and explain the functions of the frontal, parietal, occipital, temporal, insular, and limbic lobes.
- Describe the anatomy and explain the functions of the major forebrain subcortical areas: the amygdala, basal ganglia, thalamus, and hypothalamus.
- Diagram the connections among the major cortical and subcortical structures.

OVERVIEW OF THE NERVOUS SYSTEM

The mammalian nervous system has 2 major divisions: the central nervous system (CNS) and the peripheral nervous system (PNS). The general structure of the nervous system and its cellular components were provided in Chapter 1. The CNS is composed of the brain and the spinal cord. Protected on the outside by bones and the meninges, the CNS is suspended in and contains cerebrospinal fluid (CSF) and is highly vascularized. Functionally, the CNS receives and processes sensory information from the PNS and special sense organs, integrates and stores that information, and sends instructions to coordinate and control responses, activities, and movements of the body. In addition, the CNS constructs emotion, perception, and cognition. The CNS can be generally divided into the forebrain, the midbrain, and the hindbrain, which form the brainstem and cerebellum, and the spinal cord. Derived from the embryonic telencephalon and diencephalon, the forebrain encompasses the cerebral hemispheres, including the cerebral cortex, cerebral white matter, and structures located within the white matter, including the

basal ganglia, limbic system, thalamus, and hypothalamus. In this chapter, key anatomic and functional components of the forebrain are described. In the next chapter (Chapter 4), the anatomy and function of the brainstem, cerebellum, spinal cord, PNS, meninges, ventricular system, and vascular supply are further elaborated.

ANATOMIC REFERENCES & TERMS

For neuroanatomic descriptions, definitions of anatomic reference directions and terms are useful (Figure 3–1). In the human brain, anterior/rostral means toward the front of the brain and face, whereas posterior/caudal means toward the back of the cranial cavity or tail. In the brain, the direction pointing up is dorsal, and the direction pointing down is ventral. Below the midbrain and in the spinal cord, the direction pointing toward the back is dorsal, and the direction pointing toward the chest/stomach is ventral. The invisible line running down the middle of the nervous system is called the midline. Structures closer to the midline are medial; structures further away from the midline are lateral. A structure

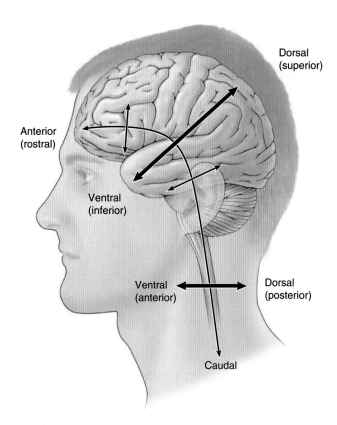

FIGURE 3–1 Anatomic reference directions and axes. The human central nervous system has a prominent flexure at the midbrain, hence the forebrain and the brainstem/spinal cord have different axes. (Reproduced with permission from Martin JH. *Neuroanatomy: Text and Atlas,* 4th ed. New York, NY: McGraw Hill; 2012.)

that is above a specific reference area is called superior, and one that is below is termed inferior. Structures that are on the same side of the midline are said to be ipsilateral to each other; structures that are on opposite sides of the midline are said to be contralateral to each other.

For postmortem brain tissue, a brain slice is called a section, and standard cuts occur in 1 of the 3 anatomic planes (Figure 3–2). The plane of section resulting from cutting the brain into equal right and left halves is called the midsagittal plane. Sections parallel to the midsagittal plane are in the

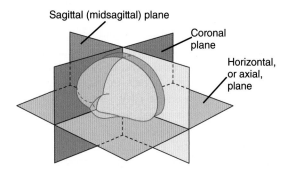

FIGURE 3–2 Planes used for brain sections. (Reproduced with permission from Waxman SG. *Clinical Neuroanatomy,* 28th ed. New York, NY: McGraw Hill; 2017.)

sagittal plane. The other 2 anatomic planes, horizontal and coronal, are perpendicular to the sagittal plane and to one another. The horizontal plane is parallel to the ground. Hence, horizontal sections separate the brain into dorsal and ventral parts. The coronal plane is perpendicular to the ground and to the sagittal plane. Thus, the coronal plane divides the brain into anterior/rostral and posterior/caudal parts.

In postmortem tissue, gray matter (which appears gray in preserved tissue, but is pink or light brown in living tissue) contains neuronal cell bodies, dendrites, synapses, and astrocytes (Figure 3–3). White matter is composed of myelinated axons, oligodendrocytes, and astrocytes. Gray matter forms the cortical layers of the brain and clusters of neurons, called nuclei, in the brain and spinal cord. Groups of nuclei form several subcortical gray matter areas. A bundle of myelinated axons (also called fibers) in the CNS is called a tract (or sometimes referred to as a nerve tract), with tracts forming the white matter regions in the brain and spinal cord.

OVERVIEW OF THE HUMAN BRAIN

The adult human brain weighs between 1200 and 1500 g (2.6 and 3.1 lb) and occupies a volume of between 1130 and 1260 cm³. Although only about 2% of the total body weight, the brain consumes 20% of the oxygen and calories supplied to the body. As described in Chapter 2, the brain and the spinal cord arise in embryonic development from the neural tube, which expands in the anterior half to form the 3 primary brain divisions: the prosencephalon (forebrain), mesencephalon (midbrain), and rhombencephalon (hindbrain). These 3 vesicles further differentiate into 5 subdivisions: the telencephalon, diencephalon, mesencephalon, metencephalon, and myelencephalon (Figure 3–4). The telencephalon forms the cerebrum, which includes the cerebral cortex, cerebral white matter, and several subcortical structures, including the amygdala and majority of the basal ganglia. The diencephalon forms the thalamus, subthalamus, hypothalamus, posterior pituitary, and epithalamus. Together, the telencephalon and diencephalon compose the forebrain. The mesencephalon forms the midbrain, the metencephalon forms the pons and cerebellum, and the myelencephalon forms the medulla. The brainstem consists of the midbrain, pons, and medulla. The cerebellum lies adjacent to the brainstem and underneath the forebrain and forms the posteriormost part of the brain. The spinal cord is continuous with the medulla.

The brain is enclosed in the cranial cavity (intracranial space), which is the space formed inside the skull (Figure 3–5). The skull is composed of 2 major parts: the neurocranium, which encases the brain, and the facial skeleton, which forms and supports the face, with the mandible being the largest component. In addition to protecting the brain, the skull fixes the distance between the eyes to allow stereoscopic vision and fixes the position of the ears to enable sound localization. Together, 8 fused cranial bones form the cavity: the frontal, occipital, sphenoid, and ethmoid bones, and 2 each of the parietal and temporal bones. The spinal cord passes through

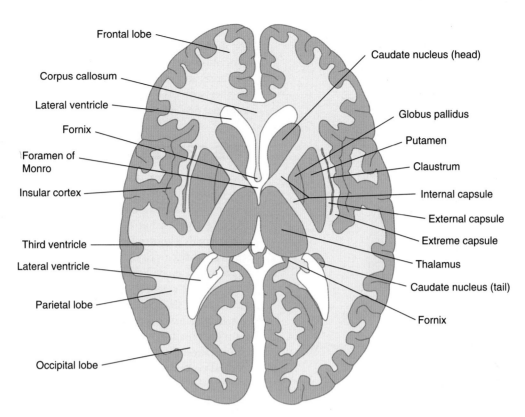

FIGURE 3–3 Illustration of gray and white matter regions in a horizontal brain section. Cerebral cortical gray matter (tan) is located at the lateral regions of the brain, adjacent to cerebral white matter (beige). The deeper subcortical gray matter regions (tan) contain nuclei and are located next to white matter (beige). (Reproduced with permission from Waxman SG. *Clinical Neuroanatomy,* 28th ed. New York, NY: McGraw Hill; 2017.)

the foramen magnum, the large opening in the occipital bone at the base of the skull, as it exits the cranial cavity.

THE CEREBRUM

Derived from the telencephalon, the cerebrum forms the largest part of the brain, is situated above the other brain structures, and consists of the 2 cerebral hemispheres that are separated by the longitudinal fissure, also called the deep sagittal fissure. The right and left sides of the brain are anatomically mirror images of each other, a characteristic known as bilateral symmetry. The right cerebral hemisphere receives sensory information from and controls the motor functions of the left side of the body. Likewise, the left cerebral hemisphere is concerned with sensations and movements on the right side of the body. Functionally, the 2 halves of the brain are not exactly alike. Some cognitive functions, such as language, are said to be lateralized, since they are more dominant on one side of the brain than the other.

The cerebral hemispheres contain the cerebral cortex, which is the thin outer layer of gray matter that covers the core of cerebral white matter. Within the cerebral white matter lie several subcortical gray matter structures, including the amygdala and basal ganglia. The cerebral hemispheres also house the lateral ventricles, where CSF is produced and circulated. The surface of the human cerebrum has many convolutions, where the brain is folded into ridges (gyri; singular: gyrus) and

grooves (sulci; singular: sulcus) (Figure 3–6). Gyri and sulci include both the cortical gray matter and a small portion of underlying white matter. The largest, primary grooves show a consistent location and are named according to their position or by the person who first described them. The locations of secondary and tertiary gyri and sulci can vary somewhat among individuals.

Each cerebral hemisphere is divided into 4 main lobes, the frontal, temporal, parietal, and occipital lobes, which are separated by primary sulci, and named according to the skull bone that overlies each (see Figure 3–6). The frontal lobe is separated from the parietal lobe by the central sulcus (also called the fissure of Rolondo), with the gyri on either side called the precentral gyrus and postcentral gyrus. The temporal lobe is separated from the frontal and parietal lobes by the lateral sulcus (Sylvian fissure). The parieto-occipital sulcus separates the parietal and occipital lobes. Two additional cortical lobes have also been described in humans. The insular lobe is formed from the insular cortex, a portion of the cerebral cortex folded deep within the lateral sulcus. The limbic lobe is an arc-shaped rim of cortex on the medial surface of each cerebral hemisphere surrounding the corpus callosum, composed of parts of the frontal, parietal, and temporal lobes.

Each of the cortical lobes is associated with 1 or a few specialized functions, although there is functional overlap between the lobes and extensive connections within and among the lobes. Within each of the cortical lobes, specific cortical areas

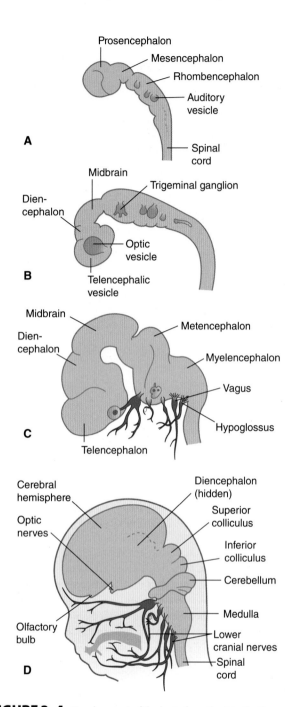

FIGURE 3–4 Development of the brain from the 3 to the 5 embryonic vesicles. Four stages in early development of the human brain and cranial nerves is illustrated (times are approximate.) **A.** 3 ½ weeks. **B.** 4 ½ weeks. **C.** 7 weeks. **D.** 11 weeks. (Reproduced with permission from Waxman SG. *Clinical Neuroanatomy,* 28th ed. New York, NY: McGraw Hill; 2017.)

called sensory, motor, and association areas are attributed with specific functions (Figure 3–7). The primary sensory areas receive inputs from the sensory tracts by way of relay nuclei in the thalamus, with the exception of the olfactory cortex. Primary sensory areas include the visual cortex in the occipital lobe, the auditory cortex and olfactory cortex in the temporal lobe, and the somatosensory cortex in the parietal lobe. The primary motor cortex, which sends axons down to motor neurons

in the brainstem and spinal cord, occupies the posterior portion of the frontal lobe. The remaining parts of each cortex are association areas. Association areas receive input from the sensory areas and subcortical structures of the brain and function together with other association areas in complex networks to construct perception, emotion, and cognitive processes.

THE CEREBRAL CORTEX

The cerebral cortex is a thin layer of gray matter between 2 and 4 mm thick and overlying the cerebral white matter. In humans, the largest part of the cerebral cortex (~90%) is the neocortex, which has 6 neuronal layers and is present only in mammals (Figure 3–8). A few small regions of human cerebral cortex (~10%) are allocortex, which has only 3 or 4 layers and is evolutionarily older, evolving in vertebrates. Although the cerebral cortex is only a few millimeters thick, it occupies a sizeable area in humans; it is estimated that the human neocortex represents approximately 75% of the total brain gray matter. It has been proposed that, in humans, gyri and sulci result from the expansion of the surface area of the cerebral cortex during fetal development, allowing a greater area of cerebral cortex to fit into the confines of the skull. The increased cortical areas have been proposed to underlie the evolution of higher cognitive functions in humans.

Although the neocortex displays a consistent 6-layer organization, different regions of the cerebral cortex are composed of distinguishably different neuronal morphologies and connections. Mapped by microscopic analysis into 52 areas by Brodmann in the early 20th century, each numbered Brodmann area has a common cytoarchitecture (Figure 3–9). At that time, Brodmann, Ramon y Cajal, and others predicted that cortical areas that look different perform different functions. Through numerous types of analyses in the past century, we now know this to be true. Because there is little difference in the thickness of the neocortex in different mammals, Brodmann also predicted that the neocortex expanded by the insertion of new areas. The neocortex contains approximately 80% excitatory glutamatergic neurons and approximately 20% inhibitory GABAergic neurons and receives inputs from neurons in all the major neurotransmitter systems. Many neuroscientists propose that the smallest functional unit of the neocortex is a cylinder of neurons approximately 2 to 3 mm in height (the distance from the white matter to the pial surface) and approximately 0.5 mm in diameter. A cortical column or hypercolumn consists of ~50-100 minicolumns and is estimated to contain ~10,000 neurons and 100 million synapses (~10,000 synapses per neuron). Cortical columns have been characterized in primary visual and somatosensory cortex, in which the neurons have similar sensory receptive fields.

THE FRONTAL LOBE

The frontal lobe is involved in voluntary motor control, production of language, and a majority of cognitive functions, including short-term working memory, attention, behavioral

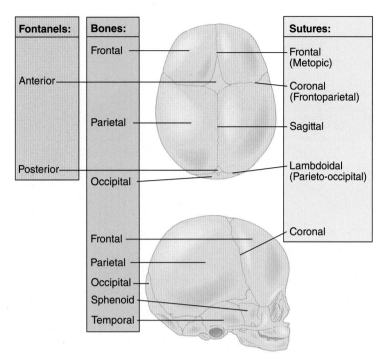

FIGURE 3–5 Components of the skull during development. The fontanels (a space between the bones of the skull in an infant), the bones, and sutures (a fibrous joint found in the skull) of the infant cranium are illustrated. Top: superior view of cranium. Bottom: lateral view of the cranium. (Reproduced with permission from Biller J, Gruener G, Brazis PW. *DeMyer's The Neurologic Examination: A Programmed Text,* 7th ed. New York, NY: McGraw Hill; 2016.)

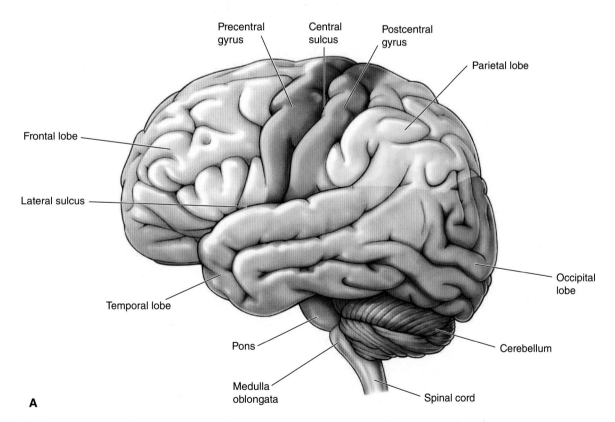

FIGURE 3–6 The main sulci, gyri, lobes, and areas of the brain. **A.** Illustration of a lateral view of the brain showing the central sulcus, lateral sulcus, and four major lobes visible from the exterior. **B.** Illustration of a lateral view of the brain showing the major gyri and sulci within the frontal, parietal, occipital, and temporal lobes. Subcortical structures are indicated within the dashed lines. (Part A, reproduced with permission from Morton DA, Foreman KB, Albertine KH. *The Big Picture: Gross Anatomy,* 2nd ed. New York, NY: McGraw Hill; 2019; part B, reproduced with permission from Martin JH. *Neuroanatomy: Text and Atlas,* 4th ed. New York, NY: McGraw Hill; 2012.)

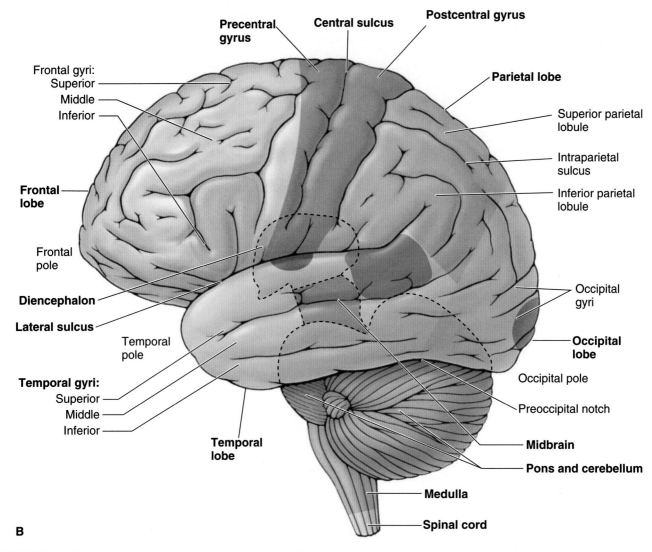

Precentral gyrus **Central sulcus** **Postcentral gyrus**

Frontal gyri:
Superior
Middle
Inferior

Parietal lobe

Superior parietal
lobule

Intraparietal
sulcus

Inferior parietal
lobule

Frontal lobe

Frontal
pole

Diencephalon

Lateral sulcus

Temporal
pole

Occipital
gyri

Occipital lobe

Occipital pole

Preoccipital notch

Temporal gyri:
Superior
Middle
Inferior

Temporal lobe

Midbrain

Pons and cerebellum

Medulla

Spinal cord

B

FIGURE 3–6 (*Continued*)

control, and executive functions. Motor areas include the motor cortex, frontal eye fields, and the Broca area. The prefrontal cortex and other areas are involved in cognitive functions. The frontal lobe also contains a small region of sensory cortex. The primary gustatory cortex, responsible for the reception of taste, consists of the frontal operculum on the inferior frontal gyrus of the frontal lobe and the anterior insula in the insular lobe.

The motor cortex is the region of the frontal lobe involved in the planning, control, and execution of voluntary movements and is composed of 3 regions: the primary motor cortex, the premotor cortex, and the supplemental motor area (SMA) (Figure 3–10). The primary motor cortex is located in the precentral gyrus immediately anterior to the central sulcus. The primary motor cortex contains upper motor neurons that send impulses via axons to the brainstem and spinal cord for the execution of movement. The premotor cortex is located anterior to the primary motor cortex and is involved

both directly and indirectly in the control of movement. The premotor cortex sends axons to the spinal cord for direct motor control of some movements, especially proximal and trunk muscles of the body, and sends inputs to the primary motor cortex for the preparation for and sensory guidance of movement. Both the primary motor and premotor cortices are somatotopically organized.

The SMA is located in the anterior paracentral lobule. Together, the premotor cortex and SMA are involved in planning of movement, selection of appropriate motor plans and sequences, and coordination of the 2 sides of the body for complex patterns of motor output. The motor cortex receives inputs from the prefrontal cortex, thalamus, primary somatosensory cortex, and posterior parietal lobe. Other brain regions including the cerebellum, basal ganglia, and brainstem nuclei are also critical in the control of motor function, but send information to the motor cortex via the thalamus.

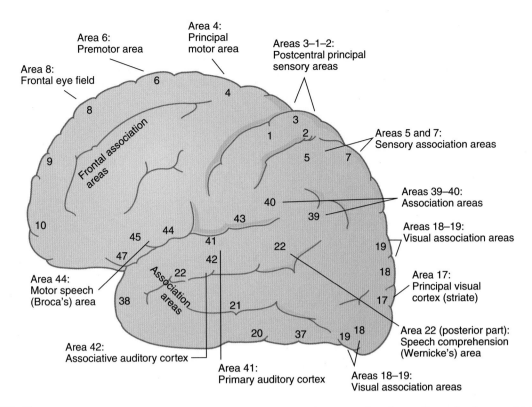

FIGURE 3-7 Illustration of a lateral view of the cerebrum showing cortical areas numbered according to Brodmann, with functional localization of sensory, motor and association areas. (Reproduced with permission from Waxman SG. *Clinical Neuroanatomy,* 28th ed. New York, NY: McGraw Hill; 2017.)

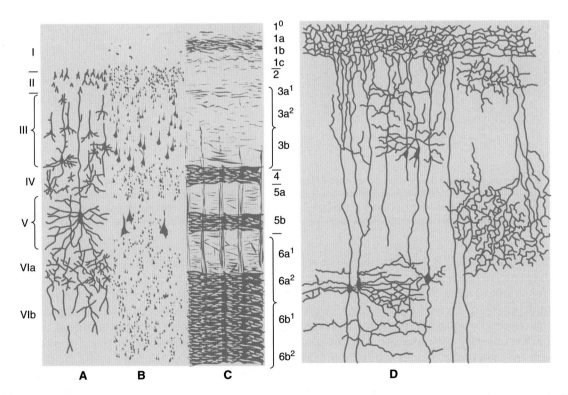

FIGURE 3-8 Diagram showing the organization of neurons and structures in the cerebral cortex. **A.** Golgi neuronal stain. **B.** Nissl cellular stain. **C.** Wigart myelin stain. **D.** Neuronal connections. Roman and Arabic numerals indicate the layers of the neocortex; 4, external line of Baillarger (line of Gennari in the occipital lobe); 5b, internal line of Baillarger. (Parts A, B, C, reproduced with permission from Ranson SW, Clark SL. *The Anatomy of the Nervous System.* 10th ed. New York, NY: Saunders/Elsevier; 1959; part D, reproduced with permission from Ganong WF. *Review of Medical Physiology,* 22nd ed. New York, NY: Appleton & Lange; 2005.)

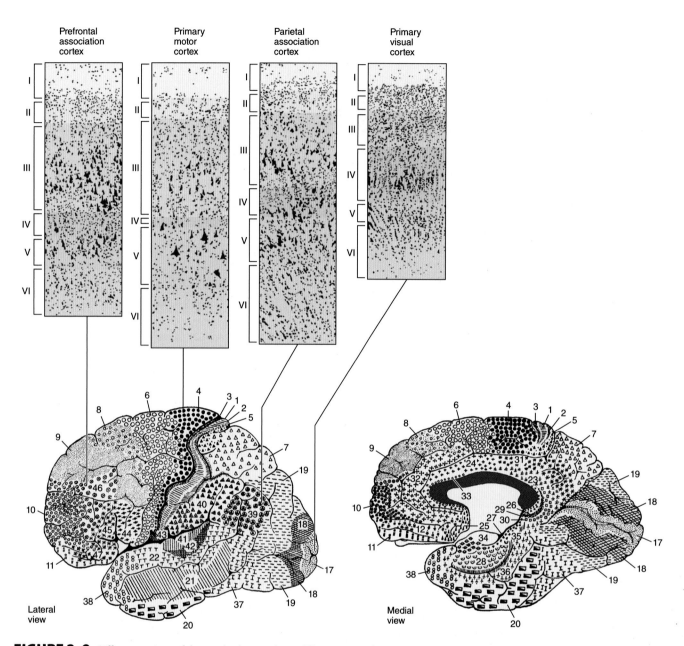

FIGURE 3–9 Different regions of the cerebral cortex have different cytoarchitecture (Top) Drawn Nissl-stained sections through various portions of the cerebral cortex. (Bottom) Brodmann's cytoarchitectural areas of the cerebral cortex. (Top, adapted with permission from Campbell AW. *Histological Studies on the Localisation of Cerebral Function*. Cambridge, United Kingdom: Cambridge University Press; 1905. Bottom, adapted with permission from Campbell 1905 and Brodmann K. Vergleichende Lokalisationslehre der Grosshirnrinde in ihren Prinzipien dargestellt auf Grund des Zellen-baues. Barth, 1909.)

The frontal eye field (FEF) is a frontal lobe motor area involved in the control of visual attention and eye movements. Located in a region around the intersection of the middle frontal gyrus with the precentral gyrus, the FEF is responsible for saccadic eye movements for visual field perception and awareness, as well as for voluntary eye movement. The FEF communicates with the extraocular muscles indirectly through the paramedian pontine reticular formation. Another motor area, the Broca area, is a small region in the frontal lobe of 1 hemisphere (usually the left in the majority of humans), with functions linked to language. Located in the inferior frontal gyrus of the dominant hemisphere, the Broca area has a key role

in various speech and language processing functions, including speech production and language comprehension. The Broca area receives substantial inputs from the other important language area, the Wernicke area, in the temporal lobe.

The other role of the frontal lobe is to produce cognitive functions that orchestrate thoughts with the selection of appropriate actions to achieve particular goals. For example, the frontal lobe constructs the ability to predict outcomes, project future consequences resulting from current activities, work toward a defined goal, make expectations based on actions and evaluate the consequences of a particular course of action, differentiate among conflicting thoughts, determine

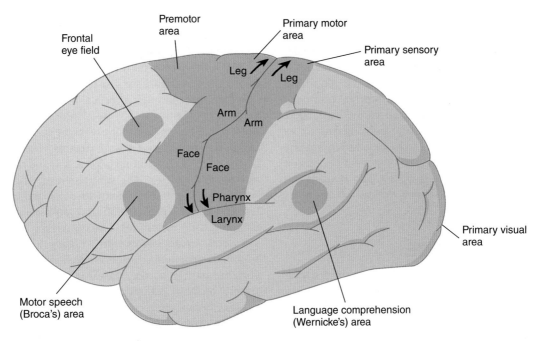

FIGURE 3–10 Lateral view of the left hemisphere illustrating several functional cortical areas. The somatotopic maps of the motor cortex in the frontal lobe, and somatosensory cortex in the parietal lobe are shown. The supplemental motor area is medial to the premotor area (not shown). (Reproduced with permission from Waxman SG. *Clinical Neuroanatomy*, 28th ed. New York, NY: McGraw Hill; 2017.)

similarities and differences between things or events, choose between good (or better) and bad (or worse) actions, suppress impulses, and override and control socially unacceptable responses.

The frontal lobe is involved in what are termed *executive functions*, including attentional control, short-term working memory, self-control and moderation of social behavior, decision making, judgment, planning, reasoning, problem solving, and abstract thinking, as well as the expression of emotion and personality. These cognitive functions require the prefrontal cortex, the region located anterior to the motor cortex, as well as other cortical and subcortical regions. The prefrontal cortex can be divided into lateral, polar, orbital, and medial domains (Figure 3–11). Each of these domains consists of a particular gyrus and has a specific function. The prefrontal cortex is highly interconnected with much of the brain, including extensive connections with other cortical, subcortical, and brainstem regions. The prefrontal cortex receives massive inputs from the somatosensory, visual, and auditory sensory association cortices and also from the thalamus. The dorsal prefrontal cortex is especially interconnected with brain regions involved with attention, cognition, and action, whereas the ventral prefrontal cortex interconnects with brain regions involved with emotion.

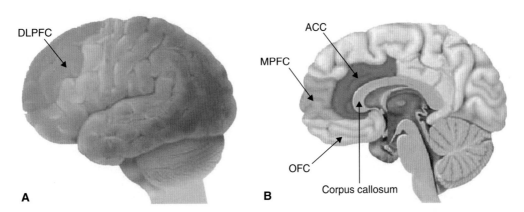

FIGURE 3–11 Regions of the prefrontal cortex involved in complex cognitive function. *Left panel*, lateral view showing the dorsolateral prefrontal cortex (DLPFC). *Right panel*, sagittal section showing the medial prefrontal cortex (MPFC), orbital frontal cortex (OFC), and anterior cingulate cortex (ACC). (Reproduced with permission from Nestler EJ, Hyman SE, Holtzman DM, et al: *Molecular Neuropharmacology: A Foundation for Clinical Neuroscience*, 3rd ed. New York, NY: McGraw Hill; 2015.)

The dorsolateral prefrontal cortex (DLPFC) is involved in executive functions, as well as motor planning. The DLPFC has connections with the orbitofrontal cortex (OFC), thalamus, basal ganglia, hippocampus, and association areas of the temporal, parietal, and occipital lobes. The OFC is considered anatomically synonymous with the ventromedial prefrontal cortex. The OFC and medial prefrontal cortex have direct connections to the thalamus, amygdala, and cingulate cortex of the limbic lobe and are thought to be involved in impulse control and to provide the emotional component to decision making, planned behavior, and memory. The ventrolateral prefrontal cortex is thought to play a critical role in motor inhibition and spatial attention.

THE OCCIPITAL LOBE

The smallest lobe, the occipital lobe, is located in the rearmost portion of the skull and is dedicated to vision. The occipital lobe contains the visual cortex and is involved in visual reception, visual-spatial processing, motion perception, and color recognition (Figure 3–12). The primary visual cortex is commonly called V1 or the striate cortex because of the prominent band of myelin in cortical layer 4. In humans, V1 is located in the posterior pole of the occipital lobe, on the medial side within the calcarine sulcus, although V1 often continues to the posterior pole of the occipital lobe. V1 receives direct input via the optic radiations from the lateral geniculate nucleus of the thalamus, which is the relay from the retina. V1 in the left hemisphere receives visual information from the right visual field, and V1 in the right hemisphere receives visual information from the left visual field. Surrounding V1 are the visual areas (V2, V3, and V4) forming the extrastriate cortex, which are specialized for different visual tasks. Each of these visual areas contains a map of the visual world. The visual association cortex extends anteriorly from the extrastriate cortex to encompass adjacent areas of the posterior parietal lobe and much of the posterior temporal lobe.

V1 is involved in the initial cortical processing of all visual information necessary for visual perception. Visual information then flows through a cortical hierarchy. In the mammalian visual system, visual sensory information is transmitted from V1 along anatomically separate and parallel streams, called the ventral and dorsal streams. The ventral stream begins with V1, goes through V2 to V4, and then to the inferior temporal cortex. The ventral stream is also called the "what" pathway, is associated with form and object recognition and object representation, and provides important information for the identification of stimuli for memory storage. The dorsal stream begins with V1, goes through V2, then to V5/middle temporal area and V6/dorsomedial area, and to the posterior parietal cortex. The dorsal stream is also called the "where" or "how" pathway and is associated with motion, spatial orientation, representation of object locations, binocular/depth perception, and guidance of behaviors to spatial locations. Originally thought to be parallel, the 2 streams are in fact heavily interconnected, and evidence suggests that both steams are essential for successful perception, especially as the stimuli take on more complex forms.

As part of visual processing, the visual system is involved in assessing distance, size, and depth; identifying visual stimuli, particularly objects and familiar faces; continually responding to changing information from the external environment; and transmitting visual information to brain regions in other lobes that encode memories, assign meaning, and guide appropriate motor and linguistic responses.

THE PARIETAL LOBE

The parietal lobe is positioned anterior to the occipital lobe, posterior to the frontal lobe, and dorsal to the temporal lobe (Figure 3–13). The parietal lobe contains the somatosensory cortex, which receives and processes touch, temperature, pain, and conscious proprioceptive information from the body and provides some motor control. The posterior parietal cortex (PPC) is important in visuospatial perception, spatial attention, and integration of somatosensory, visual, and auditory input, with connections to the motor cortex to control and plan specific movements. Several areas of the parietal lobe are also important in cognitive processing including language, learning and memory-related processes, knowledge of numbers (numerosity), categorization, and decision making.

The primary somatosensory cortex (S1) is located in the postcentral gyrus in Brodmann areas (BA) 3, 2, and 1. Area 3b in S1 receives sensory information about touch, temperature, and pain from the skin that is relayed via the thalamus from the contralateral side of the body. Neurons in 3b project to BA2 and BA1. Area 3a receives proprioceptive information via the thalamus about body position and movement. Similar to the motor cortex, which lies directly on the opposite side of the central sulcus, there is a somatotopic map in S1.

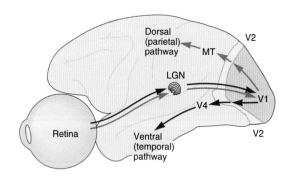

FIGURE 3–12 The visual cortex in the occipital lobe and parallel processing in visual pathways. The ventral stream is primarily concerned with object identification, carrying information about form and color. The dorsal pathway is dedicated to visually guided movement, with cells selective for direction of movement. These pathways are not strictly segregated, however, and there is substantial interconnection between them even in the primary visual cortex (V1). LGN, lateral geniculate nucleus; MT, middle temporal area; V2 and V4 are visual association areas. (Reproduced with permission from Kandel ER, Schwartz JH, Jessell TM, et al: *Principles of Neural Science*, 5th ed. New York, NY: McGraw Hill; 2013.)

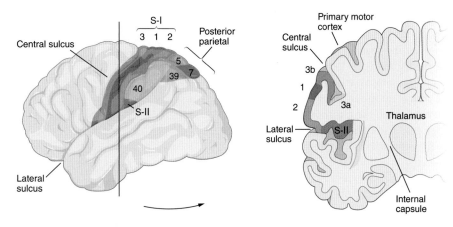

FIGURE 3-13 Functional areas in the parietal lobe. (Left) A lateral view of a cerebral hemisphere illustrates the location of the primary somatic sensory cortex in the parietal lobe. The somatic sensory cortex has three major divisions: the primary (S-I) and secondary (S-II) somatosensory cortices, and the posterior parietal cortex. (Right) A sagittal section shows the regions of S-I (Brodmann's areas 3a, 3b, 1, and 2), the adjacent posterior parietal cortex (areas 5 and 7), and motor cortex (area 4). (Reproduced with permission from Kandel ER, Schwartz JH, Jessell TM, et al: *Principles of Neural Science,* 5th ed. New York, NY: McGraw Hill; 2013.)

Area 3a is sometimes considered to be functionally part of the motor control circuitry and may contain neurons that directly control movement. S1 sends information to region S2, located in the parietal operculum on the ceiling of the lateral sulcus. Specific areas in region S2 connect to the premotor cortex, insular cortex, amygdala, and hippocampus.

An association cortex, the PPC plays an important role in transforming multisensory information into planned movements and motor commands, localization of the body and external objects in space, spatial reasoning, learning motor skills, and spatial attention. The PPC receives input from 3 sensory systems: the somatosensory, visual, and auditory systems. In turn, much of the output of the PPC projects to areas of the frontal cortex, including the motor cortex, DLPFC, and FEFs. Regions of the PPC are components of the dorsal stream (the where and how stream) in visual processing, and the PPC has been proposed to play a role in sustaining attention to spatial locations. Furthermore, the PPC is involved in ensuring that movements are targeted accurately to objects in external space. The PPC is involved in processing spatial relationships of objects in the world and in constructing a representation of external space, which allows a stable percept of the world and a representation of desired trajectories in space that are independent of viewer orientation or body position.

Human functional imaging and neuropsychological studies demonstrate that the parietal lobe and adjacent temporoparietal junction (TPJ) contribute to a variety of higher cognitive functions, including both bottom-up and top-down attention, working memory, multimodal episodic memory, and semantic cognition, which is the ability to use, manipulate, and generalize knowledge. The parietal lobe and TPJ have also been shown to function in aspects of language perception and processing, including phonology and syntax, mathematical cognition, and theory of mind, which is the ability to attribute mental states, including beliefs, intents, desires, and knowledge, to oneself and to others.

THE TEMPORAL LOBE

The temporal lobe is involved in receiving and processing auditory (sound) information and is key for humans to comprehend meaningful speech and language (Figure 3–14). The temporal

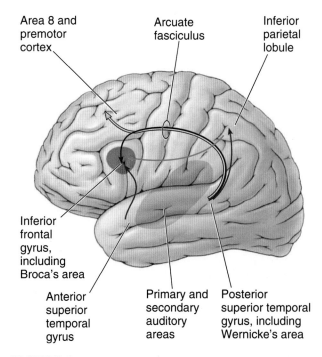

FIGURE 3-14 Auditory areas in the temporal lobe and pathways that connect linguistic areas. The C-shaped arcuate fasciculus interconnects the caudal superior temporal cortex with the inferior parietal lobule, action centers of the dorsolateral frontal cortex, and linguistic areas of the inferior frontal cortex, including Broca's area. A more direct path connects the rostral superior temporal gyrus with the inferior frontal lobe (red), and a connection from the parietal lobe to the inferior frontal lobe (green) is thought to inform frontal linguistic areas about a person's state of attention.

lobe also receives and processes olfactory information and participates in visual processing to establish object and face recognition and interpretation of the meaning of visual stimuli. Important regions in the medial temporal lobe are the hippocampus and adjacent parahippocampal, entorhinal, and perirhinal cortices, which are crucial for the encoding of long-term declarative and spatial memories and the transmission of those into long-term memory stores. Through its connections with other structures such as the amygdala in the limbic lobe, the temporal lobe is also involved in emotional processing and providing emotional content to long-term memories.

One key function of the temporal lobe is in perceiving sounds, assigning meaning to those sounds, and remembering sounds. The primary auditory cortex (A1) is located bilaterally in the superior temporal gyrus. A1 receives auditory information from the ipsilateral cochlea in the ear via the thalamus. Neurons in A1 are organized in a tonotopic map. Secondary auditory areas adjacent to A1, including A2 and areas in the superior, posterior, and lateral parts of the temporal lobes, are involved in auditory processing and perception. Secondary auditory areas process auditory information into semantic (meaningful) units such as speech and words and are involved in comprehension and verbal memory. Speech processing is lateralized, and the majority of humans have left hemisphere specialization. One such lateralized area is the Wernicke area, which spans the region between the temporal and parietal lobes, plays a key role in speech comprehension, and is highly connected with the Broca area, the speech production area in the frontal lobe. Final sound processing is performed by the parietal and frontal cortices.

The ventral regions of the temporal cortices form the ventral stream or "what" pathway of the visual system, which is involved in visual processing that aids in the assignment of meaning to visual information received and interpreting the meaning of visual stimuli, including recognizing faces and objects and reading body language. Two identified regions involved in the interpretation of complex visual stimuli are the fusiform gyrus involved in face recognition and the parahippocampal gyrus involved in interpretation of visual scenes.

The temporal lobe contains the olfactory cortex, one of the regions where olfactory information is received and processed. The olfactory cortex includes areas within the piriform (also spelled pyriform) cortex and likely involves parts of the prepyriform area, entorhinal cortex, and periamygdaloid cortex. The olfactory cortex is evolutionarily older allocortex that comprises 3 layers. Unlike the other senses, the olfactory system does not receive sensory input from the thalamus. Rather the olfactory cortex receives inputs from the olfactory bulb, a region of subcortical gray matter dorsal to the prefrontal cortex, which receives odorant information via the olfactory nerve. The olfactory bulb also sends direct inputs to the amygdala, anterior olfactory nucleus, and olfactory tubercle. The piriform cortex projects to the medial dorsal nucleus of the thalamus, which then projects to the OFC in the frontal lobe that mediates conscious perception of odor.

The medial temporal lobe contains the hippocampus and associated cortical structures that are critical for encoding

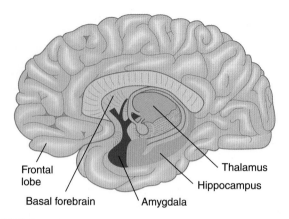

Frontal lobe

Basal forebrain

Thalamus

Hippocampus

Amygdala

FIGURE 3–15 The hippocampus and surrounding brain regions. (Reproduced with permission from Ganong WF. *Review of Medical Physiology*, 19th ed. New York, NY: Appleton & Lange; 1999.)

long-term declarative and spatial memory and transmission of memories to other cortical regions for long-term memory storage. The hippocampus has also been implicated in navigation and spatial cognition. The shape of a curved tube, the hippocampus looks similar to a seahorse or ram's horn and has functionally distinguishable anterior and posterior regions in primates (Figure 3–15). The main input to the hippocampus is from the entorhinal cortex. Located in the parahippocampal gyrus (near the perirhinal cortex), the entorhinal cortex is reciprocally connected with many cortical and subcortical structures including sensory areas, thalamic nuclei, medial septal nucleus, hypothalamus, and brainstem. The main output from the hippocampus is to the subiculum, which projects to numerous areas including the prefrontal cortex, hypothalamus, entorhinal cortex, amygdala, nucleus accumbens, septal nucleus, nucleus reuniens, and mammillary nuclei. The anatomy of the hippocampus and mechanisms of memory encoding are described in Chapters 10 and 20.

THE INSULAR LOBE

Each hemisphere of the human brain also contains the insular lobe (also called the island of Reil). The insular lobe is formed from the insula cortex, a region of cerebral cortex folded deep within the lateral sulcus between the temporal, frontal, and parietal lobes. Because it is covered by the frontoparietal and temporal operculum (meaning lid), the insular cortex is the only cortical region that is not visible on the surface of the brain. The insula has widespread bidirectional connections with the frontal, parietal, and temporal lobes; the cingulate gyrus; and subcortical structures such as the amygdala, brainstem, thalamus, and basal ganglia. These connections provide integration of autonomic, sensory, motor, and limbic functions in the insular lobe.

The insular cortex is divided into 2 parts: the larger anterior insula and the smaller posterior insula in which more than a dozen field areas have been identified. The anterior insular cortex contains part of the primary gustatory cortex, with the other part located in the frontal operculum of the frontal lobe.

In addition to taste reception and processing, the insula is believed to participate in pain perception, speech production, processing of social emotions and emotional self-awareness, interpersonal experience, compassion and empathy, consciousness, and the regulation of the body's homeostasis.

THE AMYGDALA & THE LIMBIC LOBE

The amygdala is a subcortical almond-shaped group of nuclei derived from telencephalon located deep and medially within the temporal lobes (Figure 3–16). Considered part of the limbic system, the amygdala is an integration center that is critical for the processing of emotion, including emotional reactions, emotional communication, emotional memory, motivation, and decision making. The amygdala is interconnected with numerous cortical and subcortical areas, receiving inputs from all the senses via the thalamus and cerebral cortex and from the hypothalamus and brainstem. Connections to these areas allow the amygdala to process information from sensory areas and areas associated with behavior and autonomic function. The amygdala interacts directly with other parts of the limbic system, generating autonomic emotional reactions particularly related to survival, such as fear and the fight-or-flight response. In addition, the amygdala is involved in processing of other emotions, such as anger, pleasure, and motivation, and is responsible for providing emotional content to long-term memories.

Composed of approximately 13 nuclei, the amygdala is functionally divided into 3 major interconnected regions: the basolateral complex, the corticomedial nuclear group, and the central nucleus. The largest subdivision, the basolateral complex, has reciprocal connections with the cerebral cortex, thalamus, and hippocampus. Information from the olfactory

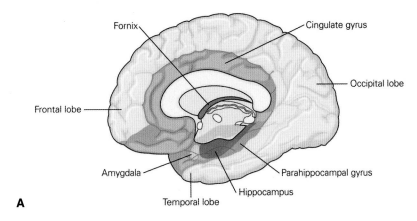

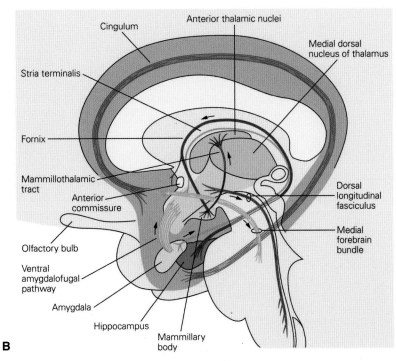

FIGURE 3–16 The amygdala and limbic lobe.

system is received by the corticomedial nuclei. The corticomedial nuclei and central nucleus provide direct outputs to the hypothalamus, and the central nucleus also provides direct output to brainstem areas that control expression of innate behaviors and associated physiologic responses.

Because the amygdala encodes information about emotional events, it participates in emotional memory, a type of implicit or unconscious form of memory. Fear conditioning and reward learning, types of conditioning responses, have been shown to involve the amygdala. In addition, through the amygdala's processing of the emotional significance of external stimuli, the amygdala is also involved in the modulation of a variety of cognitive functions, such as attention and perception. The amygdala also provides emotional content to long-term declarative memories encoded by the hippocampus. Modulation of these cognitive functions may occur through direct inputs from the amygdala to cortical areas or indirectly via the effect of hormones and/or neuromodulators that alter cognitive processing.

The amygdala is a component of the limbic system, which also includes the limbic lobe. The limbic lobe is an arc-shaped region of cerebral cortex on the medial surface of each cerebral hemisphere and includes the hippocampus, associated medial temporal lobe structures, and the cingulate gyrus and sulcus. The limbic system also includes the fornix, mammillary body, and regions of the thalamus, hypothalamus, and basal ganglia, which establish a functionally interconnected group of structures involved in emotional states, motivation and drives, affect, olfactory perception, attentional processing, time perception, autonomic regulation, arousal, consciousness, and learning and memory.

The limbic system operates by influencing the endocrine system and autonomic nervous system. Although still commonly used in neuroanatomic descriptions, the historical concept of a functionally unified limbic system has been criticized as obsolete.

THE BASAL GANGLIA

The basal ganglia, also called the basal nuclei, include a set of subcortical structures located deep within the cerebral hemispheres (Figure 3–17). Functionally, the basal ganglia are involved in the control and coordination of voluntary motor movements, decisions about which motor actions to select, eye movements, procedural learning, some behaviors and habits, cognition, and emotions such as motivation and reward. The basal ganglia are strongly interconnected with areas of the cerebral cortex, thalamus, and brainstem, as well as several other brain areas.

The basal ganglia comprise a distributed set of brain structures derived from the telencephalon, diencephalon, and mesencephalon (Figure 3–18). The largest component is the striatum (also called the corpus striatum), which includes the dorsal striatum (neostriatum) formed from the caudate nucleus and putamen and the ventral striatum formed by the nucleus accumbens and olfactory tubercle. The other regions include the globus pallidus (also called the dorsal pallidum), ventral pallidum, subthalamic nucleus, and substantia nigra in the brainstem. The caudate nucleus is a C-shaped structure that extends around and next to the lateral ventricles. The putamen and globus pallidus are separated from the lateral ventricles, the caudate nucleus, and the thalamus by the internal capsule,

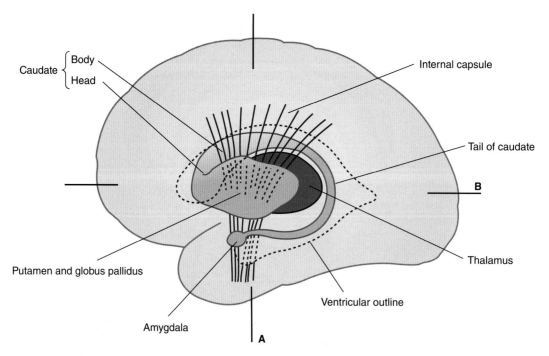

FIGURE 3–17 Relationship between the components of the basal ganglia (caudate, putamen, and globus pallidus) and the thalamus and internal capsule as viewed from the left side. (Reproduced with permission from Waxman SG. *Clinical Neuroanatomy*, 28th ed. New York, NY: McGraw Hill; 2017.)

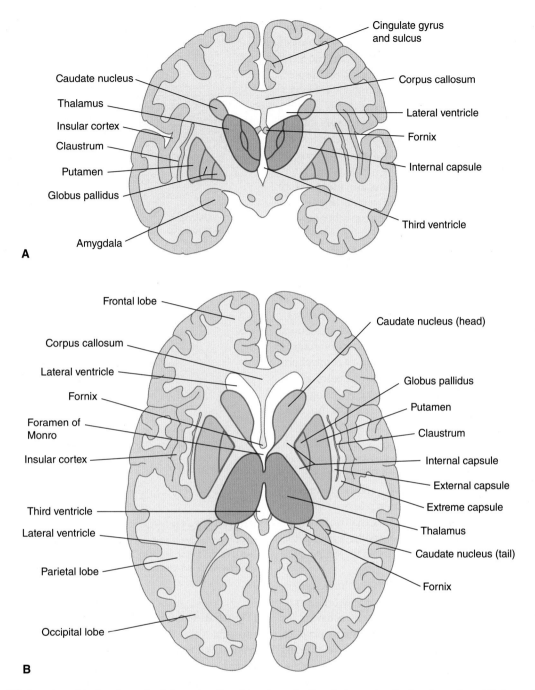

FIGURE 3–18 Location of the basal ganglia. **A.** Frontal section through cerebral hemispheres showing basal ganglia and thalamus. **B.** Horizontal section through cerebral hemispheres. (Reproduced with permission from Waxman SG. *Clinical Neuroanatomy*, 28th ed. New York, NY: McGraw Hill; 2017.)

a large white matter region containing both ascending and descending axons to and from the cerebral cortex.

Forming the neostriatum, the caudate nucleus and putamen are considered functionally equivalent to each other. The putamen is connected to the caudate head by cellular bridges that traverse the internal capsule, producing a striated appearance. The putamen and the globus pallidus are collectively called the lenticular nucleus or the lentiform nucleus. The globus pallidus is divided into 2 segments: the internal globus pallidus (GPi) and the external globus pallidus (GPe).

Located just below the thalamus is the subthalamic nucleus, a part of the diencephalon. The substantia nigra is a brainstem structure located between the red nucleus and the cerebral peduncle on the ventral part of the midbrain, composed of the pars compacta and pars reticulata. The pars compacta contains the cell bodies of dopaminergic neurons that innervate the neostriatum. A functionally analogous midbrain area is the ventral tegmental area, which contains dopaminergic neurons that project to the nucleus accumbens.

The striatum is the main recipient of inputs to the basal ganglia. Inputs to the striatum are excitatory afferents from the entire cerebral cortex and intralaminar nuclei of the thalamus. The primary motor and somatosensory cortices project mainly to the putamen, whereas the premotor cortex and SMA project to the caudate head, and other cortical areas project primarily to the caudate. The nucleus accumbens receives a large input from the limbic cortex.

The main output structures of the basal ganglia are the GPi of the globus pallidus and the substantia nigra pars reticulata (SNr). The GPi projects to a number of thalamic structures by way of 2 tracts. The circuit that processes sensorimotor information from the motor cortex and the somatosensory cortex projects to the ventral anterior (VA) and ventral lateral (VL) nuclei of the thalamus. The circuit that processes other neocortical information projects to the dorsomedial nucleus, the intralaminar nuclei, and parts of the VA nucleus of the thalamus. The SNr projects to the superior colliculus, an area involved in eye movements, as well as to the VA/VL thalamic nuclei.

Two distinct pathways process signals through the basal ganglia. Called the direct pathway and the indirect pathway, they have opposite net effects on thalamic target structures. Excitation of the direct pathway has the net effect of exciting thalamic neurons (which in turn make excitatory connections onto cortical neurons). Excitation of the indirect pathway has the net effect of inhibiting thalamic neurons (rendering them unable to excite motor cortex neurons). The normal functioning of the basal ganglia involves a balance between the activity of these 2 pathways.

The dorsal striatum contributes directly to decision making, especially to action selection and initiation, through the integration of sensorimotor, cognitive, and motivational/emotional information. The dorsal striatum primarily mediates cognition involving motor function, certain executive functions such as inhibitory control, and stimulus-response learning. It is associated with the acquisition of habits and is the main region linked to procedural memory.

The ventral striatum is associated with the limbic system and has been implicated as an essential component of the circuitry for decision making and reward-related behavior. As part of the reward system, the nucleus accumbens plays an important role in processing rewarding stimuli, reinforcing stimuli, and stimuli that are both rewarding and reinforcing such as addictive drugs.

The nucleus accumbens is often considered to be part of the basal forebrain, which lies anterior and ventral to the neostriatum. The other basal forebrain structures include the nucleus basalis, diagonal band of Broca, substantia innominata, and the medial septal nucleus. The basal forebrain is considered to be the major cholinergic output of the CNS to the striatum and neocortex, with important functions in sleep and wakefulness and learning and memory.

CEREBRAL WHITE MATTER

Three types of white matter tracts, called commissural, projection, and association tracts, connect gray matter areas in the CNS and form the majority of cerebral white matter

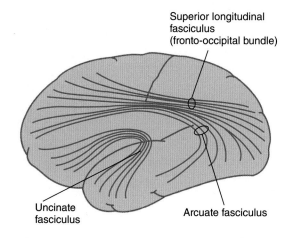

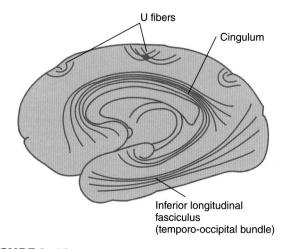

FIGURE 3–19 Diagram of the major association tracts in the brain. The fasciculi and cinculus are long association fibers while the U fibers are short association fiber. (Reproduced with permission from Waxman SG. *Clinical Neuroanatomy*, 28th ed. New York, NY: McGraw Hill; 2017.)

(Figure 3–19). The 2 hemispheres are connected by commissural tracts that span the longitudinal fissure at different regions, allowing the 2 hemispheres to communicate. The largest commissure is the corpus callosum, a broad band of about 200 million axons that join the majority of corresponding regions in the left and right hemispheres. It is the largest white matter structure in the brain. A few tracts pass through the much smaller anterior and posterior commissures. The projection tracts connect the cerebral cortex with other regions, including the striatum, thalamus, brainstem, and spinal cord. Many ascending and descending projection tracts are located in the internal capsule, which surrounds the thalamus and basal ganglia. Within the internal capsule, the largest descending projection tract is the corticospinal tract. The association tracts connect specific cortical areas within the same hemisphere. Short association tracts connect different gyri within a single lobe, whereas long association tracts connect different lobes of a hemisphere to each other. Among their many important roles, association tracts link sensory perceptual, cognitive, and memory regions of the brain. Well-characterized long association tracts include the cingulum, the fornix, and the arcuate, uncinate, occipitofrontal, and superior and inferior longitudinal fasciculi.

THALAMUS, HYPOTHALAMUS, & PITUITARY

The 2 largest structures of the diencephalon are the thalamus and the hypothalamus. Considered the gateway to the cerebral cortex, the thalamus is positioned in the center of the brain, located between the cerebral cortex and midbrain, adjacent to the basal ganglia and dorsal to the cerebellum, and has extensive connections to all 4 regions (Figure 3–20). One of the main functions of the thalamus is to transmit sensory and motor information to the cerebral cortex. However, not merely a "relay station," the thalamus is also engaged in integration and sorting of sensory and motor information that will reach the cerebral cortex and impacts cognitive functions.

The thalamus is a midline symmetrical structure of 2 halves (Figure 3–21). The medial surface of the thalamus constitutes the upper part of the lateral wall of the third ventricle and is connected to the opposite thalamus by the interthalamic adhesion. The thalamus is an organized group of approximately 60 specific nuclei, each with defined connections and roles in sensory, motor, and some cognitive functions. The lateral and posterior parts of the thalamus are continuous with the underlying midbrain; the internal capsule serves as the lateral boundary of the thalamus; the posterior commissure serves as the posterior boundary. The thalamus is separated from the frontal cortex by the anterior commissure and linea terminalis. The ventral boundary is the hypothalamic sulcus, which separates the thalamus from the hypothalamus below.

Every sensory system (with the exception of the olfactory system) involves a specific thalamic nucleus in the dorsal/sensory thalamus that receives sensory signals from ascending tracts or cranial nerves and transmits sensory information to the specific primary sensory cortex (Figure 3–22). For example, outputs from the retina, via the optic nerve, are sent to the lateral geniculate nucleus of the thalamus, which in

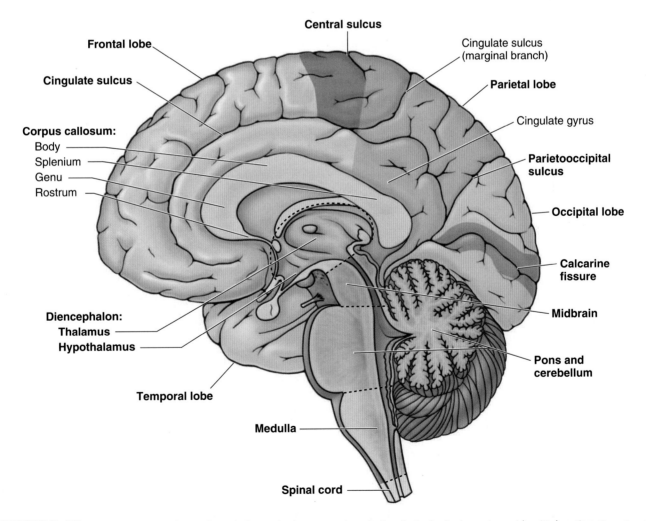

FIGURE 3–20 Location of the thalamus, hypothalamus, brainstem, and cerebellum in the brain shown in a midsagittal section. (Reproduced with permission from Martin JH. *Neuroanatomy: Text and Atlas,* 4th ed. New York, NY: McGraw Hill; 2012.)

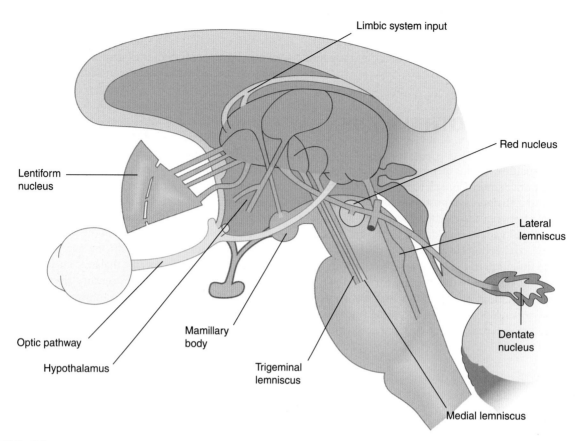

FIGURE 3–21 Location and anatomy of the thalamus, shown in a midsagittal section through the diencephalon. (Reproduced with permission from Waxman SG. *Clinical Neuroanatomy*, 28th ed. New York, NY: McGraw Hill; 2017.)

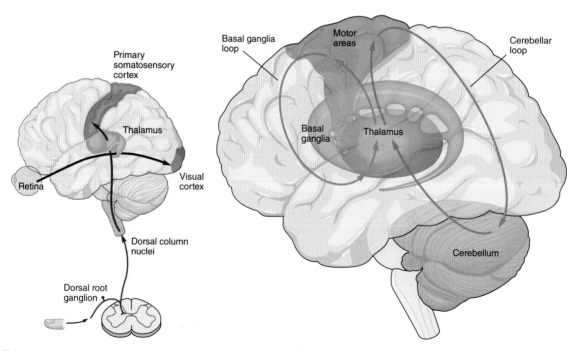

FIGURE 3–22 The thalamus functions in both sensory and motor systems. Connections with sensory systems are shown on the left; connections with areas involved in motor control are shown on the right. (Reproduced with permission from Kandel ER, Schwartz JH, Jessell TM, et al: *Principles of Neural Science*, 5th ed. New York, NY: McGraw Hill; 2013.)

turn projects to V1 in the occipital lobe. The medial geniculate nucleus relays auditory information, the ventral posterior nucleus is the somatosensory relay, and the ventral posterior medial nucleus relays gustatory sensation. The thalamus also processes sensory information and receives reciprocal connections from the sensory cortex it innervates. A current concept about the sensory thalamus is that inputs can be divided into "drivers," which provide the primary excitatory drive for the relay of information to cortex, and "modulators," which alter the gain of signal transmission.

The thalamus plays a critical role in regulation of motor function. A region of the ventral thalamus called the motor thalamus (Mthal) encompasses thalamic nuclei that are functionally positioned between cerebral cortical motor areas and 2 subcortical networks, the basal ganglia and cerebellum. Consequently, the thalamus provides specific channels from the basal ganglia and cerebellum to the cortical motor areas and receives reciprocal connections from those motor areas. Mthal receives output of the basal ganglia, the SNr, and GPi proposed to be involved in the complex cognitive control of movement. Mthal receives major inputs from the dentate nucleus and interposed nucleus, 2 deep cerebellar nuclei, which provide proprioceptive control of posture and movement. Mthal is also proposed to have a role in motor learning.

The thalamus receives inputs from the reticular thalamic nucleus, the superior colliculus, the pedunculopontine nucleus, and the somatosensory spinal cord, and has been implicated in wakefulness and sleep, awareness and alertness, and consciousness. Connections with the prefrontal cortex, hippocampus, and other cortical association areas also likely underlie the contribution of the thalamus to cognitive functions, including language processing, attention, short-term working memory, long-term memory, and decision making.

Two additional regions of the diencephalon are the subthalamus, which contains the subthalamic nucleus, and the epithalamus. Located ventral to the thalamus, the subthalamic nucleus receives inputs from the basal ganglia, specifically from the globus pallidus and substantia nigra, and sends outputs back to the basal ganglia, with a proposed function in action selection. The epithalamus, which includes the pineal gland, connects the limbic system to other parts of the brain, and has been implicated in secretion of melatonin and other neurohormones, circadian rhythm, and regulation of motor pathways and emotions.

The single hypothalamus lies beneath the thalamus and anterior to the midbrain. The overarching function of the hypothalamus is integration and control of body functions for survival and reproduction. The hypothalamus acts as an integrator to regulate basic life- and species-sustaining functions such as fluid and electrolyte balance, drinking and feeding behavior, energy metabolism, thermoregulation, stress responses, and sleep–wake cycles, as well as sexual behavior and reproduction. To produce control over so many bodily functions, the hypothalamus uses 3 major outputs: the behavioral, autonomic, and endocrine systems.

The hypothalamus receives sensory inputs necessary for the detection of changes in both the internal and external environments and controls behaviors related to those inputs. The hypothalamus receives direct sensory inputs from the visual, olfactory, gustatory, and somatosensory systems. In addition, regions within the hypothalamus contain sensors for blood sugar, temperature, and ion levels and receptors for stress hormones, such as cortisol, and appetite hormones, such as leptin and orexin. As part of the limbic system, the hypothalamus receives inputs from the hippocampus, amygdala, and cingulate cortex, which provide highly processed sensory and salience information from the rest of the cerebral cortex. These inputs to the hypothalamus contribute to a range of emotional responses, feelings, and expressions, as well as behaviors such as aggression and motivational behaviors, such as drinking, feeding, and sexual behaviors.

Well interconnected with the brainstem and spinal cord, the hypothalamus is also involved in control of the autonomic nervous system (ANS) (Figure 3–23). Hypothalamic neurons located in the paraventricular nuclei, arcuate nuclei, and lateral hypothalamic area send axons directly to the preganglionic neurons in both the sympathetic and parasympathetic ANS. Hypothalamic control of the ANS includes regulation of heart rate, blood pressure, the extent and regions of blood flow, and peristalsis. In addition, the hypothalamus has extensive outputs to adjust brainstem circuits that regulate autonomic output. Projections to the reticular formation are also involved in certain behaviors, particularly emotional reactions.

The hypothalamus links the nervous system to the endocrine system via the pituitary gland (hypophysis), which releases hormones into the bloodstream and consequently controls many physiologic functions of the body (Figure 3–24). Neurons in the paraventricular and supraoptic nuclei of the hypothalamus send their axons through the infundibulum to form the posterior pituitary (neurohypophysis) where they secrete oxytocin and vasopressin (antidiuretic hormone) directly into the circulation. Oxytocin is involved in contraction of the uterus during childbirth and lactation, whereas vasopressin regulates water retention and the control of blood pressure.

Neurons in the periventricular, paraventricular, and arcuate nuclei send axons that release hypothalamic hormones, which act on the anterior pituitary to either stimulate or inhibit the secretion of specific anterior pituitary hormones into the circulation. Hypothalamic hormones include growth hormone–releasing hormone, thyrotropin-releasing hormone, corticotropin-releasing hormone, gonadotropin-releasing hormone, somatostatin, and follistatin. The 6 anterior pituitary hormones are growth hormone, prolactin, thyroid-stimulating hormone, adrenocorticotropic hormone, follicle-stimulating hormone, and luteinizing hormone, which are released into the bloodstream.

Another key function of the hypothalamus is regulation of body functions in concert with the daily light–dark cycle. A small percentage of axons from the optic nerve go directly to a small nucleus within the hypothalamus called the suprachiasmatic nucleus, which is responsible for entraining circadian rhythms to the day–night cycle.

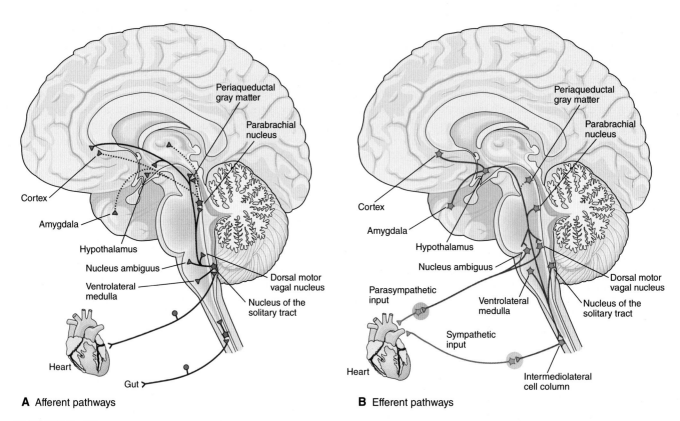

A Afferent pathways

B Efferent pathways

FIGURE 3-23 Connections among the brainstem, hypothalamus, and autonomic nervous system. **A.** Two afferent pathways are shown that provide visceral sensory information via the brainstem. **B.** Efferent pathways that provide autonomic motor control of the heart are shown. (Reproduced with permission from Kandel ER, Schwartz JH, Jessell TM, et al: *Principles of Neural Science,* 5th ed. New York, NY: McGraw Hill; 2013.)

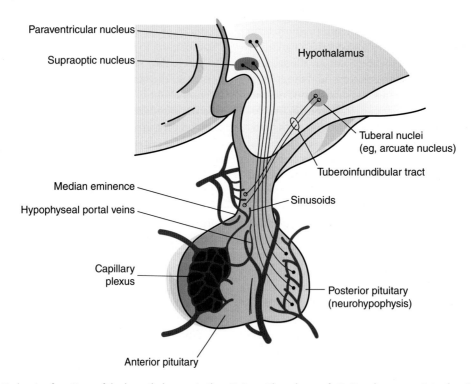

FIGURE 3-24 Endocrine functions of the hypothalamus via the pituitary. The release of pituitary hormones into the circulation by both the anterior and posterior lobes is under the control of the hypothalamus, but by different mechanisms. (Reproduced with permission from Nestler EJ, Hyman SE, Holtzman DM, et al: *Molecular Neuropharmacology: A Foundation for Clinical Neuroscience,* 3rd ed. New York, NY: McGraw Hill; 2015.)

SUMMARY

- The nervous system is composed of the CNS and PNS.

- The brain and spinal cord compose the CNS.

- Standard anatomic directional axes, such as anterior-posterior, dorsal-ventral, medial-lateral, and superior-inferior, and planes, such as sagittal, coronal, and horizontal, are useful in neuroanatomic descriptions.

- Regions of the CNS are often described in terms of gray and white matter. Gray matter contains neuronal cell bodies, dendrites, and astrocytes, whereas white matter contains myelinated axons, oligodendrocytes, and astrocytes.

- The cortex and nuclei compose the 2 types of gray matter in the CNS. White matter contains tracts, which are bundles of myelinated axons in the CNS.

- The brain develops from the 5 embryonic vesicles of the neural tube, called the telencephalon, diencephalon, mesencephalon, metencephalon, and myelencephalon. The telencephalon and diencephalon form the forebrain.

- The brain is enclosed in the cranial cavity and encased by the skull, which is formed from the fusion of 8 cranial bones.

- Developing from the telencephalon, the cerebrum comprises the left and right cerebral hemispheres separated by the longitudinal fissure.

- The cerebrum is composed of cerebral cortex, cerebral white matter, and subcortical structures.

- The cerebral cortex is a thin layer of gray matter that forms the outer surface of the brain, overlying the cerebral white matter. The 2 types of cerebral cortex are neocortex (6 layers) and allocortex (3 to 4 layers).

- The cerebral cortex forms many ridges called gyri (singular gyrus) and grooves called sulci (singular sulcus). The cerebral cortex constitutes approximately 75% of the total CNS gray matter.

- The cerebrum is separated by prominent sulci into 4 visible lobes—the frontal, parietal, occipital, and temporal lobes—which are named for the skull bone that overlies them. The insular lobe and limbic lobe are situated deeper inside the sulci.

- Different cortical regions named Brodmann areas can be distinguished by their cytoarchitecture and connections and have distinct functions.

- Identified cortical areas are called sensory, motor, and association cortices based on their function. Small functional units of neocortex are called cortical columns.

- The anteriormost lobe, the frontal lobe, contains the motor cortex, frontal eye fields, and the Broca area, which are involved in voluntary motor control, eye movements, and language production, respectively.

- The prefrontal region of the frontal lobe contains association cortex that constructs many cognitive functions, including short-term working memory, executive functions, and behavioral control.

- The posteriormost lobe, the occipital lobe, contains the visual cortex and functions in visual reception, visual-spatial processing and motion perception, and color recognition.

- The parietal lobe contains the somatosensory cortex, which receives and processes touch, temperature, pain, and conscious proprioceptive information from the body and provides some motor control.

- A main association area, the posterior parietal cortex, is involved in visuospatial perception, attention, and integration of somatosensory, visual, and auditory input, and provides output to the frontal lobe for motor control and cognitive functions.

- The temporal lobe contains the auditory cortex involved in receiving and processing auditory information. The auditory association areas include the Wernicke area, which is involved in language comprehension.

- The olfactory cortex in the temporal lobe contributes to reception and processing of olfactory information. The temporal lobe also participates in visual processing for object and facial recognition.

- The temporal lobe houses the hippocampus, entorhinal cortex, and associated cortical structures involved in encoding long-term declarative and spatial memories.

- The insular lobe is formed by the insular cortex located deep within the lateral sulcus with functions in sensory perception, processing social emotions such as compassion and empathy, emotional self-awareness, and consciousness.

- The limbic lobe is formed from the limbic cortex, which includes the cingulate cortex, hippocampus, and associated cortices in the medial temporal lobe. The limbic system comprises the limbic lobe and subcortical areas.

- The amygdala contains a group of subcortical nuclei located within each temporal lobe. Part of the limbic system, the amygdala functions in processing and communication of emotion and emotional memory.

- The basal ganglia are a set of subcortical structures involved in the control and coordination of voluntary motor movements, decisions about which motor actions to select, procedural learning, and motivation and reward.

- Three types of white matter tracts, called commissural, projection, and association tracts, connect gray matter areas in the CNS.

- Positioned in the center of the brain, the thalamus receives inputs from sensory systems, the basal ganglia, the cerebellum, and the cerebral cortex. The main functions of the thalamus are in sorting and relaying sensory and motor information to the cerebral cortex and in modulation of cognitive functions.

■ The hypothalamus regulates body functions for survival and reproduction. Through outputs that control behavioral, autonomic, and endocrine systems, the hypothalamus is involved in electrolyte balance, feeding and energy metabolism, thermoregulation, sleep–wake cycles, sexual behavior, and reproduction.

SELF-ASSESSMENT QUESTIONS

1. Which of the following statements best describes the cerebrum?
   A. The cerebrum is derived from telencephalon, forms the largest part of the brain, and consists of the left and right cerebral hemispheres, which are separated by the central sulcus.
   B. Each of the 4 main anatomic lobes—the frontal, parietal, occipital, and temporal lobes—contains a significant area dedicated to sensory and motor functions.
   C. The locations of primary, secondary, and tertiary gyri and sulci are invariant among human individuals.
   D. The right and left cerebral hemispheres are exact anatomic and functional mirror images of each other, although the right hemisphere receives sensory input from and controls the left side of the body, whereas the left hemisphere receives sensory input from and controls the right side of the body.
   E. In addition to 4 anatomic lobes, 2 functional lobes, called the insular and limbic lobes, located deep within the brain, have been characterized in humans.

2. Which of the following statements best characterizes the cerebral cortex?
   A. Human brain contains only 1 type of cerebral cortex, called neocortex, that is composed of 6 layers.
   B. Individual association areas receive substantial inputs from both primary sensory and primary motor areas.
   C. The smallest functional unit of the neocortex is a cylinder of neurons approximately 2 to 3 mm in height and approximately 0.5 mm in diameter, called a cortical column.
   D. The human neocortex represents approximately 25% of the cerebral gray matter.
   E. The cerebral hemispheres contain the cerebral cortex, which is the thin layer of gray matter that is covered by the cerebral white matter and meninges.

3. Which of the following best characterizes structures in the temporal lobe?
   A. The amygdala is an integration center that is critical for the processing of mainly pleasant emotions and euphoria.
   B. The hippocampus, entorhinal cortex, and perirhinal cortex are critical for encoding and storing all long-term declarative and spatial memories.
   C. The olfactory cortex is a type of neocortex that receives inputs from the olfactory bulb and olfactory nerve via relay from the thalamus.
   D. The auditory cortex is involved in perceiving sounds, assigning meaning to those sounds, and remembering sounds.
   E. The ventral regions of the temporal lobe form the dorsal stream, or "where" pathway involved in visual processing that aids in the processing of object location and movement.

4. Which of the following best describes the thalamus?
   A. The thalamus transmits sensory information to the cerebral cortex and is involved in cognitive functions, but is rarely involved in providing information for motor control.
   B. The gateway to the cerebral cortex, the thalamus is located between the cerebral cortex and midbrain/brainstem, adjacent to the basal ganglia, and dorsal to the cerebellum, with extensive connections with these regions and the spinal cord.
   C. The thalamus contains a single nucleus with specialized subdomains with specific connections to the cerebral cortex, basal ganglia, brainstem, and cerebellum.
   D. The thalamus regulates basic life- and species-sustaining functions such as fluid balance, energy metabolism, thermoregulation, and drinking, feeding, and reproductive behaviors.
   E. Every sensory system involves relay of information from ascending tracts or cranial nerves to the thalamus, which then transmits sensory information to the specific primary sensory cortex.

5. Which of the following statements best describes the basal ganglia (BG)?
   A. The BG are involved in the control and coordination of voluntary motor movements, decisions about motor actions, procedural learning, motivation, and reward.
   B. Anatomically, the BG include the striatum (formed from the caudate nucleus and putamen), globus pallidus, substantia nigra, hypothalamus, and thalamus.
   C. The BG form direct connections with the cerebral cortex and cerebellum for rapid exchange of motor initiation and reward information.
   D. The BG are associated with the acquisition of habits and are the main region linked to declarative memory.
   E. Loss of neurons in the BG is associated with all forms of dementia, including Alzheimer disease, Huntington disease, amyotrophic lateral sclerosis (ALS), and Parkinson disease.

Functional Anatomy of the Nervous System II: The Brainstem, Cerebellum, Spinal Cord, Peripheral Nervous System, & Supporting Systems

CHAPTER 4

Anne B. Theibert

OBJECTIVES

After studying this chapter, the student should be able to:

- Distinguish the 3 components of the brainstem and their general functions.
- Outline the cranial nerves and describe their overall motor, sensory and/or autonomic functions.
- Diagram the connections from the forebrain to and from the cerebellum and describe the functions of the cerebellum.
- Identify the gray and white matter regions of the spinal cord, explain their functions, and define the spinal cord segments.
- Outline the spinal nerves and their dorsal and ventral roots, main branches, and peripheral nerves.
- Delineate the meninges and describe its locations and 3 membrane components.
- Define the ventricular system and the flow of cerebrospinal fluid.
- Distinguish and describe the main central nervous system arteries and their origins and branches and venous drainage.

INTRODUCTION

The forebrain is highly interconnected with the midbrain, hindbrain, and spinal cord. These regions also provide the connections to the peripheral nervous system (PNS); the PNS includes the cranial nerves, spinal nerves, peripheral nerves, and ganglia located outside of the brain and spinal cord. The midbrain, pons, and medulla oblongata (hereafter medulla) compose the brainstem, which contains nuclei that are critical for survival through automatic responses such as breathing and reflexes such as coughing. The brainstem also contains nuclei for cranial nerves (CNs) III to XII. Emerging from the brainstem, CNs III to XII serve somatic and autonomic motor and sensory functions in the face, head and neck, special senses, and autonomic innervation of the heart, lungs, and other organs. The other region of the hindbrain is the cerebellum, which is connected to the rest of the brain and spinal cord via the pons. The cerebellum functions in motor functions including coordination, precision, timing, and motor learning and has been implicated in cognition and emotion.

Caudal to the medulla is the spinal cord. The spinal cord contains both ascending and descending white matter tracts and neurons involved in motor output, sensory relay, integration, and spinal reflexes. Spinal cord gray matter contains the

67

cell bodies of somatic motor neurons, preganglionic autonomic neurons, and sensory relay neurons, as well as spinal interneurons involved in integration and spinal reflexes. The spinal cord is the origin of the 31 pairs of spinal nerves and their branches, called peripheral nerves, which contain axons that innervate the skin, muscles, tendons, joints, and organs (viscera). The circuitry within the spinal cord generates spinal reflexes and contributes to central pattern generators. Another component of the PNS is the enteric nervous system (ENS); located in the gastrointestinal (GI) tract, the ENS functions in peristalsis and secretions.

The central nervous system (CNS) is protected on the outside by the skull and meninges, membranes that prevent the movement of the brain within the skull and contain cerebrospinal fluid (CSF) that helps cushion the CNS. Inside the CNS lies the ventricular system and central canal, with the main function of production and circulation of CSF. The CNS has a robust vascularization, with blood supplied from branches of the dorsal aorta and drainage via the jugular vein. The nerves are also vascularized and contain layers of protective connective tissue.

THE BRAINSTEM

Considered one of the most primitive parts of the human brain, the brainstem is the structure most important to life (**Figures 4–1** **and** **4–2**). The brainstem contains white matter tracts involved in transmission of motor impulses that control the body and head and the largest majority of sensory tracts. In addition, 10 of the 12 pairs of CNs emerge directly from the brainstem, with nuclei involved in both somatic motor and sensory functions of the head, face, and neck and in autonomic parasympathetic functions. The brainstem also contains nuclei involved in essential automatic processes,

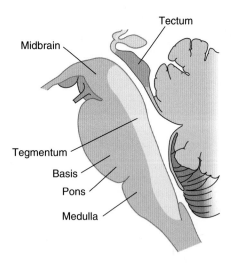

FIGURE 4–1 Illustration of the divisions of the brainstem in a midsagittal plane. The major external divisions are the midbrain, pons, and medulla. The major internal longitudinal divisions are the tectum, tegmentum, and basis. (Reproduced with permission from Waxman SG. *Clinical Neuroanatomy*, 28th ed. New York, NY: McGraw Hill; 2017.)

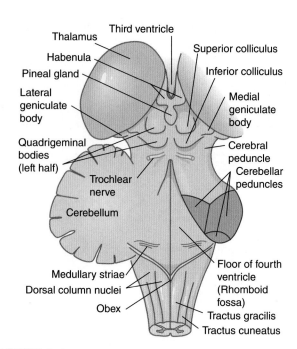

FIGURE 4–2 Illustration of the brainstem from a dorsolateral view, with most of the cerebellum hidden. (Reproduced with permission from Waxman SG. *Clinical Neuroanatomy*, 28th ed. New York, NY: McGraw Hill; 2017.)

including breathing, and encompasses the reticular formation, a group of nuclei that function in arousal, alertness, and consciousness. Anatomically, the brainstem rests on the base of the skull, known as the clivus, and ends at the foramen magnum, the large opening in the occipital bone.

THE MIDBRAIN

Rostrally, the midbrain adjoins the thalamus; caudally, the midbrain connects to the pons (**Figure 4–3**). During development, the dorsal surface of the mesencephalic vesicle becomes a structure called the tectum or roof, while the ventral region becomes the tegmentum or floor of the midbrain. The smaller tectum and larger tegmentum are separated at the midline by the narrow CSF-filled cerebral aqueduct, which connects rostrally with the third ventricle and caudally with the fourth ventricle. As the midbrain develops, large white matter regions called the cerebral peduncles form ventral to and laterally around the tegmentum.

During development, the tectum differentiates into 2 structures: the superior colliculus and inferior colliculus. Together, the superior and inferior colliculi are called the corpora quadrigemina. The superior colliculus, which is called the optic tectum in lower vertebrates, receives direct input from the retina and visual cortex and is a primary integration center that provides key output to the thalamus and nearby nuclei of the oculomotor nerve (CN III) and the trochlear nerve (CN IV). One function of the superior colliculus is to control visual reflexes, such as eye movements, lens shape, and pupil diameter. The inferior colliculus is involved in processing auditory information. It receives input from several brainstem nuclei in the auditory pathway and the auditory cortex and provides a major output to

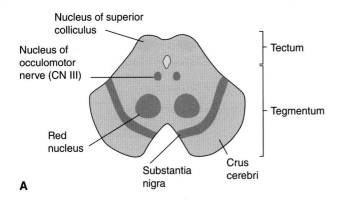

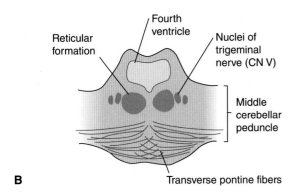

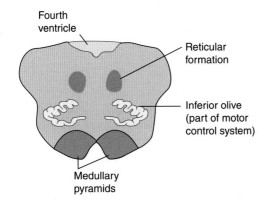

FIGURE 4–3 Illustration of brainstem transverse sections—simplified. **A.** The midbrain at the level of the superior colliculus. **B.** The pons, showing massive crossover of descending fibers in the ventral pons, which are destined for the cerebellum. **C.** The medulla oblongata, showing the large medullary pyramids ventrally, which are the site of crossover of the descending corticotracts. Several cranial nerve (CN) nuclei are shown.

the thalamus. Although the tectum is localized to the midbrain region, the tegmentum extends through the pons.

The midbrain tegmentum contains 4 regions distinguished by their pigmentation. The substantia nigra is a large highly pigmented nucleus that consists of the pars reticulata and pars compacta. The pars compacta contains dopaminergic neurons that project to the caudate nucleus and putamen, which form the striatum of the basal ganglia

involved in mediating movement and motor coordination. The striatal neurons in turn project to neurons in the pars reticulata, which, by projecting fibers to the thalamus, are part of the output system of the striatum. Located near the midline, the ventral tegmental area is the origin of dopaminergic neurons of the mesocorticolimbic dopamine system that is widely implicated in the reward circuitry of the brain. The red nucleus is a large centrally located structure that receives inputs from the motor and sensory cortices via the corticorubral tract and from the cerebellum via the cerebellar peduncles; it gives rise to the rubrospinal tract, providing motor information to the spinal cord. The periaqueductal gray functions as a primary control center for descending pain modulation.

The midbrain contains a number of other important nuclei and white matter tracts, including the mesencephalic nucleus of the trigeminal nerve (CN V) involved in proprioception of the face and a portion of the reticular formation, a neural network that is involved in arousal and alertness (see later discussion). The cerebral peduncles house the crus cerebri, which contain the descending motor axons of the corticospinal, corticobulbar, and corticopontine tracts. The ascending sensory axons from the spinothalamic and dorsal column medial lemniscus (DCML) tracts are located more dorsally, closer to the tegmentum.

THE PONS

Caudal to the midbrain is the pons (Figure 4–4). The dorsal/posterior border of the pons is separated from the cerebellum by the aqueduct of Sylvius and, more inferiorly, by the fourth ventricle. The pons appears as a broad anterior bulge rostral to the medulla that consists of 2 pairs of thick stalks called cerebellar peduncles; the specific nuclei in the pons are located in the medial regions. An important function of the pons is to relay information between the cortex and the cerebellum. The pons contains a number of other important nuclei, including those involved in automatic functions and numerous CN nuclei.

The pons can be broadly divided into 2 parts: the basilar part of the pons, located ventrally, and the pontine tegmentum, located dorsally. The ventral pons contains numerous pontine nuclei that relay signals between the cerebral cortex and the cerebellum. The pontine nuclei receive inputs from many parts of the cerebral cortex including the motor cortex and auditory, visual, somatosensory, and association regions, as well as subcortical areas. In turn, the pontine nuclei project, via the middle cerebellar peduncle, to the cerebellar cortex and interposed nucleus. Information relayed via the corticopontocerebellar tract represents a critical contribution from the cortex to the cerebellar regulation of motor function and movement. In addition, the cerebellum has been implicated in several cognitive processes (see later discussion).

The pons is involved in several automatic functions necessary for life. In the dorsal posterior pons lie nuclei that

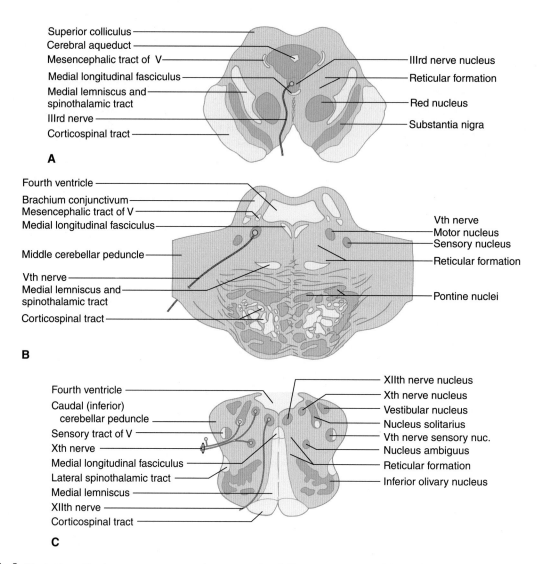

FIGURE 4–4 Illustration of brainstem transverse sections—complex. **A.** Transverse section of the midbrain at the level of the IIIrd nerve. **B.** Transverse section of the pons at the level of the Vth nerve (rostral). **C.** Transverse section of the medulla oblongata. (Reproduced with permission from Biller J, Gruener G, Brazis P. *DeMyer's The Neurologic Examination: A Programmed Text*, 7th ed. New York, NY: McGraw Hill; 2016.)

have critical functions in breathing (respiration), sleep, and swallowing. In addition, the pons contains nuclei involved in bladder control, hearing, equilibrium, taste, eye movement, facial expressions, facial sensation, and posture. The pons contains the breathing pneumotaxic center, which regulates the change from inhalation to exhalation. The pons has been implicated in sleep paralysis and rapid eye movement (REM) sleep and may also play a role in sleep cycles and generating dreams. The pons contains a number of CN nuclei, including the pontine nucleus and motor nucleus for the trigeminal nerve (CN V), the abducens nucleus (CN VI), the facial nerve nucleus (CN VII), and the vestibulocochlear nuclei (vestibular nuclei and cochlear nuclei) (CN VIII). The functions of these 4 CNs (V to VIII) include sensory roles in hearing, equilibrium, and taste and in facial sensations such as touch and pain, as well as motor roles in eye movement, facial expressions, chewing, swallowing, and the secretion of saliva and tears.

Similar to the midbrain, the pons contains the descending motor and ascending sensory white matter tracts between the forebrain, medulla, and spinal cord. Other white matter regions include the superior cerebellar peduncles, which contain the main output route from the cerebellum and extend to the red nucleus in the midbrain or to the thalamus. The inferior cerebellar peduncle is a region of the medulla that contains tracts that connect the spinal cord and medulla with the cerebellum.

THE MEDULLA

The medulla is the caudal-most region of the brainstem situated between the pons and the spinal cord and ventral/anterior to the cerebellum. The medulla merges with the spinal cord at the opening called the foramen magnum at the base of the skull. The lateral areas of the medulla form the inferior cerebellar peduncles. In the upper or superior part, the dorsal surface of the medulla is formed by the fourth ventricle. In the lower or inferior part, the fourth ventricle narrows at the obex in the caudal medulla and becomes the central canal.

Motor and sensory tracts passing between the brain and spinal cord pass through the medulla. The medulla contains the pyramids, a region where the crossing (decussation) of motor axons that form the lateral corticospinal tract occurs, and the medial lemniscus, where decussation of sensory axons of the DCML tract takes place. The medulla contains CN nuclei (Figure 4–5) and other nuclei and serves as a major

processing center involved in automatic, autonomic, and somatic functions.

Automatic functions and reflexes of the medulla include breathing, vomiting, sneezing, coughing, swallowing, and balance. Two of the major regions (the dorsal and ventral respiratory groups) of the respiratory center are located in the medulla, with the other regions located in the pons. The respiratory center receives input from chemoreceptors, mechanoreceptors, the cerebral cortex, and the hypothalamus and is responsible for generating and maintaining the rhythm and

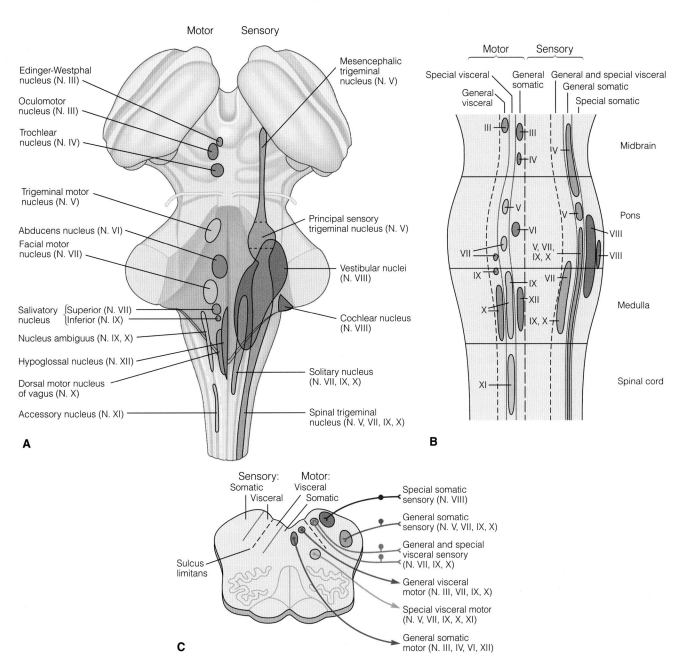

FIGURE 4–5 Organization of cranial nerve nuclei in the brainstem. The cranial nerve nuclei are organized in functional columns along the rostrocaudal axis of the brainstem. **A.** This dorsal view of the human brainstem shows the location of the cranial nerve sensory nuclei (right) and motor nuclei (left). **B.** A schematic view of the functional organization of the motor and sensory columns. **C.** The medial-lateral arrangement of the cranial nerve nuclei is shown in a cross section at the level of the medulla. (Reproduced with permission from Kandel ER, Schwartz JH, Jessell TM, et al: *Principles of Neural Science*, 5th ed. New York, NY: McGraw Hill; 2013.)

rate of respiration and adjusting those to physiologic needs. Some other reflexes may involve the raphe nucleus and the solitary nucleus (SN). The SN contains a series of sensory nuclei forming a vertical column of gray matter in the medulla. The nuclei are part of the medullary reticular formation and contain serotonergic neurons (see later discussion).

Four CNs originate from the medulla oblongata; these are the glossopharyngeal nerve (CN IX), vagus nerve (CN X), accessory nerve (CN XI), and hypoglossal nerve (CN XII), which serve both autonomic and somatic functions. Autonomic functions include maintaining blood pressure and regulation of heart rate and contraction force, with control by the cardiovascular centers. The medulla also contributes to autonomic control of the digestive system. Somatic motor and sensory functions include taste, hearing, and control of muscles of the face and neck. The SN has been implicated in regulation of autonomic functions since it receives input from the facial, glossopharyngeal, and vagus nerves. The SN projects to the reticular formation, parasympathetic preganglionic neurons, hypothalamus, and thalamus.

The medulla also contains important relay nuclei. Forming the olivary nucleus (or olive), the superior olivary nuclei form an important component of the ascending and descending auditory pathways of the auditory system, whereas the inferior olivary nuclei coordinate signals from the spinal cord to the cerebellum to regulate motor coordination and learning. The cuneate nucleus and gracile nucleus are part of DCML pathway, carrying fine touch and proprioceptive information from the upper body (cuneate) and the legs and trunk.

Phylogenetically one of the oldest parts of the brain, the reticular formation is a set of interconnected nuclei that are located throughout the brainstem, from the midbrain to the lower medulla. The reticular formation contains the raphe nuclei, which encompass the majority of serotonergic neurons in the CNS and have been implicated in mood, pain, alertness, and memory. One of its 2 components, the ascending reticular formation is called the reticular activating system (RAS), is responsible for the sleep–wake cycle, and controls various levels of alertness. The RAS projects to the thalamus, which transmits this information to the cortex. The other component, the descending reticular formation (DRF), is involved in posture and equilibrium, as well as motor movement and autonomic functions. The DRF receives information from the hypothalamus and some fibers from the corticobulbar tract that originate in the motor cortex and are involved in eye movement. Other corticobulbar fibers innervate CNs directly. Nuclei in the DRF have also been implicated in reflexes such as coughing, chewing, swallowing, and vomiting.

THE CRANIAL NERVES

The CNs are a set of 12 paired nerves that emerge from the brain. The first 2 CNs arise from the cerebrum, whereas the remaining 10 emerge from the brainstem. The CNs provide motor and sensory innervation to structures within the head, face, and neck and autonomic regulation of organs in the body. Assigned Roman numerals I to XII based on the order from which they emerge from the cerebrum or brainstem, the CNs are also named based on their function or appearance. The CNs serve functions such as smell, sight, eye movement, feeling in the face, balance, hearing, movement of the mouth and tongue for speech, chewing and swallowing, and parasympathetic control of heart rate, GI peristalsis, and sweating.

The olfactory nerve (CN I) and optic nerve (CN II) are considered CNS nerves because they emerge from the cerebrum and the tracts travel within the CNS. CNs III to XII are considered part of the PNS. The nuclei for CNs III to XII lie in the brainstem, and their axons exit or enter the skull bone and relay information between the brain and the body, primarily to and from regions of the head and neck. A thirteenth CN designated 0 in lower vertebrates does not appear to have a function in humans.

The CNs provide sensory innervation that includes general somatic sensation such as touch, temperature, and pain; visceral somatic sensation from internal regions; and special sense innervation such as smell, vision, taste, hearing, and balance. Motor function can involve somatic motor or autonomic motor innervation. Hence, CNs can include fibers for somatic sensory, visceral sensory, special sensory, somatic motor, or autonomic motor functions. Some CNs contain only 1 type of fiber. Many of the CNs contain mixtures of fiber types.

The PNS CNs (III to XII) have nuclei in the brainstem, and their axons exit or enter the skull bone via foramina and innervate regions of the head, face, neck, and body on the same side from which they originate. CNs and the axons inside travel in regions within the skull called intracranial paths; they travel outside the skull via extracranial paths. The CN nuclei in the brainstem contain the cell bodies of the neurons that send or receive the axons that form the CNs. The midbrain of the brainstem has the nuclei of CN III and IV. The pons contains the nuclei of CNs V to VIII. The medulla houses the nuclei of CNs IX to XII.

All the CNs, except CNs I, II, and IV, have associated ganglia, which are groups of neuronal cell bodies that are located outside the brainstem. The sensory ganglia are directly correspondent to dorsal root ganglia of spinal nerves and are known as cranial sensory ganglia. Sensory ganglia exist for nerves with somatic sensory components: CNs V, VII, VIII, IX, and X. Parasympathetic ganglia are present for the autonomic components of CNs III, VII, IX, and X that innervate the glands in the head and neck and include the ciliary, pterygopalatine, submandibular, and otic ganglion. In addition, the vagus nerve (CN X) supplies the output to parasympathetic ganglia that lie in the body, close to the organs they innervate in the chest and abdomen.

Considered part of the ANS, the general visceral afferent (GVA) fibers transmit sensory information about local changes in chemical and mechanical environments, including pain and reflex sensations, from the internal organs, glands, and blood vessels to the CNS. Unlike the efferent motor fibers of the ANS, the GVA fibers are not classified as sympathetic or parasympathetic. The CNs that contain GVA fibers include the facial nerve, glossopharyngeal nerve, and vagus nerve. CN GVA fibers are important in complex automatic motor acts such as swallowing, vomiting, and coughing.

CN I

The olfactory nerve conveys the sense of smell. Containing only special sensory fibers, the olfactory nerve is a purely sensory nerve in charge of transmitting olfactory sensation from the nose to the brain. The olfactory nerve originates in the olfactory epithelium and contains sensory axons (afferents) that extend to the olfactory bulb. Derived from the nasal (otic) placodes, neurons in the olfactory epithelium can be replaced and extend new axons within the nerve. Hence, the olfactory nerve is unique in that it is capable of some regeneration if damaged. The olfactory bulb extends axons via the olfactory tract, which transmits olfactory information to the primary olfactory cortex in the temporal lobe. The olfactory nerve is unmyelinated but covered with meningeal-like membranes. It is the shortest CN and does not exit the brain.

CN II

The optic nerve is dedicated to vision. Composed of axons from retinal ganglion cells, the optic nerve transsensory visual information from the retina of the eye to the brain. Emerging from the retina, the optic nerve travels through the optic canal, partially decussates in the optic chiasm and becomes the optic tract. The majority of optic tract axons terminate in the lateral geniculate nucleus of the thalamus, while a few project to nuclei in the midbrain and hypothalamus. The thalamus transmits visual perception information to the visual cortex in the occipital lobe. The few axons that terminate in the superior colliculus are responsible for reflexive eye movements and those that terminate in the pretectum control the pupillary light reflex. Axons that project to the suprachiasmatic nucleus in the hypothalamus are involved in circadian rhythms. The optic nerve is heavily myelinated by oligodendrocytes and is encased in the 3 meningeal layers. Since retinal ganglion neurons and axons do not regenerate, damage to the optic nerve can produce irreversible blindness.

CN III

The oculomotor nerve controls eye movements and pupil size. The oculomotor nerve originates in 2 nuclei in the midbrain called the oculomotor nucleus and Edinger-Westphal nucleus. The nerve enters the orbit via the superior orbital fissure to innervate muscles that enable most movements of the eye and that raise the eyelid. Located in the midbrain, the oculomotor nucleus controls striated muscle in levator palpebrae superioris and extraocular muscles except for the superior oblique muscle and the lateral rectus muscle. The Edinger-Westphal nucleus supplies parasympathetic nerve fibers via the ciliary ganglion to the eye to control the pupillae muscle for pupil

constriction and the ciliary muscle for the accommodation reflex, the ability to focus on near objects as in reading. Sympathetic postganglionic fibers join the oculomotor nerve to innervate the superior tarsal muscle, a smooth muscle. CNs IV and VI also participate in control of eye movement.

CN IV

The trochlear nerve is a somatic motor nerve that enters the orbit through the superior orbital fissure and innervates a single muscle, the superior oblique muscle of the eye. This eye muscle ends in a tendon, which passes through a fibrous loop called the trochlea that functions through a pulley-like mechanism to make the eyeballs move and rotate. The nucleus of the trochlear nerve originates in the midbrain immediately below the oculomotor nucleus. The trochlear nerve is the smallest nerve in terms of its axon number but has the longest intracranial path and is the only CN that exits from the dorsal aspect of the brainstem.

CN V

The trigeminal nerve contains both sensory and motor fibers and is responsible for sensation in the skin of the face and mouth and motor functions such as biting, chewing, and swallowing. The largest of the CNs, its name derives from the fact that it contains 3 branches, the ophthalmic nerve (V1), the maxillary nerve (V2), and the mandibular nerve (V3). The ophthalmic and maxillary nerves are purely somatic sensory, whereas the mandibular nerve supplies both somatic motor and some sensory functions.

The sensory functions of the trigeminal nerve are to provide the tactile, motion, position, temperature, and pain sensations of the top and front of the head, the face, and the mouth. Each of the 3 nerves innervates specific regions of the front of the head and face, with V1 innervating the approximate dorsal third of the face and head, V2 innervating the middle third, and V3 providing information from the approximate ventral third of the face.

The 3 trigeminal branches converge on the trigeminal ganglion, a sensory ganglion. It contains the cell bodies of incoming sensory nerve fibers from the face. From the trigeminal ganglion, a single large sensory root enters the brainstem at the level of the pons and synapses on the sensory nuclei. Immediately adjacent to the sensory root, a smaller motor root emerges from the pons at the same level. The trigeminal motor nuclei are located in the pons, and the motor fibers pass through the trigeminal ganglion en route to their muscle targets.

CN VI

The abducens nerve is also known as the abducent nerve. It is a responsible for somatic motor output to control the lateral rectus muscle of the ipsilateral eye. In humans, this allows the eyes to move horizontally and is responsible for outward, lateral gaze. The abducens nerve nucleus is present in the pons, and the nerve exits the brainstem at the junction of the pons and the medulla and ascends upward to the eye. The exact control of eye movements requires input from integration centers in the brain that coordinate the output from the oculomotor, trochlear, and abducens nuclei, which control the 6 extraocular muscles.

CN VII

The facial nerve is a mixed nerve that has 4 components with distinct functions. The facial nerve is responsible for producing facial expressions by voluntary movements, including brow wrinkling, teeth showing, frowning, eyes closing, lip pursing, and cheek puffing. It also controls the stapedius muscle of the ear. The facial nerve also functions in the transmission of taste sensations from the anterior two-thirds of the tongue and oral cavity. A somatic sensory component innervates the external ear. It also supplies preganglionic parasympathetic fibers to several head and neck ganglia and signals to the salivary, mucous, and lacrimal glands. The facial nerve's motor component originates in the facial nerve nucleus in the pons, and the sensory nuclei are located near the pons–medulla junction. The section of the facial nerve that arises from the sensory root is also known as the intermediate nerve. The geniculate ganglion contains the cell bodies of the sensory component of the intermediate nerve. The nerve traverses the facial canal, through the parotid gland, and divides into 5 branches.

CN VIII

The vestibulocochlear nerve transmits hearing (sound) information and balance (equilibrium) information from the inner ear to the brain. It contains 2 functionally separate nerves, the vestibular nerve and the cochlear nerve, which are both sensory nerves that combine in the pons. The vestibular nuclei complex, situated in the pons and medulla, receives input from 5 sensory organs in the vestibules and semicircular canal of the inner ear. The vestibular ganglion includes the cell bodies of the sensory neurons. The vestibular nerve transmits information about balance and movement and is an important component of the vestibulo-ocular reflex, which keeps the head stable and allows the eyes to track moving objects.

The ventral and dorsal cochlear nuclei, located in the inferior cerebellar peduncle, receive information from the cochlear nerve, also known as the auditory nerve, which transmits sound information for the sensation of hearing. Sound waves are detected by hair cells in the cochlea that send information to the spiral ganglia, which house the cell bodies of neurons of the cochlear nerve, and information is then transmitted to the cochlear nuclei.

CN IX

The glossopharyngeal nerve is a mixed nerve, consisting of both sensory and motor nerve fibers, and is responsible for swallowing, the gag reflex, taste sensation from the back of the tongue, and saliva production. It contains somatic sensory fibers that originate in the tonsils, pharynx, middle ear, and posterior third of the tongue. It also contains special sense fibers from the posterior third of the tongue, and GVA fibers from the carotid sinus and bodies. These various sensory fibers terminate in nuclei in the medulla. The motor fibers originate in nuclei in the medulla. Parasympathetic fibers innervate the parotid salivary gland and glands of the posterior tongue. Somatic motor fibers innervate the stylopharyngeus muscle, which provides voluntary muscle control that elevates the pharynx during swallowing and speech. GVAs synapse on neurons of the nucleus of the solitary tract.

CN X

The vagus nerve is also known as the pneumogastric nerve. The vagus nerve supplies motor parasympathetic fibers to all the organs, except the adrenal glands, from the neck down to the second segment of the transverse colon. The vagus nerve sends somatic and visceral sensory information about the body's organs to the brain, with estimates that 80% to 90% of the nerve fibers in the vagus nerve are afferent (sensory) nerves. Vagal GVAs carry information from aortic, cardiac, pulmonary, and GI receptors and synapse on neurons of the nucleus of the solitary tract.

The vagus nerve is responsible for such varied tasks as regulation of heart rate, GI peristalsis, sweating, the gag reflex, and satiation following food consumption. It also controls a few skeletal muscles, including muscles of the mouth and larynx involved in speech, swallowing, and keeping the larynx open for breathing. The vagus nerve also has a minor sympathetic function via peripheral chemoreceptors. Upon leaving the medulla between the medullary pyramid and the inferior cerebellar peduncle, it extends through the jugular foramen, then passes into the carotid sheath between the internal carotid artery and the internal jugular vein below the head, to the neck, chest, and abdomen, where it contributes to the innervation of the viscera.

CN XI

The accessory nerve is also called the spinal accessory nerve. The accessory nerve provides motor innervation from the CNS to 2 neck muscles, the sternocleidomastoid, which tilts and rotates the head, and the trapezius muscle, which has several actions on the scapula, including shoulder elevation and adduction of the scapula. Thus, the accessory nerve governs movements of the head and shoulders. Most of the fibers of the accessory nerve originate in neurons situated in the upper spinal cord. These fibers enter the skull through the foramen magnum and proceed to exit the jugular foramen with CNs IX and X. Due to its unusual course, the accessory nerve is the only nerve that enters and exits the skull. Traditional descriptions of the accessory nerve divide it into 2 components: a

TABLE 4–1 Summary of the cranial nerves.

Number of Nerve	Name of Nerve	Type	Major Function(s)
I	Olfactory	Sensory	• Smell
II	Optic	Sensory	• Vision
III	Occulomotor	Motor	• Eye movements and constriction of the pupil
IV	Trochlear	Motor	• Eye movements
V	Trigeminal • Ophthalmic division • Maxillary division • Mandibular division	 • Sensory • Sensory • Mixed	 • Cornea and skin of the forehead, scalp, nose, and eyelid • Maxillary facial skin, upper teeth, maxillary sinus, and palate • Sensory to skin over mandible, lower teeth, inside of mouth, and anterior part of the tongue • Motor to muscles of mastication
VI	Abducens	Motor	• Eye movements
VII	Facial	Mixed	• Sensory function includes taste from anterior two-thirds of the tongue • Motor to facial muscles • Parasympathetic secretomotor fibers to salivary and lacrimal glands
VIII	Vestibulocochlear • Vestibular • Cochlear	 • Sensory • Sensory	 • Position and movement of the head • Hearing
IX	Glossopharyngeal	Mixed	• Sensory to the pharynx and posterior third of the tongue; carotid sinus baroreceptor and carotid body chemoreceptor • Motor to muscles of swallowing • Parasympathetic secretomotor to salivary gland
X	Vagus	Mixed	• Major parasympathetic nerve to heart, lungs, and upper gastrointestinal system
XI	Accessory	Motor	• Spinal root: sternomastoid and trapezius muscles • Cranial root: muscles of palate, pharynx, and larynx
XII	Hypoglossal	Motor	• Muscles of the tongue

Reproduced with permission from Kibble JD, Halsey CR. *Medical Physiology: The Big Picture.* New York, NY: McGraw Hill; 2009.

spinal component and a cranial component. However, contemporary characterizations of the nerve regard the cranial component as separate and part of the vagus nerve.

CN XII

The hypoglossal nerve is a somatic motor nerve that, similar to the glossopharyngeal and vagus nerves, is also involved in tongue muscles, swallowing, and speech. A nerve with solely motor function, the hypoglossal nerve provides motor control of the extrinsic muscles of the tongue (genioglossus, hyoglossus, and styloglossus) and the intrinsic muscles of the tongue. These represent all muscles of the tongue except the palatoglossus muscle, which is innervated by the vagus nerve. These muscles are involved in moving and manipulating the tongue. The hypoglossal nerve also supplies movements including clearing the mouth of saliva and other involuntary activities. The hypoglossal nucleus interacts with the reticular formation, which is involved in the control of several reflexive or automatic motions, and several corticonuclear originating fibers supply innervation, aiding in unconscious movements relating to speech and articulation. The hypoglossal nerve (CN XII) is unique in that it is innervated from the motor

cortex of both hemispheres of the brain. See Table 4–1 for a summary of the CNs.

THE CEREBELLUM

Lying underneath the forebrain and adjacent to the brainstem is the cerebellum (Figure 4–6). The cerebellum receives substantial motor and sensory inputs via the cerebellar peduncles, directly from the brainstem and spinal cord and indirectly from the cerebral cortex. Primarily a movement control center, cerebellar functions include control of posture and balance, coordination of voluntary movements that result in smooth and balanced muscular activity of parts of the body, and learning motor behaviors. The cerebellum has also been implicated in mood and cognitive functions including language, attention, and mental imagery. Receiving extensive inputs, the cerebellar intrinsic circuits are thought to have substantial computational capacity in producing their outputs.

The cerebellum rests at the back of the cranial cavity, with the appearance of being a separate structure lying beneath the cerebral lobes, and is separated from the occipital lobes by a sheet of fibers called the cerebellar tentorium. However, the cerebellum is robustly connected with other regions of the

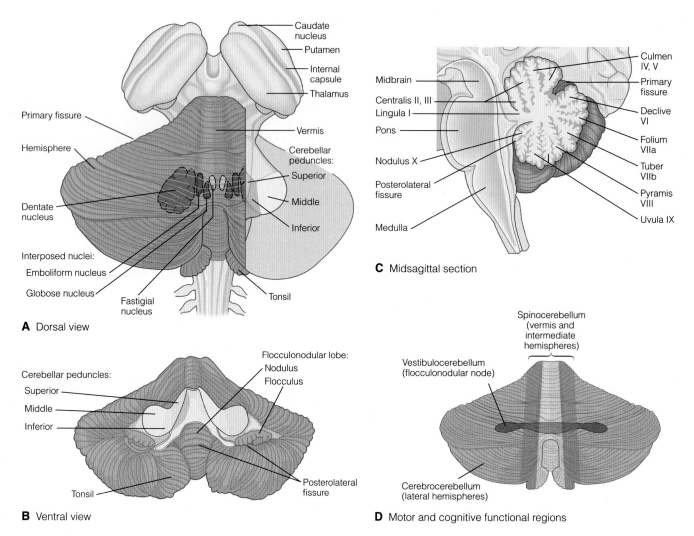

FIGURE 4–6 Gross features and functional anatomy of the cerebellum. **A.** Part of the right hemisphere has been cut away to reveal the underlying cerebellar peduncles. **B.** The cerebellum is shown detached from the brain stem. **C.** A midsagittal section through the brainstem and cerebellum shows the branching structure of the cerebellum. The cerebellar lobules are labeled with their latin names and Larsell Roman numerals. **D.** Functional regions of the cerebellum.

CNS via the cerebellar peduncles. The cerebellum has fissures that divide it into 3 lobes. The primary fissure divides the anterior lobe from the posterior lobe, which are connected in the midline by the vermis. The posterolateral fissure divides the posterior lobe from the medial flocculonodular lobe. Each of the 3 lobes has a left and right half, and each lobe consists of an inner medulla of white matter and a richly folded thin outer layer of cortical gray matter.

The continuous cortical surface contains finely spaced parallel grooves with the appearance of an accordion. Although it represents only 10% of the brain mass, the cerebellum contains as many neurons as the entire cerebrum, but many fewer types of neurons. The outer cortical layer consists of a regular 3-layer arrangement that contains Purkinje neurons and granule neurons. The majority of inputs reach the cerebellar cortex, where Purkinje neurons integrate incoming signals and send outputs to the deep cerebellar nuclei located in the white matter interior and the vestibular nuclei. Hence, the majority of outputs

from the cerebellum to the brainstem and thalamus occur via the deep cerebellar nuclei.

The cerebellum has 3 functional subdivisions and is involved in control of both conscious and unconscious movement. The flocculonodular lobe and adjacent vermis is called the vestibulocerebellum (archicerebellum) and is involved in balance and eye movements. The spinocerebellum (paleocerebellum) includes the vermis and paravermis in the anterior lobe and paramedian lobules and functions in posture and proprioception. The cerebrocerebellum (neocerebellum or pontocerebellum) makes up the lateral hemispheres of the anterior and posterior lobes and functions in control of voluntary movement.

The cerebral cortex provides the largest source of inputs to the cerebellum, although indirectly via the pons. Corticopontine fibers originate in the frontal lobe motor cortex and the parietal lobe somatosensory cortex and visual association areas, which project to the pontine nuclei in the pons. Neurons in the pons send outputs to the cerebellum by the middle cerebellar peduncles. The target of the pontine output is the cerebrocerebellum, which functions in coordination and smoothing of complex motor movements, evaluation of sensory information for action, and some cognitive functions. The cerebrocerebellum sends output via the dentate nucleus and fibers in the superior cerebellar peduncles to both the red nucleus and the ventral lateral nucleus of the thalamus. Hence, the thalamus provides the feedback to the motor cortex for the adjustment of movement.

The vestibulocerebellum is involved in maintenance of balance and coordinating eye movements. It receives direct input from the vestibular nerve and the vestibular nuclei and sends output to the medial and lateral vestibular nuclei by 2 pathways. One output pathway originates directly from the cerebellar cortex and sends fibers to the vestibular nuclear complex in the brainstem. The other output occurs via nuclei in the flocculonodular lobe. The vestibulocerebellum also receives visual input from the superior colliculus via the superior peduncles and is involved in coordinating eye movements and speech.

The spinocerebellum regulates body and limb movements involved in proprioception and posture. It receives proprioception input from the spinocerebellar tract, other dorsal columns of the spinal cord, and the trigeminal nerve nuclei. It also receives vestibular input and sensory information from visual and auditory systems. The spinocerebellum sends fibers to deep cerebellar nuclei (including the fastigial and interposed nuclei), for modulation of descending motor systems. The fastigial and interposed nuclei project to the cerebral cortex, via the thalamus, and to the brainstem, via the red nucleus, reticular formation in the pons, and vestibular nuclei in the medulla.

Numerous studies support the conclusion that the cerebellum plays an important role in some types of motor learning, in particular those voluntary motor actions that require fine adjustments for performance. In addition, a well-studied cerebellar learning task involves involuntary muscle contractions that underlie the eye blink conditioning response. Lesions or pharmacologic disruption of circuits to specific deep cerebellar nuclei or cerebellar cortical regions abolish learning in the conditioned eye blink response. Studies have identified candidate learning circuits involving Purkinje cells and their synapses, which undergo long-term plasticity.

THE SPINAL CORD

The spinal cord is a long, thin, tubular bundle of nervous tissue that is continuous with the medulla and emerges from the foramen magnum, where it enters the spinal (vertebral) canal at the beginning of the cervical vertebrae (Figures 4–7 and 4–8). It extends down to the first or second lumbar region, terminating in the conus medullaris. Between 40 and 50 cm long, the human spinal cord diameter is variable along its length, between 0.6 and 1.3 cm. Two prominent grooves, or sulci, run along its length. The posterior median sulcus is the groove in the dorsal side, and the anterior median fissure is the groove in the ventral side. The spinal cord is protected by the meninges and the bony vertebral column. In the median, the central canal is an extension of the fourth ventricle and contains CSF.

Along its length, the spinal cord connects with the spinal nerves of the PNS. The human spinal cord contains 31 segments, consisting of cervical, thoracic, lumbar, sacral, and coccygeal regions, with each region connecting to a spinal nerve on either side. The spinal nerves enter and exit the cord via roots, which then merge into bilaterally symmetrical pairs of spinal nerves. The spinal roots, nerves, and associated ganglia functionally connect the spinal cord to the skin, muscles, joints, and viscera.

Functionally, the spinal cord transmits both somatic and autonomic motor and sensory information between the brain and the body and accomplishes important integration tasks. The spinal cord white matter is found in the more lateral regions and contains ascending sensory and descending motor tracts that are often described as columns. Located more medially, spinal cord gray matter contains motor neurons, secondary sensory neurons, and interneurons (Figure 4–9). Ten regions of gray matter are named the Rexed laminae and are numbered from dorsal to ventral. The dorsal (posterior) horns are dedicated to sensory functions (laminae I to VI). The ventral (anterior) horns are involved in motor functions (laminae VIII and IX). Between the horns is the intermediate gray region (laminae VII and X).

The spinal cord plays a major role in transmission of both somatic and visceral sensory information to the brain. Axons from somatosensory neurons and GVAs enter the spinal cord via the dorsal root from the dorsal root ganglia. Depending on the sensory modality relayed, the entering axons either ascend in the cord, forming some of the sensory tracts, or synapse with sensory relay neurons, which are located in the dorsal horn and extend axons to form other sensory tracts. The 3 main ascending white matter tracts are the DCML tract, the spinothalamic tracts, and the spinocerebellar tracts.

The DCML transmits sensory information about fine touch, vibration, 2-point discrimination, and conscious proprioception. In the DCML, the primary somatosensory axons enter the cord and form the dorsal column. If an axon enters below T6, it travels in the fasciculus gracilis of the DCML. If the axon enters above T6, it travels in the fasciculus cuneatus of the DCML. For both, the primary sensory axons ascend in the dorsal column to the lower medulla, where they synapse on sensory relay neurons (called secondary sensory neurons) located in the nucleus gracilis or nucleus cuneatus. Axons from the medullary neurons form the internal arcuate fibers, which cross and ascend to become the medial lemniscus. These axons connect to neurons in the thalamus, and the thalamic neurons project to the primary somatosensory cortex.

The spinothalamic tract (also called the anterolateral system) transmits crude touch, pain, and temperature sensation. Axons from the primary somatosensory neurons enter the spinal cord and synapse on secondary sensory neurons located in the dorsal horn. The axons of the secondary sensory neurons cross over to the contralateral side of the spinal cord and form the spinothalamic tract, which ascends in the anterolateral region of the white matter and extend all the way to the

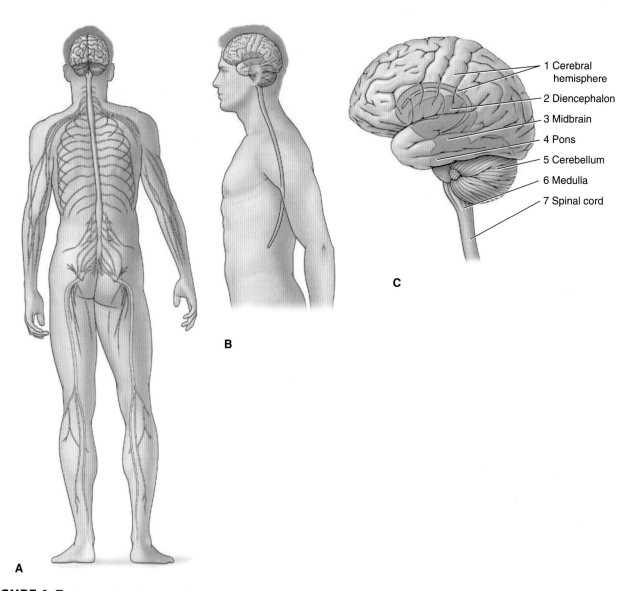

FIGURE 4–7   The central and peripheral nervous systems. **A.** Location of the central and peripheral nervous system in the body. Major cranial, spinal, and peripheral nerves are shown in yellow. **B.** The brain and spinal cord, viewed laterally. **C.** The seven major divisions of the central nervous system; the spinal cord is continuous with the brainstem. (Reproduced with permission from Martin JH. *Neuroanatomy: Text and Atlas*, 4th ed. New York, NY: McGraw Hill; 2012.)

thalamus. The thalamic neurons project to the primary somatosensory cortex, cingulate cortex, and insular cortex. Traveling along side the spinothalamic tract, the spinoreticular tract and spinotectal tracts also transmit information to the brainstem.

The spinocerebellar tracts transmit unconscious proprioception from the muscles and joints to the cerebellum. The axons from primary somatosensory neurons enter the spinal cord via the dorsal root and synapse on secondary sensory neurons in or near the dorsal horn. Depending on where the sensory information originates and enters the spinal cord, the ascending axons sort into 1 of 4 tracts called the dorsal (posterior), ventral (anterior), and rostral spinocerebellar tracts and the cuneocerebellar tract. After traversing the medulla, the axons travel via the inferior cerebellar peduncle to innervate the ipsilateral cerebellum.

Part of the ANS, GVA fibers transmit visceral sensory information about local changes in the chemical and mechanical environments from the internal organs, glands, and blood vessels to the CNS. The GVAs transmit conscious sensations, such as gut distention and cardiac ischemia, and unconscious sensations, such as blood pressure and chemical composition of the blood. Some of the key functions of GVAs are to initiate autonomic reflexes at the local, ganglion, spinal, and supraspinal levels.

Visceral sensory neuronal cell bodies are located in the dorsal root ganglia of the spinal nerves. After they enter the spinal cord, the axons branch extensively and synapse on viscerosomatic neurons in the dorsal horn and intermediate gray matter. Visceral sensation is carried primarily by the spinothalamic and spinoreticular pathways, which transmit visceral pain and sexual sensations. The DCML tract may

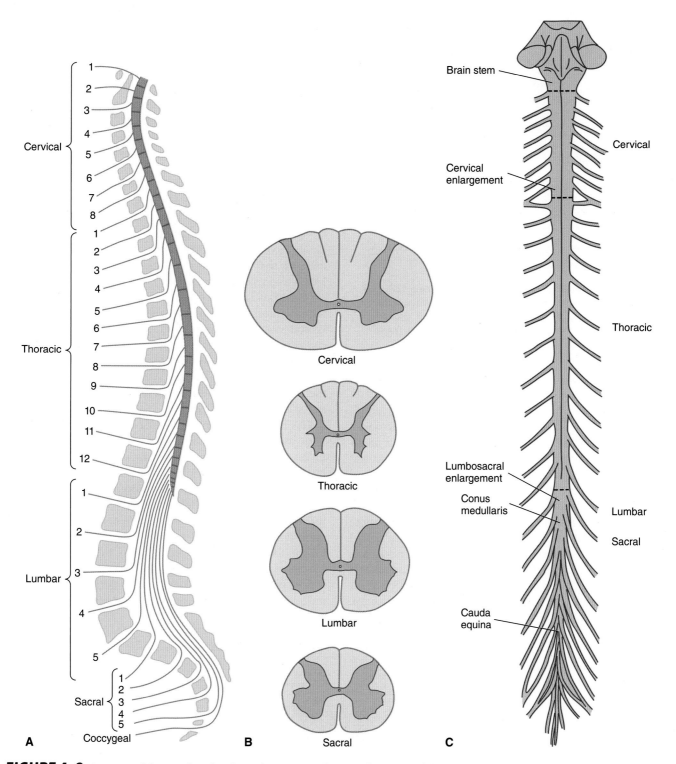

FIGURE 4-8 Anatomy of the spinal cord and spinal nerves. **A.** Schematic illustration of the relationships between the vertebral column, the spinal cord, and the spinal nerves. Note the mismatch between the location of spinal cord segments and of vertebral level where roots exit from the vertebral column. Note also the termination of the spinal cord at the level of the L1 or L2 vertebral body. **B.** Transverse sections of the spinal cord at the levels shown. **C.** Schematic dorsal view of isolated spinal cord and spinal nerves. (Reproduced with permission from Waxman SG. *Clinical Neuroanatomy*, 28th ed. New York, NY: McGraw Hill; 2017.)

relay sensations related to micturition, defecation, and gastric distention. After relay in the thalamic nuclei, viscerosensory inputs project to the insula and other cortical autonomic areas. Viscerosomatic neurons in the dorsal gray regions that receive convergent visceral and somatic inputs have been implicated in referred pain.

The spinal cord white matter contains descending somatic motor tracts involved in both voluntary and involuntary

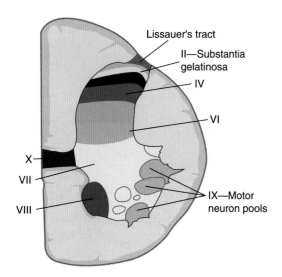

FIGURE 4–9 Illustration of the laminae of the spinal cord gray matter in the dorsal and ventral horns. The Rexed laminae of the gray matter from one half of the spinal cord are labeled. (Reproduced with permission from Waxman SG. *Clinical Neuroanatomy*, 28th ed. New York, NY: McGraw Hill; 2017.)

The VM LMNs control the large, postural muscles of the axial skeleton and are located along the length of the spinal cord.

Four additional motor tracts (called extrapyramidal tracts) extend axons down the spinal cord to LMNs and SIs. These tracts originate with upper motor neurons located in specific nuclei in the brainstem. Their tracts include the rubrospinal, vestibulospinal, tectospinal, and reticulospinal tracts. The rubrospinal tract descends with the lateral CST and synapses on cervical DL LMNs involved in voluntary control of arm muscles. The remaining 3 tracts descend with the anterior CST, synapse on VM LMNs, and are involved in involuntary muscle control for reflexes, locomotion, complex movements, and postural control.

LMNs in the dorsal horn receive descending inputs directly from the upper motor neurons. They also receive inputs from SIs, including a type of SI called propriospinal neurons that interconnect multiple spinal cord segments. LMNs also receive direct sensory signals from 1a somatosensory neurons and both excitatory and inhibitory SIs that relay sensory information. The axons of the LMNs exit through the ventral roots of the spinal cord and merge with the sensory components to form the spinal nerves, eventually emerging from the nerve to innervate its specific skeletal muscle.

For the autonomic motor system, preganglionic sympathetic neurons originate from the thoracolumbar region of the spinal cord, specifically at T1 to L2-L3 (Figure 4–11). A gray matter region in the intermediolateral nucleus of the lateral horn contains these neurons. These are analogous to somatic LMNs, with axons that leave the cord via the ventral root, but instead travel to either the paravertebral or prevertebral ganglia, where they synapse with the postganglionic sympathetic neurons, which extend their axons to their targets. Although the majority of parasympathetic motor neurons emerge from the brainstem via CNs, 3 spinal nerves in the sacral region (S2 to S4), commonly referred to as the pelvic splanchnic nerves, include parasympathetic preganglionic neurons located in the spinal cord. The targets of the splanchnic nerves include the bladder, colon, and genital organs.

control of muscle contraction (Figure 4–10). The axons in these tracts synapse on lower motor neurons (LMNs) and spinal interneurons (SIs) in the ventral horn. The 2 corticospinal tracts (CSTs) originate in the motor cortex with upper motor neurons. About 85% to 90% of the axons cross to the contralateral side at the pyramids of the medulla, forming the lateral CST. The remaining 10% to 15% of uncrossed axons descend on the ipsilateral side, forming the anterior CST, with most axons crossing to the contralateral side of the cord right before synapsing. The lateral CST axons synapse on dorsolateral (DL) LMNs in the ventral horn and control distal limb movement; these DL LMNs are located in the cervical and lumbosacral enlargements within the spinal cord. Anterior CST axons synapse on ventromedial (VM) LMNs in the ventral horn.

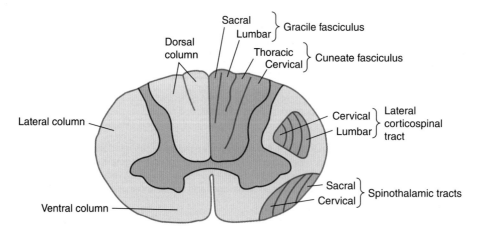

FIGURE 4–10 Somatotopic organization of several ascending sensory and descending motor tracts in the spinal cord white matter. One major descending motor tract, the lateral corticospinal tract is shown. Two major sensory tracts, the DCML composed of the gracile and cuneate fasciculus, and the spinothalamic tracts are depicted. (Reproduced with permission from Waxman SG. *Clinical Neuroanatomy*, 28th ed. New York, NY: McGraw Hill; 2017.)

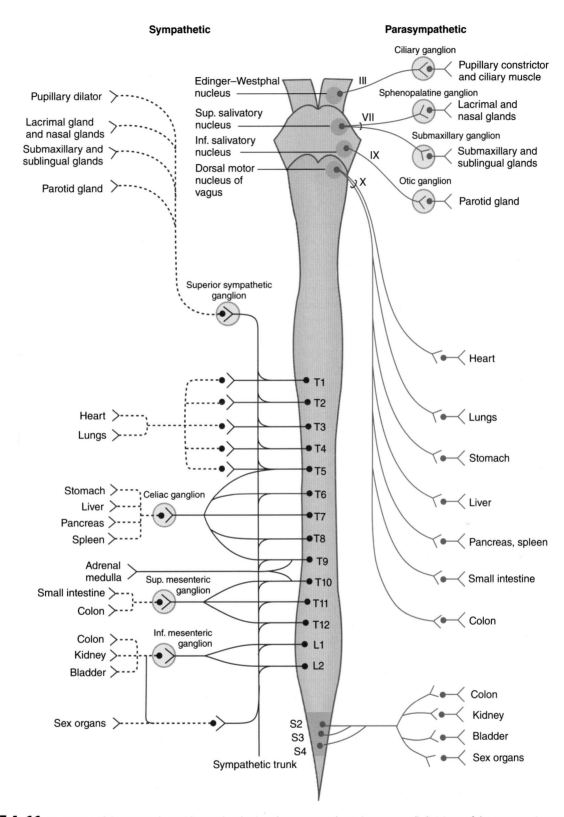

FIGURE 4–11 Overview of the sympathetic (thoracolumbar) and parasympathetic (craniosacral) divisions of the autonomic nervous system. The spinal cord and brainstem contain the preganglionic neuron cell bodies, while the spinal and cranial nerves contain the axons of these neurons, which synapse on postganglionic neurons in the autonomic ganglia shown. Inf., inferior; Sup., superior. (Reproduced with permission from Waxman SG. *Clinical Neuroanatomy*, 28th ed. New York, NY: McGraw Hill; 2017.)

In addition to motor and sensory relaying functions, the spinal cord contains neuronal circuits that generate spinal reflexes, such as the stretch reflexes involved in balance and the withdrawal reflex involved in removing a limb from a noxious stimulus. The circuits within the spine also contribute to more complex movements involving central pattern generators. For example, networks responsible for locomotion have been shown to be distributed throughout the lower thoracic and lumbar regions of the mammalian spinal cord.

THE SPINAL NERVES

The spinal nerves are components of the PNS that transmit motor and sensory signals between the spinal cord and the body. As mixed nerves, the spinal nerves include both somatic motor axons that control the actions of striated muscles and somatic sensory fibers that receive sensory information from the skin, muscles, and joints. Many spinal nerves also contain autonomic motor and visceral sensory components that provide information to and from organs, smooth muscles, and glands in the body. Humans have 31 pairs of spinal nerves, 1 on each side of the vertebral column, which arise from the spinal cord and are named for the spinal cord segment where they originate, with 8 cervical pairs, 12 thoracic pairs, 5 lumbar pairs, 5 sacral pairs, and 1 coccygeal pair. The spinal nerves branch and reorganize to form what are called peripheral nerves.

Sensory axons enter the spinal cord via small rootlets that combine to form the dorsal root (Figure 4–12). Sensory neuron cell bodies form the dorsal root ganglia that lie just outside the spinal cord. The sensory axons are called the general somatic afferents, which transmit information from the skin, muscles, and tendons, and the GVAs, which send information from the visceral organs. Motor axons leave the spinal cord via small rootlets that combine to form the ventral root. Motor neuron cell bodies lie in the ventral or lateral horn gray matter in the spinal cord itself. The motor axons include the general somatic efferents to striated muscle and the general visceral efferents, which are autonomic (sympathetic and a few parasympathetic) axons that transmit impulses to smooth muscle,

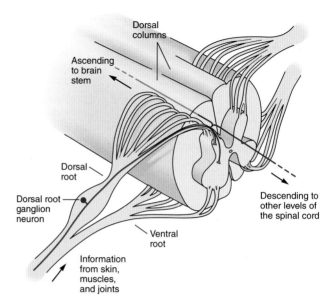

FIGURE 4–12 The spinal cord and spinal nerve roots. The cell bodies of neurons that transmit sensory information from the skin, muscles, joints, and viscera lie in the dorsal root ganglia adjacent to the spinal cord. The ventral roots contain axons from lower motor neurons. (Reproduced with permission from Kandel ER, Schwartz JH, Jessell TM, et al: *Principles of Neural Science*, 5th ed. New York, NY: McGraw Hill; 2013.)

cardiac muscle, and glands. The ventral and dorsal roots also provide the anchorage and fixation of the spinal cord to the vertebral cauda.

Spinal nerves initially form by the union of sensory axons from the dorsal root and motor axons from the ventral root. After joining, the spinal nerves exit the spinal canal and vertebral column. All spinal nerves, except the first spinal nerve C1 pair, emerge from the vertebral column through the intervertebral foramina between adjacent vertebrae. C1 emerges between the occipital bone and the first vertebra called the atlas. After it exits, each nerve then divides into branches called the dorsal ramus, the ventral ramus, and the rami communicates (Figure 4–13).

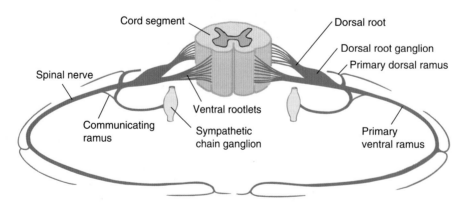

FIGURE 4–13 Schematic illustration of a spinal cord segment with its roots, ganglia, and branches. The axons from the dorsal root and ventral root merge to form a spinal nerve. Dorsal roots contain axons from somatic sensory neurons and many contain visceral sensory axons as well; ventral roots contain axons from somatic motor neurons and many contain axons from autonomic neurons as well. (Reproduced with permission from Waxman SG. *Clinical Neuroanatomy*, 28th ed. New York, NY: McGraw Hill; 2017.)

The dorsal ramus contains nerves that supply the dorsal portion of the trunk, with somatic and visceral motor and somatic sensory information relayed to and from the back muscles, dorsal muscles, and skin (Figure 4–14). The ventral ramus supplies somatic and visceral motor and sensory information to and from the ventrolateral body surface, structures in the body wall, trunk, and limbs. The rami communicantes contain autonomic axons that transmit sympathetic motor and visceral sensory information to and from the visceral organs. Additional small branches from the spinal nerves, called meningeal branches, supply nerve function to the vertebrae themselves, including the ligaments, dura, blood vessels, intervertebral disks, facet joints, and periosteum.

In the thoracic region, the ventral rami, which form the intercostal nerves, remain distinct from each other, and each innervates a narrow strip of muscle and skin along the sides, chest, ribs, and abdominal wall (Figure 4–15). In other regions, ventral rami converge with each other to form networks of nerves called nerve plexuses. Within each nerve plexus, fibers from various ventral rami branch and become redistributed such that each nerve exiting the plexus has fibers from several different spinal nerves, which travel together to their target location, mainly to the limbs. The major nerve plexuses are the cervical, brachial, lumbar, and sacral plexuses.

The cervical plexus is formed by the ventral rami from spinal nerves C1 to C4. The cervical plexus innervates muscles of the neck and diaphragm and the skin of the neck and upper chest. One branch forms the phrenic nerve, which provides motor innervation of the diaphragm. The brachial plexus is formed by ventral rami from spinal nerves C5 to T1. The brachial plexus provides almost all the innervation of the upper limb. The lumbar plexus contains ventral rami from spinal nerves L1 to L4. The sacral plexus contains ventral rami from spinal nerves L4 to S4. Together, the lumbar and sacral plexuses innervate the pelvic girdle and lower limbs.

Each spinal nerve receives a branch called a gray ramus communicans from the adjacent paravertebral ganglion of the sympathetic trunk. The gray rami contain postganglionic nerve fibers of the sympathetic neurons. The white rami communicantes exist only at the levels of the spinal cord where the intermediolateral cell column is present (T1-L2), which contain the sympathetic motor neuron cell bodies and are responsible for carrying preganglionic nerve fibers from the spinal cord to the adjoining paravertebral sympathetic ganglia. The 3 sacral parasympathetic spinal nerves in S2-S4 emerge from the spinal cord and form nerve plexuses with sympathetic fibers called the pelvic splanchnic nerves (Figure 4–16). Table 4–2 lists the peripheral nerves and their functions.

THE ENTERIC NERVOUS SYSTEM

Formerly thought to be part of the ANS, the ENS is now considered a separate component of the PNS. The ENS consists of a system of approximately 200 to 600 million neurons and glial cells distributed in many thousands of small ganglia in the

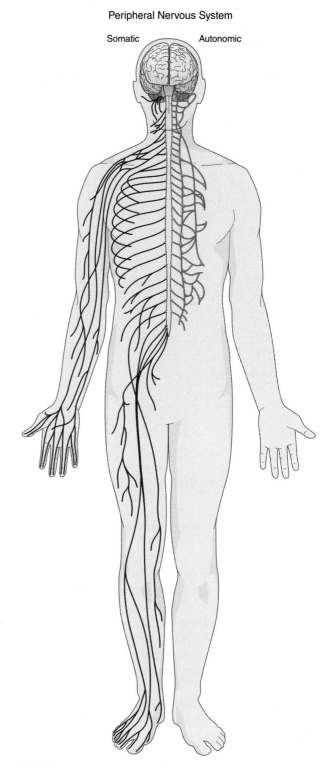

Peripheral Nervous System

Somatic   Autonomic

FIGURE 4–14 Many spinal nerves contain both somatic and autonomic components. Both somatic and autonomic components of spinal nerves branch, with branches called peripheral nerves and identified with specific names. (Reproduced with permission from Kandel ER, Schwartz JH, Jessell TM, et al: *Principles of Neural Science*, 5th ed. New York, NY: McGraw Hill; 2013.)

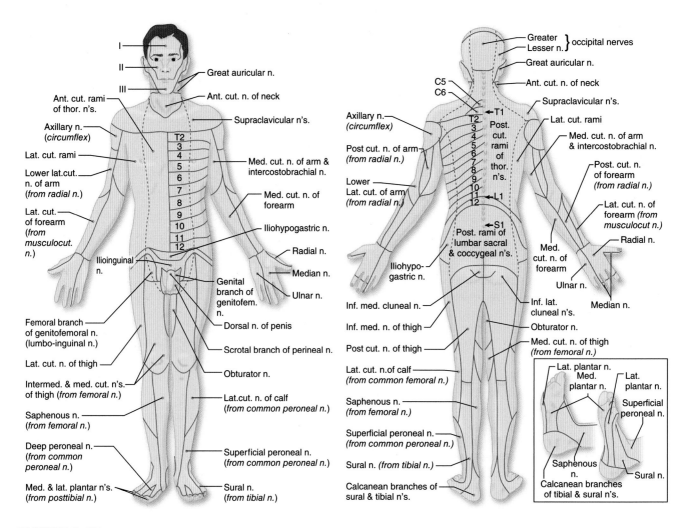

FIGURE 4–15 Dermatomes—the peripheral nerve cutaneous fields. (Reproduced with permission from Haymaker W, Woodhall B. *Peripheral Nerve Injuries*, 2nd ed. Philadelphia, PA: Saunders/Elsevier; 1953.)

lining of the GI system. Two types of ENS ganglia have been identified, called the myenteric and submucosal plexuses. The myenteric plexus forms a continuous network that extends from the upper esophagus to the internal anal sphincter. Submucosal ganglia and connecting fiber bundles form plexuses in the small and large intestines, but not in the stomach and esophagus. The ENS forms a neuronal circuitry that controls or modulates most aspects of GI function, including motility and GI transit, secretion and adsorption, water and electrolyte balance, chemical sensing, and communication between intestinal segments and the CNS.

The ENS is derived from the neural crest. A variety of different subtypes of enteric neurons and glia differentiate from neural crest progenitors that undergo proliferation and migration into the GI tract during embryonic and postnatal development. The ENS includes motor (efferent) neurons, sensory (afferent) neurons, and interneurons, all of which make the ENS capable of generating reflexes and acting as an integration center in the absence of input from the CNS or ANS. The ENS controls various types of primary GI effector cells, including epithelial cells and smooth muscle cells, which mediate GI functions. ENS sensory neurons

report on mechanical and chemical conditions. Motor neurons control peristalsis, the coordinated contraction and relaxation of intestinal smooth muscles, and churning of intestinal contents. Contact with the GI epithelium can modulate nutrient uptake. Alteration of regional blood flow can allow responses to metabolic needs. Other neurons control the secretion of enzymes. ENS interneurons coordinate the various activities.

In addition to containing the ENS, the digestive system is innervated and controlled by both the CNS and ANS. For example, movements of the striated muscles of the esophagus are determined by neural pattern generators in the CNS. Sympathetic stimulation causes inhibition of GI secretion and motor activity and contraction of GI sphincters and blood vessels. Conversely, parasympathetic stimuli typically stimulate these digestive activities. Thus, although the ENS can function as an independent system, it works in concert with CNS reflex and ANS command centers to control digestive function. Moreover, there is bidirectional information flow between the ENS and CNS and between the ENS and ANS, via the pelvic nerves and ANS pathways. Neurons also project from the ENS to prevertebral ganglia and the gallbladder, pancreas, and trachea.

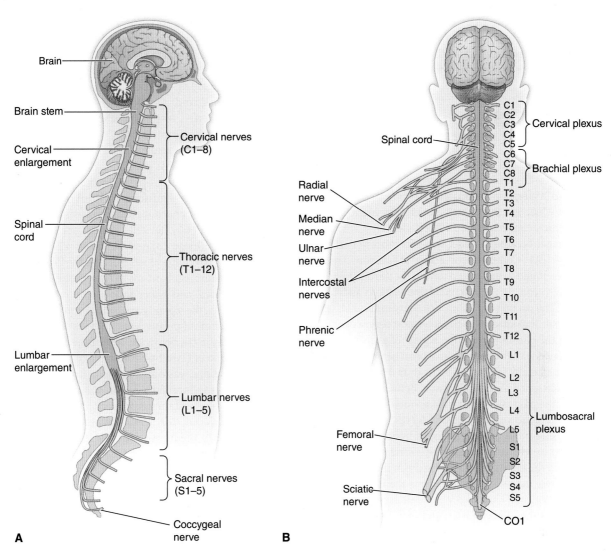

FIGURE 4-16 The nerve plexuses and peripheral nerves. **A.** Side view showing the spinal cord segments and two spinal cord enlargements. **B.** Dorsal view showing many of nerve plexus and peripheral nerves.

TABLE 4-2 The peripheral nerves and their functions.

Name	Spinal Nerves Involved	Function
Musculocutaneous nerves	C5-T1	Supply muscles of the arms on the anterior sides, and skin of the forearms
Radial nerves	C5-T1	Supply muscles of the arms on the posterior sides, and skin of the forearms and hands
Median nerves	C5-T1	Supply muscles of the forearms, and muscles and skin of the hands
Ulnar nerves	C5-T1	Supply muscles of the forearms and hands, and skin of the hands
Phrenic nerves	C3-C5	Supply the diaphragm
Intercostal nerves	T2-T12	Supply intercostal muscles, abdominal muscles, and skin of the trunk
Femoral nerves	L2-L4	Supply muscles and skin of the thighs and legs
Sciatic nerves	L4-S3	Supply muscles and skin of the thighs, legs and feet

C = cervical; L = lumbar; T = thoracic.

Approximately 30 different types of neurotransmitters have been identified in the ENS, including acetylcholine and glutamate. Interestingly more than 90% of the body's serotonin and about 50% of the body's dopamine are found in the intestine.

THE MENINGES & VENTRICULAR SYSTEM

Both the brain and spinal cord are covered and protected by the meninges (Figure 4–17), which is composed of 3 layers: the dura mater, arachnoid mater, and pia mater. The dura mater is the outermost layer, which is a thick, tough double membrane composed of collagenous connective tissue. The middle layer is called the arachnoid mater because of spider web–like processes called arachnoid trabeculae. Composed of a fine collagenous layer, regions of the arachnoid mater extend toward the third layer, the pia mater, and also contain the arachnoid granulations and villi that resorb CSF. The pia mater is a thin, delicate translucent layer of connective tissue that attaches to the outermost region of neural tissue, called the glia limitans, a thin barrier of astrocyte foot processes associated with the parenchymal basal lamina.

The arachnoid mater is attached to the dura mater, whereas the pia mater is attached to the CNS tissue. Between the arachnoid mater and the pia mater is the subarachnoid space, which contains CSF and blood vessels. The CSF serves to support the CNS and to cushion and protect it from physical shock and trauma. The falx cerebri is a double-fold of dura mater that descends through the interhemispheric fissure in the midline of the brain to separate the cerebral hemispheres and is attached to the cerebellar tentorium. The dural venous sinuses are venous channels found between the endosteal and meningeal layers of dura mater in the brain. The transverse and superior sagittal sinuses are the largest dural venous sinuses. The space between the bone and the dura mater is known as the epidural space, which is prominent in the spinal canal where it contains spinal nerve roots, connective tissue, and blood vessels.

The ventricular system is a series of interconnected, CSF-filled spaces, called ventricles, that lie in the core of the forebrain and brainstem (Figure 4–18). The ventricles produce CSF and circulate CSF. The ventricles originate as the inside or lumen of the neural tube during fetal development. The lumen of the telencephalon gives rise to the left and right lateral ventricles (formerly called the first and second ventricles). The largest of the ventricles, each lateral ventricle has a C shape that mirrors the cerebral hemisphere where it is located, and each contains a posterior horn that extends into the occipital lobe and an anterior horn that extends into the frontal lobe. The third ventricle originates from the diencephalon and is located in the midline between the left and right halves of the thalamus. CSF flows from the lateral ventricles through 2 small openings (called the interventricular foramen or foramen of Monro) into the third ventricle.

The third ventricle is continuous caudally with the cerebral aqueduct (also called the aqueduct of Sylvius). The cerebral aqueduct, which forms from the lumen of the mesencephalon, proceeds though the midbrain and then opens into the fourth ventricle. The fourth ventricle arises from the lumen of the metencephalon and myelencephalon and is located in the dorsal or roof of the pons and medulla. At the posterior region of the medulla, the fourth ventricle narrows to form the central canal of the spinal cord. As it flows from the fourth ventricle, some CSF is diverted to the subarachnoid space and some continues through the central canal.

CSF is a clear extracellular fluid that is constantly synthesized and resorbed. CSF is produced by a modified vascular structure called the choroid plexus, which is present in each of the 4 ventricles. The ventricles are lined by glial cells called ependymal cells. The choroid plexus consists of a layer of specialized choroid ependymal cells (CECs) surrounding a core of capillaries and loose connective tissue. CSF is formed as plasma is filtered from the blood through the CECs. The CECs use active transport mechanisms to transport ions and glucose into the ventricles, and water follows the resulting osmotic gradient. Hence, the ependymal cells form the blood–CSF barrier in the choroid plexus, which serves the same purpose as the blood–brain barrier in the rest of the brain. In addition to the production of CSF, the choroid plexus also acts as a filter to remove metabolic waste and excess neurotransmitters from the CSF. CSF is produced at a rate of about 600 mL/d, replacing the entire volume about once every 5 to 6 hours.

As it is produced, CSF flows from the lateral ventricles to the third and then the fourth ventricle. From the fourth ventricle, CSF can flow through the median aperture (foramina of Magendie) and 2 lateral apertures (foramina of Luschka) to the cisterna magna. From there, CSF flows to the subarachnoid space around the brain and spinal cord, where it resorbed by specialized structures called arachnoid villi and granulations and returned to the venous circulation (Figure 4–19).

In other parts of the body, circulation in the lymphatic system participates in the clearing of extracellular waste products and damaged cells from tissues and the movement of immune cells, such as white blood cells. For many years, a similar system was thought to be absent from the brain. However, recent studies have demonstrated the presence of lymphatic vessels that run parallel with blood vessels in the meninges. A potential role for brain lymphatic vessels may be to provide a route for transport of fluid and immune cells such as T cells from the CSF.

THE CNS VASCULAR SYSTEM

The CNS is highly vascularized. The adult cerebral blood flow is approximately 750 mL/min, consuming about 15% to 20% of the cardiac output. Similar to other organs and tissues, the arteries deliver oxygen, glucose, and other nutrients to the brain, and the veins carry deoxygenated blood back to the heart, removing carbon dioxide and other metabolic products. The larger arteries and veins branch to smaller arterioles and venules, and then to smaller capillaries, which supply and remove blood from the nervous tissue. Brain capillaries are lined by specialized vascular endothelial cells joined by tight junctions and covered by pericytes and astrocytic end feet, so

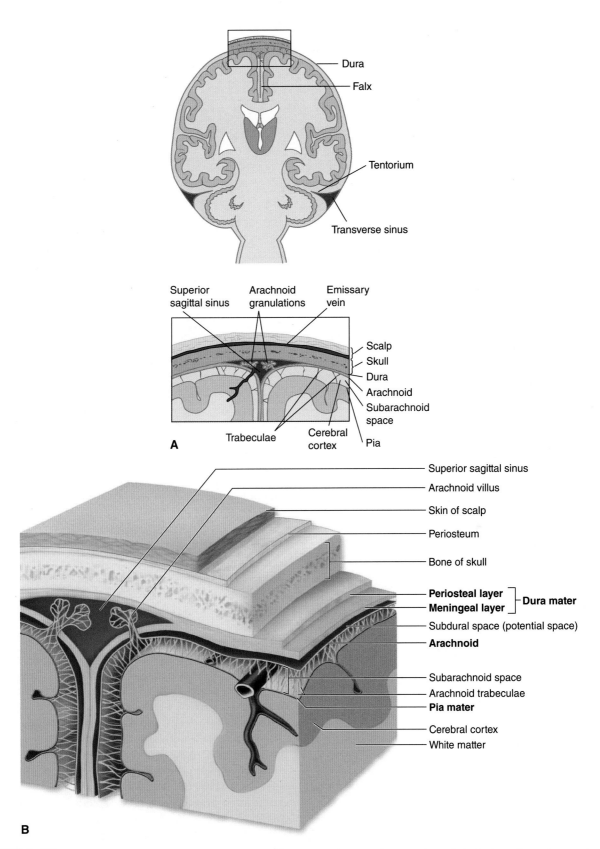

FIGURE 4–17 The meninges surround the CNS. **A.** Schematic illustration of a coronal section through the brain and coverings, and an enlargement of the area at the top showing the meninges, scull and scalp. **B.** The coverings around the cerebral cortex showing the three layers of the meninges and their spaces. (Part A, reproduced with permission from Waxman SG. *Clinical Neuroanatomy*, 28th ed. New York, NY: McGraw Hill; 2017; part B, reproduced with permission from McKinley MP, O'Loughlin VD, Bidle TS. *Anatomy and Physiology: An Integrative Approach*. New York, NY: McGraw Hill; 2013.)

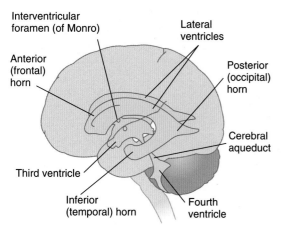

FIGURE 4–18 The brain ventricular system. (Reproduced with permission from Waxman SG. *Clinical Neuroanatomy*, 28th ed. New York, NY: McGraw Hill; 2017.)

hydrophilic molecules are unable to diffuse directly into the brain, thereby creating the blood–brain barrier. Astrocytic end feet transport specific nutrients from the blood into the brain.

The entire blood supply to the brain arises from 2 paired arteries, the internal carotid arteries and vertebral arteries,

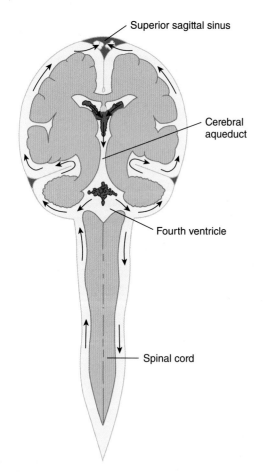

FIGURE 4–19 Schematic illustration, in coronal projection, of the circulation (arrows) of CSF. (Reproduced with permission from Waxman SG. *Clinical Neuroanatomy*, 28th ed. New York, NY: McGraw Hill; 2017.)

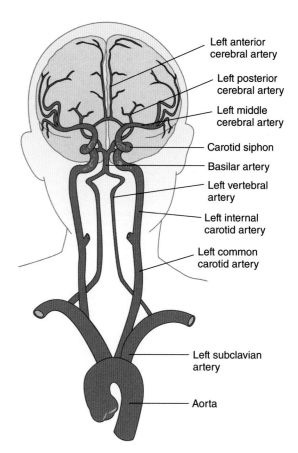

FIGURE 4–20 Major cerebral arteries. The arterial blood supply to the brain arises from the internal carotid arteries and vertebral arteries. (Reproduced with permission from Waxman SG. *Clinical Neuroanatomy*, 28th ed. New York, NY: McGraw Hill; 2017.)

which form from branches of the dorsal aorta and ascend to the cranium (Figure 4–20). The internal carotid arteries arise from the bifurcation of the left and right common carotid arteries, on each side of the head and neck, and supply blood to the front and middle regions of the brain. The vertebral arteries emerge as branches of the left and right subclavian arteries, ascend separately, and converge near the base of the pons to form the unpaired basilar artery and supply blood to the back of the brain. The blood supply to the spinal cord is via the vertebral arteries, which branch to form the anterior and posterior spinal arteries, and the medullary arteries.

The internal carotid arteries enter the cranium through the carotid canal of the temporal bone, travel through the cavernous sinus, and penetrate the dura just ventral to the optic nerve. At the level just lateral to the optic chiasm, the internal carotid artery branches to form the anterior cerebral artery and continues to form the middle cerebral artery (Figure 4–21). The left and right anterior cerebral arteries supply blood to most medial portions of the frontal lobes and anterior parietal lobes. The anterior cerebral arteries travel along the sphenoid bone of the eye socket, then upward through the insula cortex, where final branches arise. The middle cerebral artery is the larger branch of the internal carotid and continues into the

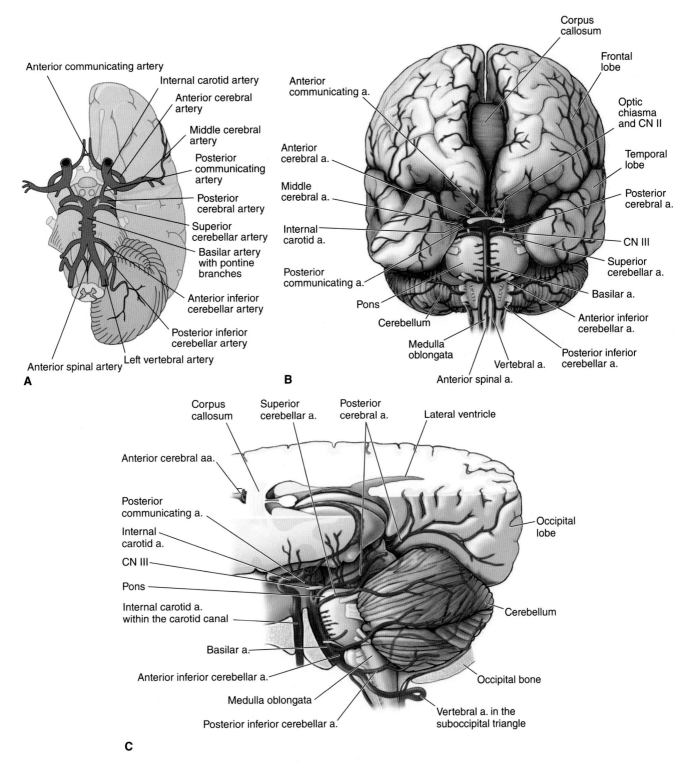

FIGURE 4–21 Arterial blood supply to different regions of the brain. **A.** Circle of Willis and principal arteries of the brainstem. **B.** Anterior view of the brain showing the arteries (a.) with the cerebral hemispheres separated. **C.** Lateral view of the brain showing the arteries (a.). (Part A, reproduced with permission from Waxman SG. *Clinical Neuroanatomy*, 28th ed. New York, NY: McGraw Hill; 2017; parts B and C, reproduced with permission from Morton DA, Foreman KB, Albertine KH. *The Big Picture: Gross Anatomy*. New York, NY: McGraw Hill; 2011.)

lateral sulcus, where it then branches and projects to lateral portions of the frontal, temporal, and parietal lobes. It also supplies blood to deeper structures of the basal forebrain and the insular cortices.

The vertebral arteries ascend upward through foramen transversarium of the cervical spine and enter the cranial cavity via the foramen magnum, emerging as 2 vessels, 1 on the left and 1 on the right of the medulla. Within the cranial vault, each vertebral artery gives off 3 branches that form the posterior inferior cerebellar artery and 2 spinal arteries. The vertebral arteries then join in front of the middle part of the medulla to form the larger basilar artery, which sends multiple branches to supply the medulla and pons, and the anterior inferior cerebellar artery. Finally, the basilar artery terminates by bifurcating into the posterior cerebral arteries and superior cerebellar artery. The posterior cerebral arteries supply the midbrain, thalamus, and subthalamic nucleus. They also travel outward, around the superior cerebellar peduncles and top of the cerebellar tentorium, where they send branches to supply the temporal and occipital lobes. The blood supply to the medulla includes the anterior spinal artery, the posterior inferior cerebellar artery, and the vertebral artery's direct branches.

The carotid and vertebral systems join together to form the cerebral arterial circle (circle of Willis), a ring of connected arteries that lies in the interpeduncular cistern between the midbrain and pons. The circle is formed by the posterior cerebral arteries, the posterior communicating arteries, and the internal carotids (from a region immediately proximal to the origin of the middle cerebral arteries, the anterior cerebral arteries, and the anterior communicating artery). Importantly, the circle of Willis provides alternative inputs to the internal carotid and posterior cerebral arteries, which is crucial in the event of stroke.

The brain is drained by a system of veins that empty into the dural sinuses, which eventually empty into the internal jugular veins (Figure 4–22). The brain has 2 main networks of veins: an exterior 3-branch network on the surface of the cerebrum and an interior network. The exterior and interior networks communicate via anastomosing (joining) veins. In the brain, the veins drain into larger cavities called the dural venous sinuses, which are typically located between the dura mater and the covering of the skull.

The great cerebral vein drains blood from the cerebellum and midbrain. The spinal veins or adjacent cerebral veins drain blood from the medulla and pons. Blood in the deep parts of the brain drains into region-specific sinuses. For the exterior network, the superior sagittal sinus, which is located at the midline at the top of the brain, receives blood from the outer portion of the brain and combines its drainage with the outflow from the straight sinus, at the confluence of sinuses, which drains into the transverse sinuses. Next, these drain into the sigmoid sinuses, which also receives blood from the cavernous sinus and superior and inferior petrosal sinuses. The sigmoid sinuses then drain into the left and right internal jugular veins.

The spinal cord is primarily supplied by 3 longitudinal arteries, the anterior spinal artery and 2 posterior spinal

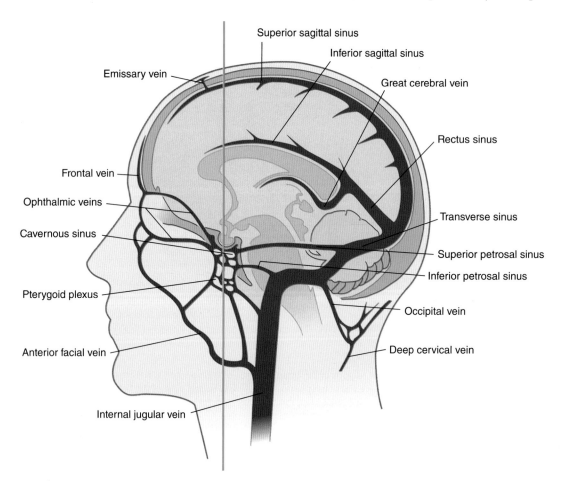

FIGURE 4–22 Organization of veins and sinuses involved in venous drainage of blood from the brain. (Reproduced with permission from Waxman SG. *Clinical Neuroanatomy*, 28th ed. New York, NY: McGraw Hill; 2017.)

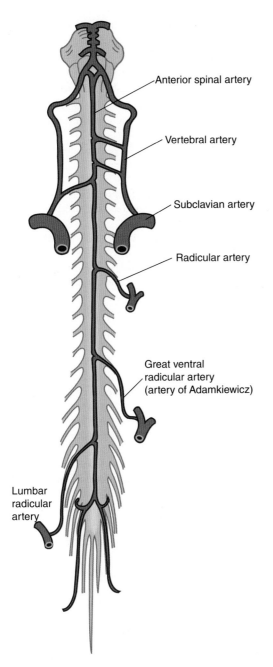

FIGURE 4–23 Vascularization of the spinal cord (ventral view). (Reproduced with permission from Waxman SG. *Clinical Neuroanatomy*, 28th ed. New York, NY: McGraw Hill; 2017.)

arteries, and the medullary arteries (Figure 4–23). In the cranium, at the medullary level, each vertebral artery branches to produce the anterior spinal artery and the posterior inferior cerebellar artery, which in about 75% of people gives rise to the posterior spinal artery. The anterior spinal artery travels along the midline of the ventral surface of the spinal cord and gives rise to the sulcal arteries, which enter the spinal cord and supply blood to the anterior two-thirds of the spinal cord. The paired posterior spinal arteries descend on the dorsolateral surface of the spinal cord slightly medial to the dorsal roots and supply blood to the posterior third of the cord.

Additional arterial supply occurs via the anterior and posterior segmental medullary arteries, which arise from the vertebral and other arteries and join with the anterior and posterior spinal arteries along the length of the cord. Venous drainage of the cord occurs via 3 anterior and 3 posterior spinal veins, which in turn empty into the systemic segmental veins. The internal vertebral plexus also empties into the dural venous sinuses. Radicular veins also contribute to venous drainage of the cord.

SUMMARY

- The brainstem and cerebellum develop from the mesencephalon and rhombencephalon vesicles of the neural tube.
- The midbrain, pons, and medulla form the brainstem, which contains nuclei for essential automatic, reflex, and autonomic functions that are critical for survival, and white matter tracks that connect the forebrain with the cerebellum and spinal cord.
- The brainstem houses the reticular formation, a set of interconnected nuclei located from the upper midbrain to the lower medulla involved in sleep and wakefulness, arousal and alertness, consciousness, and other motor and sensory functions.
- The midbrain encompasses nuclei in the superior and inferior colliculi involved in vision and hearing, nuclei for cranial nerves III and IV, and white matter regions including the cerebral peduncles.
- Also located in the midbrain are the substantia nigra and ventral tegmental area, 2 regions that contain dopaminergic neurons that contribute to the basal ganglia and are involved in motor control and the reward pathway.
- The pons contains nuclei that relay signals between the forebrain and cerebellum and nuclei involved in sleep, respiration, swallowing, and bladder control.
- The pons also houses nuclei for cranial nerves V to VIII, which are involved in hearing and taste, equilibrium, eye movement, facial expressions, and facial sensations.
- The pons includes the cerebellar peduncles, which are large white matter areas that provide the routes for all information transmitted to and from the cerebellum.
- The medulla includes nuclei involved in the automatic reflex of breathing and the autonomic regulation of heart rate and blood pressure, as well as control of several somatic functions.
- The medulla contains the nuclei for cranial nerves IX to XII and a white matter region called the pyramids, where the corticospinal tract and dorsal column medial lemniscus tract travel and decussate.
- The cranial nerves emerge from either the cerebrum or brainstem and transmit both special sense and somatic

motor and sensory information between the brain and the head, face, and neck.

■ The cranial nerves also supply parasympathetic motor control to and receive visceral sensory information from the head, neck, and organs of the body.

■ The cerebellum functions in motor control, including coordination, precision and timing of movements, and motor learning, and has been implicated in cognitive functions and emotion.

■ A component of the CNS, the spinal cord is a thin tube of nervous tissue that is enclosed in the vertebral canal, protected by meninges and the vertebral column, and divided into cervical, thoracic, lumbar, sacral, and coccygeal regions along its length.

■ The spinal cord contains white matter tracts and gray matter regions that transmit and relay motor signals from the CNS to the body and sends sensory signals from the PNS to the CNS.

■ Motor axons exit the spinal cord via the ventral roots, whereas sensory axons enter the spinal cord via the dorsal roots, forming the spinal nerves with 31 pairs along the length of the cord.

■ The peripheral nerves assemble from branches of the spinal nerves and innervate the body and limbs.

■ The enteric nervous system involves neurons and glia located in the gastrointestinal tract that function in regulation of peristalsis and secretions.

■ The meninges include the dura mater, arachnoid mater, and pia mater, which cover, protect, and cushion the brain and spinal cord.

■ The brain ventricular system unites the brain ventricles, which house the choroid plexuses that synthesize cerebrospinal fluid and circulate it within and around the brain and spinal cord.

■ The CNS arterial system arises from 2 branches from the dorsal aorta: the internal carotid arteries, which supply the anterior and middle regions of the brain, and the vertebral arteries, which supply the posterior brain, brainstem, and spinal cord.

■ The CNS venous system involves numerous venous sinuses that drain into the jugular vein.

SELF-ASSESSMENT QUESTIONS

1. Which of the following best describes the brainstem?
   A. The brainstem includes the basal ganglia, midbrain, pons, and medulla.
   B. The transmission of the majority of sensory and motor information between the cerebral cortex and spinal cord (SC) requires relay by brainstem nuclei.
   C. Functions of the brainstem include the regulation of sleep, respiration, heart rate, swallowing, and bladder control.
   D. Damage to the brainstem by injury or stroke often leads to a loss of consciousness but is not life threatening.
   E. The brainstem houses both sensory and motor white matter tracts, and half (6 of 12) of the cranial nerve nuclei.

2. Which of the following best describes the cerebellum?
   A. The cerebellum is connected to the cerebral cortices via the midbrain through 3 paired white matter tracts located in the cerebral peduncles.
   B. The main functions for the cerebellum are initiation of movements, action selection, motivation, and reward-based motor learning.
   C. The cerebellum contains 4 functional regions called the vestibulocerebellum, spinocerebellum, cerebrocerebellum, and bulbarcerebellum.
   D. Damage to the cerebellum usually leads to Parkinson-like symptoms.
   E. In the cerebellum, the cerebellar cortex receives the majority of inputs, whereas the majority of outputs occur via the deep cerebellar nuclei.

3. Which of the following statements is *not true* regarding the SC?
   A. Enclosed in the vertebral canal, the SC is protected by meninges and the vertebral column and surrounds the central canal.
   B. The SC is divided into cervical, thoracic, lumbar, sacral, and coccygeal regions along its length.
   C. The SC contains white matter tracts and gray matter regions that transmit and relay motor signals from the central nervous system (CNS) to the body and sends sensory signals from the peripheral nervous system to the CNS.
   D. Motor axons exit the SC via dorsal roots, whereas sensory axons enter the SC via ventral roots, forming 31 spinal nerve pairs along the length of the SC.
   E. The peripheral nerves assemble from branches of the spinal nerves and innervate the body and limbs.

4. Which of the following best describes the brain ventricular system and central canal (CC)?
   A. The ventricles contain the arachnoid mater and villi, which resorb cerebrospinal fluid (CSF).
   B. The lining of the ventricles and choroid plexus within them produce CSF.
   C. The third and fourth ventricles lie within the brainstem.
   D. The ventricles and CC are derived from neural crest cells during development.
   E. CSF flows from the lateral ventricles to the subarachnoid space via the cisterna magna.

5. Which of the following best describes the vasculature in the CNS?
   A. The blood supply to the brain and SC depends on 2 branches from the dorsal aorta.
   B. The vertebral arteries supply blood to the anterior part of the brain.
   C. The internal carotid arteries supply blood to the posterior part of the brain.
   D. In the brain, blood is circulated by arteries, arterioles, veins, and venules, but capillaries are absent.
   E. The main outflow from the brain is the vertebral venous plexus.

SECTION II

Cellular & Molecular Neuroscience: Electrical Signaling & Synaptic Transmission

Movement of Ions Across Biological Membranes: Ion Transporters & Channels

Robin A.J. Lester

OBJECTIVES

After studying this chapter, the student should be able to:

- Understand the structure and barrier properties of neural membranes.
- Understand how protein complexes form channels in membranes that selectively permit ion movement through the membrane.
- Know how active transporters create concentration balances for different ions.
- See how the Nernst potential equates diffusional force with electrical force on various ions.
- Understand the operation (gating) of various ion channels and their role in the electrical activity of neurons.

BIOLOGIC MEMBRANES & IONS

Although the plasma membrane is necessary for maintaining the integrity of neurons (and glial cells) by providing a barrier that keeps the cytoplasmic cellular contents separated from the extracellular space, it is also an essential element upon which all electrical signaling is based. The insulator properties of this thin lipid bilayer allow for the development of a transmembrane potential, but also impede the very movement of ions (along with other molecules) needed to establish ionic concentration gradients across the membrane, the central foundation of electrical excitability. To overcome the impermeability of the membrane to ions, complex membrane-spanning protein structures have evolved to form both ion channels and membrane exchangers, transporters, and pumps, which allow for the selective passage of ions across the bilayer. This chapter will discuss the lipid bilayer, ion channels, and various transmembrane ionic carrier systems.

Phospholipids, Fatty Acids, & Lipid Bilayers

The chief constituents of membranes are the amphipathic phospholipid molecules (>50%), which contain both a hydrophilic phosphate-containing polar head group and a pair of fatty acid chain tails. Some of the most common phospholipids are phosphatidylcholine, phosphatidylserine, and phosphatidyl ethanolymine. In the watery environment of the nervous system, a phospholipid bilayer barrier will spontaneously form, allowing the hydrophobic fatty acid tails from each monolayer to interact in the center of the bilayer, while being protected from the unfavorable aqueous extracellular (cerebrospinal fluid [CSF]) and intracellular milieu, which are in contact with the hydrophilic polar head groups (Figure 5–1).

A less plentiful component of the membrane is the glycolipid family, whose members contain polar head groups formed from straight or branched carbohydrate chains that extend into the extracellular medium, where they have a role in cell-to-cell recognition (Figure 5–2). Together with the much more abundant molecule cholesterol, these compounds contribute about 40% of the total lipid content of the mammalian plasma membrane. Cholesterol intercalates between phospholipid fatty acid chains, adding to the integrity of membranes by reducing further any permeability to ions and other biologic molecules. In addition, by immobilizing (via an interaction between the polar hydroxyl group of cholesterol and the hydrophilic head of the phospholipid) and separating phospholipids, cholesterol helps to control both the firmness and fluidity of the membrane. Overall, the fluid mosaic model posits that the plasma membrane is a dynamic structure in which both the phospholipids and embedded proteins are

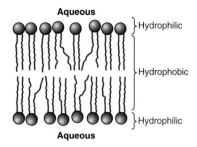

FIGURE 5–1 Diagram of a section of a bilayer membrane formed from phospholipid molecules. The unsaturated fatty acid tails are kinked and lead to more spacing between the polar head groups and hence to more room for movement. This, in turn, results in increased membrane fluidity. (Reproduced with permission from Rodwell VW, Bender DA, Botham KM, et al: *Harper's Illustrated Biochemistry*, 31st ed. New York, NY: McGraw Hill; 2018.)

able to diffuse or drift laterally (see Figure 5–2). As discussed earlier with respect to cholesterol, the fluidity of the plasma membrane is dependent on its lipid composition. Likewise, the presence of unsaturated fatty acids, by placing kinks in the tail regions of phospholipids (see Figure 5–1), decreases their ability to pack closely and increases their mobility within the bilayer.

Although the bilayer is generally uniform in nature, it possesses zones that have a different biochemical composition. One specialized region of the plasma membrane is the lipid raft (Figure 5–3). Although these structures are still able to move within the fluidity of the bilayer, they comprise functional microdomains of protein complexes anchored to the internal actin cytoskeleton and are used for a variety of purposes including regulation of synaptic transmission or

signaling. Lipids are packed more tightly in this region due to the presence of phospholipids such as sphingomyelin that contain heavily saturated fatty acid tails, which favor additional stabilizing interactions with the plentiful cholesterol.

Transmembrane Proteins

In addition to conferring electrical excitability onto neurons, the variety of cell-specific proteins associated and embedded in the lipid bilayer of the plasma membrane and membranes of other intracellular organelles allow for cell-to-cell communication through receptor–ligand interactions (see below) and for exocytosis and endocytosis of intracellular vesicles, via SNARE–protein complexes (see Chapter 7). Together, these proteins can constitute more than half of the mass, depending on the particular membrane, and can be categorized as either (1) integral membrane proteins, such as the membrane-spanning ion channels and carrier complexes associated with ion movement, or (2) peripheral proteins, such as auxiliary channel subunits, not immersed within the bilayer but in close proximity, where they can interact with other nearby proteins (see Figure 5–2). To span the distance of the lipid bilayer, integral membrane proteins, such as ion channels, must be amphipathic like the phospholipids. Their transmembrane domains (TMDs), which are embedded in the lipid core, often consist of α-helices built from nonpolar amino acid residues so that their hydrophobic side chains can interact with the fatty acid tails of the phospholipids. Portions of the proteins immersed in the cytoplasmic and extracellular environments must contain hydrophilic residues. Anchoring of peripheral membrane proteins is accomplished through lipid modifications (eg, myristylation and

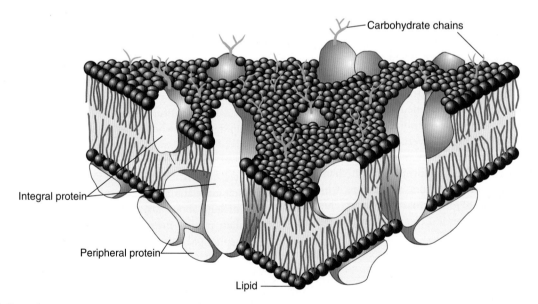

FIGURE 5–2 The fluid mosaic model of membrane structure. The membrane consists of a bimolecular lipid layer with proteins inserted in it or bound to either surface. Integral membrane proteins are firmly embedded in the lipid layers. Some of these proteins completely span the bilayer and are called transmembrane proteins, while others are embedded in either the outer or inner leaflet of the lipid bilayer. Loosely bound to the outer or inner surface of the membrane are the peripheral proteins. Many of the proteins and all the glycolipids have externally exposed oligosaccharide carbohydrate chains. (Reproduced with permission from Mescher AL. *Junqueira's Basic Histology: Text & Atlas*, 15th ed. New York, NY: McGraw Hill; 2018.)

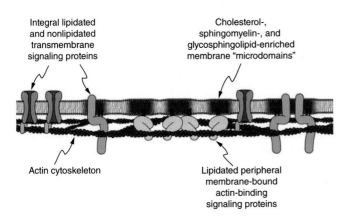

FIGURE 5–3 Schematic diagram of a lipid raft. Shown in schematic form are multiple lipid rafts (red membrane shading) that represent localized microdomains rich in the indicated lipids and signaling proteins (blue, green, and yellow). Lipid rafts are stabilized through interactions (direct and indirect) with the actin cytoskeleton (red bihelical chains). (Reproduced with permission from Owen DM, Magenau A, Williamson D, et al: The lipid raft hypothesis revisited—new insights on raft composition and function from super-resolution fluorescence microscopy, *Bioessays.* 2012 Sep;34(9):739-747.)

palmitoylation) and insertion of these fatty acid appendages into the bilayer.

Lipid Bilayer as a Barrier to Charged & Polar Molecules

In the absence of ion channels and carrier proteins, the membrane (1) is impermeable to macromolecules (eg, sugars, amino acids, neurotransmitters) due to their large size, and (2) excludes ions from the hydrophobic core of the lipid bilayer because of their charge. Moreover, ions in solution attract a number of polarized water molecules,[1] giving rise to a hydration shell surrounding the ion, which further increases its size. It is energetically highly unfavorable to strip the water shell from a hydrated ion in the aqueous extracellular or intracellular space and replace it with uncharged fatty acid chains. Although water is known to enter and exit cells by the process of osmosis, the pathway by which it does this is unclear, since water and the hydrophobic lipids do not mix. Thus, although some water (and other small polarized molecules) can directly cross the plasma membrane, a more efficient means is via the aquaporin class of water channels.

Although charged molecules cannot cross the bilayer, they can accumulate on either side of the plasma membrane. The very thin (~6 to 8 nm) nature of the membrane and its electrical insulator properties allow it to function as a good capacitor, and its ability to store and separate charges on either side gives rise to an adjustable transmembrane potential (see

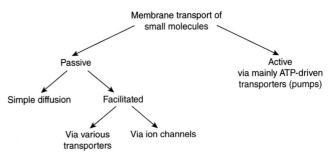

FIGURE 5–4 A schematic diagram of the 2 types of membrane transport of small molecules. (Reproduced with permission from Rodwell VW, Bender DA, Botham KM, et al: *Harper's Illustrated Biochemistry*, 31st ed. New York, NY: McGraw Hill; 2018.)

later discussion). The membrane has a net negative charge inside while at rest but can become either less negative (depolarized) during excitation or more negative (hyperpolarized) during inhibition.

PASSIVE MOVEMENT OF IONS & OTHER SMALL MOLECULES ACROSS MEMBRANES

Small uncharged molecules (eg, ethanol and gases such as oxygen, carbon dioxide, and nitric oxide) can readily move through membranes by simple diffusion (Figure 5–4) because they are small enough to move between the hydrophilic head groups and then into the fatty acid core.

A passive process is one that does not require an energy source (adenosine triphosphate [ATP] or the potential energy from an ionic concentration gradient; see later discussion). Small molecules, such as sugars and amino acids, can still move across plasma membranes from a high concentration outside the cell by facilitated transport through specific membrane carriers that recognize their molecular structure. Likewise, charged ions with their aqueous shells also require an energetically favorable pathway through the membrane, generally an ion-selective channel, to facilitate diffusion down their previously established concentration gradients (see the next section). Here, removal of their electrostatically bound water molecules is achieved by replacement with polar residues lining the pore domain of the channel protein. This latter mechanism not only allows ions to traverse the lipid bilayer, but also confers selectivity and conductance of individual ions or channels. (A discussion of the types of ion channels and transport mechanisms, including energy-dependent carriers, will be presented in later in this chapter.)

ENERGY STORED IN IONIC GRADIENTS

The difference in the concentration of an ion inside and outside of a cell generates an electrochemical potential (Nernst potential) that not only forms the basis of neuronal

---

[1]Water molecules are dipoles even though they have no net charge. Their electrons are more closely associated with the oxygen moiety, giving it a negative charge, and thus the hydrogen atom, which gives up its electrons more easily, will carry a slight positive charge. Thus, cations and anions in solution are attracted to the oxygen and hydrogen of water, respectively.

excitability, via ion movement downhill (diffusion of ions from high to low concentrations) into and out of a neuron, but also provides the free energy to drive other ions and small molecules, such as neurotransmitters, uphill (against their concentration/electrochemical gradients). The initial gradients, namely K^+ and Na^+ (but also others), that set the scene for all the standard signaling in neurons, begin with a standard source of energy, the hydrolysis of ATP, which is used to power the Na^+/K^+ pump (see later section on ion channels).

Ionic Gradients at Rest

The roots of electrical signaling in neurons are grounded in 2 essential conditions: a selectively permeable membrane (see earlier discussion in this chapter) and the concentration differences for the various ions inside and outside the cell. Table 5–1 shows the typical ionic conditions for a neuron or a muscle cell and a glial (nonexcitable) cell in the mammalian central nervous system (CNS) and also their associated Nernst equilibrium potentials. The unequal distributions of each ion are established and maintained (in the face of constant transmembrane movement of ions through "leak" channels at rest and voltage-gated channels during electrical signaling) by the ion pumps/exchangers described in the later section, "Classes of Ion Channels."

All 4 of the most abundant and biologically relevant ions for electrical signaling are distributed unequally across the membrane (see Table 5–1). Na^+ and K^+ are arranged roughly

opposite from one another, with Na^+ higher outside the cell and K^+ higher inside the cell.[2] The positive Na^+ charge is offset by Cl^-, which is also higher outside the cell, and the bulk electrical neutrality (of the intracellular environment) is maintained by the negatively charged organic anions, largely proteins and amino acids. Although the absolute concentrations may differ, the relative internal and external concentrations of each ion, known as its concentration gradient, remain qualitatively very similar across different cells and species. There are some notable exceptions in the CNS (eg, the endolymph of the specialized sensory organs of the inner ear has an unusually higher concentration of K^+ and lower amounts of Na^+; see Chapter 13 in this text). Finally, Ca^{2+}, which is important for electrical-chemical coupling in active processes such as muscle contraction and synaptic transmission, has by necessity a concentration gradient that favors rapid influx from a high extracellular concentration into a tightly buffered intracellular environment, where its sudden cytoplasmic arrival has immediate and substantial impact.

Nernst Potential

To begin to assess the impact of the concentration gradients on electrical signaling, it may help to visualize what happens when the membrane becomes permeable to a particular ion. Most descriptions of the Nernst potential begin solely by consideration of potassium ion movement across the bilayer, because these conditions approximate the resting state of the membrane (see Chapter 6). We will visualize a 2-compartment chamber, containing high and low concentrations of a potassium salt, separated by a membrane, approximating the aqueous conditions inside and outside a neuron (Figure 5–5B). Under these conditions, the transmembrane potential is zero (the concentration gradient is insufficient by itself to cause a membrane potential). Now, let us make the plasma membrane of the neuron, muscle, or glial cell selectively permeable to K^+ only (physiologically, this would be achieved by opening K^+-selective channels). The difference in concentration is the sole force initially acting on potassium ions (see Figure 5–5B; diffusion potential), and because of its high internal concentration, K^+ near the plasma membrane will tend to efflux (from inside to outside), effectively moving down its concentration gradient. As a result, a net negativity will be left behind on the cytoplasmic side of the bilayer, and a positive charge will build up on the external face. This separation and storage of charge on the membrane occur because of the capacitive properties of the lipid bilayer and result in a potential difference across the membrane (indeed, this is the basis of the resting membrane potential; see Chapter 6). The net

TABLE 5–1 Physiologic distributions of ions (Nernst potentials).

Ion	[Intracellular] mM	[Extracellular] mM	E_{Nernst} mV
Excitable cells (nerve and muscle)			
Na^+	12	145	+67
K^+	155	4.5	−95
Ca^{2+}	10^{-4}	1.0	+123
Cl^-	4	115	−89
HCO_3^-	12	24	−19
Nonexcitable cells			
Na^+	15	145	+61
K^+	120	4.5	−88
Ca^{2+}	10^{-4}	1.0	+123
Cl^-	20	115	−47
HCO_3^-	16	24	−13

Note that 61.5 mV, not 58 mV, was used to calculate the Nernst potential from the Nernst equation (see the second Nernst equation in the text that uses base 10 logarithms).

Reproduced with permission from Kibble JD, Halsey CR. *Medical Physiology: The Big Picture.* New York, NY: McGraw Hill; 2009.

[2]Analysis of freshly isolated axoplasm from the giant axon of the common squid *Loligo pealii* estimated the internal concentrations of K^+ and Na^+ as 369 and 44 mM, respectively.

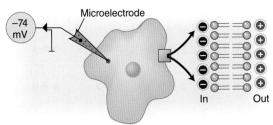

A Resting membrane potential

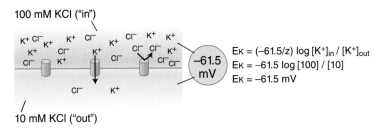

B Diffusion potentials and Nernst equation

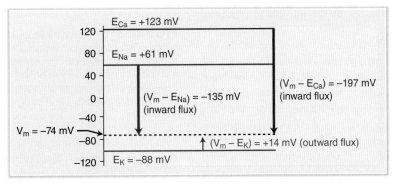

C Electrochemical gradients

FIGURE 5–5 Plasma membrane ion gradients. **A.** The resting membrane potential; all cells have a negative intracellular potential. **B.** Generation of a K^+ diffusion potential. In this example, K^+ is the only permeable ion; a small amount of K^+ diffuses to the lower compartment, creating a negative potential in the upper compartment. The Nernst equation predicts the equilibrium potential (voltage), based on the size of the K^+ concentration ratio between compartments. **C.** Electrochemical gradients. Membrane potential (V_m) is shown by the dashed line. *Downward arrows* indicate gradients for cation flux into the cell; the *upward arrow* indicates a gradient for cation efflux. (Reproduced with permission from Kibble JD, Halsey CR. *Medical Physiology: The Big Picture.* New York, NY: McGraw Hill; 2009.)

negativity left inside (largely due to organic anions) will attract back the positive potassium ions, until these opposing electrical (inward) and chemical (outward) gradients and potentials are balanced[3] and there is no further net movement of K^+. The potential across the membrane at this point (assuming a sole permeability to K^+), as measured using an intracellular electrode (shown schematically in Figure 5–5A), is called the equilibrium potential for K^+ and can be calculated using the Nernst equation:

$$E_x = \frac{RT}{zF} \ln \frac{[x]_o}{[x]_i}$$

where E_x is the Nernst potential, sometimes called the equilibrium or reversal potential for ion, x, with valence, z, and concentrations outside and inside the cell of $[x]_o$ and $[x]_i$, respectively. R and F are the ideal gas and Faraday constants, and T is the temperature. Assuming physiologic conditions,

$RT/F = 25$ mV at room temperature, the equation is often rewritten in the following approximate form using base 10 logarithms:

$$E_x = \frac{58}{z} \log \frac{[x]_o}{[x]_i},$$

where it can be seen that a 10-fold difference in the concentration of ion, x, will produce a membrane potential change of approximately 58 mV.

To calculate the Nernst potential for a given ion, it is necessary to know only its concentrations inside and outside the cell. Hence, we can find this value for all the major ions (see Table 5–1). The Nernst potential exists whether or not the membrane is permeable to a particular ion, but its impact on ion flux and ion exchange systems can only be realized when the membrane becomes permeable to that ion, and only then if the membrane potential is different from the Nernst potential (see next section).

The Electrochemical Driving Force

The Nernst potentials for each ion are important absolute values because they indicate both the direction (depolarized or hyperpolarized) and approximate value the membrane potential will achieve if the bilayer becomes selectively permeable to one particular ion. A more useful term when it comes to

---

[3]In a 50-μm neuron, efflux of only about 1 part in 10^5 total K^+ charges is required to impose a 58-mV potential across the membrane capacitance, thus having only a negligible effect on the overall ionic concentration gradients. However, a larger fraction of ions must move in a smaller neuronal process, such as a dendrite or axon, in which case alterations in the membrane potential due to electrical signaling could more rapidly have a significant influence on the concentrations of ions inside and outside the cell, and gradients will have to be continuously restored using ion pumps or exchangers.

predicting the direction of ion movement, efflux or influx, is the *net* driving force on an ion. This is a composite value obtained by relating the Nernst potential (E_x) of an ion x to the current membrane potential (V_m)

$$\text{Electrochemical driving force} = V_m - E_x$$

The approximate driving force values for Na⁺ (blue), K⁺ (red), and Ca²⁺ (purple) are shown in Figure 5–5C. For cations, a positive driving force will direct the ions out of the cell, whereas a negative value means inward movement (with the reverse holding true for anions). Under resting conditions, the (positive) driving force on K⁺ is relatively small and in the outward direction, as E_K (Nernst potential) is close to the resting membrane potential (see Chapter 6). Even so, K⁺ movement does have a stabilizing influence on the membrane potential, because any slight depolarization will increase the driving force on K⁺ and cause a concomitant increased efflux and membrane hyperpolarization. Conversely, there is a much larger (negative) driving force on Na⁺, as both its concentration and electrical gradients favor inward movement, realized only when there is an increased membrane permeability to Na⁺.

Overall the driving force determines the direction of ion flow, and together with the conductance (proportional to the number of open channels), it determines the magnitude of the current, I_x for a given ion. From Ohm's law:

$$I_x = G_x (V_m - E_x),$$

where G_x is the ionic conductance, and $V_m - E_x$ again is the electrochemical driving force. If there is either no conductance pathway for the ion (no open selective channels) and/or no driving force on the ion (equal internal and external concentrations of ion), there will be no net current flux. The ionic driving force informs us about not only the potential for diffusional movement of an ion down its concentration gradient (provided that ion channels are open), but also the amount of "potential" energy available to move other ions uphill. Perhaps it is not surprising then that cells use the large electrochemical driving force on Na⁺ to provide free energy to move other ions against their concentration gradient and facilitate the cellular uptake of neurotransmitters. Ca²⁺, which has an even larger driving force (see Figure 5–5C), cannot be used for this purpose because its cytoplasmic concentration must be tightly buffered so that any changes in intracellular Ca²⁺ can be used to drive other cellular events.

IONIC GRADIENTS ESTABLISHED BY ACTIVE TRANSPORTERS

As discussed extensively throughout this chapter, excitable and nonexcitable cells of the nervous system need to maintain, at all times, differences in the concentrations of physiologically relevant ions on either side of the plasma membrane to ensure continuity of electrical signaling (see Chapter 6). Because such conditions oppose the natural tendency for all

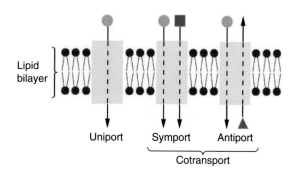

FIGURE 5–6 Schematic representation of types of transport systems. Transporters can be classified with regard to the direction of movement and whether 1 or more unique molecules are moved. A uniport can also allow movement in the opposite direction, depending on the concentrations inside and outside a cell of the molecule transported.

ions to passively diffuse down their concentration gradients through leak channels (see later section on classes of ion channels), their unchecked movement would result ultimately in equal ionic solutions inside and outside the cell. In reality, dissipation of the ion concentration gradients does not occur for 2 basic reasons. The first is the selective permeability of the membrane, which does not permit all ions to readily diffuse across the bilayer (see earlier discussion). The second is the presence of active membrane transport processes that require a source of energy (see Figure 5–4) to move ions (or other molecules) uphill against their concentration gradients, thereby offsetting any decline in normal ion concentration gradients through either passive leak or active electrical signaling (see Chapter 6). All 3 major cations, Na⁺, K⁺, and Ca²⁺, are subject to regulation by such energy-demanding pumps, whereas control of Cl⁻ (and other anions) is subject to a variety of ion exchangers (Figure 5–6).

Primary & Secondary Active Transporters

Simple and facilitated diffusion and transport help ions (and small molecules) passively traverse the impermeable lipid bilayer solely by guiding them down their concentration gradients (see earlier discussion). However, setting these gradients requires energy, either through the hydrolysis of ATP, giving rise to the primary active transporters (sometimes called pumps or ATPases), or from coupling the free energy released, as one ion moves down its own concentration gradient,[4] to the movement of a second ion by means of antiporters or symporters (see Figure 5–6). Due to its large electrochemical driving force (see previous discussion), Na⁺, rather than K⁺, is often the ion used to power these secondary active transporters.

---

[4]These transporters are called *secondary* active because of the indirect requirement of ATP consumed as energy for the pumps that initially generated the concentration gradients.

Na⁺/K⁺–ATPase

The best known of the pumps is the Na⁺/K⁺ pump (or some-times, just the Na⁺ pump). It is designed to maintain and restore the concentration gradients for the 2 major ions, Na⁺ and K⁺, involved in action potential generation and propagation in all excitable cells. Without its activity, Na⁺ and K⁺ gradients would collapse rapidly, especially after an intense period of spike activity in high surface area–to–volume neuronal compartments such as axons, as many ions repeatedly enter and exit the cell. Like many integral proteins, the Na⁺/K⁺ pump is a heteromeric structure, comprised of an α subunit, the enzymatic/exchanger part of the pump, and an accessory β subunit, which in addition to modulating pump function, allows for its correct insertion into the bilayer (Figure 5–7).

Unlike ion channels, the pump does not provide an unobstructed passage on ions through the bilayer; rather, it exists in 2 principle states, E1 and E2. The E1 conformation has the cytoplasmic binding sites accessible to 3 Na⁺, which it "carries" across the membrane while undergoing a conformational change to the E2 state, driven by the hydrolysis of ATP (also bound internally) and autophosphorylation. Due to a lowered affinity, sodium ions unbind at the extracellular face of the E2 form, to be replaced by K⁺ ions, which are transported back to the intracellular side, via a second conformational change following dephosphorylation. K⁺ ions now dissociate, and Na⁺ ions and ATP once again bind to start the cycle over. At no point are both the cytoplasmic and extracellular binding domains simultaneously accessible.

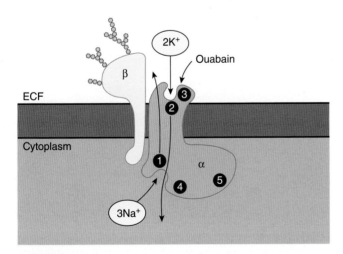

FIGURE 5–7 Na⁺/K⁺-ATPase. The intracellular portion of the α subunit has a Na⁺-binding site (1), a phosphorylation site (4), and an adenosine triphosphate (ATP)-binding site (5). The extracellular portion has a K⁺-binding site (2) and an ouabain-binding site (3). ECF, extracellular fluid. Stoichiometry of the Na⁺/K⁺-ATPase pump. This pump moves 3 Na⁺ ions from inside the cell to the outside and brings 2 K⁺ ions from the outside to the inside for every molecule of ATP hydrolyzed to adenosine diphosphate (ADP) by the membrane-associated ATPase. (Adapted with permission from Horisberger JD, Lemas V, Kraehenbühl JP, et al: Structure-function relationship of Na,K-ATPase, *Annu Rev Physiol.* 1991;53:565-584.)

Thus, its behavior approximates a ping-pong type of facilitated transport (Figure 5–8)

It makes intuitive sense that the movement of these 2 ions is paired because of their joint role in the action potential (see Chapter 6), and the cycling rate of the pump is increased as either Na⁺ increases in the cytoplasm or K⁺ accumulates outside (as would occur during action potential generation). The pump operates maximally at around 100 cycles s⁻¹, much slower than the flow of ions though channels, which occurs at rates above 10⁷ s⁻¹. As a consequence of the unequal movement of the 2 cations, the Na⁺ pump is electrogenic, transporting 1 net positive charge outside during each cycle, and because of its ongoing activity, it contributes to the negativity of the resting membrane potential. The alkaloids ouabain and digitalis (which is used therapeutically to treat cardiac conditions) bind to a site close to the extracellular K⁺ binding site and inhibit the pump (see Figure 5–7).

Ca²⁺ Pumps, Na⁺/Ca²⁺ Exchanger, & Cl⁻ Transporters

The plasma membrane Ca²⁺ pump is, like the Na⁺ pump, an E1-E2 pump or P-type ATPase (meaning that it is autophosphorylated following the hydrolysis of ATP). Together with the SERCA Ca²⁺ pump, situated on the endoplasmic reticulum membrane, they form an important component of the buffering systems that maintain nanomolar cytoplasmic concentrations of Ca²⁺. Ca²⁺ pumps transport 2 to 3 protons as counter ions in exchange for 2 Ca²⁺ (in part to neutralize the charge on the pump once Ca²⁺ unbinds), but otherwise share many of the same structural and operational features as described earlier for the Na⁺/K⁺-ATPase.

As previously discussed, secondary active transporters make use of the potential energy stored in the electrochemical gradients of various ions. For example, in addition to the Ca²⁺ ATPase, Ca²⁺ is expelled from the cell using a cotransporter (antiporter; see Figure 5–6), driven by the free energy released as Na⁺ passively moves down its own steep concentration gradient into the cell. Cl⁻ transporters are important for setting the Cl⁻ equilibrium potential of a cell, normally found just on either side of the resting membrane potentials, meaning that γ-aminobutyric acid (GABA)-ergic responses mediated via Cl⁻ channels can be either hyperpolarizing or depolarizing (see Chapter 8). There are 2 major Cl⁻ transporters, both symporters (see Figure 5–6), used to control cytoplasmic Cl⁻ levels, using the energy stored in the Nernst potentials for Na⁺ entry or K⁺ exit. The Na⁺/K⁺/Cl⁻ symporter drives Cl⁻ into the cell along with both Na⁺ and K⁺, resulting in a high intracellular Cl⁻ concentration (and an E_{Cl^-} less negative than resting membrane potential), meaning that Cl⁻ will tend to efflux when selective Cl⁻ channels are opened, resulting in depolarization. A second K⁺/Cl⁻ symporter moves both ions out of the cell, creating a lower concentration of Cl⁻ inside the cell and a resulting hyperpolarization when Cl⁻ channels open and Cl⁻ influxes down its concentration gradient. Regulation of the expression of these transporters produces an important developmental switch

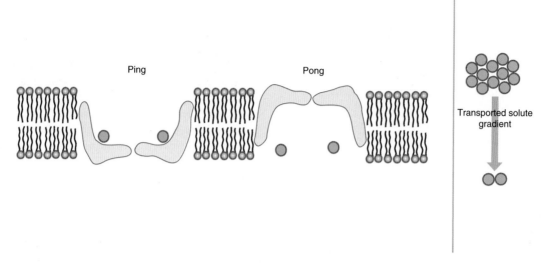

FIGURE 5-8 The "ping-pong" model of facilitated diffusion. A protein carrier (blue structure) in the lipid bilayer associates with a solute in high concentration on one side of the membrane. A conformational change ensues ("ping" to "pong"), and the solute is discharged on the side favoring the new equilibrium (solute concentration gradient shown schematically, *right*). The empty carrier then reverts to the original conformation ("pong" to "ping") to complete the cycle. (Reproduced with permission from Rodwell VW, Bender DA, Botham KM, et al: *Harper's Illustrated Biochemistry*, 31st ed. New York, NY: McGraw Hill; 2018.)

in GABAergic Cl⁻ responses from excitatory (depolarizing) to inhibitory (hyperpolarizing). Finally, Cl⁻/bicarbonate exchange across membranes is important for cellular pH regulation.

Amino Acid & Neurotransmitter Transporters

In addition to powering the movement of other ions, the free energy derived from ions flowing down their concentration gradients has been coupled to the transport of small molecules, especially neurotransmitters. Transport of chemical transmitters across lipid bilayers is physiologically important for the maintenance of synaptic transmission and is used to fill synaptic vesicles with specific neurotransmitters, as well as remove these agents from the synapse after synaptic transmission has occurred. To produce efficient postsynaptic responses, a high concentration of transmitter must be released into the synaptic cleft, which is accomplished by uploading and concentrating transmitter into vesicles through one of the families of transporters driven by the outward electrochemical proton gradient. To accomplish transmitter loading, a proton pump (or ATPase) first moves H⁺ into the vesicle, creating an acidic luminal environment and a transvesicle membrane proton gradient. All families of transporters work in a similar manner, but with some differences in ion stoichiometry and co-ions exchanged, to load vesicles with bioamines (serotonin, dopamine[5]), acetylcholine (Figure 5–9), GABA, glycine, and glutamate in presynaptic terminals.

Aside from the action of acetylcholine, which is terminated by enzymatic hydrolysis through acetylcholinesterase,[6]

most low-molecular-weight neurotransmitters rely on uptake mechanisms for removal from the extracellular space. There are 2 major categories of plasma membrane neurotransmitter transporters; the first group is responsible for clearance of

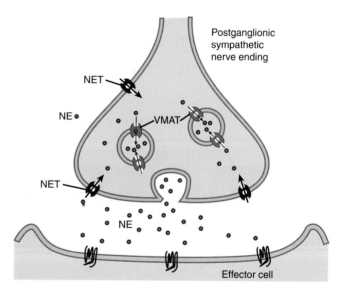

FIGURE 5-9 Fate of monoamines secreted at synaptic junctions. In each monoamine-secreting neuron, the monoamine is synthesized in the cytoplasm and the secretory granules, and its concentration in secretory granules is maintained by the 2 vesicular monoamine transporters (VMAT). The monoamine is secreted by exocytosis of the granules, and it acts on G-protein–coupled receptors. In this example, the monoamine is norepinephrine (NE) acting on adrenoceptors. Many of these receptors are postsynaptic, but some are presynaptic and some are located on glia. In addition, there is extensive reuptake of the monoamine into the cytoplasm of the presynaptic terminal via a monoamine transporter, in this case the norepinephrine transporter (NET). (Reproduced with permission from Katzung BG: *Basic & Clinical Pharmacology*, 14th ed. New York, NY: McGraw Hill; 2018.)

---

[5]Norepinephrine is synthesized from dopamine inside the synaptic vesicle.
[6]The breakdown product of acetylcholine, choline, is itself removed from the synaptic cleft through a plasma membrane uptake system.

glutamate (and other neutral amino acids), and the second group transports the bioamines (serotonin, dopamine, and norepinephrine; see Figure 5–9), along with GABA and glycine. Neurotransmitter transporters for glutamate can often be found on the plasma membrane of adjacent glial cells. Once a transmitter has diffused from the synaptic cleft, it is rapidly removed into these astrocytes, preventing the majority of glutamate from reaching other nearby synapses and reducing the potential for excitotoxicity through overstimulation of *N*-methyl-D-aspartate (NMDA) receptors. The energy for glutamate uptake is primarily derived from the Na^+ concentration gradient, and the transport is coupled to the influx of 1 Na^+ into the cell along with the extrusion of a potassium ion (other ions are also transported). The second category of transmitter transporters also makes use of the steep Na^+ gradient to uptake transmitters, with 2 or even 3 (in the case of glycine transport) sodium ions and 1 Cl^- moving downhill for each cycle of the transporter. Neurotransmitter uptake systems are important therapeutic targets for treatment of disorders involving transmitter dysregulation.

CLASSES OF ION CHANNELS: LEAK & GATED CHANNELS

The most efficient means of transporting ions across impermeable lipid bilayers is via facilitated diffusion through ion channels. These membrane-spanning proteins are comprised of an outer barrel structure, embedded in the phospholipids (through many hydrophobic residues), surrounding a water-filled pore for the passage of ions. To control the excitability of neurons, different channels have evolved exquisite selectivity, and there are channels exclusively permeable to each of the major ions, Na^+, K^+, Ca^{2+}, and Cl^-, along with a variety of channels that discriminate poorly between the cations but exclude anions. Thus, an initial selectivity is based on charge, but mechanisms other than those relying on ionic size alone are also required, because a pore diameter permitting dehydrated K^+ ions to pass would also allow permeation of the smaller Na^+. In general, single-ion selectivity is achieved by providing an energetically favorable environment for the specific ion within the pore by using the proximity of side chain groups from pore-lining residues to effectively substitute for the water molecules, which must be lost from the hydrated ion as it passes through the tight channel filter.[7] Only ions that are stabilized by the side chains can "fit" through a particular channel. More details will be considered for specific ion channels (see following sections).

The majority of, but not all, ion channel families are multi-subunit complexes, allowing for much diversity in the assembly of both homomeric and heteromeric structures. Moreover, although all channels have central aqueous pores, they vary in terms of the mechanisms governing opening and closing of the pore. We will consider the 3 major means of channel gating: (1) through changes in membrane voltage, (2) exposure to a chemical transmitter (or agonist ligand), and (3) the exertion of mechanical pressure. First, however, we will briefly consider channels that do not require a gating mechanism because they are always in an open configuration.

Leak Ion Channels

The appropriately named leak channel refers to any pore that is constitutively open or nongated and, provided there is an electrochemical driving force, will continuously allow a net flux of ions across the membrane. Indeed, in the face of ongoing activity of other ionic fluxes, it is the continuous outward movement of K^+ down its concentration gradient through potassium leak channels that largely sets the resting membrane of all excitable cells (see previous discussion and Chapter 6).[8] Members of the large group of tandem pore domain (2P) potassium channels have been assigned to the role of "leak" channels, and although these channels lack a specialized canonical voltage sensor (see later discussion), the activity of many nevertheless display at least some degree of rectification (or dependence on membrane potential).

Voltage-Gated Potassium, Sodium, & Calcium Channels

The function of many different types of ion channels is influenced by the membrane electric field, but some channels have developed exquisitely sensitive mechanisms so that they can respond extremely precisely (and contribute) to sudden changes in the membrane potential. Two of these voltage-dependent channels, those conducting Na^+ and K^+ (delayed rectifier), make use of this property and allow the rapid (and timely) influx and efflux of these ions down their respective concentration gradients, which then underlies the initiation and propagation of action potentials (see Chapter 6). Likewise, voltage-dependent calcium channels use a similar mechanism to synchronize large fluxes of Ca^{2+} to trigger processes such as fast vesicle fusion at presynaptic terminals and excitation-contraction coupling in muscle fibers.

Biochemistry, cloning, mutational analysis, modeling, and high-resolution crystallography studies have shed light on the structural organization of these channels and, in particular, formally identified the regions of the protein associated with particular functions, such as voltage-dependent activation and the ion permeation pathway. Although the full behavioral dynamics of any one channel is not fully known, there is a good understanding of their structural operation. Figure 5–10 shows the presumed secondary structure and general membrane topography of typical α subunits from each of 3 channels. Sodium and calcium channels are formed from

---

[7]Pores are not wide enough to permit fully hydrated ions to pass.

[8]Note that descriptions of the background leak conductance at resting membrane potentials imply that the bilayer is not strictly selectively permeable to K^+, and the leak of Na^+ and Cl^- partially offsets the resting K^+ flux, making the membrane potential more depolarized than the K^+ equilibrium potential.

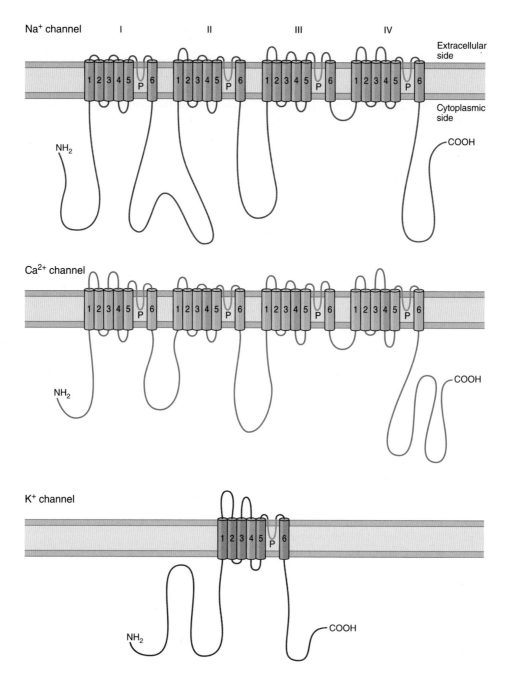

FIGURE 5–10 Diagrammatic representation of the pore-forming subunits of 3 ion channels. The α subunit of the Na⁺ and Ca²⁺ channels traverses the membrane 24 times in 4 repeats of 6 membrane-spanning units. Each repeat has a "P"-loop between membrane spans 5 and 6 that does not traverse the membrane. These P-loops are thought to form the pore. Note that span 4 of each repeat is colored in red, representing its net positive charge. The K⁺ channel has only a single repeat of the 6 spanning regions and P-loop. Four K⁺ subunits are assembled for a functional K⁺ channel.

a single protein consisting of 4 homologous repeats connected by intracellular loops, and whereas a single repeat comprises a potassium channel subunit, 4 subunits are necessary to build a functional channel, meaning its overall quaternary structure is very similar to the other 2 channels. A few important specialized functional domains can be found within each of these repeating domains.

First, as shown for voltage-gated potassium channels (Figure 5–11) the S4 transmembrane-spanning domains

(also indicated in red in Figure 5–10) form the voltage-sensing part of the channel. These α-helical structures contain conserved positively charged amino acids, which sense and respond to membrane depolarization by moving outward through the bilayer (electric field) and, in the process, initiate a conformational change in the pore region, opening the channel gate and allowing K⁺ to leave the cell. Similar activation mechanisms underlie both Na⁺ and Ca²⁺ channel gating.

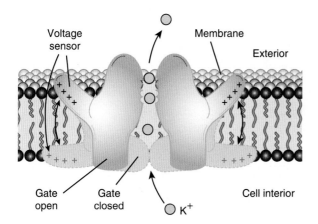

FIGURE 5–11 Schematic diagram of the voltage-gated K+ channel of *Aeropyrum pernix*. The voltage sensors behave like charged paddles that move through the interior of the membrane. Four voltage sensors (only 2 are shown here) are linked mechanically to the gate of the channel. Each sensor has 4 positive charges contributed by arginine residues. (Adapted with permission from Sigworth FJ: Structural biology: Life's transistors, *Nature*. 2003 May 1;423(6935):21-22.)

Second, the detailed structural images, including crystal structures, have revealed the precise chemistry behind ion selectivity in the narrow region of these channels. The selectivity filter is formed by the 4 "P-loop" linkers, which fold back into the membrane between TMDs S5 and S6 (see Figure 5–10). In the potassium channel, carbonyl groups lining these reentrant loops have their electronegative oxygens pointed toward the center of the lumen (helical regions in Figure 5–12), at a distance designed to stabilize a K+ after it loses its water molecules, but too far apart to coordinate the much smaller dehydrated Na+. Thus, the chemical environment in the narrow region is energetically favorable only for nonhydrated potassium ions. It is further postulated that the high channel throughput rate of K+ is mediated in part

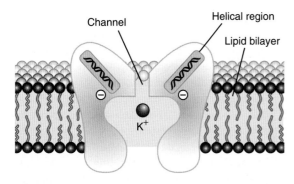

FIGURE 5–12 Schematic diagram of the structure of a K+ channel (KvAP) from *Streptomyces lividans*. A single K+ is shown in a large aqueous cavity inside the membrane interior. Two helical regions of the channel protein are oriented with their carbonyl* ends pointing to where the K+ is located. The channel is lined by carbonyl* oxygen. Asterisks indicate amendment by R. Lester.

through electrostatic repulsion by neighboring potassium ions positioned at adjacent luminal binding sites.

Third, certain voltage-sensitive channels undergo inactivation (a lasting form of channel closure) even at the depolarized membranes that initially activate them. Cytoplasmic application of the enzyme Pronase removed channel inactivation while leaving channel activation intact, demonstrating that these 2 kinetic operations have distinct molecular determinants, leading to the tethered ball-and-chain model of channel inactivation. Additional experiments using antibodies targeted against cytoplasmic domains and reconstitution of channels lacking repeat domain linkers showed that Na+ channel inactivation was dependent on the small cytoplasmic loop between the third and fourth repeats. In the rapidly inactivating Shaker A-type potassium channels, a similar inactivation mechanism exists, and following removal of inactivation by clipping the N-terminal cytoplasmic domain, it was discovered that inactivation could be restored simply by adding back a "ball" peptide made from the part of the clipped N terminus.

Ligand-Gated Ion Channels

Similar to other ion channels discussed earlier, this extensive group of channels is defined by a central ion-conducting pore formed by the circular arrangement of membrane-spanning protein subunits. However, these channels are gated by a chemical ligand (including many neurotransmitters), for which the ligand binding site is an integral part of the holoprotein (Figure 5–13). These ligand-gated ion channels or *ionotropic* receptors form 1 of the 2 major divisions of membrane receptors next to G-protein–coupled or *metabotropic* receptors (see Chapters 8 and 9). Activation by ligand confers selectivity based on the specific nature of the agonist and its interaction with amino acid side chains that make up its receptor binding site, which is generally localized to the extracellular face of the receptor. Ion selectivity, usually either mixed cation (Na+, K+, Ca2+) or Cl− preferring, then determines whether the cellular response is excitatory (depolarizing) or inhibitory (generally hyperpolarizing, but see earlier discussion), respectively. We will consider some of the many subfamilies of ligand-gated ion channels.

The acetylcholine nicotinic receptor was formally identified as the target of the South American paralytic agent *curare* in the early 1900s. Indeed, Langley first used the term *receptive substance* to define this structure, which mediated excitatory chemical transmission and muscle contraction at the neuromuscular junction (see Chapter 7). Subsequently, through purification and separation, it was discovered that the skeletal muscle receptor is composed of 5 subunits, with each contributing 4 TMDs. Two molecules of the neurotransmitter acetylcholine are required for opening of its nonselective cation channel, and although the position of the 2 binding sites at subunit interfaces is known and the TM2 pore-lining domain has been extensively mapped, questions remain about the exact locations of the gate and

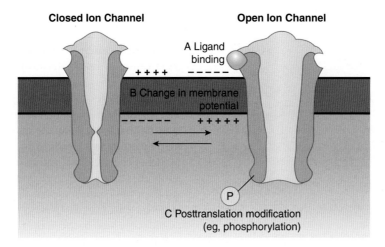

FIGURE 5–13 Regulation of gating in ion channels. Ion channels can gate open or closed in response to several environmental signals. Some typical examples are shown in an idealized channel. **A.** Ligand gating: Channel opens in response to ligand binding. **B.** Voltage gating: Channel opens in response to a change in membrane potential. **C.** Posttranslational modification: Channel gates in response to modification such as phosphorylation.

ion selectivity filter and the precise dynamics of channel opening. The large group of neuronal nicotinic acetylcholine receptors, along with the serotonin receptor, rounds out the excitatory members of the pentameric family, which also includes the ionotropic receptors for the major CNS inhibitory transmitters, GABA and glycine.

Ion selectivity in these channels, unlike K+ channels (described earlier), is determined largely by charged amino acid side groups at the entrances to the pore region. For the excitatory receptors, this includes rings of negative charges at the extracellular and cytoplasmic ends of TM2, which help to concentrate cations in the vicinity of the pore. As would be predicted, these rings of negative charges are absent in the Cl⁻ selective GABA$_A$ and glycine receptors, and additional experimental manipulation of charged residues at the intracellular end of TM2 confirms the importance of this region in cation versus anion selectivity of pentameric receptors.

Receptors for the major CNS excitatory neurotransmitter glutamate belong to their own family and include the kainate (GluK), α-amino-3-hydroxy-5-methyl-4-isoxazolepropionic acid (AMPA; GluA), and NMDA (GluN) receptors, named after their selective agonists, along with the orphan δ GluD receptors. These receptors, which share characteristics (binding sites, central aqueous ionic pore, selectivity filter, and channel gate) typical for other ligand-gated ion channels, are distinct tetrameric structures, with each of the subunits contributing a ligand binding domain, implying that 4 molecules of agonist are necessary for channel activation. Glutamate is the agonist at all 4 sites of GluA and GluK receptors, but the GluN1 subunit of NMDA receptors (which are likely composed of 2 obligatory GluN1 and 2 GluN2/GluN3 type subunits) accepts glycine, meaning that NMDA receptors are coactivated by 2 molecules each of glycine and glutamate. Activation of all glutamate receptors is thought to occur when agonist molecules bind deep into the extracellular ligand binding domains, causing closure of these "clamshell"-like structures and subsequent channel opening by pulling on linking segments. Glutamate receptors have 3 complete TMDs but can be considered a hybrid of the pentameric ionotropic receptors and *inverted* voltage-gated ion channels, because their TM2 helices are in a conformation more akin to the reentrant P-loop of K+ channels and do not fully transverse the membrane. Not surprisingly, the nature of the amino acid at the QRN[9] site, located at the apex of the P-loop, impacts both the conductance and ion selectivity of the channel and, in particular, their Ca²⁺ permeability. NMDA channels are notable for an additional voltage-dependent channel block by extracellular Mg²⁺ ions, which largely keeps the activated/open channel in a nonconducting state at near resting membrane potentials, but ion permeable during membrane depolarization. This unique property of NMDA receptors allows them to function as coincidence detectors (requiring both a presynaptic signal [transmitter] and a postsynaptic signal [depolarization] to operate) and thereby play a critical role in certain forms of associative learning. Glutamate receptors can possess large intracellular C-terminal domains, creating multiple opportunities for channel regulation through protein–protein interactions, Ca²⁺-dependent mechanisms, and phosphorylation.

P2X receptors, the ionotropic branch of the purinergic receptor tree, are the third structurally distinct family of ligand-gated ion channels. These excitatory receptors, found in the peripheral nervous system and CNS, are trimeric in nature, with each of their "dolphin-shaped" subunits contributing 2 channel-forming TMDs. Binding of 3 molecules of ATP, likely at the subunit interfaces (similar to the pentameric receptor family), is needed to open the cation-selective pore.

---

[9]Q, glutamine; R, arginine; N, asparagine. Only one of these amino acids can be present at this position.

Mechanically Gated Ion Channels

The sensory system makes use of many types of ion channels to transduce physical stimuli into electrical signals. Some of these stimuli, such as sound waves and pressure, are obviously mechanical in nature and require mechanoreceptors (mechanosensitive receptor cells) to receive and convert any mechanical energy into ion fluxes. To perform this function, these specialized cells contain mechanically gated (or mechanosensitive) ion channels (often sensitive to membrane stretch), thereby allowing them to directly engage in the perception of sound, touch, balance, pain, and proprioception.

Although many types of channels are sensitive to mechanical stimulation, only those for which mechanical stimulation is the primary mode of activation should be considered mechanosensitive. Despite this restrictive condition, true mechanosensitive channels likely encompass a diverse group or proteins, including transient receptor potential (TRP) cation channels, a variety of K[+] channels (eg, tandem pore domain), and the more recently discovered Piezo[10] channels. It is thought that some of these channel candidates, including the TREK1 and TRAAK potassium channels and Piezo channels, may sense changes in membrane tension directly, through interactions with membrane lipids, without the need for accessory proteins or intermediate messengers. Conversely, force may be conveyed through structural proteins such as the intracellular cytoskeleton or, as in the case of hair cells in the inner ear, extracellular "tip links" that couple channel opening to movement of stereocilia (see Chapter 13). In some situations, the mechanical forces may be first captured by a mechanically sensitive protein and transferred to separate ion channels via second messengers. To date, unambiguous determination of mechanisms of activation for many mechanically gated ion channels and assignment of specific mechanosensitive channels to specific roles (eg, electrical transduction in hair cells) have been difficult.

SUMMARY

- The lipid bilayer plasma membrane maintains the integrity of neurons by keeping the cytoplasmic cellular contents separated from the extracellular space.
- The plasma membrane is the substrate for electrical signaling in neurons.
- Electrical signaling in neurons occurs via the activity of ion channels composed of membrane-spanning protein structures that form both membrane exchangers/transporters/pumps and ion channels.
- Ion channels allow the passage of selected ions across the bilayer.

- Ion transporters selectively change the concentration of ions, such as sodium, potassium, chloride, and calcium, inside the cell versus outside.
- Ion channels may be constituently open (leakage) or gated by ligand binding, voltage, mechanical stimulation, or binding by intracellular molecules.
- The Nernst potential allows the calculation of the balance between diffusional force created from inside versus outside concentration differences for each type of ion and the voltage across the membrane.
- Electrical activity in neurons is the result of the modulation of ion channel conductances that drive the membrane potential toward or away from the Nernst potential for each ion.

SELF-ASSESSMENT QUESTIONS

1. Why is the concentration of chloride in virtually all neurons lower inside than outside?
    A. All neurons have chloride transporters that reduce the intracellular concentration.
    B. The hyperpolarizing phase of action potentials pushes chloride outside the cell.
    C. The negative potential inside neurons causes exiting of chloride ions through leakage channels.
    D. Chloride accompanies the exit of sodium in the sodium/potassium active transporter.
    E. None of the above are correct.

2. What active ion transporter in neurons is necessary for the ionic concentration differences underlying the action potential?
    A. Na[+]/K[+] ATP pump
    B. Ca[2+] pump
    C. Na[+]/Ca[2+] exchange pump
    D. Cl[−] transporter pump
    E. Na[+]/Cl[−] ATP pump

3. What other molecules beside ions are transported across neural membranes by active pumps?
    A. Glucose and dextrose
    B. Amino acids and neurotransmitters
    C. RNA
    D. Molecules with phenyl rings
    E. Enzymes

4. What voltage-gated ion channel causes the relative refractory period?
    A. Na[+]
    B. Cl[−]
    C. Ca[2+]
    D. K[+]
    E. Mg[2+]

5. What does the term *ligand-gated* mean?
    A. Opened by stretch
    B. Open only transiently
    C. Opened by concentration differences
    D. Opened by liganic ions
    E. Opened by binding a neurotransmitter.

---

[10]Piezo channels have no homology to other known proteins and can contain upwards of 14 transmembrane domains.

Resting Membrane Potential & Action Potential

Franklin R. Amthor

- Understand the phospholipid structure of neural membranes and the protein complexes therein that compose ion channels and transporters.
- Know how the Na^+/K^+ ATP pump creates the ionic basis for the neural resting potential and electrical responses to stimulation.
- Understand how the Nernst potential calculates the balance between the tendency for ions to traverse the membrane due to concentration differences versus the tendency to move via electrical potential across the membrane.
- See that the neuron can be modeled as an equivalent electrical circuit composed of batteries derived from ionic concentration differences across the membrane and variable resistors capturing the action of ion channels.
- Understand how the action potential is created by the opening and closing of voltage-gated Na^+ and K^+ channels.
- Understand the absolute and relative refractory periods of the action potential.
- See why action potentials are necessary for long-distance neural potential propagation.

OVERVIEW

Neurons, like all cells, carry out metabolic, synthesis, and reproductive functions. In their evolution from nonneuronal precursor cells, neurons elaborated on several existing cellular processes to promote intra- and intercellular communication. Three of the most important communication functions considered here are (1) ion channel–mediated membrane potential and (2) membrane receptor recognition of exogenous molecules, and (3) secretion. The existence of a modifiable membrane potential allows intracellular communication between the dendritic tree and the cell soma via the flow of electrical currents. Membrane receptors that recognize exogenous molecules cause currents to flow through the membrane (and sometimes other, more long-lasting effects). Exocytosis of neurotransmitter molecules at synapses, a modified form of secretion, enables specific cell–cell communication in defined functional circuits.

NEURAL MEMBRANES

Virtually all cells, including those of plants, maintain a negative potential inside with respect to outside. Although this potential may have originated merely as a by-product of the predominance of negatively charged proteins inside cells, it enabled the possibility of electrical control of the flow of ions through membrane channels due to the voltage gradient across the membrane.

Single-cell organisms express a variety of receptors that recognize desirable versus toxic substances in their environment. Early in the evolution of multicellular life-forms, some cells began to express receptors for the exocytosis of substances from other cells in the organism rather than from the external environment. These substances may have originally been waste products from other cells, but, eventually, some cell began secreting molecules whose existence and detection constituted intercellular signaling (hormones). Neurons evolved to elaborate hundreds of specific ion channel types whose activation modulates their membrane potential. The summated membrane potential at the neural cell soma or axon initial segment causes action potentials via the action of voltage-gated ion channels. These action potentials travel to the end of the axon where they generate the release of neurotransmitters targeted at other neurons (or muscles or glands) by a secretory process.

Neural membranes, like those of other animal cells, consist of a relatively impervious phospholipid bilayer into which

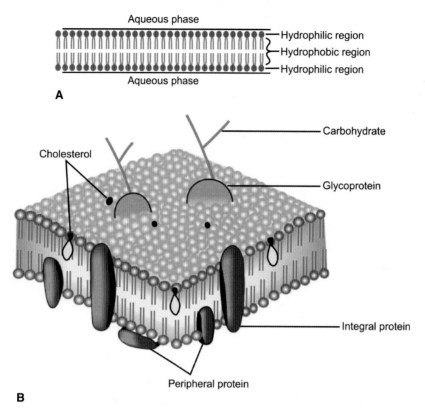

FIGURE 6-1 **A.** Basic structure of the phospholipid bilayer that forms the membrane of neurons (and other animal cells). Because phospholipids have a hydrophilic head and hydrophobic tail, they spontaneously assemble in aqueous solutions in a bilayer with the heads pointing out and bound to water molecules and the hydrophobic tails pointing inward. **B.** Three-dimensional structure of the phospholipid bilayer that also shows that various other substances such as cholesterol and protein complexes are typically incorporated in the phospholipid membrane. (Adapted with permission from Naik P: *Biochemistry*, 3rd edition, Jaypee Brothers Medical Publishers (P) Ltd., 2009.)

various protein complexes are inserted. These protein complexes mediate the recognition of endogenous ligands (neurotransmitters and hormones), which activates ion channels that allow ion flow through the membrane, modifying membrane potential.

Phospholipid Membrane Structure

Neurons, like other animal cells, are enclosed by a membrane that separates inside from outside. This membrane is composed of phospholipid molecules. Figure 6–1A shows a diagram of a linear section of membrane formed from phospholipid molecules. These molecules are amphipathic, meaning one end (the "head") is hydrophilic, while the other (the "tail") is hydrophobic. Hydrophobicity depends on whether charge is localized to parts of the molecule or distributed equally throughout it. If the charge is localized to one end of the molecule, it becomes a dipole. Water (H_2O), for example, is a dipole because, although it is overall electrically neutral, negative charge is localized near the oxygen atom, and positive charge is localized near the hydrogens. The dipole charge distribution in the head area of the phospholipid binds water molecules, whereas the nonpolar tail end does not. Phospholipids thus spontaneously form bilayers in water oriented with the hydrophilic heads on the outside bound to water molecules and the hydrophobic tails on the inside.

Figure 6–1B shows a 2-dimensional representation of a phospholipid bilayer. These phospholipid bilayers are almost totally impervious to the movement of water or ions dissolved in the water, as well as most larger molecules. Inserted within this bilayer are proteins and other molecules important for cellular function, specifically, for controlling the movement of ions and other molecules across the membrane. In carefully prepared laboratory conditions, phospholipid bilayers can be made to form sheets extending for millimeters. However, normally, phospholipid bilayers close upon themselves to form spheres, which are the cell membranes.

Functional Molecules in Membranes

As shown in Figure 6–1B and Figure 6–2, proteins and other molecules such as cholesterol synthesized by neurons are present in neural membranes. This synthesis occurs under the control of DNA and involves the Golgi apparatus and endoplasmic reticulum, by which synthesized molecules such as proteins are transported to the cell membrane throughout the neuron. Complexes of proteins in neural membranes form ion channels, transporters, and receptors that mediate neural function.

Neural signaling via activation of membrane receptors is accomplished via a variety of mechanisms. Figure 6–3 shows 5 transmembrane signaling mechanisms. Some lipophilic

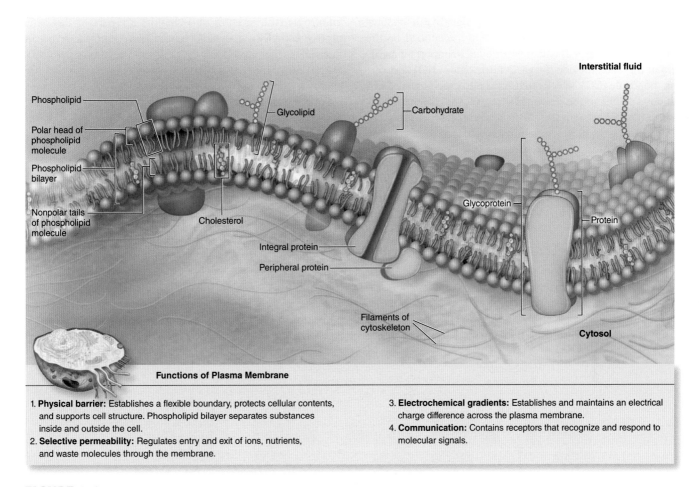

FIGURE 6–2 Structure of the phospholipid membrane enclosing the cell with incorporated ion channels and receptors in the membrane. (Reproduced with permission from McKinley MP, O'Loughlin VD, Bidle TS. *Anatomy and Physiology: An Integrative Approach.* New York, NY: McGraw Hill; 2013.)

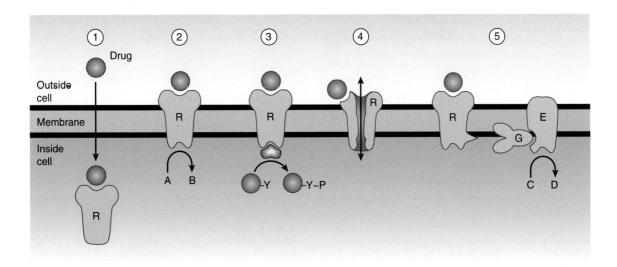

FIGURE 6–3 Transmembrane signaling mechanisms: (1) some lipid soluble molecules traverse the membrane, (2) reception of a ligand on the extracellular side of a receptor activates a biochemical cascade initiated by a receptor conformational change on the cytoplasmic side, (3) extracellular domain binding activates a tyrosine kinase (phosphorylation) cascade, (4) ionotropic channels are opened by ligand binding, and (5) ligand binding to the extracellular domain initiates a G-protein cascade that may open or close nearby channels from the cytoplasmic side. E, endogenous channel activated by intracellular messenger; G, G-protein cascade; R, receptor complex. (Reproduced with permission from Katzung BG: *Basic & Clinical Pharmacology,* 14th ed. New York, NY: McGraw Hill; 2018.)

substances that function as interneural signals can dissolve directly into the membrane (mechanism 1, identified by the number 1 in Figure 6–3) and move through it. Important members of this class include the gases nitric oxide (NO) and carbon monoxide (CO), which often act as retrograde signals from the postsynaptic to the presynaptic cell. Other exogenous substances bind to and activate specific receptors (mechanisms 2 to 4, see Figure 6–3), such as ionotropic or metabotropic receptors (see Chapters 10 and 11). Mechanism 5 (see Figure 6–3) shows an intracellular signaling mechanism in which a neurotransmitter binds a metabotropic receptor that initiates G-protein–mediated control of other membrane protein complexes that control metabolic pathways within the cell.

Ion Channels & Transporters

Neural signaling function is based on the control of ion movement through channels in the neural membrane. Figure 6–4 shows several of the most important types of ion channels found in neurons, including voltage-gated and ligand (neurotransmitter-gated) channels that can be either ionotropic (the receptor and channel are part of the same protein complex) or metabotropic (the receptor activates an internal biochemical cascade such as a G-protein mechanism). Neural membranes also have transporters or pumps that use energy (typically adenosine triphosphate [ATP]) to move ions into or out of the cell, typically in a fixed ratio. One of the most important of these for neural function is the sodium/potassium (Na^+/K^+) transporter discussed in the next section.

Active Transport via the Na^+/K^+ Pump

Neurons use protein complexes called ion transporters to create different concentrations of several important ions inside the cell versus outside. The 4 most important ions in neural function are sodium (Na^+), potassium (K^+), chloride (Cl^-), and calcium (Ca^{2+}).

Na^+/K^+ Pump

The operation of the Na^+/K^+ transporter (sometimes called a pump) and several similar transporters is shown in Figure 6–5. Note that the Na^+/K^+ pump (in the upper left of Figure 6–5)

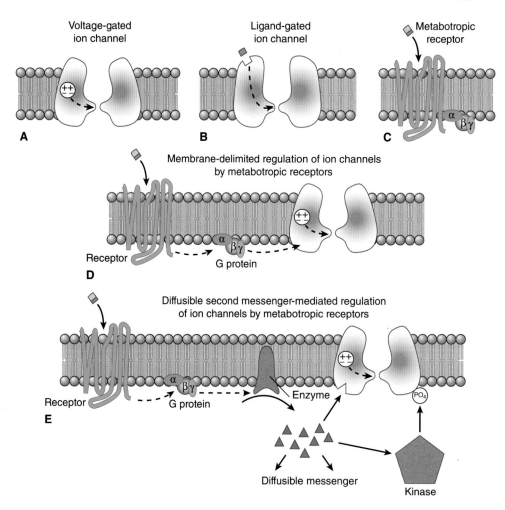

FIGURE 6–4 Types of ion channels and receptors: (**A**) voltage-gated; (**B**) ionotropic ligand gated; (**C**) metabotropic ligand gated via G-protein cascade within the membrane; (**D**) metabotropic channel activated via intracellular diffusible messengers; and (**E**) amplification of metabotropic receptor function by enzymes and kinase channel phosphorylation. (Reproduced with permission from Katzung BG: *Basic & Clinical Pharmacology*, 14th ed. New York, NY: McGraw Hill; 2018.)

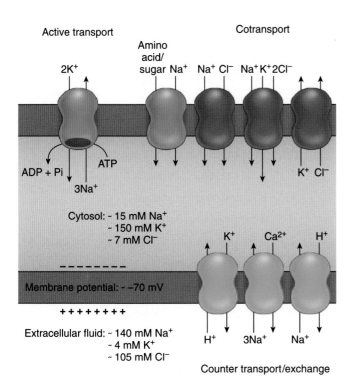

FIGURE 6–5 Several types of transporters (ion pumps) that are common in neural membranes. One of the most important is the Na⁺/K⁺ transporter shown in the upper left that uses energy from adenosine triphosphate (ATP) to cyclically pump 3 Na⁺ ions out per 2 K⁺ ions in. These pumps run constantly and produced the Na⁺/K⁺ concentration differences shown in Figure 6–3. Several other transporters for Na⁺, K⁺, Cl⁻, Ca²⁺, and H⁺ are shown. (Reproduced with permission from Barrett KE, Barman SM, Brooks HL et al: *Ganong's Review of Medical Physiology*, 26th ed. New York, NY: McGraw Hill; 2019.)

operates in a cycle in which 2 potassium ions are brought into the cell and 3 sodium ions are removed. This means that not only does the pump create concentration differences for these 2 ions inside versus outside the cell, but also the pump generates a net electrical current that makes the inside of the cell more negative (3 sodium ions out per 2 potassium ions in).

The 2 most important ions whose concentration differences control the membrane potential and electrical signaling are sodium and potassium. The ionic constitution of extracellular fluid outside cells in animals is similar to seawater, which is composed primarily of dissolved sodium chloride, with much less potassium chloride and several divalent cations such as calcium, magnesium (Mg^{2+}), and manganese (Mn^{2+}). Neurons use membrane pumps powered by ATP to selectively remove sodium and bring in potassium ions so that the internal concentrations of these ions are very different from that outside, as shown in Figure 6–6. Neural membranes have many of these pumps that run constantly to produce and maintain these concentration differences, also called gradients.

Establishing the Neuronal Resting Membrane Potential

When experimenters insert microelectrodes inside neurons, the voltage measured inside with respect to the outside is for most neurons on the order of –65 to –70 mV

Ion	Concentration	
	Inside	Outside
Na^+	18 mM	145 mM
K^+	135 mM	3 mM
Cl^-	7 mM	120 mM
Ca^{2+}	100 nM	1.2 mM

FIGURE 6–6 The inside versus outside concentration of 4 significant ions for electrical behavior of neurons: sodium (Na^+), potassium (K^+), chloride (Cl^-), and calcium (Ca^{2+}).

(see Figure 5-5). This is the voltage across the cell phospholipid bilayer, or plasma membrane. Many treatments of membrane potential suggest that this is due primarily to the charge imbalance (3 Na^+ out to 2 K^+ in) of the Na^+/K^+ transporter. This is not really the case, however. The current produced by the Na^+/K^+ transporter only amounts to a few millivolts in most neurons. What then brings about the –65 mV membrane potential?

Electrical & Diffusional Forces Experienced by Ions

How ions in solution on either side of the neural membrane flow through the membrane depends on 3 factors, 2 of which are forces (illustrated in Figure 6–7). The third is the type of channel through which they can flow.

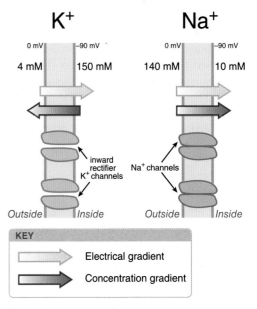

FIGURE 6–7 The electrical and concentration gradients for Na^+ and K^+. Both gradients favor entry of Na^+ into the cell, whereas the electrical force for K^+ is for motion inward, while the diffusional force is outward. (Reproduced with permission from Brunton LL, Hilal-Dandan R, Knollmann BC: *Goodman & Gilman's the Pharmacological Basis of Therapeutics*, 13th ed. New York, NY: McGraw Hill; 2018.)

The first force is the diffusional force due to the concentration differences created by the Na⁺/K⁺ transporter pump. Because the concentration of sodium is higher inside the cell than outside, the diffusional force for sodium will tend to make it move outside the cell when any channel is open that is "permeable" to sodium, that is, allows sodium to move through the membrane. The diffusional force is the opposite for potassium, however, because it has a higher concentration inside the cell than outside, so the diffusional force for potassium tends to cause a net movement from inside to outside.

The second force is the potential difference or voltage across the membrane. This voltage is about –65 to –70 mV in most neurons, what is called the resting state, when only leakage channels are conducting current (we have not yet indicated quantitatively how this voltage exists or what "leakage" channels are, which is to follow). The potential difference (voltage) causes positive ions such as Na⁺ and K⁺ to be attracted to the negative interior of the cell.

How and whether ions move through the membrane is also controlled by the third factor, the type of ion channel. The phospholipid membrane is impermeable to water and dissolved ions, so ions can only move through the membrane through channels, which are molecular "holes" in the membrane created by protein complexes synthesized by the nucleus of the cell and transported to various locations on its plasma membrane. There are many types of ion channels in neurons (and other cells). The 2 types of ion channels most important for controlling the neural membrane potential are the sodium and potassium channels.

If a sodium-selective channel is open, both the voltage force and diffusional force tend to make the highly concentrated positively charged sodium ions outside the cell move toward the low sodium concentration, negatively charged interior of the cell, as shown schematically on the right in Figure 6–7. For potassium, however, these 2 forces point in opposite directions, as shown on the left in Figure 6–7. What tells us which way potassium ions will move (net flow)?

The Nernst equation (Figure 6–8) gives the voltage produced by the concentration difference for each ion, which can be regarded as being equivalent to a battery. Figure 6–9 shows that typical intracellular ion concentrations created by the Na⁺/K⁺ pump result in values for E_K in neurons of about –80 mV and for E_{Na} of +55 mV. The Nernst equation can also be interpreted as giving the balance point between voltage and diffusional force, the voltage at which the next current would be 0. Thus, for potassium, if the inside voltage of the neuron were made to equal the potassium Nernst potential (–80 mV), there would be no net flow of potassium through the membrane when potassium channels were opened because the diffusional flow would equal the voltage-induced flow. At potentials more negative than –80 mV, net movement would be inward; at more positive intracellular potentials, net movement would be outward. Because both voltage and diffusional forces for sodium are inward, it would require making the inside of the cell strongly positive (+55 mV) for the electrical repulsion of sodium ions to counterbalance the diffusional force from the much higher concentration outside than inside.

The Nernst equation for an ion X in solution is given by:

$$E_X = \frac{RT}{Z_X F} \ln \frac{[X]_o}{[X]_i}$$

Where:

$[X]_o$ is the concentration of **X** outside the cell

$[X]_i$ is the concentration of **X** inside the cell

E_X is the equilibrium potential of **X**

R is the universal gas constant

T is the temperature (degrees Kelvin)

Z_X is the ion's valence (⁺1 for Na⁺ & K⁺, ⁻1 for Cl⁻)

F is Faraday's constant

$\ln$ is the natural logarithm (base)

At a warm mammalian body temperature, combining term and converting to a base 10 log the equation can be rewritten:

$$E_X \approx \frac{60}{Z_X} \log_{10} \frac{[X]_o}{[X]_i}$$

FIGURE 6–8 The Nernst equation for calculation of the electromotive force (E) due to a concentration gradient across a neural membrane.

Current Flowing Through Ion Channels: Ohm's Law

The Nernst equation indicates that the concentration differences between the inside and outside of the neuron create a voltage difference, which is modeled as a battery in an electrical circuit. Ions flow across the membrane through channels, and many important ion channels are selective for a particular ion. The quantity of ionic current through the membrane depends on the number of channels through which the ion can flow and the permeability (electrical conductance) of

$E_K = 60 \log_{10} (K_o/K_i)$

For K_o =   20 mM (concentration outside)
K_i = 400 mM (concentration inside)

$E_K = 60 \log_{10} (20/400) = -78$ mV

$E_{Na} = 60 \log_{10} (Na_o/Na_i)$

For Na_o = 400 mM (concentration outside)
Na_i =   50 mM (concentration inside)

$E_{Na} = 60 \log_{10} (440/50) = +56.7$ mV

FIGURE 6–9 The Nernst potentials for sodium (Na) and potassium (K).

these channels. In electrical terms, the conductance of the channel is given in the units siemens, which is the reciprocal of the electrical resistance in ohms.

Equivalent Electrical Circuit of the Neuron

Figure 6–10 shows an equivalent circuit for a "typical" neuron membrane area with the associated sodium and potassium batteries and conductances. Conductances (the electrical equivalent of permeabilities) are modeled as resistors in the electrical circuit, where conductance in siemens is the reciprocal of resistance in ohms. In membrane models like this, the extracellular voltage is assumed to be 0, and the intracellular voltage is the net current across the membrane multiplied by the membrane resistance. In this example, the calculated intracellular potential would be about –69 mV.

K⁺ Leak Channels & Chloride

The electrical potential measured inside a neuron is always the result of the current flowing across the membrane. When the neuron is not strongly depolarized, such as when producing

action potentials, most of the membrane permeability is due to constituently open potassium and chloride channels. These are often called "leakage" channels because they are not gated but always open. As we saw before, the Nernst potential for potassium is about –80 mV, so open potassium channels tend to push the neuron's intracellular potential toward that value.

The other constituently open channels are chloride channels. Although there are chloride transporters in many neurons, typically leakage chloride channels allow the chloride concentration to follow the membrane potential set by potassium leakage. Because the resting potential voltage inside the neuron is on the order of –65 mV, negatively charged chloride will tend to move out of the cell through the leakage channels, resulting in a much lower concentration inside the cell than outside. Active chloride transport outside the cell may reduce its inside concentration even further. The Nernst potential for chloride in most neurons is typically, therefore, very close to the resting potential, or slightly more hyperpolarized.

Many inhibitory synapses (eg, γ-aminobutyric acid A receptor [GABA_A] and glycine) open chloride channels. Although such synapses themselves produce small direct hyperpolarization, their major effect is to counteract the depolarization of excitatory synapses by forcing the membrane potential back toward the resting potential. Another inhibitory effect of increasing chloride conductance is that their reduction of the membrane resistance, by Ohm's law, reduces the depolarization produced by current flowing through sodium channels. This effect is sometimes called silent or shunting inhibition.

The actual voltage across the membrane is produced by a combination of currents associated with the different conducting ion channels and depends on their Nernst potentials and conductances (permeabilities). The transmembrane voltage can be calculated from these parameters using the Goldman equation (see Figure 6–10B). The P values are the total channel permeabilities for each specific ion, and the bracketed values are the concentrations inside or outside the cell. Note that if there is significant permeability (conductance) for only 1 ion, the Goldman equation reduces to the Nernst equation for that ion.

Synaptic Potentials

The effect of synapses depends on their location on the dendritic tree. Neurotransmitters released by presynaptic neurons open ion channels that are usually selective for specific ions. Excitatory synapses usually open channels that allow the passage of sodium through the membrane, while inhibitory synapses allow the flux of chloride or potassium. The time that the released neurotransmitters are bound to the postsynaptic ion channels determines the duration of the postsynaptic potential, which is usually on the order of a few milliseconds. This decay, due to the decay of neurotransmitter concentration, is due to (1) diffusion of the neurotransmitter molecules out of the synaptic cleft, (2) enzymatic degradation of some neurotransmitter molecules (eg, the destruction of acetylcholine

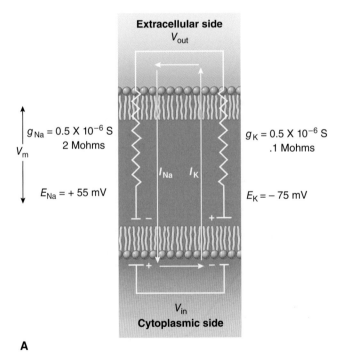

A

Goldman equation:

$$V_m = \frac{RT}{F} \ln \frac{P_k[K^+]_o + P_{Na}[Na^+]_o + P_{Cl}[Cl^-]_i}{P_k[K^+]_i + P_{Na}[Na^+]_i + P_{Cl}[Cl^-]_o}$$

B

FIGURE 6–10 **A.** Equivalent membrane circuit for sodium and potassium channel conductances and batteries. **B.** Goldman equation for calculating membrane potential based on Nernst voltages and specific ion permeabilities.

by the enzyme acetylcholinesterase), and (3) active uptake (transport) of neurotransmitters by the presynaptic neuron by which they are removed from the synaptic cleft. Some postsynaptic receptors also desensitize, that is, close or stop conducting after some open time even when the neurotransmitter is still bound to the recognition site.

Current flows along the dendrite due to the difference between the voltage across the membrane at the synapse, versus elsewhere. The magnitude of depolarization produced by an excitatory input at 1 dendritic tree location is attenuated as one moves farther and farther from the input locus. This is due to 2 effects: (1) the loss of current through the membrane and (2) the voltage drop along the dendritic process due to axial resistance. This makes the voltage across the membrane at the synapse different from that away from the synapse along the dendritic process. The situation is like a garden hose when the faucet is turned on. The faucet at one end of the hose corresponds to voltage. If the hose has lots of holes in it (leakage channels), very little water will reach the opposite end. If the

hose has a very small diameter (analogous to a high dendritic resistance per unit length), there will also be attenuated water flow.

Figure 6–11 shows several aspects of synaptic dynamics. Figure 6–11A illustrates the attenuation of the transmembrane voltage between the synapse and a dendritic location closer to the soma, where integration of all synaptic current occurs. Figure 6–11B shows a second feature of the distant membrane potential produced away from a synapse that is also seen in the garden hose analogy. This is the fact that, although the faucet may be turned from off to full on very quickly, the effect at the opposite end of the hose is delayed. The fast turn-on pulse at the faucet is smoothed to a more gradual build up farther away. This phenomenon in neurons is due to membrane capacitance and would be modeled by a very elastic water hose. Thus, away from the synapse, the voltage across the membrane induced by the synaptic current has a lower amplitude and longer, delayed time course compared to that at the synapse.

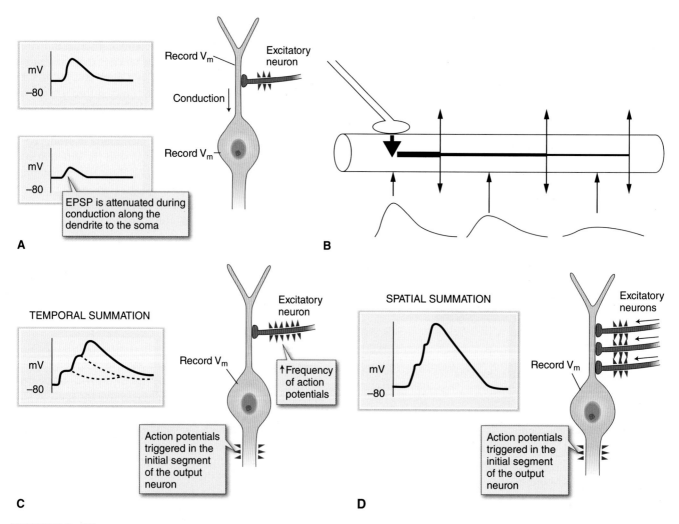

FIGURE 6–11 **A.** Attenuation of transmembrane potential away from the synapse. **B.** Passive electrotonic spread of membrane potential showing both attenuation and time delay. **C.** Temporal summation. **D.** Spatial summation. (Reproduced with permission from Kibble JD, Halsey CR. *Medical Physiology: The Big Picture.* New York, NY: McGraw Hill; 2009.)

Synaptic inputs also demonstrate temporal (Figure 6–11C) and spatial (Figure 6–11D) integration. Temporal integration occurs when multiple action potentials (spikes) in a presynaptic neuron are close enough together in time so that the synaptic potential from earlier spikes has not decayed completely before the effect of the next spike. This increases the total membrane potential induced by a volley of spikes. A similar effect occurs when multiple spikes from different synapses arrive within a short time interval (Figure 6–11D).

THE ACTION POTENTIAL

Typical neuronal processes have membrane and axial resistances and membrane capacitance such that synaptic signals can travel at most a few hundred micrometers before being attenuated. This limits the length of most neuronal dendrites to a few hundred micrometers from the soma. However, neurons communicate over much longer distances than this via their axons. To do this, something else is required that can amplify the electrotonic signal so that it can travel these longer distances. This amplifier is the action potential.

Activation of Voltage-Gated Na⁺ Channels: Depolarization

A typical neuron shown in this and other textbooks has a compact dendritic tree spanning a few hundred micrometers and a single long axon that may extend for a meter or more; for example, some upper motor neurons in your primary motor cortex send an axon down the length of the spinal cord to the lumbar segments to innervate lower motor neurons that drive muscles in the legs and feet. Passive electrotonic spread is adequate for current injected by synapses on distal dendrites a few hundred micrometers away from the soma to reach it, but these currents would be negligible at the end of the axon a meter away from the soma.

Neurons solve the distant transmission problem via the production of action potentials. Action potentials depend on the existence of 2 specialized types of channels that, instead of being ligand (neurotransmitter) gated, are gated by voltage. These are the voltage-gated sodium and potassium channels found in virtually all neuronal axons.

Voltage-gated channels are opened by membrane depolarization. When the neuron is not depolarized, but in its "resting" state at about –65 mV inside with respect to outside, these channels are closed. However, if the neuron is depolarized by sufficient excitatory input, a threshold is reached at which the channels open. This behavior is shown in **Figure 6–12**. Here, low-amplitude depolarizing or hyperpolarizing currents injected into the neuron, such as at a synapse or with a microelectrode, produce passive, quickly declining changes in membrane potential that would only be propagated a few hundred micrometers along the dendrite. However, when a depolarizing current reaches the threshold (here about –55 mV), a self-sustaining all-or-none action potential is generated.

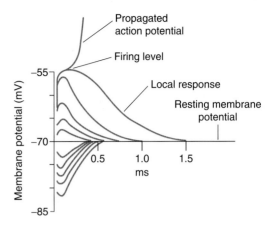

FIGURE 6–12 Threshold for the action potential. (Reproduced with permission from Barrett KE, Barman SM, Brooks HL et al: *Ganong's Review of Medical Physiology*, 26th ed. New York, NY: McGraw Hill; 2019.)

This action potential is produced by the voltage-gated sodium and potassium conductances.

The shape of the action potential is controlled by the time course of the sodium and potassium voltage-gated channels. The sodium channel is the dominant mechanism underlying the action potential. It opens and closes more quickly than the potassium channel, as shown in **Figure 6–13**. The solid line in Figure 6–13 shows the membrane potential changes during the action potential, whereas the dashed and dotted lines show the sodium and potassium conductance changes that cause the membrane potential to change.

The traces start when the neuron has been at the resting potential (or at least below threshold for an action potential) for at least several milliseconds and the voltage-gated sodium and potassium channels are in their closed state. Once threshold is reached or passed by depolarizing inputs to the neuron, the voltage-gated sodium channels (dashed line) open rapidly, the second state. But note that, even though the membrane potential is depolarized and therefore above threshold, the voltage-gated channels close. This state is a distinct state from the closed state in which they began, because they are not openable by depolarization in this state. This closure arises from biophysical properties of the channels themselves.

As the voltage-gated sodium channels close, the membrane potential declines. At about this time, the slower voltage-gated potassium channels also have been triggered by the previous depolarization, and they begin to open (dotted line). Figure 6–13 shows that the peak of the potassium channel conductance is during the falling phase of the sodium channel conductance. At the point where the sodium conductance has returned to 0 (near the intersection of this trace with the membrane potential), the potassium channels are still open and remain open for several milliseconds. In this phase of the action potential, the voltage-gated potassium channels, but not the voltage-gated sodium channels, are open. This increases the membrane potassium conductance beyond the level from constituently active potassium channels that

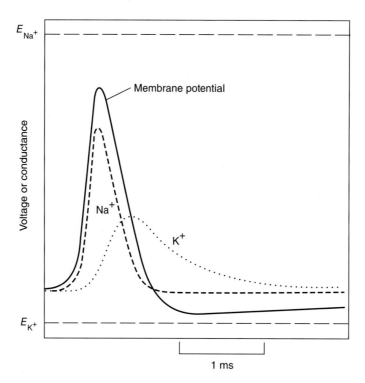

FIGURE 6–13 Ionic conductances that mediate the action potential. (Reproduced with permission from Toy EC, Weisbrodt N, Dubinsky WP, et al: *Case Files: Physiology*, 2nd ed. New York, NY: McGraw Hill; 2009.)

are open when the membrane is hyperpolarized, driving the membrane potential even farther toward the potassium equilibrium potential.

Refractory Periods & Time Course

The period of time composed of several milliseconds after the peak voltage-gated sodium channel conductances is called the refractory period (Figure 6–14). The refractory period has 2 major phases: the absolute and relative refractory periods. The absolute refractory period is the time during which the sodium channels are in the closed but unopenable state. No second action potential can be retriggered in this state because the sodium channels are desensitized to opening by voltage. Thus, the voltage-gated sodium channels have 3 states—transition from the resting potential closed-openable, open, to closed-unopenable, then back to the original closed-openable. The closed-unopenable state lasts for less than a millisecond, with the transition from closed-unopenable to closed-openable being silent and having no effect on membrane potential.

After the sodium channel transition from closed-unopenable to closed-openable occurs, the potassium channels are still conducting for several milliseconds. This is the relative refractory period. During this time, it is possible for input depolarization to produce another action potential, but it is more difficult for 2 reasons: (1) the membrane potential is hyperpolarized below the normal resting potential by the remaining potassium conductance, and (2) the potassium conductance

reduces the membrane resistance and, by Ohm's law, reduces any depolarizing voltage generated across the membrane by synaptic currents.

Introduction to the Neural Code

The generation of action potentials allows us to summarize the basic operation of neurons. Thousands of excitatory and inhibitory inputs on the neuron's dendritic tree and soma transiently open ion channels in a complex spatiotemporal pattern. Currents flow through these channels and travel throughout the dendritic tree. A crucial location in the neuron is the beginning of the axon where it leaves the soma, called the initial segment or axon hillock. These few hundred microns of axon have a large concentration of voltage-gated sodium and potassium channels and are where the action potential is first generated in most neurons. The complex spatiotemporal pattern of synaptic inputs to the neuron produces a constantly changing voltage across the membrane at the initial segment. This voltage is translated into a rate of action potentials. Strong depolarizations from many active excitatory inputs may produce firing rates as high as 800 spikes per second, at least for short periods of time, while strong inhibition may keep the initial segment membrane below threshold so that there are no action potentials. Thus, the net balance of excitatory and inhibitory input leads to a net analog voltage at the initial segment that becomes a firing rate. The action potentials produced at the initial segment travel down the axon to its terminals where neurotransmitter molecules are released onto

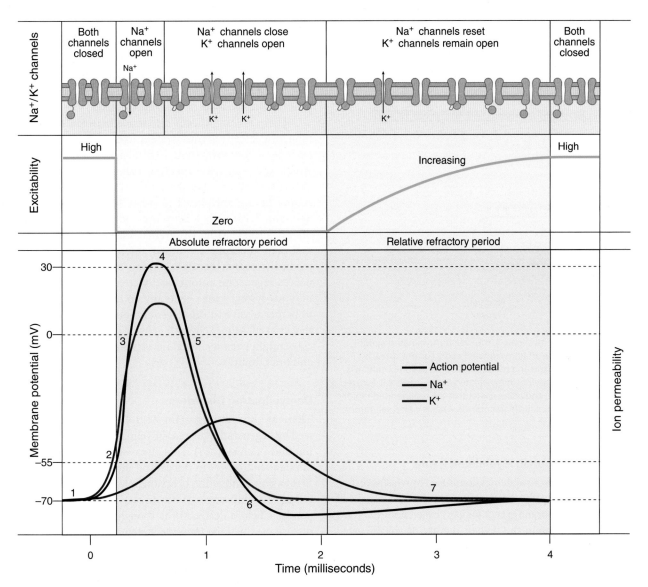

FIGURE 6-14 The action potential and its phases showing sodium and potassium conductance time courses and absolute and relative refractory periods. (Silverthorn, Dee Unglaub: *Human Physiology: An Integrated Approach*, 5th Ed., ©2010. Reprinted by permission of Pearson Education, Inc., New York, New York.)

other neurons, forming a complex neural circuit. The neural code for the time-varying input to the neuron is the rate and pattern of the action potentials it produces.

Action Potential Conduction

The action potential, once initiated at the initial segment, is conducted without decrement to the axon's terminals where other neurons (or muscles or glands) are contacted. This conduction occurs because the depolarization in one area of the axon membrane depolarizes adjacent areas. These areas also have voltage-gated sodium and potassium channels that regenerate the action potential so that it propagates down the length of the axon. There are 2 main mechanisms by which this occurs depending on whether the axon is unmyelinated or myelinated.

Continuous Conduction in Unmyelinated Axons

Invertebrates and cold-blooded vertebrates have nervous systems dominated by unmyelinated axons. The membranes of these axons have a continuous density of voltage-gated sodium and potassium channels. Once the action potential is initiated at the axon initial segment, depolarizing current flows along the axon and depolarizes adjacent patches of axonal membrane, inducing a spreading action potential that propagates without attenuation or significant change in shape from the initial segment to the axon terminals centimeters or more distant from the soma. The action potential only moves in 1 direction (orthograde) because the refractory period prevents back-propagation in the retrograde direction toward the soma from the current active region.

Unmyelinated axon

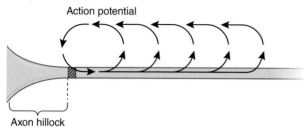

Myelinated axon

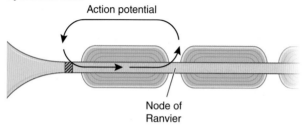

FIGURE 6–15 Unmyelinated (top) versus myelinated action potential conduction. In an unmyelinated axon, current spreads diffusely through the axon and production of the action potential is continuous and slow moving. In myelinated axons, current is focused at the nodes of Ranvier, and action potentials are regenerated rapidly and discontinuously from node to node via what is called salutatory conduction.

Saltatory Conduction in Myelinated Axons

The mammalian nervous system is dominated by what are called myelinated axons. Myelinated axons are "wrapped" by layers of fatty insulating membrane except for gaps called nodes of Ranvier. These gaps contain the highest density of voltage-gated sodium channels. There are few channels where the myelin wrapping exists except for potassium channels at the edges of the nodes of Ranvier. In Figure 6–15, the bottom figure shows how the current in a myelinated axon generated at one node of Ranvier is concentrated at the next node. This means that the

action potential is quickly regenerated at the next node but not in the myelin wrapping region. The action potential thus jumps from node to node rapidly in what is called saltatory conduction. Saltatory conduction makes action potential conduction speed approximately 10 times faster in a myelinated axon than an unmyelinated axon of the same diameter.

There is a significant difference between myelin wrapping in central nervous system axons versus those in the peripheral nervous system. Central nervous system axons are wrapped by oligodendrocytes, with 1 oligodendrocyte providing the myelin covering for several axons (Figure 6–16). Axons in the peripheral nervous system are wrapped by Schwann cells, with 1 Schwann cell wrapping the segment of only a single axon. Differences between oligodendrocytes and Schwann cells are under intense scrutiny in modern medical research because, among other things, peripheral nerves regenerate automatically after being cut, but central nervous system axons generally do not. Schwann cells seem to be permissive to this regeneration, leading to some hope that transplanting Schwann cells or modifying oligodendrocytes might permit central nerve regeneration in spinal cord and brain injuries.

Demyelinating Disorders

There are several important neurologic disorders characterized by degeneration of axon myelination. The most notable is multiple sclerosis (MS). This disease arises from degeneration of oligodendrocytes in the central nervous system, leading at first to slow conduction of action potentials and finally to total failure. The end stages of the disease include extensive motor paralysis before death. MS is thought to be an autoimmune disease in which the immune system attacks the myelin coating of axons, possibly after being triggered by an infectious agent containing proteins that mimic myelin.

Other demyelinating diseases of the central nervous system include Devic disease, myelinoclastic disorders, and leukodystrophic disorders. There are also demyelinating

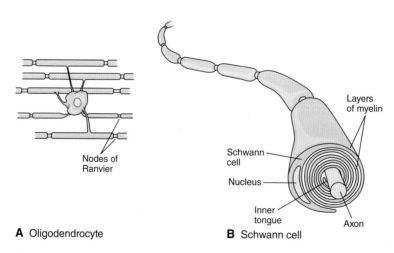

A Oligodendrocyte   **B** Schwann cell

FIGURE 6–16 Oligodendrocytes versus Schwann cells. (Part A, reproduced with permission from Kandel ER, Schwartz JH, Jessell TM, et al: *Principles of Neural Science*, 5th ed. New York, NY: McGraw Hill; 2013.)

disorders of the peripheral nervous system such as Guillain-Barré syndrome, Charcot-Marie-Tooth disease, and progressive inflammatory neuropathy.

CONCLUSION

Ion transporters (pumps) establish concentration gradients between the interior of neurons and the extracellular space for sodium and potassium. Neurons can be modeled as electrical devices in which these concentration gradients comprise batteries whose voltage is given by the Nernst equation. The actual transmembrane voltage can be calculated from the Goldman equation based on the Nernst potentials and channel permeabilities for each ion. Synaptic inputs on neural dendritic trees exhibit complex, location-dependent dynamics in which attenuation, delay, and temporal and spatial summation occur. The net current crossing the axon initial segment produces action potentials when the transmembrane voltage there exceeds threshold. Action potentials depend on voltage-gated sodium and potassium channels. These channels allow the spike to be propagated without attenuation from the axon initial segment to the axon terminals where neurotransmitter is released onto other neurons. The speed of spike transmission along the axon is faster for myelinated than unmyelinated axons. Central versus peripheral nervous system axons have different glial cells producing the myelin wrapping. There are distinct central versus peripheral nervous system neuropathies associated with demyelination.

SUMMARY

- Neural cell membranes, like all animal cells, are made of a phospholipid bilayer that isolates the cell's contents from the extracellular space by being generally impervious to the movement of water and solutes.

- Neurons manufacture proteins that are inserted into their membranes that allow the movement of some specific ions through the membrane.

- The control of ion movement through neural membranes may be dependent on binding of extracellular ligands (neurotransmitters), transmembrane voltage, or active, energy-driven pump mechanisms, among other mechanisms.

- The sodium-potassium active pump mechanism in neural membranes creates an ionic imbalance between the cell's interior versus exterior whereby the neural interior is very low in sodium compared to outside but high in potassium.

- The transmembrane voltage in neurons is set primarily by the conductances of sodium, potassium, and chloride.

- The resting potential of a neuron when few sodium channels are open (usually in the range of –70 to –55 mV) is determined primarily by leakage conductances for potassium and chloride.

- Action potentials are created by the rapid opening and closing of voltage-gated sodium and potassium channels following depolarization of the neuron by neurotransmitter-gated opening of sodium channels.

- Action potentials are characterized by an approximately 0.5-millisecond depolarization to about +50 mV, followed by an absolute refractory period in which the voltage-gated sodium channels are closed but inactivatable by voltage and a relative refractory period in which the voltage-gated potassium channels remain open, driving the neuron toward a more hyperpolarized membrane potential and reducing the impedance across the membrane.

- The neural code for the representation of information in action potential firing consists of both firing rate and firing pattern components.

- Neural action potentials are transmitted in unattenuated form by regeneration along the axon by voltage-gated sodium and potassium channels.

- Myelin wrapping of axons enhances action potential conduction speed by about a factor of 10.

SELF-ASSESSMENT QUESTIONS

1. The resting membrane potential is characterized by which of the following?
   A. Passive fluxes of Na^+ and K^+ are balanced by an active pump that derives energy from enzymatic hydrolysis of adenosine triphosphate (ATP).
   B. A membrane is depolarized when the differences between the charges across the membrane are increased.
   C. As the inside of the cell is made more negative with respect to the outside, the cell becomes depolarized.
   D. In a cell whose membrane possesses only K^+ channels, the membrane potential cannot be determined.
   E. The resting membrane potential is unrelated to the separation of the charge across the membrane.

2. After the occurrence of an action potential, there is a repolarization of the membrane. Which of the following is the principal explanation for this event?
   A. Potassium channels have been opened.
   B. Sodium channels have been opened.
   C. Potassium channels have been inactivated.
   D. The membrane becomes impermeable to all ions.
   E. There has been a sudden influx of calcium.

3. Where in the neuron is the trigger zone that integrates incoming signals from other cells and initiates the signal that the neuron sends to another neuron or a muscle cell?
   A. Cell body
   B. Dendritic trunk
   C. Dendritic spines
   D. Axon hillock and initial segment
   E. Axon trunk

4. The equilibrium potential for potassium, as determined by the Nernst equation, differs from the resting potential of the neuron. Which of the following best accounts for this difference?

    A. An active sodium-potassium pump makes an important contribution to the regulation of the resting potential.
    B. The membrane is selectively permeable only to the potassium ion.
    C. The Nernst equation basically considers only the relative distribution of potassium ions across the membrane.
    D. The resting potential is basically dependent upon the concentration of sodium but not potassium ions across the membrane.
    E. The Nernst equation fails to account for local changes in temperature that influence the resting membrane potential.

5. To which of the following does the term **all-or-none response** most closely relate?

    A. The resting potential
    B. Increased-conductance presynaptic potentials
    C. Increased-conductance postsynaptic potentials
    D. The generator potential
    E. The action potential

Mechanisms of Synaptic Transmission

Anne B. Theibert

OBJECTIVES

After studying this chapter, the student should be able to:

- Define neurotransmission types: synaptic and volume transmission.
- Distinguish synaptic transmission at electrical and chemical synapses.
- Identify the morphologic features of chemical synapses.
- Categorize the different types of neurotransmitters (NTs).
- Diagram the mechanisms of NT synthesis, storage. and release.
- Describe the types of NT receptors and their functions.
- Compare and contrast fast/direct and slow/neuromodulatory synaptic transmission.
- Diagram the mechanisms for NT removal from the synapse.
- Illustrate how synaptic transmission responses are integrated.
- Explain how volume transmission can influence neuronal function.
- Identify psychoactive drug targets in neurotransmission.

OVERVIEW OF NEUROTRANSMISSION & SYNAPTIC TRANSMISSION

Neurotransmission includes the processes by which neural cells communicate with other neural or target cells. The term *neurotransmission* is often used synonymously with *synaptic transmission*, where a neuron communicates with its target cell at a specialized junction called the synapse. Classical synaptic transmission is also called wiring or point-to-point or wired transmission, and involves neurotransmitter (NT) release by a presynaptic neuron and generation of a rapid response in the target cell. However, neurotransmission and synaptic transmission are much more complex than originally envisioned. Neurotransmission includes both synaptic/wiring and volume transmission. In volume transmission, signaling molecules, called neuromodulators, released by neuronal, glial, or endothelial cells into the extracellular fluid (ECF) or cerebrospinal fluid (CSF), undergo short- or long-distance diffusion and activate receptors found on many regions of neural cells. Synaptic/wiring transmission includes both fast/direct electrical responses and also slow/indirect responses called neuromodulation that produce short-term changes in membrane

potential and long-term changes in metabolism, excitability, and gene expression, as well as feedback to the presynaptic axon.

Synaptic transmission mediates many different effects, from the generation of electrical responses in target neurons, to activation of muscle contraction, to secretion of hormones from glands. Investigated for over a century, synaptic transmission is a major focus of basic and clinical neuroscience research today. Errors in synaptic transmission have been implicated in many nervous system disorders. In addition, dynamic and long-term changes in synaptic transmission, called synaptic plasticity, have been proposed to underlie learning and memory. This chapter will concentrate primarily on synaptic transmission but also highlights several current concepts in volume transmission and how synaptic activities during neurotransmission can be integrated.

As described in the previous chapters, the output signal from most neurons is the action potential (AP), an electrical signal that is conducted along the axon to the presynaptic terminus or bouton. In some special sensory neurons that lack axons, the output signal is a graded potential. All synapses possess a gap, between 20 and 40 nm in diameter, called the synaptic cleft. Two different mechanisms are used by neurons to transmit the presynaptic signal to the postsynaptic target. At electrical synapses, the presynaptic and postsynaptic membranes are connected by gap junction channels, where the presynaptic current flows directly to the postsynaptic neuron. At chemical synapses, depolarization of the presynaptic terminus induces release of NTs, which diffuse across the synaptic cleft and bind to and activate receptors on the postsynaptic cell, producing electrical and other responses. In the mammalian nervous system, chemical synapses are much more common than electrical synapses and have been studied extensively for their roles underlying nervous system function and dysfunction.

In the CNS, chemical synapses occur between a presynaptic axon and another neuron. In the PNS, a chemical synapse occurs between a neuron and its target muscle or gland cell and is often called a junction. Synaptic transmission at chemical synapses involves common features. NTs are packaged into vesicles. Depolarization of the presynaptic terminus increases the presynaptic $[Ca^{2+}]$, which induces fusion of vesicles, releasing NTs into the cleft. NTs diffuse across the cleft, bind to NT receptors, and induce a response in the postsynaptic cell. Following release, NT is rapidly removed or degraded at the cleft to terminate synaptic transmission.

NT receptors convert the NT signal into a response in the postsynaptic cell. Responses depend on the NT released, the type of receptor that detects the NT, as well as the cellular context, and can be excitatory, inhibitory, or modulatory (hereafter neuromodulatory), with a short-term or long-lasting time course. In general, the flow of information proceeds from the presynaptic neuron to the postsynaptic cell, although several types of feedback mechanisms can provide information back to the presynaptic neuron. Axons are often branched, where branches transmit signals to many neurons that may be connected in elaborate networks called neural circuits. Neurons can receive inputs from many thousands of synapses, and responses are integrated to determine whether the postsynaptic neuron generates an AP. The common mechanisms and general features of synaptic transmission are described in this chapter. In the next 2 chapters, individual NT systems, NT receptors, and responses are discussed in greater detail.

TYPES AND FEATURES OF SYNAPTIC TRANSMISSION

The simplest and fastest type of synaptic transmission occurs at electrical synapses (Figure 7–1). Discovered in invertebrates where they are involved in escape and defense responses, electrical synapses have been identified in the mammalian hypothalamus, retina, and hippocampus, where they are proposed to synchronize groups of neurons. In an electrical synapse, the synaptic cleft contains 1 or more domains where the presynaptic and postsynaptic plasma membranes are closely apposed (~3–4 nm), forming a gap junction. Gap junctions interconnect many types of cells in the body and contain gap junction channels. In electrical synapses, a transmembrane protein complex called a connexon in the presynaptic membrane binds

a connexon in the postsynaptic membrane, forming the gap junction channel that connects the cytoplasm of the 2 cells. These connexon channels allow current (ions) and second messengers to flow directly from the presynaptic to the postsynaptic neuron and vice versa. Because small ions diffuse rapidly, there is only a short delay (~0.1 millisecond) between the presynaptic and postsynaptic responses. Although extremely rapid, synaptic transmission at electrical synapses has limitations. Signaling is restricted to the small gap junction regions, and since there is no gain or conversion, the postsynaptic response is always smaller than and the same sign as the presynaptic response.

Chemical synapses are the most abundant synapses in the adult mammalian nervous system, and therefore, the rest of this chapter will focus primarily on transmission at chemical synapses. Morphologically, chemical synapses are distinguished by the presence of the synaptic cleft; presynaptic vesicles near the active zones, which are the sites of NT release; and postsynaptic membrane specializations. Many chemical synapses contain extracellular matrix proteins in the cleft, and transmembrane proteins expressed by the presynaptic neuron can bind partners across the synapse on the postsynaptic cell. In chemical synapses, the presynaptic electrical signal is converted into a chemical signal (the NT), which binds to postsynaptic receptors and produces a response in the postsynaptic cell, often an electrical signal. Because there are several biochemical steps, synaptic transmission is slower at chemical synapses, involving a delay of between approximately 0.5 and 3.0 milliseconds. However, the advantage of having biochemical steps is that chemical synapses are more adaptable. The response can be boosted, the sign of the electrical response can be inverted, responses can involve second messengers, and responses can be short term or long lasting.

Two major types of transmission can occur at chemical synapses (Figure 7–2). Fast/direct synaptic transmission involves NT binding to ionotropic receptors that leads to rapid changes in the postsynaptic membrane potential. Slow/indirect transmission (also called neuromodulation) involves NT binding to metabotropic receptors, leading to activation of G proteins and second messengers that can modulate ion channels and/or produce long-lasting changes in metabolism, excitability, and gene expression. Many NTs function in both types of transmission because neurons express both ionotropic and metabotropic receptors for that NT, whereas other NTs act through only metabotropic receptors. In this chapter, the terms *neuromodulator* and *neuromodulation* apply to signaling molecules, cascades, and effects that involve metabotropic receptors. Although many neuromodulators are released at synapses and are therefore classified as conventional NTs, many other classes of neuromodulators have been identified, including unconventional NTs, neurohormones, growth and trophic factors, immune mediators, and neurosteroids. Many neuromodulators can also be released from other regions of neurons, glial cells, or endothelial cells and function as retrograde messengers or in volume transmission (see later section titled "Volume Transmission").

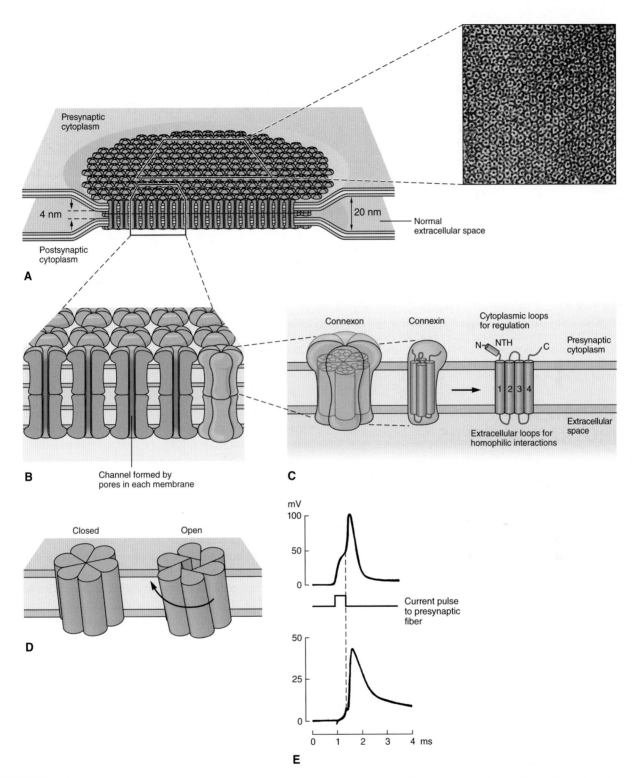

FIGURE 7–1 An electrical synapse and electrical synaptic transmission. **A.** An electrical synapse is composed of multiple gap junction channels. The array of channels shown in the electron micrograph (right) was isolated from the membrane of rat liver. Magnification × 307,800. **B.** A GAP junction channel is formed by a pair of hemichannels, one in each apposite cell that connects the cytoplasm of the two cells. **C.** Each hemichannel, or connexon, is made up of six identical subunits called connexins. **D.** The connexins are arranged in such a way that a pore is formed in the center of the structure. The resulting connexon, with a pore diameter of approximately 1.5 to 2 nm, has a characteristic hexagonal outline. In some gap junction channels the pore is opened when the subunits rotate approximately 0.9 nm at the cytoplasmic base in a clockwise direction. **E.** Transmission at an electrical synapse is nearly instantaneous, with the postsynaptic response following presynaptic stimulation in a fraction of a millisecond. The dashed line shows how the responses of the two cells correspond in time. (Part C, reproduced with permission from Kandel ER, Schwartz JH, Jessell TM, et al: *Principles of Neural Science*, 5th ed. New York, NY: McGraw Hill; 2013.)

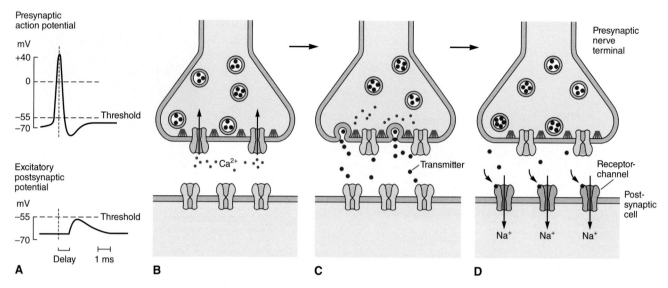

FIGURE 7–2   Synaptic transmission at a chemical synapse. **A.** At chemical synapses there is a short delay between the pre- and postsynaptic potentials. **B.** An action potential arriving at the presynaptic terminus causes voltage-gated Ca^{2+} channels to open. Gray filaments represent the active zone. **C.** The Ca^{2+} channel opening produces a high concentration of intracellular Ca^{2+} near the active zone, causing synaptic vesicles to fuse with the presynaptic cell membrane and release NT into the synaptic cleft. **D.** NTs diffuse across the cleft and bind specific receptors on the postsynaptic membrane. An ionotropic receptor is depicted. (Reproduced with permission from Kandel ER, Schwartz JH, Jessell TM, et al: *Principles of Neural Science,* 5th ed. New York, NY: McGraw Hill; 2013.)

CATEGORIES OF NEUROTRANSMITTERS

Acetylcholine was the first diffusible molecule discovered to function in mediating synaptic transmission. In the decades after that discovery, the following criteria were developed for defining a chemical as an NT. The chemical must be endogenously synthesized or present at the presynaptic neuron. When a neuron is electrically stimulated, the chemical must be released and produce a response in its target cell. The response must be mimicked by exogenous application of the chemical, and the chemical must be endogenously removed at the synapse. By these criteria, conventional NTs were identified and include small-molecule NTs and neuropeptides (NPs). Conventional NTs are packaged into vesicles, are released by the presynaptic neuron, and bind to receptors on the target cell. A brief overview of conventional NTs is provided here.

Conventional small-molecules NTs (Figure 7–3) can be grouped into 3 main categories based on their chemistry: the amines, which include acetylcholine and the monoamines (MAs), the amino acids, and the purines. The MAs include dopamine, norepinephrine, epinephrine, serotonin, and histamine. The amino acid NTs are glutamate, aspartate, γ-aminobutyric acid (GABA), and glycine. Adenosine triphosphate (ATP) and adenosine compose the purines. In the peripheral nervous system (PNS), acetylcholine is released by somatic and preganglionic autonomic motor neurons and produces excitatory responses. Postganglionic parasympathetic neurons use acetylcholine. In the central nervous system (CNS), a few populations of cholinergic neurons are present in the basal forebrain, which have neuromodulatory functions in memory, arousal, and reward. Glutamate is the most abundant

NT in the CNS and mediates the majority of fast excitatory synaptic transmission in the CNS. GABA and glycine are the NTs that produce fast inhibitory synaptic transmission in the CNS. In the CNS, MAs are produced by subsets of neurons whose cell bodies are located primarily in the brainstem and produce neuromodulatory responses important in cognition, emotion, and behavior. In the PNS, postganglionic sympathetic neurons use norepinephrine as their NT. The purine adenosine has a central role in sleep. More detailed information about specific NTs is provided in the next 2 chapters, Chapters 8 and 9, on neurotransmitter systems.

Small-molecule NTs are synthesized and packaged into small (~40 to 50 nm) synaptic vesicles at the presynaptic terminus. Synaptic vesicle lipid and transmembrane components are synthesized by the smooth and rough endoplasmic reticulum (ER) in the cell body and transported to the presynaptic terminus via fast axonal transport. At the presynaptic terminus, synaptic vesicles are generated by a specialized endosome called the synaptic endosome. Small-molecule NTs are synthesized by enzymes at the presynaptic terminus from readily available precursors and involve 1 or a few steps in their biosynthesis. After synthesis, NTs are transported into synaptic vesicles by vesicular NT transporters. A type of secondary active transporter, vesicular NT transporters are selective for their specific category of NT and use the H^+ gradient produced by the H^+ ATPase to transport NT into the vesicle. Once filled, distinct pools of synaptic vesicles, the readily releasable, recycling, and resting pools, are located in the presynaptic terminus.

The other group of conventional NTs, NPs, are synthesized as precursors in the cell body in the rough ER, traffic through the Golgi, are packaged into secretory vesicles at the trans-Golgi network (TGN), and are transported via fast

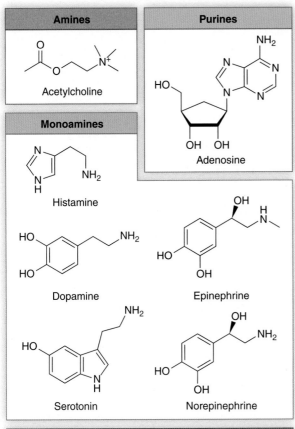

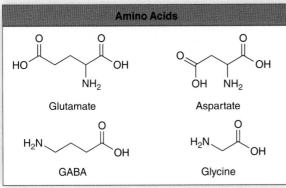

FIGURE 7–3 Conventional small molecule neurotransmitters. GABA, γ-aminobutyric acid.

chemistry, such as opioid peptides. Many NPs are co-released with a small-molecule NT, and subpopulations of neurons can be distinguished by the specific NPs they coexpress with their small-molecule NT. Implicated in responses ranging from analgesia, to food intake, to reproductive and social behaviors, NPs produce slow/indirect neuromodulatory responses in neurons.

Over the past few decades, another category of NTs, the unconventional NTs, has been identified. Unconventional NTs are also considered neuromodulators and include the gasotransmitters, such as nitric oxide (NO), carbon monoxide, and hydrogen sulfide (H_2S), and lipid metabolites, such as the endocannabinoids. Unconventional transmitters are not packaged into vesicles or released by exocytosis. Rather, they are rapidly synthesized or released during synaptic transmission, in many cases in response to a conventional NT. Because hydrophobic molecules can diffuse directly across the plasma membrane, unconventional NTs can interact with protein targets in the presynaptic or postsynaptic neuron and function to modulate synaptic transmission. Unconventional NTs are also candidate retrograde messengers, molecules proposed to provide feedback to the presynaptic terminus about activity in its postsynaptic neuron, and neuromodulators in volume transmission.

CHEMICAL SYNAPTIC TRANSMISSION: MECHANISM OF NEUROTRANSMITTER RELEASE

An AP arrives at the presynaptic terminus, or the presynaptic neuron produces a graded potential in response to a sensory stimulus (Figure 7–5). In both cases, depolarization activates voltage-gated (VG) Ca^{2+} channels. VG Ca^{2+} channels are structurally related to VG Na^+ and VG K^+ channels, which contain a voltage sensor transmembrane domain that moves in response to depolarization and pore-forming domains that allow Ca^{2+} ions to move through the channel, down its electrochemical gradient. The N and P/Q types of VG Ca^{2+} channel genes function in the presynaptic terminus. The threshold to activate the VG Ca^{2+} channels is between −45 and −40 mV. The large depolarization produced by the AP is sufficient to activate the VG Ca^{2+} channels, which are localized to a presynaptic region called the active zone. When Ca^{2+} enters the presynaptic neuron, it forms a Ca^{2+} microdomain around the active zone, where the $[Ca^{2+}]$ is relatively high (about 10 μM). The active zone is also the region where a number of synaptic vesicles are docked close to the plasma membrane.

The increase in presynaptic $[Ca^{2+}]$ stimulates the fusion of docked synaptic vesicles with the presynaptic membrane, via a process called exocytosis, followed by NT release into the synaptic cleft. The fusion of synaptic vesicles requires SNARE proteins found on both the synaptic vesicle membrane (v-SNAREs) and presynaptic plasma membrane (t-SNAREs) (Figure 7–6). Following the activation of VG Ca^{2+} channels, the influx of Ca^{2+} is detected by a Ca^{2+} binding protein, a Ca^{2+} sensor on the synaptic vesicle called synaptotagmin. When

axonal transport to the presynaptic terminus (Figure 7–4). In some neurons, NP-containing secretory vesicles are called dense core granules (~100 to 150 nm in diameter) because of their appearance in electron microscopy. NP precursors are packaged together with peptidases at the TGN, which cleave the precursors during maturation as the vesicles travel along the axon. At the presynaptic terminus, NP-containing vesicles are localized farther away from the active zones, which impacts the requirements for exocytosis and release of NPs (Table 7–1). Approximately 100 NPs have been identified and can be classified based on their locations, such as the brain–gastrointestinal peptides and hypothalamic peptides, or their

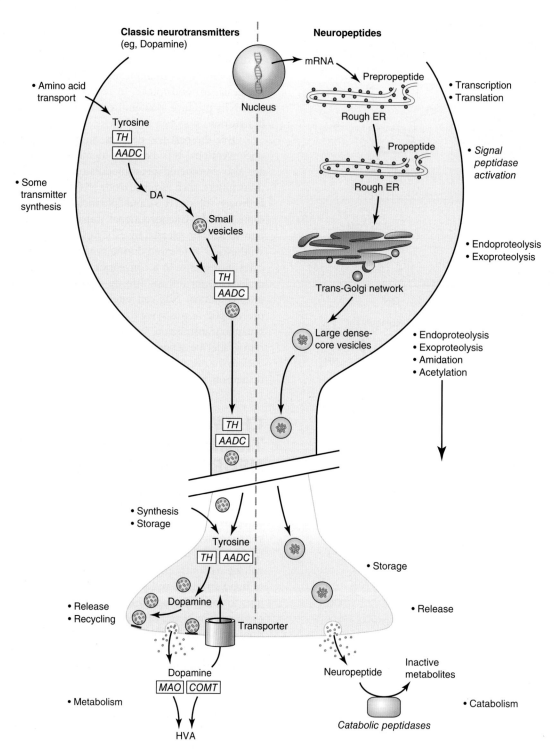

FIGURE 7–4 Comparison between conventional small molecule and neuropeptide (NP) neurotransmitter (NT) in synthesis, release, and removal. A dopaminergic neuron is used for illustration. The majority of dopamine is synthesized in the axon terminal and transported into synaptic vesicles. In contrast, NP synthesis occurs in the cell body in the rough ER. NPs are packaged into secretory or dense core granules in the Golgi, and maturation occurs in vesicles as they are transported down the axon. Small molecule NTs are typically released close to the active zone while NPs are often released far from the active zone. Dopamine is transported back into the nerve terminal whereas NPs are not. AADC, aromatic amino acid decarboxylase; COMT, catechol-*O*-methyltransferase; DA, dopamine; ER, endoplasmic reticulum; HVA, homovanillic acid; MAO, monoamine oxidase; TH, tyrosine hydroxylase. (Reproduced with permission from Nestler EJ, Hyman SE, Holtzman DM, et al: *Molecular Neuropharmacology: A Foundation for Clinical Neuroscience*, 3rd ed. New York, NY: McGraw Hill; 2015.)

TABLE 7–1 Examples of co-localization of small-molecule transmitters with neuropeptides.

Small-Molecule Transmitter	Neuropeptide
Glutamate	Substance P
GABA	Cholecystokinin, enkephalin, somatostatin, substance P, thyrotropin-releasing hormone
Glycine	Neurotensin
Acetylcholine	Calcitonin gene-related protein, enkephalin, galanin, gonadotropin-releasing hormone, neurotensin, somatostatin, substance P, vasoactive intestinal polypeptide
Dopamine	Cholecystokinin, enkephalin, neurotensin
Norepinephrine	Enkephalin, neuropeptide Y, neurotensin, somatostatin, vasopressin
Epinephrine	Enkephalin, neuropeptide Y, neurotensin, substance P
Serotonin	Cholecystokinin, enkephalin, neuropeptide Y, substance P, vasoactive intestinal polypeptide

GABA, γ-aminobutyric acid.

Reproduced with permission from Barrett KE, Barman SM, Brooks HL et al: *Ganong's Review of Medical Physiology*, 26th ed. New York, NY: McGraw Hill; 2019.

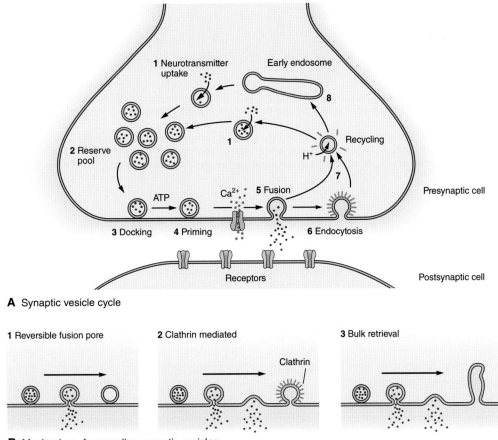

A Synaptic vesicle cycle

B Mechanisms for recycling synaptic vesicles

FIGURE 7–5 Mechanism of synaptic transmission at chemical synapses and the synaptic vesicle cycle. **A.** Synaptic vesicles are filled with NT by vesicular NT transporters (step 1) and join the reserve pool (step 2). Synaptic vesicles dock at the active zone (step 3) where they undergo a priming reaction (step 4) that makes them competent for Ca2+ stimulated fusion (step 5). After releasing NT, synaptic vesicles are recycled (see part B) via clathrin-mediated endocytosis (step 6), directly (step 7) or by synaptic endosomes (step 8). **B.** Retrieval of vesicles after NT release can occur via three mechanisms. 1. A reversible fusion pore is the most rapid mechanism where the synaptic vesicle membrane does not completely fuse with the plasma membrane and NT is released through the fusion pore. 2. In the classical pathway excess membrane is retrieved through endocytosis by means of clathrin-coated pits. 3. In the bulk retrieval pathway, excess membrane reenters the terminal by budding from uncoated pits at the active zones.

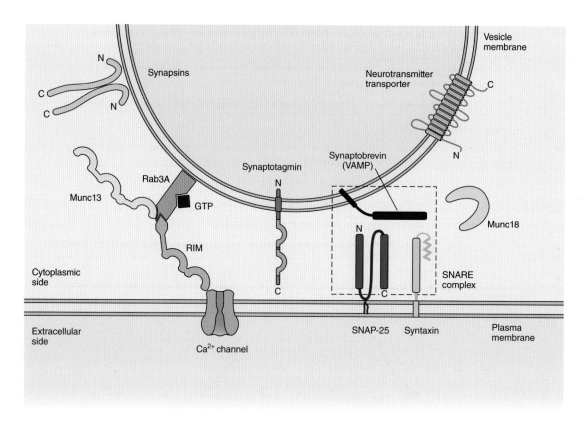

FIGURE 7-6   Proteins involved in synaptic vesicle exocytosis. Synaptic vesicles contain vesicular NT transporters necessary for NT uptake. Exocytosis is mediated by the formation of the SNARE complex (dotted lines), which results from the tight interaction between the protein synaptobrevin (VAMP) in the vesicle membrane and the proteins syntaxin and SNAP-25 in the plasma membrane. The vesicle protein synaptotagmin serves as the Ca^{2+} sensor for exocytosis. When Ca^{2+} binds to synaptotagmin, it interacts with the SNARE complex and Munc 18 to induce synaptic vesicle fusion and exocytosis. Other key synaptic vesicle proteins are involved in regulating vesicle docking at the active zone or interactions among the SNARE complex proteins. (Reproduced with permission from Kandel ER, Schwartz JH, Jessell TM, et al: *Principles of Neural Science*, 5th ed. New York, NY: McGraw Hill; 2013.)

Ca^{2+} binds to synaptotagmin, this enhances the interaction between the v-SNAREs and t-SNAREs, forming the trans-SNARE complex that brings the synaptic vesicle in close proximity to the plasma membrane, allowing the membranes to fuse, and inducing exocytosis of the synaptic vesicle. Many neurotoxins work by targeting SNARE protein components. For example, botulinum toxin is a proteolytic enzyme, and tetanus toxin is an endopeptidase, and each toxin cleaves a specific SNARE protein. By preventing the normal release of NT or synaptic vesicle recycling, these toxins result in poor muscle control, spasms, paralysis, and even death.

During fusion, the inside of the synaptic vesicle gains access to the ECF, and NTs quickly diffuse into the synaptic cleft. Synaptic vesicles can undergo partial or full fusion with the presynaptic membrane. In partial fusion, also called kiss-and-run, the synaptic vesicle membrane only transiently fuses with the presynaptic plasma membrane, and then is rapidly taken back in to reform an intact synaptic vesicle, which will be refilled with NT. In full fusion, also called full collapse, the synaptic vesicle fuses completely with plasma membrane. Following full fusion, patches of presynaptic plasma membrane undergo endocytosis to form endocytic vesicles that fuse with the synaptic endosome, where new synaptic vesicles will be

generated and then refilled with NT. This recycling of synaptic vesicles is crucial for normal synaptic transmission.

Exocytosis of docked synaptic vesicles and release of NT are extremely fast because VG Ca^{2+} channels are colocalized with the docked synaptic vesicles at the active zones. After docked vesicles fuse, the increased presynaptic $[Ca^{2+}]$ also enhances the mobilization of additional synaptic vesicles in the readily releasable pool, so they can dock at the membrane and undergo exocytosis. Multiple mechanisms are present in the presynaptic terminus that rapidly extrude or sequester Ca^{2+}, so the Ca^{2+} microdomains are small and transient when a single AP arrives at the presynaptic terminus. However, if a high-frequency train of APs arrives at the presynaptic terminus, the VG Ca^{2+} channels will be activated and open until the AP train ceases. The increased Ca^{2+} influx produces larger Ca^{2+} microdomains that extend farther into the presynaptic terminus for longer periods of time, inducing more synaptic vesicle fusion and NT release. As a result, information encoded in the frequency, number, and/or pattern of presynaptic APs can be translated into the magnitude, duration, and/or pattern of NT release by the presynaptic neuron.

Similar to synaptic vesicles, NP release by secretory vesicle exocytosis also involves the Ca^{2+} sensor synaptotagmin and SNARE proteins. However, secretory vesicles are located much farther way from the active zones. Consequently, fusion of secretory vesicles and release of NPs require larger Ca²⁺ microdomains that extend farther into the presynaptic terminus. As described, the production of large Ca²⁺ microdomains requires high-frequency trains of AP and time to develop. Therefore, release of NPs requires greater presynaptic stimulation than does the release of small-molecule NTs. In addition, NP release is slower and usually occurs outside the active zones, in some cases releasing NP outside the synaptic cleft.

CHEMICAL SYNAPTIC TRANSMISSION: NEUROTRANSMITTER RECEPTORS

Following their release, NTs diffuse across the cleft, bind to receptors, and activate responses in the postsynaptic cell. Over 100 different NT receptor genes have been identified, which fall into 2 main functional categories: the ionotropic and metabotropic receptors (Figure 7–7). Ionotropic receptors are also called ligand-gated or NT-gated ion channels. Metabotropic receptors, so called because they produce metabolic effects, are G-protein–coupled receptors. Both receptor types bind their ligands reversibly and with high affinity and specificity, but they use different mechanisms to produce postsynaptic responses. Ionotropic receptors mediate fast/direct synaptic transmission. Metabotropic receptors mediate slow/indirect synaptic transmission, also called modulatory transmission or neuromodulation. Many small-molecule NTs, including acetylcholine, glutamate, GABA, serotonin, and purines, bind to and activate receptors in both receptor categories and, therefore, can mediate fast/direct and slow/indirect neuromodulatory synaptic transmission. Other NTs, such as norepinephrine, epinephrine, dopamine, and histamine, as well as all the NPs, activate only metabotropic receptors and, therefore, function in slow/indirect neuromodulatory transmission.

Ionotropic receptors contain both an extracellular ligand binding domain and a transmembrane ion channel domain.

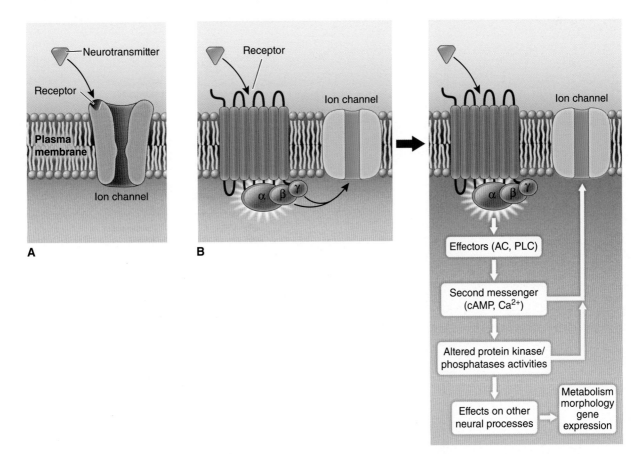

FIGURE 7–7 Two types of neurotransmitter receptors. **A.** Ionotropic receptors are ligand-gated channels that contain both an NT binding domain and an integral ion channel domain. Most ionotropic receptors are composed of four or five subunits. **B.** Metabotropic receptors are composed of a single subunit with seven membrane-spanning α-helical regions that bind the ligand and activate an associated G protein. G proteins can directly modulate ion channels (panel B left) or activate an effector (panel B right) such as AC or PLC. G protein effectors activate second-messengers, which can regulate ion channels directly, or control protein kinases and phosphates that modulate phosphorylation of ion channels, receptors, metabolic enzymes, cytoskeletal proteins, and/or proteins that control gene expression. AC, adenylyl cyclase; cAMP, cyclic adenosine monophosphate; PLC, phospholipase C.

In ionotropic receptors, the channel is closed in the absence of NT. Binding of NT induces a conformational change, opening the channel. After the NT binds, it dissociates, leading to closing of the channel. By opening ion channels, ionotropic receptors conduct ionic currents that produce fast/direct changes in the membrane potential. In neurons, NT-mediated depolarization responses produced by Na^+ influx are called excitatory postsynaptic potentials (EPSPs) because they bring the membrane potential toward threshold for generating an AP. Hyperpolarization responses produced by Cl^- influx are called inhibitory postsynaptic potentials (IPSPs) because they move the potential away from threshold for firing an AP. In skeletal muscle, the response is called an end-plate potential (EPP) and is a large depolarization. In addition to producing changes in membrane potentials, some ionotropic receptors allow Ca^{2+} to flow into the postsynaptic cell, which, acting as a second messenger, regulates proteins that control metabolism, morphology, and gene expression.

Distinguishable by their morphology, synapses that mediate EPSPs are called Gray type I synapses, whereas those that produce IPSPs are called Gray type II synapses (Figures 7–8 and 7–9). In general, Gray type I synapses are excitatory and glutamatergic, contain round synaptic vesicles

in electron microscopy (EM) analysis, and are asymmetric with an electron-dense region at the presynaptic membrane and an even larger dense region in the postsynaptic membrane called the postsynaptic density (PSD). Gray type II synapses are usually inhibitory and GABAergic, contain oval or flattened synaptic vesicles in EM micrographs, and are symmetric with less obvious presynaptic and PSD membrane specializations.

Metabotropic receptors bind NTs and activate G proteins, called heterotrimeric G proteins, composed of an α, β, and γ subunit. When a metabotropic receptor binds its NT, it stimulates the binding of guanosine triphosphate (GTP) to the α subunit and dissociation of the α subunit–GTP from the β/γ subunit. Both the α–GTP and β/γ subunits activate specific effector proteins, including ion channels and enzymes that produce second messengers. Second messengers such as cyclic adenosine monophosphate (cAMP) regulate downstream signaling pathways, most involving protein kinases. Because they require G proteins and second messenger pathways, metabotropic receptors mediate slow/indirect synaptic transmission. Second messenger pathways can lead to the regulation of ion channels, with resulting slow changes in membrane potential, as well as modulation of neuronal morphology, metabolism,

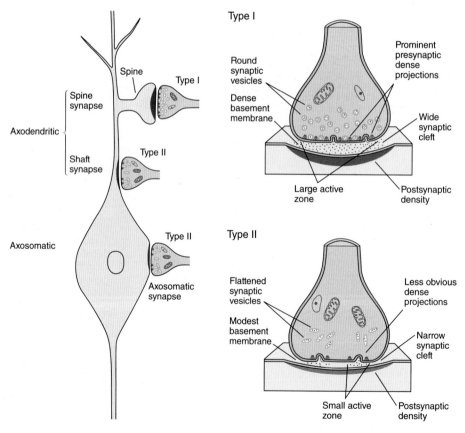

FIGURE 7–8 Localization and morphology of type I and type II synapses. Type I synapses are typically excitatory glutamatergic synapses. Type II synapses are typically GABAergic or glycinergic inhibitory synapses. Type I synapses characteristically form on dendritic spines and less commonly contact the shafts of dendrites. Type II synapses often contact the cell body and dendritic shaft. Differences include the shape of vesicles, prominence of presynaptic densities, total area of the active zone, width of the synaptic cleft, and presence of a dense basement membrane. (Reproduced with permission from Kandel ER, Schwartz JH, Jessell TM, et al: *Principles of Neural Science*, 5th ed. New York, NY: McGraw Hill; 2013.)

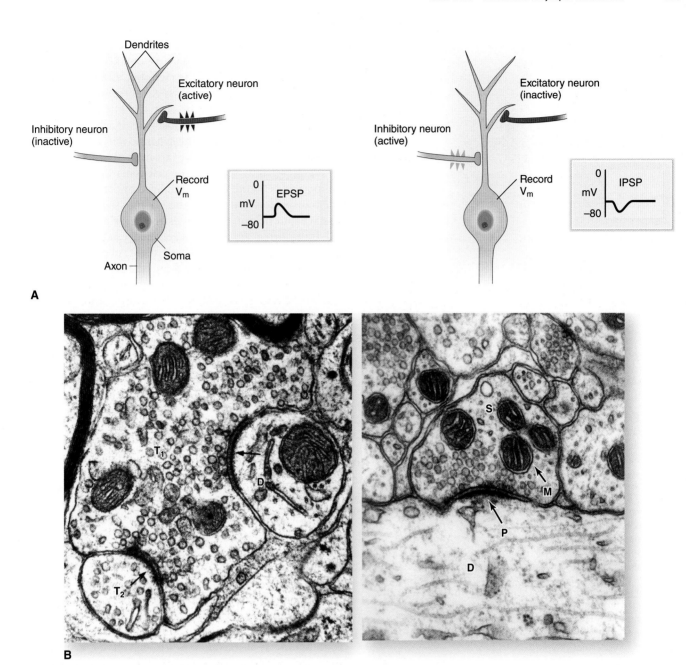

FIGURE 7–9 Electrical responses and ultrastructure of excitatory and inhibitory synapses. **A.** An input from an excitatory neuron leads to an excitatory postsynaptic potential (EPSP), which is a depolarization. Input from an inhibitory neuron causes an inhibitory postsynaptic potential (IPSP), which is a hyperpolarization. **B.** (Left panel) Electron micrograph showing a large excitatory (type I) asymmetric synapse with a presynaptic terminal (T$_1$) filled with synaptic vesicles close to the 20- to 30-nm-wide synaptic clefts (arrows). The postsynaptic membrane is part of a dendrite (D), with a large postsynaptic density suggesting this is an excitatory axodendritic synapse. Another presynaptic terminal (T$_2$) suggests an axoaxonic synapse with a role in modulating activity of the other terminal. (X35,000). (Right panel) An electron micrograph of a presynaptic ending (S) on the shaft of a dendrite (D) in the CNS. The asymmetrical synapse also suggests a type I synapse. P, postsynaptic density; M, mitochondrion (×56,000). (Part A, reproduced with permission from Kibble JD, Halsey CR. *Medical Physiology: The Big Picture*. New York, NY: McGraw Hill; 2009; part B (left), reproduced with permission from Mescher AL. *Junqueira's Basic Histology: Text & Atlas*, 15th ed. New York, NY: McGraw Hill; 2018; part B (right), reproduced with permission from Barrett KE, Barman SM, Brooks HL et al: *Ganong's Review of Medical Physiology*, 26th ed. New York, NY: McGraw Hill; 2019.)

and/or gene expression. Thus, metabotropic receptors mediate neuromodulatory responses.

Numerous NTs function through activation of both ionotropic and metabotropic NT receptors, and at many synapses, both receptor types are coexpressed. Consequently, fast/direct and slow/indirect postsynaptic responses can be produced at the same synapse. Ionotropic receptors are often concentrated directly across from the presynaptic active zones, whereas metabotropic receptors can be localized in the synapse and also in the perisynaptic and extrasynaptic regions (Figure 7–10). Both ionotropic and metabotropic receptors can be located at the presynaptic membrane as well. Often referred to as

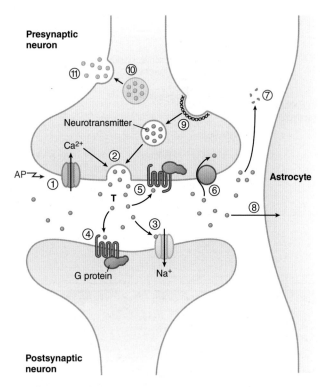

FIGURE 7–10 Summary of the stages of synaptic transmission. Depolarization by the action potential opens voltage-gated Ca²⁺ channels in the presynaptic terminus (1). The influx of Ca²⁺ triggers (2) the exocytosis of synaptic vesicles. Released neurotransmitter (T) interacts with postsynaptic ionotropic receptors which affect the membrane potential (3) or metabotropic receptors which function through G proteins (4). Ionotropic and metabotropic receptors in the presynaptic membrane (5) can inhibit or enhance subsequent exocytosis. Released neurotransmitter is inactivated by uptake into the presynaptic neuron (6), degradation (7) or by (8) uptake and metabolism by nearby astrocytes (glutamate). The synaptic vesicle membrane is recycled by endocytosis (9). Neuropeptides are stored in (10) larger, secretory/dense core granules within the nerve terminal, which can be released from sites (11) distinct from active zones after repetitive stimulation. (Reproduced with permission from Brunton LL, Hilal-Dandan R, Knollmann BC: *Goodman & Gilman's the Pharmacological Basis of Therapeutics*, 13th ed. New York, NY: McGraw Hill; 2018.)

autoreceptors, presynaptic receptors provide feedback to the presynaptic neuron about NT levels at the synapse. NPs can be released from secretory vesicles at the presynaptic terminus and from regions farther away from the synapse. In addition, after some NTs are released, they can diffuse out of the synapse into the ECF. As a result, NPs and small-molecule NTs in the ECF can influence not only the postsynaptic region, but also other nearby synapses, neurons, and astrocytes that express receptors for those NTs. This type of communication is considered volume transmission (see later section titled "Volume Transmission").

NEUROTRANSMITTER REMOVAL: UPTAKE & DEGRADATION

The time during which the NT is present at the cleft is critical in determining the magnitude and duration of the postsynaptic response. NT is cleared from the synaptic cleft by both passive diffusion and active uptake or inactivation. All NTs can diffuse out of the cleft, but different NTs have different mechanisms for their specific removal at the cleft. Acetylcholine is degraded by acetylcholine esterase localized within the synaptic cleft. Likewise, inactivation of NPs involves endopeptidases in the synaptic cleft. Consequently, acetylcholine and NPs must be replenished by new synthesis in the presynaptic terminus or cell soma, respectively. All amino acid NTs and MAs are removed by plasma membrane NT transporters that uptake the NT into the presynaptic or postsynaptic neuron or nearby astrocytes. Plasma membrane NT transporters are a type of secondary active transporter that depend on the Na⁺ and Cl⁻ gradients to drive the uptake of NT. NTs that are transported into the presynaptic neuron can be directly reincorporated into synaptic vesicles. NTs that are transported into nearby astrocytes are converted to intermediates, which are then shuttled back to nearby neurons.

SUMMATION OF POSTSYNAPTIC RESPONSES

Most CNS neurons receive thousands of inputs from synapses, located throughout the neuron, on dendrites, dendritic spines, the cell soma, and axons, with different combinations of ionotropic and metabotropic receptor responses. The postsynaptic electrical signals are integrated to produce a simple output, the AP, by the postsynaptic neuron. Integration and transformation of synaptic inputs to a single neuronal output is a type of neural computation. One of the simplest types of integration is summation (Figure 7–11), the algebraic processing of electrical responses (EPSPs and IPSPs); the brain carries out billions of such neural computations every second. In temporal summation, repeated inputs at the same synapse are summated, whereas in spatial summation, multiple simultaneous inputs from different synapses are summated. Summation occurs continuously at all membranes throughout the neuron, but the place where summation is critical is at the initial segment of the axon, the region where the AP is generated. Thus, the output AP is dependent on both spatial and temporal summation, which are affected by the relative number, magnitude, location, and timing of the excitatory and inhibitory synaptic inputs.

VOLUME TRANSMISSION

The concept of volume transmission was first introduced in the 1980s to explain the mismatch between the localization of NT release sites and their receptors for some brain NT systems, including MAs and several NPs. It is now well established that communication between cells in the CNS is not limited solely to synaptic connections. Volume transmission involves the release of neuromodulators by neuronal, glial, and CNS vascular endothelial cells, which diffuse in the ECF

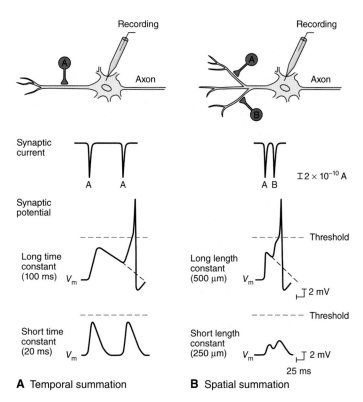

A Temporal summation   **B** Spatial summation

FIGURE 7-11 Integration of postsynaptic responses by temporal and spatial summation. **A.** Temporal summation involves the integration of responses from an individual synapse and depends on the time constant of the response. In a cell with a *long* time constant the first EPSP does not fully decay by the time the second EPSP is triggered. Therefore, the depolarizing effects of both potentials are additive, bringing the membrane potential above the threshold and triggering an action potential. In a cell with a *short* time constant the first EPSP decays to the resting potential before the second EPSP is triggered. The second EPSP alone does not cause enough depolarization to trigger an action potential. **B.** Spatial summation involves integration of responses from different synapses and depends on the location of synapses and length constant of the response. If the distance between the site of synaptic input and the trigger zone in the postsynaptic cell is only one length constant, then summation of the two potentials results in enough depolarization to exceed threshold, triggering an action potential. If the distance between the synapse and the trigger zone is equal to two length constants, summation will not be sufficient to trigger an action potential. (Reproduced with permission from Kandel ER, Schwartz JH, Jessell TM, et al: *Principles of Neural Science*, 5th ed. New York, NY: McGraw Hill; 2013.)

or CSF and activate receptors on nearby or distant neurons. Likewise, neurons, glia, and endothelial cells release other signaling molecules that modulate glial and endothelial functions. Volume transmission in the CNS involves conventional small-molecule and NP NTs, unconventional NTs, neurohormones, neurotrophic factors, immune modulators, and neurosteroids. Thus, volume transmission encompasses a wide variety of chemical signals, cells, and effects, including modulation of synaptic transmission, plasticity, and crosstalk, as well as nonsynaptic neurotransmission, neuronal survival, glial functions, and immune and hemodynamic responses.

In one type of volume transmission, the NT is released by a presynaptic neuron at the synapse, but as a result of high levels of NT release, lower NT uptake, or the morphology of the synapse, NT can diffuse away from the synapse to activate receptors located in regions outside the synapse, nearby neurons, and on glial cells (Figure 7–12). Studied in several brain regions, including the cerebellum and hippocampus, a process called glutamate spillover provides a mechanism for synapses to communicate with other synapses and neurons.

Glutamate spillover from the synapse leads to the activation of metabotropic and ionotropic glutamate receptors located in the presynaptic, perisynaptic, and extrasynaptic membranes of the same and nearby synapses to regulate processes including NT release by both excitatory and inhibitory synapses, neuronal excitability, and possibly even neuronal survival. Glutamate spillover can be impacted by astrocytes and can modulate astrocytes as well (see the next section on Astrocyte Modulation of Neurotransmission).

Besides the enigma of the release/receptor mismatch, another puzzle about MAs is how such a small number of monoaminergic neurons can modulate activities in so many neurons throughout the brain (Figure 7–13). In a similar manner, it has been shown that NPs can regulate activities in groups of neurons acting at some distances from their sites of release. Both MAs and NPs can be released at synapses, but they can also be released from nonsynaptic regions of the axon by dendrites and by the cell soma, meaning they can be released directly into the ECF or CSF. NTs in the ECF are not as rapidly taken up or inactivated as NTs at the synapse. Furthermore, MA and NP receptors are localized to the perisynaptic

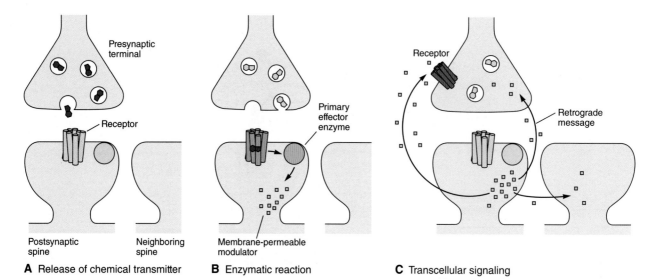

FIGURE 7–12 Retrograde messengers and transcellular signaling in synaptic transmission. **A.** A presynaptic terminal releases NT at the synapse, which activates a metabotropic receptor in a postsynaptic dendritic spine. **B.** The receptor activates enzymes that produce a membrane-permeable modulator. **C.** The modulator is released from the postsynaptic spine and diffuses to neighboring postsynaptic spines as well as presynaptic terminals. In this transcellular signaling, the modulator is called a retrograde messenger and it can produce either first-messenger effects, by acting on receptors in the surface membrane, or second-messenger-like effects, by entering the cell to act within. Ionotropic receptors, such as the NMDA receptor, which increase postsynaptic Ca^{2+} levels, can also activate second messenger cascades that lead to the release of retrograde messengers. (Reproduced with permission from Kandel ER, Schwartz JH, Jessell TM, et al: *Principles of Neural Science*, 5th ed. New York, NY: McGraw Hill; 2013.)

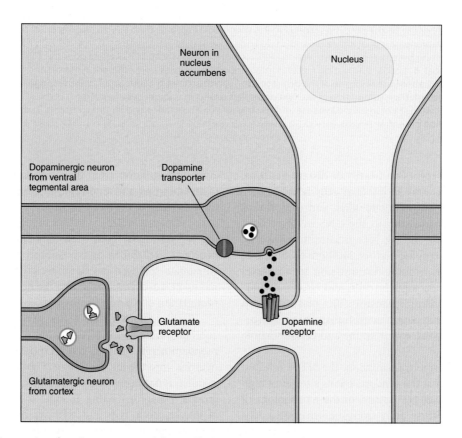

FIGURE 7–13 Monoamines function as neuromodulators. Glutamatergic neurons that transmit sensorimotor information from the cerebral cortex and dopaminergic neurons that transmit reward-related information from the ventral tegmental area form connections with the same medium spiny neurons in the dorsal striatum and nucleus accumbens. The glutamatergic neurons make excitatory synapses on the heads of dendritic spines and the dopaminergic neurons make en passant connections at the necks of spines. (Reproduced with permission from Kandel ER, Schwartz JH, Jessell TM, et al: *Principles of Neural Science*, 5th ed. New York, NY: McGraw Hill; 2013.)

region, nearby synapses, and somatodendritic areas, where these metabotropic receptors typically display higher affinity than ionotropic receptors. Thus, MAs and NPs possess all the features that make them ideal participants in volume transmission for signaling at extrasynaptic regions, at neighboring synapses, and at long distances as well.

Unconventional NTs, such as NO and endocannabinoids, and other hydrophobic signaling molecules, such as prostaglandins and neurosteroids, can function in volume transmission by direct diffusion across membranes and modulation of targets on the cell surface and inside cells. NO and endocannabinoids, which are candidate retrograde messengers at synapses, may also diffuse to nearby synapses and act in volume transmission. NO produced by neurons and prostaglandins (and other arachidonic acid metabolites) produced by astrocytes can also affect vasodilation in vascular endothelial cells and control blood flow. Endocannabinoids bind to presynaptic metabotropic receptors to control NT release. Neurosteroids include a variety of steroids synthesized by neurons and glia and have been implicated in development, neuronal plasticity, cognition, mood control, social and sexual behavior, and myelination. Neurosteroids can affect neuronal excitability and neurotransmission through direct effects on GABA and N-methyl-D-aspartate (NMDA) receptors, in addition to their functions through classic intracellular steroid receptors. Recently, another mechanism involving extracellular vesicles (EVs), including exosomes and shedding vesicles, has been implicated in volume transmission. Molecules released from EVs include proteins, lipids, messenger RNA, microRNA, and mitochondrial DNA. EVs have also been implicated in the spread of neurodegenerative disorders and brain cancer.

ASTROCYTE MODULATION OF NEUROTRANSMISSION

Astrocytes are important support cells for neurons, providing structure and metabolic support. Through their astrocytic end feet, astrocytes take up essential nutrients from the circulation and provide neurons with energy substrates and regulate blood flow. In addition, evidence supports the existence of dynamic, bidirectional, and active regulation of synaptic transmission by astrocytes, which surround the synapse and form what is called the tripartite synapse. By the expression of ion channels and NT transporters, astrocytes can modulate extracellular ionic concentrations, as well as NT levels and duration at the synaptic cleft. Astrocytes also express metabotropic and ionotropic receptors, so they may be affected by NTs released during synaptic transmission at nearby synapses. Astrocytes themselves release signaling molecules called gliotransmitters. In the example in discussed earlier, astrocytes have been implicated in glutamate spillover, through regulation of glutamate levels at the synapse, by providing gliotransmitters such as ATP, and also by being a target of the glutamate spillover by expression of glutamate receptors. Astrocytes may also release neurotropic factors that may contribute to modulation of synaptic transmission and synaptic plasticity.

SYNAPTIC TRANSMISSION IS NOT FIXED, BUT CHANGES VIA SYNAPTIC PLASTICITY

Since the discovery of synaptic transmission, one of the most exciting developments in neuroscience is that synaptic transmission is not fixed, but can change, increasing or decreasing over time. Synaptic transmission is also called synaptic strength, and the process of changing synaptic strength is called synaptic plasticity. Many propose that synaptic plasticity is central to the mechanisms underlying learning and memory. Furthermore, because synaptic plasticity has been documented during development and at synapses throughout the CNS, many sensory, motor, and cognitive systems are expected to involve synaptic plasticity. Accordingly, many types of synaptic plasticity have been identified with different computational functions anticipated. Synaptic plasticity can be short term, lasting a few seconds to minutes, or long term, lasting minutes to hours and longer. Synaptic plasticity can lead to increases in synaptic transmission, called facilitation or potentiation, or decreases in synaptic transmission, called depression. Plasticity depends on the timing of inputs, the history of synaptic activity at the synapse, and in many synapses, the activity in adjacent or neighboring synapses. In this chapter, the description of biochemical mechanisms involved in chemical synaptic transmission highlights presynaptic and postsynaptic mechanisms that can contribute to the induction, expression, and maintenance of synaptic plasticity. In Chapter 10, "Synaptic Plasticity," current ideas about specific types, mechanisms, and functions of synaptic plasticity are described.

NEUROPHARMACOLOGIC TARGETS: SYNAPTIC TRANSMISSION

A psychoactive drug is defined as a chemical substance that changes brain function and results in alterations in perception, mood, consciousness, or behavior. Practically all psychoactive drugs, including both therapeutic drugs and drugs of abuse, exert their effects by targeting components in chemical synaptic transmission (Figure 7–14). Consequently, basic research in synaptic transmission intersects with the field of neuropharmacology, the study of how drugs affect neurons and behavior, with the united goal of developing drugs that produce beneficial effects on neurologic and/or psychiatric functions.

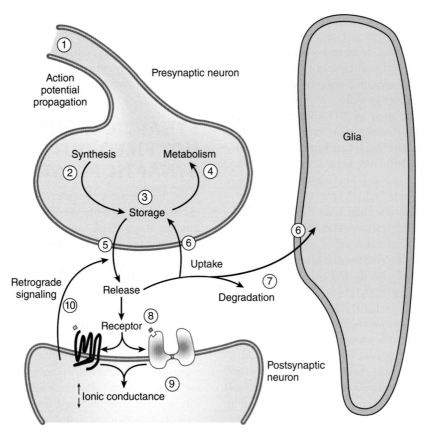

FIGURE 7-14 Sites of psychoactive drug action. Schematic drawing of steps at which drugs can alter synaptic transmission. (1) Action potential in presynaptic axon; (2) synthesis of transmitter; (3) transport of transmitter into synaptic vesicles; (4) metabolism; (5) release; (6) reuptake into the nerve ending or uptake into a glial cell; (7) degradation; (8) receptor for the transmitter; (9) receptor-induced increase or decrease in ionic conductance; (10) retrograde signaling. (Reproduced with permission from Katzung BG: *Basic & Clinical Pharmacology*, 14th ed. New York, NY: McGraw Hill; 2018.)

SUMMARY

- Neurotransmission involves 2 major complementary modes of intercellular communication, namely synaptic transmission and volume transmission.

- In synaptic transmission, also called wiring or point-to-point or wired transmission, communication occurs at the synapse, a specialized junction where neurons signal to their target neuron, muscle, or gland.

- Volume transmission is a widespread type of neural communication where neuromodulators are released into the extracellular fluid or cerebrospinal fluid and affect targets at short or long distances.

- Synaptic transmission at electrical synapses is rapid and involves gap junction channels that mediate the direct flow of current between cells.

- Synaptic transmission at chemical synapses involves NT release, NT binding to receptors, and activation of postsynaptic responses.

- Conventional NTs are small molecules or neuropeptides that are packaged into vesicles and released from the presynaptic neuron.

- Small-molecule NTs are synthesized and packaged into small (~40 to 50 nm) synaptic vesicles in the presynaptic neuron and localized near active zones.

- Neuropeptides are synthesized in secretory vesicles at the cell soma and transported to the presynaptic terminus by fast axonal transport.

- In synaptic transmission, depolarization of the presynaptic membrane activates voltage-gated Ca^{2+} channels and increases presynaptic $[Ca^{2+}]$, which stimulates fusion of synaptic vesicles with the presynaptic plasma membrane by exocytosis, and NT release.

- NTs bind to NT receptors on the postsynaptic membrane.

- Ionotropic NT receptors produce fast excitatory or inhibitory postsynaptic potentials.

- Metabotropic NT receptors activate second messenger pathways that mediate slower changes in postsynaptic potentials and/or excitability, metabolism, gene expression, and morphology, in a process called neuromodulation.

- NTs are removed from the synapse by degradation, inactivation, or uptake, terminating the postsynaptic response.

- Summation of postsynaptic responses determines whether the postsynaptic neuron will fire an action potential.

- Volume transmission involves the release of neuromodulators, including small-molecule NTs, neuropeptides, unconventional NTs, neurotrophic factors, and neurosteroids, which diffuse and activate receptors at extrasynaptic regions, the axon, dendrites, and/or cell soma, producing neuromodulatory responses.

- Astrocytes participate in neurotransmission by removal of NTs, regulation of the extracellular fluid, and release of gliotransmitters.

- Chemical synaptic transmission can be modified in synaptic plasticity, which is a proposed mechanism underlying learning and memory.

- The majority of psychoactive drugs function by targeting components of neurotransmission.

SELF-ASSESSMENT QUESTIONS

1. Which of the following best describes a basic property of synapses in the central nervous system (CNS)?
   A. Synaptic vesicles constitute important features for transmission in both chemical and electrical synapses.
   B. A postsynaptic neuron typically receives input from different presynaptic axons that are either excitatory or inhibitory, but it cannot receive inputs from both types.
   C. Synaptic delay is approximately the same for both chemical and electrical synapses.
   D. Neurotransmitter (NT) receptors can regulate the gating/opening of an ion channel either directly (ionotropic receptor) or indirectly (metabotropic receptor)
   E. The mechanism of indirect gating of ions normally does not involve the activation of G proteins.

2. Which of the following events directly determines the release of NTs from the terminal of the presynaptic neuron?
   A. Activation of voltage-gated Na^+ channels and Na^+ influx
   B. Activation of voltage-gated Na^+ channels and Na^+ efflux
   C. Activation of voltage-gated K^+ channels and K^+ influx
   D. Activation of voltage-gated K^+ channels and K^+ efflux
   E. Activation of voltage-gated Ca^{2+} channels and Ca^{2+} influx

3. The level and duration of NT release are determined predominantly by which of the following?
   A. The magnitude and duration of the presynaptic action potential
   B. The inactivation of the presynaptic voltage-gated Na^+, K^+, and Ca^{2+} channels
   C. The frequency and pattern of presynaptic action potentials
   D. The rate of recycling and refilling of synaptic vesicles
   E. The extent of synaptic delay

4. Which of the following best describes NT removal from the synaptic cleft? NTs are removed by
   A. astrocytic end feet located in nearby capillaries.
   B. channels that open in response to depolarization.
   C. transporters or degradative enzymes.
   D. endocytosis by the presynaptic plasma membrane.
   E. oxidation and diffusion out of the cleft.

5. Following exocytosis, lipids and transmembrane proteins of the synaptic vesicles that fuse with the plasma membrane can be recycled by
   A. endocytosis and trafficking to the early/synaptic endosome.
   B. release into the synaptic cleft and uptake by nearby astrocytes.
   C. secretory trafficking via the rough endoplasmic reticulum and Golgi complex.
   D. degradation through the lysosomal pathway.
   E. trafficking back to the trans-Golgi network (TGN) in the cell soma.

Neurotransmitter Systems I: Acetylcholine & the Amino Acids

CHAPTER

8

Anne B. Theibert

OBJECTIVES

After studying this chapter, the student should be able to:

- Diagram the synthesis, packaging, and degradation of acetylcholine (ACh).
- Distinguish the 2 types of ACh receptors and describe their mechanisms of action.
- Identify the main types and location of cholinergic neurons in the central and peripheral nervous systems.
- Illustrate the mechanisms of glutamate packaging, interconversion with glutamine, and glutamate uptake.
- Describe the different types of ionotropic and metabotropic glutamate receptors and their modes of regulation and function.
- Identify the general types and locations of glutamatergic neurons.
- Diagram the synthesis, packaging, and uptake of γ-aminobutyric acid (GABA) and glycine.
- Identify the locations where GABAergic and glycinergic neurons function.
- Distinguish the types of ionotropic and metabotropic GABA receptors and the glycine receptor.
- Describe the mechanisms of GABA and glycine-mediated synaptic inhibition.
- Define glutamate excitotoxicity and the excitation/inhibition (E/I) ratio, and identify the importance of each.

NEUROTRANSMITTERS IN NEURONAL TRANSMISSION

The previous chapter provided an overview of synapses and general mechanisms of neurotransmitter (NT) packaging, release, and receptors. In this chapter, the specific NT systems involving acetylcholine (ACh) and the amino acids glutamate (Glu), γ-aminobutyric acid (GABA), and glycine (Gly) are described. For these NT systems, neurotransmission between the presynaptic neuron that releases the NT and its target can be complex (Figure 8–1). Synaptic/wiring transmission involves activation of NT receptors in the postsynaptic and presynaptic regions. Volume transmission involves receptors in the perisynaptic or extrasynaptic regions and/or adjacent neurons. Fast synaptic transmission involves ionotropic NT receptors, which produce rapid changes in the postsynaptic membrane potential. Slow synaptic transmission involves metabotropic G-protein–coupled receptors (GPCRs), which

produce slow changes in the membrane potential. GPCRs also act as neuromodulators to alter the cellular or synaptic properties of neurons so that synaptic transmission between them is modified. Many target neurons express both ionotropic and metabotropic receptors for the same NT, and the NT receptors can be localized postsynaptically, presynaptically, perisynaptically, and/or extrasynaptically. Consequently, using NTs, the presynaptic neurons can excite, inhibit, and/or modulate their postsynaptic targets, with short-term effects on membrane potential and/or longer lasting effects on neuronal excitability, synaptic transmission, metabolism, morphology, and gene expression.

ACh & ACh RECEPTORS

The first NT discovered, ACh is synthesized, packaged, and released by cholinergic neurons. ACh is synthesized in the presynaptic region from acetyl-coenzyme A (CoA) and

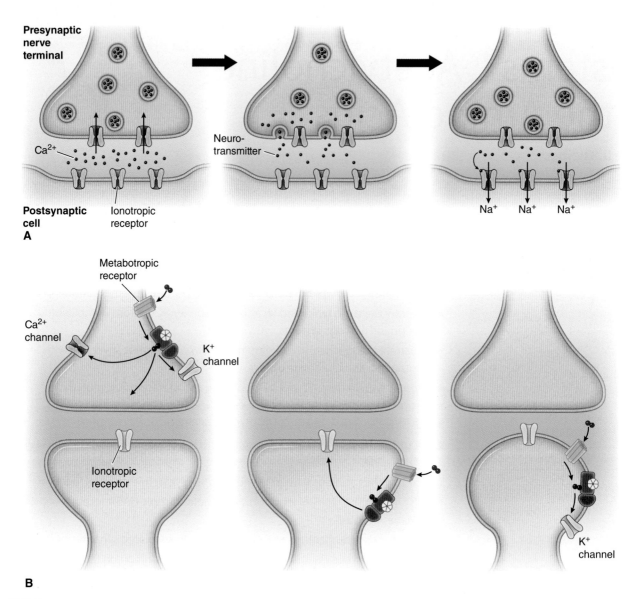

FIGURE 8–1 Types of synaptic transmission at chemical synapses. **A.** In fast, direct transmission, a presynaptic action potential activates voltage-gated Ca²⁺ channels, influx of Ca²⁺ (red spheres) and release of neurotransmitter (purple spheres) into the synaptic cleft. Neurotransmitters bind to ionotropic receptors leading to changes in the postsynaptic membrane potential. **B.** In slow, indirect transmission, released neurotransmitters (blue spheres) can diffuse inside and outside the synaptic cleft and activate receptors located at different sites. Left, activation of presynaptic metabotropic receptors leads to regulation of neurotransmitter release. Middle, activation of postsynaptic metabotropic receptors leads to modulation of ionotropic receptors. Right, activation of metabotropic receptors in the cell body or nearby synapses or neurons, can lead to effects on multiple targets including ion channels and other activities.

choline provided by the choline transporter (CT), by the enzyme choline acetytransferase (ChAT) (Figure 8–2). Following synthesis, ACh is transported into synaptic vesicles by the vesicular ACh transporter (VAChT). VAChT is a member of the solute carrier (SLC) transporter superfamily. All vesicular NT transporters are antiporters that require the proton gradient produced by the proton ATPase to transport the NT inside the synaptic vesicle. In histologic studies, expression of ChAT and/or VAChT is a criterion that identifies neurons as cholinergic. Synaptic vesicles loaded with ACh are localized to the presynaptic active zone, where release of ACh into

the synaptic cleft is activated by the action potential and subsequence increase in presynaptic [Ca²⁺]. After release, ACh is degraded by the enzyme ACh esterase to acetate and choline at the synaptic cleft. The released choline is transported back into the presynaptic neuron by the CT. Choline is rate limiting for the ChAT enzyme, and for several disorders in which cholinergic synaptic transmission is impaired, treatment includes choline supplements. The effects of ACh are mediated by 2 main categories of ACh receptors, the nicotinic ACh receptors (nAChR) and muscarinic ACh receptors (mAChR).

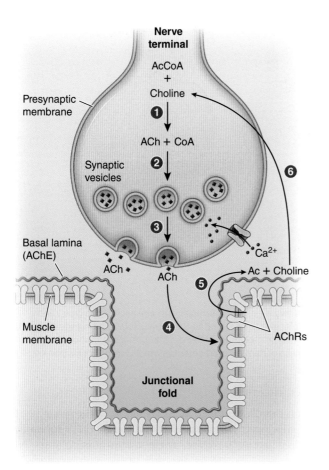

Nerve terminal

Presynaptic membrane

AcCoA + Choline

ACh + CoA

Synaptic vesicles

Basal lamina (AChE)

ACh

ACh

Muscle membrane

Junctional fold

Ca²⁺

Ac + Choline

AChRs

FIGURE 8–2 Transmission at the neuromuscular junction. 1. Choline and acetyl CoA are converted to acetylcholine (ACh) via choline acetyl transferase. 2. ACh is transported into synaptic vesicles via the vesicular ACh transporter. 3. In response to an action potential, synaptic vesicles fuse and release ACh into the synaptic cleft. 4. ACh binds to ionotropic ACh receptors called nicotinic ACh receptors, producing the end plate potential. 5. ACh is degraded to choline and acetate by ACh esterase. 6. Choline is transported to the presynaptic neuron by the choline transporter.

The nAChRs are ionotropic receptors that can be activated by nicotine, a tobacco plant alkaloid, and there are 2 main types, the muscle-type and neuronal-type nAChRs (Figure 8–3). nAChRs are assembled from 5 subunits. A total of 17 different subunit genes ($\alpha 1$ to $\alpha 10$, $\beta 1$, $\beta 2$, δ, γ, and ε) are expressed in humans. Muscle-type nAChRs contain 2 α, 1 β, 1 γ, and 1 δ or ε subunit, whereas neuronal nAChRs contain 4 α and 1 β subunit. The 2 types of nAChRs have different properties and synaptic localization. Neuronal-type nAChRs are approximately 50-fold more sensitive to nicotine than are the muscle-type nAChRs. All nAChRs are nonselective cation channels that are permeable to Na⁺ and K⁺. A few rare neuronal receptor assemblies are also permeable to Ca²⁺. Binding of ACh to the 2 α subunits in the nAChR induces a conformational change, opening the channel and allowing cations to flow down their electrochemical gradient, which produces a depolarization of the postsynaptic membrane (ie,

an excitatory response). The nAChR antagonists include the chemicals hexamethonium and dextromethorphan, tubocurarine from the curare plant, and α-bungarotoxin, a component of krait snake venom.

mAChRs are metabotropic GPCRs that can be distinguished pharmacologically using the agonist muscarine, a toxin from the mushroom *Amanita muscaria*, or the agonist drug carbachol (Figure 8–4). Muscarinic receptors are inhibited by atropine, a toxin antagonist derived from the *Atropa belladonna* plant. As metabotropic receptors, mAChRs function through the activation of G proteins. Five subtypes of mChRs have been identified. The M2 and M4 subtypes couple to $G\alpha_{q/11}$ and activate phospholipase C (PLC), whereas the M1, M3, and M5 subtypes couple to $G_{i/o}$, which inhibits adenylyl cyclase. The pathways downstream of these G proteins are described in Chapter 7. Through G-protein regulation of ion channels and second messenger pathways that modulate kinases and phosphatases, mAChRs can control a variety of downstream effects. Activation of mAChRs can influence short-term and/or long-term changes in the membrane potential and neuronal excitability, NT synthesis and release mechanisms, cytoskeletal proteins and morphology, metabolic pathways, and gene expression. In the peripheral nervous system (PNS), mCHRs are expressed by the targets of all postganglionic parasympathetic neurons and a few sympathetic neurons. In the central nervous system (CNS), mAChRs have widespread expression, with highest levels in the cerebral cortex.

CHOLINERGIC NEURONS IN SOMATIC MOTOR & AUTONOMIC SYSTEMS

Cholinergic neurons are found in the somatic motor system and autonomic nervous system (Figure 8–5). All somatic lower motor neurons that innervate skeletal muscles are cholinergic. Alpha motor neuron cell bodies are located in the CNS, either in the ventral horn of the spinal cord or brainstem cranial nerve nuclei, and extend their axons outside the CNS, forming the motor efferents of spinal or cranial nerves, part of the PNS. Groups of α motor neurons called motor pools coordinately control contraction of a single muscle, wherein each branch of an α motor axon innervates a single muscle fiber. The junction between the presynaptic axon from the lower motor neuron and skeletal muscle is called the neuromuscular junction (NMJ), and the region on the muscle cell that is innervated by the motor neuron is called the motor end plate.

The best-characterized chemical synapse, the NMJ is an excitatory synapse where ACh produces the end-plate potential (EPP) and induces skeletal muscle contraction. At the NMJ, the action potential (AP) reaches the presynaptic motor neuron axon terminal, activating voltage-gated Ca²⁺ channels, and Ca²⁺ flows in, causing the fusion of synaptic

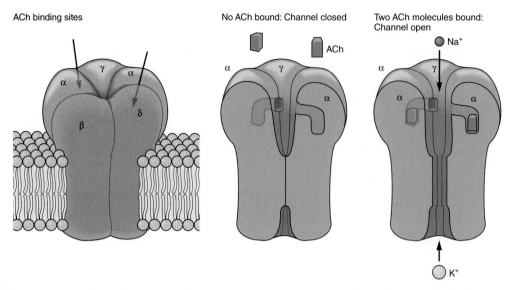

FIGURE 8–3 Nicotinic ACh receptors are ionotropic receptors. Composed of two identical α-subunits, and one each of the β-, γ-, and δ-subunits, the nicotinic receptor is a non-selective cation channel. When two molecules of ACh bind to the extracellular binding sites located at the interface between the α-subunits and the adjacent γ-, and δ-subunits, the receptor-channel molecule changes conformation that leads to opening of the pore region, through which both K⁺ and Na⁺ flow down their electrochemical gradients. (Reproduced with permission from Kandel ER, Schwartz JH, Jessell TM, et al: *Principles of Neural Science*, 5th ed. New York, NY: McGraw Hill; 2013.)

vesicles, and ACh is released into the synaptic cleft. Binding of ACh to the muscle-type nAChRs results in an initial influx of Na⁺, which produces the EPP, a large depolarization (to about –40 mV) of the muscle membrane potential. This depolarization by the EPP travels passively along the muscle membrane to the adjacent regions where it activates voltage-gated Na⁺ channels, which initiate and conduct an AP in the muscle membrane.

The muscle AP leads to an increase in Ca²⁺ in the muscle cell, triggering a sequence of steps that leads to muscle contraction. As the EPP becomes more depolarized, the driving force for K⁺ increases and K⁺ flows out of the nAChRs, helping to repolarize the muscle membrane. After release,

ACh is rapidly degraded by ACh esterase at the synaptic cleft. mAChRs located on the presynaptic membrane of motor neurons regulate ACh release. Synaptic transmission at the NMJ (Figure 8–6), as well as disorders of the motor systems and NMJ targets of therapeutic drugs, are described in greater detail in Chapters 16 and 31.

In the autonomic motor system, the preganglionic neuron cell bodies are located in the CNS (spinal cord or brainstem) and send axons that innervate the postganglionic neurons located in the autonomic ganglia. Postganglionic neurons project their axons to their target muscles or glands. All preganglionic neurons are cholinergic, and the postganglionic neurons respond rapidly to ACh via nAChRs. In addition,

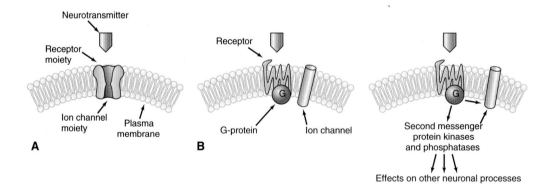

FIGURE 8–4 Comparison of ionotropic and metabotropic receptor mechanisms. **A.** Ionotropic receptors contain both neurotransmitter binding domains and ion channel domains. **B.** Metabotropic receptors function through the activation of G proteins. The effectors of G proteins include ion channels and enzymes that produce second messengers, which regulate protein kinases and phosphatases. (Reproduced with permission from Nestler EJ, Hyman SE, Holtzman DM, et al: *Molecular Neuropharmacology: A Foundation for Clinical Neuroscience*, 3rd ed. New York, NY: McGraw Hill; 2015.)

Sympathetic nervous system

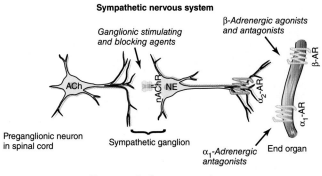

Parasympathetic nervous system

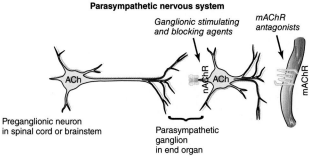

Adrenal medulla

Somatic motor nervous system

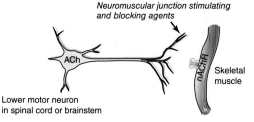

FIGURE 8–5 Cholinergic neurons in the autonomic and somatic motor nervous systems. In the autonomic nervous system (top three panels), all preganglionic neurons are cholinergic and act through nicotinic receptors on their postganglionic neurons. The majority of postganglionic sympathetic neurons are noradrenergic, while all postganglionic parasympathetic neurons are cholinergic. In both systems, effects are mediated by metabotropic receptors on target organs. The adrenal medulla is innervated by preganglionic sympathetic neurons, which stimulate adrenal chromaffin cells to release epinephrine and norepinephrine into the circulation. Somatic lower motor neurons (bottom panel) are cholinergic and act by activation of nicotinic receptors on skeletal muscle cells. (Reproduced with permission from Nestler EJ, Hyman SE, Holtzman DM, et al: *Molecular Neuropharmacology: A Foundation for Clinical Neuroscience*, 3rd ed. New York, NY: McGraw Hill; 2015.)

the hyperpolarization and slow depolarization that represent the recovery of postganglionic neurons from stimulation are mediated by mAChRs.

All postganglionic parasympathetic neurons are cholinergic, projecting to their targets in many organs that respond to ACh via mAChRs. Depending on the type of G protein and second messenger pathways activated, ACh can mediate slow excitatory, inhibitory, or modulatory responses in the target smooth and cardiac muscles or glands. As a competitive antagonist of muscarinic receptors, atropine is used to modulate several autonomic responses. A small percentage of postganglionic sympathetic neurons are cholinergic, but the great majority are noradrenergic. Specific information about target receptors and responses in the autonomic nervous system is found in Chapter 18.

The enteric nervous system (ENS) is regulated by the autonomic nervous system but is also considered a separate division of the PNS because it consists of neurons that function autonomously to control the gastrointestinal (GI) tract. In the ENS, cholinergic motor neurons within the enteric plexuses control GI motility and secretion. In performing these functions, ENS motor neurons act directly on a large number of effector cells, including smooth muscle cells, secretory cells, and GI endocrine cells, with responses mainly through mAChRs.

CHOLINERGIC NEURONS IN THE BRAIN

The 3 main brain areas that contain the cell bodies of cholinergic neurons are the basal forebrain, basal ganglia, and brainstem (Figure 8–7). In the basal forebrain, cholinergic cell bodies are located in the basal nucleus of Meynert, which project to the neocortex, and the medial septal nucleus and diagonal band of Broca, which project to the hippocampus and neocortex. Loss or dysfunction of basal forebrain cholinergic neurons and their projections is one of the earliest pathologic changes in Alzheimer disease (AD) and is implicated in the early memory deficits in AD. In the basal ganglia, cholinergic interneurons in the striatum are proposed to play a role in motor function. In the brainstem, cholinergic neurons originate from the pedunculopontine nucleus and laterodorsal tegmental area, known as the pontomesencephalotegmental complex, which project to other brainstem nuclei, deep cerebellar nuclei, thalamus, basal ganglia, and basal forebrain. In the spinal cord, a population of cholinergic interneurons gives rise to the "C boutons," which regulate excitability of ventral horn alpha motor neurons.

Both nAChRs and mAChRs are expressed in many areas of the brain, including most regions of the cerebral cortex, hippocampus, and brainstem. Moreover, both nAChRs and mAChRs are located both presynaptically and postsynaptically throughout the brain, and mAChRs are also localized extrasynaptically. Cholinergic transmission in the CNS often involves neuromodulation, including alterations of neuronal excitability,

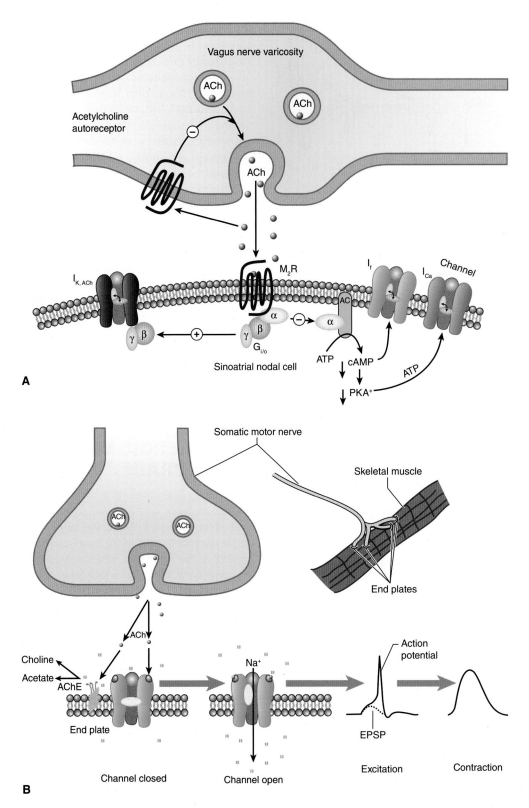

FIGURE 8–6 Comparison of cholinergic synaptic transmission in the autonomic and somatic nervous systems. **A.** ACh released from a varicosity of a postganglionic parasympathetic axon interacts with a heart sinoatrial node cell muscarinic receptor (M_2R) linked via $G_{i/o}$ to K^+ channel opening, which causes hyperpolarization, and to inhibition of cAMP synthesis. Reduced cAMP affects pacemaker channels (I_f) and L-type Ca^{2+} channels (I_{Ca}). Released ACh also acts on an axonal muscarinic autoreceptors to inhibit ACh release. **B.** ACh released from a somatic motor axon terminal at the neuromuscular junction binds and opens the nicotinic receptor channel allowing Na^+ influx to produce an end plate potential, a type of excitatory postsynaptic potential (EPSP), triggering a muscle action potential and muscle contraction. ACh esterase (AChE) hydrolyzes ACh. (Reproduced with permission from Katzung BG: *Basic & Clinical Pharmacology*, 14th ed. New York, NY: McGraw Hill; 2018.)

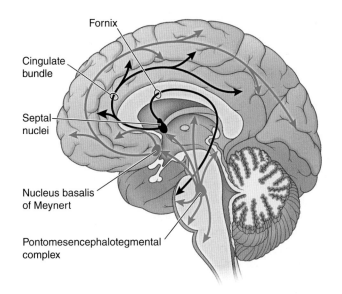

FIGURE 8-7 Localization of cholinergic neurons in the brain. Cholinergic neuron cell bodies are located in nuclei in the basal forebrain (purple and green), striatum (not highlighted) and the brainstem (blue). Cholinergic axons project throughout the CNS.

presynaptic NT release, and coordination of the firing patterns of neuronal groups (Figure 8–8). In addition to its roles in synaptic plasticity and memory, ACh has a variety of well-supported functions in cognition, arousal, attention, concentration, cue detection, reward, motor learning, and sleep. ACh has also been implicated in modulation of hypothalamic functions, including thermoregulation, sleep patterns, food intake, metabolism, stress, and endocrine functions. The antagonist scopolamine, which is used to treat motion sickness and postoperative nausea and vomiting, blocks neuronal mAChRs, whereas the addictive properties of the agonist nicotine derive from its effects on nAChRs expressed in the brain reward systems. Specific mAChR agonists and antagonists are being investigated for potential treatment of cognitive symptoms associated with several CNS disorders, including schizophrenia and mood disorders.

Inhibition of ACh esterase prevents the breakdown of ACh, allowing ACh levels to remain elevated at the synapse and prolonging cholinergic signaling. Reversible ACh inhibitor drugs are used to treat (1) the cognitive (memory and learning deficit) symptoms in AD, Lewy body dementia,

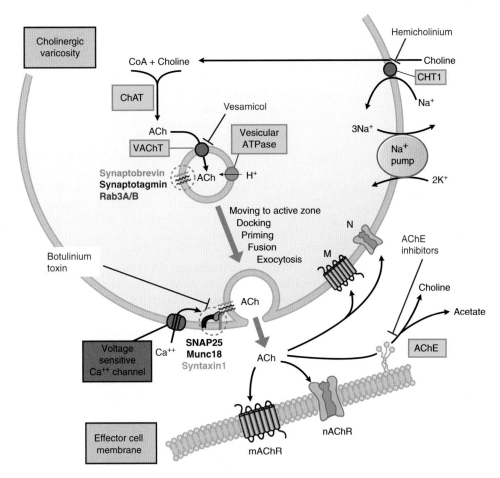

FIGURE 8-8 Cholinergic transmission in the CNS. Released ACh can activate postsynaptic nicotinic receptors (N and nAChR), and/or muscarinic receptors (M and mAChR) in the CNS. ACh can also act on presynaptic mAChRs or nAChRs to modify its own release. The action of ACh is terminated by ACh esterase (AChE), which is the target of several therapeutic drugs used to treat some neurological disorders. (Reproduced with permission from Brunton LL, Hilal-Dandan R, Knollmann BC: *Goodman & Gilman's the Pharmacological Basis of Therapeutics*, 13th ed. New York, NY: McGraw Hill; 2018.)

and Parkinson disease (PD); (2) the psychotic symptoms in schizophrenia and PD; (3) glaucoma; and (4) muscle weakness in myasthenia gravis, an autoimmune disorder involving loss of nAChRs at the NMJ. ACh esterase is also the target of insecticides and nerve gases, including sarin gas. Acute effects of these poisons include marked decreases in heart rate and blood pressure, with irreversible inhibition of ACh esterase typically resulting in respiratory paralysis.

GLU & GLUTAMATERGIC NEURONS

The most abundant NT, Glu is an amino acid NT involved in excitatory synaptic transmission in the CNS (Figure 8–9). The NT Glu is the same nonessential L-amino acid used in protein biosynthesis in all cells that is obtained from the diet or synthesized from glucose via glycolysis and the Krebs cycle. Glu can also be converted to and generated from glutamine by the enzymes glutamine synthase and glutaminase, respectively. At the presynaptic terminus, Glu is transported into synaptic vesicles by the vesicular Glu transporter (vGLUT). In the CNS, most glutamatergic synapses are excitatory, with a characteristic asymmetric morphology resulting from the concentrated postsynaptic density.

Glutamatergic neurons are the most abundant type of neuron in the brain, estimated to represent approximately 80% of total brain neurons, found in nearly every region of the CNS. For example, glutamatergic neurons are the most abundant neurons in the neocortex (pyramidal and spiny stellate neurons), cerebellum (cerebellar granule neurons), hippocampus (hippocampal granule and pyramidal neurons), and retina (photoreceptor, bipolar, and retinal ganglion cells); they are also located in the thalamus, hypothalamus, basal ganglia, limbic system, brainstem, and spinal cord. Glutamatergic neurons have been implicated in most aspects of normal brain functions and vital processes, including relaying of sensory information, encoding of information, brain motor control and coordination, cognition, formation and retrieval of memories, emotion, spatial recognition, and consciousness. Glutamatergic synapses on dendritic spines mediate the majority of excitatory synaptic transmission in the mammalian brain. In the hippocampus, neocortex, cerebellum, and other parts of the brain, glutamatergic synapses have been shown to undergo synaptic plasticity, involving changes in synaptic transmission known as long-term potentiation (LTP) and long-term depression (LTD), discussed in Chapter 10.

GLU RECEPTORS & GLU UPTAKE

Glu binds to and activates 2 main categories of receptors, the ionotropic Glu receptors and metabotropic Glu receptors (mGluRs) (Figure 8–10). Ionotropic Glu receptors are ligand-gated nonselective cation channels that produce fast excitatory responses. The ionotropic Glu receptors can be distinguished pharmacologically by their affinities for the Glu agonists kainite, α-amino-3-hydroxy-5-methyl-4-isoxazolepropionic acid (AMPA), and N-methyl-D-aspartic acid (NMDA). mGluRs are GPCRs, which produce neuromodulatory responses by activating G proteins that control ion channels and second messenger signaling pathways. Both ionotropic and metabotropic receptors have been shown to localize on the presynaptic and postsynaptic membranes, and mGluRs are also located perisynaptically and extrasynaptically. Many synapses express multiple types of Glu receptors. Glu functions not only as a point-to-point transmitter at excitatory synapses, but also through the process of volume transmission, in which spillover of Glu into the extracellular fluid can influence extrasynaptic receptors and nearby synapses.

All ionotropic Glu receptors are tetrameric protein complexes that form nonselective cation channels, but they have different properties. Composed of 4 subunits containing GluR1 to GluR4, AMPA receptors (AMPARs) are selectively activated by the Glu agonist AMPA. Most AMPARs are assembled as dimers of dimers, with the vast majority containing 2 GluR2 subunits and a dimer of either GluR1, GluR3, or GluR4. AMPARs interact with several regulatory proteins, including transmembrane AMPAR regulatory proteins (TARPs) that control the membrane trafficking and conductance of AMPARs. AMPARs and TARPs can bind to the PDZ domain

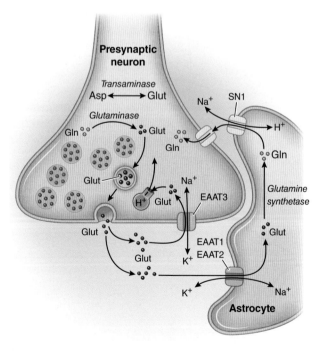

FIGURE 8–9 Glu synthesis, packaging and uptake. Glu (glut) is synthesized in the presynaptic neuron; synaptic vesicles are filled by vesicular glut transporters. Glut is removed from the synapse by plasma membrane glut transporters (EEATs) on the presynaptic neuron and nearby astrocytes where it is converted to glutamine, released and taken up by the presynaptic axon.

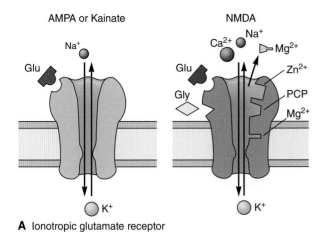

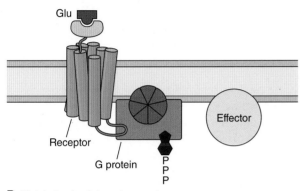

FIGURE 8–10 Categories of Glu receptors. **A.** The main types of ionotropic Glu receptors and their differences are illustrated. **B.** Metabotropic Glu receptors function through G proteins that control effectors. (Reproduced with permission from Kandel ER, Schwartz JH, Jessell TM, et al: *Principles of Neural Science*, 5th ed. New York, NY: McGraw Hill; 2013.)

containing scaffolding proteins that contribute to their localization at the synapse.

When AMPARs bind Glu, the channel domain opens, allowing Na^+ and K^+ to flow down their electrochemical gradients. A rare tetramer of AMPAR lacking the GluR2 dimer is also permeable to Ca^{2+}. AMPARs activate rapidly and many undergo rapid desensitization. Therefore, AMPARs open and close quickly, on the order of a few milliseconds, producing fast excitatory postsynaptic potentials (EPSPs), which are usually small depolarizations on the order of a few millivolts. The most commonly found NT receptor in the CNS, AMPARs are expressed in most regions of the brain and are responsible for mediating most of the fast excitatory synaptic transmission in the CNS. AMPAR-generated EPSPs are transmitted passively along dendrites or the cell body where they can summate with other responses (Figure 8–11). If enough excitatory synapses are activated concomitantly, the summated EPSPs will reach threshold at the axon initial segment, and the neuron will fire an AP.

Kainate receptors (KaRs) were identified as a distinct receptor type through their selective activation by the agonist kainate, a drug first isolated from the red alga *Digenea*

simplex. Kainate is a convulsant that induces seizures, in part, by activation of KaRs and also probably via AMPARs. KaRs are similar to AMPARs in many respects, although they are much less abundant and not as well characterized. KaRs allow Na^+ and K^+ to permeate the channel pore, are formed via tetramers containing GluK1 and GluK2 subunits, but open and close more slowly than AMPARs. However, given their similar properties and function, AMPARs and KaRs are often grouped together into a single category of ionotropic Glu receptors (Glu Rs).

NMDA receptors (NMDARs) are tetramers that assemble from 4 GluN1 to GluN3 subunits and are selectively activated by the Glu agonist NMDA. NMDARs differ from AMPARs and KaRs in 3 important ways. First, in addition to binding Glu, NMDARs require coactivation by binding another ligand: either Gly or D-serine. Second, in addition to Glu and coagonist binding, NMDA receptors require depolarization of the postsynaptic membrane to allow cations to permeate through the channel. Third, all NMDARs are permeable not only to Na^+ and K^+, but also to Ca^{2+}, and mediate postsynaptic Ca^{2+} increases in response to Glu binding.

NMDARs have an internal binding site for a Mg^{2+} or Zn^{2+} ion, creating a voltage-dependent block of the channel at the resting membrane potential. Depolarization of the membrane dislodges and repels the Mg^{2+} or Zn^{2+}, allowing the pore to permeate Na^+, K^+, or Ca^{2+}. Therefore, in order to be activated, NMDARs require Glu, a coagonist, and membrane depolarization produced by AMPARs or other excitatory NT response. Indeed, a majority of synapses that express NMDARs also express AMPARs, with levels of colocalization varying between 40% and 100%, depending on neuronal type (Figure 8–12). Similar to AMPARs, NMDARs interact with PDZ domain containing scaffolding proteins at the synapse, which also provide platforms for the tethering of intracellular signaling proteins.

NMDARs are affected by endogenous neurosteroids and psychoactive drugs such as phencyclidine (PCP), ketamine, ethanol, and dextromethorphan. In dendritic spines, both NMDARs and AMPARs are involved in LTP and LTD, which are types of long-term synaptic plasticity proposed to underlie learning and memory and are described in detail in Chapter 10. In several pathologic conditions of the nervous system, excessive Glu and NMDAR activation contributes to Glu excitotoxicity, a process that can cause neuronal injury and death (see below). Glu excitotoxicity can result from hypoxic injury, hypoglycemia, stroke, epilepsy, or traumatic brain injury. Increased release of Glu or diminished Glu uptake, or both, leads to the persistent activation of AMPAR and NMDAR pathways and membrane depolarization. Through NMDARs and voltage-gated Ca^{2+} channel activation, the resulting prolonged intracellular Ca^{2+} levels can activate phospholipases, endonucleases, and proteases, leading to damage of organelles, the cytoskeleton, membrane, and DNA. Current research seeks to develop NMDAR antagonists that can selectively block excitotoxic NMDAR activation without disrupting NMDAR activity required for normal excitatory synaptic transmission and plasticity.

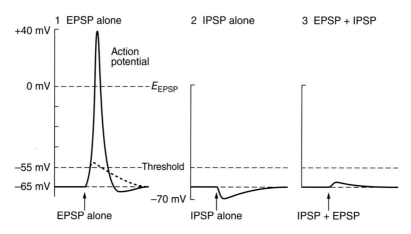

FIGURE 8–11   Ionotropic Glu receptors produce excitatory postsynaptic potentials (EPSPs) involved in summation with other postsynaptic responses. 1. Glu typically produces small EPSPs, which can summate to produce larger EPSPs (dashed line) that can induce an action potential. 2. An inhibitory postsynaptic potential (IPSP) produced at an inhibitory synapse. 3. When EPSPs and IPSPs occur together in time and space, the effectiveness of the EPSP is reduced, preventing the neuron from reaching the threshold for an action potential. (Reproduced with permission from Kandel ER, Schwartz JH, Jessell TM, et al: *Principles of Neural Science*, 5th ed. New York, NY: McGraw Hill; 2013.)

mGluRs are metabotropic GPCRs involved in slow synaptic transmission and neuromodulation, functioning in the hippocampus, cerebellum, cerebral cortex, and other parts of the brain and in the PNS (Figure 8–13). Eight different subtypes of mGluRs are expressed. Group I mGluRs (mGluR1 and mGluR5) activate the $G\alpha_{q/11}$ family, which stimulates PLC located mostly on postsynaptic regions. Groups II (mGluR2 and mGluR3) and III (mGluR4 and mGluR6 to mGluR8) mGluRs couple through $G\alpha_{i/o}$ to inhibit adenylyl cyclase and are mainly involved in presynaptic inhibition. The scaffolding protein homer binds to mGluRs and contributes to their localization at the synapse. mGluRs can modulate NMDARs, as well as dopaminergic and adrenergic neurotransmission. mGluRs have been implicated in learning and memory, the perception of pain, and transmission of visual information in the retina. Dysregulation of mGluRs has been implicated in the pathogenesis of fragile X mental retardation/autism

disorder, anxiety, schizophrenia, and neurodegenerative disorders including PD. Development of selective mGluR agonists and antagonists for the treatment of these disorders is another goal of current clinical research.

Astrocytes within the tripartite synapse are exposed to elevated Glu levels during synaptic transmission. mGluRs are expressed in different types of glial cells, including astrocytes, oligodendrocytes, and microglia, although their functions have not yet been clearly elucidated. Glutamatergic synaptic activity can evoke Ca^{2+} signals in astrocytes, which may lead to the release of gliotransmitters that modulate synaptic transmission. mGluRs also have a widespread distribution in the periphery, where they mediate diverse functions, including roles in cardiorespiratory, endocrine, immune, and reproductive systems. Specific roles for peripheral mGluRs include regulation of hormone production in the adrenal gland and pancreas, modulation of heart rhythm and blood pressure,

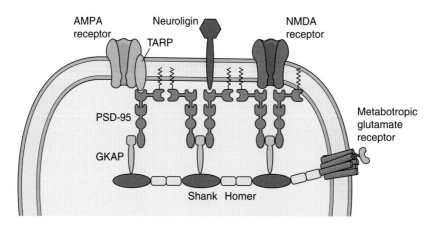

FIGURE 8–12   Illustration of the postsynaptic density. The scaffolding protein PSD-95 binds directly to the NMDA receptor, neuroligin, and GKAP. PSD-95 binds indirectly with AMPA receptors (via TARP) and with Shank. The metabotropic Glu receptor is localized in the perisynaptic region where it interacts with the Homer, which in turn binds Shank. (Reproduced with permission from Kandel ER, Schwartz JH, Jessell TM, et al: *Principles of Neural Science*, 5th ed. New York, NY: McGraw Hill; 2013.)

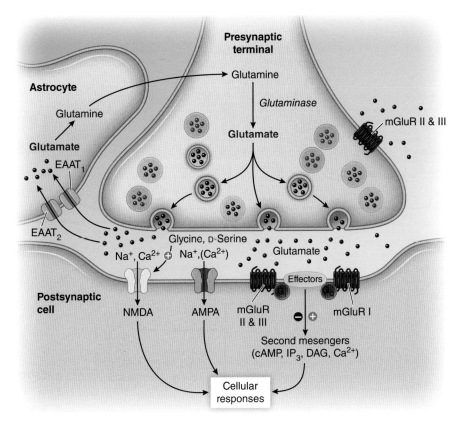

FIGURE 8–13 Diagram of a glutamate synapse. AMPA, NMDA and metabotropic Glu receptors can be co-expressed at excitatory synapses, including many synapses on dendritic spines. This implies that both fast excitatory responses EPSPs and slow modulatory responses via Ca²⁺ influx and G proteins can occur at the same synapse. Though depicted at the postsynaptic region, metabotropic receptors are thought to be localized outside the synapse at peri- or extra-synaptic sites. Presynaptic ionotropic and metabotropic receptors can also modulate synaptic transmission.

mineralization in developing cartilage, lymphocyte cytokine production, differentiation in embryonic stem cells, and GI secretory functions.

Glu is removed from the synaptic cleft and extracellular fluid via Glu transporters expressed in neurons or nearby astrocytes at the synapse. Plasma membrane Glu transporters are a family of Na⁺- and K⁺-dependent NT transporter proteins called excitatory amino acid transporters (EAATs). EAATs can also transport aspartate and are expressed in the CNS, PNS, and most peripheral tissues. Five EAAT genes are expressed in the CNS, with differential expression in neurons and glia. It has been estimated that the predominantly astrocyte-expressed EEAT2 is responsible for approximately 90% of the Glu uptake in the brain. The activity of Glu transporters not only terminates Glu responses, but also allows Glu to be recycled for repeated release. Glu taken up by astrocyte cells is converted to glutamine, which is released from astrocytes into the extracellular fluid and taken up by presynaptic neurons, which convert glutamine back to Glu. Overactivity of Glu transporters is observed in schizophrenia, whereas decreased Glu transporter activity has been implicated in Glu excitotoxicity (**Figure 8–14**) in ischemia, traumatic brain injury, and neurodegenerative disorders, including AD, PD, and amyotrophic lateral sclerosis.

ASPARTATE

It has long been debated whether the amino acid aspartate serves as an NT and, possibly, as a cotransmitter with Glu at glutamatergic synapses. Although aspartate satisfies many of the criteria required to have a role as an NT, a major role for aspartate as an NT in the mammalian brain is not unequivocally supported. Aspartate is a selective agonist for NMDARs, but does not activate AMPARs. The vesicular Glu transporters VGLUT1 to VGLUT3 do not transport aspartate, so it would require a separate, yet-to-be-identified NT transporter. However, if aspartate is a cotransmitter, variation in the vesicular content of Glu and aspartate could have a significant effect on the relative contribution of AMPARs and NMDARs to synaptic transmission and plasticity. Thus, the debate in this area continues.

GABA & GABAERGIC NEURONS

The amino acid derivative γ-aminobutyric acid (GABA) is the major inhibitory NT in the brain. In the spinal cord, both GABA and the amino acid Gly are the main inhibitory NTs. Neurons that synthesize and release GABA are termed GABAergic. GABA is synthesized via the GABA shunt, in

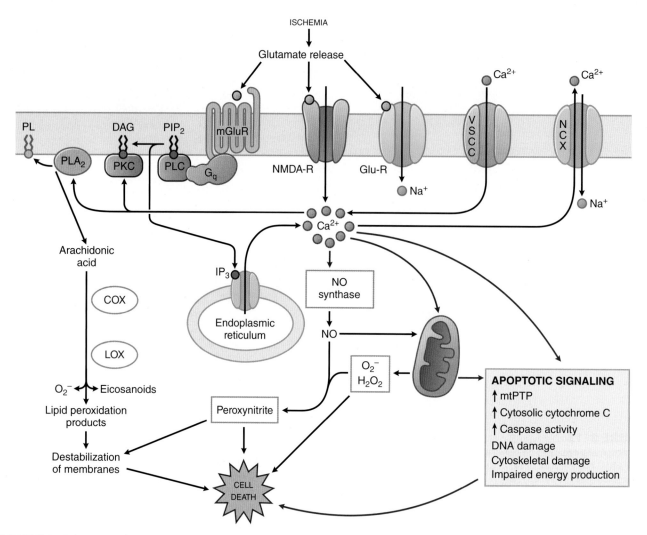

FIGURE 8–14 Glu excitotoxicity. Increased extracellular Glu activates pathways that lead to neuronal injury and death, with excess cytosolic Ca^{2+} playing a central role. COX, cyclooxygenase; DAG, diacylglycerol; GluR, AMPA/kainate Glu receptors; IP3, inositol trisphosphate; LOX, lipoxygenase; mGluR, metabotropic glutamate receptor; mtPTP, mitochondrial permeability transition pore; NCX, NA^+/Ca^{2+} exchanger; NMDA-R, NMDA receptor; O_2^-, superoxide radical; PIP_2, phosphatidylinositol 4,5-bisphosphate; PKC, protein kinase C; PL, phospholipids, PL phospholipase; VSCC, voltage-sensitive Ca^{2+} channel. (Reproduced with permission from Siegel GS, Albers RW, Brady S, et al: *Basic Neurochemistry: Molecular, Cellular, and Medical Aspects.* 7th ed. Burlington, MA: Elsevier Academic Press; 2006.)

which α-ketoglutarate is transaminated to Glu by GABA α-oxoglutarate transaminase, followed by decarboxylation of Glu by glutamic acid decarboxylase (GAD) to GABA (Figure 8–15). GABA is transported into synaptic vesicles at the presynaptic terminus by the vesicular GABA transporter (vGAT), also called the vesicular inhibitory amino acid transporter (VIAAT). vGAT/VIAAT can also transport Gly, and in some inhibitory spinal neurons, both GABA and Gly function as cotransmitters.

GABAergic neurons represent the majority of inhibitory neurons, with a principal role in controlling neuronal excitability throughout the CNS. GABAergic transmission is also thought to set the spatiotemporal conditions required for the various patterns of network oscillations that may be critical for information processing. Given its widespread presence, GABA is implicated in a majority of

functions in the CNS, with roles in motor control, sensorimotor processing, anxiety, emotions, learning and memory, pain, and sleep.

GABAergic neurons are located in most CNS regions, including the cerebral cortex, hippocampus, thalamus, brainstem, retina, and spinal cord. Examples include GABAergic medium spiny neurons, which represent approximately 95% of neurons within the striatum. Stellate and basket cells are local GABAergic neurons in the cerebellum. Approximately 20% to 30% of neurons in the cerebral cortex and 10% to 20% of neurons in the hippocampus are GABAergic interneurons, local circuit neurons that can be distinguished by their morphologies and proteins they coexpress. In the spinal cord, local GABAergic neurons include Ia and Ib inhibitory interneurons and Renshaw cells that synapse onto motor neurons to coordinate muscle contraction, especially important in spinal

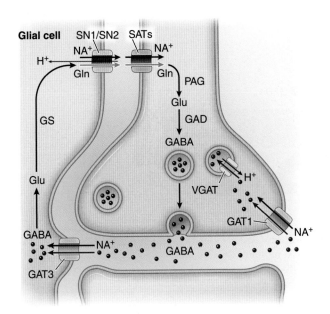

FIGURE 8–15 γ-Aminobutyric acid (GABA) synthesis, packaging and uptake. GABA is synthesized in the presynaptic neuron via glutamate decarboxylase (GAD); synaptic vesicles are filled by vesicular GABA transporters (vGAT). GABA is removed from the synapse by plasma membrane GABA transporters (GAT) on the presynaptic neuron and nearby astrocytes, where it is converted first to Glu and then glutamine, which is released and taken up by the presynaptic axon and converted to Glu via phosphate activated glutaminase (PAG).

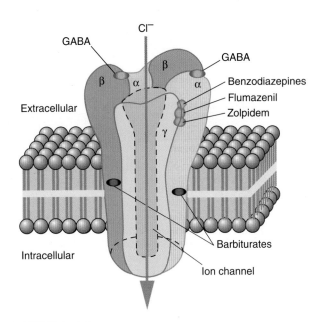

FIGURE 8–16 A model of the ionotropic γ-aminobutyric acid (GABA$_A$) receptor. The receptor complex consists of two α, one β, and one γ subunit. GABA binds at two sites between α and β subunits, induces opening of the channel domain, and allows Cl⁻ to flow into the neuron, causing inhibition. Benzodiazepines, hypnotic drugs such as zolpidem, and barbiturates bind at sites distinct from the GABA binding site, and their effect is to facilitate the process of Cl⁻ channel opening, enhancing inhibition. (Reproduced with permission from Katzung BG: *Basic & Clinical Pharmacology*, 14th ed. New York, NY: McGraw Hill; 2018.)

reflexes. Spinal GABAergic interneurons play a role in the regulation of sympathetic activity.

The majority of GABAergic neurons are local interneurons that function within specific regions to modulate excitability. Although the majority of projection neurons in the CNS are glutamatergic, a few populations of projection neurons are GABAergic. These include Purkinje neurons, which provide the sole output from the cerebellar cortex, and neurons in the ventral pallidum that provide an important output of the basal ganglia to the thalamus. Recent studies have identified GABAergic projection neurons in the cerebral cortex and hippocampus.

GABA RECEPTORS & GABA UPTAKE

GABA exerts its effects by binding to 2 receptor types, the ionotropic and metabotropic GABA receptors (Figure 8–16). The ionotropic receptors, called GABA$_A$ receptors (GABA$_A$R), are ligand-gated Cl⁻ channels. For GABA$_A$Rs, 19 different subunit genes have been identified, with subunits grouped into α, β, γ, δ, ε, and σ according to sequence homology. Individual GABA$_A$Rs are composed of 5 subunits, containing at least 1 α and 1 β subunit and 3 additional subunits; the most common GABA$_A$R in the brain is formed by 2 α subunits, 2 β subunits, and 1 γ subunit. When activated by

GABA binding, GABA$_A$Rs allow Cl⁻ to flow down its electrochemical gradient, usually into the cell, which often leads to a hyperpolarization of the membrane potential called a fast inhibitory postsynaptic potential (IPSP). However, because the typical reversal/Nernst potential for Cl⁻ is approximately –65 mV, which is close to the resting membrane potential, activation of GABA$_A$Rs does not always produce a detectable IPSP. Instead GABA can mediate a type of inhibition called shunting inhibition. If a neuron receives excitatory inputs that depolarize the neuron, coincident activation of GABA$_A$Rs at GABAergic synapses produces Cl⁻ influx that can reduce or reverse the depolarization response produced at excitatory synapses. Consequently, shunting inhibition can override the excitatory effect of depolarizing glutamatergic inputs, resulting in overall inhibition, even if the membrane potential remains the same or becomes slightly less negative. Importantly, GABAergic transmission can prevent the neuron from firing an AP (Figure 8-11).

Therapeutic drugs that affect GABA$_A$Rs are used clinically to treat a variety of disorders, including epilepsy, anxiety, and insomnia, and are used as sedatives and muscle relaxants. Drugs that bind to the GABA binding site in the GABA$_A$R are called orthosteric agonists, such as muscimol, and antagonists, such as bicuculline. In contrast, allosteric modulators bind at allosteric sites distinct from the GABA binding site, to indirectly increase or decrease Cl⁻ conductance in response to GABA. Allosteric agonists include barbiturates, ethanol,

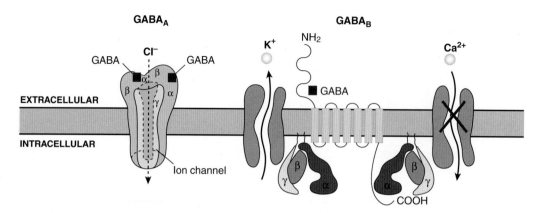

FIGURE 8–17 Mechanisms of γ-aminobutyric acid (GABA) receptor action. GABA$_A$ receptors are inotropic receptors where GABA binding opens the Cl⁻ channel domain. GABA$_B$ receptors are metabotropic receptors, which regulate G proteins (α, β, γ) that can inhibit Ca²⁺ channels or activate K⁺ channels. GABA$_B$ receptors, acting through G proteins, can also inhibit adenylyl cyclase, leading to decreases in cAMP signaling (not shown). (Adapted with permission from Bowery NG, Brown DA: The cloning of GABA(B) receptors, *Nature.* 1997 Mar 20;386(6622):223-224.)

benzodiazepines such as diazepam (Valium) and alprazolam (Xanax), Z-drugs such as zolpidem (Ambien), anesthetics, and neurosteroids. Allosteric drugs that enhance GABA receptor activation typically have anxiolytic, anticonvulsant, amnesic, sedative, hypnotic, euphoriant, and muscle relaxant properties. Some, such as muscimol and the Z-drugs, may also be hallucinogenic. Allosteric GABA$_A$R antagonists such as flumazenil are used for counteracting overdoses of sedative drugs. Picrotoxin is a GABA$_A$R channel blocker used in laboratory research.

GABA$_B$ receptors (GABA$_B$R) are metabotropic GPCRs (Figure 8–17). Expressed throughout the brain, GABA$_B$Rs have been implicated in development, regulation of oscillatory activity in neuronal networks, and learning and memory. Dysregulation of GABA$_B$Rs has been documented in behavioral pathologies such as substance abuse, anxiety, and depression. Baclofen is a GABA$_B$R agonist, a CNS depressant used as a skeletal muscle relaxant and to treat spasticity, and is under investigation to treat addiction. GABA$_B$Rs exist as heterodimers consisting of the GABA$_{B1}$R and GABA$_{B2}$R subunits and are localized presynaptically and postsynaptically. GABA$_B$Rs couple to the Gα$_{i/o}$ protein, which regulate 3 effectors. Presynaptic GABA$_B$R activation inhibits voltage-gated Ca²⁺ channels and adenylyl cyclase, which decreases NT release, and depending on the NT, this effect can be excitatory or inhibitory. Postsynaptically, GABA$_B$Rs stimulate the opening of the GIRK channels, bringing the neuron closer to the equilibrium potential of K⁺ and hyperpolarizing the neuron. Postsynaptic inhibition of adenylyl cyclase can control gene expression. The overall result of these processes is often a slow, long-lasting hyperpolarization and inhibition of the postsynaptic neuron.

GABA is removed from the synaptic cleft and extracellular fluid by GABA transporters (GATs) located on presynaptic neurons and astrocytes, decreasing the concentration of GABA at the synapse (Figure 8–18). GATs are widely distributed throughout the entire CNS in neurons and astrocytes, and their activity is crucial to regulate the extracellular concentration of GABA under basal conditions and during ongoing synaptic events. Experimental evidence indicates that the distribution of GATs in the membrane is highly dynamic and can be modified in an activity-dependent manner. A number of GAT reuptake inhibitors are currently being developed as potential anticonvulsant and antiepilepsy drugs.

Gly & GLYCINERGIC NEURONS

The amino acid glycine (Gly) is the other major NT that mediates fast inhibitory synaptic transmission in the CNS (Figure 8–19). Gly is formed from serine by the enzyme serine hydroxymethyltransferase and packaged into synaptic vesicles by vGAT and VIAAT. Some spinal interneurons use both Gly and GABA as cotransmitters. In addition, as described earlier, Gly also functions also a coagonist with Glu at the NMDAR, where it promotes the actions of Glu. Consequently, Gly subserves both fast inhibitory and excitatory functions within the CNS.

Located in the spinal cord, brainstem, caudal brain, and retina, glycinergic neurons have been proposed to control fluxes of sensory and motor information between the periphery and the CNS. Glycinergic neurons are involved in a variety of sensory functions, including vision, audition, and pain, and in diverse motor activities including locomotion, respiration, and vocalization. In the brainstem, glycinergic neurons are scattered along diverse nuclei such as the pontine, reticular, and auditory nuclei. In the cerebellum, glycinergic fastigial neurons project to vestibular and reticular neurons in the brainstem and influence motor outputs. In the retina, glycinergic amacrine cells are involved in processing visual information. In the spinal cord, glycinergic interneurons located mainly in the deep dorsal horn have been implicated in pain processing and pain gating.

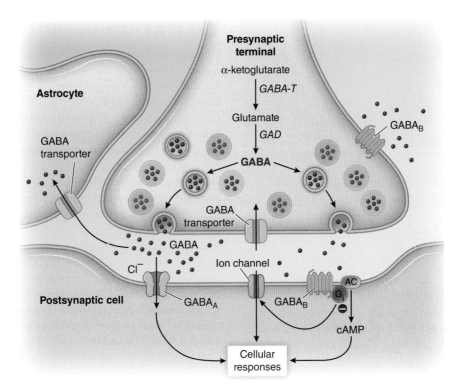

FIGURE 8–18 Diagram of a GABA synapse. GABA$_A$ and GABA$_B$ receptors may be co-expressed at inhibitory synapses, which suggests that both fast inhibitory responses (IPSPs) and slow modulatory responses via G proteins, may occur at the same synapse. Both types of receptors may also be expressed in the presynaptic region, which could modulate GABA release at the synapse.

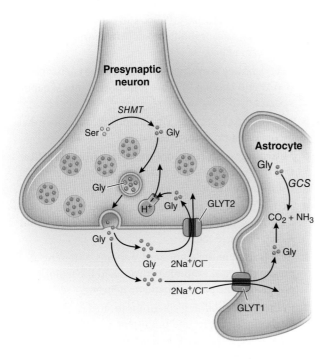

FIGURE 8–19 Glycine (Gly) synthesis, packaging and uptake. Gly is synthesized in the presynaptic neuron from by serine hydroxymethyltransferase (SHMT), packaged into synaptic vesicles via the vesicular Gly transporter, and removed from the synapse through uptake by the plasma membrane Gly transporter (GlyT) on the presynaptic terminus or nearby astrocytes.

Gly RECEPTORS & Gly UPTAKE

Gly functions through only 1 category of receptor, the ionotropic Gly receptor (GlyR) (Figure 8–20). Functional GlyRs are heteropentamers composed of subunits GlyRα1 to GlyRα4 and GlyRβ. The most commonly expressed adult GlyRs contain 3 or 4 α1 subunits and 1 or 2 β subunits and are localized throughout the brainstem and spinal cord. GlyRs are similar to GABA$_A$Rs in that they are ligand-gated Cl⁻ channels that produce either hyperpolarizing IPSPs or shunting inhibition. The plant alkaloid strychnine is a potent antagonist at the GlyR, whereas caffeine and bicuculline are weak antagonists; alanine and taurine are GlyR agonists. In the spinal cord, Gly and GABA may function as cotransmitters. Consistent with this, GlyRs have been shown to colocalize with the GABA$_A$Rs, in the spinal cord and, interestingly, on some hippocampal neurons. GlyRs, as well as GABA$_A$Rs, bind the scaffolding protein gephrin, which helps localize and cluster the receptors at the postsynaptic membrane and recruit signaling and cytoskeletal proteins.

The reuptake of Gly is mediated by plasma membrane Gly transporters (GlyT). GlyTs are expressed in the brainstem and spinal cord in regions where there are also high densities of GlyRs. In the short term, GlyTs reduce the levels of Gly in the synaptic cleft and decrease glycinergic transmission or NMDAR-dependent glutamatergic transmission. In the long term, because the rate of synthesis of Gly in the presynaptic

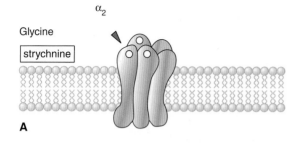

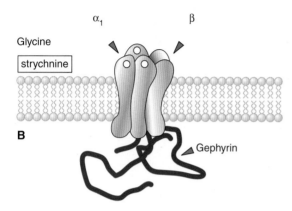

FIGURE 8–20 Glycine (Gly) receptors are similar to GABA$_A$ receptors. Gly binding opens the Cl⁻ channel domain, Cl⁻ flows down its electrochemical gradient, typically leading to Cl⁻ influx and inhibition in adult neurons. **A.** In embryonic tissue, glycine receptors comprise only α$_2$ subunits. **B.** Adult Gly receptors typically comprise 3α$_1$ and 2β subunits, which allows the glycine receptor binding to gephyrin, that links it to tubulin. Strychnine is an antagonist for both forms of Gly receptors. (Reproduced with permission from Nestler EJ, Hyman SE, Holtzman DM, et al: *Molecular Neuropharmacology: A Foundation for Clinical Neuroscience*, 3rd ed. New York, NY: McGraw Hill; 2015.)

neuron is modest, GlyTs are key for recycling Gly into the presynaptic neuron where it can replenish the Gly synaptic vesicle pool. GlyT1 is primarily an astrocytic Gly transporter expressed near glutamatergic neurons where it regulates Gly levels in the vicinity of the NMDARs. GlyT2 is expressed predominantly by glycinergic neurons, where it functions acutely to decrease synaptic Gly concentrations, but chronically, it is required to replenish presynaptic Gly stores.

Mutations in the GlyRs, gephrin, or GlyT genes have been implicated in hyperekplexias, a set of genetic disorders characterized by pronounced startle responses to tactile or acoustic stimuli and hypertonia. Mutations in the *GLRα1* gene are associated with hereditary hyperekplexia type 1, whereas mutations in the *GlyRβ* gene are associated with hereditary hyperekplexia type 2. A mutation in the gephrin gene has been identified in a sporadic case of hyperekplexia. A third form of inherited hyperekplexia of presynaptic origin (hereditary hyperekplexia type 3) results from mutations in the *GlyT2* gene. Defects within the *GlyT2* gene are expected to reduce the presynaptic concentrations of Gly necessary for normal glycinergic transmission.

EXCITATION/INHIBITION RATIO

Glutamatergic excitatory and GABAergic inhibitory neurons are immensely interconnected, forming networks of feedforward and feedback circuits whereby inhibitory neurons modulate the activity of excitatory neurons and vice versa. In the cerebral cortex, the interplay of cortical excitation and inhibition is a fundamental feature of cortical information processing. For example, a subset of GABAergic cortical interneurons drive gamma rhythms and promote cortical circuit performance and cognitive flexibility. A balance between neural excitation and neural inhibition is crucial to normal cognition and behavior. Disturbances in the balance between excitatory and inhibitory transmission (the E/I balance) are proposed to underlie a number of disorders. For example, excessive excitation or diminished inhibition can result in seizures and epilepsy, whereas decreased excitation or enhanced inhibition can result in coma. E/I imbalances have been implicated in schizophrenia, which has been correlated with a low E/I ratio caused by weakly active Glu receptors, and in autism, in which a high E/I ratio caused by decreases in active GABA receptors have been documented.

SUMMARY

- Neurotransmitter-dependent communication between a presynaptic neuron and its target can be complex, involving synaptic (wiring) transmission and/or volume (nonsynaptic) transmission and ionotropic receptors and/or metabotropic GPCRs, and can be excitatory, inhibitory, and/or modulatory, with short- and/or long-term effects.

- Acetylcholine is synthesized from acetyl-coenzyme A (CoA) and choline. NTs are transported into synaptic vesicles by NT transporters.

- Nicotinic ACh receptors are ionotropic receptors that mediate fast excitatory responses.

- Muscarinic ACh receptors are metabotropic GPCRs that mediate slow synaptic transmission and neuromodulation.

- ACh is the NT used in the somatic motor system at the neuromuscular junction between motor neurons and skeletal muscle cells.

- ACh is used in the autonomic nervous system by all preganglionic autonomic neurons and the majority of postganglionic parasympathetic neurons.

- In the CNS, cholinergic neurons located in the basal forebrain, striatum. and brainstem are involved in memory, arousal, attention, reward, and sleep.

- ACh is removed from the synapse by ACh esterase, a target of several therapeutic drugs, pesticides, and nerve gas.

- Glutamate is the major excitatory NT in the CNS. Glutamatergic neurons have been implicated in nearly every aspect of normal brain function, including motor control, sensory relay and processing, emotion, cognition, and memory.

- Three types of ionotropic receptors, AMPA, and kainite, and NMDA receptors, mediate fast excitatory synaptic transmission.

- NMDA receptors require glutamate, a coagonist such as glycine, and membrane depolarization to be active; they are permeable to Ca^{2+}.

- Metabotropic glutamate receptors are GPCRs that mediate slow synaptic transmission and neuromodulation.

- Glutamate is removed from the synapse by EAATs expressed by astrocytes and neurons.

- Excessive glutamate signaling can produce excitotoxicity that can lead to neuronal injury and death.

- γ-Aminobutyric acid is the major inhibitory NT in the brain; both GABA and glycine are the main inhibitory NTs is the spinal cord.

- $GABA_A$ and glycine receptors are ionotropic receptors that produce fast inhibitory postsynaptic potentials or shunting inhibition.

- $GABA_B$ receptors are metabotropic GPCRs, with generally inhibitory effects.

- GABA and glycine are removed from the synapse by GABA transporters and glycine transporters, respectively.

- The balance between excitation and inhibition, the E/I ratio, is crucial in normal cortical circuit activities; E/I imbalances have been implicated in several nervous system disorders.

SELF-ASSESSMENT QUESTIONS

1. The cell bodies for neurons that synthesize and release acetylcholine (ACh), called cholinergic neurons, are located in
   A. only the brainstem and spinal cord.
   B. only the autonomic nervous system.
   C. only the central nervous system (CNS).
   D. only the peripheral nervous system (PNS).
   E. both the CNS and PNS.

2. A neurologist selects a drug that has properties similar to γ-aminobutyric acid (GABA) for the treatment of temporal lobe epilepsy. This neurotransmitter (NT) serves important functions within the CNS. Which of the following accurately characterizes a basic property of this NT?
   A. GABA is known to have equal inhibitory and excitatory properties in the adult CNS.
   B. The associated receptor channel is permeable to Cl^- ions.
   C. GABA is formed directly from serine.
   D. Increased GABA is associated with the generation of seizure activity.
   E. GABA is present mainly in the spinal cord.

3. A patient with a history of depression is treated with a novel compound that acts mainly upon *N*-methyl-D-aspartate (NMDA) receptors. Which of the following best describes a basic property associated with the NMDA receptor?
   A. The NMDA receptor–associated channel is blocked by the presence of Mg^{2+} at the resting membrane potential.
   B. It controls a high-conductance anion channel.
   C. NMDA is selective for metabotropic receptors.
   D. Insufficient amounts of glutamate, acting through NMDA receptors, may cause neuronal cell death.
   E. Current flow is blocked in the presence of glutamate, leading to hyperpolarization of the postsynaptic cell.

4. Which of the following best describes neurons in the cerebral cortex?
   A. Cortical local circuit neurons release monoamines that modulate projection neurons.
   B. Cortical projection neurons are mainly GABAergic and send axons to other CNS regions.
   C. Cortical neurons receive inputs from other cortical regions but not other brain areas.
   D. Cortical neurons are either glutamatergic or GABAergic.
   E. The majority of cortical glutamatergic neurons are local circuit neurons.

5. Summation in neurons refers to the addition of all the
   A. driving forces for all the ions.
   B. action potentials.
   C. inhibitory postsynaptic potentials (IPSPs) and excitatory postsynaptic potentials (EPSPs).
   D. Na^+ currents.
   E. Nernst/equilibrium potentials for all the ions.

Neurotransmitter Systems II: Monoamines, Purines, Neuropeptides, & Unconventional Neurotransmitters

Anne B. Theibert

OBJECTIVES

After studying this chapter, the student should be able to:

- Diagram the synthesis, packaging, and transport of the monoamine neurotransmitters (NTs) dopamine, norepinephrine (NE), epinephrine (EP), serotonin, and histamine.
- Identify the localization of monoaminergic neuron cell bodies in the brainstem or hypothalamus and their projections in the brain and spinal cord.
- Describe the functions of the monoamine NTs.
- Distinguish the types of purine NTs and their metabolism, receptors, and functions.
- Illustrate the synthesis, packaging, and removal of neuropeptides (NPs).
- Identify the main categories of NPs and outline their general functions.
- Define unconventional NTs, gasotransmitters, and endocannabinoids.
- Diagram the synthesis and targets of unconventional NTs.

MONOAMINES

Monoamine neurotransmitters (NTs) are a subgroup of biogenic amines that contain an amino and aromatic group and function as NTs. The 3 categories of monoamine NTs are the catecholamines, which include dopamine (DA), norepinephrine (NE), and epinephrine (EP); the indolamine serotonin (abbreviated by its chemical name 5-hydroxytryptamine [5-HT]); and the imidazolamine histamine (HA) (Figure 9–1). Monoamine neuron cell bodies are located in the brainstem or hypothalamus, with their axons projecting throughout the brain and spinal cord. Although they represent only a small percentage of the total number of neurons in the brain, monoaminergic neurons function in important processes, including emotion, arousal, mood, reward, sleep, and memory. Therapeutic drugs that modulate monoamine transmission are used to treat depression, bipolar disorder, attention deficit hyperactivity disorder (ADHD), anxiety disorders, posttraumatic stress disorder (PTSD), schizophrenia, and

Parkinson disease (PD). Several addictive drugs of abuse, including cocaine and methamphetamine, lead to alteration of neuronal circuits involving monoamines. In the peripheral nervous system (PNS), monoamines are synthesized and released by postganglionic sympathetic neurons, adrenal chromaffin cells, and neurons in the gastrointestinal (GI) tract. All monoamines function via specific metabotropic G-protein–coupled receptors (GPCRs); 5-HT also employs an ionotropic receptor (Figure 9–2). Given their mechanisms of action through G proteins and second messenger pathways, monoamines function in slow synaptic transmission and neuromodulation.

DOPAMINE

Catecholamines are defined by containing an amino group and the aromatic catechol group. All 3 catecholamine NTs are derived from the amino acid tyrosine, which is obtained from the diet or synthesized in the liver from phenylalanine by

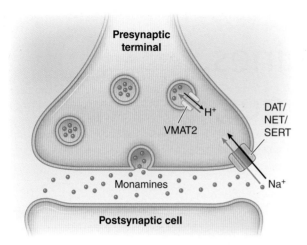

FIGURE 9-1 Schematic of a presynaptic monoaminergic neuron. All monoamines are transported into synaptic vesicles by a vesicular monoamine transporter (VMAT1 or VMAT2). Following release into the synaptic cleft, monoamines are transported back into the presynaptic neuron or nearby astrocytes by the selective transporters for dopamine (DAT), norepinephrine (NET) or serotonin (SERT).

the enzyme phenylalanine hydroxylase. The first step in catecholamine NT biosynthesis involves the conversion of tyrosine to L-3,4-dihydroxyphenylalanine (L-DOPA) by tyrosine hydroxylase (Figure 9–3). L-DOPA is then converted to DA by aromatic L-amino acid decarboxylase (AAAD). After synthesis in dopaminergic neurons, DA is transported into synaptic vesicles by the vesicular monoamine transporter (VMAT) isoform VMAT2.

Dopaminergic neurons are located in the midbrain region of the brainstem in the substantia nigra (SN) and ventral tegmental area (VTA) and in the hypothalamus. The SN derives its name from the expression of melanin, which produces a dark bluish-black pigmentation in neurons. Dopaminergic neurons project to nearly every region of the brain (Figure 9–4). DA is involved in executive functions, motivation, arousal, reward, and motor control, as well as lower level functions including lactation, sexual gratification, and nausea.

Projection of dopaminergic neurons from the SN pars compacta to the dorsal striatum (the caudate nucleus and putamen), termed the *nigrostriatal pathway*, plays significant

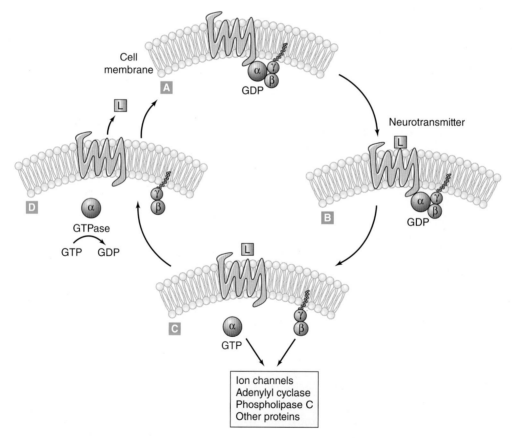

FIGURE 9-2 Monoamines function through metabotropic G-protein–coupled receptors. **A.** Under basal conditions, the α subunit is bound to GDP and the G protein exists in a heterotrimer complex composed of a single α, β, and γ subunit. **B.** After the receptor (R) is activated by its ligand (e.g., a monoamine), R associates with the α subunit, causing the α subunit to release the bound GDP. Subsequently GTP (present in higher concentrations than GDP) binds to the α subunit. **C.** GTP binding causes the dissociation of the α subunit from its βγ subunits and from the receptor. Free α subunit, bound to GTP, directly regulates effector proteins, such as adenylyl cyclase and phospholipase. Free βγ subunits can also directly regulate some of the same effector proteins as well as ion channels. **D.** Intrinsic GTPase activity in the α subunit hydrolyzes GTP to GDP and causes reassociation of the α and βγ subunits, restoring the basal state. (Reproduced with permission from Nestler EJ, Hyman SE, Holtzman DM, et al: *Molecular Neuropharmacology: A Foundation for Clinical Neuroscience*, 3rd ed. New York, NY: McGraw Hill; 2015.)

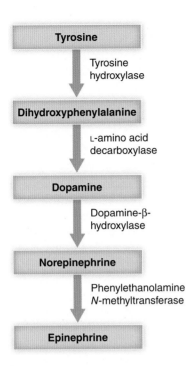

FIGURE 9-3 Steps in the biosynthesis of catecholamines. Dopamine, norepinephrine, and epinephrine are derived from the multistep processing of tyrosine, a dietary amino acid that is actively transported across the blood–brain barrier and concentrated in catecholaminergic neurons. Neuron-specific expression of the enzymes shown here determines which neurotransmitters are synthesized in a given neuron.

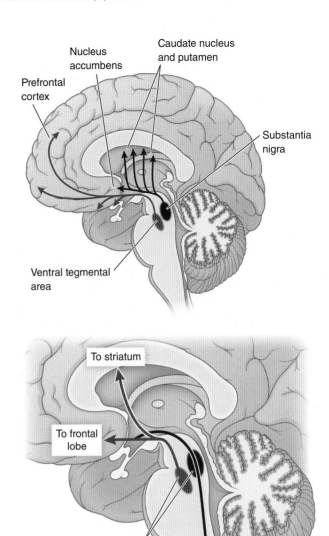

FIGURE 9-4 Localization of dopaminergic neurons in the brain. Dopaminergic neuron cell bodies are located in the midbrain in the substantia nigra and ventral tegmental area, and in the hypothalamus (not illustrated). Axons from dopaminergic neurons project to cortical, subcortical, brainstem, and spinal cord regions.

roles in the regulation of motor control and in learning motor skills. These SN neurons are especially vulnerable to damage, and when a large number degenerate, the result is PD. The nigrostriatal pathway is also partially involved in reward and procedural memory. VTA dopaminergic neurons project to the prefrontal cortex via the mesocortical pathway, which is involved in cognitive control, executive functions, motivation, and emotional responses. Another smaller group from the VTA projects to the nucleus accumbens (NA) via the meso-limbic pathway. Sometimes referred to as the reward pathway, the mesolimbic pathway is involved in motivation, incentive salience (an increased motivation for rewarding stimuli), reinforcement and reward-related motor function learning, and fear. The VTA also sends dopaminergic projections to the amygdala, cingulate gyrus, hippocampus, and olfactory bulb. The fourth dopaminergic pathway is the tuberoinfun-dibular system, which originates in the arcuate nucleus of the hypothalamus, projects to the median eminence, and controls secretion of prolactin by the pituitary.

DA receptors are metabotropic GPCRs. Five sub-types of DA receptors (D1R to D5R) have been identified, which can be divided into the D1-like and D2-like fami-lies. D1-like receptors (D1R and D5R) are predominantly expressed postsynaptically where they couple through $G\alpha_s$ to stimulation of adenylyl cyclase, which synthesizes cyclic adenosine monophosphate (cAMP), leading to activation

of protein kinase A (PKA). D1-like effects can be excitatory or inhibitory. D2-like receptors (D2R, D3R, and D4R) are located both presynaptically and postsynaptically, where they couple through $G\alpha_{i/o}$ to inhibition of adenylyl cyclase and decreased cAMP and PKA activity. Activation of D2-like receptors usually produces inhibition. The signal-ing pathways downstream of DA receptors can be complex, with effects on several mitogen-activated protein (MAP) kinase pathways reported.

D1Rs are the most abundantly expressed DA receptors in humans, with highest levels in the striatum, NA, SN, olfactory bulb, amygdala, and frontal cortex, and lower levels in the hippocampus, cerebellum, thalamus, and hypothalamus. D5Rs are expressed in the prefrontal cortex, hippocampus, SN, and hypothalamus. D2R expression occurs in the striatum, NA, olfactory tubercle, SN, NA, VTA, hypothalamus, cortex, septum, amygdala, and hippocampus. Consistent with the proposal that dysregulation of DA signaling contributes to symptoms in schizophrenia and bipolar disorder, D2-like receptor antagonists are the main receptor targets for antipsychotic drugs. In addition, some typical and atypical antipsychotics are antagonists of D1-like, 5-HT, and HA receptors as well.

DA is synthesized by neurons and nonneuronal cells in the periphery, where it exerts many local effects. In the GI tract, dopaminergic neurons reduce GI motility and protect intestinal mucosa. DA inhibits insulin synthesis in the pancreas and increases Na+ excretion and urinary output by the kidneys. In the immune system, DA reduces activity of lymphocytes. A substantial amount of DA circulates in the bloodstream in the conjugated form DA sulfate, with low levels of free DA. In blood vessels, DA inhibits NE release and acts as a vasodilator.

DA is removed from the synapse by uptake via the specific DA transporter (DAT) or the nonselective plasma membrane monoamine transporter (PMAT). Dysfunction of DAT is implicated in a number of disorders, including ADHD, bipolar disorder, clinical depression, and alcoholism. DAT is a target for addictive drugs of abuse and therapeutic drugs, which are predicted to enhance dopaminergic signaling by increasing DA levels at the synapse. Cocaine, methylphenidate (Ritalin) prescribed for ADHD, and bupropion prescribed for depression block DAT by binding directly and reducing the rate of DA transport. Amphetamine and methamphetamine work by a less direct mechanism. They enter the presynaptic neuron, compete for reuptake with DA, and stimulate the reverse transport (efflux) of intracellular DA. Within the presynaptic neuron, DA is degraded by the sequential activity of monoamine oxidase (MAO), catechol-O-methyltransferase (COMT), and aldehyde dehydrogenase (ALDH). Drugs that block these enzymes are used to treat depression and PD, but are nonselective, with some diet and drug interactions and significant side effects. The other important drugs, including L-DOPA, used in the treatment of PD are described in Chapter 28.

NOREPINEPHRINE & EPINEPHRINE

NE is synthesized from DA by the enzyme DA β-hydroxylase (DBH). Both soluble and membrane-associated DBH isoforms exist. After synthesis by soluble DBH, NE is transported into synaptic vesicles in the central nervous system (CNS) by VMAT2. In neurosecretory cells such as chromaffin cells in the PNS, NE is transported by VMAT1 into a specialized type of secretory vesicle called a dense core vesicle, which is larger than a synaptic vesicle and contains adenosine triphosphate (ATP) and the protein chromogranin. NE can also be synthesized from DA by DBH located inside synaptic or dense core vesicles. NE is also called noradrenaline, and neurons that synthesize and release NE are called noradrenergic neurons. In the CNS, noradrenergic neurons are located in 3 brainstem areas and project throughout the CNS. The largest population of noradrenergic neurons is located is the locus coeruleus (LC) in the pons, which send projections to every major part of the brain and spinal cord (Figure 9–5). Noradrenergic neurons located in the caudal ventrolateral part of the medulla play a role in the control of body fluid metabolism. Noradrenergic neurons located in the nucleus tractus solitarius (NTS) in the medulla function in control of food intake and responses to stress.

LC noradrenergic (LCN) neurons are involved in sleep and dreaming. During sleep, LCN activity is low and decreases even further during rapid eye movement (REM) sleep. During wakefulness, LCN neurons are involved in attentiveness, memory, and emotion. LCN activity increases transiently when presented with attention-drawing stimuli. NE enhances attention, processing of sensory inputs and perception, modulation of synaptic plasticity, and formation and retrieval of both long-term and working memory. Unpleasant stimuli, such as pain, difficulty breathing, bladder distension, or noxious temperature, or stimuli that produce fear generate larger increases in LCN activity. In general, situations that activate LCN neurons are similar to those that activate the sympathetic nervous system. Consequently, as the LCN system mobilizes the brain to respond, the sympathetic system mobilizes the body for action.

In the PNS, postganglionic sympathetic neurons (except those that innervate sweat glands and some blood vessels) are noradrenergic. Sympathetic neurons innervate tissues in most organ systems, providing regulation of a diversity of functions, including pupil constriction, gut motility, mobilization of energy, urinary system output, activity in the heart, and regulation of blood flow. Preganglionic sympathetic innervation of the adrenal medulla stimulates adrenal chromaffin cells to release NE and EP into the circulation, which causes blood vessel constriction to divert blood from nonessential organs and increases in heart rate.

EP (also known as adrenaline) is synthesized from NE by the enzyme phenylethanolamine N-methyltransferase (PNMT). Similar to NE, EP is transported into synaptic vesicles by VMAT2 or into dense core vesicles by VMAT1. Adrenergic neurons identified in the CNS by the expression of PNMT are located in several nuclei in the medulla oblongata, including the dorsal part of the NTS and dorsomedial reticular formation. Adrenergic neurons in the brain are involved in sexual arousal and sexual behavior, control of appetite, and metabolic control, and may contribute to some functions

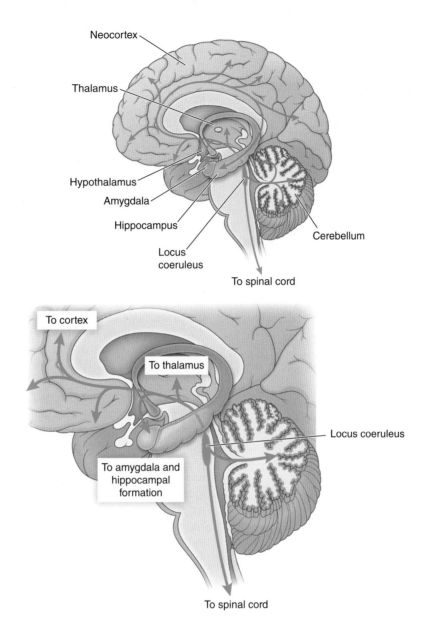

FIGURE 9–5 Localization of noradrenergic neurons in the brain. Noradrenergic cell bodies are located in the pons in the locus coeruleus as illustrated, and project axons to many cortical and subcortical regions of the brain, the brainstem and to the spinal cord. Noradrenergic neuron cell bodies are also located in the medulla (not shown) where they contribute to autonomic control.

ascribed to NE, including attentiveness, arousal, cognition, and mental focus. In the periphery, adrenal chromaffin cells are the major source of EP. In response to sympathetic activation, EP and NE are released into the circulation and act as adrenal stress hormones.

Both NE and EP function through metabotropic GPCRs called α- and β-adrenergic receptors. The α1 receptor subtypes (α1A, α1B, and α1D) are $G\alpha_{q/11}$-coupled receptors that activate phospholipase C (PLC), resulting in increases in inositol triphosphate, Ca^{2+}, and diacylglycerol. The α2 receptors (α2A to α2C) are $G\alpha_{i/o}$-coupled receptors that inhibit adenylyl cyclase, reducing levels of cAMP and decreasing PKA activity. Phenylephrine is a selective agonist of the

α1 receptor, whereas clonidine is a nonselective α2 receptor agonist. Three subtypes of β receptors (β1, β2, and β3) are linked to the $G\alpha_s$ proteins that activate adenylyl cyclase, which increase cAMP and PKA activity. The β2 isoform can also couple to $G\alpha_{i/o}$. Isoproterenol is a nonselective β receptor agonist, whereas propranolol, one of the "β-blockers," is a β receptor antagonist.

Both α- and β-adrenergic receptors are expressed in many brain regions including the cerebral cortex, hippocampus, brainstem, thalamus, and cerebellum, where they produce a variety of neuromodulatory effects. Coexpressed in most brain regions, β1 receptors predominate in the cerebral cortex, whereas β2 receptors predominate in the cerebellum.

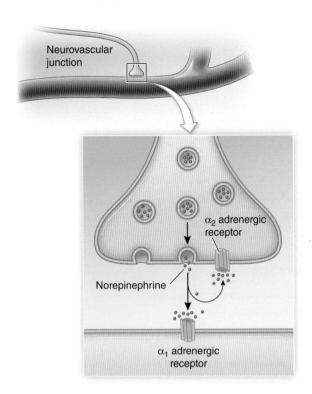

FIGURE 9–6 Illustration of a synapse between a sympathetic neuron and its target blood vessel, called a neurovascular junction. The presynaptic sympathetic neuron releases norepinephrine, which can bind to α-adrenergic receptors localized at the postsynaptic (α1) and presynaptic (α2) regions.

α2 receptors are located postsynaptically and presynaptically, where they mediate inhibition of NT release (Figure 9–6). In the periphery, responses to postganglionic sympathetic neurons involve α- or β-adrenergic receptors. For example, α receptors mediate smooth muscle contraction, whereas β receptors mediate heart muscle contraction, smooth muscle relaxation, and gluconeogenesis. A large number of important therapeutic drugs exert their effects by interacting with adrenergic systems in the brain or body, including treatment of cardiovascular disorders, shock, and a variety of psychiatric conditions. For CNS disorders, the α2-adrenergic agonist clonidine is used to treat ADHD and anxiety disorder. Recently, α1-adrenergic antagonists have emerged in treatment of PTSD, dementia-related agitation, and alcohol, cocaine, and nicotine dependence.

In the CNS, NE is taken up by the NE transporter (NET). Although NET expression appears to be restricted to noradrenergic neurons, NETs can also take up DA. NETs are targets of many antidepressant drugs, including 5-HT–NE reuptake inhibitors (SNRIs), NE-DA reuptake inhibitors (NDRIs), NE reuptake inhibitors (NRIs or NERIs), and the tricyclic antidepressants (TCAs). Moreover, although originally thought to be selective DAT modulators, cocaine, amphetamine, methylphenidate, and bupropion are also inhibitors of reuptake by NETs and 5-HT transporters as

well. Consequently, NETs are also the target of addictive drugs of abuse and therapeutic drugs. Polymorphisms in NETs have been implicated in several clinical disorders, including ADHD, postural tachycardia, and orthostatic intolerance. A selective EP transporter has yet to be identified, and EP transport may involve PMAT and/or the organic cation transporter 3 (OCT3).

SEROTONIN & HISTAMINE

The indolamine 5-HT is synthesized from the amino acid tryptophan by the enzymes tryptophan hydroxylase and AAAD (Figure 9–7). 5-HT is one of the oldest NTs in evolution. In the presynaptic neuron, 5-HT is transported into synaptic vesicles via VMAT2. In the brain, serotonergic neurons are localized in 9 nuclei in the median and dorsal raphe nuclei in the reticular formation (Figure 9–8). From this brainstem region, serotonergic neurons project to nearly every region of the CNS, including the hippocampus, amygdala, hypothalamus, thalamus, neocortex, brainstem, and basal ganglia.

Serotonergic neurons are involved in the regulation of mood, reward, anger, aggression, anxiety, sleep, nausea, sexuality, sensorimotor functions including pain processing, and cognition including learning and memory. Dysregulation of serotonergic systems has been implicated in the pathogenesis of depression, bipolar disorder, anxiety disorders, neuropathic pain, and schizophrenia. 5-HT is also involved in homeostatic mechanisms including appetite, thermoregulation, modulation of energy balance, and the hypothalamic-pituitary-adrenal axis. In addition, roles for 5-HT in the control of breathing and respiratory drive have been revealed by studies showing serotonergic abnormalities in roughly half of infants who have died from sudden infant death syndrome. In nonhuman primates, levels of 5-HT are correlated with social hierarchy and with risk-sensitive decision making.

The 2 main categories of 5-HT receptors (5HTRs) are the ionotropic 5HTRs and metabotropic GPCR 5HTRs. A total of 15 5HTR genes grouped into 7 families ($5HT_{1-7}R$) have been

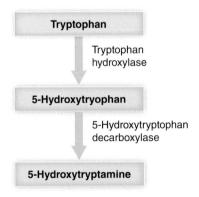

FIGURE 9–7 Biosynthetic pathway of serotonin. Serotonin, also known as 5-hydroxytryptamine (5-HT), is derived from the multistep processing of the dietary amino acid tryptophan.

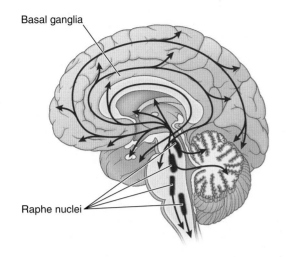

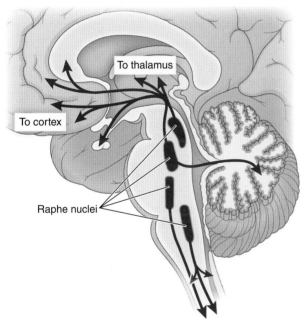

FIGURE 9-8 Localization of serotonergic neurons in the brain. Serotonergic neuron cell bodies are located in the raphe nuclei in the reticular formation. Serotonergic axons project to the majority of regions in the brain and spinal cord.

identified, with numerous subtypes within each family. The 5HT$_3$R genes encode the ionotropic receptors. All the rest are GPCRs. 5HTRs are expressed throughout the CNS, including the cerebral cortex, amygdala, basal ganglia, thalamus, hypothalamus, hippocampus, brainstem, cerebellum, and spinal cord. Located both postsynaptically and presynaptically, many effects of 5HTRs are mediated through effects on the release of other NTs, including glutamate (Glu), γ-aminobutyric acid (GABA), DA, EP, NE, and acetylcholine (ACh), and neurohormones.

As an ionotropic receptor, the 5HT$_3$R consists of 5 subunits, which forms a nonselective cation channel permeable to Na$^+$, K$^+$, and Ca^{2+}. Binding of 5-HT to the 5HT$_3$R opens the channel and leads to a fast excitatory postsynaptic potential (EPSP). 5HT$_3$Rs are localized to brainstem regions that control the vomiting reflex. Accordingly, 5HT$_3$Rs antagonists are the current gold standard for treatment of postoperative, chemotherapy-induced, and radiation-induced nausea and vomiting. 5HT$_3$Rs are expressed in many other brain regions, including the neocortex and amygdala. Mutations in 5HT$_3$R subunits have been associated with bipolar disorder, depression, anxiety, anorexia, and irritable bowel syndrome (IBS). Postsynaptic 5HT$_3$Rs are preferentially expressed on interneurons where they may play a role in the formation and function of cortical circuits. Consistent with this, 5HT$_3$Rs have also been implicated in susceptibility to seizures.

5HT$_1$R and 5HT$_5$R inhibit adenylyl cyclase through Gα$_{i/o}$, and as neuromodulators, 5HT$_1$R and 5HT$_5$R generally produce inhibitory effects. 5HT$_{1A}$Rs are expressed in high densities in the cerebral cortex, hippocampus, septum, amygdala, and raphe nucleus, whereas lower levels are located in the medulla, basal ganglia, and thalamus. 5HT$_{1A}$Rs have been implicated in the central control of blood pressure and heart rate and have been demonstrated to affect specific aspects of memory, probably through their modulation of other NT levels. 5HT$_{1A}$R agonists such as buspirone have shown efficacy in relieving anxiety, depression, and migraine and cluster headaches. Some atypical antipsychotics such as aripiprazole are partial agonists at the 5HT$_{1A}$R and are sometimes used in combination with 5-HT reuptake inhibitors to treat depression.

5HT$_2$Rs activate PLC through Gα$_{q/11}$ and generally mediate excitatory effects. However, because an important target of 5HTRs is NT release, enhancing GABA release can produce inhibitory effects. The 5HT$_2$Rs were first noted for their importance as targets for the psychedelic drugs lysergic acid diethylamide (LSD) and mescaline, which are 5HT$_2$R agonists. 5HT$_{2A}$Rs are widely distributed in the brain, including the neocortex and cerebellum. 5HT$_{2A}$R antagonists have antipsychotic, antidepressant, and anxiolytic properties and may be useful in treating drug addiction and disorders that affect memory. 5HT$_{2C}$Rs are distributed throughout the brain and regulate anxiety, reward processing, locomotion, appetite, and energy balance.

5HT$_4$Rs and 5HT$_6$Rs activate adenylyl cyclase through Gα$_s$. 5HT$_4$Rs are expressed throughout the brain, with the highest levels in the basal ganglia. Evidence supports a role for 5HT$_4$R s in the pathogenesis of depression, and other studies on animal models show that modulation of 5HT$_4$Rs produces effects on memory and feeding. Based on its abundance in extrapyramidal, limbic, and cortical regions, it has been suggested that 5HT$_6$R plays a role in motor control, emotion, cognition, and memory. Recent studies report cognitive enhancing properties of a 5HT$_6$R antagonist in patients with moderate Alzheimer disease (AD).

Several lines of evidence indicate that 5-HT and 5HTRs are involved in cognition and memory. Serotonergic neurons project to, and 5HTRs are robustly expressed in, brain regions and neuronal populations essential for learning and memory. Reductions in brain 5-HT concentrations impair contextual fear memory and object memory in rodents and declarative memory in humans.

Decreased expression of 5HTRs has been observed in postmortem AD brains. Polymorphisms in the human 5HT$_{2A}$R gene are associated with altered memory processes. Agonists of 5HT$_2$Rs and 5HT$_4$Rs, and antagonists of 5HT$_1$Rs and 5HT$_3$Rs prevent memory impairment and facilitate learning in situations involving a high cognitive demand. Likewise, antagonists for 5HT$_2$R and 5HT$_4$R or agonists for 5HT$_1$R or 5HT$_3$R have the expected opposite effects on learning and memory.

After release, 5-HT is transported back into the presynaptic neuron by the specific 5-HT transporter (SERT) and possibly via PMAT, reducing the levels of 5-HT at the synapse. Inhibition of 5-HT reuptake at synapses is the target of therapeutic drugs including selective 5-HT reuptake inhibitors (SSRIs) and TCAs. SSRIs are usually the first-line treatment option for depression and some of the most widely prescribed antidepressants. SSRIs are also frequently prescribed for anxiety disorders, such as social anxiety disorder, panic disorders, obsessive-compulsive disorder, eating disorders, chronic pain, and, occasionally, PTSD. Several addictive drugs of abuse, including cocaine, amphetamine, and dextromethorphan, also modulate 5-HT levels at the synapse by effects on SERT.

The highest concentrations of 5-HT are found in the body, produced by enterochromaffin cells of the GI tract, where 5-HT regulates intestinal movements, and by platelets in the blood. 5HT$_3$R and 5HT$_4$R antagonists are used to treat symptoms in IBS. The effects of 5-HT are also prominent in the cardiovascular system, with additional effects on the peripheral respiratory and genitourinary system. 5-HT can cause either vasoconstriction or vasodilation of blood vessels, depending on which subtypes of receptors are involved.

The imidazolamine histamine (HA) functions as an NT in the CNS and as a mediator released by cells in the immune system and GI tract. HA is synthesized from the amino acid histidine by the enzyme L-histidine decarboxylase and is transported into synaptic vesicles by VMAT. The cell bodies of histaminergic neurons are found in the tuberomammillary nuclei in the posterior hypothalamus (**Figure 9–9**). Passing through the medial forebrain bundle, histaminergic neurons project to several regions throughout the brain, including the cortex. In the periphery, mast cells and basophils of the immune system and enterochromaffin-like cells of the GI system are the major HA-producing cells.

Four HA receptors, identified as H1R, H2R, H3R, and H4R, are metabotropic GPCRs. Expressed in the CNS in the tuberomammillary nucleus and in many peripheral tissues, H1R is coupled to G$\alpha_{q/11}$ and activation of PLC (**Figure 9–10**). In their central action, the H1Rs participate in modulation of the circadian cycle and sleep. H2R is coupled to Gα_s and increased cAMP and is expressed in the brain. The H3R protein is coupled to a G$\alpha_{i/o}$ and PLC. Expression of the HRH3 gene occurs predominantly in the basal ganglia, cortex, hippocampus, and striatum, where it decreases ACh, 5-HT, and NE production and release. HA neurons increase wakefulness and prevent sleep. Antihistamines (H1R receptor antagonists),

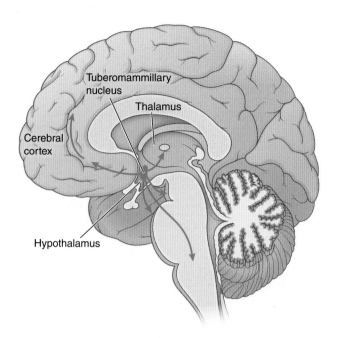

FIGURE 9–9 Localization of histaminergic neurons in the brain. Histaminergic neuron cell bodies are located in the tuberomammillary nuclei in the hypothalamus. Histaminergic axons project to regions in the forebrain, brainstem, and spinal cord.

which cross the blood–brain barrier, produce drowsiness and impair the ability to maintain vigilance. Histaminergic neurons have a wakefulness-related firing pattern. They fire rapidly during waking, fire slowly during periods of relaxation/tiredness, and completely stop firing during REM and non-REM sleep. They also have possible roles in learning and memory. After release, HA can be metabolized by oxidation involving diamine oxidase or by methylation via HA *N*-methyltransferase, producing *N*-methylhistamine that is further metabolized by MAO. HA can also be taken up via the transporters PMAT and OCT3.

PURINES

By numerous criteria, purines are considered NTs and have emerged as important neuromodulators in the CNS and PNS. Purine NTs contain an adenine group and include ATP, adenosine diphosphate (ADP), and adenosine (Ado). ATP is released from synaptic vesicles and often functions as a cotransmitter. In contrast, ADP and Ado are not released from synaptic vesicles but are derived from ATP. At the synapse and extracellular fluid, ATP is rapidly metabolized by ectonucleoside triphosphate diphosphohydrolases to ADP and AMP, which is further metabolized by ecto-5′-nucleotidase to form Ado. Extracellular Ado can be removed by a nucleoside transporter or by metabolism by Ado deaminase and Ado kinase. Purines act through specific purinergic receptors, which are expressed in neurons, glial cells, and PNS targets.

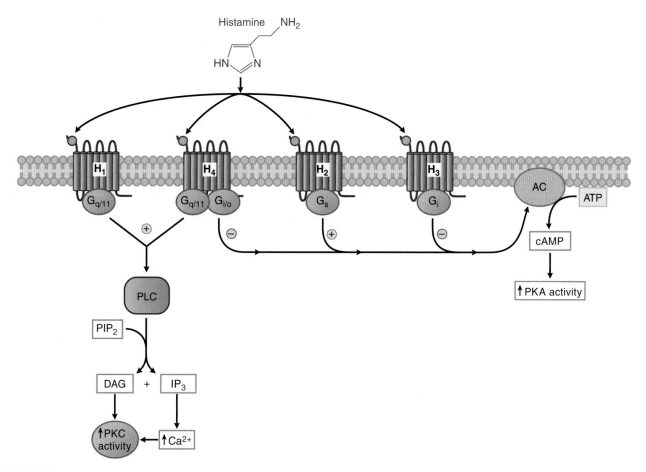

FIGURE 9–10 Different histamine receptor types couple to different G protein signal transduction pathways. H_1 receptors activate phosphatidylinositol turnover via $G_{q/11}$. The other receptors couple either positively (H_2 receptor) or negatively (H_3 and H_4 receptor) to adenylyl cyclase activity via G_s and $G_{i/o}$, respectively. Signaling pathways affected by histamine provide both immediate and long-term regulation of cell function. (Reproduced with permission from Brunton LL, Hilal-Dandan R, Knollmann BC: *Goodman & Gilman's the Pharmacological Basis of Therapeutics*, 13th ed. New York, NY: McGraw Hill; 2018.)

Two main categories of receptors are activated by purines, the ionotropic receptors and metabotropic GPCRs. The P2X receptors (P2XRs) are ionotropic receptors that are considered ATP receptors because P2XRs exhibit a much higher affinity for ATP compared with other purines (Figure 9–11). Seven P2XR isoform genes have been cloned, and they likely form heterotrimer channels. P2XRs are nonselective cation channels with high Ca^{2+} permeability that are expressed in neurons both presynaptically and postsynaptically and in glial cells throughout the CNS and PNS.

P2Y receptors (P2YRs) and P1 receptors (P1Rs) are metabotropic GPCRs. The P2Ys have high affinity for ATP, ADP, or uridine-5′-triphosphate (UTP). Eight different P2YRs have been identified. $P2Y_1R$, $P2Y_2R$, $P2Y_4R$, $P2Y_6R$, and $P2Y_{11}R$ couple through $G\alpha_{q/11}$ proteins to activation of PLC. $P2Y_{12}R$, $P2Y_{13}R$, and $P2Y_{14}R$ couple through $G\alpha_{i/o}$ to inhibition of adenylyl cyclase. P2YR signaling may be complex because $P2Y_{11}R$ can also couple to $G\alpha_s$ and $P2Y_{14}R$ may couple to $G\alpha_q$. P2YRs are expressed throughout the CNS by neurons, astrocytes, oligodendrocytes, and microglia. Localized both presynaptically and postsynaptically in neurons, P2YRs are

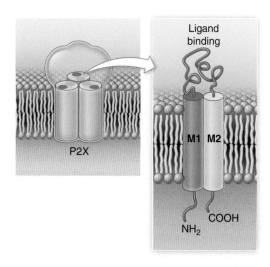

FIGURE 9–11 Ionotropic purinoreceptor (P2X). P2X is an ATP-gated cation channel that is similar in structure to the epithelial Na^+ channel (ENAC). It binds ATP in the extracellular ligand binding domain and is permeable to Na^+, K^+, and Ca^{2+}. Separate genes coding for P2X subunits have been identified, named $P2X_1$ through $P2X_7$.

anticipated to modulate synaptic transmission and plasticity by effects on a number of ion channels, receptors, and gene expression.

P1Rs have a high affinity for Ado compared with other purines and are considered Ado receptors. Four Ado receptor subtypes (A1R, A2AR, A2BR, and A3R) have been identified. The A1Rs and A3Rs couple to $G\alpha_{i/o}$ to inhibition of adenylyl cyclase, inhibit Ca^{2+} conductance, and activate K^+ channels. A2ARs and A2BRs couple to $G\alpha_s$, which stimulates adenylyl cyclase (Figure 9–12). A2BRs and A3Rs may also couple to $G\alpha_{q/11}$ to activation of PLC activity. A1Rs are highly expressed by neurons in many brain regions including the neocortex, hippocampus, cerebellum, and brainstem. Expressed by both neurons and glial cells and displaying a more restricted localization, A2ARs are highly expressed in the striatum and olfactory bulb but show lower expression in other brain regions. Both presynaptic A1R and A2ARs are linked to modulation of NT release. Low levels of A2BR and A3R expression occur in most CNS areas.

ATP functions as an NT in both the CNS and PNS. In postganglionic sympathetic and parasympathetic neurons, ATP is coreleased with NA and ACh, respectively. In both neuronal types, ATP acts at postjunctional P2X1Rs to enhance smooth muscle contraction, often synergizing with NA or ACh. ATP is also coreleased with ACh from motor neurons at the neuromuscular junction, where it may function in regulating postjunctional gene expression and nicotinic ACh receptor clustering. In the periphery, nonneuronal cells release ATP after tissue damage in response to pressure, heat, or chemicals. Released ATP can activate purinergic receptors on receptor regions of somatosensory neurons and transmit nociceptive responses. Sensory axons also release ATP at terminals in the dorsal horn of the spinal cord. In the GI tract, ATP is released from enteric neurons where it acts as an inhibitory NT, mediating descending muscle relaxation during peristalsis.

In the gustatory system, ATP is released by taste receptor cells in response to tastants, most likely through a nonvesicular mechanism involving ATP release channels. The released ATP

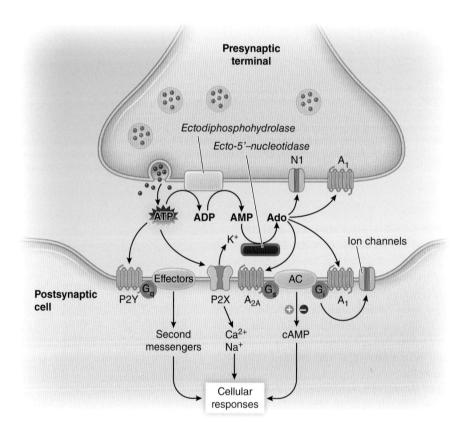

FIGURE 9–12 Diagram of a purinergic synapse. Adenosine triphosphate (ATP) is typically colocalized with a small molecule neurotransmitter and is released into the synaptic cleft in a Ca^{2+}-dependent manner. After release, ATP can directly activate P2Y and P2X receptors. P2Y receptors are coupled to G proteins and activate second messenger systems. Most are coupled to $G_{q/11}$ and activate phospholipase C (PLC) and the phosphatidylinositol pathway. P2X receptors are ligand-gated cation channels that depolarize the postsynaptic membrane and increase Ca^{2+} levels. ATP remaining in the synapse is rapidly converted into adenosine (Ado) by the actions of an ectodiphosphohydrolase and an ecto-5′-nucleotidase. Subsequently, Ado can activate presynaptic and postsynaptic G-protein–coupled P1 receptors (A_1 and A_2) and regulate adenylyl cyclase (AC) and the cAMP pathway, and in turn can be recycled into the presynaptic cell by means of a Na^+-dependent transporter (N1). (Reproduced with permission from Nestler EJ, Hyman SE, Holtzman DM, et al: *Molecular Neuropharmacology: A Foundation for Clinical Neuroscience*, 3rd ed. New York, NY: McGraw Hill; 2015.)

activates purinergic receptors on second-order taste neurons to mediate sensory transmission. In the CNS, although a few small populations of neurons in the hippocampus, brainstem, and cortex may use ATP in fast excitatory synaptic transmission, in general, ATP is a cotransmitter and neuromodulatory in its effects, through both P2X and P2Y receptors. Disruption of purine-regulated responses has been linked to a variety of disorders, including anxiety, stroke, and epilepsy, and has prompted the development of new therapies to target specific purinergic receptors.

As a neuromodulator, Ado plays an important role in neuronal excitability, with a general inhibitory effect and a central role in sleep. Activation of presynaptic A1Rs inhibits the release of the majority of NTs including Glu, ACh, NE, 5-HT, and DA, whereas stimulation of A2ARs facilitates the release of Glu and ACh and inhibits release of GABA. The concentration of Ado in the brain, most notably in the basal forebrain, increases during waking periods and decreases during sleep. The Ado antagonists caffeine and theophylline are stimulants that act through A1R and A2AR to increase wakefulness and decrease sleep. Ado is involved in regulation of slow wave activity expressed during slow wave sleep. A population of cells in the brainstem and basal forebrain arousal centers has been identified that have activity that is both tightly coupled to thalamocortical activation and under tonic inhibitory control by Ado. Ado regulates numerous NT systems involved in sleep and wakefulness. A1Rs and A2ARs are thought to act in various areas of the brain to decrease neural activity and facilitate sleep. Ado receptors have also been implicated in neuroprotection following brain injury, cognition, and memory.

NEUROPEPTIDES

Neuropeptides (NPs) are small polypeptides containing between 3 and 40 amino acids that are neuromodulatory NTs. NPs represent the most diverse class of signaling molecules in the brain. The human genome contains about 90 genes that encode precursors of NPs, which can be processed to form about 100 identified NPs, although estimates of the total number of candidate NPs are much greater. Most neurons synthesize both a small-molecule NT, such as Glu or GABA, and 1 or more NP, which together function as cotransmitters (Figure 9–13). NPs are similar to peptide hormones released by endocrine cells and neurohormones released by neuroendocrine cells but are released into the synapse or extracellular fluid rather than into the blood. In fact, a number of NPs that function at synapses also function as hormones or neurohormones in the periphery. NPs are involved in a wide range of brain functions including neuroendocrine regulation, analgesia, food and water intake, thermoregulation, circadian rhythms, energy homeostasis and metabolism, sleep-wake states, sexual and reproductive behaviors, social behaviors, mood, reward and motivation, and learning and memory.

In the neuronal soma, NPs are synthesized and packaged as precursor peptides in the rough endoplasmic reticulum and traffic to the Golgi where they are sorted and packaged into secretory vesicles that then travel along the axon. NP precursors undergo maturation as they are transported down the axon via fast axonal transport to the presynaptic terminus. Inside the secretory vesicles, prohormone convertases and carboxypeptidases selectively cleave the NP precursors to generate bioactive NPs, in some cases giving rise to several NPs with distinct functions. Secretory vesicles containing NPs are distinguishable as 100- to 200-nm dense core vesicles (DCVs) that are so named for their electron-dense appearance by electron microscopy. In contrast, synaptic vesicles containing small-molecule NTs are smaller (40 to 50 nm) and are electron lucent.

NP-containing DCVs coexist in the presynaptic neuron with synaptic vesicles but in different locations, with important consequences. Whereas synaptic vesicles are localized close to the presynaptic active zone near the voltage-gated Ca^{2+} channels, DCVs are often located far away from the active zone. Thus, DCVs require a higher rate of presynaptic APs for their Ca^{2+}-dependent fusion and release of NP. NPs can be released near the synapse, but also outside the synapse where they can diffuse some distance. Hence, released NPs tend to be found in lower concentrations but can have access to receptors located extrasynaptically and even on nearby neurons. Once released, NPs are not recycled back to the presynaptic neuron but are cleaved by extracellular peptidases that either inactivate the NP or produce modified NPs with different receptor properties. Therefore, NPs may have more prolonged actions than small-molecule NTs.

Many NPs were originally discovered in the context of regulation of hormone release, and their NP name may reflect that functional link. For example, somatostatin (SS) released by the hypothalamus acts on the anterior pituitary to decrease growth hormone release into the circulation, but SS released by cortical or hippocampal neurons is not involved in hormone regulation. Likewise, vasopressin released by the posterior pituitary into the circulation acts in the kidney as an antidiuretic hormone and on blood vessels to regulate blood pressure, but within the CNS, vasopressin has different functions, including regulation of social behaviors. NPs can be categorized based on different criteria, including their functions, or where the NP is also used as a hormone in the periphery (Table 9–1). Some NPs are synthesized by small populations of neurons, whereas other NPs are synthesized throughout the brain. For several NPs, neurons that use NPs in one brain region may have no anatomic or functional connection with neurons that use that NP in another brain region.

NPs function via the activation of metabotropic GPCRs and are neuromodulatory in their action. Depending on which G protein is involved, NPs can produce different modulatory effects. In addition, because NPs usually act as cotransmitters, NP modulation is intricately linked with fast or slow synaptic transmission mediated by small-molecule NTs. NPs can exert effects on the membrane potential or neuronal excitability within seconds to minutes, but can also modulate gene

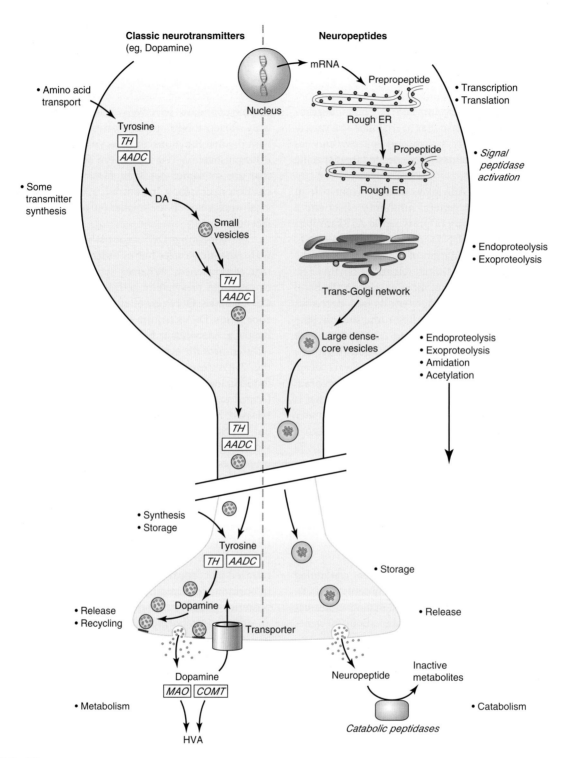

FIGURE 9–13 Comparison between small molecule neurotransmitter and neuropeptide synthesis and localization at the same synapse. Here dopamine represents the small molecule neurotransmitter. Although some dopamine is synthesized in the cell body, the majority of dopamine is synthesized in the presynaptic terminals where it is transported into small clear synaptic vesicles which are located closer to the active zones. In contrast, neuropeptide synthesis occurs in the cell body in the rough ER, and neuropeptides are packaged into large dense core vesicles at the trans Golgi network, transported down the axon and are located further away from the active zone. Both dopamine and the neuropeptides can be degraded at the synapse, but only dopamine is transported back into the nerve terminal. Note that MAO is also located in the presynaptic terminus. AADC, aromatic amino acid decarboxylase; COMT, catechol-O-methyltransferase; DA, dopamine; ER, endoplasmic reticulum; HVA, homovanillic acid; MAO, monoamine oxidase; TH, tyrosine hydroxylase. (Reproduced with permission from Nestler EJ, Hyman SE, Holtzman DM, et al: *Molecular Neuropharmacology: A Foundation for Clinical Neuroscience*, 3rd ed. New York, NY: McGraw Hill; 2015.)

TABLE 9–1 Examples of neuropeptides.

- **Calcitonin family**
  - Calcitonin
  - Calcitonin gene–related peptide
- **Hypothalamic hormones**
  - Oxytocin
  - Vasopressin
- **Hypothalamic releasing and inhibitory hormones**
  - Corticotropin-releasing factor (CRF or CRH)
  - Gonadotropin-releasing hormone (GnRH)
  - Growth hormone-releasing hormone (GHRH)
  - Somatostatin
  - Thyrotropin-releasing hormone (TRH)
- **Neuropeptide Y family**
  - Neuropeptide Y (NPY)
  - Neuropeptide YY (PYY)
  - Pancreatic polypeptide (PP)
- **Opioid peptides**
  - β-Endorphin (also a pituitary hormone)
  - Dynorphin peptides
  - Leu-enkephalin
  - Met-enkephalin
- **Pituitary hormones**
  - Adrenocorticotropic hormone (ACTH)
  - α-Melanocyte-stimulating hormone (α-MSH)
  - Growth hormone (GH)
  - Follicle-stimulating hormone (FSH)
  - Luteinizing hormone (LH)
- **Tachykinins**
  - Neurokinin A (substance K)
  - Neurokinin B
  - Neuropeptide K
  - Substance P
- **VIP–glucagon family**
  - Glucagon
  - Glucagon-like peptide-1 (GLP-1)
  - Pituitary adenylate cyclase–activating peptide (PACAP)
  - Vasoactive intestinal polypeptide (VIP)
- **Some other peptides**
  - Agouti-related peptide (ARP)
  - Bradykinin
  - Cholecystokinin (CCK; multiple forms)
  - Cocaine- and amphetamine-regulated transcript (CART)
  - Galanin
  - Ghrelin
  - Melanin-concentrating hormone (MCH)
  - Neurotensin
  - Orexins (or hypocretins)
  - Orphanin FQ (or nociceptin) (also grouped with opioids)

The traditional families of peptides listed here are based partly on other functions of the peptides (eg, hypothalamic releasing and inhibitory hormones), partly on amino acid sequence (eg, NPY family), and partly on pharmacology (opioids peptides), and must be considered at best a rough and incomplete guide to relationships among peptides. For example, β-endorphin is traditionally counted among the opioid peptides, and ACTH and α-MSH as pituitary hormones, but all 3 are derived from the same gene, proopiomelanocortin (POMC).

Reproduced with permission from Nestler EJ, Hyman SE, Holtzman DM, et al: *Molecular Neuropharmacology: A Foundation for Clinical Neuroscience*, 3rd ed. New York, NY: McGraw Hill; 2015.

expression over the course of hours to days. NP receptors are expressed heterogeneously throughout the brain and can be localized to neuronal cell bodies, dendrites, and axon terminals. Numerous NP receptors have been identified, and some NPs act on several different isoforms, suggesting that hundreds of NP receptors may be encoded in the genome. Adding to their complexity, NP receptors can interact by heteromerization, with mosaic formation between different subtypes and subfamilies of NP GPCRs.

The release of NPs outside of the synapse raises an important question about the distances over which NPs work and has sparked debates about whether NPs function as local and/or long-distance neuromodulators. Complicating this debate, DCVs are also found in and released by the soma and dendrites. In many CNS regions, the expression patterns of NP-containing axons and their NP receptors correspond, consistent with a local action ascribed to NPs, meaning that the activity of an NP would be exerted on its synaptic partner and nearby cells. For some NPs, anatomic expression of the NP and its receptors may occur in different regions of the brain. Perhaps this mismatch represents a vestigial feature that was important during evolution but is no longer relevant. Alternately, a robust coordinated release of NP by a group of neurons could elevate the extracellular NP to a level that NPs could diffuse and act far away from the release site. This type of longer distance signaling has been proposed for oxytocin. Thus, there is evidence that most NPs function locally, but in a few cases, NPs may act in longer distance signaling.

NPs have been most extensively characterized in the hypothalamus, an ancient and conserved forebrain area. However, recent studies have also focused on the role of NPs in the neocortex and hippocampus, where GABAergic inhibitory interneurons differentially express NP cotransmitters, including SS, vasoactive intestinal peptide, cholecystokinin, neuropeptide Y (NPY), and substance P. Inhibitory interneurons also differentially express Ca^{2+} binding proteins such as parvalbumin and the $5HT_{3A}R$, which are used to distinguish inhibitory neuronal subtypes. Because local GABAergic inhibitory interneurons are proposed to play fundamental roles in shaping neocortical circuits, specific interneuron subtypes that differ in their NPs and responses may contribute to dynamic alterations in brain states and behavioral context. Moreover, given the importance of the excitation/inhibition ratio, dysregulation of specific subtypes of inhibitory interneurons has been examined for its contribution to disorders, including epilepsy, schizophrenia, and autism.

NPY & THE OPIOID PEPTIDES

One of the most abundant NPs, NPY is a 36–amino acid NP that functions in both the CNS and PNS. In the PNS, NPY is produced by sympathetic neurons and, together with NE, serves as a strong vasoconstrictor; it also enhances growth of fat tissue and affects immune cells. In the CNS, NPY is produced at highest levels in the hypothalamus and at lower levels in the pituitary, retina, hippocampus, neocortex, thalamus, amygdala, basal ganglia, and brainstem. Five NPY receptors (Y1R to Y5R) have been identified. All NPY receptors are GPCRs that couple through $G\alpha_{i/o}$ protein to inhibition of adenylyl cyclase and decreased cAMP production, depressed Ca^{2+} channel, or enhanced GIRK currents. NPY has numerous functions. It is a potent orexigenic hypothalamic NP that increases food intake and storage of energy as fat. NPY is also involved in anxiety and stress reduction, pain perception reduction, and memory processing and cognition; it also affects the circadian rhythm and has central effects on blood pressure. Dysregulation of NPY has also been implicated in several human disorders including obesity, alcoholism, and depression.

Three well-characterized families of endogenous opioid peptides are the endorphins, enkephalins, and dynorphins, produced by proteolytic cleavage of precursor proteins (proopiomelanocortin, proenkephalin, or prodynorphin). Opioid peptides are so named because they bind the opioid receptors, the same receptors that bind the opiates morphine and heroin, which mimic the effects of endogenous opioid peptides. Opioid peptides play a central role in pain processing and regulate many other aspects of behavior, including stress responses, mood, motivation and reward, emotion, and control of food intake, as well as functions in the endocrine, respiratory, GI, and immune systems.

Neurons that produce opioid peptides are found in specific populations of projection neurons in the hypothalamus, which project to limbic forebrain and midbrain areas, and in the medulla, which project to other areas of the brainstem and spinal cord. Opioid peptides are synthesized and released by local neurons distributed throughout the CNS, including the neocortex, hippocampus, thalamus, basal ganglia, brainstem, and spinal cord. In many neurons, opioid peptides are coexpressed with small-molecule NTs. Opioid peptides colocalize with GABAergic, glutamatergic, dopaminergic, and serotonergic neurons in several CNS regions.

The opioid receptor family includes μ, δ, and κ opioid receptors, which are GPCRs defined pharmacologically by their blockade by naloxone and differential affinities for different opioid peptides. Activation of opioid receptors leads to coupling through $G\alpha_{i/o}$ to inhibition of adenylyl cyclase, inhibition of presynaptic voltage-gated Ca^{2+} channels, activation of GIRK channels, and regulation of several MAP kinase pathways. Opioids exert a variety of neuromodulatory effects, depending on whether they act on presynaptic or postsynaptic receptors and in projection neurons or local neurons. Opioid receptors often lead to inhibition of NT release, postsynaptic inhibition, and decreased neuronal excitability. Although generally inhibitory, opioid peptides can also produce excitatory effects by inhibition of GABA release. Opioid receptors are widely but differentially expressed throughout the CNS, including the cerebral cortex, thalamus, limbic system, basal ganglia, brainstem, and dorsal horn, and in the PNS in the dorsal root ganglion and enteric nervous system.

The endogenous opioid systems are fundamental components of the central pain-modulatory network and potentially in peripheral mechanisms of analgesia. Events or stimuli that are perceived as traumatic, painful, and/or stressful often induce release of endogenous opioid peptides. Networks that involve endogenous opioid peptides are also involved in reward systems, mood control, and drug addiction. Endogenous opioids have been implicated in the pathophysiology of PD and seizures and may have roles in neuroprotection and immune modulation. The opiate drugs, including morphine, heroin, and oxycontin/oxycodone, produce potent analgesic and euphoric effects via their actions on opiate receptors. However, because opioids are major addictive drugs of abuse, opiate use represents a major public health problem worldwide. Hence, intense efforts are focused on developing selective drugs that target specific opioid receptors in order to enhance therapeutic efficacy, especially as analgesics, while reducing side effects, including addiction.

UNCONVENTIONAL NTS

Unconventional NTs include gasotransmitters and endocannabinoids, which are not synthesized, stored, or released from the presynaptic neuron. Rather, they are hydrophobic molecules that are synthesized in response to conventional NT activity and diffuse directly across membranes to regulate their targets in the presynaptic, postsynaptic, and/or adjacent neurons. Gasotransmitters are small molecules of gas that are freely permeable to membranes, endogenously and enzymatically generated in a regulated manner, with specific functions at physiologic concentrations that can be mimicked by exogenous application of the gas. With specific molecular targets, the cellular effects of gasotransmitters may or may not be mediated by second messengers and can be endocrine, paracrine, and/or autocrine. Nitric oxide (NO), carbon monoxide (CO), and hydrogen sulphide (H_2S) have been proposed to function as gasotransmitters.

The best-characterized gasotransmitter, NO is synthesized from arginine by the enzyme nitric oxide synthase (NOS) (**Figure 9–14**). NOS is localized to the postsynaptic regions, chaperoned there by scaffolding proteins. NOS is activated by Ca^{2+}/calmodulin following Glu activation of N-methyl-D-aspartic acid (NMDA) receptors. NO can diffuse into the cytoplasm and across the membrane to the presynaptic cell and nearby neurons, where it modifies its targets. Presynaptic NOS has also been identified. One well-studied target of NO is guanylyl cyclase (GC). NO binds to the heme at the active site of GC, enhancing its activity. GC synthesizes cyclic guanosine monophosphate (cGMP), a messenger that regulates cGMP-dependent protein kinase G (PKG) and the opening of the cyclic nucleotide–gated channel. Similar to PKA, PKG phosphorylates and regulates a myriad of neuronal substrates involved in synaptic transmission.

In a redox-mediated reaction, NO can be covalently attached to sulfhydryl residues of proteins, called

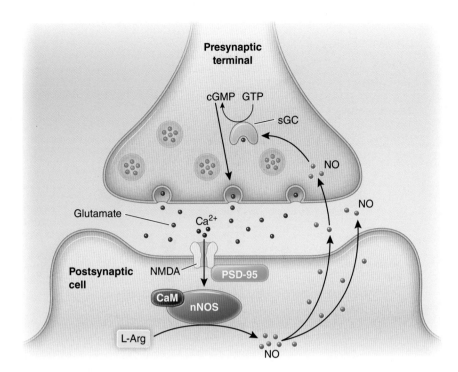

FIGURE 9–14 Nitric oxide can function as a gasotransmitter. Activation of NMDA receptors leads to the production of nitric oxide (NO) that can function as a retrograde messenger. The entry of Ca^{2+} via NMDA glutamate receptors activates neuronal nitric oxide synthase (nNOS) that converts L-arginine to NO. nNOS is localized next to NMDA receptors by the scaffolding protein PSD-95. Since it is a small gas, NO can diffuse directly from the postsynaptic cell into the presynaptic terminus and activate soluble guanylyl cyclase (sGC) that produces cGMP, a second messenger that modulates several presynaptic targets. (Reproduced with permission from Nestler EJ, Hyman SE, Holtzman DM, et al: *Molecular Neuropharmacology: A Foundation for Clinical Neuroscience*, 3rd ed. New York, NY: McGraw Hill; 2015.)

S-nitrosylation, with numerous potential neuronal targets, including ion channels and receptors, scaffolding proteins, cytoskeletal proteins, metabolic enzymes, and transcriptional regulators. Depending on the target, *S*-nitrosylation can induce conformational changes, activate or inhibit protein activity, modulate protein–protein interactions, or affect protein localization, or do a combination of these. In the CNS, NO has been implicated in synaptic plasticity, including long-term potentiation and long-term depression, learning, memory, neurogenesis, the central regulation of blood pressure, and the homeostatic regulation of sleep. In the periphery, many smooth muscle tissues are innervated by nitrergic nerves that generate and release NO. NO can also react with reactive oxygen species such as superoxide to form peroxynitrite, which can lead to protein nitration and lipid peroxidation. Abnormal NO signaling may contribute to neurodegenerative pathologies such as those that occur in excitotoxicity following stroke or epilepsy, and in multiple sclerosis, AD, and PD. CO is generated in neurons by the enzyme heme oxygenase (HO). Similar to NO, CO stimulates GC and increases cGMP second messenger pathways.

The endocannabinoids (ECs) anandamide and 2-arachidonoylglycerol (2-AG) are lipids produced in the postsynaptic neuron in response to NTs that increase postsynaptic Ca^{2+} levels. Anandamide synthesis involves conversion of the membrane phospholipid phosphatidylethanolamine by transacylase into *N*-acyl-phosphatidylethanolamine, followed by phospholipase D cleavage to yield anandamide. The mechanism of 2-AG synthesis is not as well characterized. ECs are released into the extracellular space by a putative EC transporter (Figure 9–15).

ECs and tetrahydrocannabinol (THC), the psychoactive component in cannabis, bind to cannabinoid receptors, which are metabotropic GPCRs. Two cannabinoid receptor isoforms have been identified; CB1 receptors are expressed in the CNS, whereas CB2 receptors are expressed in the PNS. CB1 activation couples through $G\alpha_{i/o}$ to inhibition of adenylyl cyclase and also activation of several MAP kinase and phosphoinositide 3-kinase pathways. A well-studied function for CB1 receptors at presynaptic membranes is inhibition of NT release. CB2 receptors also function in the immune system.

Anandamide, 2-AG, and THC have been implicated in the regulation of appetite, eating and feeding behavior, sleep, pain relief, motivation, and pleasure. Anandamide and THC have been shown to impair memory and enhance adult neurogenesis in the hippocampus in rodent models. ECs are taken up by a transporter on glial cells and possibly neurons and are degraded by hydrolases or lipases to arachidonic acid and other products. Arachidonic acid is a substrate for leukotriene and prostaglandin synthesis, although it has not been determined whether this product has a role in cannabinoid signaling.

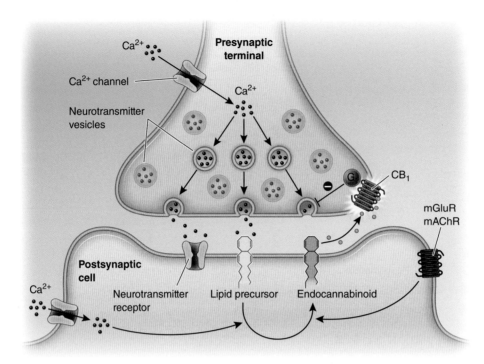

FIGURE 9–15 Endocannabinoids can function as retrograde messengers. Activation of voltage-dependent Ca^{2+} channels, metabotropic glutamate receptors (mGluR), or muscarinic acetylcholine receptors (mAChR) in the postsynaptic cell can increase the synthesis of endocannabinoids from a lipid precursor. Endocannabinoids diffuse or are transported out of the postsynaptic cell and activate presynaptic CB_1 receptors, which inhibit neurotransmitter release. (Reproduced with permission from Nestler EJ, Hyman SE, Holtzman DM, et al: *Molecular Neuropharmacology: A Foundation for Clinical Neuroscience*, 3rd ed. New York, NY: McGraw Hill; 2015.)

SUMMARY

■ Monoamines, purines, and NPs are NTs that function predominantly in slow synaptic transmission and neuromodulation.

■ Monoamine NTs include the catecholamines dopamine, NE, and EP; the indolamine serotonin; and the imidazolamine histamine.

■ Monoamines are synthesized from amino acids and are packaged into synaptic vesicles or dense core vesicles by the vesicular monoamine transporter.

■ Monoamine cell bodies are located in the brainstem or hypothalamus, and they project throughout the brain and spinal cord.

■ Dopamine functions in reward-motivated behavior and motor control.

■ NE and EP are involved in arousal and alertness.

■ Serotonin acts in mood, appetite, and sleep, whereas histamine is involved in wakefulness and sleep.

■ Monoamine NTs also play roles in cognitive functions including learning and memory.

■ Monoamines are removed from the synapse by specific plasma membrane NT transporters, which are targets of therapeutic drugs and addictive drugs of abuse.

■ As a purine NT, ATP is released from synaptic vesicles, whereas the purine NTs ADP and adenosine are derived from ATP by metabolism at the synapse.

■ Purine NTs function via ionotropic and metabotropic receptors in the CNS and PNS.

■ Adenosine plays an important role in sleep.

■ NPs are released from dense core or secretory granules at and around synapses and act via metabotropic receptors in neuromodulation.

■ At many synapses, small-molecule NTs and NPs are often coreleased and act as cotransmitters.

■ Unconventional NTs include the gasotransmitters, which are small gases, and the endocannabinoids, which are phospholipid derivatives.

■ Synthesized in response to conventional NTs, unconventional NTs diffuse or are transported across membranes and regulate targets in the postsynaptic, presynaptic, and adjacent neurons.

SELF-ASSESSMENT QUESTIONS

1. In the central nervous system (CNS), all monoamine (biogenic amine) cell bodies are found in the
   A. cerebral cortex or cerebellum.
   B. spinal cord or brainstem.

C. brainstem or hypothalamus.

D. hypothalamus or basal forebrain.

E. sympathetic or parasympathetic ganglia.

2. Monoamine (biogenic amine) neurons project to and synapse onto neurons in

A. only the autonomic nervous system.

B. only the brainstem.

C. predominantly the basal ganglia, thalamus, and cerebellum.

D. many areas of the cerebral cortex, subcortical regions, and spinal cord.

E. mainly the brainstem, hypothalamus, and basal forebrain.

3. A patient was treated with a drug whose basic mechanism involves the activation of second messengers. Which of the following statements is correct regarding second messengers within neurons?

A. They most frequently generate a marked hypersensitization of most types of receptors.

B. They regulate gene expression that controls the levels and types of proteins synthesized.

C. They generally do not affect the opening or closing of ion channels.

D. Glutamate typically generates inhibitory effects upon metabotropic receptors.

E. They are directly involved in the gating of nonselective cation channels by N-methyl-D-aspartic acid (NMDA) receptors.

4. Which of the following best describes neuropeptides (NPs)?

A. NPs are usually released by the presynaptic terminus at the active zone.

B. NPs function by activating both ionotropic and metabotropic receptors.

C. NPs are transported into small synaptic vesicles at the presynaptic terminus.

D. NPs are released following low-frequency action potential trains in the presynaptic axon.

E. NPs are cleaved by proteases in vesicles during maturation along microtubules.

5. Which of the following best explains how nitric oxide differs from other "classical" neurotransmitters?

A. Nitric oxide is a gaseous transmitter.

B. Nitric oxide has both excitatory and inhibitory functions.

C. Nitric oxide release by neurons occurs predominantly in response to injury.

D. The distribution of nitric oxide is limited to the peripheral nervous system.

E. Nitric oxide is packaged into vesicles.

10

Synaptic Plasticity

Cristin F. Gavin & Anne B. Theibert

OBJECTIVES

After studying this chapter, the student should be able to:

- Define neuroplasticity and describe Hebbian plasticity.
- Distinguish between short-term and long-term plasticity and describe the general features of each.
- Diagram the main neuronal populations and synaptic connections in the hippocampus.
- Identify the phases and parts of long-term potentiation (LTP) and long-term depression (LTD) and describe the features of each.
- Describe the biochemical and molecular mechanisms underlying early and late LTP.
- Define a silent synapse and how it becomes unsilenced.
- Diagram the synaptic morphologic changes during LTP and LTD.
- Outline the mechanisms of cerebellar and hippocampal LTD.
- Identify other regions where plasticity has been documented, and distinguish the type of memory proposed for each.

OVERVIEW OF NEUROPLASTICITY

Neuronal circuits are considered the primary mediators of the brain's diverse and varied functional abilities. Defined as groups of interconnected neurons or networks of interconnected brain regions, neuronal circuits execute specific brain functions and behavior and are responsible for integrating information and performing complicated cognitive tasks. During development and throughout life, neuronal circuits form and reorganize by a process called neuroplasticity. Neuroplasticity is proposed to be the process by which permanent learning and memory take place in the brain and also enables the brain to recover from injury and disorders. In prenatal and postnatal developmental periods, neuroplasticity involves the differentiation of new neurons from progenitor cells, axonal and dendritic outgrowth, and the formation, pruning, and reorganization of synapses. In the adolescent and adult brain, neuroplasticity involves the ability of the brain to form and reorganize synaptic connections (called synaptic plasticity) and modulate excitability, especially in response to experience or following injury. It is now clear that modifications to neural circuits are ongoing, as existing circuits are structurally and functionally remodeled in response to experience throughout the life span of an organism.

Three main categories of synaptic plasticity mechanisms are considered candidate processes that mediate or contribute to changes in neuronal circuits during development and in the adult brain. One well-studied category, referred to as Hebbian or associative plasticity, is an activity-dependent and synapse-specific change in the synaptic response; furthermore, it includes both short- and long-term mechanisms of plasticity. Another more recently characterized category is homeostatic plasticity, a type of synaptic plasticity that is not synapse specific but involves more global and compensatory changes in neuronal excitability and synaptic responses that act to stabilize neuronal and circuit activity. A third category was defined by the discovery that synaptic plasticity is itself modifiable; that is, synaptic plasticity is plastic. Referred to as metaplasticity, synaptic plasticity can be governed by and adapt as a function of the previous activity of the postsynaptic neuron or neural network. This chapter will focus mainly on Hebbian plasticity because research over 4 decades has provided a wealth of information about its physiologic features, functions, and underlying molecular mechanisms.

Understanding how all 3 categories of synaptic plasticity cooperate to produce the important changes in neuronal circuits underlying brain functions, including control of behavior and learning and memory, is an exciting area of current and future neuroscience research.

SYNAPTIC PLASTICITY IN THE DEVELOPING BRAIN

The development of neural circuits involves the intricate orchestration of multiple developmental events, including cell fate specification, cell migration, axon guidance, and dendritic growth, which are described in Chapter 2 of this book. Neuronal circuits first require synapse formation, and later, refinement to establish and ultimately define the functional circuit. In the developing human brain, the first synaptic connections are formed at approximately 5 gestational weeks, and robust synaptogenesis continues until birth. At its peak, nearly 40,000 new synapses are formed every second, and synaptogenesis continues into perinatal/early postnatal periods. Synaptogenesis occurs at different temporal windows in different brain regions and at different subcellular localizations (eg, on the dendrite or dendritic spines) at different stages. Synaptogenesis continues in the adolescent and adult brain, although at reduced levels in adulthood compared to development.

When an axonal growth cone arrives at a target cell, a series of biochemical and structural changes mediate the formation of a functional synapse. Three major stages of synaptogenesis have been identified: cell adhesion, pleomorphic clustering, and pre- and postsynaptic differentiation and specialization. These processes involve an elaborate bidirectional exchange of signals between the axon growth cone and target, in which each cell induces the differentiation of its partner. Cell adhesion and signaling receptors include activities of the cadherins, integrins, neuronal cell adhesion molecules (nCAMs), neurexin-neuroligins, and ephrin (Eph)-Eph receptors. Differentiation of the presynaptic element by formation of synaptic vesicle clusters in close proximity to postsynaptic contact zones is one of the first detectable events in synaptogenesis. Synapsins, which are synaptic vesicle–associated proteins, appear to play an integral role in this process. Several presynaptic and postsynaptic scaffolding proteins preassemble into protein complexes and can then be recruited to the differentiating synapse. Differentiation on the postsynaptic side includes formation of the postsynaptic density (PSD), a protein-dense specialization that in glutamatergic synapses contains localized glutamate receptors, scaffolding, and signaling proteins (**Figure 10–1**).

The developing nervous system overproduces both neurons and synaptic connections in excess during development. As many as a third to a half of the neurons produced during prenatal neurogenesis die in the process of apoptosis, or naturally occurring cell death. Likewise, by the end of adolescence, some brain regions will contain roughly twice as many synaptic connections as will be maintained into adulthood. Once axons reach their appropriate target, they form weak synaptic contacts that subsequently remodel as some inputs strengthen and others are functionally eliminated. The process of synapse elimination, also called synaptic pruning or refinement, is an activity-dependent removal of excess, inappropriate, or unused synapses and is a crucial step in the refinement in functional connectivity of synaptic networks and neural circuits. Pruning processes begin in late gestation and become increasingly active postnatally. As with synaptogenesis, the time course for pruning differs across brain regions, with sensory and motor cortices undergoing dramatic fine-tuning after birth, followed by association cortices and the corpus callosum, and later by regions that subserve higher cognitive functions. Semaphorins, the transcription factor MEF2 and its regulator FMRP, the proteasome system, and components of the classical complement cascade, phagocytosis by glial cells, and exosomes

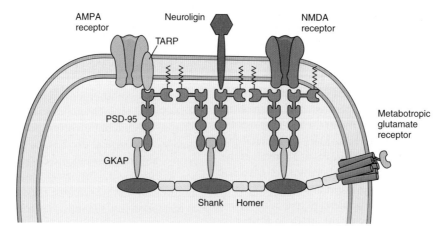

FIGURE 10–1 Illustration of the network of receptors and their interacting proteins in the postsynaptic density (PSD) specialization of an excitatory synapse. The PSD involves protein–protein interactions between neurotransmitter receptors (NMDA, AMPA, and metabotropic glutamate receptors) and scaffolding (PSD-95), cytoskeletal, cell adhesion (neuroligin), and signaling proteins (guanylate kinase associated protein-GKAP).

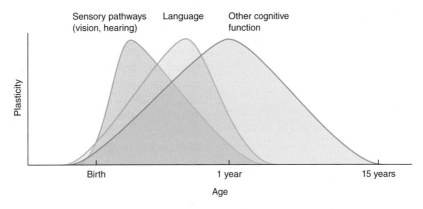

FIGURE 10–2 The proposed timing of critical periods for sensory and cognitive skills varies with brain function. These critical periods are estimated based on experience dependent synaptogenesis in specific human cortical regions. (Reproduced with permission from Hensch TK: Critical period plasticity in local cortical circuits, *Nat Rev Neurosci*. 2005 Nov;6(11):877-888.)

have all been implicated in the elimination of central nervous system (CNS) synapses. Many of the molecular processes, proteins, and mechanisms involved in synaptogenesis and synaptic refinement during development are recapitulated during synaptic plasticity in the adult brain.

Experience-driven activity and plasticity play essential roles in the development of brain circuitry during "sensitive periods" and "critical periods" of early postnatal life. Experience during these early periods has a profound effect on the wiring of skills and behaviors, such as language, music playing, visual processing, and emotional processing. A sensitive period is a window of time in development during which effects of experience on the brain are unusually strong. During a sensitive period, the brain circuitry is particularly sensitive to specific environmental or other stimuli, and this is a time when changes in the environment can alter pre-existing neuronal connections. A critical period is a special class of sensitive periods, such that if the organism does not receive the appropriate stimuli during the critical period for that process, function, or skill, it may be difficult or impossible to develop that function after the critical period closes (Figure 10–2). Research in this field suggests that sensitive and critical period windows may extend beyond those originally defined and seeks to identify mechanisms to reopen sensitive and critical periods to treat visual system, language, and neurodevelopmental disorders.

SYNAPTIC PLASTICITY IN THE MATURE BRAIN

In 1898, Santiago Ramon y Cajal suggested that learning results from changes in the strength of synaptic connections between neurons, laying a foundation for contemporary plasticity research that still stands as a guiding principle after more than 100 years. In the 1940s, Donald Hebb further refined this idea by introducing a model of synaptic modification as a cellular mechanism of learning. Hebb's rule or postulate was that when a presynaptic axon is active and at the same time its postsynaptic neuron is stimulated, then the synapse from that presynaptic axon is strengthened. A mechanism such as

the one Hebb proposed could act to stabilize specific neuronal activity patterns in the brain, thus establishing neuronal activity to underlie behavior such as that during learning. Thus, for more than a century, scientists have hypothesized that persistent changes in synaptic connections among neurons may be involved in the formation and maintenance of long-term memory. Studies over the past 40 years have identified and characterized activity-dependent modifications of synaptic transmission at the physiologic, biochemical, and molecular levels in a number of brain regions.

SHORT-TERM SYNAPTIC PLASTICITY

Short-term plasticity involves activity-dependent processes that modulate synaptic efficacy on very short time scales, on the order of tens of milliseconds to a few minutes. Short-term plasticity reflects the recent history of presynaptic activity and involves modulation of the presynaptic neurotransmitter release machinery, with activity returning to its baseline level after a brief duration. Despite its transitory nature and abbreviated time course, short-term plasticity has been implicated in important brain functions and behavioral tasks, including motor control, speech regulation, decision making, and working memory. These tasks and others can be influenced by transient, short-term increases or decreases in synaptic transmission. Short-term synaptic enhancement has been well characterized at hippocampal synapses and can be divided into the following categories: posttetanic potentiation, synaptic augmentation, and paired pulse facilitation. All 3 likely involve enhanced probability of synaptic vesicle fusion, although they work on different time scales and through different mechanisms. The opposite process, short-term depression (also called synaptic fatigue), is attributed to the depletion of the readily releasable synaptic vesicle pool or diminished synaptic vesicle fusion. With the potential roles for short-term plasticity in working memory, it is anticipated that this will be an important area of research.

LONG-TERM SYNAPTIC PLASTICITY: LONG-TERM POTENTIATION & LONG-TERM DEPRESSION

A breakthrough experiment by Bliss and Lomo in 1973 demonstrated that high-frequency stimulation (HFS) of axons from the entorhinal cortex (EC) to the dentate gyrus (DG) in the rabbit hippocampus led to a persistent and enduring increase in synaptic transmission; subsequently, they described the phenomenon as long-term potentiation (LTP). Ito and colleagues then described a complementary but opposite decrease in synaptic transmission in cerebellar Purkinje neurons following stimulation of climbing fiber (CF) and parallel fiber (PF) axons, and aptly coined it long-term depression (LTD). LTP and LTD are types of long-term plasticity, which is defined as a persistent, activity-dependent change in synaptic transmission that lasts for longer than 30 minutes and can last for hours, days, or weeks. Long-term plasticity has been documented in vivo and ex vivo (acute brain slices) across various brain regions, including the hippocampus, cerebellum, amygdala, striatum (basal ganglia), and sensory cortices. Although we lack a complete understanding of the connections that underlie most forms of mammalian learning and memory, especially the means by which complex memories are stored and recalled at the level of the neural circuit, the evidence supports a role for long-term plasticity as the cellular and molecular basis underlying hippocampal and cerebellar dependent learning.

The hippocampal circuit is an ideal preparation with which to study synaptic plasticity. Often referred to as the trisynaptic circuit, the hippocampal circuitry is composed of a largely unidirectional cell-to-cell relay encompassing 4 distinct cellular populations and 3 named axon tracks between them (Figure 10–3). The main input into the hippocampus is via pyramidal neurons in EC, which project axons that synapse on the granule neurons in the DG, termed the *perforant pathway* (PP) (Figure 10–3). The DG granule neurons extend axons that synapse on pyramidal neuron dendrites in the CA3 region, called the mossy fibers (MFs). Finally, the CA3 neurons send axons that synapse on dendrites in the CA1 neurons, through the Schaffer collaterals (SC). All of these neuronal populations are glutamatergic, and the synapses they form on their targets are excitatory and occur predominantly on dendritic spines.

While recording from granule cells in the DG, Bliss and Lomo measured control synaptic responses of DG dendrites to a single-pulse stimulation of the presynaptic input from the EC along the PP. When they delivered an HFS (called a tetanus) to the presynaptic axons of the PP, they observed enhanced responses in the DG dendrites to the single-pulse stimuli that lasted for more than 30 minutes and up to 6 hours. A similar effect was demonstrated in the CA3-CA1 SC synapses, which can also be easily manipulated and recorded in rodent brain slices (Figure 10–4). Probably the most well-characterized

synaptic circuit in the brain, the CA3-CA1 SC synapse has been investigated in electrophysiologic studies combined with pharmacologic, biochemical, and genetic analyses to yield a remarkable amount of information about the cellular and molecular changes that occur in long-term plasticity. In addition, LTP serves a cellular model for long-term memory formation, because many of the manipulations characterized in brain slice recordings also disrupt learning and memory processes in behaving animals.

In a similar but opposite fashion to LTP, LTD was first documented by Ito and colleagues in the cerebellum. Cerebellar Purkinje neurons are the main output from the cerebellar cortex and are themselves inhibitory γ-aminobutyric acid (GABA)-ergic neurons. Purkinje neurons receive 2 major forms of excitatory inputs, from CFs and PFs. When both inputs are simultaneously activated, LTD is observed at the PF–Purkinje cell synapses. In addition, recent reports show a decrease in the CF synaptic transmission. Like LTP, LTD can also be induced at hippocampal synapses; indeed, LTD is observed at both CA3-CA1 SC synapses and at the EC-DG PP synapses. In the hippocampus, LTD is induced by low-frequency stimulation (LFS) of the inputs. Many experimental preparations use paradigms to induce long-term plasticity using artificial and synchronous presynaptic activations of a large number of synapses. However, it is anticipated in their endogenous environment that some synapses will be strengthened while others will be weakened, and a given synapse itself may experience LTP or LTD, facilitating activity-dependent changes in neuronal circuitry.

Although they lead to opposite effects on synaptic transmission, LTP and LTD share a number of common features. Both (1) depend on specific recent electrical patterns of activity; (2) involve specific time courses with temporal phases involving distinct biochemical mechanisms; (3) involve postsynaptic Ca^{2+}-dependent mechanisms; (4) involve changes in presynaptic and postsynaptic components, including a key change in postsynaptic α-amino-3-hydroxy-5-methyl-4-isoxazolepropionic acid (AMPA) receptors (AMPARs) and currents; (5) are synapse specific; (6) are reversible and saturable; and (7) are associative and cooperative (Figure 10–5). Indeed, the presence of many of these features, together with information from a variety of pharmacologic, biochemical, and genetic studies, further supports the argument that long-term plasticity underlies learning and memory.

A concept that encompasses the bidirectionality of LTP and LTD in activity-dependent plasticity is spike-timing-dependent plasticity (STDP). STDP is proposed to modify the strength of synaptic connections as a direct result of the relative timing of a particular neuron's output and input; specifically, the order and precise temporal interval between presynaptic and postsynaptic action potentials determines the sign and magnitude of LTP or LTD. For example, during STDP, synapses will become potentiated (increased magnitude of response) if, and only if, a postsynaptic neuron is depolarized in a specific temporal window following an upstream

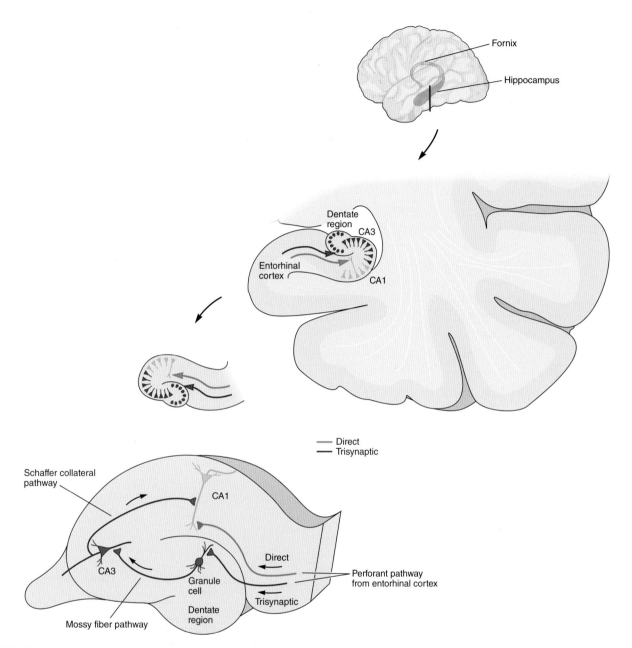

FIGURE 10-3 Hippocampal anatomy and the trisynaptic circuit. The upper three figures illustrate the human hippocampus; the lower figure illustrates the rodent hippocampus. In the indirect *trisynaptic pathway,* neurons in the entorhinal cortex transmit information along their axons (perforant pathway) to excitatory synapses on granule cells of the dentate gyrus. The granule cells transmit information along their axons (mossy fiber pathway) to excitatory synapses on pyramidal cells in area CA3. The CA3 neurons transmit information along their axons (Schaffer collateral pathway) to synapses on pyramidal cells in CA1. In the *direct pathway* neurons in the entorhinal cortex send information along the perforant pathway to excitatory synapses on CA1 pyramidal neurons. The CA1 pyramidal neurons are the major output neurons of the hippocampus. (Reproduced with permission from Kandel ER, Schwartz JH, Jessell TM, et al: *Principles of Neural Science,* 5th ed. New York, NY: McGraw Hill; 2013.)

action potential (~40 milliseconds). This specific pattern of LTP induction mimics the physiologic event of firing of the postsynaptic cell in response to a presynaptic action potential, which facilitates local membrane depolarization and activation of key signaling events to sustain long-term plasticity. In contrast, if a postsynaptic cell fires *before* the upstream action potentials arrive, LTD is induced in the postsynaptic cell. Because of its simplicity, STDP is widely used in computational

models of associative plasticity and neural network plasticity and in models of learning. However, the dependence on STDP varies across synapses, and other factors are likely to be important in associative plasticity as well.

Another concept that incorporates the bidirectionality and the dynamic nature of LTP and LTD is metaplasticity. Theoretically, metaplasticity serves to maintain synapses within a dynamic range of plastic states where they are still

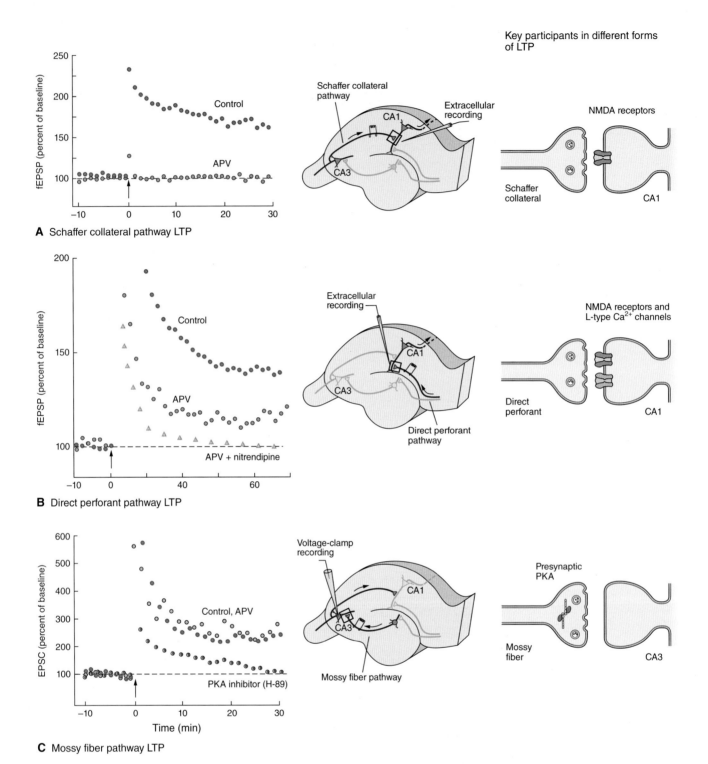

FIGURE 10–4 Long-term potentiation (LTP) at 3 synaptic pathways in the hippocampus. **A.** Tetanic stimulation of the Schaffer collateral pathway induces LTP at the synapses between CA3 axons and their postsynaptic CA1 dendrites. Field excitatory postsynaptic potential (fEPSP) responses are expressed as a percent of pre-LTP baseline fEPSP. LTP is blocked by the NMDA receptor antagonist 2-amino-5-phosphonopentanoic acid (APV). **B.** Tetanic stimulation of the direct pathway from entorhinal cortex to CA1 dendrites generates LTP that depends partially on activation of the NMDA receptors and L–type voltage-gated Ca^{2+} channels. Addition of APV and nitrendipine, an L–type channel blocker, fully inhibits LTP. **C.** Tetanic stimulation of the mossy fiber pathway induces LTP at the synapses in the CA3 dendrites, as measured by the excitatory postsynaptic current (EPSC). This LTP does not require NMDA receptors, but requires activation of protein kinase A (PKA) since it is blocked by the kinase inhibitor H-89. (Part A, adapted with permission Morgan SL, Teyler TJ. Electrical stimuli patterned after the theta-rhythm induce multiple forms of LTP, *J Neurophysiol.* 2001 Sep;86(3):1289-1296; part B, adapted with permission from Remondes M, Schuman EM: Molecular mechanisms contributing to long-lasting synaptic plasticity at the temporoammonic-CA1 synapse, *Learn Mem.* 2003 Jul-Aug;10(4):247-252; part C, reproduced with permission from Zalutsky RA, Nicoll RA: Comparison of two forms of long-term potentiation in single hippocampal neurons, *Science.* 1990 Jun 29;248(4963):1619-1624.)

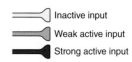

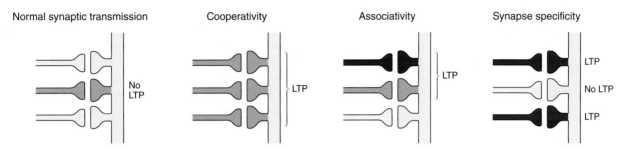

FIGURE 10–5 Characteristics of hippocampal LTP in CA1 pyramidal neurons. A single action potential in one or a few axons (weak input) leads to a small EPSP that is insufficient to induce LTP. Concomitant activation of several weak inputs leads to a summed EPSP that results in LTP in all pathways (cooperativity). Stimulation of strong and weak inputs together causes LTP in both pathways (associativity). An unstimulated synapse does not undergo LTP in spite of strong stimulation of neighboring synapses (synapse specificity). (Reproduced with permission from Kandel ER, Schwartz JH, Jessell TM, et al: *Principles of Neural Science*, 5th ed. New York, NY: McGraw Hill; 2013.)

able to respond to relevant stimuli, never reaching a state of saturation or elimination. Via metaplasticity, the dynamical context of the synapse and neuron can modify the ability of subsequent activity to alter synaptic efficacy. For example, synapses that undergo LTP will be more likely to drive downstream action potentials and consequently strengthen all synaptic connections within a given trace. Over time, those synapses would reach a "ceiling" of potentiation and no longer respond to salient stimuli. Thus, metaplastic processes serve to "reset" a potentiated circuit to respond dynamically without reaching a point of saturation.

MOLECULAR MECHANISMS UNDERLYING LONG-TERM POTENTIATION IN THE HIPPOCAMPUS

LTP can be divided into stages or phases based on modalities of time, molecular mechanisms, and pharmacologic targets (Figure 10–6). Although the terms are useful to divide LTP conceptually, they are largely descriptive and subject to change based on experimental parameters. Most contemporary models divide long-lasting LTP (5 to 6 hours) into at least 3 phases: short-term potentiation (STP), early LTP (E-LTP), and late LTP (L-LTP). LTP exhibiting all 3 phases can be induced with repeated trains of HFS stimulation in CA3-CA1 SC synapses, and the phases are expressed successively over time. The first stage of LTP, generally referred to as STP, is independent of protein kinase activity for its induction and lasts approximately 30 minutes. At present, mechanisms for STP are largely unknown. E-LTP includes biochemical changes that occur between about 30 minutes and 2 to 3 hours and involves activated protein kinases and modification of preexisting proteins.

L-LTP comprises mechanisms that develop during E-LTP, but are persistent, lasting for many hours or even days, and requires changes in gene expression and de novo protein synthesis.

LTP can also be subdivided into phases called induction, expression, and maintenance, based on conclusions drawn from pharmacologic studies. Induction refers to the transient events that signal the formation of LTP. Expression includes the activities that produce the increase in synaptic transmission. Maintenance refers to the persisting biochemical signals that are ongoing in the cell and are driven by induction of LTP. During maintenance, signals act on effectors or targets, such as the machinery regulating presynaptic glutamate release and postsynaptic glutamate receptors, resulting in the persistent expression of LTP.

LTP encompasses changes in both the presynaptic and postsynaptic neuron. Extensive research in the 1990s focused on identifying the molecular mechanisms involved in each phase of LTP, with lively debates concerning the locus and mechanism of LTP expression. It now appears that LTP is not a single phenomenon, but rather a group of plasticities, displaying neuron and synapse specificity. Even at excitatory glutamatergic synapses, not only have several different mechanisms of LTP induction been identified, but whereas postsynaptic changes underlie expression and maintenance of LTP in many systems examined, presynaptic changes are involved in LTP expression in some types of synapses. In addition, LTP is likely to be even more complex than this, with the emerging concept of LTP mediators and modulators. A mediator is a molecule whose activity is required for generating LTP under most conditions, whereas a modulator is a molecule that can modify LTP but is not essential for LTP generation or expression. Thus, even where presynaptic or postsynaptic effects have been clearly shown to be mediators of LTP, activities on the opposite side of the synapse and/or activity from other synapses function as modulators that

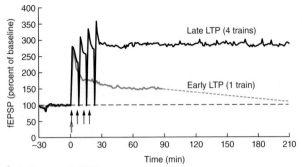

A Late vs early LTP

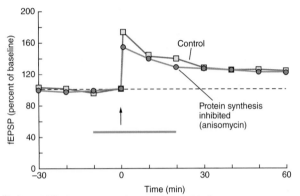

B Early LTP does not require protein synthesis

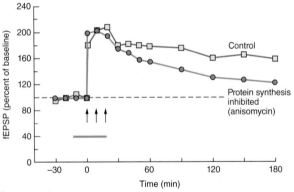

C Late LTP requires protein synthesis

FIGURE 10-6 Early and late phases of LTP in the hippocampal CA1 region. **A.** Early LTP is induced by 1 tetanus lasting 1 second at 100 Hz. Late LTP is induced by 3 or 4 tetani given 10 minutes apart. Early LTP of the fEPSP lasts only 1 to 2 hours, whereas late LTP lasts more than 8 hours (only the first 3.5 hours are shown). **B.** Early LTP induced by 1 tetanus is not blocked by anisomycin applied during LTP induction. **C.** Late LTP induced by 3 trains of stimulation is blocked by anisomycin. (Part A, reproduced with permission from Kandel ER: The molecular biology of memory storage: a dialog between genes and synapses, *Biosci Rep.* 2001 Oct;21(5):565-611; parts B and C, reproduced with permission Huang YY, Kandel ER: Recruitment of long-lasting and protein kinase A-dependent long-term potentiation in the CA1 region of hippocampus requires repeated tetanization, *Learn Mem.* 1994 May-Jun;1(1):74-82.)

contribute to LTP, which is exactly what would be expected for Hebbian plasticity.

LTP expression at CA3-CA1 SC synapses requires predominantly postsynaptic mechanisms (**Figure 10-7**).

At these synapses, HFS or theta burst stimulation leads to robust presynaptic glutamate release. The initial responses are excitatory postsynaptic potentials (EPSPs) and membrane depolarization mediated by AMPAR activation. Strong stimuli that induce LTP are also likely to drive a postsynaptic neuron to fire an action potential. This creates a wave of depolarization that extends both forward down the axon as well as backward into the dendrites and is thus called a back-propagating action potential. Subsequently, *N*-methyl-D-aspartate (NMDA) receptors (NMDARs) are activated by simultaneous glutamate binding and local membrane depolarization to remove the Mg^{2+} block from the pore, allowing ions to pass through the channel. NMDARs are permeable to Na^+, K^+, and Ca^{2+}, and not only produce EPSPs but, importantly, also lead to an increase in postsynaptic Ca^{2+} levels. Both NMDAR activation and Ca^{2+} are required for LTP induction. LTP can also be induced by coincident LFS paired with depolarization of the postsynaptic neuron. Under physiologic plasticity conditions, NMDAR activation and the consequent Ca^{2+} increase are most likely mediated by coincident presynaptic glutamate release and postsynaptic depolarization produced by other concomitant synaptic inputs and/or dendritic spikes. It is also likely that postsynaptic voltage-gated Ca^{2+} channels (VGCCs) and release of Ca^{2+} from dendritic Ca^{2+} stores contribute to the magnitude and duration of the Ca^{2+} signal during induction.

The elevated postsynaptic Ca^{2+} levels activate the ubiquitous Ca^{2+} binding protein calmodulin, which has many downstream targets. One key target in LTP is the calmodulin-dependent protein kinase 2 (CaMKII). Following activation, CaMKII undergoes autophosphorylation, becomes localized to the PSD, and plays a central role in LTP expression. In addition, through other Ca^{2+}-activated signaling pathways, cyclic adenosine monophosphate (cAMP)-dependent protein kinase A (PKA), protein kinase C (PKC), the MAP kinases Erk1/2, and tyrosine kinases are also activated. The elevated Ca^{2+} also leads to activation of protein phosphatases, lipid kinases, and the Ca^{2+}-dependent protease calpain, all of which have been implicated as modulators of LTP. Although the elevated postsynaptic Ca^{2+} is transient (lasting from a few hundreds of milliseconds to seconds), it triggers a cascade of sustained biochemical events that leads to LTP expression and subsequently to LTP maintenance.

Immediately after induction, the activation of protein kinases drives early mechanisms of LTP expression in which phosphorylation of a number of substrates controls the localization, trafficking, and activity of AMPARs. This is the E-LTP phase, which develops around 30 minutes, is transient (lasting about 2 hours), involves activation of protein kinases, and does not require new protein or mRNA synthesis (**Figure 10-8**). The major consequence of the activated kinases is increased synaptic AMPAR number/density and enhanced conductance that underlies the increased synaptic transmission (ie, the potentiation). LTP expression continues throughout the time course of both E-LTP and L-LTP, wherein additional mechanisms contribute to enhanced AMPAR activity and increased synaptic transmission.

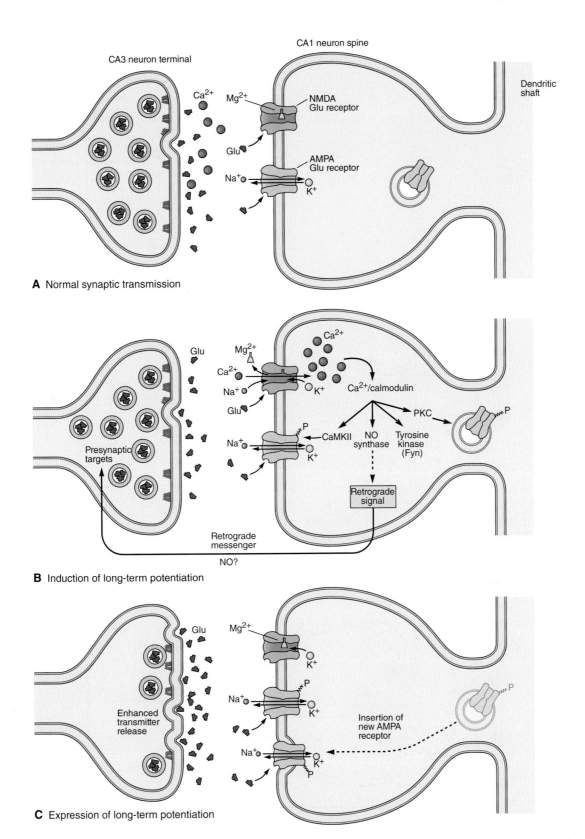

FIGURE 10–7   Model of mechanisms underlying induction and expression of LTP in CA3-CA1 synapses. **A.** During normal, low-frequency transmission glutamate released from CA3 leads to Na⁺ and K⁺ flow through AMPARs but not NMDARs because their pores are blocked by Mg²⁺ at negative membrane potentials. **B.** During high-frequency tetanus, strong activation of AMPARs leads to a large depolarization, which relieves the Mg²⁺ block of the NMDARs, allowing Na⁺, K⁺, and Ca²⁺ to flow through NMDAR channels. Increased Ca²⁺ in dendritic spines activates CAMKII and PKC. **C.** Phosphorylation by activation of protein kinases enhances current through AMPARs and leads to insertion of new AMPARs and retention of AMPARs at spine synapses. The postsynaptic neuron produces retrograde messengers, such as NO, that activate protein kinases in the presynaptic terminal to enhance subsequent transmitter release. See text for abbreviations. (Reproduced with permission from Kandel ER, Schwartz JH, Jessell TM, et al: *Principles of Neural Science*, 5th ed. New York, NY: McGraw Hill; 2013.)

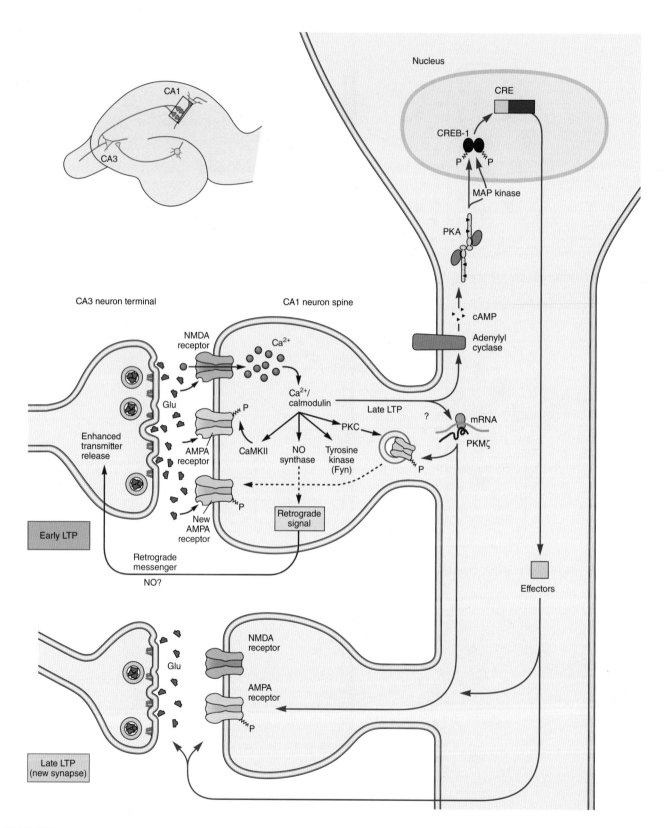

FIGURE 10–8 Model for molecular mechanisms involved in early and late LTP. A single tetanus induces early LTP by activating NMDA receptors, triggering Ca²⁺ influx into the postsynaptic spine and the activation of protein kinases. With repeated tetani the Ca²⁺ influx also recruits adenylyl cyclase, which generates cAMP that activates PKA. These lead to the activation of MAP kinase, which translocates to the nucleus where it regulates kinases that phosphorylate CREB-1 and Elk-1. CREB-1 and Elk-1 activate transcription and the mRNAs are translated. Repeated stimulation also activates translation in the dendrites of PKMζ, an isoform of PKC. Together, these effectors lead to enhanced AMPAR responses, and growth of spines and synapses. A retrograde signal, perhaps NO, diffuses from the postsynaptic cell to the presynaptic terminal to enhance transmitter release. See text for abbreviations.

(Reproduced with permission from Kandel ER, Schwartz JH, Jessell TM, et al: *Principles of Neural Science*, 5th ed. New York, NY: McGraw Hill; 2013.)

In a widely accepted mechanism of LTP induction, protein kinases activated downstream of Ca^{2+} regulate AMPARs via both direct and indirect mechanisms. Direct phosphorylation of AMPARs by CaMKII, PKA, and/or PKC increases the conductance of the AMPAR channel and efficiency in responding to glutamate. AMPARs are transmembrane proteins that undergo constitutive and activity-dependent translocation to, recycling at, and removal from synapses, and can undergo lateral diffusion between the extrasynaptic and synaptic spine regions. AMPARs bind tightly to scaffolding proteins called transmembrane AMPAR proteins (TARPs), which regulate activity of AMPARs, as well as their membrane trafficking and tethering at the PSD. When TARPs are phosphorylated, this enhances their binding to other scaffolds such as PSD-95 at the PSD, resulting in the tethering of the AMPAR-TARP complex at the PSD and preventing AMPAR movement out of the synapse. Activated kinase-dependent phosphorylation of trafficking proteins has been shown to lead to insertion of AMPARs at the plasma membrane. Changes in AMPAR subunit composition also occurs during E-LTP, leading to AMPARs with different channel and trafficking properties.

The increase in AMPAR number also involves a concerted structural reorganization of the PSD, synapse, and dendritic spine. CaMKII activation promotes remodeling of the F-actin cytoskeleton within the synapse and spine, leading to their physical enlargement, which permits an increase in the number of available sites in the PSD that can accommodate and tether more AMPARs. In one model, before LTP, a network of F-actin forms the framework of the dendritic spine, which is stabilized in bundles by CaMKII. Activation of CaMKII leads to its release from F-actin, wherein it regulates the activity of members of the Rho GTPase family, which then control actin-binding proteins to promote actin polymerization, severing, and stabilization, resulting in synapse and spine expansion and enlargement. Not only can the reorganized synapse accommodate more AMPARs, but also the spine contains F-actin–based cytoskeletal tracts that facilitate vesicle trafficking, which is important for insertion of vesicles containing AMPARs.

Another important mechanism in LTP expression involving CaMKII and activated kinases that control AMPAR trafficking is the activation of silent synapses. Silent synapses contain an active presynaptic neuron that releases glutamate but that postsynaptically contains only NMDARs and no, or very few, AMPARs. Therefore, such synapses are functionally silent in synaptic transmission under baseline conditions. It has been estimated that a significant number of synapses in the hippocampus are silent. Following LTP induction, these synapses become unsilenced and functional through the insertion of AMPARs into their postsynaptic membrane (Figure 10–9). Because silent synapses do not initially contain AMPARs, their NMDAR activation must depend on depolarization (to remove the Mg^{2+} block) by other mechanisms, such as EPSPs from other synaptic inputs or receptors, or dendritic spikes. Once NMDARs are activated, Ca^{2+} influx activates CaMKII and kinases that regulate the trafficking machinery and lead to the insertion of vesicles containing AMPARs.

Thus, LTP at both silent synapses and synapses already containing AMPARs involves the insertion of more AMPARs into the synapse. In addition, newly added AMPARs are liable to undergo enhanced tethering and the impact of cytoskeletal rearrangements in the synapse and spine.

In addition to these postsynaptic LTP expression mechanisms, the CA3-CA1 SC synapse is accompanied by a presynaptic increase in glutamate release, which has been proposed to be an important modulator of LTP expression. One hypothesis is that enhanced presynaptic glutamate release requires persistent postsynaptic CaMKII activity during E-LTP that leads to release or presentation of a retrograde messenger to the presynaptic neuron (Figure 10–10). Candidate retrograde messengers include small molecule gases, such as nitric oxide (NO); lipid-derived molecules such as endocannabinoids; growth and trophic factors such as brain-derived neurotrophic factor (BDNF); and proteins that span the synapse such as Eph and the Eph receptor. The mechanism of enhanced synaptic glutamate may involve an increase in neurotransmitter vesicle number, probability of vesicle release, and/or mechanisms that modulate the levels of glutamate at the synapse. In addition, a morphologic expansion of the presynaptic area has been shown to accompany the postsynaptic enlargement described earlier.

Late LTP involves mechanisms that ensure the persistence of synaptic potentiation through additional biochemical mechanisms and morphologic changes to the synapse. This phase requires new mRNA and protein synthesis brought about by sustained activation of protein kinases activated during E-LTP and persists for more than 5 hours to several days. Structural remodeling of both the pre- and postsynaptic compartments can be observed during L-LTP and may involve the formation of new synapses. It is during this phase that the process of synaptic consolidation takes place.

L-LTP is initiated by protein kinases persistently activated during E-LTP, where their critical functions for L-LTP are to regulate translation, transcription factor activities, and epigenetic modifications that combine to control gene expression in the postsynaptic neuron participating in LTP, and ensure persistent morphologic changes in the synapse and spine. One such E-LTP kinase is PKMζ, an atypical PKC member that has been implicated in the maintenance of L-LTP by directing the trafficking and reorganization of proteins in the synaptic scaffolding. The other important E-LTP kinases are the MAP kinases ERK1/2, PKA, and CaMKIV, which regulate transcription of a set of genes called plasticity-related proteins or products (PRPs). A subset of PRP genes, known as immediate early genes (IEGs), have been implicated in L-LTP because of their rapid and transient responsiveness less than 15 minutes after initial synaptic activation. Transcription and expression of PRP genes, including IEGs, are controlled by the regulation of transcription factors and through epigenetic alterations, including covalent DNA methylation and histone modifications by acetylation, phosphorylation, and/or methylation, that have been shown to play an important role in learning and memory.

Neurons that express IEGs in response to a relevant stimulus are thought to encode and store information that is

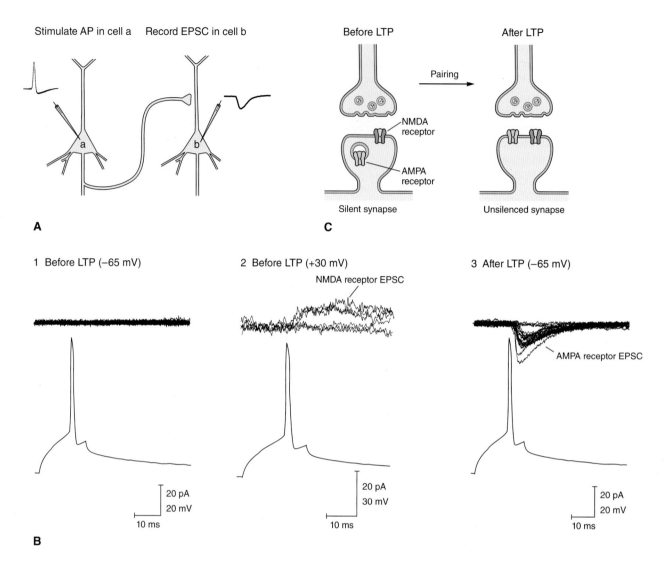

Stimulate AP in cell a   Record EPSC in cell b

Before LTP   After LTP

Pairing

NMDA receptor

AMPA receptor

Silent synapse   Unsilenced synapse

A

C

1 Before LTP (−65 mV)

2 Before LTP (+30 mV)

NMDA receptor EPSC

3 After LTP (−65 mV)

AMPA receptor EPSC

20 pA
20 mV

10 ms

20 pA
30 mV

10 ms

20 pA
20 mV

10 ms

B

FIGURE 10–9 Mechanisms of unsilencing of silent synapses during LTP. **A.** An AP is triggered in neuron *a* by a depolarizing current pulse and an excitatory postsynaptic current (EPSC) produced in neuron *b* is recorded. **B.** Before LTP induction there is no EPSC in cell *b* in response to an AP in cell *a* when the membrane potential of neuron *b* is at resting levels of −65 mV (1). However, slow NMDAR-mediated EPSCs are observed when neuron *b* is depolarized by the voltage step to +30 mV *(2)*. LTP is then induced by pairing APs in neuron *a* with postsynaptic depolarization in neuron *b* to relieve the Mg^{2+} block of the NMDARs. After pairing fast AMPAR-mediated EPSCs are observed at −65 mV (3). **C.** Prior to LTP the dendritic spine contains only NMDARs. Following LTP induction, vesicles containing AMPARs fuse with plasma membrane, adding new AMPARs at the spine. (Reproduced with permission from Kandel ER, Schwartz JH, Jessell TM, et al: *Principles of Neural Science*, 5th ed. New York, NY: McGraw Hill; 2013.)

required for memory consolidation and recall, suggesting that they may be involved in forming the memory trace. Importantly, IEGs also represent a transcriptional mechanism that is activated at the time of learning but before new proteins are synthesized; in fact, IEG activation is independent of short-term memory processes. Although a functionally diverse set of genes, IEGs contain common DNA elements, called promoters, in their 5′ noncoding gene regions that bind specific transcription factors and can undergo epigenetic modifications. Three promoters common in IEGs are cAMP response element (CRE), synaptic activity response element (SARE), and serum response element (SRE).

The promotor CRE binds the transcription factor CRE binding protein (CREB), which can be phosphorylated directly by PKA or CaMKIV or indirectly via Erk1/2, through regulation of ribosomal S6 kinase (RSK) or mitogen and serum activated kinase (MSK), which phosphorylate CREB. When phosphorylated, CREB stimulates transcription by activating CREB-binding protein (CBP), a histone acetyl transferase that enhances recruitment of the RNA polymerase machinery. CREB also binds to the SARE. The promotor SRE binds the transcription factor Elk-1, a direct substrate of Erk1/2.

IEGs include 2 main categories: transcription factors and effector genes. The transcription factor IEGs include c-fos, jun, and egr-1 (zif268/krox-24), which function to regulate the subsequent transcription of additional plasticity-related genes. The effector genes include several well-characterized PRPs, including AMPARs, BDNF, Homer 1a, and Arc.

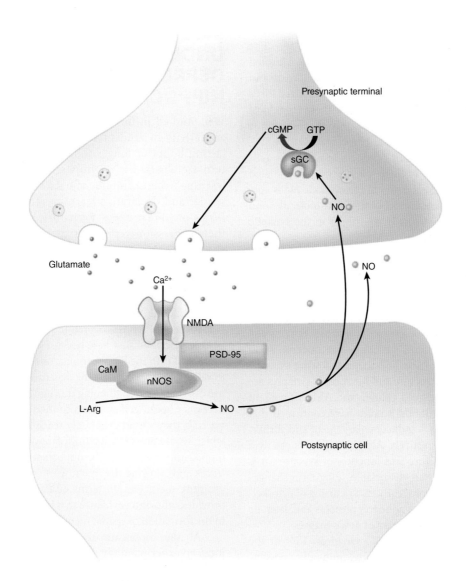

FIGURE 10–10 Long-term potentiation may involve retrograde messengers. Activation of NMDARs by glutamate leads to the influx of Ca²⁺, which activates neuronal nitric oxide synthase (nNOS) that converts L-arginine (L-Arg) to NO. nNOS is localized near NMDARs by the scaffolding protein PSD-95. NO can diffuse across the synapse and activate the presynaptic soluble guanylyl cyclase (sGC), which produces cGMP that can lead to several effects, including increased glutamate release. AMPARs are often co-expressed with NMDARs at many spine synapses. See text for other abbreviations. (Reproduced with permission from Nestler EJ, Hyman SE, Holtzman DM, et al: *Molecular Neuropharmacology: A Foundation for Clinical Neuroscience*, 3rd ed. New York, NY: McGraw Hill; 2015.)

AMPAR expression is increased during L-LTP, which contributes a direct effect on LTP expression by increasing AMPAR protein levels. BDNF is a neurotrophic factor that is translated and released by synapses during LTP. BDNF, acting through presynaptic and postsynaptic receptors (TrkB) that produce numerous effects on synaptic proteins, has been shown to be required for LTP. Homer 1a is a scaffolding protein that contributes to the tethering of ionotropic receptors at the PSD. Arc is an activity-regulated cytoskeleton-associated protein that is localized to dendrites and the PSD, where it regulates endocytosis of AMPRs, Notch signaling, and spine volume and is required for memory consolidation.

To summarize, persistently activated protein kinases during E-LTP lead to phosphorylation of transcription factors and changes in epigenetic modifications that regulate transcription of IEG genes and other PRP genes during L-LTP. Many of these E-LTP kinases also regulate translation and both mRNA and protein trafficking factors that lead to enhanced translation during L-LTP, mRNA localization, and vesicle trafficking. In addition, several protein phosphatases activated during E-LTP have also been implicated in L-LTP. Furthermore, several genes, called memory suppressor genes, show decreased expression during L-LTP. A current hypothesis is that LTP also involves a decrease in memory suppressor proteins that need to be downregulated for memory formation.

An important feature of Hebbian plasticity is synapse specificity. How is it that only active synapses are strengthened while gene products emerge from a central nucleus? This conceptual disconnect has led to the suggestion of a "synaptic tag." The idea proposes the existence of a molecular tag at the activated synapse that serves as a marker for potential consolidation and leading to a mechanism that can tether newly synthesized PRPs produced and trafficked from the nucleus, or those from local dendritic protein synthesis. Furthermore, this phenomenon is observed in both L-LTP and the late phase of LTD (L-LTD), with a common pool of protein products available to activated synapses independent of their state change (potentiated or depressed). Although the identity of the synaptic tag is currently unknown, there are many viable candidate molecules and mechanisms that could potentially contribute to the synaptic tag, including include PKMζ and CaMKII.

It has long been postulated that changes in the physical connections between neurons could serve as a mechanism for information storage; specifically, the remodeling of synaptic structure could encode information about previous experience. In support of this, one of the key modifications during L-LTP is the morphologic reorganization of the synapse. Structurally speaking, synapses are dynamic structures that undergo rapid and dramatic alterations of size and shape following synaptic stimulation. In addition, structure and function of synapses are intimately related, as spine head volume and AMPAR content are tightly correlated. Additional studies have confirmed that the induction of LTP or LTD induces enlargement and shrinkage of existing spines, respectively. Although there is clearly a relationship between structure and function of synapses, it is important to note that they are dissociable. Long-term changes in synaptic morphology involve early restructuring of cytoskeletal elements and expression of adhesion proteins and, later, de novo protein synthesis and formation of new synapses.

In contrast to the CA3-CA1 SC synapses, LTP in the DG-CA3 MF synapses involves predominantly presynaptic mechanisms and is largely NMDAR independent. MF DG-CA1 LTP can be induced by various HFS protocols, or endogenous granule cell firing patterns can trigger a long-lasting increase in presynaptic release probability and a potentiation of the excitatory synaptic response. There is agreement that the presynaptic enhancement of glutamate release is a key component in the development of DG-CA3 MF LTP. Studies have reported an increase in presynaptic Ca^{2+} currents, presynaptic kainate-type glutamate receptors, a role for VGCC and Ca^{2+} release from internal stores, and activation of the adenylyl cyclase–cAMP–PKA cascade. These mechanisms could converge on an increase in presynaptic Ca^{2+} levels, resulting in an enhanced probability of glutamate release and/or an effect on the synaptic vesicle release machinery. Consistent with Hebbian LTP, whereby plasticity is induced by both presynaptic activity that releases glutamate to activate a postsynaptic component in LTP induction, it has also been proposed that there is a postsynaptic component that produces a retrograde signal. Involvement of postsynaptic Ca^{2+} regulation via VGCCs, metabotropic glutamate receptors (mGluRs), and postsynaptic Eph receptors binding presynaptic Eph has been reported.

MOLECULAR MECHANISMS UNDERLYING LONG-TERM DEPRESSION IN THE HIPPOCAMPUS & CEREBELLUM

Well studied in the cerebellum and hippocampus, LTD is an activity-dependent decrease in synaptic transmission lasting hours or longer following a specific stimulus pattern. Cerebellar LTD is proposed to be important for motor learning, whereas hippocampal LTD has been implicated in spatial and declarative learning. These well-characterized forms of LTD occur at excitatory, glutamatergic synapses; their expression represents the inverse of LTP, and they share the same characteristics of input specificity, reversibility, saturability, and associativity with LTP. It is anticipated that an individual synapse may undergo both LTP and LTD depending on its input stimulation pattern and other neuronal activities.

Although first discovered in the cerebellum, hippocampal LTD is described first here because of its parallels with hippocampal LTP. In the hippocampus, one function for LTD may be to selectively weaken specific synapses in order for productive use of synaptic strengthening during LTP to occur. LTD may be necessary because, if synapses continued to increase in strength via LTP, they would eventually reach a ceiling level of activity, which would prevent encoding of new information. Thus, in the hippocampus, LTD may be important for clearing old memory traces and allowing the resetting of synapses for the formation of future memories. In terms of a specific role, recent studies provide compelling evidence that hippocampal LTD is involved in the formation of spatial memories (Figure 10–11).

At the hippocampal CA3-CA1 SC synapse, LTD is induced experimentally using persistent weak synaptic stimulation, typically LFS (1 to 3 Hz) for 5 to 15 minutes. Similar to LTP, LTD at the CA3-CA1 SC synapses depends on AMPARs, NMDARs, and postsynaptic Ca^{2+} influx. Consequently, it is the magnitude and duration of the postsynaptic Ca^{2+} signal that determine whether LTD or LTP occurs. LFS leads to release of glutamate, which activates AMPARs and subsequently, NMDARs. Because the block of NMDARs by Mg^{2+} is incomplete even at resting potentials, some Ca^{2+} enters the spine in response to LFS, which leads to small, slow rises in postsynaptic Ca^{2+} levels. LTD arises from activation of Ca^{2+}-dependent phosphatases, calcineurin (protein phosphatase 2B [PP2B]) and protein phosphatase 1 (PP1), which dephosphorylate AMPARs, and AMPAR-associated scaffolding and trafficking proteins. The activation of these postsynaptic phosphatases causes internalization of synaptic AMPARs into the postsynaptic spine by endocytosis, thereby decreasing synaptic transmission. This early phase of LTD is transient, lasting 3 to 4 hours, and is protein synthesis independent.

Hippocampal LTD can also involve activation of different types of G–protein-coupled receptors, in particular mGluRs and muscarinic acetylcholine receptors, which couple to

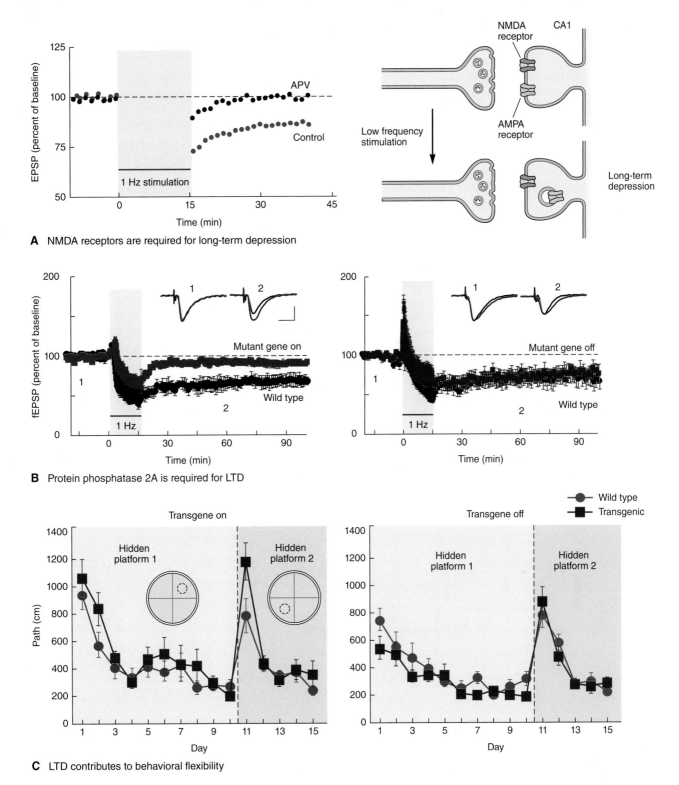

A NMDA receptors are required for long-term depression

B Protein phosphatase 2A is required for LTD

C LTD contributes to behavioral flexibility

FIGURE 10–11 Hippocampal long-term depression (LTD). **A.** Prolonged low-frequency stimulation (1 Hz for 15 minutes) of Schaffer collaterals produces a long-term decrease in the size of the field excitatory postsynaptic potentials (fEPSP) in hippocampal CA1 region. LTD is prevented when NMDARs are blocked with APV. Schematic proposing LTD results from removal of AMPARs from the postsynaptic membrane by endocytosis. **B.** LTD requires protein phosphatases. The plots compare LTD in the CA1 region of wild-type mice and transgenic mice that express an inhibitor of phosphoprotein phosphatase 2A (PP2A). In the absence of doxycycline, when the phosphatase inhibitor is expressed, induction of LTD is inhibited (left plot). When inhibitor expression is turned off by doxycycline, normal-sized LTD is induced (right plot). **C.** Inhibition of PP2A alters behavioral flexibility. Transgenic mice expressing the PP2A inhibitor learn the location of the submerged platform in the Morris maze at the same rate as wild-type mice (days 1 through 10), shown by the daily decrease in the path length the mice traverse as they search for the platform during training. After 10 days the mice are retested (days 11-15) with a new platform location. Transgenic mice require significantly longer path lengths to find the platform on the first day of retesting. When transgene expression is turned off with doxycycline, the transgenic mice display normal learning. (Panels B and C, repdroduced with permission from Nicholls RE, Alarcon JM, Malleret G, et al: Transgenic mice lacking NMDAR-dependent LTD exhibit deficits in behavioral flexibility, *Neuron*. 2008 Apr 10;58(1):104-117.)

phospholipase C via tyrosine kinases. Similar to L-LTP, L-LTD is de novo protein synthesis dependent and lasts for at least 8 hours, although much less is known about the mechanisms underlying L-LTD. However, just as LTP is correlated with increases in spine volume and density, LTD is also associated with the shrinkage of dendritic spines and possibly their loss.

In the cerebellum, LTD at excitatory synapses between PFs and their target Purkinje cells is considered a key cellular mechanism for associative motor learning, including adaptation of the horizontal vestibulo-ocular reflex, eye blink conditioning, locomotion learning on the Erasmus Ladder, hand reaching, and cursor tracking (Figure 10–12). LTD is induced by coincident activation of PFs and CFs that both innervate a Purkinje cell dendrite. Compelling evidence shows that cellular and molecular processes underlying LTD are mediated postsynaptically, although as with many forms of LTP, presynaptic modulation occurs as well. Underlying LTD are a series of complex signal transduction processes triggered by PF and CF inputs that converge in Purkinje dendritic spines. Eventually, these signaling cascades, acting through protein kinase regulation, affect AMPARs, which are removed by internalization (endocytosis), resulting in a decrease in the number of AMPARs on the postsynaptic membrane. Physiologically, this is represented by a persistent decrease of PF stimulation–evoked excitatory postsynaptic responses in Purkinje neurons (ie, LTD).

PF and CF synapses work together in a positive feedback loop for invoking LTD. At CF synaptic inputs onto Purkinje dendrites, release of glutamate leads to activation of AMPARs and depolarization, which induces a regenerative action potential that spreads to the dendrites that leads to activation of VGCC and a resulting Ca^{2+} increase in Purkinje dendrites. Concomitant activation of PF leads to glutamate activation of AMPARs and metabotropic glutamate receptor type 1 (mGluR1). mGluR1 in turn activates phospholipase C (PLC) to generate inositol trisphosphate (IP_3) and diacylglycerol (DAG). IP_3 induces the release of Ca^{2+} from intracellular stores, thus boosting the dendritic Ca^{2+} increase. The most robust Ca^{2+} increase involves PF activation a few hundred milliseconds before CF activity. In the Purkinje dendrites, Ca^{2+} and DAG activate PKC, whereas Ca^{2+} stimulates cytosolic phospholipase A2 (cPLA2) and CaMKII. Activated PKC phosphorylates AMPARs, which promotes their dissociation from scaffold proteins in the PSD and subsequent internalization underlying LTD. Note that phosphorylation in hippocampal

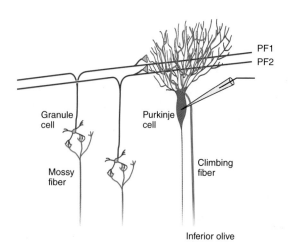

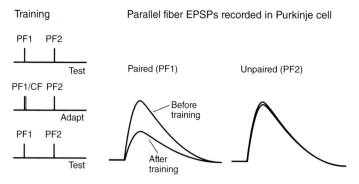

FIGURE 10–12 Long-term depression (LTD) in the cerebellum. In the cerebellar cortex, Purkinje neurons receive synaptic inputs from neurons in the inferior olive via climbing fibers and inputs from granule neurons via parallel fibers. Repeated stimulation of one set of parallel fibers (PF1) at the same time as the climbing fibers (CF) produces a long-term reduction in the excitatory postsynaptic potential (EPSP) responses in Purkinje neurons to subsequent stimulation by PF1. The responses to a second set of parallel fibers (PF2) are not depressed because they are not stimulated simultaneously with the climbing fibers.

LTP leads to AMPAR insertion, whereas phosphorylation in cerebellar LTD leads to AMPAR internalization.

Activated cPLA2 produces arachidonic acid, which in turn activates cyclooxygenase-2 that generates prostaglandin D2 or E2, which is required for LTD induction. One function of CaMKII is in suppression of phosphodiesterase 1, which subsequently facilitates the cGMP/protein kinase G (PKG) cascade. Activated PKG phosphorylates the G-substrate (GS), a protein that inhibits the protein phosphatases PP1 and PP2A. Because PP1 and PP2A function to dephosphorylate AMPARs and normally antagonize the actions of PKC, when the cGMP-PKG-GS cascade is activated, PP1 and PP2A are inhibited, leading to enhanced phosphorylation of AMPARs and internalization.

PF activation also leads to stimulation of presynaptic nitric oxide synthase (NOS). The produced NO diffuses to the postsynaptic side of Purkinje cell synapses, where during early postnatal development, it can modulate both CaMKII and the cGMP–PKG–GS–protein phosphatase pathway. Interestingly, NO has also been implicated as a retrograde messenger in LTP, leading to the proposal that CaMKII and NO may switch LTD to LTP and vice versa. PKC and cPLA2 also regulate a MAP kinase cascade, which has been shown to function in LTD. These signal transduction, lipid, kinase, and phosphatase pathways converge on AMPARs to control their trafficking, and overall, the magnitude of the LTD correlates with AMPAR phosphorylation. In addition, LTD has been correlated with gradual and persistent synapse elimination, with corresponding PC spine loss. Recent studies demonstrating lack of motor deficits in mice that lack LTD suggest there may also be compensatory plasticity mechanisms involved in motor learning.

SYNAPTIC PLASTICITY IN THE AMYGDALA, STRIATUM, & SENSORY CORTICES

Synapses in several other adult brain regions have been shown to undergo LTP, LTD, or other types of synaptic plasticity. Research in the amygdala demonstrates that fear conditioning, a simple form of associative (Pavlovian) emotional learning, is correlated with changes in synaptic strength at sensory inputs to the lateral amygdala (LA) (see Chapter 20 for more details). During auditory fear conditioning, sensory information from both an auditory cue and the coincident foot shock reaches the LA by inputs from the thalamus and the cortex, with both projecting excitatory, glutamatergic inputs directly onto dendrites in the LA. Learned fear produces a persistent enhancement in synaptic strength by both thalamo- and cortico-amygdala pathways measured in vivo. In ex vivo brain slices, LTP in the LA can be induced by stimulation to cortical or thalamic afferents. LA LTP involves NMDARs and VGCC, with both leading to postsynaptic Ca²⁺ influx. Thalamo-LA LTP expression is mediated by mainly postsynaptic mechanisms involving increased AMPAR levels via insertion, as well as ubiquitin pathway–mediated protein turnover. Cortico-LA LTP involves a presynaptic mechanism involving PKA and

may include modulation of presynaptic NMDARs. The neurotrophin BDNF, identified as a key gene in hippocampal LTP maintenance, is also implicated in amygdala-dependent fear learning, memory, and synaptic plasticity. In addition to the glutamatergic excitatory inputs, GABAergic inhibitory control is crucial for fear conditioning. Norepinephrine and dopamine may modulate LTP in the amygdala by affecting GABAergic inhibitory circuits (Figure 10–13).

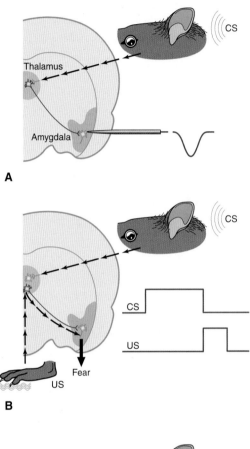

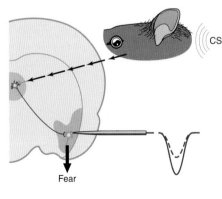

FIGURE 10–13 The occurrence of LTP during fear conditioning. **A.** An auditory conditioned stimulus (CS) evokes a synaptic response (generated by way of the thalamus) in the amygdala. **B.** The CS is paired with a foot shock, which is referred to as the unconditioned stimulus (US). **C.** After repeated training (pairing of the CS and US), the CS causes a larger synaptic response in the amygdala and is capable of eliciting fear.

The basal ganglia are critically important in motor planning and control, motor skill learning, and reinforcement learning. The major input nucleus of the basal ganglia, the striatum, is composed predominantly of GABAergic medium spiny neurons. Striatal synaptic plasticity has been implicated in information processing and learning. Depending on the electrode location and stimulation pattern, striatal subregion (dorsomedial or dorsolateral), and age of the rodent, stimulation can induce either LTD or LTP at corticostriatal synapses, with both involving postsynaptic Ca^{2+} (**Figure 10–14**). HFS-induced LTD is the most common plasticity studied in rodent corticostriatal slices, where LTD induction requires postsynaptic membrane depolarization, dopamine, G-protein–coupled mGluRs, VGCC, and the release of endocannabinoids for retrograde signaling. LTD is expressed through a presynaptic reduction in glutamate release. For LTP, it has been proposed that glutamatergic (via NMDARs) and dopaminergic synaptic transmission trigger intracellular signaling cascades involving Ca^{2+} and protein kinases such as PKA, PKC, ERK, and Cdk5. Presynaptic BDNF release has been implicated in striatal LTP, where expression appears to involve postsynaptic mechanisms.

During development, experience-dependent plasticity is a critical feature of mammalian sensory cortical wiring. In

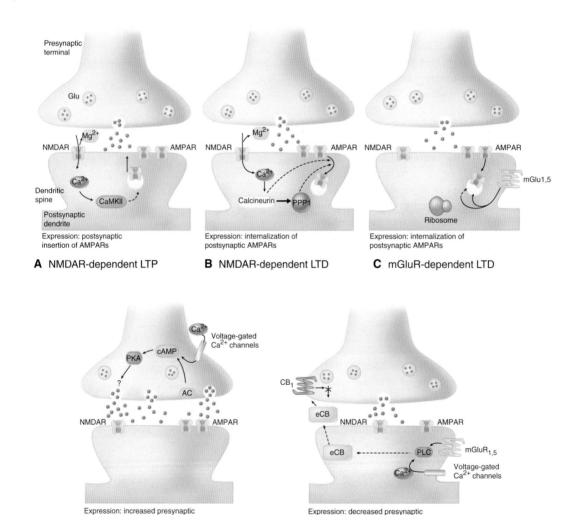

FIGURE 10–14 Comparison of different types of LTP and LTD. **A.** NMDAR-dependent LTP involves postsynaptic NMDAR activation, increased Ca^{2+} and CaMKII, leading to AMPAR insertion into the postsynaptic membrane. **B.** In presynaptic LTP, repetitive synaptic activity leads to increased presynaptic Ca^{2+}, activation of adenylyl cyclase (AC), increased cAMP and the activation of PKA, which leads to long-lasting increases in glutamate release. **C.** NMDAR-dependent LTD is triggered by Ca^{2+} entry through postsynaptic NMDARs, increased activity of protein phosphatases, internalization of postsynaptic AMPARs and decreased NMDARs. **D.** In metabotropic glutamate receptor (mGluR)-dependent LTD, activation of postsynaptic mGluR1/5 triggers internalization of postsynaptic AMPARs. **E.** In endocannabinoid (eCB) LTD, mGluR1/5 activation of phospholipase C (PLC) or increased Ca^{2+} (or both), in the postsynaptic neuron initiates synthesis of eCB. The eCB travels retrogradely and activates presynaptic cannabinoid 1 receptors (CB1R) leading to decreased neurotransmitter release. See text for other abbreviations. (Reproduced with permission from Kauer JA, Malenka RC: Synaptic plasticity and addiction, *Nat Rev Neurosci.* 2007 Nov;8(11):844-858.)

the adult visual system, cortical circuits can be modified by a range of manipulations, such as perceptual learning and sensory deprivation. For example, in the visual cortex, a type of plasticity called stimulus-specific response potentiation (SRP) of the cortical visual-evoked potential occurs in response to brief daily presentation of a particular visual stimulus. SRP resembles LTP in that it is input specific, long lasting, requires NMDARs, and involves AMPA insertion. Visual cortical plasticity is thought to be important for improvements in visual performance. In addition, because the visual cortex provides a key sensory input to the hippocampus, the fact that it undergoes dynamic synaptic plasticity suggests it may also be essential in information processing and spatial memory in the hippocampus.

SUMMARY

- Neuroplasticity occurs during development and throughout life and can lead to lasting changes in the structure and function of brain circuitry underlying behavior.

- Hebbian synaptic plasticity is activity dependent and synapse specific, whereas homeostatic plasticity affects the excitability of neurons and neural network activities, and metaplasticity refers to the plasticity of synaptic plasticity.

- During development, synaptogenesis and synaptic refinement lead to local and distributed neural circuit formation and tuning.

- Short-term plasticity involves presynaptic mechanisms and has been implicated in working memory.

- Long-term plasticity includes activity-dependent LTP and LTD.

- Hippocampal LTP has been implicated in explicit/declarative memory.

- In the hippocampal CA3-CA1 Schaffer collateral synapse, LTP depends on NMDA receptors and Ca^{2+}-dependent and other protein kinases and is expressed as an increase in synaptic AMPA receptor levels and activity.

- Cerebellar LTD is important in associative motor learning and involves metabotropic glutamate receptors and AMPA receptor regulation.

- Hippocampal LTD has been implicated in spatial learning and involves Ca^{2+}-dependent protein phosphatases and decreased synaptic AMPA receptor levels and activity.

- Late LTP and late LTD require gene expression and protein synthesis that are controlled by transcription factors and epigenetic modifications.

- Long-term plasticity has also been observed in the amygdala, striatum, and visual cortex, where it has been implicated in fear, procedural learning, and perceptual learning, respectively.

SELF-ASSESSMENT QUESTIONS

1. Which of the following statements best describes neuroplasticity?
   A. Neuroplasticity takes place during development but not in the adult brain.
   B. Neuroplasticity is the process that prevents the brain from becoming rewired after injury and disorders.
   C. Neuroplasticity is synonymous with neurotransmission.
   D. Neuroplasticity is proposed to be the mechanism whereby learning and memory take place.
   E. Neuroplasticity involves modification of individual synapses but not neuronal circuits.

2. Which of the following best describes synapses?
   A. Synapses form predominantly during prenatal synaptogenesis but can be weakened or strengthened postnatally.
   B. Synapses occur only between axons and dendrites but involve astrocytes that regulate neurotransmitter uptake.
   C. Synaptogenesis occurs robustly during the critical period, and the majority of those synapses are stable in adulthood.
   D. A typical interneuron receives between 1 and 10 synapses.
   E. Synapses can be modified postnatally by experience and activity.

3. Changes in synapse number and strength in the adult brain are usually called
   A. synaptogenesis.
   B. synaptic plasticity.
   C. synaptic transmission.
   D. synaptic integration.
   E. adult neurogenesis.

4. Which of the following best describes the process of long-term potentiation (LTP) as studied in the Schafer collateral (SC CA3-CA1 neurons) in the hippocampus?
   A. LTP occurs in the hippocampal Schaffer collaterals (SCs), but not in other neuronal circuits.
   B. LTP expression is mainly a presynaptic effect that involves an increase in presynaptic α-amino-3-hydroxy-5-methyl-4-isoxazolepropionic acid (AMPA) receptors and glutamate release.
   C. Protein kinase activity, transcription, and translation are required for LTP.
   D. In LTP, regulation of gene expression involves the control of transcription factors but does not involve epigenetic mechanisms.
   E. LTP requires the silencing of synapses.

5. Which of the following best describes a likely function of long-term depression (LTD) in the hippocampus?
   A. LTD resets synapses following synaptic and system consolidation so the hippocampus can be used for future encoding.
   B. LTD releases plasticity molecules so they can be recycled and used by other nearby synapses.
   C. LTD transfers information to other subregions of the hippocampus.
   D. LTD decreases synaptic transmission at synapses that receive high synaptic activity and prevent excitotoxicity.
   E. LTD quickly reverses the effects of LTP so that irrelevant information is forgotten.

Systems Neuroscience: Sensory & Motor Systems

Visual System I: The Eye

Franklin R. Amthor

- Describe the optical functions of the cornea and lens, problems that occur in focus, and the correction of these problems.
- Describe the process of phototransduction from photon capture to neurotransmitter release.
- Diagram the neural circuit of the retina, and outline the function of each major cell class.
- List the central projection targets of retinal ganglion cells and describe the functions of these brain areas.

IMAGING & CAPTURING LIGHT

Vision begins with light passing through the cornea and lens, the optical elements that refract, focus, and transmit light to the innermost layer of the eye, the retina, the region that transduces light information to electrical signals and transmits them to the brain. Because the cornea is at the interface between air (index of refraction close to 1.0) and the corneal tissue (index of refraction about 1.38), the cornea does most of the focusing. The lens, with a slightly higher index of refraction than the aqueous humor (variable, but about 1.4 in its center), fine tunes the focus. Ciliary muscles modulate refraction by the lens, controlling focus. This process is called accommodation. Because the cornea and lens are converging and positive lenses, they project an inverted image on the retina.

Anatomy of the Eye

The main structural elements of the eye are shown in Figure 11–1.

The eye is composed of 3 main layers that enclose 3 transparent structures. The outermost layer, composed of the cornea and sclera, is called the fibrous tunic. The middle layer, composed of the choroid, ciliary body, and iris, is called the vascular tunic (uvea). The inner layer is the retina, which obtains its blood supply from the choroid and retinal vessels. Within these layers are 3 transparent structures: (1) the aqueous humor, filling the anterior and posterior chambers between the lens and cornea; (2) the gelatinous vitreous humor (vitreous body),

filling the bulk (80%) of the eyeball between the lens and the retina; and (3) the flexible lens. The overall structure of the eye is illustrated in the section view in Figure 11–1A.

Figure 11–1B shows a magnified section of the anterior portion of the eye. Approximately 70% of the focusing of the light is done at the cornea at the air–tissue interface. The lens fine-tunes this focus by changing its shape, illustrated in Figures 11–1C and 11–1D. The control of focus is called accommodation. The pupil is an adjustable hole in the iris that controls the amount of light entering the eye. The pupil size is controlled by the third cranial nerve, the oculomotor nerve. This nerve arises from 2 nuclei in the anterior mesencephalon (midbrain): the oculomotor nucleus and the Edinger-Westphal nucleus. The Edinger-Westphal nucleus projects to the eye via the ciliary ganglion as part of the parasympathetic system. It controls pupil constriction via the sphincter pupillae muscle and accommodation via the ciliary muscle. The oculomotor nucleus also controls eye movements (see later discussion).

The Formation of Images on the Retina

The optical elements of the eye are critical for normal vision, and thus, dysfunction, aging, or errors in development of these elements can require corrective lenses or surgery. Conditions affecting the eye include the following:

1. Opacities in the cornea or lens (cataracts) that block or scatter light, resulting in degradation of image quality.
2. Asphericity in the cornea reducing focusing quality, called astigmatism. There are 2 types of astigmatism: meridional

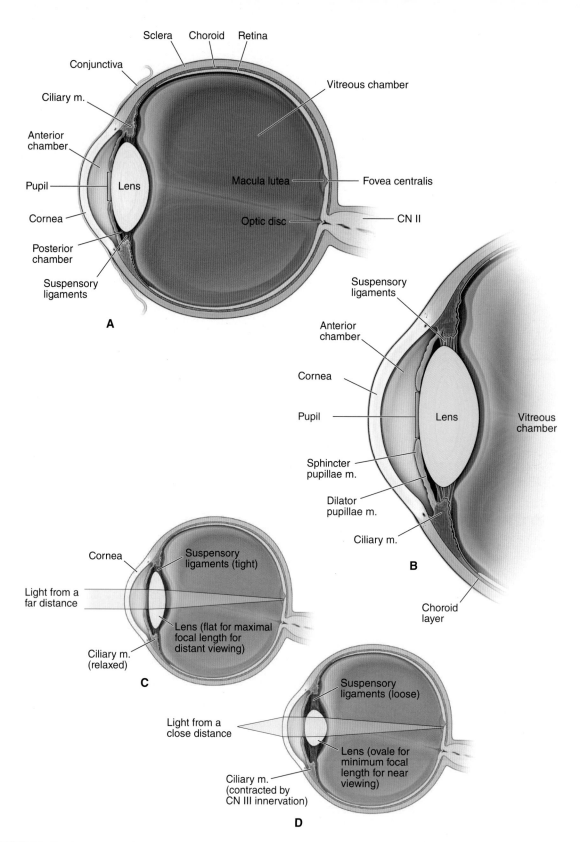

FIGURE 11-1 The anatomy of the eye. **A.** An axial cross-section of the eye. The outer surface of the eye is the sclera. Inside that is the choroid containing blood vessels that nourish the retina and pigment epithelium. Inside the choroid is the retina. The vitreous (from the Latin for glass) is a gel-like substance that fills the inside of the eye. The area of highest acuity in the eye is the macula lutea. Within the macula is the small area of ultra-high acuity found only in mammals and some birds, the fovea centralis. The optic disk is where the ganglion cell axons leave the optic nerve. There are no photoreceptors there, so it constitutes the "blind spot" in the retina. **B.** Close-up of the anterior portion of the eye. The cornea does approximately 70% of the focusing. Between the cornea and lens is the aqueous humor. Just in front of the lens is the pupil made by the iris. Pupil size is controlled by the ciliary muscle, which is driven by the ciliary nerve. **C.** How accommodation, the control of focus, works: The lens fine-tunes the focusing of light entering the eye. Light from a distance is refracted a small amount by the stretched, flat lens to strike the retina in focus. **D.** Light from a source nearby is refracted more by the relaxed, more convex lens to be focused on the retina. This is controlled by the third cranial nerve (CN), the oculomotor nerve. m., muscle. (Reproduced with permission from Morton DA, Foreman KB, Albertine KH. *The Big Picture: Gross Anatomy*, 2nd ed. New York, NY: McGraw Hill; 2019.)

and nonmeridional astigmatism. Meridional astigmatism is characterized by a corneal surface that is slightly cylindrical rather than spherical, making its focusing power in 1 axis different than off that axis. If, for example, the cornea/lens optical system is set for proper vertical but not horizontal focus, vertical lines can be resolved, but horizontal lines would be blurry. Nonmeridional astigmatism, in contrast, occurs when the corneal surface is irregular in a complex way such that there is not even a single axis of good focus.

3. Conditions that affect focus, such as myopia and hyperopia. The eye is said to be emmetropic if the match between the focusing power of the cornea and lens and the length of the eye is such that light from distant objects is correctly focused on the retina when the lens is in its flattest, lowest power state. During normal development, the growth of the eye matches changes in the eye's optics, but errors in this process result in either myopia, where the length of the eye is too long for the front of the eye optics, or hyperopia, where it is too short (Figure 11–2). In myopia, the power of the cornea/lens system is too high for the length of the eyeball, so that myopes cannot focus on distant objects. However, myopes can focus on objects closer to the eyes than those with normal emmetropic eyes. A negative lens (Figure 11–2A, bottom) is used to reduce the cornea/lens power and achieve normal focus. In hyperopia, the cornea/lens system has insufficient power for the length of the eye. In mild cases, lens accommodation may allow distant objects to be focused, but then there is no remaining accommodative power to focus near objects. This is corrected with a positive lens (Figure 11–2B, bottom).

4. Presbyopia (literally "old eye") arising during aging, in which the lens hardens and can no longer be made to bulge to increase its optical power. If one is emmetropic prior to the onset of presbyopia, then distance vision, where the lens is flat, is normally unaffected, but lens power cannot be increased to see closer objects, requiring, for example, reading glasses. Someone who is not emmetropic prior to presbyopia onset may require different compensation lenses for distant versus close vision, such as bifocals.

Eye Movements

Our eyes move continually. Eye movements can be voluntary or involuntary and are essential for acquiring, fixating, and tracking visual stimuli. About 3 to 4 times a second, the eyes make large movements, called saccades, that shift the fovea to a new area of attention. The fovea is the small specific pit-like region of the retina, located within a disk called the macula that is involved in sharp central vision (see Figure 11–1).

Figure 11–3 shows eye movements recorded during free fixation of a photograph of a girl's face. In between saccades, during fixation, our eyes make several types of small movements, called microsaccades, drift, and tremor, which are necessary for vision. Eye movements are controlled by 3 cranial nerves. The oculomotor nerve controls the majority of eye muscles, with the exception of the superior oblique, which is

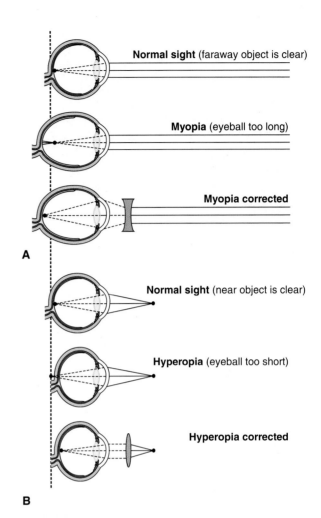

FIGURE 11–2 Refractive error in the eye and its correction. **A.** In normal sight (top) the optics of the eye match its length, so that when the lens is at its flattest, parallel rays from very distant objects are focused on the retina. In myopia (middle), the eyeball grows too long for the eye's optics, and distant parallel rays are focused in front of the retina, producing blurry vision at distance. Close objects may be in focus, however, because their diverging rays require more power in the lens. Hence, the popular name for myopia is "near-sightedness." Myopia is corrected with a negative curvature (concave) lens (bottom). **B.** In hyperopia, the eyeball is too short for the eye's optics, and parallel rays from distant objects are focused behind the retina. Normally people with hyperopia will accommodate to see distant objects. This leaves no accommodation for near objects, however, so they are called "farsighted." Hyperopia is corrected with a positive (convex) lens (bottom). (Reproduced with permission from Widmaier EP, Raff H, Strang KT. *Vander's Human Physiology*, 11th ed. New York, NY: McGraw Hill; 2008.)

controlled by the trochlear nerve, and the lateral rectus, controlled by the abducens nerve.

If images are artificially stabilized on the retina, after a few seconds, all vision disappears because the retina adapts to constant light and only responds to changes. The brain takes into account the eye movements it commands with the associated image movements so that when you are tracking a bird moving across the sky and the image on the retina is relatively stationary, your brain knows that the bird is moving because it knows your eyes are moving with it. When we move, the

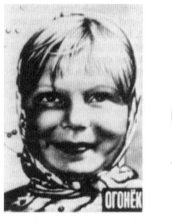
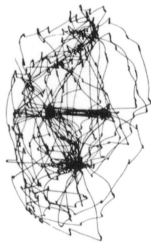

FIGURE 11–3 The pattern of eye movements for an observer looking at the face of a young girl. Eye movements are characterized by a sequence of fixations lasting about one-quarter of a second followed by rapid eye movements called saccades to new location. Fixations tend to occur at points in the scene of particular interest, which in this case are the girl's eyes and mouth. (Reproduced with permission from Yarbus AL. *Eye Movements and Vision*. New York, NY: Plenum Press; 1967.)

output of the vestibular system (the semicircular canals in the ear) is stimulated by self-movement. This signal is combined with visual information so that we perceive movement of ourselves rather than that of things around us.

THE RETINA

Images transformed by the cornea and lens are projected onto the retina, the neural tissue in the innermost lining of the eye. The retina and optic nerve are derived from the optic vesicle of the prosencephalon of the neural tube and are considered part of the central nervous system (CNS) and brain. The retina is a component of the CNS that is located outside the skull or vertebral column, for the obvious reason of allowing light to be imaged by the transparent anterior eye components.

The retina is nourished by 2 main sources of vasculature. The first of these is the central retinal artery and vein, which enter through the optic nerve. These blood vessels ramify a capillary bed across the retinal surface everywhere except in the macular area of highest visual acuity. The other source of blood supply is the choroidal vasculature, which is just distal to the retinal pigment epithelium (RPE). These vascular structures are illustrated in Figure 11–4A. This figure

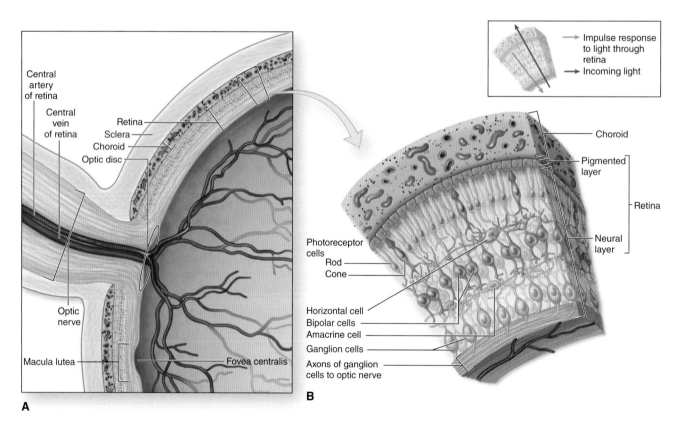

FIGURE 11–4 Detailed view of the optic disk, macula, fovea, and retina. **A.** A cross-section through the eye at the optic nerve head and fovea shows important structures of the eye. The central retinal artery and vein enter the eye from the optic nerve and produce the blood circulation in the choroid, located just distal to the retinal pigment epithelium. Below the optic nerve head is the central region of high acuity, the macula lutea. Within this region is the region of ultra-high acuity, the fovea centralis. **B.** A cross-section through the retina showing the 5 major cell types and their relationship to the surrounding tissues. (Reproduced with permission from McKinley MP, O'Loughlin VD. *Human Anatomy*, 3rd ed. New York, NY: McGraw Hill; 2012.)

also shows the macula lutea and fovea centralis, structures at the center of the retina that enable the highest visual acuity. The macula is blood vessel free and exhibits a high density of cones and rods. The fovea, in the center of the macula, has an ultra-high density of cones and is rod free. The fovea receives input from the central one-half degree of visual angle, which is about the size of the moon. The center of the fovea has only red and green cones, but no blue cones.

A typical region of the retina outside the fovea is illustrated in Figure 11–4B. Because the retina more or less lines the inside of the spherical eyeball, vision scientists use the center of the eye as the main reference point and the terms *proximal* and *distal* to refer to cell and synaptic layers closer to and farther from, respectively, this center point. The most proximal illustrated structure is a capillary on the proximal surface of the retina (next to the vitreous) from the central retinal artery. Distal to this is the ganglion cell axon layer, then the retinal neurons and synaptic layers, the RPE, and finally, the choroid. Light passes through all the cell and synaptic layers before reaching the photoreceptor outer segments at the top of Figure 11–4. To prevent scattering, light not absorbed by the photoreceptor outer segments is absorbed by the dark RPE.

Two nonneural cell types are important in the function of the retina. Figure 11–5 shows, on the left, a photomicrographic cross-section of the retina stained for cell bodies rather than processes. This reveals the neural cell layers. On the right of the figure is a depiction that includes 2 important nonneural cells: the RPE cell, discussed earlier, and the Müller cell. Radial Müller cells are glia that extend throughout the entire radius of the retina. Their end feet form the inner limiting membrane at the vitreal surface.

The relationship between the photoreceptor outer segments and the RPE is shown in Figure 11–6. Photoreceptor health and function are dependent on the RPE, which supplies vitamin A for production of retinal, the photon-absorbing molecule associated with the photoreceptor opsin. Lysosomal enzymes within the RPE also digest the rod outer segment tips that are constantly shed as their light-absorbing pigment is used up. Dark melanosomes within the RPE prevent scattered light and image blurring. Blindness in diseases such as retinitis pigmentosa (RP) stem from RPE dysfunction.

Retinal Neurons: Organization & Function

There are 5 major classes of retinal neurons whose location and connectivity are illustrated in Figure 11–7. The initial process of seeing, as mediated by the retina, starts with the capture of light photons by photoreceptor cells, which are specific types of sensory neurons. Light capture controls the release of glutamate by the photoreceptors. This glutamate modulates the activity of bipolar and horizontal cells to which they are connected in the outer plexiform layer. Bipolar cells, in

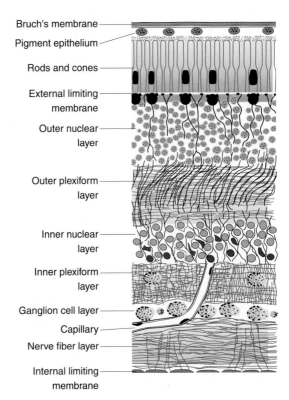

FIGURE 11–5 Diagram of the layers of the retina from Bruch's membrane at its outermost extent to the inner limiting membrane next to the vitreous. Layers with cell bodies include the outer nuclear layer containing photoreceptor somas, the inner nuclear layer containing the somas of horizontal, bipolar and amacrine cells, and the ganglion cell layer with somas of ganglion cells and some amacrine cells. The two major synaptic layers are the outer plexiform layer where photoreceptor terminals contact bipolar and horizontal cell dendrites, and the inner plexiform layer where bipolar cell terminals contact ganglion and amacrine cell dendrites. (Reproduced with permission from Riordan-Eva P, Augsburger JJ: *Vaughan & Asbury's General Ophthalmology*, 19th ed. New York, NY: McGraw Hill; 2018.)

turn, activate amacrine and retinal ganglion cells in the inner plexiform layer. The result of this process is the conversion of the optical image to several neural images represented in the firing of different ganglion cell classes whose axons form the optic nerve and project to visual processing centers in the brain. This is discussed in more detail later.

1. **Retinal layers and cells.** The retina is an ordered, layered, hierarchical structure with distinct cell body and synaptic layers. Starting from the most proximal layer at the vitreal surface (where light enters) is the optic nerve fiber layer. This layer contains the axons of retinal ganglion cells that will gather at the optic nerve head and exit the retina on their way to the optic chiasm and retinal recipient zones in the brain. Distal to that is the ganglion cell layer that contains the cell bodies of the retinal ganglion cells (2 types are shown: midget and diffuse). Within the ganglion cell layer are also several types of amacrine cells, which are interneurons that do not project to the brain (and are not shown in the ganglion cell layer in Figure 11–7). These are

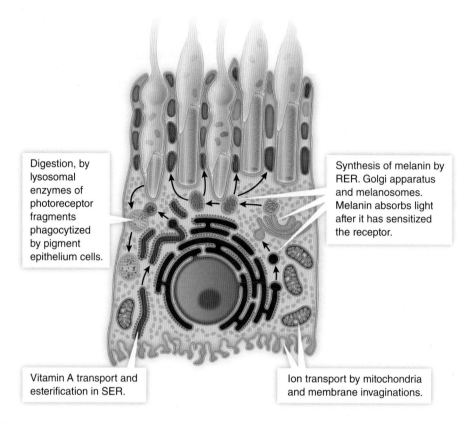

Digestion, by lysosomal enzymes of photoreceptor fragments phagocytized by pigment epithelium cells.

Synthesis of melanin by RER. Golgi apparatus and melanosomes. Melanin absorbs light after it has sensitized the receptor.

Vitamin A transport and esterification in SER.

Ion transport by mitochondria and membrane invaginations.

FIGURE 11–6   The retinal pigment epithelium (RPE). Photoreceptor health and function are dependent on the RPE. The RPE supplies vitamin A for production of retinal, the photon-absorbing molecule associated with the photoreceptor opsin. Lysosomal enzymes within the RPE also digest the constantly shed rod outer segment tips. Dark melanosomes within the RPE prevent scattered light and image blurring. Blindness in diseases such as retinitis pigmentosa stem from RPE dysfunction. RER, rough endoplasmic reticulum; SER, smooth endoplasmic reticulum.

called "displaced" amacrine cells. Distal to the ganglion cell layer is the inner plexiform (plexiform = synaptic) layer, which contain the output terminals of bipolar cells that release glutamate onto the dendrites of amacrine and ganglion cells.

Distal to the inner plexiform layer is the inner nuclear layer that contains the cell bodies of bipolar (midget, rod, and flat bipolar), horizontal, and amacrine cells. Distal to that is the outer plexiform layer, which contains the photoreceptor terminals that synapse onto bipolar cell and horizontal cell dendrites. Beyond that is the outer nuclear layer containing the photoreceptor cell bodies (rod and cone), and beyond that the photoreceptor inner and outer segment layers.

2. **Major neuronal cell classes.** The 5 major neuronal cell classes in the retina are photoreceptors, bipolar cells, horizontal cells, amacrine cells, and ganglion cells. The main pathway through the retina is the sequence of photoreceptor to bipolar cell to ganglion cell. Horizontal cells modulate the signals from photoreceptors to bipolar cells, and amacrine cells modulate the output of bipolar cells to ganglion cells.

3. **Müller cells.** Müller cells are radially oriented glial cells that provide the initial scaffolding for retinal development and provide metabolic support for the neurons in the developed retina (see Figure 11–5).

4. **Pigment epithelial cells.** RPE cells not only reduce the scattering of unabsorbed photons, but are also important in nourishing the photoreceptor cells and in phagocytosis and recycling photopigment (see Figure 11–6).

PHOTORECEPTORS: ANATOMY, DISTRIBUTION, & FUNCTION

Anatomy of Rods and Cones

The first step in seeing is the capture of photons by photoreceptors. The 2 major types of photoreceptors, rods and cones, function in dim and bright light, respectively. **Figure 11–8** shows a typical rod (left) and cone (right). A major structural difference between rods and cones is that, in rods, the photopigment is contained in disks that are completely internal to the outer segment of the receptors, whereas in cones, the cell membrane itself is folded into a comb-like membrane process that contains the photopigment. Rods and cones also differ in their distribution within the retina.

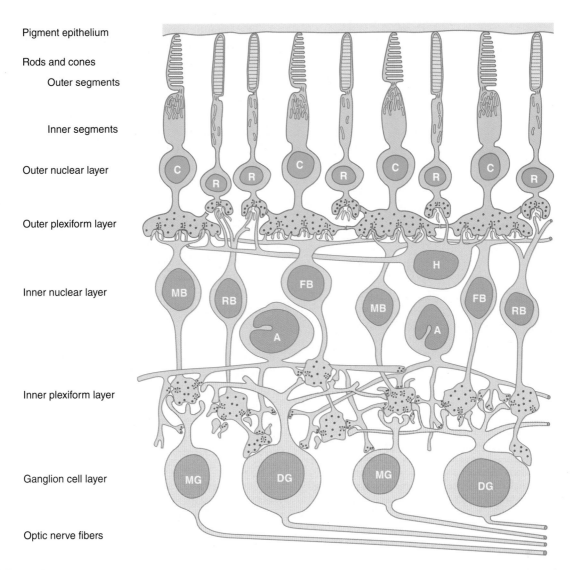

Pigment epithelium

Rods and cones

Outer segments

Inner segments

Outer nuclear layer

Outer plexiform layer

Inner nuclear layer

Inner plexiform layer

Ganglion cell layer

Optic nerve fibers

FIGURE 11–7 The 5 major cell classes of the retina and their organization. This view shows the retinal cells in the orientation they occupy in the superior retina. The photoreceptor cell labels are C for cone and R for rod. Horizontal cells are labeled as H, and amacrine cells are labeled as A. The 3 types of bipolar cell are midget (MB), rod (RB), and flat bipolar (FB) cells. Two major ganglion cell classes are diffuse and midget, labeled DG and MG, respectively. Light passes through the inner retina (ganglion cell axons, then ganglion cells, and so forth), reaching the photoreceptor outer segments last, where the photons are absorbed). Photons not captured by photopigment molecules in the photoreceptors are absorbed by the pigment epithelium to prevent scattering and image blurring. Retinal processing involves a 3-neuron chain in the major throughput pathway, namely, photoreceptors, bipolar cells, and ganglion cells. Ganglion cells are the output of the retina via their axons that exit at the optic disk and make up the optic nerve. These axons are unmyelinated within the retina to avoid light scattering because light passes through the axon layer before reaching the photoreceptor outer segments. Horizontal cells modulate the signal from photoreceptors to bipolar cells. Amacrine cells modulate the signal from bipolar to ganglion cells. There are 3 main cell soma layers: the outer nuclear layer (photoreceptor somas), the inner nuclear layer (somas of horizontal, bipolar, and amacrine cells), and the ganglion cell layer. There are 2 major synaptic layers: the outer plexiform and inner plexiform layers. (Reproduced with permission from Dowling JE, Boycott BB: Organization of the primate retina: electron microscopy, *Proc R Soc Lond B Biol Sci.* 1966 Nov 15;166(1002):80-111.)

Photoreceptor Anatomy

Photoreceptors convert light into a modulation of the release of the neurotransmitter glutamate. This process is called phototransduction. Photoreceptors have 3 main structural parts, as illustrated in Figure 11–8:

1. **The outer segment** contains the photon-absorbing photopigment in an array of disk-like membrane structures. The plasma membrane of the outer segment has a high concentration of cyclic nucleotide–gated sodium/calcium channels.

2. **The inner segment** contains mitochondria and biochemical machinery for transporting the photopigment, such as rhodopsin, to the outer segment from its sites of synthesis in the cell body. Within the inner segment is the cell body that contains the nucleus and protein-manufacturing machinery.

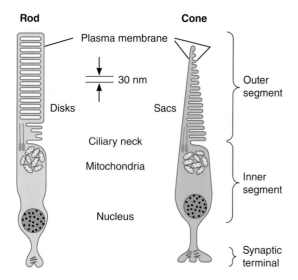

FIGURE 11–8   Rod and cone photoreceptors. The 2 major types of photoreceptors are the rod (left) and cone (right). Rods function in dim light, responding to <10 photons. Cones operate in bright daylight, requiring hundreds of photons per second. The rod photopigment is contained in disks that are completely internal to the outer segment of the receptors, whereas in cones, the photopigment lies in the cell membrane that is folded into a comb-like membrane process. Both rods and cones have 3 main structural elements: The outer segment contains the photon-absorbing photopigment in an array of disk-like membrane structures. The inner segment contains mitochondria and biochemical machinery for transporting the photopigment, such as rhodopsin, to the outer segment from its sites of synthesis in the cell body. Within the inner segment is the cell body that contains the nucleus and protein-manufacturing machinery. The synaptic terminal is where glutamate is released to regulate second-order cells (bipolar and horizontal cells).

3. **The synaptic terminal** is where glutamate is released to regulate second-order cells (bipolar and horizontal cells).

The outer segments of rods and cones interdigitate into the RPE, which provides essential metabolic support, such as resupplying new photopigment after it is bleached by light. The RPE also has a phagocytic function to degrade the distal tips of the rod and cone outer segments that are constantly being shed (see Figure 11–6). RPE dysfunction may cause photoreceptor death. This is a frequent cause of blindness, such as in RP.

Distribution of Rods & Cones

Unlike the imaging chip in a camera, which typically has a uniformly dense detector array, the retina has a much higher density of receptors in the center than in the periphery. Moreover, the mix of receptors also differs as a function of retinal location. Several aspects of the receptor density function are shown in **Figure 11–9**.

The horizontal axis of Figure 11–9 is eccentricity, in units of visual angle. What this refers to is the projection of the visual world onto the retina along a horizontal line that runs through the fovea and extends from the periphery of the retina closest to the nose (nasal retina) to the periphery closest to the cheek (temporal retina). The density of cones is strongly peaked within the central retina, which corresponds to just a few degrees of visual angle. This area is the fovea (see Figures 11–1 and 11–4), and the immediately surrounding region is the parafovea. Outside this region, the cone density is relatively constant out to the far periphery of the retina. Of the approximately 6.5 million cones in the retina, more than half are in the foveal region.

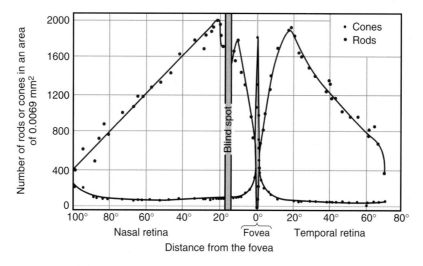

FIGURE 11–9   Distribution of photoreceptors in the retina. Cones are concentrated in the fovea and parafovea and then have a relatively constant distribution throughout the rest of the retina. Rods are absent from the fovea and parafovea, but peak in density just outside this region. Their density falls off more slowly toward the retinal periphery. The blind spot at the optic nerve head where the ganglion cell axons leave the eye has no cones or rods. (Reproduced with permission from Barrett KE, Barman SM, Brooks HL et al: *Ganong's Review of Medical Physiology*, 26th ed. New York, NY: McGraw Hill; 2019.)

Not shown in this diagram is that fact that within the fovea center there are only green and red cones, but no blue cones. Blue cone density relative to green and red cones peaks slightly just outside the fovea in the parafovea, and then constitutes a relatively constant percentage of all cones throughout the rest of the retina, where the relative percentages are about 64% red, 32% green, and 2% blue. There are approximately 6.5 million cones in the human retina. Cones mediate daylight vision, including color.

The rod distribution is quite different from that of the cones. The fovea and parafoveal region are virtually rod free. Rod density peaks just outside this region, and then gradually declines out to the retinal periphery. Because rods mediate vision in dim light, it has long been known that in trying to locate a very dim object, such as a faint star, one should not look directly at the assumed location but just to the side of that location. Rods greatly outnumber cones across the retina except in the central foveal region. The retina contains approximately 120 million rods. The vertical density function follows a similar, but not identical, eccentricity profile for both rods and cones.

The blind spot is the retinal area where the ganglion cell axons become myelinated and exit the retina to form the optic nerve. There are no photoreceptors there. Generally, we are not aware of the blind spot for 2 reasons: (1) the blind spots in the 2 eyes are at different visual field locations; and (2) the brain "fills in" the lack of input based on surrounding neural activity. This also occurs during the slow onset of blindness; patients may lose considerable vision before they become consciously aware that there is any problem.

Rods & Night Vision

Rods mediate vision in dim light. The vast majority of mammals, including humans, have a single type of rod whose maximum sensitivity is to a wavelength of approximately 500 nm. Figure 11–9 shows that there are many more rods everywhere in the retina except the fovea, where they are completely absent. The human retina contains approximately 120 million rods. Rods are specialized to operate in very low light levels. Under ideal circumstances, a brief flash can usually be detected if approximately 5 to 7 rods each capture a single photon of light at about the same time. Individual rod cells are more sensitive to light because they express more photopigment and have higher amplification in the phototransduction cascade. Vision at low light levels mediated by rods is called scotopic vision.

Cones & Color Vision

Humans, like many primates, have 3 types of cones, called short-wavelength (blue), middle-wavelength (green), and long-wavelength (red) cones. When photoreceptors capture a photon of visible light, their response is the same regardless of its wavelength, because the molecular cascade that modulates glutamate release is the same regardless of the wavelength of the photon that is absorbed. This means that

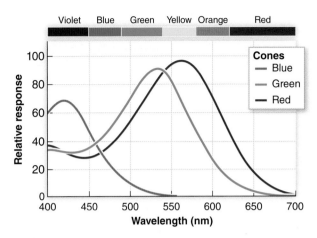

FIGURE 11–10 Spectral sensitivities of human cones and rods. Human vision operates based on absorption of photons from just below 400 to nearly 700 nm. The 3 cone types and rods have different absorption curves. For the cones, the peaks are at 420, 534, and 564 nm for the blue, green, and red cones, respectively. Human rods have an absorption maximum at about 498 nm. The wavelength of the absorbed photon only affects its probability of absorption, not the receptor's electrical response. Because of this, color vision depends on having multiple receptor types with different spectral sensitivity curves whose ratio of activity codes for wavelength. In dim light, only rods are active, so there is no color vision, but during the day, the 3 cones give us what is called trichromatic vision.

in dim light, where only rods are sensitive enough to generate visual signals, there is no color vision (vision is scotopic) because nothing about the wavelength of the absorbed photon is communicated to higher order retinal neurons. In bright light, however, retinal cells are sensitive to the ratio of activity of different cones, which varies with wavelength, and vision is photopic. Vision at high light levels mediated by cones is called photopic vision. Figure 11–10 shows the relative absorption efficiency for the short-, middle-, and long-wavelength cones (and rods) as a function of wavelength. Photons of any wavelength of light produce a unique ratio of activity of the 3 cones, allowing color to be identified independently of light intensity level. There is a regime at middle light levels in which both cones and rods operate to some extent. This is called mesopic vision.

PHOTOTRANSDUCTION

The Phototransduction Second Messenger Cascade

The absorption of a light photon by the photopigment in the photoreceptor outer segment (Figure 11–11A) initiates a cascade of intracellular events that leads to the modulation of glutamate release by the photoreceptors on to bipolar and horizontal cells. Key aspects of this cascade (described in the following text) are illustrated in Figure 11–11B:

1. The photopigment is formed by the protein opsin, which is bound to a molecule of *retinal*. Opsins are transmembrane

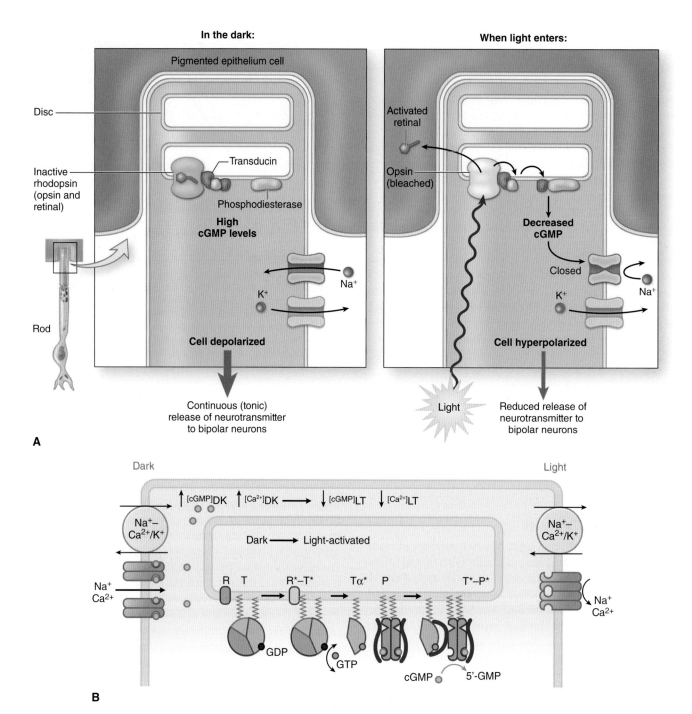

FIGURE 11–11   Phototransduction. **A.** The photopigment molecules reside in internal disks in rods but in the cell membrane in cones. In rods, as shown, the photopigment is formed by the protein opsin, bound to a molecule of retinal. **B.** When the photopigment molecule absorbs a photon, the retinal unit changes its stereoisomer form from the kinked structure called 11-*cis* retinal to a straighter form called all-*trans* retinal. All-*trans* retinal separates from the protein opsin to which it was bound, allowing the opsin to be active. The released opsin then activates transducin, a type of G protein, which dissociates its bound guanosine diphosphate (GDP) and binds to guanosine triphosphate (GTP). The transducin-GTP complex activates phosphodiesterase (PDE), the enzyme that breaks down cyclic guanosine monophosphate (cGMP) into 5′-GMP. cGMP is a second messenger that promotes the opening of the cyclic nucleotide–gated (CNG) sodium/calcium channels in the outer segment of the photoreceptor. The reduction in the levels of cGMP reduces the number of open CNG channels, which flux sodium primarily, depolarizing the cell when open, but closure of CNG channels causes hyperpolarization of the photoreceptor. The hyperpolarization of the photoreceptor causes its synaptic terminal to release less glutamate, the photoreceptor neurotransmitter. The modulation of glutamate release drives bipolar and horizontal cells. (Part A, reproduced with permission from Mescher AL. *Junqueira's Basic Histology: Text & Atlas*, 15th ed. New York, NY: McGraw Hill; 2018; part B, reproduced with permission from Zhang X, Cote RH. cGMP signaling in vertebrate retinal photoreceptor cells, *Front Biosci*. 2005 May 1;10:1191-1204.)

proteins in the G-protein–coupled receptor family. When the photopigment molecule, such as rhodopsin in rods (or photopsins in cones), absorbs a photon, the retinal changes its stereoisomer form from the kinked structure called 11-*cis* retinal to a straighter form called all-*trans* retinal.

2. All-*trans* retinal separates from the protein opsin to which it was bound, allowing the opsin to be active.

3. The released opsin then activates transducin, a type of G protein. When activated, transducin dissociates its bound guanosine diphosphate (GDP) and binds to guanosine triphosphate (GTP).

4. The transducin-GTP complex activates phosphodiesterase, the enzyme that breaks down cyclic guanosine monophosphate (cGMP) into $5'$-GMP. cGMP is a second messenger that promotes the opening of the cyclic nucleotide–gated (CNG) sodium/calcium channels in the outer segment of the photoreceptor. The reduction in the levels of cGMP reduces the number of open CNG channels (see Figure 11–11). Note that only sodium moving through this channel is depicted in Figure 11–11, but some other cations also transit this channel.

5. Closure of CNG channels causes hyperpolarization of the photoreceptor. Hyperpolarization is also contributed by the potassium current in the inner segment that pulls the membrane potential down toward the equilibrium potential for potassium (E_K). The sodium-potassium transporter pump works to counteract the effect of the dark current and maintain the normal cell low sodium–high potassium concentration gradients.

6. The hyperpolarization of the photoreceptor causes its synaptic terminal (see Figure 11–8; also called the pedicle) to release less glutamate, the photoreceptor neurotransmitter.

7. The modulation of glutamate release drives other cells in the retina. Specifically, the outputs of photoreceptors drive 2 main types of cells, called bipolar and horizontal cells.

Dark Currents & Synaptic Glutamate Release

cGMP concentrations in photoreceptor outer segments are high in the dark, and this ensures that the percentage of open CNG sodium/calcium channels is high. A large number of potassium channels are continuously open in the inner segment. Thus, in the dark, the simultaneous entry of sodium and calcium in the outer segment and exit of potassium in the inner segment produce the dark current. The dark current holds the membrane potential at about –40 mV, so glutamate release is high in the dark. Closure of the outer-segment CNG sodium/calcium channels by the light, from reduction of cGMP concentration, allows the excess potassium current in the inner segment to hyperpolarize the photoreceptor to approximately –60 mV. This hyperpolarization reduces the release of glutamate from the photoreceptor terminal. Hyperpolarization in response to light occurs in the photoreceptors of all vertebrates. However, many invertebrates operate in an opposite mode and have photoreceptors that depolarize to light via photochemical mechanisms.

Photoreceptor Adaptation

The visual system has evolved to function from light levels at which single rods absorb a few photons per second, to levels where cones absorb millions. This dynamic range is mediated by 3 types of adaptation: (1) the use of rods in dim light and cones in bright light; (2) light and dark adaptation by rods and cones themselves within their operating range; and (3) adaptation by other retinal neurons. Cones function in light levels from daylight shadows to reflection off snow, which constitutes a range of about 8 log units of light intensity. Rods adapt over a range from a few photons per second to hundreds, or about 2 log units of background intensity. Adaptation allows the photoreceptors to generate relatively large signals for small changes in light level or the mean illumination at that time of day. Adaptation involves processes within photoreceptors and within the retinal circuitry. Schematically, regardless of the locus, adaptation depends on detecting the mean light level and dividing or subtracting that level from the direct response to light intensity, as illustrated in Figure 11–12.

One important place this is done is at the photoreceptor to bipolar cell synapse, mediated by horizontal cells. Horizontal cells summate input from neighboring photoreceptors and, via inhibition, reduce the photoreceptor to bipolar cell drive in a proportional manner. The result is a shift of the operating curve of the bipolar cell, so that its response range is adjusted to be centered at the current overall light level (illustrated in Figure 11–12).

Photoreceptor Diseases

Most blindness in the developed world is caused by photoreceptor degeneration (the major exception is glaucoma, in which retinal ganglion cells degenerate). Photoreceptors are highly specialized cells with intense metabolic and protein trafficking demands placed on them by the processing of visual pigments. Photoreceptors also depend on metabolic support by the pigment epithelium, into which their outer segments interdigitate, so that pigment epithelium dysfunction can secondarily produce photoreceptor degeneration.

1. **Macular degeneration.** Macular degeneration refers to a loss of vision in the center of the visual field (the macula) because of damage to the photoreceptors in this central region of the retina. It can be differentiated into so-called "dry" and "wet" types. Dry macular degeneration (often called age-related macular degeneration) is associated with the accumulation of drusen (a kind of cellular debris) that accumulates between the choroid (blood vessel network distal to the pigment epithelium that nourishes the retina) and the retina (see Figures 11–4 and 11–5). Death of photoreceptors mediating central vision occurs. Dry age-related macular degeneration is more prevalent in the elderly and typically has a slow progression. Its progression can sometimes be slowed with dietary modification.

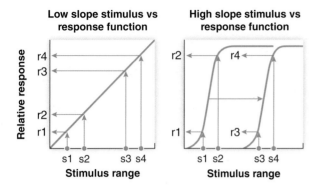

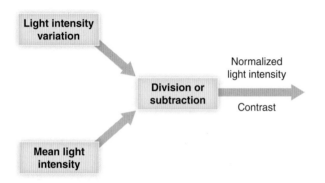

FIGURE 11–12 Sensory adaptation. Adaptation involves changing the response range of a retinal neuron, such as a bipolar cell, depending on the mean light level. If the stimulus versus response function spanned the entire stimulus range, as on the left, the response difference for typical light excursions about any mean level would be quite small. On the other hand, having a highly sloped response versus stimulus function, as on the right, leads to saturation at higher light levels. The solution is to shift the highly sloped function so that it is always centered at the average light level. This is done by a divisive or subtractive process that estimates the mean light level and moves the function to that level. At the photoreceptor to bipolar cell synapse this is done by horizontal cells that summate input from neighboring photoreceptors and, via inhibition, reduce the photoreceptor to bipolar cell drive in a proportional manner to shift the bipolar response operating curve to be centered at the current overall light level.

Wet macular degeneration occurs when blood vessels sprout (neovascularization) from the choroid behind the retina. These neovascular vessels often leak, leading to retinal scarring and cell death. The retina can also become detached, with the detached portion also dying. It is sometimes treated with laser photocoagulation therapy to limit neovascularization.

2. **Retinitis pigmentosa.** Retinitis pigmentosa is a progressive degenerative, inherited pathology caused either by genetic defects in the rod photoreceptors or the RPE. It typically begins with loss of night vision due to rod death and progresses to tunnel vision from death of all peripheral photoreceptors. Ultimately, total blindness can occur. Mutations in >35 genes have been linked to RP, with mutation in the rhodopsin gene responsible for approximately 25% autosomal dominant RP.

3. **Color blindness and anomalies.** Color vision is possible when there are different receptor types with different spectral sensitivities, which is the probability of absorbing light as a function of the wavelength (see Figure 11–10). Humans with normal color vision are called trichromats because they have 3 distinct cone types. However, most mammals and many partially colorblind humans have only 2 cone types and are called dichromats. Dichromacy is usually caused by a pigment allele mutation in which either the green cone is switched to a red pigment (deuteranope) or the red cone is switched to green (protanope), so that the dichromat has about the normal number of cones but no red-green opponency. It is also possible to lose the blue cone system altogether, although that is rarer (tritanope). Calling humans who are missing a cone type "colorblind" is a misnomer because these people are color deficient in only part of the spectrum. Colorblindness is an X-linked recessive disorder. The genes for the red and green cones are located on the X chromosome. Because women have 2 X copies, they need 2 defective genes to have this colorblindness. But because men have only 1 X chromosome, 1 mutation gives the defect to a man. Red-green color blindness occurs in approximately 5% of men, but only 0.25% of women. Tritanopes who are missing a blue cone do not see well at all in the blue end of the spectrum because they lack the blue cone that is sensitive there. Some hereditary conditions and retinal degenerations, such as RP, result in retinas with no rods. These people are night blind. Anomalous (abnormal) color vision occurs when a person has cones with a different spectral sensitivity than a "normal" person. This produces poorer color vision in most cases, but some cases result in better color vision. For example, because a woman has 2 X chromosomes, if she has 2 different genes for the same cone but with different spectral sensitivities, she can be effectively a tetrachromat (4 colors).

RETINAL VISUAL PROCESSING: RETINAL CIRCUITS

The end effect of the absorption of photons by photoreceptors, which communicate via graded potentials, is the modulation of the release of glutamate at the photoreceptor synaptic terminal. This modulated glutamate release activates the network of neurons in the retina that culminates in the firing of action potentials by retinal ganglion cells, whose axons form the optic nerve and project to several retinal recipient zones in the brain, most notably the lateral geniculate nucleus of the thalamus and the superior colliculus.

Photoreceptor Synaptic Release

The glutamate release from photoreceptor synaptic terminals occurs at what is called a ribbon synapse. This synapse, which involves robust release of glutamate due to its morphology, is common in the retina but rare elsewhere in the CNS. The postsynaptic receptors for glutamate released by the photoreceptors are found on the dendrites of 2 major classes of cells—bipolar and horizontal cells—with the synapses located in the outer plexiform layer (see Figure 11–7). Bipolar cells transmit the photoreceptor signal from the outer plexiform layer to the inner plexiform layer, where they synapse onto the dendrites of amacrine and ganglion cells. Horizontal cell processes modify the photoreceptor to bipolar cell message in a lateral inhibitory network.

Bipolar & Horizontal Cells

Horizontal Cells & Lateral Inhibition

Horizontal cells receive inputs from multiple photoreceptor cells and synapse back onto those photoreceptors. Their role in retinal signal processing is to modulate the signal from photoreceptor to bipolar cells via lateral inhibition. Horizontal cells are activated by photoreceptors over a large region. This produces an estimate of the average local light intensity, a percentage of which is then subtracted from the output of the central photoreceptor that activates a particular bipolar cell. Thus, horizontal cells cause photoreceptors to communicate to bipolar cells the difference between the light they receive and the surrounding light. This is called local contrast, which is relatively independent of overall luminance level (see Figure 11–12). Horizontal cells contact only photoreceptors and other horizontal cells and do not send outputs to ganglion or amacrine cells.

Because photoreceptors are hyperpolarized by light and inhibited by horizontal cells activated by surrounding photoreceptors, more glutamate is released for areas of the image that are darker than the local average, and less glutamate is released for areas brighter than the local average. At all but the lowest light levels, objects are represented by a small modulation around the ambient light level that is either above or below that level. Object detection based on detecting this modulation is robust and independent of the ambient light level. Horizontal cell lateral inhibition reduces redundancy in retinal signals. Thus, the bipolar cell signals the difference between the activation it receives from photoreceptors connected directly to it and the surrounding average intensity.

Bipolar Cells

Different bipolar cell types receive synaptic input from either rods or cones and are distinguished as rod or cone bipolar cells. Cone photoreceptors can synapse onto bipolar cells having 2 different types of response, hyperpolarizing or depolarizing, thus splitting the photoreceptor signal at the first synapse in the retina between depolarizing (on) and hyperpolarizing (off) pathways. This is accomplished by the presence of 2 main types of bipolar cells, which are called depolarizing (on) and hyperpolarizing (off), depicted in Figure 11–13. Hyperpolarizing (off) bipolar cells express AMPA (α-amino-3-hydroxy-5-methyl-4-isoxazolepropionic

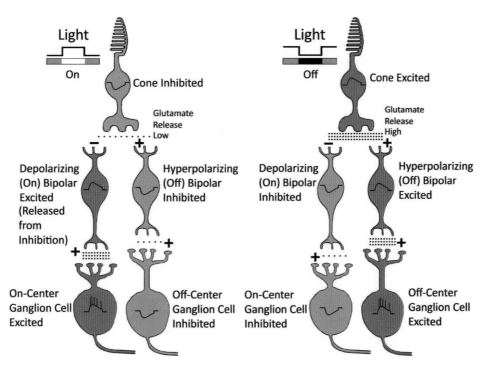

FIGURE 11–13 Depolarizing and hyperpolarizing bipolar cells transmit high and low local contrast in 2 parallel pathways. On the left, when the light level is high, the photoreceptors are hyperpolarized and release less glutamate. This reduces the inhibitory input to depolarizing bipolar cells, whose MGluR6 receptors are potassium selective, and they depolarize. These bipolar cells typically make excitatory synapses onto the dendrites of on-center ganglion cells, exciting them for light increases. On the other hand, hyperpolarizing bipolar cells have AMPA (α-amino-3-hydroxy-5-methyl-4-isoxazolepropionic acid)/kainite excitatory receptors for glutamate, so they hyperpolarize to light when the photoreceptors do the same, as do the off-center ganglion cells. At light offset, on the right, the photoreceptors are depolarized, inhibiting depolarizing bipolar cells and on-center ganglion cells, but exciting hyperpolarizing bipolar cells and off-center ganglion cells.

acid)/kainite–type receptors for glutamate and depolarize when their photoreceptors do, in the dark, and hyperpolarize in response to light. Depolarizing (on) bipolar cells have an inhibitory receptor for glutamate (metabotropic MGluR6) that inverts the signal from photoreceptors so that these bipolar cells hyperpolarize to dark and depolarize to light. In summary, in the dark, a photoreceptor cell releases glutamate, which hyperpolarizes (and inhibits) "on" bipolar cells and depolarizes (excites) "off" bipolar cells. In the light, photoreceptor cells release less glutamate; this causes the on bipolar cell to lose its inhibition and become active (depolarized), whereas the off bipolar cell loses its excitation (becomes hyperpolarized) and becomes silent. Similar to the photoreceptors, bipolar cells also use glutamate and graded responses to communicate to their targets, amacrine cells and retinal ganglion cells. (In Figure 11–13, the bipolar cells are referred to as on-center and off-center.) Most mammalian retinas actually have about 10 distinct types of bipolar cells. These include a depolarizing and hyperpolarizing bipolar cell type for each of the 2 or 3 cone types and at least 1 bipolar cell type that receives inputs from rods. Bipolar cells also vary regarding whether they receive input from either a large or small number of photoreceptors.

The bipolar cell situation is different for rods compared to cones. Rods connect only to depolarizing rod bipolar cells. These bipolar cells make gap junction contacts with depolarizing cone bipolar cells and thus activate on-center ganglion cells (and amacrine cells) through the depolarizing cone bipolar cell terminals. The depolarizing rod bipolar cells also have inhibitory, glycine-mediated outputs to hyperpolarizing cone bipolar cells. By disinhibiting these cells for light increases, they activate them for light decrements.

Amacrine Cells

The 2 major bipolar cell types establish 2 parallel pathways in the retina that respond to stimuli lighter than the background (on bipolar cells) or darker than the background (off bipolar cells). Bipolar cell terminals connect to the dendrites of 2 kinds of postsynaptic cells: amacrine and ganglion cells.

Bipolar Cell Inputs to the Inner Plexiform Layer

Bipolar output synaptic terminals end in separate layers of the inner plexiform layer, with depolarizing on bipolar cells terminating in the proximal part of the inner plexiform layer and hyperpolarizing off bipolar cells terminating in the distal inner plexiform layer. These parallel on and off pathways are maintained through the connections to the retinal ganglion cells and to the thalamus.

Laterally Inhibitory Amacrine Cells

Amacrine cells are laterally interacting interneurons. Some have a similar function in the inner plexiform layer to that of horizontal cells in the outer plexiform layer. These amacrine cells conduct inhibitory signals from the surrounding

bipolar cells, so that the ganglion cell responds to the difference between the light in its central area and the surrounding area. This action reduces the amount of redundant information that ganglion cells must transmit.

Amacrine Cells Generate Complex Receptive Field Properties

Some amacrine cells generate complex receptive field properties. Other amacrine cells sculpt the bipolar cell output to ganglion cells to produce a variety of ganglion cell classes that respond to particular features of the visual input, such as motion, edges, or colors. Most amacrine cells use the neurotransmitter γ-aminobutyric acid (GABA), but others use glycine, neuropeptides, and even acetylcholine to produce complex ganglion cell response properties. Thus, from a limited number of bipolar cell types, there emerge ganglion cell classes that respond to different colors, movement, or the presence of long edges or corners. Over 30 classes of amacrine cells help to create all these ganglion cell classes.

Ganglion Cells

Retinal ganglion cells are the sole output from the retina. Their axons form the optic nerve that conducts action potentials to approximately 15 retinal recipient zones in the brain. The most important of these for visual acuity and perception is the projection to the lateral geniculate nucleus (LGN) of the thalamus. Important projections are also made to the hypothalamus and midbrain areas such as the pretectal and accessory optic system nuclei.

Thalamic Layer-Projecting Ganglion Cell Classes

On and off bipolar cells are connected to similarly responding ganglion cells called on-center and off-center ganglion cells, respectively (Figure 11–14). The 2 major ganglion cell classes project to distinct layers within the dorsal LGN of the thalamus. These ganglion cell classes are called parvocellular (which means small) and magnocellular cells, although they may also be called midget and parasol cells, respectively. Both parvo- and magnocellular ganglion cells have so-called "concentric" receptive fields. Concentric means that there is an excitatory central region, usually coextensive with the ganglion cell dendritic tree, in which light-on stimulation produces an excitatory response in on-center ganglion cells, whereas light-off stimulation produces and excitatory response in off-center ganglion cells. Usually the best response occurs when the light increment or decrement exactly matches or fills the excitatory receptive field center region.

Concentric receptive field ganglion cells have regions surrounding the excitatory center that have the following 2 main characteristics. (1) Stimulation with spots larger than the receptive field center, that is, invading the inhibitory surround, produces a weaker response than stimulation confined to the center; hence the name, inhibitory surround. (2) The surround also has a property called "antagonistic." An antagonistic surround is one in which surround stimulation in an on-center

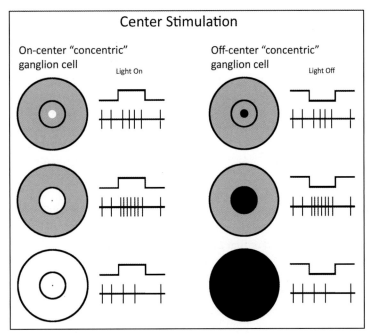

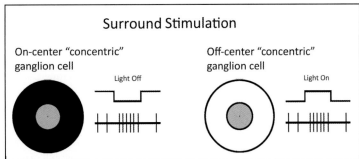

FIGURE 11–14 Ganglion cell receptive field sensitivity. Most ganglion cells that project to the thalamus have "concentric" receptive fields. This means that the optimal stimulus just fills what is called the excitatory receptive field center, with spots smaller or larger producing weaker responses. The surrounds of concentric ganglion cells are also antagonistic, which means that light offset is excitatory in the surround of on-center ganglion cells (bottom left), whereas light onset is excitatory in the surround of off-center ganglion cells (bottom right).

ganglion cell produces light-offset excitation, whereas light-onset stimulation produces an excitatory response in off-center ganglion cells (see bottom of Figure 11–14). Both parvo- and magnocellular ganglion cells that form the main projection to the LGN of the thalamus have antagonistic surrounds, but many other ganglion cells have only inhibitory surrounds.

Parvocellular/Midget Ganglion Cells

In the fovea, all ganglion cells are a particular type of parvocellular ganglion cell in a neural circuit called the midget system, in which a single photoreceptor (a cone) activates a single bipolar cell, which feeds a single ganglion cell. However, outside the fovea, there are generally many photoreceptors (rods or cones) that are connected to 1 bipolar cell and several bipolar cells are input to 1 parvocellular ganglion cell. The responses of parvocellular ganglion cells resemble their respective depolarizing or hyperpolarizing bipolar cell input, except that the ganglion cell excitatory postsynaptic

potential produces action potentials that will transmit the ganglion cell message via its axons to the brain. Parvocellular ganglion cells have brisk-sustained responses, meaning that they have high action potential firing rates that are well modulated by small changes in light intensity. These are the most numerous ganglion cells in the human retina, constituting approximately 1 million of the approximately 1.2 million total ganglion cells. They form the main projection to the upper 4 layers of the LGN of the thalamus, called the parvocellular layers, which is a relay in the high-acuity, conscious visual pathway. Parvocellular ganglion cells code for color and fine detail. Their small size and small receptive fields mediate very high acuity in the human fovea.

Magnocellular/Parasol Ganglion Cells

Virtually all mammalian retinas also have the magnocellular ganglion cell class. Although absent from the fovea itself, these ganglion cells range from just outside the immediate fovea to the extreme periphery. Magnocellular ganglion cells respond more transiently than parvocellular cells, and they have larger integration areas (receptive fields) than parvocellular cells at any given eccentricity. Magnocellular ganglion cells have relatively more amacrine inputs than parvocellular ganglion cells and respond well to changes in the visual image, such as motion, even at low contrast. They project to the bottom 2 layers of the LGN of the thalamus, the magnocellular layers, in primates.

Other Ganglion Cell Classes

The network of amacrine cells also gives rise to ganglion cell classes that respond only to specific features of the visual input. Some of these ganglion cell classes project to the thalamus, but others project to different brain areas. Bistratified retinal ganglion cells project to the koniocellular layers of the LGN and are proposed to function in color vision. Directionally selective ganglion cells are not only sensitive to movement, but also to its direction. These cells project to a variety of brain nuclei that enable target tracking and using vision to maintain balance and orientation. A small percentage of ganglion cells are intrinsically light sensitive. This means that they express their own photopigment that causes them to respond directly to light, without photoreceptor input. These intrinsically photoreceptive ganglion cells are sensitive to the overall light level, and they project to the suprachiasmatic nucleus in the hypothalamus and control circadian rhythms. Other intrinsically photoreceptive ganglion cells project to the Edinger-Westphal nucleus and control the pupillary light reflex.

Chromatic Processing

The visual system is thought to interpret color in an antagonistic way, with antagonism occurring at the level of ganglion cells. A range of wavelengths stimulate each of the cone types to varying degrees. Color vision requires that the signals from different cone types be kept separate until color-opponent ganglion cells can compare the ratio of activity between cones. The activity of red cones is typically opposed to the activity of green cones in some color-opponent ganglion cells. The other main type of color-opponent ganglion cell has blue opposed to the combination of red and green. Color opponency is another parallel visual pathway, like on versus off in the bipolar and ganglion cells.

Glaucoma

The major disease of ganglion cells is glaucoma, one of the leading causes of blindness. Glaucoma is an optic neuropathy associated with elevated intraocular pressure in the aqueous humor, in which retinal ganglion cells die due to damage to their axons. However, glaucoma causing optic nerve damage can also occur in individuals with normal intraocular pressure. Retinal ganglion cells tend to be lost in a characteristic pattern with an associated expanding visual field loss that often progresses to blindness. There

are 2 main categories of glaucoma: open-angle and closed-angle. Open-angle glaucoma is chronic, typically symptomless, and of slow progression until significant vision has been lost. It is associated with poor drainage of the scleral venous sinus that builds up pressure in the anterior chamber and then the vitreous.

Closed-angle glaucoma refers to the situation where the iris sticks to the lens, preventing fluid from escaping from the vitreous to the anterior chamber. It often has a sudden painful onset. Treatment can involve using a laser to make a hole in in the iris to allow drainage, but without treatment, vision can rapidly deteriorate.

In both types of glaucoma, ganglion cell axons in the periphery tend to die first so that visual field loss tends to progress from the periphery to the center, yielding a stage near the end of the disease characterized as "tunnel vision."

What Does the Human Eye Tell the Human Brain?

Although the exact number of distinct ganglion cell classes in the human eye is unknown, the number is likely to be at least 20, as is the case with other mammals in which this issue has been investigated. How are these ganglion cell classes distributed across the retina? Like the photoreceptors, ganglion cells show an eccentricity factor: Ganglion cell somas and dendritic trees are smaller in and near the fovea than in the periphery. At each locus (eccentricity) in the retina, each ganglion cell class appears to tile the retina, with no gaps between dendritic trees and little overlap. However, the size of each ganglion cell class at each eccentricity varies as a function of class.

Figure 11–15 illustrates how, at 1 particular retinal location, 6 to 7 parvocellular ganglion cells might tile the interior of 1 magnocellular ganglion cell. The magnocellular ganglion cells themselves form a similar tiling on a larger scale. If there are 20 ganglion cell classes and each tiles the retina, then every point on the retina is within the receptive field of 1 of each of the 20 different ganglion cell classes, each of which extracts some particular information from the visual scene for projection to the brain (where there are at least 15 different retinal recipient zones). Some of these ganglion cells care about color, others about edges, and still others about movement. The retina does not transmit a picture of the visual scene for the brain to analyze; rather, it transmits 20 transforms of the visual scene that are used by the brain for perception and visually guided behavior in many different ways. This must be clear from the numbers: There are >120 million photoreceptors but only approximately 1.2 million ganglion cells. Only in the midget/parvocellular system within the fovea does the retina approach the idea of sending the output of a single cone via a single ganglion cell to the brain. Elsewhere, each parvocellular ganglion cell extracts some average chromatic signal from the photoreceptors that influence it, and other ganglion cells extract more complex information.

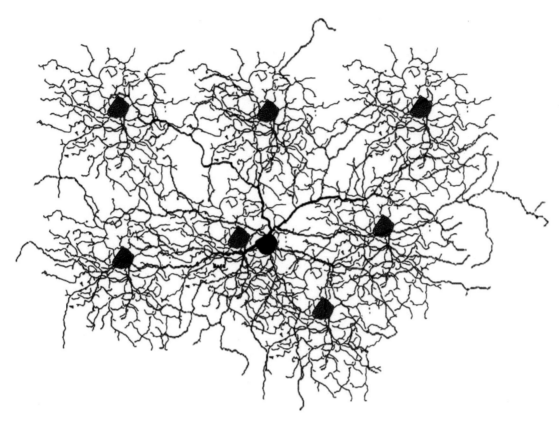

FIGURE 11–15 Tiling by parvocellular ganglion cells within the receptive field of a magnocellular cell. At any given retinal location, 6 to 7 parvocellular ganglion cells might tile the interior of 1 magnocellular ganglion cell. The magnocellular ganglion cells themselves form a similar tiling on a larger scale. The more numerous parvocellular ganglion cells with smaller receptive fields constitute the highest acuity visual pathway for perceptual acuity. These cells may also be more important in color vision than magnocellular ganglion cells.

SUMMARY

- Vision is a hierarchical process.
- Mechanical elements of the eye, such as the lens and pupil, control the focus and intensity of light reaching the retina.
- Eye movements are an integral part of visual processing.
- Retinal photoreceptors convert captured photons to modulated glutamate release.
- Retinal bipolar cells communicate positive and negative excursions around the mean light level to the inner retina.
- Amacrine and ganglion cells in the inner retina sculpt and transmit extracted aspects of the changing light distribution for transmission to the brain.
- Retinal ganglion cells project to 15 different retinal recipient zones in the brain.
- The most important retinal recipient zone is the lateral geniculate nucleus of the thalamus.
- Blindness and visual deficits occur primarily in the retina, but also in higher visual processing centers.

SELF-ASSESSMENT QUESTIONS

1. An individual is diagnosed with retinitis pigmentosa (RP). Which of the following is the most likely cause of this disease?

   A. Degeneration of area 17 of the cerebral cortex
   B. Degeneration of bipolar cells of the retina
   C. Degeneration of amacrine cells
   D. Degeneration of retinal ganglion cells
   E. Degeneration of photoreceptors

2. A 21-year-old man, who previously had normal vision, suddenly becomes blind. A detailed examination and analysis indicate that he was infected by a virus that selectively attacked and destroyed the same retinal cells that are attacked in felines as determined from experimental studies. In such studies, the cells attacked by the virus are ones that produce action potentials in response to changes in position of selective objects presented to the visual field of a cat. Which of the following retinal cells are destroyed by this virus?

   A. Amacrine cells
   B. Rods
   C. Cones
   D. Ganglion cells
   E. Horizontal cells

3. A patient is diagnosed by the same optometrist as being farsighted. To correct this defect, which of the following lenses should the doctor recommend be put into his eyeglasses?

   A. Cylindrical
   B. Concave
   C. Convex
   D. Neutral
   E. Spherical

4. A patient presents with a selective vision loss for movement and low contrast but appears to have normal color vision at high contrast levels. This is indicative of a selective loss of what type of retinal neurons?

   A. Parvocellular ganglion cells
   B. Magnocellular ganglion cells
   C. Bipolar cells
   D. Horizontal cells
   E. Dopaminergic amacrine cells

5. A patient presents with headaches and sudden-onset pain in the eyes. Visual field tests show a loss of peripheral vision in 1 eye. What is the diagnosis?

   A. Retinitis pigmentosa
   B. Open-angle glaucoma
   C. Closed-angle glaucoma
   D. Macular degeneration
   E. Diabetic retinopathy

Visual System II: Central Visual Pathways

Franklin R. Amthor

THE OUTPUT OF THE RETINA: WHAT THE EYE TELLS THE BRAIN

The common metaphor that the eye is like a camera works reasonably well for some of the optical components of the eye such as the lens and pupil but fails dramatically in describing the output of the retina. A camera is a recording device whose purpose is to register (and, in the video case, transmit) a true rendition of the light distribution focused on the film or detector. Virtually all cameras have a homogeneously dense pixel array, whereas the photoreceptor density in the retina varies markedly from center to periphery. More importantly, a camera records or transmits the light intensity at each pixel, but in the retina, most ganglion cells receive inputs from many photoreceptors, and many ganglion cells extract a highly processed signal from these photoreceptor inputs, such as motion occurring in a particular direction or the presence of an edge.

A Review of Ganglion Cell Classes

The mammalian retina, including that of primates such as humans, contains at least 20 to 25 classes of ganglion cells whose axons terminate in at least 15 different retinal recipient zones. The responses of these different ganglion cells mediate many different types of visual functions by virtue of their receptive field properties (what causes them to respond) and central projections (where in the brain the ganglion cell axons terminate). Many retinal ganglion cells terminate in multiple retinal recipient zones and thus participate in multiple visual processing pathways.

Functions of Visual Output

There are several visually mediated functions of which we are conscious, and many of which we are not conscious. Conscious visual functions include perception, identification, and visually controlled movement guidance. Unconscious

visually mediated processes include the control of eye position and pupil size and circadian rhythms. These processes are mediated by different ganglion cell classes in different visual pathways.

Ganglion Cell Response Selectivity

Different ganglion cell classes differ considerably in their response selectivity, which is related to the function of the visual circuit to which they project. At one extreme are the midget or parvocellular ganglion cells of the fovea whose input arises primarily from a single bipolar cell, which in turn is driven mostly by a single red or green cone. The intracellular voltage response of these midget ganglion cells closely resembles that of the single bipolar cell driving them. In the case of off-center ganglion cells, the hyperpolarizing bipolar cell response itself resembles that of the cone to which it connects. Because the spike output of the midget ganglion cell follows its intracellular potential fairly faithfully, this spike output is a reliable index of the photoreceptor response as though passed through a voltage to frequency converter. The bipolar cell connected to the on-center midget ganglion cell has an inhibitory mGluR6 receptor for glutamate, so its response is the reverse of that of the hyperpolarizing bipolar cell. The on-center midget ganglion cell thus signals light increases fairly faithfully, whereas the off-center midget ganglion cell signals light decreases.

Many retinal ganglion cells, in contrast, have response characteristics that depend on complex spatiotemporal characteristics of the light distribution over the thousands of photoreceptors and hundreds of bipolar cells to which they are connected. Notable examples include selectivity for direction of motion or the presence of edges. Many of these ganglion cells exhibit memory dependence in their responses such that the pattern of light stimulation many seconds previously strongly influences current responses, which underlies phenomena such as contrast gain control.

Overview of Ganglion Cell Retinal Recipient Zones

Conscious vision is mediated almost exclusively via the ganglion cell projection to the thalamus, specifically, the lateral geniculate nucleus of the thalamus. The next most important projection is to the superior colliculus (SC) for visual orienting and eye movement control, especially voluntary eye movements called saccades. Retinal ganglion cells also project to several pretectal and accessory optic nuclei, to the hypothalamus, and to several other less well-understood retinal recipient zones.

Thalamus

All sensory systems except for olfaction involve a projection to a sensory modality–specific region of the thalamus that in turn projects to what is called a *primary* cortex for that sense. The thalamic pathway is always crucial to conscious awareness of sensory input for that sensory modality. In the visual system, the visual thalamus region is called the lateral genicular nucleus (LGN). Two ganglion cell classes, called parvocellular and magnocellular ganglion cells, form the major projection to the LGN. Several other ganglion cell classes, usually termed koniocellular due to their smaller soma sizes, also project there. Sparser projections from the retina are also made to the ventral geniculate nucleus and possibly the pulvinar, which is an integrating and visual attention control thalamic area.

Superior Colliculus

The SC receives axons from almost all ganglion cell classes except the parvocellular cells. The SC evolved from its homolog in nonmammalian vertebrates, the optic tectum.

Pretectum

The pretectum is a set of midbrain nuclei that receive direct retinal projections. The main pretectal nuclei are the nucleus of the optic tract (NOT), the olivary pretectal nucleus (ON), and the anterior, medial, and posterior pretectal (PP) nuclei. The pretectum is involved in mediating visual reflexes such as optokinetic nystagmus (the cycle of tracking and saccadic return elicited by a stimulus such as a moving grating) and pupillary reflexes.

Accessory Optic System

The accessory optic system (AOS) consists of several retinal recipient nuclei that are involved in attention, eye movements, and vestibular coordination with visual input for balance. The AOS includes the medial terminal nucleus, lateral terminal nucleus, and dorsal terminal nucleus. Many ganglion cells projecting to the AOS are directionally selective in their responses.

The Hypothalamus & Other Specialized Recipient Areas

The suprachiasmatic nucleus of the hypothalamus, Edinger-Westphal nucleus, and other specialized recipient areas receive inputs from specialized retinal ganglion cells such as intrinsically photoreceptive ganglion cells.

VISUAL PROCESSING IN THE BRAIN: THE THALAMUS

Approximately 80% of all retinal ganglion cells, including the important midget system that comprises the fovea, project to the LGN of the thalamus. Virtually all magnocellular ganglion cells also project there, as well as several additional cell classes called koniocellular cells. By virtue of the optics of the eye, there is a correspondence between visual field angular location and retinal location, a topology. This topology is not retained within the optic nerve, but it is reconstituted in a layer- and class-specific manner in the LGN. This involves a sorting of fibers in the changeover from the optic nerve to the optic tract at the optic chiasm.

The Optic Nerve & Optic Chiasm

The output of the retina, the optic nerve, consists of the axons of all ganglion cells that exit the eye there. A few centimeters after the axons leave the eye, they enter a structure called the optic chiasm, which means "optic crossing," where some of the ganglion cell axons from each eye cross at the chiasm and go to the other side of the brain and some do not. Figure 12–1 shows that ganglion cells from the part of the right retina farthest from the nose (called the temporal retina) project ipsilaterally to the LGN on the right side. This portion of the retina receives input from the left visual field. The other half of the retina (closest to the nose, called the nasal retina) projects contralaterally to the left LGN. The nasal retina of the right eye receives input from the right visual field. The nasal left retina, which receives input from the left visual field, projects to the right thalamus with the temporal right retina. Thus, the right LGN receive inputs from both eyes from the left visual field, and similarly, the left LGN receives axons from both eyes, which receive visual input from the right visual field. The nerves leaving the optic chiasm are called the optic tracts. The major destination of the optic tracts is the LGN, but ganglion cells also project to >10 other retinal recipient zones in the brain.

The Thalamic "Relay"

In the LGN, each thalamic relay cell receives inputs from 1 or a few similar ganglion cells that are either parvo- or magnocellular, depending on the layer. For this reason, and because LGN relay cells respond very much like their parvocellular or magnocellular ganglion cell inputs, LGN cells have often been called relay cells. The ratio of retinal input to LGN output is approximately 1:1, consistent with the idea that each retinal ganglion cell mostly drives a single LGN cell. However, other inputs to the LGN from other parts of the brain (including visual cortex) allow gating functions that are associated with attention. These inputs modulate the strength of a neuron's

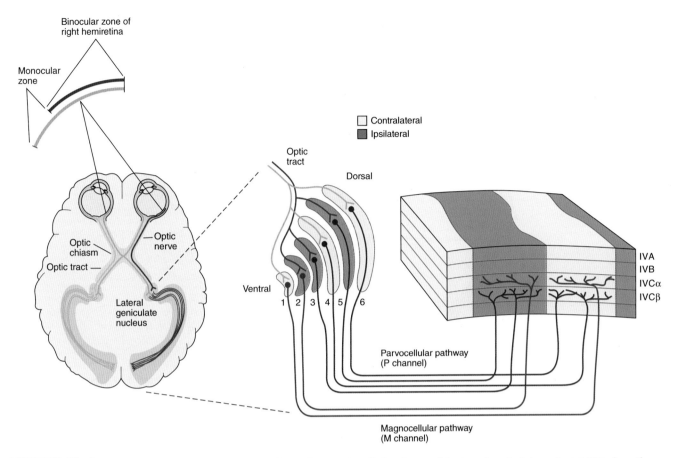

FIGURE 12–1 Parvocellular and magnocellular ganglion cells project to distinct layers of the lateral geniculate nucleus (LGN) where they are spatiotopically organized and segregated into different layers by ganglion cell class. Parvocellular ganglion cells project to layers 3 to 6, whereas magnocellular ganglion cells project to layers 1 and 2. The LGN layers alternate receiving projections from ipsilateral and contralateral eyes and project to alternate layers, except parvocellular layer 3 and magnocellular layer 2, which are both ipsilateral. The LGN projects via the optic radiation to visual cortex in the occipital lobe. (Reproduced with permission from Kandel ER, Schwartz JH, Jessell TM, et al: *Principles of Neural Science*, 5th ed. New York, NY: McGraw Hill; 2013.)

responses to any particular stimulus based on the contextual importance of that stimulus. There are actually more reciprocal inputs to the LGN from the visual cortex, which feeds information back and modifies it, than from the retina going up to the LGN.

Note that no LGN cells are binocular, but the LGN on each side receives inputs from the portions of both eyes viewing the opposite side visual hemifield. Damage to the LGN on 1 side or to 1 optic tract, but not 1 optic nerve, produces a visual field scotoma (blind area) under binocular viewing. A different result occurs if there is damage to the upper 4 versus lower 2 layers of the LGN. Damage to the upper 4 parvocellular layers results in a loss of color and fine detail perception. Damage to the bottom 2 magnocellular layers reduces the ability to respond to changes in the visual image, such as motion, particularly at low contrast.

The main output of all LGN layers is to visual cortex in the occipital lobe via a fiber pathway called the optic radiation. There are also LGN cells between the 6 main layers called interlaminar cells, which project to visual cortex. The overall projection scheme from the retina to

visual cortex is shown in Figure 12–2, with the scotoma (visual field loss) associated with damage to various loci in the pathway.

The LGN is located at the lateral inferior edge of the thalamus, just lateral to the medial geniculate nucleus that similarly relays auditory information, as shown in Figure 12–3. The LGN is also close to the midbrain inferior and superior colliculi, which relay auditory and visual information, respectively.

An important principle of cortical organization with respect to its representation of the sensory periphery is shown in Figure 12–4. This is the so-called *cortical magnification factor*, in which the foveal representation of the retina occupies a much larger cortical area than other retinal areas. The explanation for this is simple and fundamental, however. The neocortex neural circuitry is fundamentally similar throughout its extent (with important exceptions to be discussed elsewhere). This implies that its processing capabilities are similar per unit area, which is reflected in the fact that the number of thalamic inputs to a given cortical area is relatively constant for a given sensory modality. Because the density of retinal ganglion cells

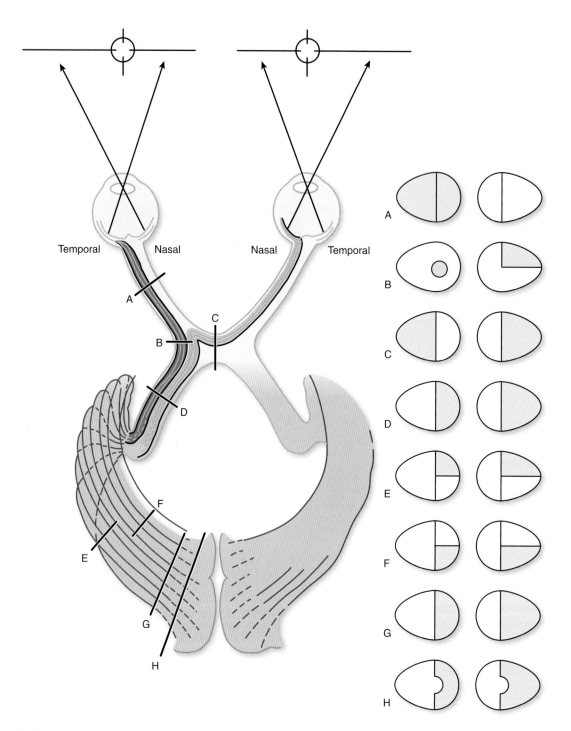

FIGURE 12–2 The pathway from retina to visual cortex. Visual signals are conducted by retinal ganglion cell axons through the optic nerve, optic chiasm, and optic tracts to the lateral geniculate nucleus of the thalamus, where they terminate on thalamic relay cells. These cells project via the optic radiation to the occipital lobe in area V1, the primary visual cortex, also called striate cortex. The visual field loss associated with damage to various parts of the pathway is shown. (Reproduced with permission from Ropper AH, Samuels MA, Klein JP: *Adams and Victor's Principles of Neurology,* 11th ed. New York, NY: McGraw Hill; 2019.)

and thalamic relay cells is much higher in the center than the periphery of the retina, as shown in the top of Figure 12–4, this relatively small retinal area projects to a much larger cortical area than the periphery, keeping the number of retinal ganglion cells and thalamic relay cells relatively constant per unit of cortical area.

THE SUPERIOR COLLICULUS & EYE MOVEMENTS

Most ganglion cell classes except the parvocellular cells project to the SC in the midbrain. SC layers exhibit a retinotopic map of the surrounding space. This structure is the mammalian

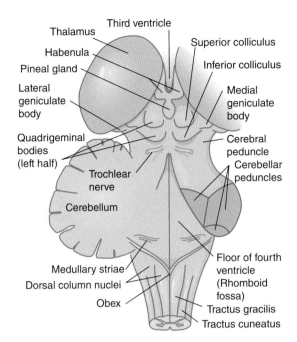

FIGURE 12–3 Posterior view of the brainstem showing the location of the superior colliculus and lateral geniculate nucleus of the thalamus in relation to other brainstem structures. (Reproduced with permission from Waxman SG. *Clinical Neuroanatomy*, 28th ed. New York, NY: McGraw Hill; 2017.)

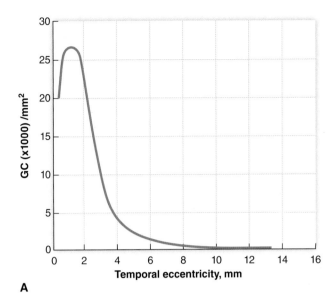

A

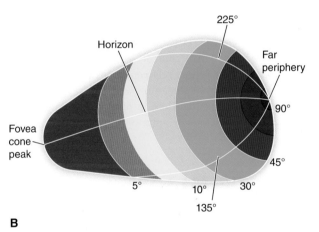

B

FIGURE 12–4 Graph of ganglion cell (GC) density versus temporal eccentricity (data from Curcio and Allan) and topographic organization of V1. The area of V1 devoted to different regions of the retina follows ganglion cell count.

analog of the optic tectum in nonmammalian vertebrates who generally lack any significant visual cortex. In such animals, the optic tectum is the main visual processing center for controlling visually guided behavior. In mammals, however, the SC controls orienting and eye movements, and visually guided behavior and perception are mediated by thalamic pathways to the cortex. The superficial layers project to deeper layers that encode saccade targets. Thus, the output of the deep layers of the colliculus controls eye movements to visual targets. Neural activation at a specific locus in the SC evokes a response directed toward the corresponding spatial location. Lesions to the SC reduce or eliminate orienting eye and head movements to peripheral objects.

The main class of eye movements controlled by the SC are called saccades. Saccades are large jumps in eye position from one fixation point to another. Voluntary saccades occur at a rate of about 3 to 4 times per second. Involuntary saccades also occur when something appears in the visual periphery and we direct our gaze to place the central fovea at the peripheral target. Our eyes also constantly make smaller movements called microsaccades, drift, and tremor. One function of these movements is to prevent image fading, because artificially stabilizing images on the retina invokes adaptation mechanisms that eliminate neural firing and cause vision to disappear.

THE PRETECTUM

The pretectum is a set of midbrain nuclei that receive direct retinal projections and mediate visual reflexes such as optokinetic nystagmus (the cycle of tracking and saccadic return

elicited by a stimulus such as a moving grating) and pupillary reflexes. The main pretectal nuclei are the NOT, ON, and the anterior, medial, and PP nuclei. These nuclei are located anterior to the SC, posterior to the thalamus, and above the periaqueductal gray. The NOT and ON receive inputs from intrinsically photosensitive ganglion cells. These ganglion cells have their own photopigment and respond directly to overall light levels.

Pretectal nuclei send their outputs to the thalamus, SC, reticular formation, pons, and inferior olive. The ON and PP nucleus project to the Edinger-Westphal nucleus, which controls pupil diameter. There are also pretectal projections to the pulvinar, a thalamic integration and control area for visual attention. The NOT receives inputs from directionally selective ganglion cells that mediate its involvement in smooth pursuit. Some pretectal nuclei may have roles in nociception and sleep regulation.

ACCESSORY OPTIC SYSTEM

Other retinal ganglion cell projection areas include the AOS, whose nuclei include the medial terminal nucleus, lateral terminal nucleus, and dorsal terminal nucleus. These areas are concerned with attention, eye movements, and vestibular coordination with visual input for balance. AOS nuclei receive projections from directionally selective retinal ganglion cells to mediate these functions.

THE HYPOTHALAMUS & OTHER SPECIALIZED RECIPIENT AREAS

Intrinsically photoreceptive retinal ganglion cells respond directly to light via their own membrane photopigment. These cells respond slowly at high firing rates to overall changes in average luminance, which is quite different from the complex, center-surround structure of most retinal ganglion cells. The intrinsically photoreceptive ganglion cells send their outputs to nuclei such as the suprachiasmatic nucleus, which controls circadian rhythms, and the Edinger-Westphal nucleus, which controls pupil dilation. There are indications of other retinal recipient areas of the brain such as the pulvinar, ventral thalamus, and Raphe about which little is known except that these projections are likely to be involved in unconscious or autonomic processing of visual information.

THE OCCIPITAL LOBE

As in all sensory systems with the exception of part of olfaction, the projection to visual cortex is primarily from a specific region of the thalamus. In the case of vision, the thalamic relay cells are in the LGN. Cells there send their axons to the visual area of the neocortex at the pole of the occipital lobe via a fiber tract called the optic radiation (see Figure 12–2). The recipient area of the occipital lobe is called visual area 1 (V1), as well as area 17 (from the Brodmann map) and the striate cortex, because of a dense cell layer that appears in histologic stains. This pathway mediates almost all the vision of which a person is conscious (versus vision functions, such as pupil contraction and dilation, which a person is neither conscious of nor able to control voluntarily).

Representation of the Visual Field

The 1 million LGN relay cells project in a topographic manner to primary visual cortex (V1) at the pole of the occipital lobe and within the calcarine sulcus. The left visual field is represented on the right visual cortex, and the right visual field on the left visual cortex.

Retinotopy

The cortical cells driven from each LGN form a map of visual space distorted by the higher retinal ganglion cell

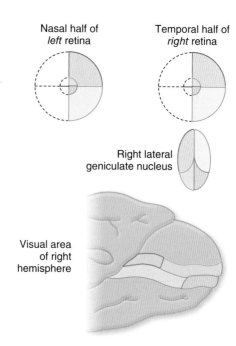

FIGURE 12–5 Sagittal section of the calcarine fissure in visual cortex showing the mapping between visual field regions and occipital location.

representation in the center versus the periphery. Figure 12–5 shows how the visual field and LGN thalamic representation are mapped onto the inner surface of the right visual cortex within the calcarine sulcus. Central visual areas, including the large foveal representation, occupy the most posterior regions of the sulcus, with the peripheral representation extending anteriorly.

Processing Expansion

The projection from the LGN to the visual cortex consists of approximately 1 million axons, similar to the number of ganglion cell axons that project to each LGN from the retina. However, this million-cell input from the LGN drives approximately 200 million cortical cells in V1. However, cells in V1 are more specialized for stimulus parameters such as orientation and movement direction. This results in a sparser representation of the visual stimulus in cortex than retina or LGN. Whereas in retina and LGN, most visual stimuli cause some change in firing of most cells in that area of the visual field, in visual cortex, only a small percentage of more selective cells respond well to any stimulus, depending on specific aspects of the stimulus such as its orientation or motion direction. Thus, V1 neurons extract local stimulus features from a restricted region of the retina.

Columnar Organization of V1

Organization of Inputs   The cellular architecture of V1, or striate cortex, is similar to that of neocortex throughout the brain in that it has 6 layers with a characteristic input/output pattern. Figure 12–6 illustrates the layers, the types of cells (pyramidal

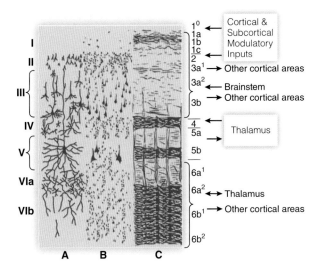

FIGURE 12–6 The layers of neocortex and their typical input and output pattern.

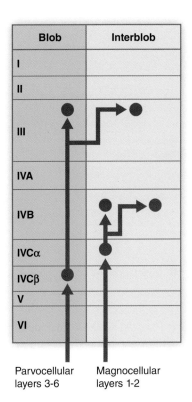

FIGURE 12–7 The pattern of projection of parvocellular and magnocellular axons from lateral geniculate nucleus to layer IV of the visual cortex.

and local) that occupy the layers, and the characteristic inputs and outputs. The general plan for visual cortex is that thalamic inputs terminate in layer IV, and in this regard, the visual cortex is similar to other sensory cortices, and, in fact, all cortices. However, the visual cortex differs from other cortical areas in the density of inputs. There are >2 million LGN inputs in the visual pathway, versus, for example, a few tens of thousands of auditory inputs to the auditory cortex. The result in the visual cortex is a thickening of layer IV compared to other cortical areas with a very high cell density. This high-density, thickened layer IV makes the cytoarchitecture of layer IV stand out compared to other cortical areas and leads to the name "striate" cortex for V1. Layer IV in the striate cortex is so thick that it has been subdivided into sublayers A to C, and layer C is further subdivided in the sub-sublayers α and β, as shown in Figure 12–7.

The input to visual cortex from the LGN is different for parvocellular versus magnocellular layers and still partially segregated. Figure 12–7 shows that the parvocellular layer (layers 3 to 6) axons from LGN terminate in visual cortical layer IVCβ. Cells in this layer project upward to layer III. Magnocellular inputs arrive in cortical layer IVCα, however. There is also a horizontal regional specialization in striate cortex, referred to as "blobs" and "interblobs," which are areas of high and low cytochrome oxidase staining, respectively. The cytochrome oxidase staining differentiates areas of relatively high versus low metabolic activity. Input to the blob areas is almost exclusively parvocellular. Input to the interblob areas, however, comes directly from the magnocellular input and secondarily through a cortical projection in layer III from parvocellular cells.

Cell Physiology As mentioned earlier, each visual LGN relay cell drives, on average, several hundred V1 cells. The cells in V1 have more specificity in their responses than retinal ganglion cells or LGN relay cells. As Hubel and Weisel famously showed, V1 cells are almost all sensitive to the orientation of an extended

stimulus on the retina and do not fire action potentials unless there is an edge, represented by several collinear ganglion cells. Many of these cells are also sensitive to direction of motion, and others are sensitive to edge length. Cells that are purely orientationally selective are called simple cells. Cells that are both orientationally selective and direction of motion selective are called complex cells, which also differ from simple cells in several other response properties. An additional class, called hypercomplex or end-stopped cells, is orientationally selective, directionally selective, and selective for stimulus length.

Electrophysiologic recordings made in V1 show that the orientation selectivity in V1 has a specific horizontal organization in sync with the blob and interblob regions. At any location in visual cortex, all cells at various depths have the same orientation selectivity, and the preferred orientation changes systematically as one moves the electrode horizontally across the cortical surface. A region whose extent includes all orientations is termed a *column* and tends to extend from one cytochrome oxidase blob to the next.

At the same time, V1 cells are the first in the visual pathway to be binocularly driven. The binocularity of cells also systematically changes with cortical horizontal position, such that as one moves a microelectrode, one sees a systematic change from cells totally driven by the left eye, to equal eye contribution, to right eye dominance. At any given cortical location, ocular dominance and orientation selectivity change at relatively right angles, leading to the idea of a 2-dimensional

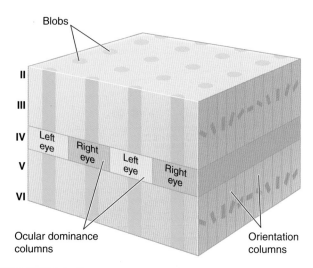

FIGURE 12–8 Orientation and ocular dominance columns in V1.

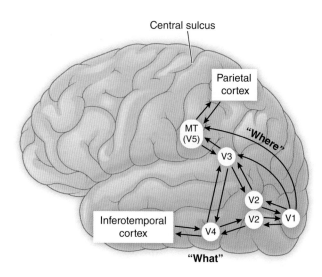

FIGURE 12–9   Dorsal and ventral stream visual processing pathways with important visual areas delineated. MT, middle temporal.

column (Figure 12–8) in which ocular dominance changes from left to equal to right and orientation selectivity changes from horizontal to vertical.

HIGHER CORTICAL PROCESSING AREAS

V1, at the posterior pole of the occipital lobe, contains an entire representation of the retina, and therefore the visual world, onto which orientation, motion direction, edge length selectivity, and ocular dominance are grafted onto the position map. V1 sends its outputs to several other cortical areas and back to the thalamus. The thalamic return projection modulates the input V1 itself receives in ways that are not completely understood but appear to contribute to the selectivity of V1 cells and serve as a basis for visual attention.

V1 projects to adjacent cortical areas such as V2 and V3. Neurons in these areas have similar response properties to those in V1, and the additional processing done in V2 and V3 is not well understood. After these areas, however, the visual cortical output diverges into 2 anatomically differentiated streams whose functions are relatively well understood and that have important clinical ramifications. An outline of this dual projection system is shown in Figure 12–9.

VENTRAL STREAM FOR OBJECT PERCEPTION

The V2-V3 complex forms 1 projection via the inferior longitudinal fasciculus into the inferior portion of the temporal lobe (also called inferotemporal cortex). This cortical analysis system is dominated by parvocellular input. It specializes in object identification and related aspects of perception and is sometimes called the *what pathway*. Cortical areas in the what pathway include the TE (temporal; also called PIT [posterior inferior temporal]) and TEO (temporal occipital; also called

anterior inferior temporal) areas. The beginning stage for this pathway is usually taken to be area V4, where most neurons are color selective. More anterior neurons in this pathway (TEO) respond only to very complex patterns such as the shape of a hand. In the fusiform gyrus (fusiform face area) near this area are many neurons that are face selective. The output of the ventral processing stream includes the hippocampus and anterior areas of the frontal lobe.

Dorsal Stream & Visually Guided Behavior

A second processing stream from the V2-V3 complex passes through area V5 into the parietal lobe via the superior longitudinal fasciculus. Neurons in V5 (also called MT [middle temporal]) are almost all directionally selective, and this pathway is dominated by magnocellular input. Major areas in the dorsal stream include the middle temporal and medial superior temporal areas. The dorsal pathway has been termed the *where pathway* because of its involvement in the use of vision for navigating in space. Some researchers believe, however, that a better term would be the *how to pathway* because of its necessity for visually guided behaviors, such as catching a ball or running through an obstacle course. Damage to this area causes apraxia, which is the inability to skillfully conduct tasks such as manipulating objects based on visual information.

Dorsal-Ventral Crosstalk

Despite the fact that the ventral stream is dominated by parvocellular input and the dorsal stream by magnocellular input, there is crosstalk between them. In the structure-from-motion phenomena, a few visible spots on a moving object are sufficient to give away its shape identity during movement. In this case, dorsal motion-detecting neurons must communicate with object-detecting neurons in the ventral pathway. Depth perception is another example of a holistic perception that may be derived from ventral pictorial cues or dorsal motion parallax.

Blindness, Agnosias, & Visual Field Deficits

Blindness

Blindness typically originates from damage or cell loss early in the visual pathway, including retina, thalamus, and V1. Because of the parallelized processing at higher levels, losses there tend to be selective and are called agnosias, which is the loss of a specific visual ability without the loss of other abilities, and are usually due to damage to a high order cortical visual area. The term *agnosia* was coined by Sigmund Freud.

Most blindness originates in the retina. Photoreceptor retinopathies, such as macular degeneration, retinitis pigmentosa, and diabetic retinopathy, are caused by photoreceptor death. The other major retinopathy, glaucoma, is caused by death of retinal ganglion cells, usually associated with excessive pressure within the eye.

The cause of retinitis pigmentosa is a hereditary degeneration of retinal rod photoreceptors, progressing to loss of all vision due to secondary death of cones. The retinitis pigmentosa sequence starts with night blindness from rod death; later, all peripheral vision is lost, leading to tunnel vision. Central vision is spared for some time because there are no rods in the fovea. In the last phase, the fovea also degenerates, and all vision is lost. There is no treatment for retinitis pigmentosa, and the resulting blindness is irreversible.

Photoreceptors die in macular degeneration and diabetic retinopathy because of metabolic disorders that lead to neovascularization or inadequate retinal nutrition. The sequence typically begins with photoreceptor death and then is followed by death of other retinal neurons. Retinal death can also occur if the retina detaches from the underlying pigment epithelium after a blow to the head.

Glaucoma is caused by the death of retinal ganglion cells and is typically associated with excessive pressure within the eye restricting axonal trafficking at the optic nerve head. There are 2 major subtypes. Closed-angle glaucoma occurs when the iris obstructs drainage canals from the vitreous in the middle of the eye to the aqueous chamber behind the cornea, allowing vitreal pressure to build up. This type of glaucoma is the rarer of the 2 types and is treatable using laser surgery to blast small holes in the iris. Open-angle glaucoma usually has a heritable component and is often associated with high blood pressure. It can often be controlled with medication. In either glaucoma subtype, however, once the ganglion cells have died, the blindness is irreversible.

Amblyopia is a dysfunction in which 1 eye appears to be blind, but the eye itself presents as being neutrally normal. Its origin is often a congenital optical problem in the eye such as severe astigmatism or a cataract that degrades the neural output of the eye during the critical developmental period from birth to about 6 years. Cortical synapses are taken over almost completely by the better eye, and after the plastic critical period, the damage is irreversible, even if at a later age the optical problem with the amblyopic eye is corrected.

Dorsal/Ventral Stream Damage

Damage from a tumor or stroke to areas in the dorsal stream causes apraxias or loss of ability to use vision to manipulate objects. A well-known agnosia called akinetopsia was experienced by a patient with bilateral damage to V5. This patient was unable to avoid cars crossing the street or pour a cup of tea because she could not estimate time to impact or time to full cup from the motion signal. Her visual experience is something like that in a strobe light. Damage to the parietal lobe, particularly on the right side of the brain, results in hemineglect, in which people are inattentive to objects in their left visual field.

Ventral stream damage is often associated with loss of pattern perception. One example is achromatopsia, occurring from damage to V4 in the ventral stream. This is the loss of the ability to identify colors and is distinct from color blindness. Color blindness occurs because of the loss of 1 or more cone types, so that the person cannot see any difference between some colors. In achromatopsia, however, the person sees a difference between color patches, but they do not seem to have any quality of color but, rather, appear as different dirty shades of gray.

Face & Complex Perception

Although the ventral visual processing stream has no final output or highest level area, the most complex neural selectivity known in that stream is undoubtedly the face-selective cells in the fusiform face area. Many cells recorded in this area in nonhuman primates respond well only to faces, and this area is activated in functional magnetic resonance imaging scans in humans when they view faces. Patients with damage to this area also may lose the ability to visually recognize another's face while still being able to identify the person by the sound of the person's voice or the way he or she walks.

SUMMARY

- Vision is a hierarchical process.
- Retinal ganglion cells project to 15 different retinal recipient zones in the brain.
- The most important retinal recipient zone is the LGN of the thalamus.
- The LGN projects to the visual cortex, which engages in complex analysis of the visual scene, and projects to other brain areas.
- Visual areas of the brain produce neural images that represent different aspects of the visual world based on factors such as color, the location of edges, and movement.
- Blindness and visual deficits occur primarily in the retina, but also occur in higher visual processing centers.

SELF-ASSESSMENT QUESTIONS

1. A routine magnetic resonance imaging scan reveals the presence of a tumor situated in the left optic tract proximal to the lateral geniculate nucleus. The patient complains of a reduction in his field of vision. Which of the following best characterizes the likely visual deficit?

   A. Total blindness of the left eye
   B. Bitemporal hemianopsia
   C. Right homonymous hemianopsia
   D. Left homonymous hemianopsia
   E. Left homonymous quadrantanopia

2. After a stroke, a patient appears to have normal visual acuity but is unable to recognize faces. Where is the lesion likely to be?

   A. Left parietal lobe
   B. Right parietal lobe
   C. Inferior left temporal lobe
   D. Inferior right temporal lobe
   E. Occipital lobe

3. A patient shows up in clinic with only the right side of his face shaved and complains that he ran into the left side of his garage when parking his car at home the previous evening. Where is the lesion likely to be?

   A. Left parietal lobe
   B. Right parietal lobe
   C. Inferior left temporal lobe
   D. Inferior right temporal lobe
   E. Occipital lobe

4. A patient's wife complains that the patient tends to stare fixedly at the same spot for long periods of time and ignores gestures made by her when she is not directly in front of him. Examination shows that the patient does not orient well to stimuli in the periphery, making neither eye or head movements when peripheral objects move toward him. What is the probable location of the lesion?

   A. Superior colliculus
   B. Left parietal lobe
   C. Right parietal lobe
   D. Left temporal lobe
   E. Right temporal lobe

5. A poor, elderly patient is brought to clinic who appears to be nearly totally blind. His relatives suspect glaucoma because it runs in his family but remark that he wakes up at sunrise like he always has. This last fact suggests that

   A. the glaucoma diagnosis is probably correct.
   B. the glaucoma diagnosis is probably incorrect.
   C. continuing to wake up at sunrise is irrelevant.
   D. the damage is central, not retinal.
   E. the blindness is psychosomatic.

Auditory & Vestibular Systems

Franklin R. Amthor

OVERVIEW

The sense of hearing allows us to capture sound energy from the environment and informs us about the identity of the sound emitter and its location. Complex sounds are also an essential means of complex communication for biological organisms, reaching their pinnacle in human language. Sound consists of a sequence of air pressure pulses created by vibrating objects such as vocal cords. Vibrations cause compression and rarefaction of the air, which result in the characteristics of frequency, the number of cycles per second, amplitude, and sound intensity, which is usually measured in decibels, a log scale. The sensitivity of the auditory system is very close to the absolute threshold created by random movement of air molecules. Sound reception begins with mechanical modification and transduction in the outer and middle ear and neural coding in the inner ear at the cochlea. Relays in the brainstem and thalamus pass the encoded auditory input to the auditory cortex in the mid-superior temporal lobe, where higher auditory processing allows us to understand language and appreciate music.

Near the cochlea of the auditory system are the semicircular canals of the vestibular system. Hair cells in those canals respond not to external sound input but to motion along 3 axes of rotation. The neural output of the vestibular system is essential for maintaining balance and works with motion-detecting cells from the retina in central pathways that code our motion in space and allow the performance of complex, balanced motion.

PROPERTIES OF SOUND

As any object vibrates, it compresses air on the side it is moving toward and rarefies air on the other side. These pressure pulses are transmitted and spread by collisions of the molecules in the air as longitudinal waves. This is illustrated in Figures 13–1 and 13–2. Most objects have a natural frequency at which, when struck, they vibrate. Objects will also typically vibrate at various amplitudes at all the integral multiples (harmonics) of that frequency.

Intensity & Loudness

Sound waves have the physical properties of intensity, which we perceive as loudness, and frequency, which we perceive as pitch. Figure 13–1A shows a sinusoidal pressure oscillation at a particular frequency on an arbitrary time and amplitude scale. If the amplitude is increased, the vertical pressure excursions are larger (Figure 13–1B). If the frequency is increased, the wavelength is shorter (Figure 13–1C).

There is a million-fold range of sound amplitudes to which our ears respond. A compact notion used to describe this range is the decibel scale, named after Alexander Graham Bell. Figure 13–3 shows the how the decibel varies logarithmically with sound pressure. The decibel scale is usually referenced to a basis pressure p_0 of 20 µPa, close to the threshold of hearing, and is then referred to as the sound pressure level in decibels.

The human hearing threshold is not the same for all frequencies. Figure 13–4 shows the audibility curve for human

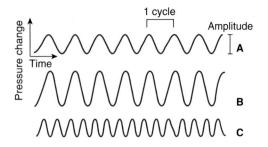

FIGURE 13–1 Sound has the properties of frequency and amplitude. **A.** A representation of the changes in sound pressure over time for a pure tone, which is a single frequency. **B.** An increase in amplitude. **C.** An increase in frequency. (Reproduced with permission from Barrett KE, Barman SM, Brooks HL et al: *Ganong's Review of Medical Physiology*, 26th ed. New York, NY: McGraw Hill; 2019.)

hearing, which shows the threshold, and the perceived loudness above threshold, as a function of frequency. Our threshold is lowest for frequencies of a few thousand hertz (hertz is sinusoidal cycles per second, after Heinrich Hertz). This frequency range is approximately the same as that of human speech, the range at which telephones work. The bass and treble controls on music stereo amplifiers are there to boost low and high frequencies that are below threshold when music is played at low

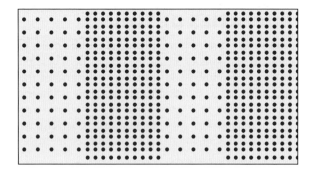

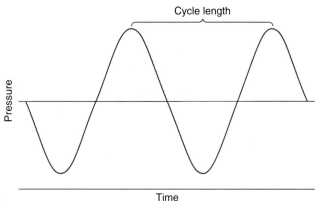

FIGURE 13–2 Vibrating objects that produce sounds do so by causing the air (or other conductive medium, such as water) to be alternately compressed and rarefied. These regions of high and low pressure are conducted longitudinally by collisions among air molecules. (Reproduced with permission from Hagan AD, DeMaria AN. *Clinical Applications of Two-Dimensional Echocardiography and Cardiac Doppler.* 2nd ed. Boston, MA: Little, Brown; 1989.)

dB in decibels = 20 logarithm $\dfrac{p}{p_0}$	

Where p is the sound pressure of the stimulus, and p_0 is a standard sound pressure, The dB scale is called the SPL (Sound Pressure Level) when p_0 is set to a "standard" 20 micropascals, close to the hearing threshold

Pressure ratio ($\dfrac{p}{p_0}$)	dB SPL
1	0
10	20
100	40
1,000	60
10,000	80
100,000	100
1,000,000	120
10,000,000	140

Adding 20 dB means multiplying the sound pressure by a factor of 10

FIGURE 13–3 The decibel scale for sound is a logarithmic scale that condenses the 10 million–fold range of sound pressures from threshold to hearing damage to a scale of 0 to 140 dB. It is obtained by taking the logarithm of the sound pressure to a reference pressure of 20 µPa, multiplied by 20.

volume. At higher sound pressure levels, the audibility curve is flatter and the compensation needed is much less. The level of 140 dB is the threshold of pain or feeling, and rapid damage occurs to the auditory hair cells at such levels. Prolonged exposure to levels of 120 dB or even lower can also damage hearing.

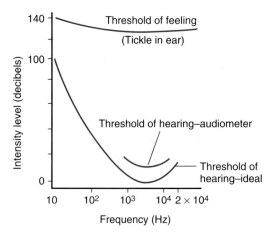

FIGURE 13–4 Sounds of different frequencies are not equally audible, and the audibility curve changes with sound level. Human hearing is most sensitive to frequencies of a few thousand hertz, the dominant frequency band used in speech. This sensitivity is very large near absolute threshold but becomes less pronounced for higher sound amplitudes. (Reproduced with permission from Barrett KE, Barman SM, Brooks HL et al: *Ganong's Review of Medical Physiology*, 26th ed. New York, NY: McGraw Hill; 2019.)

Frequency, Pitch, & Harmonics

Most real-world sounds are not simple sine waves, but neither are they arbitrary combinations of frequencies. Objects can generally sustain vibrations whose wavelengths fit an integral number of times within the length of the object. Figure 13–5 illustrates this phenomenon for the 1-dimensional case of a vibrating string. A plucked string may initially be excited by a range of frequencies, as shown in Figure 13–5A. However, because the 2 ends of the string are clamped, only frequencies whose wavelength is such that the amplitude is 0 at those points will be sustained. Other frequencies whose amplitudes would not be 0 at the clamped ends are quickly damped out.

Figure 13–5B shows that the set of sustainable frequencies begins with f1, whose wavelength is half the distance between the fixation points, and includes all integral multiples of f1, the harmonics of f1. The summation of all these frequencies at various amplitudes may look like Figure 13–5C, which is not a pure sine wave. Natural 3-dimensional objects emit sounds with different frequencies corresponding to different resonant lengths of the object along 3 axes and may be quite complicated. Later we will see that the auditory cortex is sensitive to such complex frequency sets and can distinguish them from randomly assembled sets of frequencies.

ANATOMY OF THE EAR

The first stages of auditory processing are mechanical transformations of the sound pressure variations reaching the ear in the outer and middle ear. Then, in the inner ear, sound pressure is transformed into neural impulses sent to the brain.

The Outer Ear & Localization: Tuning & Directing

The outer ear consists of 3 main elements: the pinna, auditory canal, and eardrum. The pinna is what people colloquially refer to as the ear. This structure filters the sound waves as it directs them into the auditory canal. The filtering changes the sound composition as a function of the elevation of the sound emitter, allowing localization of sounds in elevation by decoding this frequency alteration. The pinna and the nomenclature of its structures are shown in Figure 13–6.

Sounds then traverse the auditory canal on the way to the eardrum. The overall structures of the outer, middle, and inner ear are shown in Figure 13–7. The auditory canal has a resonant frequency of approximately several kilohertz that enhances the frequency range of best human hearing. The auditory canal ends at the tympanic membrane or eardrum, which is set in motion by the sound pressure as modulated by the pinna and auditory canal.

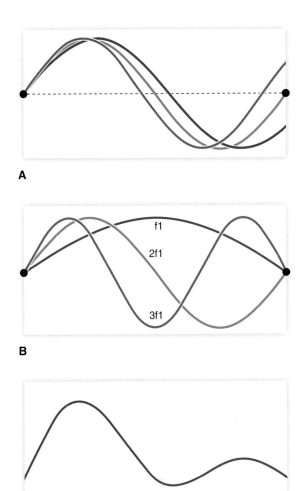

FIGURE 13–5 Natural objects sustain vibrations for certain frequencies and their harmonics. **A.** A representation of the response to a plucked string fixed at each end. Although the plucking excites the string at many frequencies, only those frequencies whose amplitudes are near 0 at the string ends will have their vibrations sustained. **B.** Sustainable vibrations occur for the fundamental frequency and all integral harmonics of that frequency. Properties of the vibrating object determine the relative amplitudes of the harmonics. **C.** The resulting total vibration consisting of the fundamental and various harmonics can have a complicated waveform.

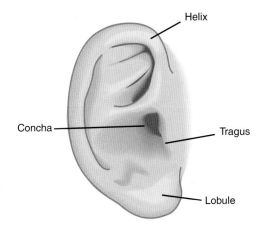

FIGURE 13–6 Nomenclature for structures of the external ear (pinna). (Reproduced with permission from Doherty GM: *Current Diagnosis & Treatment: Surgery*, 14th ed. New York, NY: McGraw Hill; 2015.)

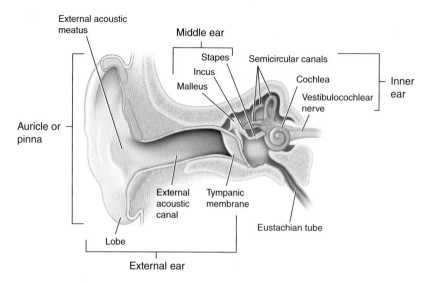

FIGURE 13–7 Cross-section through the various structures of the outer, middle, and inner ear. The outer ear consists of the external ear (pinna), auditory canal, and eardrum. The middle ear consists of the malleus, incus, and stapes bones. The inner ear begins where the stapes connects to the oval window and includes the cochlea and neurons associated with it. (Reproduced with permission from Jameson JL, Fauci AS, Kasper DL, et al: *Harrison's Principles of Internal Medicine*, 20th ed. New York, NY: McGraw Hill; 2018.)

The Middle Ear Bones & Amplification

Figure 13–8 shows a more detailed view of the middle ear, which is composed of 3 bones called the malleus, incus, and stapes, the smallest bones in the human body. The movement of the tympanic membrane drives the malleus, which moves the incus, which in turn moves the stapes that is attached to the cochlear entrance at the oval window. The arrangement of this system performs a force amplification to translate a larger, weaker movement of the tympanic membrane in air to a stronger, smaller movement of the oval window bounding the fluid-filled cochlea.

The force amplification by the middle ear system is accomplished in 2 ways: (1) the tympanic membrane has a larger area than the oval window, and therefore, force is concentrated from a large to a small area; and (2) the arrangement of the middle ear bones forms a lever, with the tympanic membrane on the long arm and oval window on the short arm. The total force multiplication is on the order of 100 times.

The Inner Ear: Cochlea & Organ of Corti

Sound is transduced into neural signals in the cochlea, whose relation to the rest of the structures of the ear can be seen in Figure 13–7 and Figure 13–9. Situated near the cochlea are the

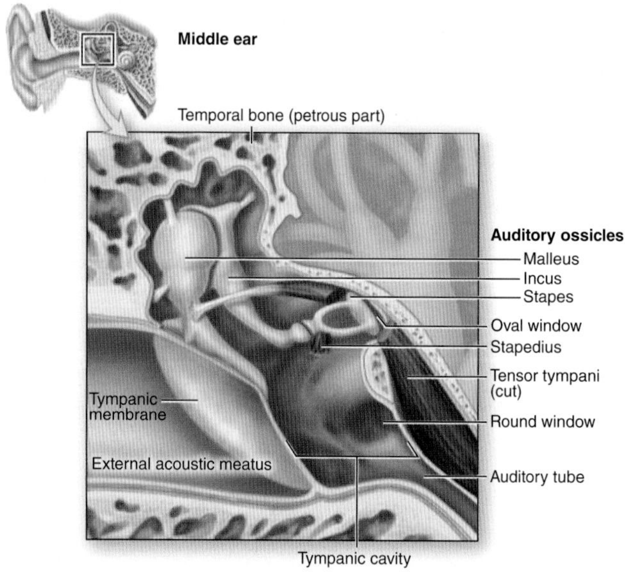

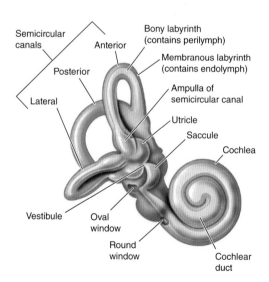

FIGURE 13–8 Detailed structure of the middle ear and its coupling to the eardrum (tympanic membrane) and oval window of the cochlea. (Reproduced with permission from McKinley MP, O'Loughlin VD, Bidle TS. *Anatomy and Physiology: An Integrative Approach.* New York, NY: McGraw Hill; 2013.)

FIGURE 13–9 The cochlea and surrounding structures. The cochlea is proximal to the semicircular canals, which also contain sensory transducer hair cells. (Reproduced with permission from Jameson JL, Fauci AS, Kasper DL, et al: *Harrison's Principles of Internal Medicine*, 20th ed. New York, NY: McGraw Hill; 2018.)

semicircular canals that transduce head orientation and movement into neural signals. The output of both of these inner ear structures travels to the brain via the vestibulocochlear nerve, which is cranial nerve VIII.

THE COCHLEA & SOUND TRANSDUCTION

Sound Wave Transduction & Place Coding

A cross-section of the Organ of Corti within the cochlea is shown in Figure 13–11B. The cochlea has 3 fluid-filled chambers: (1) the scala vestibuli above the organ of Corti in which pressure waves are induced by the oval window, (2) the scala tympani below the organ of Corti, and (3) the cochlear duct containing the organ of Corti with the tectorial and basilar membranes and auditory hair cells. The leverage changes in the middle ear allow the larger, low-impedance vibrations of the tympanic membrane to produce smaller more forceful vibrations of the oval window to transmit pressure pulses into the fluid-filled cavity called the scala vestibuli.

The way sound energy is localized by frequency along the cochlea is shown schematically in Figure 13–10, with the cochlea schematically "unrolled." The selectivity for vibration frequency along the length of the cochlea is called a *place code*. High frequencies cause large displacements of the basilar membrane at the oval window entrance to the cochlea, but not farther along its extent. Medium frequencies cause the maximal vibration in the middle of the cochlea, and low frequencies at the end of the cochlea, called the helicotrema, which is actually in the center of the coiled structure (shown in Figure 13–911A).

The place selectivity along the basilar membrane is much greater for high than low frequencies, shown in the bottom panel of Figure 13–10. High-frequency activation of the basilar membrane is restricted to small regions near the oval window, but very low frequencies vibrate almost the entire membrane. This place restriction difference is related to the way the nervous system encodes frequency. Because neural action potential and refractory periods last on the order of 2 milliseconds, neurons cannot generally fire >500 action potentials per second. At sound frequencies <500 Hz, a large percentage of neurons in the cochlear can fire every sound cycle, encoding sound frequency by their firing frequency. However, at higher frequencies, neurons cannot fire at the sound frequency, but at separated sound pressure peaks. Frequency is then encoded by which neurons along the basilar membrane are firing—a place code.

A more detailed, less schematic illustration of the cochlea and the organ of Corti within it is shown in Figure 13–11. In Figure 13–11A, the oval window is at the extreme left, underneath the text "Scala vestibuli." The cochlea is coiled such that it traverses about 2.5 turns between the oval window and helicotrema. A cross-section of the cochlea is shown in Figure 13–11B, showing the scala vestibuli, scala tympani, and organ of Corti. The basilar and tectorial membranes are in the organ of Corti, as are the auditory hair cells that convert sound pressure changes in the fluid-filled scala into neural action potentials. Figure 13–11B also shows the location of the spiral ganglion that contains the cell bodies of the neurons whose axons make up the auditory nerve and cochlear branch of cranial nerve VIII. The spiral ganglion cells are bipolar neurons whose dendrites contact auditory hair cells and whose axons project to the cochlear nucleus.

Auditory Hair Cells

A detailed cross-section of the organ of Corti showing the auditory hair cells is shown in Figure 13–11C (Figure 13–11D shows an actual photomicrograph of this structure). The pressure changes at the oval window are transmitted to the scala vestibuli and tympani to produce a shearing action between the basilar and tectorial membranes. This deflects the stereocilia of the hair cells whose movement is transduced into action potentials in the auditory nerve. This is accomplished by specialized channels at the hair cell base that open when the cilia bend. This takes place for hair cell deflections as small as the width of an atom.

At the base of the hair cells are the endings of neurons whose somas are located in the spiral ganglia. Depolarization of the hair cell produces action potentials in the spiral ganglia neurons, which in turn project via cranial nerve VIII to the cochlear nucleus in the brain.

There are 2 major classes of hair cells: inner and outer. The inner hair cells are responsible for the majority of auditory transmission to the brain. These are contacted by myelinated axon-like processes of several spiral ganglion cells. The major function of the more numerous outer hair cells is to control the stiffness of the membrane at their base, enhancing hair cell output at low volume, but decreasing it and protecting the hair cells at higher volumes. Each outer hair cell is contacted by a single, usually unmyelinated spiral ganglion cell ending.

The transduction mechanism of auditory hair cells is shown in Figure 13–12. Potassium (K^+) channels in the stereocilia are opened by deflection in one direction and closed for the other. The net effect of opening the potassium channels at the tips of the stereocilia is to open nonselective cation channels permeable to sodium, potassium, and calcium in the cell body of the hair cell. This depolarizes the hair cell, causing the release of an excitatory neurotransmitter (probably glutamate) onto receptors on the end process of the spiral ganglion cell.

The Spiral Ganglion Cell

Spiral ganglion cells are bipolar neurons whose somas or cell bodies are located next to the scala tympani in the bony part of the cochlea. The proximal process of the spiral ganglion cell is a conventional myelinated axon that projects to the cochlear nucleus. The distal process, sometimes referred to as a dendrite, has axonal properties such as the ability to conduct action potentials and being myelinated. In this regard, there is at least a superficial resemblance to dorsal root ganglion cells outside the spinal cord, which are pseudo-unipolar cells

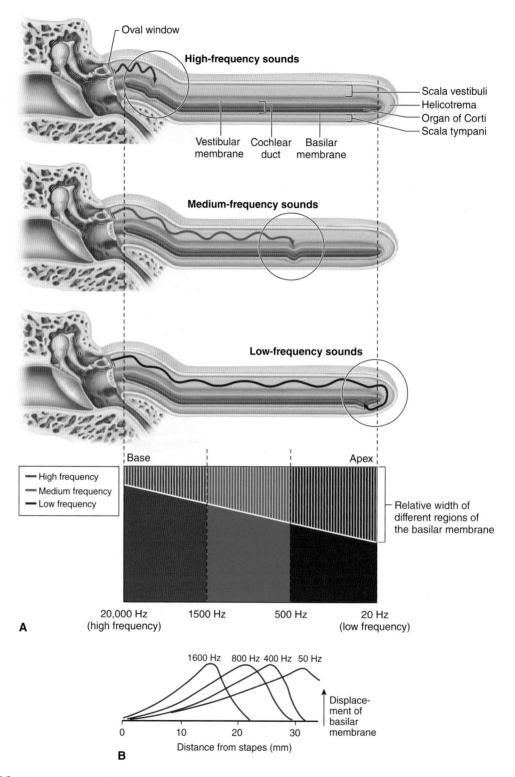

FIGURE 13–10 Illustration of sound localization by frequency in the basilar membrane (**A**) and amplitude distribution along the basilar membrane for sounds of 4 different frequencies (**B**). High-frequency sounds produce maximal displacement of the basilar membrane at the oval window entrance and little displacement elsewhere. Low-frequency sounds produce a maximal displacement at the end of the cochlea (the helicotrema). Note that high-frequency sounds are more localized in their displacement. (Part A, reproduced with permission from McKinley MP, O'Loughlin VD, Bidle TS. *Anatomy and Physiology: An Integrative Approach.* New York, NY: McGraw Hill; 2013; part B, reproduced with permission from Barrett KE, Barman SM, Brooks HL et al: *Ganong's Review of Medical Physiology,* 26th ed. New York, NY: McGraw Hill; 2019.)

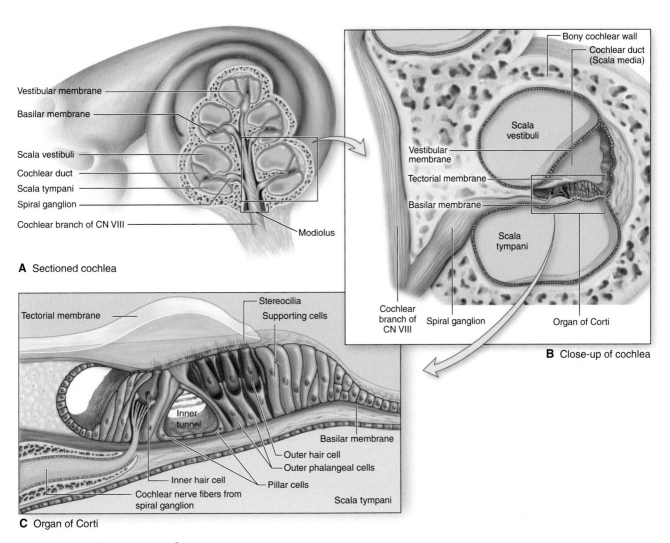

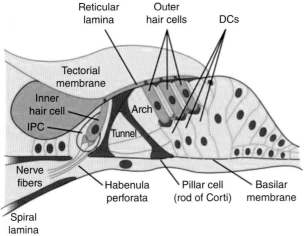

FIGURE 13–11 Detailed structure of the organ of Corti in the cochlea. **A.** A section through the entire cochlea and surrounding structures. **B.** An expanded view of a single cochlear coil with the 3 cavities: the scala vestibuli, scala tympani, and scala media (cochlear duct). Below the scala media is the organ of Corti, shown in more detail in **C** with associated neural structures including the inner and outer hair cells and cochlear branch of cranial nerve VIII. **D.** A photomicrograph of a section through the organ of Corti. (Parts A, B, and C, reproduced with permission from McKinley MP, O'Loughlin VD, Bidle TS. *Anatomy and Physiology: An Integrative Approach.* New York, NY: McGraw Hill; 2013; part D, reproduced with permission from Pickels JO: *An Introduction to the Physiology of Hearing,* 2nd ed. Philadelphia, PA: Academic Press; 1988.)

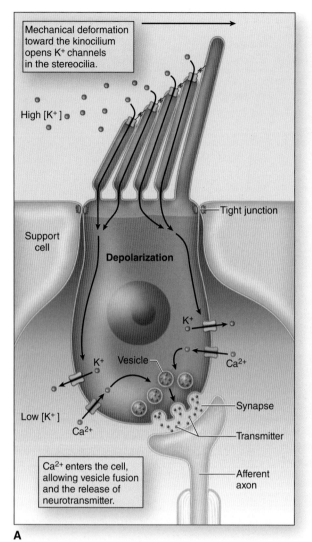

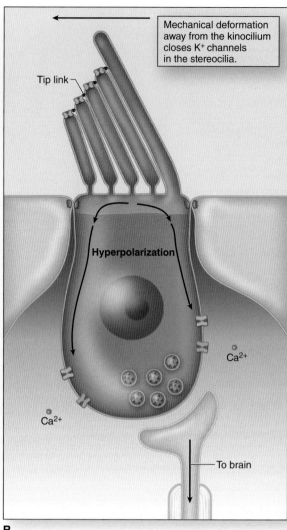

FIGURE 13–12 Auditory hair cells with their stereocilia that transduce sound into action potentials in the cochlear nerve. Bending of the cilia by sound waves opens potassium ion channels at the ends of the cilia, which depolarizes the cell body and brings about the release of glutamate, which in turn causes an action potential in the cochlear nerve. (Reproduced with permission from Mescher AL. *Junqueira's Basic Histology: Text & Atlas,* 15th ed. New York, NY: McGraw Hill; 2018.)

with 1 "conventional" axonal segment projecting centrally and another projecting peripherally at whose tip mechanotransduction produces action potentials that travel retrogradely toward the soma and beyond it to the spinal cord. The distal end of the spiral ganglion cell at the base of the auditory hair cell has receptors for the neurotransmitter (probably glutamate) released by the auditory hair cell base that has performed the mechanical transduction via its stereocilia.

Spiral ganglion cell distal processes make 2 different types of connections with auditory hair cells, called type I and type II, illustrated in Figure 13–13. Type I hair cells receive an enveloping spiral ganglion afferent nerve terminal (nerve calyx), which itself has a connection to an efferent nerve terminal. Type II hair cells receive an afferent axon-like nerve terminal from a spiral ganglion cell with an adjacent efferent nerve terminal on the hair cell itself. The efferent nerve terminals are

from the lateral olivocochlear region of the brainstem. Details of the stereocilia and their mechanical linkage are shown in Figure 13–13B.

Auditory Nerve Representation

There are approximately 30,000 spiral ganglion cells contacting approximately 3500 inner and 12,000 outer hair cells. The auditory nerve is composed of these 30,000 spiral ganglion cell axons whose inputs come mostly from inner hair cells. This nerve also contains axons from the vestibular system. Axons from the spiral ganglia project to the cochlear nucleus, located in the dorsolateral brainstem at the border between the pons and medulla. Individual auditory nerve fibers are sensitive to particular frequency ranges, especially for higher frequencies, reflecting the frequency map of their position in the basilar membrane.

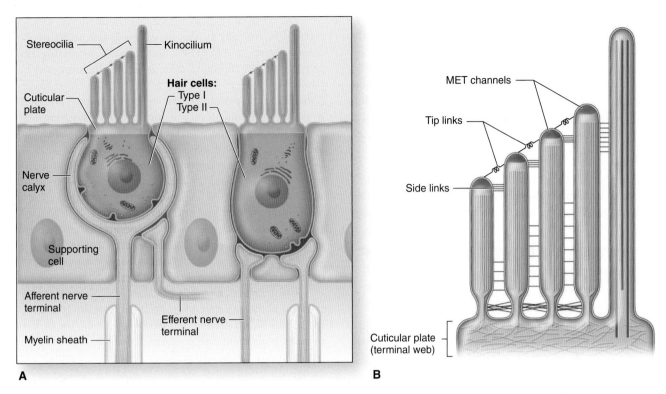

FIGURE 13–13 Structural differences between type I and type II auditory hair cells (left) and details of the structure of the stereocilia (right). (Reproduced with permission from Mescher AL. *Junqueira's Basic Histology: Text & Atlas*, 15th ed. New York, NY: McGraw Hill; 2018.)

Conduction Versus Neural Hearing Loss

Hearing loss is called conductive when sound is not mechanically transmitted from the eardrum to the cochlea, usually due to damage to the eardrum itself or the middle ear bones. The eardrum can be damaged by diving into deep water or by sharp objects entering the auditory canal. Inner ear infections that literally erode the middle ear bones are a common cause of conductive hearing loss. Infections that reach the middle ear sometimes cause otosclerosis, or remodeling of the middle bones that reduces their ability to transmit sound from the eardrum to the cochlea. German measles (rubella) contracted during pregnancy can be passed to the fetus, in many cases causing the infant to be born deaf.

Neural hearing loss is due to neural damage, usually loss of auditory hair cells in the cochlea. This can occur from exposure to loud noise and commonly occurs in aging at the high-frequency end of the sound spectrum. At higher levels in the auditory system along the projection to auditory cortex, tumors or strokes can damage cells.

Hearing loss also occurs during aging (called presbycusis), much of which is associated with exposure to loud environmental sound. The frequency range for young people ranges from 20 to 20,000 Hz, but the elderly are relatively insensitive to sounds above approximately 15,000 Hz. Continuous exposure to moderately loud sounds or single exposures to very loud sounds can damage hearing. Male hearing loss with aging tends to be worse than that for females because of exposure to high-level workplace sound, such as in manufacturing.

Hearing aids are external audio amplifiers that compensate for the mechanical signal attenuation caused by conductive hearing loss. They can also compensate for low to moderate neural loss of cochlear hair cells. Because hearing loss usually is much higher for some frequencies than others (typically high frequencies), hearing aids must be customized to selectively amplify the attenuated frequencies without overwhelming the user with high-volume amplification of frequencies the person can still hear.

Cochlear Implants

If large-scale hair cell loss is present, external hearing aids are ineffective. The current best solution for this situation is the cochlear implant, which consists of approximately 30 electrodes on a flexible polymer tube threaded into the cochlea. These electrodes are driven by an external microphone and electronics to electrically stimulate the cochlear nerve fibers. Over 100,000 cochlear implants have been implanted worldwide. Many users with these devices have experienced considerable hearing restoration. Damage at higher levels in the auditory pathway cannot be treated with cochlear implants. Current research focuses on using microelectrode arrays implanted in nuclei along the auditory pathway past the side of damage.

Ringing & Tinnitus

Tinnitus is the perception of ringing in the ears in the absence of actual sound. It may arise from exposure to loud noises, ear infections, and allergies. However, in many cases, its cause is unknown. Tinnitus is divided into objective and subjective types. Objective tinnitus is often associated with movement spasms within the cochlea that actually produce sound, which can be detected by diagnostic instruments. Subjective tinnitus can result from known and unknown causes and is difficult to treat. It is often associated with some hearing loss and can occur and improve on its own over a period of months or years. One treatment involves the use of noise-producing earphones that mask the ringing sound. Extreme cases of tinnitus can be debilitating and have been associated with suicide. In some of these cases, surgical destruction of the auditory nerve has been done to produce relief, but this also causes loss of normal hearing.

AUDITORY PROJECTIONS TO THE BRAINSTEM

The Cochlear Nucleus

The spiral ganglion axons and those from the semicircular canals of the vestibular system project via cranial nerve VIII (vestibulocochlear nerve) to the ipsilateral cochlear nucleus (Figure 13–14). This nerve passes through the skull via the internal acoustic (auditory) meatus in the temporal bone. The cochlear nucleus has distinct dorsal and ventral nuclei, shown in Figure 13–15. The ventrolateral dorsal cochlear nucleus and anteroventral ventral cochlear nucleus receive axons from lower frequency sensitive auditory fibers that synapse on auditory hair cells distant from the oval window, whereas the dorsomedial portion of the dorsal cochlear nucleus and dorsal ventral cochlear nucleus receive inputs from high-frequency fibers originating near the oval window. This tonotopic organization of the cochlear nucleus is maintained in higher projection areas all the way to the primary auditory cortex in the superior temporal lobe.

The cochlear nucleus projects both ipsilateraly and contralaterally rostrally to the superior olivary nuclei on both sides (Figure 13–14). The contralaterally projecting fibers cross by passing through a structure called the trapezoid body (shown in Figures 13–14 and 13–15). The ascending fibers on both sides then project via the lateral lemniscus on each side to the inferior colliculus, a major auditory processing center. A cochlear projection called the dorsal acoustic stria ascends to nuclei of the lateral lemniscus.

Cochlear axons convey frequency and amplitude information explicitly and sound localization implicitly in their firing, because there is no explicit representation of sound location in the cochlea. Auditory neurons tend to fire at the peak of sound pressure waves. Sound amplitude is encoded by the number of spikes that are generated at each peak and the number of fibers that fire (fibers sensitive to particular frequencies have somewhat different thresholds).

The inferior colliculi and all later projection areas receive bilateral auditory input from both ears, which is important for sound localization. The inferior colliculus on each side projects ipsilaterally to the medial geniculate in the thalamus, which in turn projects to auditory cortex in the middle of the superior temporal lobe (superior temporal gyrus).

The Superior Olive, Lateral Lemniscus, & Directional Localization

There is no explicit representation of sound location in the cochlea, but rather a tonotopic or frequency representation along the basilar membrane. The superior olive is an important structure for sound localization in azimuth (horizontally) because it receives inputs from both cochlear nuclei that can be used to compute azimuth via interaural time difference and interaural intensity difference. Time difference computations are thought to be computed in the medial

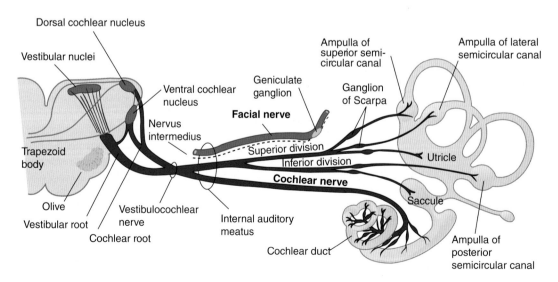

FIGURE 13–14 Axons of the spiral ganglion cells of the cochlea project via cranial nerve VIII (vestibulocochlear nerve) with those from the semicircular canals of the vestibular system to the ipsilateral dorsal and ventral cochlear nuclei. This nerve passes through the skull via the internal acoustic (auditory) meatus in the temporal bone. (Reproduced with permission from Waxman SG. *Clinical Neuroanatomy,* 28th ed. New York, NY: McGraw Hill; 2017.)

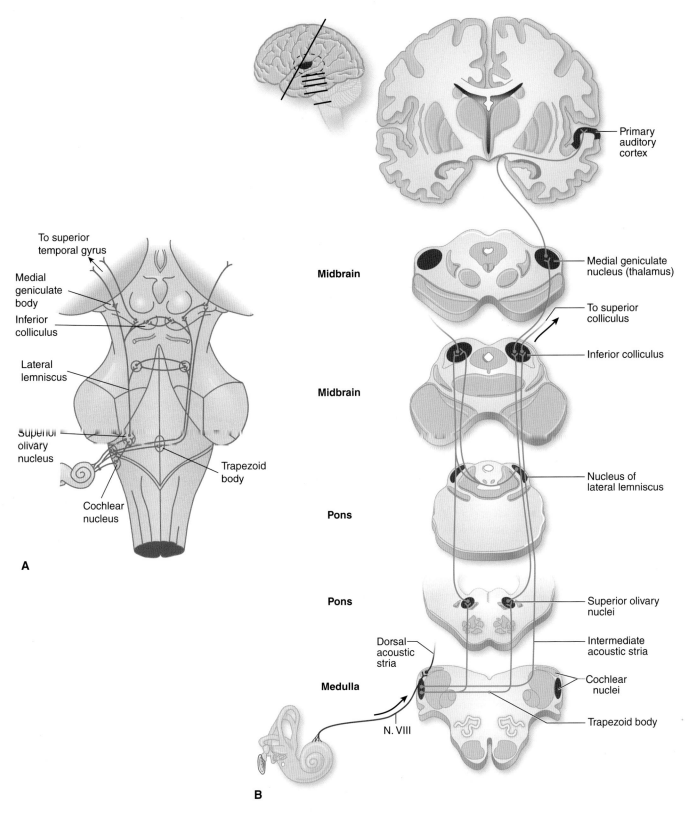

FIGURE 13–15 **A.** Details of cochlear projections to the brainstem. Ipsilateral cochlear axons project to the ipsilateral superior olive in the brainstem. The olive projects via the lateral lemniscus to the nucleus of the lateral lemniscus and inferior colliculus. The inferior colliculus projects to the medial geniculate nucleus. Some cochlear nerve fibers also project contralaterally by relaying through a structure called the trapezoid body before projecting to higher centers. **B.** Cochlear projections to the brainstem, thalamus, and cortex. (Part A, reproduced with permission from Waxman SG. *Clinical Neuroanatomy*, 28th ed. New York, NY: McGraw Hill; 2017.)

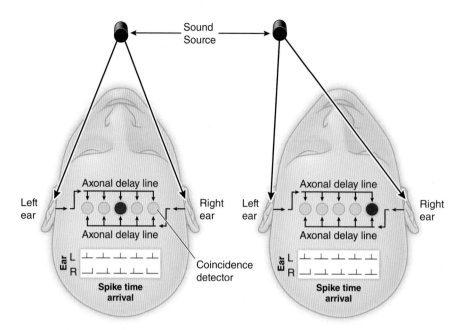

FIGURE 13–16 Neural delay line mechanism for interaural time difference localization. L, left; R, right.

superior olive, whereas intensity difference is registered in the lateral superior olive.

The method by which the brain accomplishes interaural time difference discrimination for azimuth sound localization is shown schematically in Figure 13–16. Neural coincidence detectors are arrayed along axonal delay lines carrying spikes from the left and right ears. For a sound source directly ahead, spikes will reach only the middle coincidence detector at the same time. Sounds located to the left or right of this middle position will arrive synchronously at different coincidence detectors.

The time sensitivity of this system is extraordinary. A "back of the envelope calculation" using the speed of sound as 1000 ft/s and the distance between the ears as 6 in (0.5 ft) yields a maximum delay for a sound source directly to the left or right of 0.5 milliseconds, or 500 microseconds. Because the neural action potentials last about 1 millisecond, this means that the interaural time difference neural system can discriminate arrival time differences much less than the width of 1 action potential. The basis for this capability is the phase locking of auditory nerve firing in each ear to the exact peak of the sound wave. Interaural time difference works best for low frequencies where phase differences yield the largest absolute time differences and where shadowing by the head does not reduce the amplitude as much in 1 ear compared to the other. The neural structure and mechanism for interaural time difference sound localization have been demonstrated in the barn owl, a bird that can locate and strike prey in complete darkness using this type of mechanism. In humans, similar circuits exist in the superior olive and may be the reason why the cochlear nucleus projects both ipsilaterally and contralaterally close to the initial sound transduction.

The other mechanism for azimuth sound localization is interaural intensity difference. Sound amplitude will be greater on the side of the head closer to the sound source because of shadowing by the skull. This effect is greater for higher than lower frequencies. Different neuronal types in the lateral superior olive are sensitive to the sum of excitation (EE) from the 2 ears or the difference between the firing from each ear (EI). Dividing the EI output by the EE output (neurally) will give a normalized representation of the distance from the middle position.

Localizing elevation is more complicated because the 2 ears are in the horizontal plane and no difference in arrival time or intensity occurs at the ears because of pure elevation changes. However, one of the functions of the complex shape of the pinna or external ear (see Figure 13–6) is that it alters the frequency spectrum of complex sounds reflected into the auditory canal as a function of elevation. Specifically, the middle-frequency spectrum of complex sounds reflected by the pinna into the auditory canal is attenuated for sources at high elevations compared to middle or low elevations. During development, the nervous system "learns" the change in transfer function for familiar complex sounds generated by the pinna, which permits localization in elevation. However, the precision of this elevation localization is poorer than for azimuth.

The Inferior Colliculus

Neurons in the medial superior olive and lateral superior olive project to the inferior colliculus in the midbrain. The inferior colliculus consists of a central nucleus surrounded by a dorsal cortex and a lateral external cortex. Elevation- and azimuth-detecting cells in the superior olive converge on colliculus neurons that thus represent location in both horizontal and vertical angles. The inferior colliculus receives reciprocal innervation from the medial geniculate nucleus of the thalamus to which it projects, as well as the auditory cortex. It also receives input from the somatosensory system. The colliculus is thus an integration center for spatial location and reflexive orientation for auditory inputs in the startle reflex.

The Medial Geniculate Nucleus of the Thalamus

The inferior colliculus projects to the medial geniculate nucleus of the thalamus above it in the midbrain (see Figure 13–15). As for vision, somatosensation, and taste, auditory information is relayed through a sensory modality–specific thalamic nucleus that, in turn, projects to a specific "primary" cortical area for that sense. The medial geniculate nucleus consists of 3 main subdivisions: ventral, dorsal, and medial. The ventral nucleus of the medial geniculate contains a tonotopic map with low frequencies being lateral and high frequencies being medial. Neurons in the ventral nucleus represent amplitude and binaural localization information as well as frequency. The dorsal nucleus contains cells that respond to complex environmental stimuli as well as somatosensory input. Neurons in the medial nucleus receive input from intensity and duration coding cells that appear to be part of the azimuth localization pathway.

High Order Auditory Processing

Neurons in the medial geniculate nucleus project to primary auditory cortex in the mid-posterior superior sulcus of the temporal lobe. The primary auditory cortex includes the Heschl gyrus and extends into the lateral fissure of the temporal lobe, including the planum temporale and planum polare. In the Brodmann map of cortex, the auditory cortex comprises areas 41 and 42 and part of area 22. Neurons projecting to the primary auditory cortex explicitly encode frequency, intensity, and some aspects of sound location. The auditory cortex refines discrimination in these dimensions and enables more complex sound identification.

Primary Auditory Cortex

The predominant organization of the primary auditory cortex is a tonotopic map. This map represents the preservation of the initial auditory transduction by the place code of spiral ganglion cell axons along the basilar membrane from oval window to helicotrema. In the auditory cortex, low frequencies are represented anteriorly and high frequencies posteriorly. However, there are multiple maps in the auditory cortex besides frequency, including binaurality (related to localization), intensity, and latency.

Auditory Association Cortex

Neurons in the primary auditory cortex project to other cortical areas for higher order sound processing. Figure 13–17 shows higher order or "association" areas of the auditory

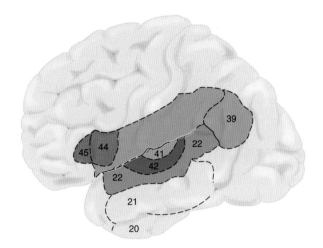

FIGURE 13–17 Cortical auditory areas. (Reproduced with permission from Ropper AH, Samuels MA, Klein JP: *Adams and Victor's Principles of Neurology*, 11th ed. New York, NY: McGraw Hill; 2019.)

cortex and also its projection to the Broca area (44 and part of 45) and other frontal lobe areas. Language and complex sounds are processed in the Wernicke area in the vicinity of Brodmann area 39.

Understanding Language

Language sits at the top of the hierarchy of sound processing and is unique to humans. Other animals can recognize and respond to complex sounds such as keys jangling or doors creaking, but only humans use a complex grammar for communication. Language reception and recognition involve all the early stages of sound processing from the cochlear to auditory primary and association cortical areas, but then extend into the Wernicke area at the junction of the temporal and parietal areas (Figure 13–18). This area projects to the frontal lobe via a tract called the arcuate fasciculus to the Broca area, which is just anterior to the primary motor areas for the larynx, pharynx, and other vocalization apparatus of the mouth, tongue, and lips.

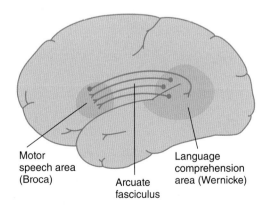

FIGURE 13–18 Major language areas of the cortex. (Reproduced with permission from Waxman SG. *Clinical Neuroanatomy*, 28th ed. New York, NY: McGraw Hill; 2017.)

Language processing is also unique in its extreme lateralization. Virtually all right-handers and a majority of left-handers process language primarily in the left temporal lobe and show major deficits from brain damage only on the left side. Language output, or speech, is also controlled by the Broca area on the left side.

THE VESTIBULAR SYSTEM

The vestibular system is responsible for informing us about our orientation in space and acceleration through space and for maintaining balance. The initial sensory transduction in the vestibular system originates close to the cochlea and shares many similarities with it. The transduction mechanisms of the vestibular system for rotation are composed of the semicircular canals (see Figure 13–9). Linear accelerations are transduced by otoliths. The output of the vestibular system is via cranial nerve VIII (see Figure 13–14).

The Vestibular Labyrinth

The cochlea, semicircular canals, and otoliths compose what is called the vestibulum of the labyrinth of the inner ear. Some details of these structures are illustrated in **Figure 13–19**.

Otolith Organs: Utricle & Saccule

The otolith consists of 2 suborgans called the utricle and saccule, which are oriented at 90 degrees to each other, illustrated in Figure 13–19. The receptors in both of these organs are called maculae, which consist of cilia on whose tips are calcium crystals called otoconia. The individual cilia within each otolith are oriented in multiple directions so that there will be an output from either organ or both organs for acceleration in any direction for any head position. The otoliths sense linear forces.

The Semicircular Canals

There are 3 semicircular canals oriented at right angles to each other. These structures, via their cilia, sense head tilt and rotary accelerations. The output of the semicircular canals

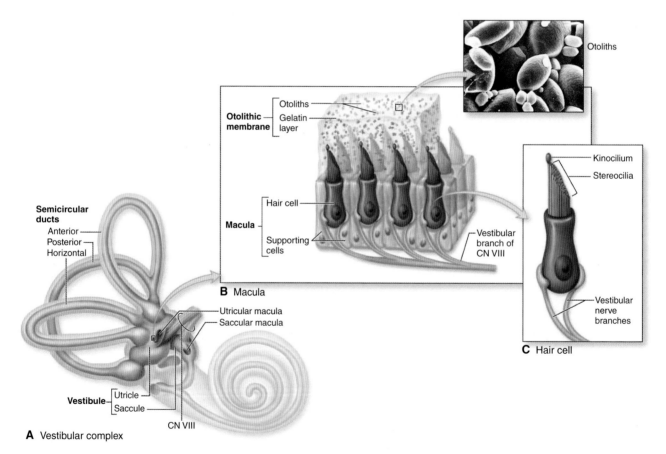

FIGURE 13–19 **A.** Two sensory areas called maculae occur in the membranous labyrinth of the vestibular utricle and saccule, both specialized for detecting gravity and endolymph movements. **B.** A more detailed diagram of a macular wall shows that it is composed of hair cells, supporting cells, and endings of the vestibular branch of the eighth cranial nerve. The apical surface of the hair cells is covered by a gelatinous otolithic layer or membrane, and the basal ends of the cells have synaptic connections with the nerve fibers. Scanning electron microscopy shows otoliths embedded in this membrane. These mineralized structures make the otolithic membrane heavier than endolymph alone, which facilitates bending of the kinocilia and stereocilia by gravity or movement of the head. **C.** Detailed structure of auditory hair cell showing kinocilium, sterocilia, and contacts with vestibular nerve endings. (Reproduced with permission from McKinley MP, O'Loughlin VD, Bidle TS. *Anatomy and Physiology: An Integrative Approach.* New York, NY: McGraw Hill; 2013.)

is combined in the brainstem with visual information about movement to yield information about movement and rotation in space. This information is used to program compensatory eye movements, such as the vestibulo-ocular reflex, and to control postural compensation for balance.

Vestibular Hair Cells

The transduction mechanisms of the vestibular system are based on hair cells similar to those in the cochlea for both the otolith and semicircular canals.

Vestibular Pathways to Thalamus & Cortex

The output of the vestibular system is via cranial nerve VIII (see Figure 13–14) through the internal auditory meatus with the cochlear nerve, which enters the brainstem at the border between the medulla and pons. The axons project to 4 vestibular nuclei and the cerebellum (via the inferior cerebellar peduncle). The outputs of the vestibular nuclei project via the medial longitudinal fasciculus to several oculomotor nuclei to control eye movements, as well as to the cerebellum.

Balance Problems

Vestibular system dysfunction can lead to balance problems. Infections of the inner ear can cause labyrinthitis, leading to dizziness and balance difficulties. Ménière disease, which is associated with dysregulation of fluid volume in the vestibular system, exhibits symptoms such as dizziness and vertigo. The vestibular nerve itself can become inflamed from viral infections, leading to vestibular neuronities and vertigo. Less severe vestibular problems include benign paroxysmal positional vertigo, which occurs transiently with any rapid change in head position.

SUMMARY

- Sound consists of air vibrations that have the properties of frequency and amplitude.
- Sound is mechanically modified and transduced in the outer and middle ear.
- Sound frequency and amplitude are converted into neural codes in the cochlea.
- The cochlea is tonotopically organized with auditory hair cells transducing sound to neural firing.
- Brainstem nuclei process auditory information and begin coding for location.
- The auditory thalamus relays auditory information to the primary auditory cortex in the temporal lobe.
- Primary and higher order auditory areas in the temporal and parietal lobes further process auditory information.
- The vestibular system originates with the transduction of self-motion by 3 semicircular canals used for balance and spatial orientation.

SELF-ASSESSMENT QUESTIONS

1. A patient complains of hearing loss, and a test reveals the following results. A vibrating tuning fork is placed along the midline of the top of the head, and sound is localized toward the left ear. Then, a tuning fork is placed around the mastoid process of the skull, and the tuning fork is held in the air next to each of the ears at separate times. The sound is perceived as being louder when placed near the right ear. It is concluded that the patient suffers from which of the following?
   A. Conduction loss involving the left middle ear
   B. Conduction loss involving the right middle ear
   C. Sensorineural deficits most likely involving the left cochlear nerve
   D. Sensorineural deficits most likely involving the right cochlear nerve
   E. Tumor proximal to the cerebellar vermis

2. A woman visits her physician after experiencing attacks of vertigo, some hearing loss, nausea, vomiting, fullness of pressure in 1 ear, and tinnitus. Tests of cerebellar function are normal. This constellation of symptoms can best be accounted for by the presence of a lesion in which of the following regions?
   A. Cochlea
   B. Vestibular labyrinth
   C. Middle ear
   D. Dorsolateral medulla
   E. Medial longitudinal fasciculus

3. After a viral infection, a patient complains about difficulty in being able to detect tones. An audiology examination further confirms this deficit, indicating that the patient is unable to discriminate among different tones. Damage to which of the following structures by the viral infection would account for the loss of this patient's ability to discriminate tones?
   A. Basilar membrane
   B. Tympanic membrane
   C. Otolithic membrane
   D. Superior olivary nucleus
   E. Middle temporal gyrus

4. An elderly male school teacher complains that his students were pranking him by alerting each other to phone text messages via a high-frequency beep that they could hear but he could not. This selective high-frequency loss in an elderly man is indicative of what?
   A. Onset of Parkinson disease
   B. Onset of Huntington disease
   C. Conduction deafness
   D. Common age-related presbycusis
   E. Herpes infection of the temporal lobe

5. Auditory hair cells in the cochlea contact which neurons to relay their information to the brain?
   A. Superior olivary cells
   B. Inferior colliculus cells
   C. Medial geniculate cells
   D. Medullary pyramidal cells
   E. Spiral ganglion cells

Chemical Senses: Olfactory & Gustatory Systems

Franklin R. Amthor

- Outline the transduction of molecules received by olfactory receptors into signals sent to the olfactory bulb.
- Diagram the olfactory bulb and indicate its organization.
- Describe the olfactory projection system involving direct and indirect routes to cortex.
- Describe the major taste dimensions and their transduction mechanisms.
- Diagram the taste projection pathway cortex.

OVERVIEW

Smell and taste are called chemical senses because molecules activate the receptors in these systems rather than energy, such as photons in vision and vibrations in hearing. Smell and taste have important gateway functions in approach/withdrawal behaviors. The smell given off by a ripe pineapple induces us to consider eating it, and the ripe, sweet taste prompts consumption of the fruit. However, we are repulsed by the smells and tastes of many bitter and sour substances. Those chemical qualities are often (but not always) associated with spoilage or toxicity. Taste receptors, found mostly on the tongue, exist for sweet, sour, salt, bitter, and, according to some researchers, umami, the savory taste induced by the additive monosodium glutamate (MSG). Taste is also strongly influenced by smell because mastication of food also activates olfactory receptors in the nose. The combination of smell and taste gives rise to the complex perception of flavor. The message encoded by receptors for taste relays through several subcortical structures before reaching the thalamus and then the cortex. Olfaction is the exception among the senses in that neurons in the olfactory bulb project directly to cortex in a pathway whose activation is largely subconscious. However, there is an olfactory projection from cortex back to the thalamus, and then back to cortex. This projection reaches, among other loci, the orbitofrontal cortex, where smell and taste inputs are combined to mediate complex olfactory perceptions such as flavor.

ORGANIZATION OF THE OLFACTORY SYSTEM

The nose has a number of functions besides smell, such as filtering, warming, and humidifying the air you breathe. However, here we concentrate on its function of detecting odorants and reporting their characteristics to the brain. Olfactory receptors exist in the roof of the nose. Figure 14–1 shows the overall internal structure of the nose.

The Nose & Olfactory Epithelium

Internally the nose is divided in the middle by a cartilaginous structure called the septum. On each side of the septum are 3 cavities called "turbinates," shown in Figure 14–1. Within the superior turbinate at the top rear of the nose's internal chamber is the olfactory mucosa located on its lateral wall. This is where the olfactory cilia sit that transduce odorants into neural signals. These cilia are extensions of the olfactory receptor cells, which are located below the lamina propria, which is below a bone called the cribriform plate, as shown in Figure 14–2.

One basis for the difference in odor sensitivity between animals such as humans and dogs is the vastly different number of olfactory receptors in various species. There are approximately 5 to 10 million olfactory receptor neurons in humans versus approximately a billion in dogs.

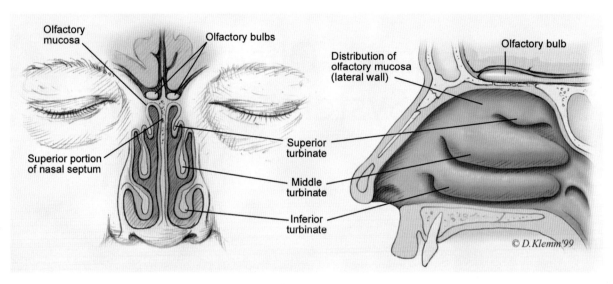

FIGURE 14–1　General structures of the nasal cavities and olfactory mucosa. On the left is a frontal cutaway view of the main nasal chambers (turbinates). The olfactory mucosa is in the uppermost turbinate just inferior to the olfactory bulb. On the right is a side view of the same structures. (Used with permission from David Klemm, Faculty and Curriculum Support, Georgetown University Medical Center, Washington, DC.)

Olfactory Receptors

Olfactory cells extend approximately 5 to 10 processes called cilia into the mucous layer where odor molecules entering the nose are entrapped. Olfactory receptors reside on these cilia. In this regard, they resemble receptors for other senses such as sight and hearing. The photoreceptor outer segments that contain the photon-absorbing pigment also are derived from cilia. Auditory hair cells in the organ of Corti are also modified cilia. Olfactory receptors are like G-protein–coupled metabotropic receptors for neurotransmitters, except that they are activated by a molecule from the external world rather than a neurotransmitter released from another neuron. Although

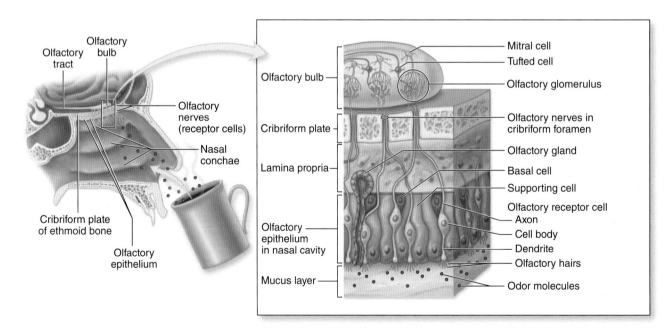

FIGURE 14–2　Detailed views of the olfactory mucosa, cribriform plate, and olfactory bulb. On the left is a side view of the olfactory mucosa and cribriform plate above. On the right is a more detailed view of the mucosa, cribriform plate, and olfactory bulb showing several of the main neural types. (Reproduced with permission from McKinley MP, O'Loughlin VD, Bidle TS. *Anatomy and Physiology: An Integrative Approach.* New York, NY: McGraw Hill; 2013.)

there are approximately 1000 distinct olfactory receptor types (and corresponding genes that code for them), a single olfactory receptor cell expresses only 1 of these receptor types. With 5 to 10 million olfactory receptor cells, this means that there are approximately 5000 to 10,000 different receptor cells of each receptor type.

The Transduction of Olfactory Signals

Figure 14-3 shows how the process of smell works. An odorant molecule that has crossed the mucosa binds a receptor recognition site on the olfactory receptor, which is located on one of the olfactory receptor neuron's cilia. The receptor, like

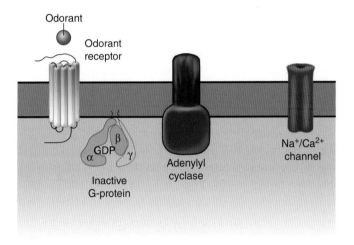

A

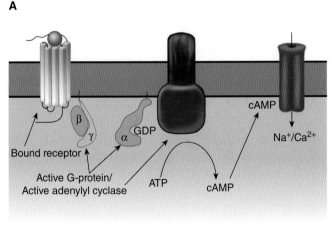

B

FIGURE 14-3 Signal transduction in olfactory receptors. Olfactory receptors use a G-protein–adenyl cyclase cyclic adenosine monophosphate (cAMP) system with 3 G-protein subunits. The top figure shows the state of the receptor and adenylyl cyclase system prior to odorant binding. Below, after odorant binding to the receptor, the alpha G-protein subunit is released. This subunit activates adenylyl cyclase to convert adenosine triphosphate (ATP) to cAMP, which acts as a second messenger that opens cation channels permeable to Na^+ and Ca^{2+}, depolarizing the cell. GDP, guanosine diphosphate. (Reproduced with permission from Barrett KE, Barman SM, Brooks HL et al: *Ganong's Review of Medical Physiology*, 26th ed. New York, NY: McGraw Hill; 2019.)

other G-protein–coupled receptors, is a 7-membrane domain spanning molecule. On the external side of the membrane is the recognition site for a specific odorant, whereas on the internal side, the molecule is associated with a G-protein complex. This G-protein complex is in an inactive state when no odorant is bound to the external portion of the receptor. Upon binding an odorant, however, the receptor structure undergoes a conformational change that activates the G-protein complex by causing the subunits to dissociate. The free alpha G-protein subunit binds to and activates adenylyl cyclase, catalyzing the conversion of adenosine triphosphate to cyclic adenosine monophosphate (cAMP). Finally, the cAMP binds to a site on the internal side of Na^+/Ca^{2+} cation channels that open.

Olfactory receptors constantly turn over, living only a few months. This is the longest known case of adult neurogenesis. In the past, some researchers have attempted to repopulate other brain areas that have experienced cell death with olfactory receptor cells hoping they would multiply and integrate into damaged neural circuits in a manner similar to the use of neural stem cells more recently. Within the past few decades, adult neurogenesis has also been shown in the hippocampus.

The Olfactory Bulb & Olfactory Coding

The odorant-induced cation flux in the olfactory cilia depolarizes the olfactory receptor, generating action potentials that travel down the receptor axons through the cribriform plate to the olfactory bulb. This axon tract is cranial nerve I. The axon terminals of these cells contact the dendrites of mitral and tufted cells, releasing of the excitatory neurotransmitter glutamate. The olfactory receptor axon terminals cluster in several thousand distinct structures called glomeruli, each of which receives input primarily from olfactory receptors of a given odorant receptor type. Glomeruli having similar receptor type inputs tend to be close together, so their organization forms a multidimensional spatial map of odor properties. Dimensions of this map are thought to include properties such as molecular carbon chain length and functional group similarity. Figure 14–4 shows the basic projection scheme from olfactory receptors to the olfactory bulb. In addition to the direct feedforward connections from olfactory receptor cells to mitral and tufted cells, there are also lateral inhibition neurons such as granule cells that mediate mutual inhibition between mitral and tufted cells by releasing γ-aminobutyric acid (GABA). Glomeruli inhibit each other via interneurons called periglomerular cells.

Mitral and granule cells contact each other via dendrodendritic synapses, with the mitral cell dendrites releasing glutamate to the granule cells, and the granule cells releasing GABA onto the dendrites of mitral cells. The net result of this is a feedback inhibition for the mitral cells mediated via their connections to granule cells, as well as mutual inhibition between mitral cells.

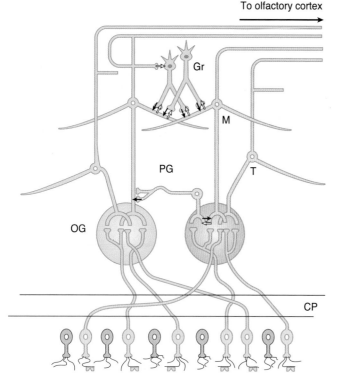

FIGURE 14–4 The projection system from the olfactory receptors to the olfactory bulb and thence to the olfactory cortex. There are several thousand distinct types of olfactory receptor cells, each of which responds to a specific set of odorants. Although receptors of each odorant recognition type are scattered across the olfactory mucosa, each type projects primarily to 1 specific olfactory glomerulus (OG). The axons of tufted (T) and mitral cells (M) whose dendrites are in the glomeruli project to olfactory cortex. The feedforward excitatory pathway from olfactory receptors to glomeruli to cortex is mediated by the neurotransmitter glutamate at each synapse. GABA-mediated lateral inhibitory interactions between glomeruli are mediated by granule cells (Gr) and periglomerular cells (PG). (Adapted with permission from Mori K, Nagao H, Yoshihara Y: The olfactory bulb: coding and processing of odor molecule information, *Science*. 1999 Oct 22;286(5440):711-715.)

The Vomeronasal Organ & Pheromones

Many mammals, including humans, have another distinct olfactory organ toward the front of the septum within the nose called the vomeronasal organ. Olfactory receptors in this organ are involved in the detection of intraspecies communication odors called pheromones. Although pheromones are best known in insects for functions such as trail marking, they also exist in mammals as mediators of social and sexual communication and behavioral triggering. Their detection is usually unconscious, mediating behavioral changes such as menstrual synchrony in women. Vomeronasal receptors project to a structure distinct from the olfactory bulb called the accessory olfactory bulb, which in turn projects to the amygdala and hypothalamus.

CENTRAL PROJECTIONS OF THE OLFACTORY BULB

Direct Projections

The olfactory system is the exception among the major senses in projecting directly to the cortex without a relay in the thalamus (although there is a thalamic circuit in the olfactory system). Specifically, the olfactory bulb projects directly to the pyriform cortex in the frontal lobe and the entorhinal cortex outside the hippocampus (Figure 14–5). Both of these cortical areas are ancient mesocortex, rather than neocortex. Details of the olfactory bulb projections can be seen in Figure 14–6, which shows that the olfactory bulbs on each side of the nose project to each other via the anterior commissure (just anterior to the corpus callosum) and the important direct projections to the amygdala and anterior olfactory nucleus.

(Figure 14–7) shows the overall projection scheme for the olfactory bulb. Of particular note is that several cortical and subcortical structures project olfactory information to the thalamus, which in turn projects to the orbitofrontal cortex. Activity in the orbitofrontal cortex underlies our conscious

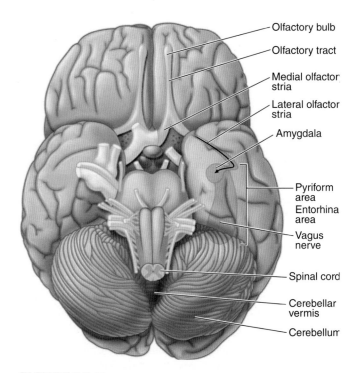

FIGURE 14–5 Ventral view diagram of the main brain areas mediating olfaction. The pyriform and entorhinal cortical areas are medial to the amygdala. (Reproduced with permission from Ropper AH, Samuels MA, Klein JP: *Adams and Victor's Principles of Neurology*, 11th ed. New York, NY: McGraw Hill; 2019.)

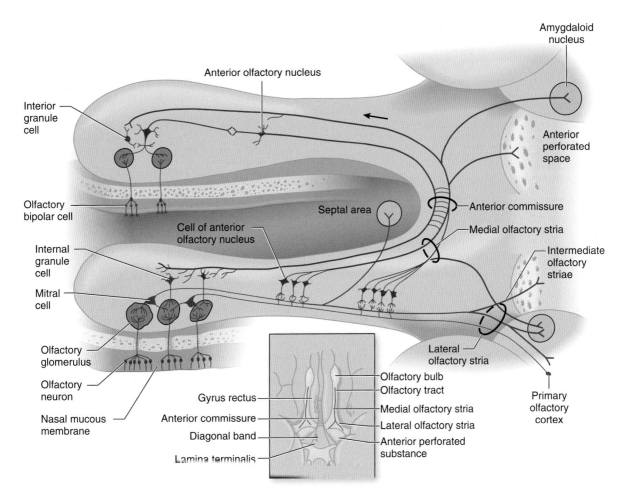

FIGURE 14–6 Overall organization of the projections from the olfactory mucosa to the bulb and then to the olfactory cortex. Olfactory bulb mitral output cells make synapses with anterior olfactory nuclei. Cells in these nuclei project centrally via medial, intermediate, and lateral olfactory stria. Olfactory bulb glomeruli, mitral cells, and neurons of the anterior olfactory nuclei project directly to the amygdala and septum. Note that there are projections between the 2 olfactory bulbs mediated by neurons of the anterior olfactory nuclei through the anterior commissure. (Reproduced with permission from Kandel ER, Schwartz JH, Jessell TM, et al: *Principles of Neural Science*, 5th ed. New York, NY: McGraw Hill; 2013.)

perception of odor. Activation of the hippocampus is important in forming episodic memories associated with odors, that is, memories associated with a particular event and its context. In addition, neurons in the orbitofrontal cortex that also receive input from the tongue mediate the combination of smell and taste often referred to as flavor.

Olfactory projections to the hippocampus via the entorhinal cortex mediate learning and memory functions associated with smell, whereas the projection to the amygdala adds emotional content to this learning and memory via the amygdala's projections to both the orbitofrontal cortex and the hippocampus. The amygdala is important in the learning process that associates positive valence with odors that have had positive consequences and negative valence with those that predict negative outcomes. It is particularly important in fear conditioning, for example, as might be the case for the smell of gunpowder for traumatized soldiers.

Projections to the Orbitofrontal Cortex & Olfactory Contributions to Taste

Taste is heavily dependent on smell. When food is masticated, molecules of the injected substance reach the nasal pharynx via what is called the retronasal route from the mouth, where they activate olfactory receptors in a manner similar to odorants. If the nose is pinched shut during chewing, many otherwise easily distinguishable foods are indistinguishable. A major brain locus for the combination of taste and smell is the orbitofrontal cortex, where multimodal neurons occur that have inputs from both the taste and olfactory systems. The sensory addition of olfaction to taste is often referred to as flavor.

The firing of neurons in the orbitofrontal cortex is also influenced by hunger and satiety. As food is consumed, hunger decreases. This phenomenon is called alliesthesia, and it is based on central nervous system mechanisms that receive inputs from receptors in the stomach. A faster acting satiety

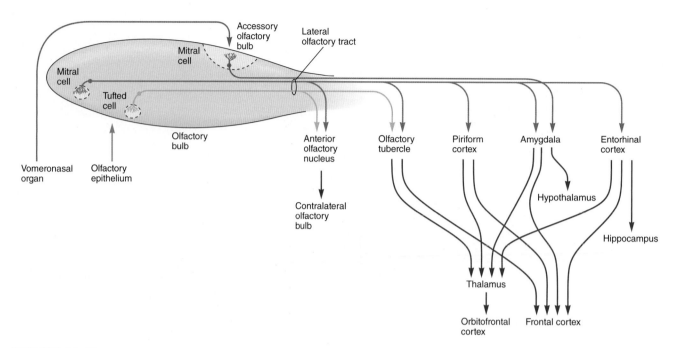

FIGURE 14–7 Summary diagram of the olfactory pathways. Mitral and tufted olfactory bulb neurons project via the lateral olfactory tract to the anterior olfactory nuclei and thence to the contralateral olfactory bulbs. The lateral olfactory tract also projects to the olfactory tubercle, pyriform cortex, amygdala, and entorhinal cortex. The pyriform cortex projects to the thalamus, which in turn projects to the orbitofrontal cortex. Thus, like other senses, there is a thalamocortex pathway in olfaction. The amygdala projects to the hypothalamus and frontal cortex, whereas the olfactory projection to the entorhinal cortex relays to the hippocampus. (Reproduced with permission from Jameson JL, Fauci AS, Kasper DL, et al: *Harrison's Principles of Internal Medicine*, 20th ed. New York, NY: McGraw Hill; 2018.)

mechanism is called sensory-specific satiety, which is specific to the food consumed and depends on receptors on the tongue and in the mouth.

Clinical Aspects of Smell

Smell loss can be caused by peripheral or central mechanisms. Chronic rhinosinusitis or other insults to the nasal cavity can kill olfactory receptor cells. Because the olfactory cortex is in the frontal lobe, frontal lobe dysfunctions can affect olfactory processing. Neurodegenerative diseases that impact the sense of smell include schizophrenia and Parkinson, Huntington, and Alzheimer disease. People with Down syndrome also have smell impairment.

TASTE

Humans are probably the most omnivorous vertebrates on the planet, eating almost anything that can be found that has nutritional potential. Our taste receptors, combined with the act of smelling what we masticate, give us sophisticated sensitivity to quickly discriminate nutritious from toxic substances we have ingested.

Classically, taste has been thought to be based on a set of 4 receptor types, namely, sweet, salt, bitter, and sour. However, there is general agreement now for a fifth basic taste, usually referred to as *umami* (from the Japanese meaning "pleasant and savory taste"), typified by the taste of MSG. The existence

of umami as a basic taste is based primarily on the existence of a receptor that responds very specifically to this class of taste substances, such as the amino acid L-glutamate.

Taste receptors are found primarily on the tongue, although a few reside on the roof of the mouth in the pharynx. Taste receptors reside in bump-like structures called papillae. Figures 14–8 and 14–9 show that there are 4 major types of papillae on the tongue: filiform, fungiform, foliate, and circumvallate (vallate). The filiform papillae, which are found across the dorsal tongue surface, particularly in the tongue's central region, do not contain taste buds, but the other types of papillae do. In some species, filiform papillae make the tongue rough and function mechanically to rasp ingested food.

Humans have several thousand papillae that contain taste cells, that is, taste buds. Each taste bud has >50 cells that include both taste receptor cells and supporting epithelial cells (Figure 14–10). Fungiform papillae tend to be found toward the front of the tongue, foliate on the side toward the rear, and circumvallate at the very rear across the dorsal surface. There are only approximately 10 circumvallate cells at the back of the tongue. Taste substances contact the taste receptor neurons through the taste pore. Within most taste buds are receptor cells for several tastes. There are receptors for all 5 basic tastes throughout the tongue, and these receptors occur in each of the 3 taste bud morphologies (fungiform, foliate, and circumvallate), although the front of the tongue is slightly more sensitive to sweet tastes and the back

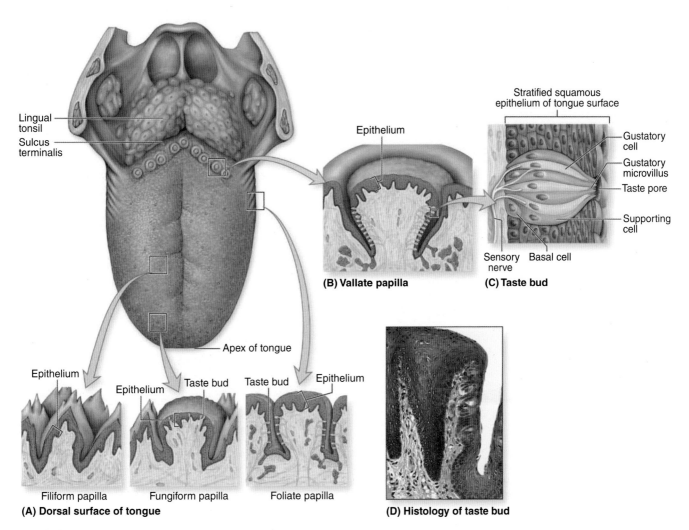

FIGURE 14–8 Location and structure of taste buds on the tongue. There are 4 major types of "bumps" or papillae on the tongue: filiform, fungiform, foliate, and vallate (circumvallate). The filiform papillae, which are found across the dorsal tongue surface, do not contain taste buds, but the other papillae do. Fungiform papillae tend to be found toward the front of the tongue, foliate on the side toward the rear, and vallate at the very rear across the dorsal surface. Cross-sections of filiform, fungiform, and foliate papillae are shown in **A** and vallate in **B**. Diagram **C** shows a cross-section of a taste bud with gustatory and supporting cells. Taste substances contact the taste receptors through the taste pore, and sensory signals exit the tongue via axons projecting from the taste cells. **D.** Histology of a taste bud at low magnification. (Reproduced with permission from McKinley MP, O'Loughlin VD, Bidle TS. *Anatomy and Physiology: An Integrative Approach.* New York, NY: McGraw Hill; 2013.)

to bitter. Sensory signals exit the tongue via the chorda tympani and glossopharyngeal axons projecting from the taste cells (see Figure 14–9).

The receptor mechanisms underlying the 5 basic tastes of sweet, salt, bitter, sour, and umami are shown in Figure 14–11. Salt and sour are associated with specific ion channels. Salt (NaCl) is detected by the flux of external Na^+ through sodium channels. The sour taste is primarily due to acidity, or the presence of H^+ ions. The detection of acidity is complex and not well understood but may ultimately involve K^+ flux.

Sweet, bitter, and umami are associated with second messenger receptor systems (see Figure 14–11). The sweet taste, exemplified by glucose, also operates via an MGluR4-like metabotropic receptor via a G-protein second messenger system that causes the release of intracellular calcium from internal stores. Bitter substances, exemplified by quinine,

are detected by TAS2R receptors containing a protein called gustducin the activation of which lowers intracellular cyclic nucleotide concentrations and may also activate the IP3-DAG second messenger cascade. These second messenger systems are believed to cause the release of internal calcium from stores and open ion channels. The umami taste is mediated by a receptor that activates an Na^+/Ca^{2+} cation channel via a G-protein second messenger system.

Taste receptor cells synapse with axon-like processes (see Figure 14–10) in either the chorda tympani or glossopharyngeal nerves that extend from sensory ganglion called the geniculate and petrosal ganglia, respectively (Figures 14–12 and 14–13). There are also a few taste receptors in the pharynx that project to the brain via processes of cells in the nodose ganglion. This arrangement bears some similarity to the connection scheme of sensory dorsal root

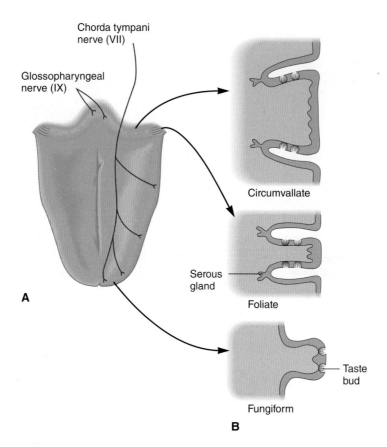

FIGURE 14–9 Taste buds of the tongue and central projections. **A.** Locations of fungiform, foliate, and circumvallate taste buds on the tongue. Fungiform and foliate buds project the medulla via the chorda tympani nerve. Circumvallate buds project via the glossopharyngeal nerve. **B.** Diagrammatic sections of the 3 taste buds. (Reproduced with permission from Kandel ER, Schwartz JH, Jessell TM, et al: *Principles of Neural Science*, 5th ed. New York, NY: McGraw Hill; 2013.)

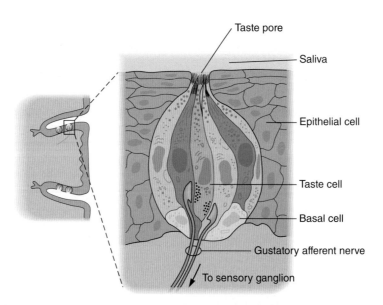

FIGURE 14–10 Cross-section of a circumvallate taste bud and higher magnification details of cells within. Note that the projection to the brain is made via the taste receptor cell by a process that resembles an axon coming from a sensory ganglion. This arrangement bears some similarity to the connection scheme of sensory dorsal root ganglion cells and auditory hair cells. (Reproduced with permission from Royer SM, Kinnamon JC: HVEM serial-section analysis of rabbit foliate taste buds: I. Type III cells and their synapses, *J Comp Neurol.* 1991 Apr 1;306(1):49-72.)

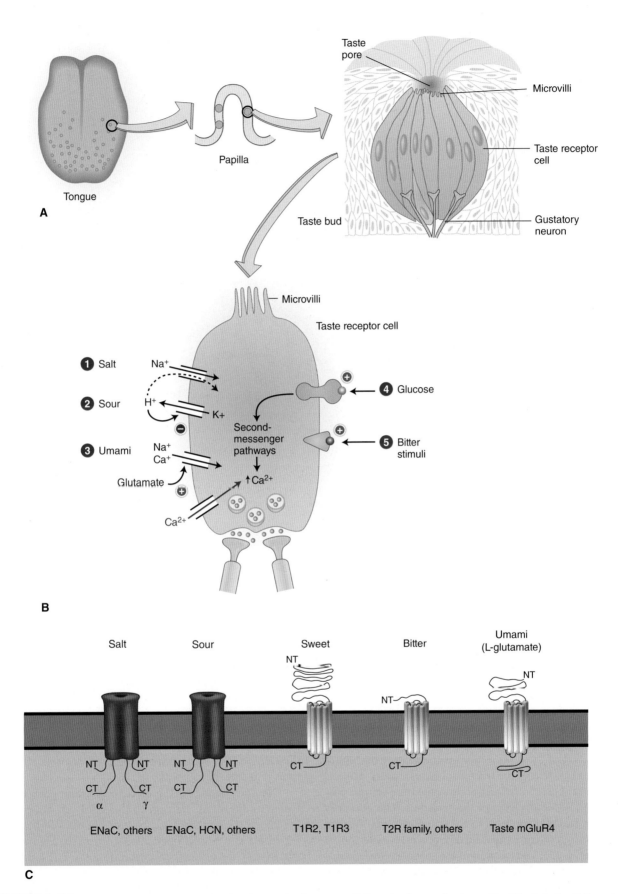

FIGURE 14-11 Mechanisms of taste. **A.** Taste bud and internal cell structure. **B.** Transduction mechanisms of the 5 basic tastes. **C.** Receptor details for taste mechanisms. (Parts A and B, reproduced with permission from Kibble JD, Halsey CR. *Medical Physiology: The Big Picture*. New York, NY: McGraw Hill; 2009; part C, reproduced with permission from Barrett KE, Barman SM, Brooks HL et al: *Ganong's Review of Medical Physiology*, 26th ed. New York, NY: McGraw Hill; 2019.)

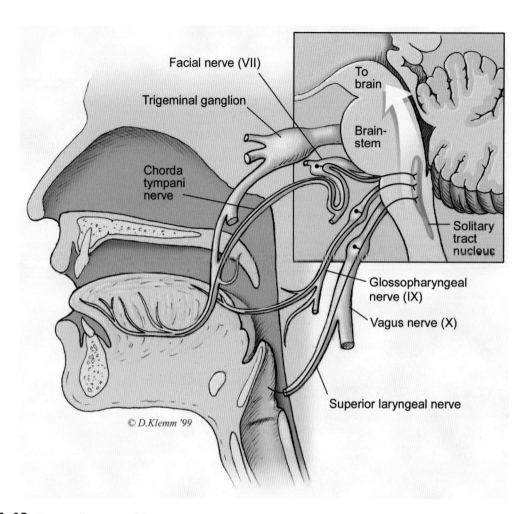

FIGURE 14–12 Cutaway illustration of the taste projection pathways via the chorda tympani and glossopharyngeal nerves to the solitary nucleus of the medulla. Note that these nerves join other cranial nerves in route to the brain. (Used with permission from David Klemm, Faculty and Curriculum Support, Georgetown University Medical Center, Washington, DC.)

ganglion cells and auditory hair cells. Taste messages from most of the front of the tongue (mainly fungiform papillae) project to the brain via the chorda tympani nerve, whereas the glossopharyngeal nerve carries messages from foliate, circumvallate, and fungiform papillae. The chorda tympani and glossopharyngeal nerves join other cranial nerves en route to the brain (see Figure 14–12). A few taste receptors in the larynx and mouth project to the medulla via the vagus nerve.

The target of these projections is the solitary nucleus of the medulla (nucleus of the tractus solitarius), which projects to the ventral posterior nucleus (also called the ventral posteromedial [VPM] nucleus) of the thalamus. The gustatory area of the thalamus projects to the anterior insula—frontal operculum area of cortex that further processes taste signals (see Figure 14–13). The location of the gustatory area of neocortex in the area of the insula is illustrated in the coronal section diagram of Figure 14–14.

Axonal endings of fibers in the chorda tympani nerve receive inputs from a number of taste cells in a variably selective manner. Some fibers are activated nearly exclusively by a single receptor type (labeled line coding), such as salt, but others have mixed receptor input (distributed coding). One of the functions of cortical processing is to identify specific tastes from the activation occurring across multiple fibers. However, before reaching the cortex, taste messages are modulated in the nucleus of the solitary tract (NST) in the medulla and in the thalamus. Neurons in the NST receive satiety inputs that modulate their activity. Eating sweet substances will reduce the responses of sweet-responding NST neurons after some time, reducing their appeal.

Neurons in the NST project to the taste portion of the thalamus, the VPM. Damage to the VPM can cause ageusia, the loss of the sense of taste. Neurons in the VPM project to the insula and frontal operculum cortex (see Figures 14–13 and 14–14), the primary cortical taste areas. The insula lies at the junction of the parietal, frontal, and temporal lobes with the opercular cortex (operculum means "lid") just above it. These 2 evolutionarily old primary gustatory areas are affected by olfactory and visual inputs.

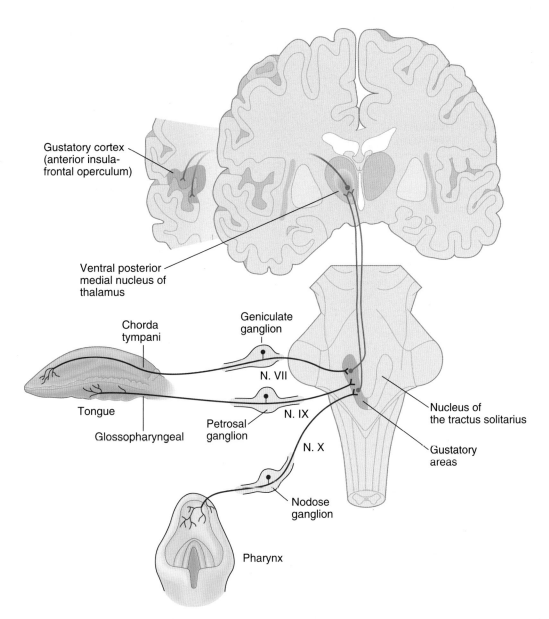

FIGURE 14–13 Central projections for taste. Cells of origin for the axon-like processes in the chorda tympani and glossopharyngeal nerves are in the geniculate and petrosal ganglia, respectively. There are also a few taste receptors in the pharynx that project to the brain via processes of cells in the nodose ganglion. The target of these projections is the solitary nucleus of the medulla (nucleus of the tractus solitarius), which projects to the ventral posterior nucleus of the thalamus. The gustatory area of the thalamus projects to the anterior insula–frontal operculum area of cortex that further processes taste signals. (Reproduced with permission from Kandel ER, Schwartz JH, Jessell TM, et al: *Principles of Neural Science*, 5th ed. New York, NY: McGraw Hill; 2013.)

The primary insula and opercular cortical areas project to the amygdala and orbitofrontal cortex. Taste information is combined with olfactory input in the orbitofrontal cortex to represent what is called flavor, the combination of taste and smell. The projection to the amygdala mediates memory for emotionally salient tastes. The amygdala sends a projection to the orbitofrontal cortex, perhaps functioning in its learning function with the orbitofrontal cortex like the hippocampus does with other parts of the frontal lobe. This learning function mediates the association between the sight, smell, and taste of very specific foods and the experience after ingesting it, forming the basis of learned food preferences

and various sensory-mediated triggers for hunger. The pleasure derived from eating goes beyond smelling and tasting to include food texture, which is transmitted to the brain by activation of mechanoreceptors while chewing. Despite the fact that some people congenitally lack the senses of taste and smell, they still enjoy eating because of this mechanical component. Texture manipulation is an important aspect of food preparation.

The total lack of taste is called ageusia. More common than ageusia is a poor sense of taste, called hypogeusia, which may be due to damage to the olfactory mucosa that causes partial anosmia. Some cancer chemotherapies temporarily cause

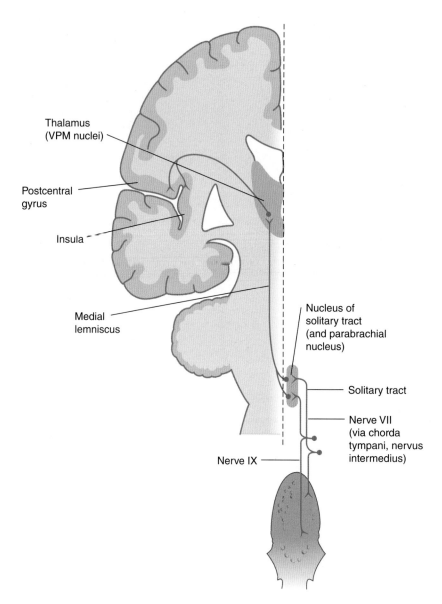

FIGURE 14-14 Simplified cross-section (coronal) view of the main anatomic areas subserving taste, from the tongue to the solitary tract of the medulla, to the ventral posteromedial (VPM) nucleus of the thalamus, to the cortex insula. (Reproduced with permission from Waxman SG. *Clinical Neuroanatomy*, 28th ed. New York, NY: McGraw Hill; 2017.)

hypogeusia. Anosmia, the lack of sense of smell, which can affect taste or flavor, can be congenital or result from brain damage or damage to the olfactory mucosa such as from exposure to noxious substances. Sensitivity to bitter tastes declines with age. Schizophrenia is often associated with deficiencies in smell, which are thought to be linked to generalized frontal lobe neuropathy.

Two main satiety mechanisms modulate the sense of taste, one in the central nervous system and central brain mechanism and the other in the taste receptors. The central mechanism, called alliesthesia ("changed taste"), is a brain mechanism that indicates you are getting full. The mechanism is mediated by reduced firing of orbitofrontal taste and smell neurons to the specific odor of an ingested substance after a substantial consumption, causing a loss

of general appetite. The peripheral mechanism is called sensory-specific satiety. Its mechanism involves reduced output in taste and olfactory receptors themselves. This mechanism suppresses appetite specifically for the taste of what is being consumed and acts on a faster time scale than the alliesthesia "fullness" mechanism.

Alliesthesia is mediated by the action of several gastrointestinal hormones, including insulin, ghrelin, and pancreatic polypeptide. The digestion process causes the release of these hormones into the bloodstream, where they act on areas of the hypothalamus and brainstem. These hormones also modulate the transmission of taste information by the vagus nerve to the NST in the medulla. Interactions between the orbitofrontal cortex and the amygdala mediate taste learning.

SUMMARY

- Molecular receptors for smell are found in the nose in the olfactory epithelium.
- There are approximately 1000 distinct types of olfactory receptors.
- Olfactory signals are transduced by several molecular mechanisms.
- Olfactory axons project to the olfactory bulb into structures called glomeruli.
- The olfactory bulb projects directly to cortex and indirectly to other areas of neocortex.
- Taste receptors are found mostly on the front, sides, and back of the tongue in papillae.
- Axons of taste receptors project to the NST, which in turn projects to thalamus.
- Taste and smell inputs are combined in orbitofrontal cortex to produce the complex perception of flavor.

SELF-ASSESSMENT QUESTIONS

1. An individual loses his sense of smell. After receiving a medical examination, it is determined that the reason for his loss of sensation is due to degeneration of primary afferent fibers that enter the olfactory glomerulus. In a healthy individual, upon which of the following structures do these primary afferent fibers terminate?

   A. Granule cell dendrites forming axodendritic synapses
   B. Granule cell axon terminals forming axoaxonic synapses
   C. Mitral cell dendrites forming axodendritic synapses
   D. Mitral cell axon terminals forming axoaxonic synapses
   E. Axon terminals of fibers arising from the olfactory tubercle, forming axoaxonic synapses

2. A middle-aged man is involved in an automobile accident that causes brain damage affecting a region of the cerebral cortex, resulting in loss of the conscious perception of smell. Which of the following regions of the cortex is most likely affected?

   A. Temporal neocortex
   B. Posterior parietal lobule
   C. Cingulate gyrus
   D. Prefrontal cortex
   E. Precentral gyrus

3. A 45-year-old woman who has difficulty in sensing different odors is examined by her primary physician and then by a neurologist. A magnetic resonance imaging scan is negative, and the neurologist concludes that the loss of the sense of smell is due to damage to the olfactory receptor mechanism that initially responds to an olfactory stimulus. Which part of the olfactory receptor mechanism that normally responds to an olfactory stimulus is presently unresponsive to such a stimulus?

   A. Mitral cell
   B. Granule cell
   C. Sustentacular cell
   D. Basal cell
   E. Olfactory cilia

4. A 47-year-old man who had been working in a factory for many years where a strong chemical odor was present finds it now difficult to discriminate different types of odorants. Following a neurologic examination, it is concluded that the neural basis of olfactory discrimination is significantly impaired. Which of the following neural properties underlying the patient's ability to discriminate odorants is now disrupted?

   A. Specific activation of different cell groups within the amygdala
   B. Specific activation of different groups of olfactory glomeruli that are spatially organized and segregated within the olfactory bulb
   C. Specific activation of different groups of cells within the olfactory tubercle
   D. Temporal summation of olfactory signals in the anterior olfactory nucleus
   E. Temporal summation of olfactory signals in the mediodorsal thalamic nucleus

5. A patient suffers damage to the olfactory bulb and its output pathways, resulting in the loss of smell. Which of the following combinations of structures is deprived of this direct (monosynaptic) olfactory input?

   A. Hypothalamus and prefrontal cortex
   B. Amygdala and pyriform cortex
   C. Hippocampus and amygdala
   D. Prefrontal cortex and medial thalamus
   E. Septal area and prefrontal cortex

Somatosensory System

Franklin R. Amthor, Stacie K. Totsch, & Robert E. Sorge

OBJECTIVES

After studying this chapter, the student should be able to:

- Understand how the skin elaborates a variety of receptors that sense various kinds of touch, temperature, and pain.

- See how receptors for various skin sensations have different anatomic morphologies and physiologic transduction mechanisms.

- See the relationship between different mechanoreceptor types and the ensuing perceptions, such as vibration or pressure, associated with stimulation of that receptor type.

- Understand how the spatial resolution of touch is related to the density of receptors in any skin area and inversely related to receptive field (RF) size.

- Follow the pathway for transmitting touch, temperature, and pain perception from sensory neurons in the dorsal root ganglia of the spinal cord, up through spinal cord pathways to the brainstem and thalamus, and then to somatosensory cortex in the most anterior portion of the parietal lobe.

- See how transient receptor potential (TRP) channels mediate temperature sensation.

- Understand psychological aspects of pain perception and the role of endorphins.

- Learn what regions of the brain process somatosensory information.

- See how proprioception and kinesthesis (joint position, movement, and force) are mediated by receptors similar to mechanoreceptors.

OVERVIEW

Embedded in the skin are receptors for touch, temperature, and pain. These receptors are at the axon endings of neurons whose soma are in the dorsal root ganglia outside the spinal cord, or other ganglia outside the brain for cranial nerves mediating somatosensation in the head. Action potentials produced by somatosensory receptors travel retrogradely past the axonal bifurcation in the dorsal root ganglion to synapses in the spinal gray area. Somatosensory synapses in the spinal gray area participate in local circuits that mediate reflexes and project to the thalamus and other brain areas.

CUTANEOUS & SUBCUTANEOUS SOMATIC SENSORY RECEPTORS

The skin is the boundary between the body and the world, enclosing the body's tissue, retaining water, excluding bacteria and dirt, and providing thermal insulation. The skin detects the world through the sense of touch, which is called cutaneous or somatosensory perception. The kinds of touch that we can perceive include various kinds of mechanical sensations (pressure, movement, and flutter), as well as temperature and pain. These different kinds of perceptions arise from the activation of different kinds of receptors in the skin.

Detecting something as a skin sensation without or before perceiving what has made this contact is called passive touch. Touch has another, more active function, called haptic perception, which enables us to perform complicated manipulations of objects whose shape and orientation are perceived through touch. This type of perception (active touch) is particularly important for tool use and dexterity skills involving the fingers and fingertips. It has been shown, for example, that people blind from birth who have no visual input to the occipital visual cortex experience activation in the visual cortex during their finger manipulations when reading Braille. Both active and passive touch depend on the activation of a variety of cutaneous receptor types.

The skin has 2 main layers that allow it to perform its functions, the epidermis and dermis, shown in Figure 15–1. The epidermis is the outermost layer of the skin (*epi* means "above" or "on"; *dermis* means "skin"). The epidermis consists of layers of dead cell ghosts that provide an insulating barrier to the outside. There are virtually no tactile receptors in the epidermis and none in the superficial epidermis, so moderate abrasions of the skin surface do not kill any living cells and are not felt as painful. The epidermis is formed by the division of cells in the dermis below it that are continually dividing and migrating outward to replace the dead layers as they wear off. As these cells reach the epidermis, they flatten, die, and form the inert epidermis barrier. The dermis is the living layer of skin below the epidermis that includes virtually all the somatosensory receptors. Hairs from hair follicles in the dermis pass through the epidermis before appearing on the skin surface. Below the dermis is the subcutaneous layer that contains vasculature and fat cells.

For all the skin below the neck, somatosensory receptors are specializations of the axons of sensory neurons whose cell bodies are in the spinal cord dorsal root ganglia. The other end of the axons of these cells enters the spinal cord at the dorsal root and makes synapses with local and projection neurons. Cutaneous information is relayed by spinal cord projection neurons to the ventral posterior nucleus of the thalamus, and then to a strip in the parietal lobe where a "touch" map of the body exists. Cutaneous sensation in the face and neck is mediated by cranial nerves in functionally similar pathways.

Mechanoreceptors for Touch

The skin has receptors for several kinds of touch, warm and cold temperature, and several types of pain. Touch receptors are called mechanoreceptors. Four types of mechanoreceptors with distinct transducer structures are specialized to receive tactile information: Pacinian corpuscles, Ruffini endings, Merkel disks, and Meisner corpuscles (Figure 15–2). In addition to these receptor morphologies, different types of so-called "free nerve endings" respond to pain stimuli and temperature. Mechanical displacement of the skin or skin hairs is also detected by free nerve endings in the hair follicle at the hair root.

Mechanoreceptors signal various kinds of touch or mechanical skin displacement. There are 4 main types of mechanoreceptor morphology: Meissner corpuscles, Merkel disks, Ruffini endings, and Pacinian corpuscles (see Figure 15–2). The response properties of these different receptor types fall along 2 major axes, receptive field (RF) size and response transience, illustrated in Figure 15–3. The RF size dimension is related to depth in the skin. The effect of a punctate displacement on the surface of the skin extends farther out laterally for deep versus shallow skin locations. Thus, deep mechanoreceptors (Ruffini endings and Pacinian corpuscles) tend to have larger RFs than shallow ones (Meissner corpuscles and Merkel disks).

The second mechanoreceptor response dimension is how sustained their responses are to a continuous stimulus. The Merkel disk is a shallow, small RF, sustained-responding fiber, whereas the Ruffini ending is a deep, large RF, sustained unit. Meissner corpuscles are shallow, small RF, transiently responding receptors, whereas Pacinian corpuscles have large RF, transient responses.

There is 1 additional response dimension beyond RF size and sustained/transient responsiveness: frequency response. There is a considerable difference among the fibers in the frequency of stimulation to which they respond, which translates into the resulting cutaneous perception. Merkel disks, the small RF sustained units, respond only to very low frequencies, so they tend to report constant force on the skin. The small RF transient Meissner corpuscles respond over a range of 3 to 40 Hz, and their activation is felt as "flutter." The large RF sustained Ruffini endings respond to stimulus frequencies from 15 to 400 Hz, with their firing interpreted as stretch. Pacinian corpuscles have large RFs and transient responses over a frequency range of 10 to 500 Hz and signal vibration. These frequency ranges overlap, so that at most stimulus frequencies >1 fiber class is active, and the perception of the stimulus is based on the firing of several cutaneous receptor types.

Mechanotransduction

The receptor structures of mechanoreceptors are composed of mechanically gated ion channels in the axonal membranes of dorsal root ganglion cells. The unusual "pseudo-unipolar" morphology of these cells is shown schematically in Figure 15–4. These neurons are composed of a cell body located in the dorsal root ganglion just outside the spinal cord. These cells have no dendrites (typically) and only a single axon. This axon bifurcates close to the cell body in the ganglion and gives rise to 2 processes: 1 projecting out to the periphery in the skin, forming the receptor, and the second axon process extending into the dorsal spinal cord gray area.

The mechanoreceptor at the axonal ending typically consists of a number of mechanically gated channels and, in some types, an enclosing corpuscle that modulates the properties of the transduction. Figure 15–5 shows a highly schematic drawing of a mechanically gated ion channel. Stretch or deflection of the neural membrane in which the channel is embedded causes that channel to open and allow

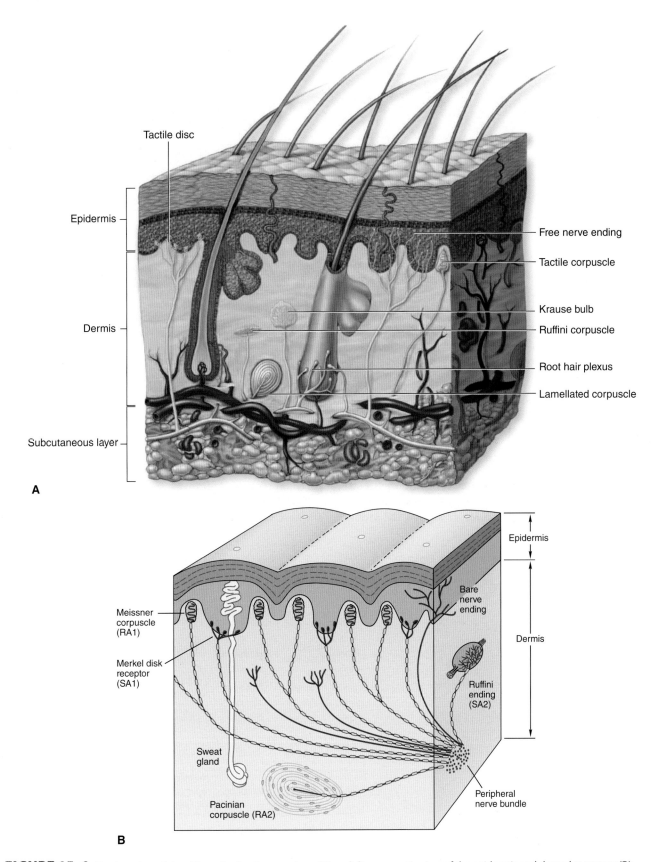

FIGURE 15–1 Section view of the skin and subcutaneous layer (**A**) and diagrammatic view of the epidermis and dermal receptors (**B**). Cutaneous receptors are almost exclusively in the living dermis, although a few free nerve endings sometimes extend into the deep epidermis.

(Part A, reproduced with permission from McKinley MP, O'Loughlin VD, Bidle TS. *Anatomy & Physiology: An Integrative Approach*. New York, NY: McGraw Hill; 2013; part B, reproduced with permission from Kandel ER, Schwartz JH, Jessell TM, et al: *Principles of Neural Science*, 5th ed. New York, NY: McGraw Hill; 2013.)

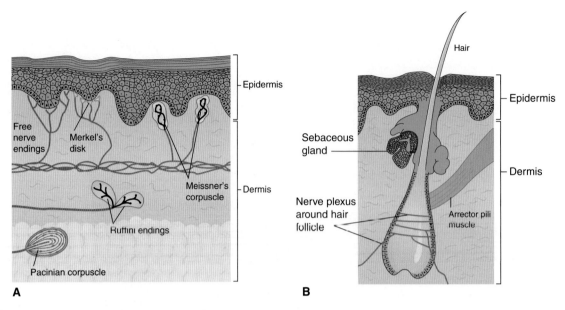

FIGURE 15–2 Section view of the main cutaneous receptor morphologies. **A.** Free nerve endings, a Merkel disk, a Meissner corpuscle, a Ruffini ending, and a Pacinian corpuscle are shown. Merkel disks and Meissner corpuscles are close to the skin surface and have small receptive fields. These mechanoreceptors are important for active or manipulative touch. Deeper Ruffini endings signal stretch, and Pacinian corpuscles encode vibration. **B.** A nerve plexus formed of axonal endings surrounding the base of a hair follicle signals displacement of the hair or skin near the hair. Cutaneous receptors around hair follicle bases are activated by movement of the hairs. (Reproduced with permission from Kibble JD, Halsey CR. *Medical Physiology: The Big Picture.* New York, NY: McGraw Hill; 2009.)

the flux of ions, usually sodium, thus depolarizing the axon and generating action potentials. The corpuscle enclosure in mechanoreceptors such as Pacinian corpuscles mechanically modulates the mechanical input to the axonal ending. The ending by itself responds in a sustained manner, but the corpuscle flexes under pressure so that the axonal ending within experiences a deflection at the onset and offset of applied force, thus becoming an on-off responding receptor despite being based on a sustained on-responding mechanoreceptor within.

The mechanically induced action potentials initiated in the dorsal root ganglion peripheral axon travel in what would

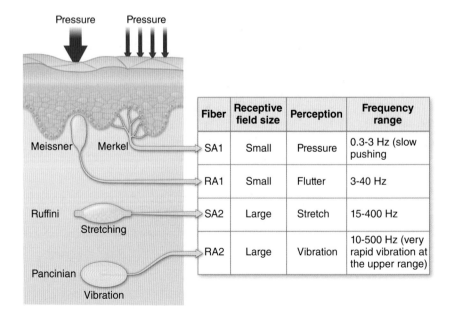

FIGURE 15–3 The 4 major types of mechanoreceptors and their receptive field sizes, perceptual attributes, and response frequency range. Meissner corpuscles and Merkel disks are located near the surface of the skin and have small receptive fields. The responses of Meissner corpuscles are transient (rapidly adapting), whereas Merkel disks respond in a more sustained manner. The deeper, larger receptive field mechanoreceptors are Ruffini endings and Pacinian corpuscles. Ruffini endings have sustained responses, but Pacinian corpuscles are transient.

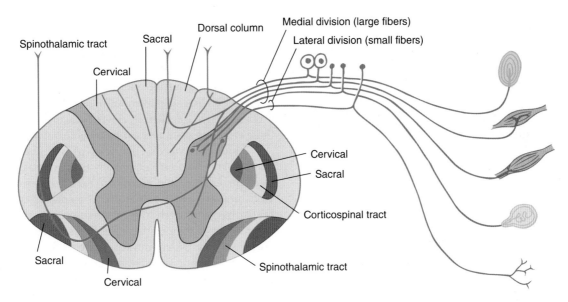

FIGURE 15–4 Diagrammatic cross-section through the spinal cord showing major tracts in the white matter and the layout of sensory neurons whose cell bodies are in the dorsal root ganglion. Cutaneous receptors are at the axonal endings of neurons whose cell bodies are located in the dorsal root ganglia outside the spinal cord or in various brain ganglia for cranial nerves that mediate head somatosensation. The axonal endings of somatosensory neurons elaborate various kinds of receptors sensitive to mechanical, temperature, or pain perception. The other end of the axon enters the spinal cord through the dorsal root and synapses on interneurons, motor neurons, and projection neurons in the central spinal gray area. (Reproduced with permission from Waxman SG. *Clinical Neuroanatomy*, 28th ed. New York, NY: McGraw Hill; 2017.)

be classically considered a retrograde manner toward the cell body and the axonal bifurcation point in the dorsal root ganglion. These action potentials simply continue past the axon bifurcation point now in an orthograde direction into the dorsal root of the spinal cord (see Figure 15–4) to synapse on neurons in the spinal gray area. The second-order neurons can be either spinal interneurons or projection neurons that relay somatosensory information to the thalamus.

Receptive Fields, Sensory Maps, & Dermatomes

The RF of a cutaneous fiber is the area of skin that, if mechanically stimulated, will influence the firing of that fiber. The RF concept can be extended to a particular spinal cord segment dorsal root ganglion as the skin area that influences firing of any of the cells in that ganglia. This is of clinical significance because injury to a specific spinal cord dorsal root will be associated with sensory dysfunction over a particular skin area, called a dermatome. Skin dermatomes associated with particular spinal cord segments (cervical, thoracic, lumbar, sacral) are illustrated in Figure 15–6.

Differences in Mechanosensory Discrimination Across the Body Surface

The ability to resolve small differences in the location of a mechanical stimulus to the skin varies considerably across the body, being very high in locations such as the fingertips and face and low on the body trunk. This resolution ability is related to receptor density and inversely to receptor RF size. The minimum distance needed to distinguish 1 from 2 stimulus points is as high as 2 mm on the fingertips and face, but may exceed 40 mm on the trunk, as shown in Figure 15–7. Mechanoreceptors on high-acuity skin areas such as the

fingertips and skin have small RFs and are located very close to each other compared to low somatosensory acuity areas. Because a given area of somatosensory cortex processes information from about the same number of peripheral receptors, the cortical map will be enlarged for high-acuity versus low-acuity areas, as will be seen later in this chapter.

Trigeminal Ganglion & Nerve

The general plan of spinal nerves, as shown in Figure 15–8, is for sensory inputs to enter the dorsal horn and motor outputs to exit the ventral root. These nerves merge into a single bundle peripheral to the dorsal root ganglia (where the cell bodies of the sensory nerves reside) to form what is called a "mixed" sensory and motor nerve. Above the spinal cord, some cranial nerves follow a similar plan, although rather than emanating from the spinal cord, they arise in brainstem areas such as the medulla. The processing of cutaneous perception from the face is mediated largely by the trigeminal nerve, shown in Figure 15–9. The cell bodies of the sensory axons are located in a ganglion outside the brainstem called the trigeminal ganglion. The sensory messages from facial stimulation are conveyed to what is called the main (principle) nucleus in the pons (rather than the spinal gray area for spinal nerves), which in turn relays to the thalamus via the dorsal and ventral trigeminothalamic tracts.

Active Tactile Exploration & Joint Receptors

There is another type of mechanoreceptor that is similar to cutaneous mechanoreceptors but mediates the senses of proprioception (limb position) and kinesthesis (limb motion). Many of these receptors are similar to some of the skin mechanoreceptors such Ruffini corpuscles but are located either in tendons

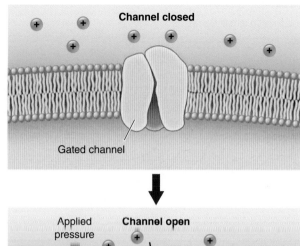

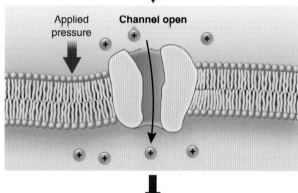

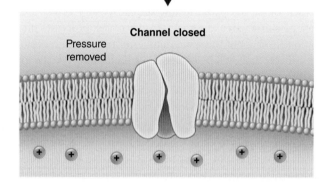

FIGURE 15–5 Schematic diagram of a mechanically gated ion channel such as found in mechanoreceptor nerve endings. Flexion of the axonal membrane opens channels permeable to sodium, causing action potentials to originate in the axonal ending.

(Golgi tendon organs) or muscles (muscle spindles), as well as in ligaments and joints. Activation of these receptors informs the brain about limb position and movement for motor control. Proprioceptors tend to have sustained responses, whereas kinesthesis receptors tend to be more transient. These receptors allow you to do things such as touch your nose with your eyes closed. Limb movement also stretches the skin around joints in various ways that activate cutaneous mechanoreceptors. This activity is also used by the brain for motor control.

Temperature Receptors

Temperature receptors have the morphology called free nerve endings, which are similar to axon terminals without

myelination or other enveloping structures around them. There are 2 basic types of temperature receptors: "warm" receptors that respond with an increase in firing to temperatures above body temperature (37°C), and "cold" receptors that respond with an increase in firing to temperatures below body temperature. The free nerve endings that form warm receptors are unmyelinated C fibers that have a relatively slow conduction velocity, whereas those of cold receptors are a mixture of C and Aδ fibers.

Temperatures below the range of cold fibers and above that of warm fibers are potentially tissue damaging and activate temperature pain receptors. Temperatures below about 10°C or above about 45°C to 50°C are felt as cold pain and heat pain, respectively. These sensations are mediated by a different set of temperature-pain fibers, discussed in the following section. Different warm and cold fibers have different peak temperature sensitivities. Figure 15–10 shows a diagrammatic distribution of the responses of cold, warm, cold pain, and heat pain fibers. The peak of the cold fiber population response is between 20°C and 30°C, but individual fibers respond maximally at temperatures above and below this. The warm fiber population maximum is between 40°C and 50°C, with individual fibers having peak responses over a broader range. Note the minimum response of the entire population at 35°C to 37°C (normal body temperature). As with the broad spectral sensitivity curves for cones in color vision, temperature perception can be quite precise when derived from the ratio of activity of broadly tuned temperature receptors.

The transduction of temperature is mediated primarily by channels called transient receptor potential (TRP) protein complexes. TRPV1 provides the sensation of scalding heat, whereas cold is mediated by TRPM8, whose conductance for Na+ and Ca2+ is temperature dependent. TRPV1 is also activated by capsaicin, the active ingredient in chili peppers. Interestingly, the TRPA1 (painful cold) and TRPV1 receptors can be found on the same populations of nociceptors, resulting in the "burning cold" sensation with very cold temperatures (<17°C). The percept of cooling can arise from ligands such as menthol that bind the channel and modulate its conductance. Temperature also affects the kinetics of other membrane channels, such as potassium channels.

Pain Receptors & Transduction

There are a variety of stimulus modalities that cause pain, such as extreme temperatures, pressures, or chemical acids and bases. The modalities that are sensed by peripheral pain fibers and interpreted by the brain as pain have the common property of being associated with tissue damage.

Pain Receptor Anatomy & Physiology

Pain neurons, known as nociceptors, have the morphology of free nerve endings. However, unlike thermoreceptors, nociceptors only respond to noxious stimuli. Under normal circumstances, nociceptors are generally responsible for the initiation of pain processing. Two major types of nociceptive fibers are Aδ and C fibers. Aδ fibers are myelinated and

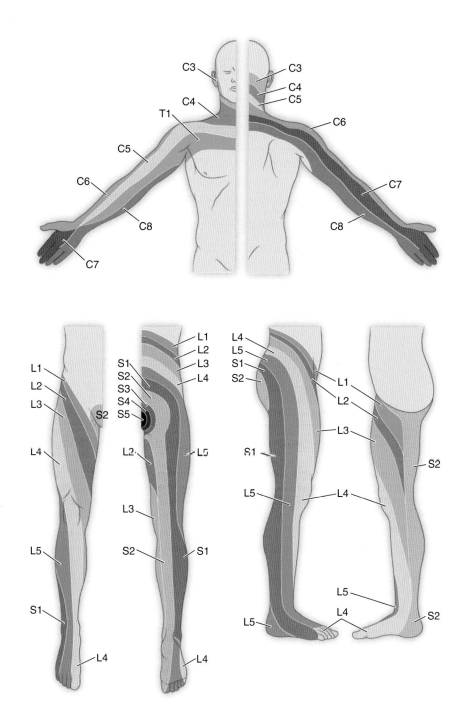

FIGURE 15–6 Dermatomes of the trunk are the skin areas innervated by receptors whose cell bodies are in the dorsal root ganglia of the indicated spinal segments (cervical, thoracic, lumbar, and sacral). Dermatomes are significant clinically because spinal injury at a particular segment will affect somatosensation and motor output of that segment's dermatome.

have a fast conduction speed. Therefore, they are responsible for the first, sharp pain. As mentioned earlier, C fibers are unmyelinated with slow transmission. Therefore, their activation results in throbbing and burning second pain. Some pain fibers respond by firing action potentials exclusively to stimuli near and above the level of damage, whereas other skin receptors report a nonpain sensation at low stimulus intensities, but pain at intensities above a threshold. An example of this dual function is seen in receptors with the

aforementioned TRP channels. In addition, the specific modality that a nociceptor responds to is determined by the expression of ion channels.

Complex Aspects of Pain Perception

There are important differences between pain and other cutaneous senses. Pain activates neurons in many areas of the brain beyond the somatosensory cortex, and compared to other cutaneous senses, the perception of pain is strongly modified

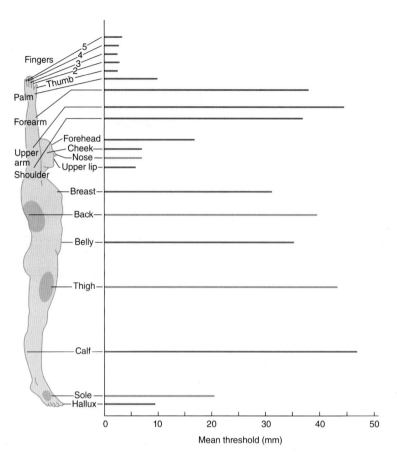

FIGURE 15-7 The minimum distance needed to distinguish 1 from 3 stimulus points on various areas of the body. Two-point resolution is as high as 2 mm on the fingertips and face, but may exceed 40 mm on the trunk, more than an order of magnitude difference. Where receptors have small receptive fields, there is usually a much higher receptor density. This is reflected in the cortical somatosensory map where a given area of cortex processes about the same number of receptors, which is a small skin area in places such as the fingertips and face. (Reproduced with permission from Kenshalo DR, ed. *The Skin Senses*. Springfield, IL: Charles Thomas; 1968.)

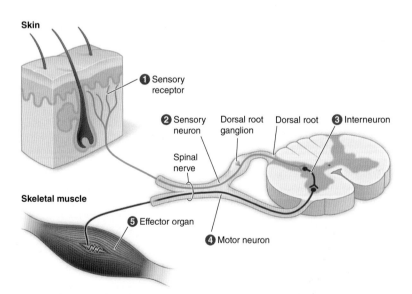

FIGURE 15-8 Neural circuit of a sensory mediated spinal reflex. A painful or potentially painful stimulus to the skin, such as contact with a hot or sharp object, sends an action potential into the spinal gray area. Typically, a monosynaptic contact may be made with motor neurons mediating flexion (withdrawal). Additional synapses on inhibitory interneurons reduce the firing of the antagonist extensor muscle and also mediate intra- and intersegment projections for coordinated multimuscle movements. Synapses are also made on central projection neurons that report the painful stimulus, but the withdrawal reflex can be entirely carried out independently and before conscious awareness.

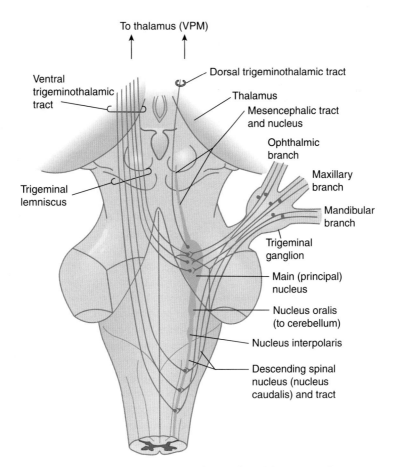

FIGURE 15-9 Trigeminal ganglion and nerve. Above the spinal cord, several cranial nerves mediate somatosensation with a similar organization to that of the dorsal root ganglia of the spinal cord. The largest cranial nerve is nerve V, the trigeminal nerve, which mediates somatosensation for the face. The trigeminal nerve has, as its name implies, 3 divisions: the ophthalmic nerve, the maxillary nerve, and the mandibular nerve. The cell bodies of these nerves are located in a ganglion outside the brainstem called the trigeminal ganglion, with axons splitting into peripheral and central projecting branches in a manner similar to that of the dorsal root ganglia of the spinal cord. Unlike the spinal nerves peripheral to the dorsal root ganglia, however, the ophthalmic and maxillary nerves are purely sensory. The mandibular nerve, on the other hand, has both sensory and motor axons. VPM, ventral posteromedial nucleus. (Reproduced with permission from Waxman SG. *Clinical Neuroanatomy*, 28th ed. New York, NY: McGraw Hill; 2017.)

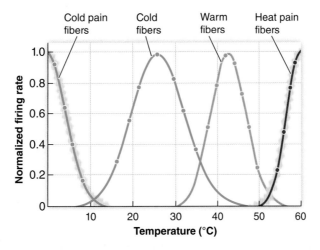

FIGURE 15-10 Activity of cold and warm receptors as a function of temperature. Temperature receptors are generally free nerve endings that fire at temperatures either above or below body temperature (37°C). Fibers exist with peak activities at different parts of the cold or warm curves (*filled circles*). As in color vision, higher level neurons can resolve temperature much more accurately than the response width of a given temperature receptor by comparing activity of receptors with different temperature tuning curves. Temperatures colder or hotter than the ranges of temperature fibers are potentially damaging and signaled by additional pain fibers.

by and can alter the mental state. Cognitive factors can strongly mitigate the sensation of pain, such as seen during childbirth or when soldiers ignore significant wounds. Pain can also produce long-lasting changes in mood. For example, chronic pain, or pain that remains after an injury has healed, is often clinically associated with depression. Although pain exists to warn of imminent body damage, it can become disabling in disease conditions such as cancer, for which no behavior can reverse the damage or reduce the pain. The current understanding of chronic pain is that the input to the spinal cord becomes sensitized such that previously nonpainful stimuli elicit a pain response. This process is termed central (as part of the central nervous system) sensitization and is thought to be mechanistically similar to the process of long-term potentiation studied as the basis for memory in the hippocampus.

The attempt to understand the nociceptor and the complex phenomenon that is pain has resulted in a number of theories over the past century. The *specificity theory* was the belief that there were nociceptors that responded to painful stimuli and only this type of stimulation. This was later replaced by the *intensity theory*, which stated that a stimulus can be painful or not based on the intensity of the stimulation at the nociceptor. An example would be something akin to a heat stimulus—not painful in the short term, but more painful as the intensity increases. As more neurons were identified in the skin (A and C fibers), the *pattern theory* emerged, wherein the pattern of cellular activation was the signal to determine whether or not a stimulus was painful. However, none of the previous theories took cognitive factors into account (mentioned earlier). Currently, the only theory that takes both physical and psychological aspects of pain into account is the *gate control theory*. Briefly, this theory states that nonpainful stimuli can prevent the sensation of pain from traveling to the central nervous system by closing the "gate" to painful stimuli. Put another way, signals from nonpain fibers can block signals from pain fibers, leading to an inhibition in pain. This theory explains why rubbing an area that is in pain seems to provide relief and is a "natural" response to injury. The theory also allows for input from the brain to "close the gate," and we know that this process is referred to as descending inhibition of pain.

The pain system in the brain uses a unique set of neurotransmitters and antagonists so these receptors can specifically reduce pain without affecting the ability to perceive other sensations. An important class of pain neurotransmitters are the so-called endogenous opioids (opioids generated within the body), such as the endorphins (an abbreviation of endogenous morphine). Endorphins are produced in pain-stress situations, such as running the last few miles of a marathon.

Endorphins contribute to the placebo effect, where patients experience pain relief when given an inert substance they believe will block pain. Opiates such as morphine and heroin reduce pain because they bind the same receptors that endorphins bind; however, when injected in large doses, these drugs produce a "high" and are addictive. The drug naloxone antagonizes the effects of these opioids and is often given to addicts to reverse the effects of heroin they have injected. Naloxone also blocks much of the placebo effects.

There are notable individual and group differences in pain tolerance. Pain tolerance generally increases with age, for example. Some data suggest that men are more tolerant of acute pain but less tolerant of chronic pain than women. Athletic training enhances pain tolerance. Cultures that encourage expression of emotions in general tend to be associated with lower thresholds for reporting pain, but it is not clear that such differences reflect anything but a labeling, rather than an experiential threshold.

An important brain area for processing pain is the anterior cingulate cortex, an anterior mesocortical area immediately above the corpus callosum. This structure has an executive role in allocating cortical processing and priorities according to current goals and results. Consistent with its function of arbitrating between taking different strategies in response to experience, the anterior cingulate is activated by pain, the anticipation of pain, and the production of errors in goal pursuit.

In terms of the brain's control of pain, an important brain region is the periaqueductal gray (PAG). This area is involved in descending modulation, which ultimately leads to the inhibition of a pain signal before it reaches the brain. This mechanism underlies the gate control theory and is supported by the fact that when the PAG is stimulated, it produces analgesia. The rostral ventromedial medulla receives input from the PAG and is considered the final output pathway for the descending inhibition of pain. Importantly, the dopaminergic, serotonergic, and noradrenergic projection areas also send axons down to the spinal cord to reduce the transmission of pain.

CENTRAL PROCESSING OF CUTANEOUS SENSATION

Skin receptors convey information about skin contact to neural circuits, mediate somatosensory perception, and enable responses to cutaneous stimuli. The touch, temperature, and pain messages encoded by cutaneous receptors are sent via synapses to neurons within the same spinal cord segment, to other spinal cord segments, and to the brain. Somatosensory axons synapse in the spinal gray area, illustrated schematically in Figure 15–4. The neurotransmitter for most mechanoreceptors is glutamate, but pain neurons may also release the neurotransmitter substance P.

Cutaneous Synapses in the Spinal Cord

Local spinal cord circuits mediate reflex arcs through spinal interneurons such as the withdrawal reflex (eg, flexion of the bicep to move the hand away from something hot or an otherwise painful stimulus that has been touched), shown in Figure 15–8. A spinal withdrawal reflex such as this typically consists of monosynaptic and polysynaptic pathways. Recall that cutaneous receptors are the axonal endings of sensory neurons located in the dorsal root ganglia just outside the spinal cord. Action potentials travel in what in most neurons would be considered a retrograde manner from the receptor ending to the axonal bifurcation near the cell body (see Figure 15–4) and then into the spinal cord via the dorsal "root" or axon bundle. The cutaneous axon may synapse directly on lower (α) motor neurons that drive flexor muscles such as the biceps. At the same time, some of these cutaneous axons also synapse on spinal cord interneurons in the gray cell body area of the spinal cord. These interneurons simultaneously inhibit the extensor motor neurons whose relaxation allows the flexor muscle to move the hand away from the painful stimulus. The cutaneous input also projects (sometimes through interneurons) to the contralateral side of the same spinal segment and other spinal segments to allow coordinated withdrawal. For example, in an encounter with a very painful stimulus, not only is the stimulated arm involved in withdrawal, but also the trunk and legs,

and this activity is coordinated to maintain balance during the evasive maneuver.

Cutaneous Projections to the Brain

Cutaneous inputs to the spinal cord also synapse on centrally projecting neurons. Projection neurons in the spinal gray area send axons to the thalamus (ventral posterolateral nucleus) and other brain areas via 2 major tracts: the medial lemniscus and spinothalamic tract (illustrated in Figure 15–11). The medial lemniscus is composed of large-diameter

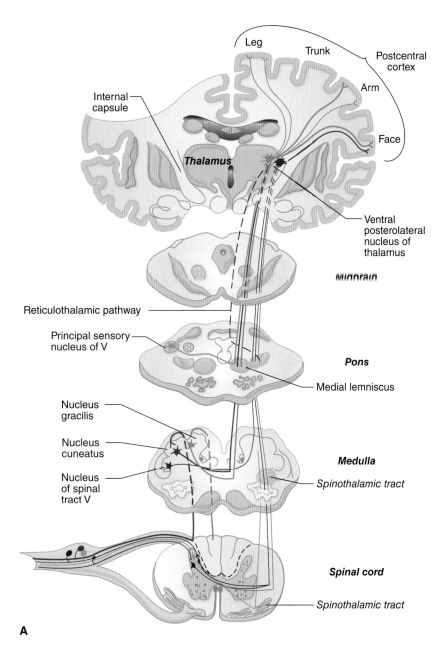

FIGURE 15–11 **A.** Cutaneous projections from the spinal cord to the brain. Cutaneous signals travel along 2 major pathways: the medial lemniscus tract, which carries large mechanoreceptor axons, and the spinothalamic tract, which carries smaller diameter axons of temperature and pain perception. **B.** Coronal section showing the relation between some somatosensory afferent projections and basal ganglia and corticospinal tracts. (Part A, reproduced with permission from Ropper AH, Samuels MA, Klein JP: *Adams and Victor's Principles of Neurology*, 11th ed. New York, NY: McGraw Hill; 2019; part B, reproduced with permission from Waxman SG. *Clinical Neuroanatomy*, 28th ed. New York, NY: McGraw Hill; 2017.)

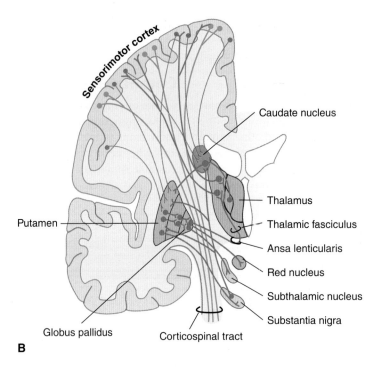

FIGURE 15–11 (*Continued*)

mechanoreceptor axons. The spinothalamic tract consists of smaller diameter temperature and pain axons that project to, in addition to the thalamus, the reticular formation. Central projection axons cross within the spinal cord before ascending to the thalamus so that the left side of the brain receives information from the right side of the body and the right side of the brain receives information from the left side of the body. The target of these central projections is the ventral posterolateral nucleus of the thalamus, which in turn relays to Brodmann areas 1, 2, and 3 in the postcentral gyrus of the parietal lobe.

Somatosensory Cortex

From each thalamus, somatosensory signals travel to the somatosensory cortex, which is located just anterior to the central sulcus (Figure 15–12) in the most anterior portion of the parietal lobe (the central sulcus is the border between the frontal and parietal lobes). Somatosensory cortex consists of at least 3 subdivisions (S1, S2, and S3). Although it was once thought that these areas composed a hierarchy in which S1 projected to S2 and S2 to S3, it is now clear that there are direct projections from the thalamus to S2 and S3, which also may receive projections from S1. Thus, consistent with the tradition of referring to all cortical areas that receive direct thalamic sensory projections as "primary," S1, S2, and S3 would all be considered to be primary somatosensory cortex. These 3 somatosensory areas project to more posterior loci in the parietal lobe, where somatosensory information is linked in terms of location with respect to self and to that from other senses, particularly vision and audition.

This body map in the somatosensory cortex is sometimes called a "homunculus," and it is very similar to the motor output map just anterior to the central sulcus in the frontal lobe. The somatosensory map or homunculus has several odd features. One is that, contrary to what one might expect, distal, peripheral areas of the body such as the feet are located medially, on the wall of the medial longitudinal fissure, whereas central facial and mouth structures such as the lips and face are laterally located. A second odd feature of the representation is its distortion: Small skin areas of the face and fingertips, for example, occupy cortical areas as large as the entire trunk. This distortion generally follows the principle that each unit of cortical area processes inputs from a relatively constant number of peripheral receptors. In Figure 15–7, one can see that since fingertip skin has 50 to 100 times the receptor density as trunk areas, fingertip representation per skin area will be larger on the somatosensory cortex by that ratio. This constant receptor density per cortical area principle also extends to other senses.

A third oddity of the cortical somatosensory representation is that it exhibits several discontinuities. For example, although, in moving along the skin, the fingers are quite distant from the forehead, their representation in somatosensory cortex is adjacent. This feature of the map has implications for some types of phantom limb pain, where amputees may report pain or touch they perceive to be felt in a limb they no longer have when their faces are touched. Another discontinuity is that there is a small representation of the head near that of the upper trunk, but a separate, much larger discontinuous representation of the face more laterally in the cortex along with the representation of the vocal apparatus.

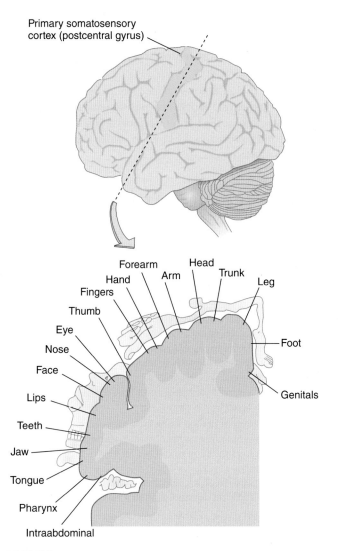

FIGURE 15–12 Somatosensory cortex homunculus (hemisphere coronal section). Top: The location of the primary somatosensory area in the postcentral gyrus just posterior to the central sulcus. This is the most anterior area of the parietal lobe. Below: The body map on somatosensory cortex, which is the area that receives input from the illustrated part of the body. This map has several kinds of distortions. Proportional area distortion occurs because the density of peripheral receptors varies by more than an order of magnitude across various parts of the body, and each unit cortical area tends to process inputs from about the same number of receptors, yielding larger areas representing the fingers and face than the trunk. There are also discontinuities in the representation of parts of the head and genitals compared to nearby skin areas. (Reproduced with permission from Kibble JD, Halsey CR. *Medical Physiology: The Big Picture.* New York, NY: McGraw Hill; 2009.)

It is not currently clear the extent to which mechanosensation and other cutaneous senses such as temperature and pain have anatomically segregated representations in somatosensory cortex. Pain sensation is projected from the spinal cord not only through the thalamus, but also via the reticular formation. This latter pathway allows pain inputs to generate autonomic responses such as tachycardia and sweating independent of conscious awareness. Pain inputs to the brain can also activate midbrain descending pathways that module its character, often via opioid neurotransmitters that act within the dorsal gray area of the spinal cord.

Proprioception & Kinesthesis Are Mediated by Tendon & Joint Receptors

Throughout the body are mechanoreceptors whose structure and physiologic characteristics are similar to cutaneous receptors, but whose function is to report limb location (proprioception) and limb movement and force (kinesthesis). Although these topics are treated more fully in the chapters on motor control, it is appropriate to consider some as aspects of proprioception and kinesthesis with cutaneous senses for several reasons: (1) the sensory transducers for proprioception and kinesthesis such as Golgi tendon organs and muscle spindles are mechanoreceptors with similarities in their physiology and morphology to cutaneous mechanoreceptors; (2) the cell bodies for these receptors are located in the dorsal root ganglia, like other mechanoreceptors; (3) the central projections follow a similar scheme; and (4) some information about joint position and movement is obtained from skin cutaneous receptors because skin around joints is stretched during movement. Proprioception and kinesthesis receptors also participate in spinal reflex loops that react to changing loads to maintain limb position, rather than withdrawing a limb in reaction to a painful stimulus, for example.

CONCLUSION

The cutaneous senses inform the brain about what contacts the skin. There are 4 major mechanical transduction pathways for various types of touch. Other fibers mediate cold and hot temperature perception. Pain is transmitted by a variety of other fibers sensitive to extreme mechanical pressure, temperature, or chemical activity (eg, acids and bases). The somatosensory system follows a common sensory plan in which peripheral receptors relay to synapses in a specific area of the thalamus (ventral posterolateral nucleus), which in turn projects to the postcentral gyrus of the cortex. The cortical "primary" receiving areas are comprised of Brodmann areas S1, S2, and S3. These areas in turn project to more posterior areas of the parietal lobe. The perception of pain is more complex, with projection paths reaching the reticular formation. Pain pathways also use endorphin neuropeptide neurotransmitters, and can be modulated by central cognitive states. The anterior cingulate is an important brain area in the perception and modulation of pain.

SUMMARY

- Skin, besides its function in isolating the body from the environment, has receptors for various kinds of touch (mechanoreceptors), as well as receptors for temperature and pain.

- The skin continuously produces new cells below the dermis that migrate, flatten, and eventually die on the surface of the skin in a layer called the epidermis.

- Virtually all skin receptors are found in the dermis with the exception of occasional receptors located in the transition zone between dermis and epidermis.

- Somatosensory receptors originate from dorsal root ganglion cells whose axons bifurcate, with one end going to the skin and elaborating the receptor and the other end entering the spinal dorsal root and synapsing in the spinal gray area on local circuit and thalamic transmission neurons.

- Four types of mechanoreceptors with distinct transducer structures are specialized to receive tactile information: Pacinian corpuscles, Ruffini endings, Merkel disks, and Meisner corpuscles.

- The response properties of different tactile receptor types fall along 2 major axes, RF size and response transience.

- The RF size dimension is related to depth in the skin, such that deep mechanoreceptors (Ruffini endings and Pacinian corpuscles) tend to have larger RFs than shallow ones (Meissner corpuscles and Merkel disks).

- The Merkel disk and Ruffini endings are sustained-responding fibers, whereas the Meissner and Pacinian corpuscles are transiently responding.

- The 4 major tactile receptors also have different stimulation frequency response properties that mediate different perceptual sensations such as stretch, pressure, or vibration.

- Temperature receptors are mostly of the free nerve ending structure and are called cold receptors if their optimum response is below body temperature or heat receptors if their optimum response is above body temperature.

- Pain receptors are primarily free nerve endings but respond to different inputs (pressure, temperature, chemical) whose commonality is immanent tissue damage.

- Local spinal cord circuits mediate reflex arcs through spinal interneurons such as the withdrawal reflex that triggers flexion of the bicep to move the hand away from something hot.

- Cutaneous inputs to the spinal cord synapse on centrally projecting neurons in the spinal gray area that project to the thalamus (ventroposterolateral nucleus) and other brain areas via 2 major tracts: the medial lemniscus and spinothalamic tract.

- The somatosensory thalamic areas project to the most anterior part of the parietal cortex in Brodmann areas 1, 2, and 3.

- Somatosensory cortex is organized in a body map sometimes called a homunculus, which is distorted such that areas of the skin with a high density of receptors project to larger cortical areas than those with low density; to a first approximation, any unit area of somatosensory cortex processes inputs from the same number of receptors.

- Receptors similar to some mechanoreceptors in tendons and muscles that signal limb position, movement, and muscle force, called proprioceptors and kinesthesis receptors, project to the brain in similar pathways as the mechanoreceptors.

SELF-ASSESSMENT QUESTIONS

1. A 49-year-old woman complains about loss of accuracy in identifying and localizing sensation (in particular, conscious proprioception, tactile sensation, and pressure) from the appropriate sites along her right hand and leg. A magnetic resonance imaging (MRI) scan indicates the presence of a tumor in the region of the right dorsal columns at the level of the spinal cord–medulla border. The presence of the tumor could account for both loss of sensation and loss of accuracy in identifying the sites on the limbs associated with the respective sensation because of a general property of inhibition associated with dorsal column functions. Which one or more of the following types of inhibition have been identified within the dorsal column nuclei that are disrupted by the tumor?

   A. Feedforward inhibition using local interneurons only
   B. Feedback inhibition using local interneurons only
   C. Descending inhibition from fibers arising in the cerebral cortex only
   D. Feedforward, feedback, and descending inhibition
   E. Feedforward and descending inhibition only

2. A 57-year-old man is referred to a neurologist after he complains about difficulties in determining the directionality and orientation of movement of stimuli along his right arm. An MRI is taken of the patient, and a central nervous system (CNS) tumor is noted. Where in the regions listed below is the tumor most likely to be present?

   A. Left spinal cord
   B. Medial half of thalamus
   C. Ventral pons
   D. Internal capsule
   E. Cerebral cortex

3. A patient has been seeing a physician for almost a year because she complains of pain in her shoulder. After extensive analysis, the physician determines that the pain in her shoulder reflects referred pain that is arising from another source. In this case, which of the following best explains the basis for the referred pain?

   A. Inhibitory fibers that block transmission of pain impulses along a given pathway and then transfer the impulses to a different pathway associated with a different part of the body
   B. A massive discharge along a given pathway that results in the activation of a separate pathway because of the principle of divergence
   C. A convergence of primary afferent fibers from a given region onto second-order neurons that normally receive primary afferents from a different body part
   D. The disruption of lateral spinothalamic fibers
   E. The blockade of substance P from primary afferent terminals

4. A car door is accidentally closed on the hand of a teenage boy. As a result, he experiences significant pain that persists for a while. In terms of the neurochemical events that take place at the afferent terminals of the first-order pathway that conveys the pain sensation to the spinal cord, which of the following transmitters will be released onto dorsal horn neurons of the spinal cord from these primary afferent fibers?

   A. Enkephalins alone
   B. Glutamate alone
   C. Substance P alone
   D. Glutamate and substance P
   E. Enkephalins, substance P, and glutamate

5. A patient is experiencing severe pain. If it were possible to place an electrode into the gray matter around the cerebral aqueduct of the midbrain and stimulate the cells in this region, it would induce an analgesic response. Which of the following best explains such an effect?

   A. Activation of a pathway that ascends directly to the cortex and mediates analgesia
   B. A descending pathway that blocks nociceptive inputs at the level of the dorsal horn
   C. Activation of local interneurons that block ascending nociceptive signals at the level of the midbrain
   D. Activation of an ascending inhibitory pathway that projects to the ventral posterolateral nucleus of the thalamus
   E. Activation of cholinergic neurons in the basal forebrain

Pyramidal Motor System

Franklin R. Amthor

OBJECTIVES

After studying this chapter, the student should be able to:

- See how control of movement is instantiated in a hierarchical control system, much of which appears to involve the evolution of higher levels of more sophisticated control using lower levels as subsystems.
- Understand how the pyramidal motor system originating in primary motor cortex permits learning of complex and subtle motor sequences.
- See how goal execution proceeds from the most abstract planning stages in prefrontal cortex, through the supplementary motor and premotor global organizational areas to primary motor cortex.
- Follow motor commands from primary motor cortex via upper motor neurons to the lower motor neuron spinal cord output.
- See how the cortical motor output control of the body is laid out in a body map called a homunculus in a manner similar to that of the somatosensory system just across the central sulcus in neocortex.
- Understand the role of the thalamus and other subcortical structures in motor control.

HIERARCHICAL CONTROL OF MOVEMENT

Movement distinguishes animals from plants. The sea squirt begins life as a free-swimming larva with sensory receptors like eyes, muscles that enable it to swim, and a small brain that mediates its behavior. At the end of the larval stage, it permanently adheres to a spot on the ocean bottom and commences to digest its eyes and nervous system. The nervous system exists to control movement. Movement must be directed toward some goal (planning), and the component muscles must be controlled to act in concert to achieve that goal.

Muscles, which produce movement by contraction, are called effectors. Different types of movement are subserved by 3 different primary muscle types: striated muscles for voluntary movement of skeletal bones around joints via attachments by tendons, smooth muscle that contracts the walls of organs like the stomach and esophagus, and unique cardiac muscle that has hybrid properties between striated and smooth muscle.

This chapter will focus on the cortical control of striated muscle underlying voluntary control of limb movement. All vertebrate striated muscles are activated by receipt of acetylcholine from motor neurons. Each motor neuron spike releases sufficient acetylcholine to elicit an action potential in the muscle cell. The rate of muscle cell action potentials is generally proportional to the contractile force the muscle generates. The motor neurons emanating from the spinal cord that activate muscles that control the limbs and limb appendages (hands and feet) are called lower or α motor neurons. Lower motor neurons are controlled, in turn, by neural circuits in the spinal cord, brainstem, and motor cortex.

Direct activation of lower motor neurons by neurons in primary motor cortex (upper motor neurons) is phylogenetically new and permits the learning of novel and complex motor sequences such as associated with manual praxis. In contrast, basic, highly evolutionarily conserved movement sequences such as walking and running are controlled by circuits in the spinal cord, with compensation for rough terrain and other perturbations mediated by circuits in the brainstem and cerebellum that receive vestibular and visual input.

The control of movement is done by a hierarchy of neural circuits ranging from the spinal cord to the brainstem to primary motor cortex and prefrontal areas. The focus of this chapter will be on movement control via primary motor cortex. Because the axons of the upper motor neurons emanate from pyramidal cells in layer 5 of this cortical area, it has been named the pyramidal tract, but it is also referred to as the corticospinal tract.

Neocortical Areas Mediating Motor Control

The cerebral neocortex is composed of 4 major lobes: frontal, parietal, temporal, and occipital (Figure 16-1). The parietal, temporal, and occipital lobes are primarily sensory, processing

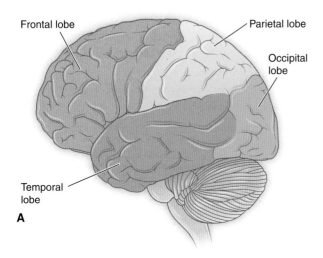

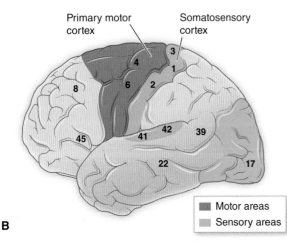

FIGURE 16-1   Lateral view of the left human brain hemisphere. **A.** Areas corresponding to the frontal (blue), parietal (green), occipital (orange), and temporal (beige) lobes. **B.** Immediately posterior to the central sulcus is the primary sensory cortex (purple), comprised of Brodmann areas 1, 2, and 3. Anterior to this sulcus is primary motor cortex (red), Brodmann area 4. Anterior to this are the two main premotor areas (Brodmann area 6, also red): the supplementary motor area (SMA) medially and the premotor cortex (PMC) laterally.

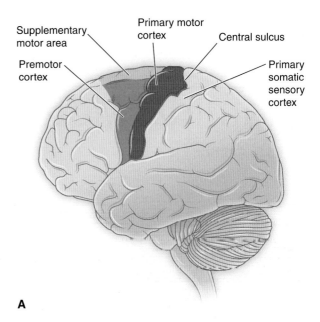

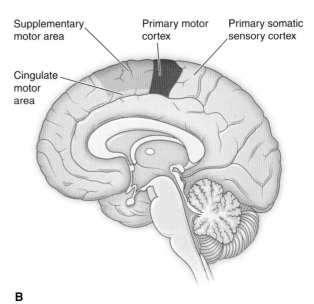

FIGURE 16-2   Supplementary motor area (SMA) and premotor cortex (PMC) viewed from outside on the left (**A**) and in sagittal section (**B**).

inputs from the 5 major senses. The frontal lobe is concerned with movement. Anterior parts of the frontal lobe, called prefrontal, are involved in goal generation and motor planning for set goals. Middle areas of the frontal lobe (Brodmann area 6), particularly the supplementary motor area (SMA) and premotor cortex (PMC), organize and generate complex motor sequences involving the movement of many limbs in a coordinated manner through time. These areas are shown in more detail in Figure 16-2. SMA is largely more medial and anterior than PMC. The primary motor cortex (Brodmann area 4) is the output of this system via the pyramidal or corticospinal tract.

The Motor Control Hierarchy

The hierarchical nature of motor control is best appreciated from an evolutionary perspective. The behavior of primitive, low-cephalic animals is primarily reflexive, driven by immediate stimuli and basic limbic system–level drives such as hunger and predator avoidance. In developing complex, internal goal–driven behavior, high-cephalic animals, such as humans, have retained many of the circuits and competencies of previously evolved lower level systems but have layered more complex long-range, goal-driven behavior on top of these.

Figure 16–3A is a simplified illustration of the main components of the mammalian motor control system. Prefrontal goal-setting neural circuits project to SMA and PMC, which in turn drive primary motor cortex. The primary motor cortex, via projections of its axons through the corticospinal tract, can directly drive lower motor neurons or indirectly drive them through the brainstem. The primary motor cortex also receives sensory feedback information from the limbs and cerebellar input that helps coordinate multilimb movement.

Spinal Cord Segment Circuits

The lowest level of the control hierarchy is illustrated in Figure 16–3B. At the spinal cord level, the maintenance of limb position uses feedback between sensors for limb position (projected via Ia afferent fibers) to drive α (lower) motor neurons to generate restoring force to perturbation within a single spinal cord segment. However, the motor neuron efferent can be driven directly by upper motor neuron axons from primary motor cortex.

The pyramidal or corticospinal tract is shown in Figure 16–4, along with sensory tracts that send information from the skin, joints, and muscles to the sensory homunculus in somatosensory cortex. This tract of upper motor neurons first passes through the cortical white matter. Upper motor neuron axons that will innervate lower motor neurons in the spinal cord then travel down the brainstem where they cross ("decussate") in the medulla to the opposite side of the body. The area of the medulla where this occurs is called the medullary pyramid. Some references suggest the name *pyramidal tract* comes from this fact rather than from the tract's origin in giant Betz pyramidal cells in motor cortex.

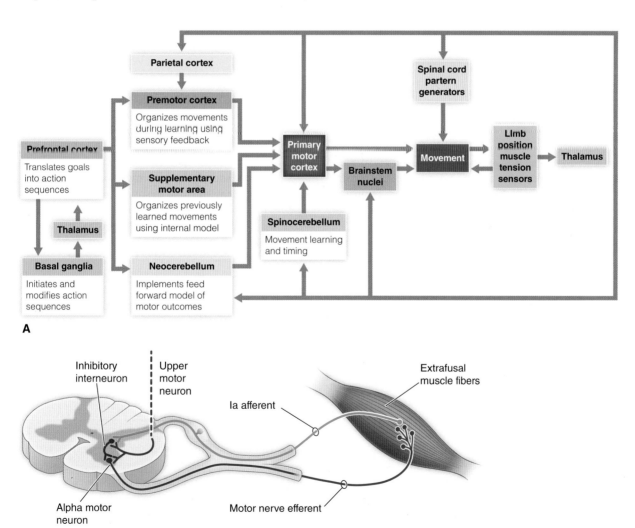

FIGURE 16–3 **A.** Hierarchical organization of the motor control system. **B.** Neural circuit mediating the spinal reflex. Upper motor neurons can enhance or inhibit the spinal reflex via their connections to lower motor neurons, or inhibitory interneurons in the spinal cord, respectively.

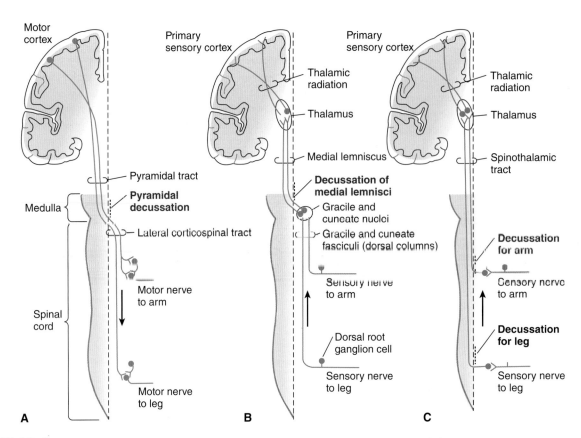

FIGURE 16–4 The pyramidal or corticospinal tract shown in relation to dorsal column and spinothalamic sensory systems. (Reproduced with permission from Waxman SG. *Clinical Neuroanatomy*, 28th ed. New York, NY: McGraw Hill; 2017.)

Primary motor neuron axons that will innervate muscles above the spinal cord in the neck and head enter tracts called corticobulbar tracts that terminate on nuclei in the brainstem. Axons emanating from these brainstem nuclei compose the cranial nerves that control muscles of the face and mouth.

Within the spinal cord, the corticospinal axons run in 2 tracts, shown in Figure 16–5. The largest of these is the lateral tract, whereas there is also a ventromedial tract called the ventral tract.

Integrated Control

At the next level of the hierarchy, basic motor behaviors, such as walking or running, can be generated by spinal cord mechanisms embodied across many spinal cord segments that generate motor stimulus patterns. Above that, brainstem mechanisms that receive vestibular and visual input add balance and rough terrain compensation. Above that is direct and indirect control by the primary motor cortex, which receives input from frontal and prefrontal lobe complex goal-action sequence plans. The corticospinal tract not only passes through the brainstem on the way to the spinal cord, but it also innervates several motor control nuclei within the brainstem. These form the nonpyramidal tracts and are discussed in more detail in Chapter 17.

At the top of the hierarchy, motor sequences consequent to goal pursuit are initiated in an interaction between the basal ganglia and prefrontal cortex (see Chapter 17).

Prefrontal cortex is the locus of interaction between limbic system goals and working memory. Its output is the choice among the many possible means of accomplishing that goal, gating neural circuits that lead to organized coherent muscle command sequences. This is accomplished in multiple stages through feedforward projections between prefrontal areas and the basal ganglia. The output of these prefrontal computations is sent to cortical areas just anterior to primary motor cortex, namely the SMA and PMC. The output of these areas is to the primary motor cortex, whose output axons (upper motor neurons via the corticospinal tract) drive α or lower motor neurons in the spinal cord. This output is modulated by inputs from the cerebellum (see Chapter 17), which participates in motor learning of timing sequences and in the formation of an internal model of the skeleton-muscle system.

The pyramidal or corticospinal tract originating in the primary motor cortex can bypass lower level motor control circuits that evolved to control basic functions such as balance while standing, movement gaits such as walking, and whole-hand grasping (see Figure 16–3B). Direct primary motor cortex control allows complex, arbitrary learned sequences to be generated, such as typing, which involve movement of the fingers individually and sometimes in opposite directions. Sophisticated motor sequences such as typing or playing a musical instrument could not have evolved as genetically embedded capabilities like grasping have. The ability to control individual muscles through primary motor

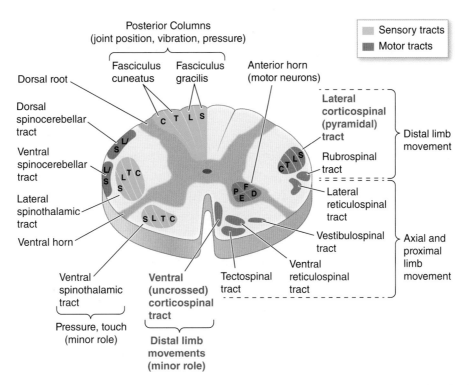

FIGURE 16-5 The location of the lateral and medial pyramidal tracts in a spinal cord cross-section. The spinal cord, unlike neocortex, has its cell body area located medially with fiber tracts running laterally. These tracts include the pyramidal and other afferent motor tracts as well as ascending efferent sensory tracts. (Reproduced with permission from Jameson JL, Fauci AS, Kasper DL, et al: *Harrison's Principles of Internal Medicine*, 20th ed. New York, NY: McGraw Hill; 2018.)

cortex requires some sort of map that can allow the muscle movement goal generated in the prefrontal cortex to project to and act on that muscle's upper motor neuron. That map is called a homunculus.

Cortex & Motor Homunculus

Primary sensory cortical areas are typically those that receive a direct input from the area of the thalamus that receives a direct input from the physiologic sensor array, such as the retina for vision or the cochlea for hearing. These primary cortical areas form a map that usually conforms to the sensor layout. In the case of skin senses, the layout is the skin surface. Underneath the skin at various joints and in muscles are receptors for joint position and acceleration and muscle force. The various types of cutaneous and proprioceptive transducers form a map called a homunculus in somatosensory cortex just posterior to the central sulcus. Several kinds of distortions and discontinuities in this map, and the reasons for them, are discussed in Chapter 15 on skin senses.

Anterior to the central sulcus is a very similar map for motor output from the primary motor cortex, shown in Figure 16–6, which strongly resembles the sensory homunculus across the central sulcus in parietal cortex. The proximity of the sensory and motor representations allows direct, fast interactions between cutaneous and proprioceptive inputs from a particular part of the body with motor projections from primary motor cortex. Similar distortions in the 2 maps indicate that muscles that receive many upper motor neuron

inputs, for precise control, also tend to have many associated sensory outputs.

Layer V pyramidal cells in the primary motor cortex send their axons through the white matter and then through the brainstem to the spinal cord via the pyramidal or corticospinal tract. Some, but not all, corticospinal tract axons originate from very large pyramidal cells called Betz cells, which are unique to the primary motor cortex. A section of motor cortex is shown in Figure 16–7. The large Betz pyramidal cells are unique to layer V in motor cortex so that it is sometimes called agranular, meaning not dominated by uniformly smaller cells. A small minority of corticospinal axons originate not in the primary motor cortex (Brodmann area 4), but in the supplemental motor cortex (SMA: area 6).

CORTICAL CONTROL OF VOLUNTARY MOVEMENT

Highly evolutionary motor behaviors such as walking, running, and grasping are controlled primarily via subcortical mechanisms. With the addition of vestibular and visual input, balance can be maintained and obstacles avoided through brainstem integrative mechanisms. However, more complex behaviors, such as digging and manual manipulation of seeds, nuts, and eventually tools, were enabled by the neocortex and the prefrontal, frontal, and primary motor cortex systems, which together compose nearly half of the entire human brain.

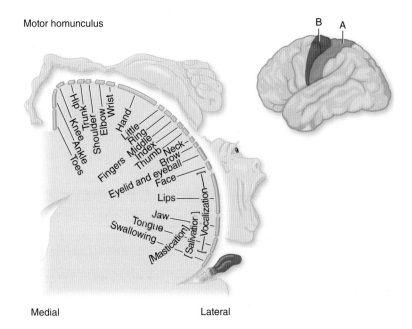

Motor homunculus

Medial   Lateral

FIGURE 16–6   The motor homunculus. On the left, details of the muscle location control are shown in a schematic cross-section of 1 hemisphere. This map parallels the somatosensory map across the central sulcus in the parietal lobe. Notable features include distortions due to higher innervation of motor control for particular skeletal locations, such as the fingers; discontinuities, such as the finger representation being located near the face; and some counterintuitive orientation features, such as the toes being represented medially, while the tongue and chin representations are lateral. (Reproduced with permission from Ropper AH, Samuels MA, Klein JP: *Adams and Victor's Principles of Neurology*, 10th ed. New York, NY: McGraw Hill; 2014.)

Premotor Cortex Organizes Muscle Groups During Learned Sequences

The output of the prefrontal–basal ganglia motion selection system is a projection to areas just anterior to the primary motor cortex that encode activation of coordinated groups of muscles, namely the SMA and PMC. These systems have parallel functions that differ primarily in organizing novel versus well-learned tasks and are shown in Figure 16–8. The PMC is

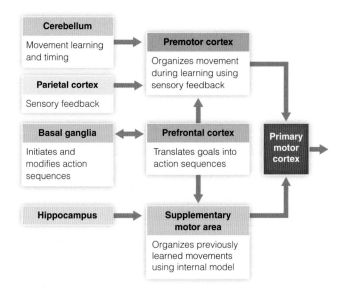

FIGURE 16–8   The division of frontal input to primary motor cortex between the supplementary motor area (SMA) and premotor cortex (PMC). This division is based primarily on whether the task is novel and requires sensory feedback, in which case it is driven by the PMC, or well learned, depending on memory via the hippocampus. Both the PMC and SMA receive input from the basal ganglia–prefrontal cortex goal path selection system. The final common output of both systems is the primary motor cortex. The SMA, however, unlike the PMC, contributes a minority of fibers to the pyramidal corticospinal tract.

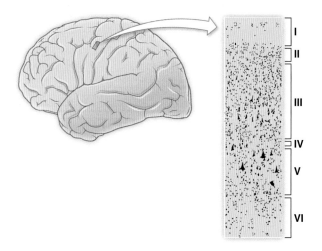

FIGURE 16–7   Section view of primary motor cortex. Unique to this cortical area are very large soma pyramidal cells called Betz cells from which the descriptive name "agranular" was derived for this cortical area. (Reproduced with permission from Martin JH. *Neuroanatomy: Text and Atlas*, 4th ed. New York, NY: McGraw Hill; 2012.)

activated primarily for coordinating activation of the primary motor cortex for novel tasks, that is, while they are being learned. In doing so, it requires feedback about the state of the limbs from the parietal somatosensory and proprioceptive areas and the state of the motor program sequence from the cerebellum.

Supplementary Motor Cortex Organizes During Monitored Movement

The SMA is activated for task performance when tasks are well-learned, including imagining performing a motor task. Memory input to this system comes from the hippocampus, and there may also be input from multimodal sensory areas at the junction of the parietal, temporal, and occipital lobes. The output of the SMA, like the PMC, is almost entirely to the primary motor cortex, where a map of individual muscles exists. However, unlike the PMC, there are some direct projections into the corticospinal tract. These projections are different from those from the primary motor cortex, however, because virtually all corticospinal axons that are monosynaptic on α (lower) motor neurons arise from primary motor cortex.

Motor Learning & Population Coding

The primary motor cortex is more than just an excitation map for the muscles of the body. It is also involved in learning motor sequence behaviors. Its plasticity is evident in changes in the sizes of areas associated with specific muscles or muscle groups following training, with areas associated with extensive limb use becoming larger with practice. Task learning is also associated with initial increases in motor cortex activity, followed by decreases as the task is mastered, paralleling the switch from PMC- to SMA-dominated input control.

Neurons in the primary motor cortex fire according to the direction a limb is moved. The tuning of individual neurons is broad, however, so that it has been proposed that the limb movement direction is generated by a population code whereby the actual movement is a vector sum of all firing neurons weighted by their activity. Such a code is thought to provide robustness against noise and greater computational speed than rate coding by a smaller number of neurons.

FRONTAL & SUPPLEMENTARY EYE FIELDS

Anterior to SMA and PMC in the frontal lobe is Brodmann area 8, called the frontal eye fields (FEFs). This frontal area appears to receive direct input from the superior colliculus via the medial dorsal nucleus of the thalamus. This area also receives input from the medial pulvinar, an area of the thalamus associated with visual attention. The FEF and the more medial supplemental eye fields (SEFs) are involved in the voluntary control of eye movement, particularly saccades and slow pursuit.

PREFRONTAL CORTEX INSTANTIATES OVERALL MOVEMENT GOALS

In most current function maps of neocortex, the prefrontal area is the most undifferentiated. It is unclear whether this reflects our present ignorance of its distinct functional prefrontal subareas or if perhaps the prefrontal cortex operates somewhat like the "association cortex" postulated in the early 20th century. It is clear, however, that this area is proportionately larger in primates than other mammals and in humans compared to other primates. Research and examination of clinical cases of prefrontal damage show clearly that it is the seat of working memory, where the representation of objects and goals is maintained during the pursuit of a task when the direct sensory input is no longer present.

Why has the prefrontal lobe become so large in primates, particularly humans? One hypothesis is that this enlargement instantiates more levels in the goal-motion control hierarchy that translates into a higher level of abstraction in goal pursuit. For example, if you want to sit down and there is nothing to sit on, you may need to get a job to buy a chair. Another possibility is suggested by the fact that humans perform more varied and more complex motion sequences than any other animal, and virtually all of these are learned.

Primates in general and humans in particular have among the most complex social organizations of any animals. Damage to prefrontal cortex typically results in deficits in working memory, specifically as applied to maintaining contingencies in complex social situations. The appropriateness of human behavior is uniquely dependent on multiple facets of the identity of the person with whom one is interacting. Patients with considerable prefrontal damage can retain higher than normal test-measured intelligence quotients while having extremely poor social function and engaging in inappropriate behavior, such as excessive gambling and treatment of other humans as objects. Appropriate behavior in complex societies clearly places high demands on the use of episodic memory to select the best ends and means in pursuit of limbic system–generated needs.

CONCLUSION

The pyramidal motor system is the most recently evolved circuit in the motor control hierarchy. Lower motor control levels in the spinal cord and brainstem mediate balance, basic gaits such as walking and running, and elementary manual praxis such as grasping. The pyramidal system, through the corticospinal tract and feedback from thalamus and cerebellum, allows frontal control of individual muscles in complex, novel, learned sequences such as dancing the tango or playing the violin.

SUMMARY

- Motor control is mediated by a hierarchical control system, with spinal level reflexes at the lowest level and cortical control via the pyramidal (corticospinal) tract from primary motor cortex at the highest.

- At the spinal cord level, the maintenance of limb position uses feedback between sensors for limb position to drive α (lower) motor neurons to generate restoring force to perturbation within a single spinal cord segment.

- At the intermediate level, brainstem nuclei such as the red nucleus control and modulate stereotyped behavior such as gait.

- The evolutionarily newest level of control is that of direct muscle activation by primary motor cortex via the pyramidal tract.

- Primary motor cortex is organized in a body map sometimes called a homunculus, which is similar in layout to the somatosensory map just across the central sulcus in the parietal lobe.

- The pyramidal tract permits complex motor control of learned motor sequences via projections it receives from the immediately anterior motor regions (supplementary motor and premotor areas), which in turn are sequenced and modulated by the basal ganglia and cerebellum.

- The prefrontal cortex, which is the locus of the most general representation of action goals, projects to supplementary and premotor cortical areas that in turn project to primary motor cortex and the pyramidal tract to activate specific action sequences to meet current goals.

- The pyramidal motor system, as the most recently evolved circuit in the motor control hierarchy, works with lower motor control levels in the spinal cord and brainstem to mediate balance, basic gaits such as walking and running, and elementary manual praxis such as grasping, whereas the pyramidal system, through the corticospinal tract and feedback from the thalamus and cerebellum, allows frontal control of individual muscles in complex, novel, learned sequences such as dancing the tango or playing the violin.

SELF-ASSESSMENT QUESTIONS

1. A 74-year-old woman is brought to the hospital after she suffered a stroke. Several days later, a neurologic examination reveals that she is unable to perform certain types of learned, complex movements (referred to as apraxia). Which of the following regions of the cerebral cortex is most likely affected by the stroke?
   A. Precentral gyrus
   B. Postcentral gyrus
   C. Premotor cortex (PMC)
   D. Prefrontal cortex
   E. Cingulate gyrus

2. A patient with motor disturbances presents with the following signs and symptoms: The patient is unable to maintain a posture when the eyes are closed and the arms outstretched and is unable to exert a steady contraction; the speed of tapping of the hand is diminished; and manipulation of small objects is reduced and so are the exploratory movements. Based on these observations, a lesion of which of the following sites could account for these deficits?
   A. Medial aspect of prefrontal cortex
   B. Primary region of visual cortex
   C. Posterior aspect of middle temporal cortex
   D. Medial half of postcentral cortex
   E. Far lateral aspect of precentral cortex

3. A patient is referred to a neurologist because he is unable to perform certain acts. The neurologist tests the patient by observing how he performs routine tasks such as washing, dressing, and using eating utensils. Then, the patient is asked how he would brush his teeth, hammer a nail, comb his hair, or perform the more complex act of opening a soda bottle and pouring the contents into a glass. The patient is unable to follow the command of taking a pen out of his pocket, yet sometime later, he is able to execute the same task when not prompted. A magnetic resonance imaging scan of this patient is taken, and a lesion is detected. From the following list of structures, which one would correspond to the region most closely associated with this patient's deficit?
   A. Medial precentral gyrus
   B. Lateral precentral gyrus
   C. Posterior parietal cortex
   D. Superior temporal gyrus
   E. Lateral prefrontal cortex

4. A patient presents with paralysis and the inability to make voluntary movements of her left lower leg, from the hip through the toes. Spinal reflexes in this region are intact. The lesion is likely to be located where?
   A. Medial right primary motor cortex
   B. Lateral right primary motor cortex
   C. Medial right supplementary motor area (SMA)
   D. Medial left SMA
   E. Medial right PMC

Extrapyramidal Motor Systems: Basal Ganglia & Cerebellum

Franklin R. Amthor

OBJECTIVES

After studying this chapter, the student should be able to:

- Understand how the basal ganglia, through the thalamus, control motor sequences by selecting a particular motor sequence pathway from abstract goal representation in prefrontal cortex to specific muscle output in primary motor cortex.

- Relay how the basal ganglia are organized, with the caudate and putamen forming the striatum input and the globus pallidus as the main output to the thalamus.

- See how the substantia nigra (SN) and subthalamic nucleus (STN) interact with the globus pallidus in the basal ganglia complex.

- Understand the direct and indirect pathways through the basal ganglia to the globus pallidus.

- Comprehend how disorders of the basal ganglia are associated with the important neurologic disorders of Parkinson disease and Huntington disease.

- Understand how the cerebellum mediates feedforward control and refinement of movement sequences.

- Relay the 3 major functional subdivisions of the cerebellum: neocerebellum, spinocerebellum, and vestibulocerebellum.

- Understand the projection pathways into the cerebellum, the circuit processing within it, and the projections from it.

BASAL GANGLIA INITIATE MOVEMENT

What structures in the brain cause movement? Bacteria and plants exhibit phototaxis, movement toward or away from the sun. Virtually all animals execute reflex movements such as moving a limb away from a painful stimulus. Vertebrate animals clearly have higher, limbic system types of goals such as pursuit of food, water, and mates and avoidance of predators and temperature extremes. Humans are thought to consciously make movement decisions based on high-level goals. The likely locus of these high-level goals and their translation into motor sequences were postulated in Chapter 16 to be the prefrontal cortex. However, as any Parkinson disease sufferer can tell you, an intact prefrontal cortex alone is not sufficient to initiate and control movement.

The initiation and modulation of movement in vertebrates generally depends on 2 phylogenetically old systems: the basal ganglia and cerebellum. In mammals, the basal ganglia system interacts with the frontal lobe to produce motor behavior (Figure 17–1). The large, complex frontal neocortex provides the basal ganglia with a wealth of behavioral options. The basal ganglia, acting through the thalamus, act as a central program that calls frontal and cerebellar subroutines that contain the expertise for specific, complex motor sequences. Much of this high-level control relies on lower level motor expertise in the brainstem and spinal cord that controls balance and limb alteration and other basic locomotion procedures.

Organization of the Basal Ganglia: Nuclei

Figure 17–2 shows a pseudo-3-dimensional rendering of the basal ganglia on the top left and a coronal (frontal) section through the basal ganglia and thalamus on the right.

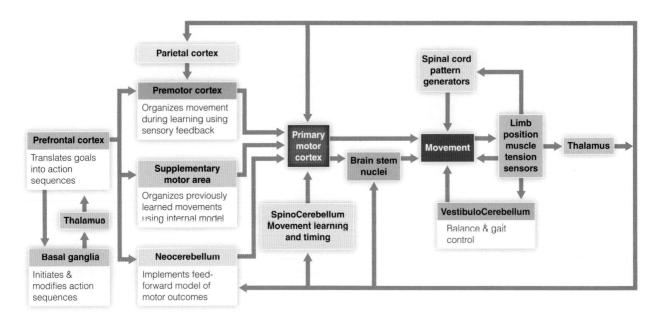

FIGURE 17–1 Hierarchical organization of the motor control system with the basal ganglia–frontal cortex subsystem in green and the cerebellar modulation systems in blue. The basal ganglia receive inputs from virtually the entire frontal lobe and project back to it through the thalamus. The cerebellum consists of 3 main substructures: the vestibulocerebellum, spinocerebellum, and neocerebellum.

The basal ganglia proper consist of an interconnected system of several nuclei. The main processing nuclei of the basal ganglia are structures called the globus pallidus, which is composed of internal and external segments (GPi and GPe). The globus pallidus is lateral to the thalamus. Lateral to the globus pallidus is the putamen, an input area to the globus pallidus. The caudate nucleus passes above the thalamus and has direct inputs to the globus pallidus and indirect inputs through the putamen. The caudate and putamen together are called the striatum. Associated with the basal ganglia and often described as part of it are 2 midbrain nuclei: the substantia nigra (SN) and subthalamic nucleus (STN), both of which project to the globus pallidus.

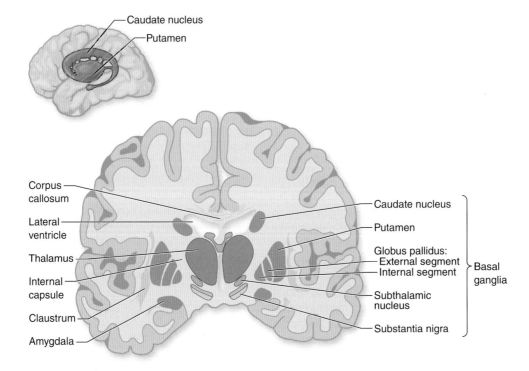

FIGURE 17–2 Three-dimensional rendering of the basal ganglia (top left) and coronal section through the basal ganglia (bottom). (Reproduced with permission from Ropper AH, Samuels MA, Klein JP: *Adams and Victor's Principles of Neurology*, 11th ed. New York, NY: McGraw Hill; 2019.)

Basal Ganglia Connections

The basal ganglia receive inputs from virtually the entire frontal lobe through the striatum (caudate and putamen) and project back to the frontal lobe via the thalamus. The basal ganglia and frontal lobe together are involved in initiating and controlling movement both through the pyramidal motor system (Chapter 16) and the extrapyramidal motor system. Like the pyramidal motor system, the basal ganglia nonpyramidal system interacts with the cerebellum.

Inputs via the Striatum (Caudate & Putamen)

The striatum, consisting of the caudate and putamen, composes the primary input to the basal ganglia. Figure 17–3B shows the cortical input-output connections between frontal cortex and the basal ganglia. The frontal lobe has the job of translating motivations into general goals, and general goals into specific sets of actions to accomplish those goals. Goal and goal-instantiation details exist in the frontal lobe, while the control and steering are done by the basal ganglia in a feed-forward projection system. The basal ganglia receive extensive projections from prefrontal and frontal cortical areas, including the frontal eye fields (Brodmann area 8), as well as proprioceptive information from the parietal lobe.

Figure 17–4 is a schematic of how the basal ganglia select a motor path from the prefrontal cortex to the cortical output at M1, the primary motor cortex. This selection is via their projection to the thalamus, which functionally inhibits all motor pathways except the selected one. The basal ganglia are crucial for both initiating the motor sequence and for maintaining or altering the sequence during its execution. Parkinson patients, for example, have trouble both initiating motor activity and accommodating minor necessary changes in that activity demanded by sensory feedback, such as stepping over a low 2 × 4–inch board while walking down the hall.

Sensory, proprioceptive, and kinesthetic information from mechanoreceptors, Golgi tendon organs, and muscle spindles reaches the somatosensory cortex in the anterior parietal lobe via the corticospinal tracts, as shown in Figure 17–5. These areas make excitatory projections to both the caudate and putamen, which in turn project to the globus pallidus. The globus pallidus also receives inputs from the midbrain SN and subthalamic nuclei.

The striatal areas (caudate and putamen) receive reciprocal projections from thalamic intralaminar nuclei and the SN. The striatum also receives projections from the hippocampus, amygdala, and Raphe serotonergic nuclei in the midbrain. Most of the neurons within the striatum are GABAergic.

Basal Ganglia Outputs

Figure 17–3B illustrates the fact that the primary output of the basal ganglia is from the GPi to the ventral anterior (VA) and ventrolateral (VL) nuclei of the thalamus. These thalamic areas also receive projections from the SN, STN, and cerebellum. There is also a significant output to the red nucleus in the brainstem.

The ventrolateral thalamus in turn projects to motor and premotor areas to control movement. This control is primarily inhibitory; all thalamic relays except the selected current motor sequence are gated out so that the selected sequence alone is allowed to progress. Thus, there is a reciprocal circuit

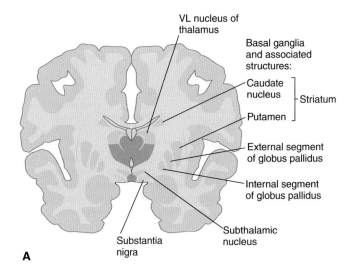

A

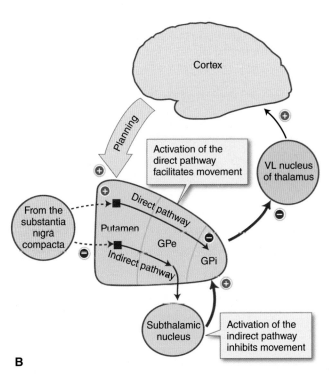

B

FIGURE 17–3 **A.** Coronal section showing the basal ganglia and related structures. **B.** Essential input and output circuitry of the basal ganglia and related input and output structures. Inputs to the basal ganglia come from the caudate (not shown), putamen, substantia nigra, and subthalamic nucleus. The processing by the basal ganglia can be divided into a direct and indirect pathway to the output nucleus, the globus pallidus internal segment (GPi). The major output of the basal ganglia is from the GPi to the ventrolateral (VL) thalamus. (Reproduced with permission from Kibble JD, Halsey CR. *Medical Physiology: The Big Picture.* New York, NY: McGraw Hill; 2009.)

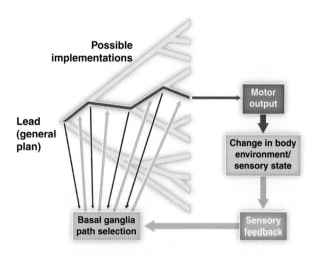

FIGURE 17–4 Reciprocal feedforward selection scheme between the basal ganglia and frontal lobe. Within the frontal lobe are details of goal implementation procedures. There are multiple general ways of accomplishing any goal and multiple subprocedures for each general way. The basal ganglia reciprocally choose the next path step in the motor procedure using, as input, the current motor state and sensory feedback from the environment.

between the frontal lobe and basal ganglia, with frontal (and parietal) lobe areas projecting to the basal ganglia and the basal ganglia projecting to thalamic nuclei, which in turn project back to the frontal lobe. As Figure 17–4 indicates, however, this is primarily a feedforward rather than a feedback system. The cortex informs the basal ganglia of the state of the current motor program and sensory feedback resulting from its execution, and the basal ganglia facilitate the next portion of the motor program and inhibit all other options.

The basal ganglia thalamic areas (VA and VL thalamus) also project back to sensorimotor areas of the parietal lobe and other nuclei in the limbic system.

Neural Circuits of the Basal Ganglia

The general organizational structure of a normal basal ganglia system and a basal ganglia system affected by Parkinson disease is shown in Figure 17–6. The globus pallidus nuclei are divided into internal and external segments. The external segment (see also Figure 17–2) receives input from the putamen and feedback from the internal segment (GPi). The major output of GPi is to VL thalamus and is primarily inhibitory.

The pharmacology of the projection system to, from, and within several areas of the basal ganglia is shown in Figure 17–7. γ-Aminobutyric acid (GABA) is the dominant neurotransmitter between many areas of the basal ganglia system. Glutamate is an important excitatory transmitter used by the thalamic output of the GPi and cortical projection to the striatum. It is also the transmitter of the projection from the midbrain subthalamic nucleus to the GPi. Dopamine, notably, is the transmitter from the portion of the midbrain SN called the pars compacta (SNPC) to the striatum. The loss of these

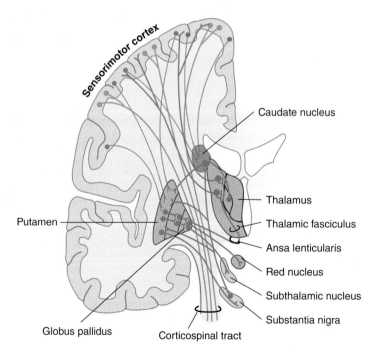

FIGURE 17–5 Important input/output tracts of the basal ganglia. Sensory information about the body and muscle state is projected from the periphery to the parietal lobe via the thalamus, which in turn is sent to the caudate, which projects to the putamen, which then projects to globus pallidus, substantia nigra, and subthalamic nucleus. The globus pallidus internal segment (GPi) projects to the ventrolateral (VL) thalamus and to the red nucleus in the brainstem, which controls some stereotypical motor behavior via the rubrospinal tract (not shown). The pyramidal or corticospinal tract from the primary motor cortex (M1) to the spinal cord is also shown (orange). (Reproduced with permission from Waxman SG. *Clinical Neuroanatomy*, 28th ed. New York, NY: McGraw Hill; 2017.)

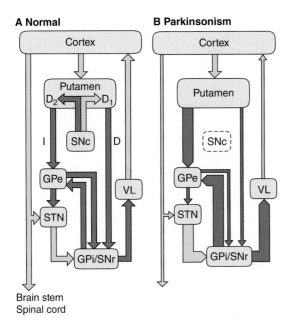

FIGURE 17–6 Circuit activity in the normal (**A**) and Parkinson-affected (**B**) basal ganglia. Excitatory connections are green, and inhibitory connections are red. In Parkinson disease, the dopaminergic output of the substantia nigra is reduced or absent, reducing the excitatory drive in the putamen onto dopamine D_1 receptors (direct pathway) and the inhibitory drive onto dopamine D_2 receptors (indirect path). Both result in increased output from the subthalamic nucleus (STN) to the globus pallidus internal segment (GPi) that increases its inhibitory output to the thalamus, compromising the ability to execute and modify motor behavior. GPe, globus pallidus external segment; SNc, substantia nigra pars compacta; SNr, substantia nigra pars reticulata. (Reproduced with permission from Wichmann T, Vitek JL, DeLong MR: Parkinson's disease and the basal ganglia: Lessons from the laboratory and from neurosurgery. *Neuroscientist.* 1995 July 1;1(4):236-244.)

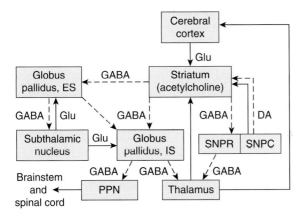

FIGURE 17–7 Pharmacology of the basal ganglia circuit. Most inhibition is mediated by γ-aminobutyric acid (GABA). Long-distance excitatory pathways are generally glutamatergic, with the notable exceptions of the dopamine (DA) projection from the substantia nigra pars compacta (SNPC) to the striatum, which contains cholinergic interneurons (among other types) within it. ES, external segment; Glu, glutamine; IS, internal segment; PPN, pedunculopontine nucleus; SNPR, substantia nigra pars reticulata. (Reproduced with permission from Barrett KE, Barman SM, Brooks HL et al: *Ganong's Review of Medical Physiology*, 26th ed. New York, NY: McGraw Hill; 2019.)

dopamine-releasing cells underlies Parkinson disease. There is also a direct inhibitory GABAergic pathway from the portion of the SN called the pars reticulata to the thalamus.

Thus, the SN has reciprocal connections with the caudate and putamen via dopamine projections from the SNPC to the striatum and GABAergic projections from the striatum back to the SN. The dopaminergic SNPC neurons act on both excitatory D_1 receptors and inhibitory D_2 receptors in the striatum. The GABAergic inhibitory projections from the striatum to the SN complete a feedback loop between the SN and caudate and putamen.

The SN projection to the basal ganglia is generally thought to be organized in 2 main pathways, called direct and indirect (see Figure 17–3B and Figure 17–8). The direct pathway is mediated by D_1 receptor neurons in the putamen projecting to GPi. The indirect pathway involves D_2 neurons in putamen projecting to GPe, which projects to GPi and to the STN to inhibit nonselected movements. In this pathway, the STN is inhibited by the globus pallidus. The direct pathway (SNPC GPe to GPi to VL thalamus) also inhibits nonselected movements but facilitates selected ones.

There is also a direct output from the basal ganglia to the cerebellum, shown in Figure 17–8, via a projection in the central tegmental tract that relays to the contralateral cerebellum. The basal ganglia also project to the red nucleus in the brainstem that also receives cerebellar and motor cortex inputs.

DISEASES OF THE BASAL GANGLIA

Basal ganglia disorders arise primarily from damage to nuclei or tracts in this complex reciprocally connected system. Generally, these disorders are associated with compromised motor function, either deficient (hypokinesia), as in Parkinson disease, or excessive (hyperkinesia), as in Huntington. These dysfunctions typically reflect aberrations in the final common output of the basal ganglia to the thalamus, where appropriate motor sequences are enabled and inappropriate ones inhibited. There can also be cognitive dysfunctions associated with these disorders, particularly in their late stages.

Parkinson Disease

Parkinson disease is caused by the loss of dopaminergic projecting neurons from the SN (SNPC) to the basal ganglia. Figure 17–6 shows the contrasting activity in the various projection branches of the normal (Figure 17–6A) versus parkinsonian (Figure 17–6B) basal ganglia. In Parkinson disease, the input from the SN is reduced or eventually absent. The lowered activation of the inhibitory D_2 receptors in the putamen results in a disinhibitory increase in the putamen's inhibition of the GPe segment, producing a disinhibitory increase in the output of the STN, whose larger excitatory

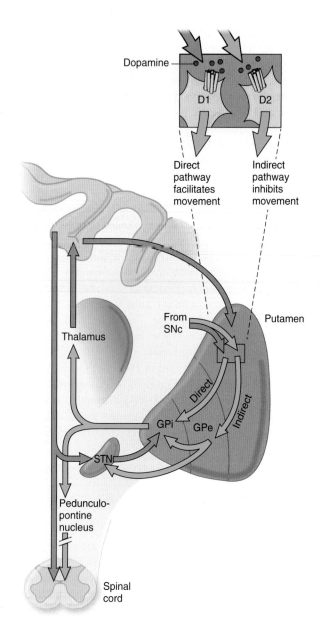

FIGURE 17–8 Details of the direct versus indirect pathway from the substantia nigra to putamen to globus pallidus. Excitatory connections are in orange, and inhibitory connections are in green. Within the putamen (magnified cutaway at top) are dopamine D_1 and D_2 receptors that mediate the direct and indirect pathways to the globus pallidus. In the direct pathway, D_1 receptor–mediated activity in putamen projects directly to the globus pallidus internal segment (GPi), whereas the indirect pathway from D_2 receptor–mediated activity in the putamen involves a projection first to the globus pallidus external segment (GPe) that in turn projects to GPi. GPi also receives input from the subthalamic nucleus (STN). The output of the basal ganglia is primarily that of GPi to thalamus (inhibitory toward nonselected movements with some [not shown] facilitation of selected ones). GPi also projects to the brainstem. SNc, substantia nigra pars compacta. (Reproduced with permission from Kandel ER, Schwartz JH, Jessell TM, et al: *Principles of Neural Science*, 5th ed. New York, NY: McGraw Hill; 2013.)

output overinhibits the VL thalamus. The loss of input from the SN also produces the larger inhibitory output of the GPi via the direct pathway.

Patient symptoms include difficulty in initiating and modifying motion sequences such as walking, balance problems, tremor, and muscle rigidity. Parkinson patients may also experience mild cognitive impairment early in the disease progression that becomes more severe as the disease progresses. These cognitive impairments mirror, at a high level, some of the lower level motor problems such as difficulty making and following through on plans and being overwhelmed by distractions.

Huntington Disease

Huntington disease is in many ways the opposite of Parkinson disease, being a hyperkinesia rather than a hypokinesia and stemming from a different basal ganglia degeneration. Figure 17–9 compares normal, Parkinson, and Huntington basal ganglia operation. Whereas in Parkinson disease there is reduced input from the SN, Huntington disease is associated with degeneration of the striatum (caudate and putamen). Decreased inhibition from the degenerated striatum causes a reduced inhibition of the GPi in the direct pathway. The reduced striatal input causes reduced excitation of GPi via the indirect pathway. Both lead to reduced inhibitory output to the thalamus, which is unable to then inhibit multiple cortical movement commands, resulting in hyperkinesia.

Unlike Parkinson disease, whose ultimate cause (degeneration of the SN) is unknown, Huntington disease has a clear molecular origin. Huntington patients have, on chromosome 4, an extended CAG repeat that produces a long polyglutamine repeat sequence in the huntingtin protein (whose normal function is not yet currently known).

Huntington disease is associated with other impairments besides hyperkinesia, including cognitive effects. These include problems with memory, reasoning, and decision making and difficulties in awareness and focusing attention. As in Parkinson disease, cognitive symptoms are usually mild early in the course of the disease, but become more severe later.

Other Basal Ganglia Disorders

There are a number of disorders traditionally classified as basal ganglia disorders that may involve the basal ganglia without the origin of the dysfunction being within the basal ganglia. Dystonia, for example, is characterized by involuntary movement and reduced velocity in intentional movement. Dystonia can be a side effect of Parkinson disease but may also occur after cerebellar degeneration.

Hemiballismus is uncontrolled movement on 1 side of the body, frequently associated with damage to the STN. This causes a reduced inhibitory output from GPi and, therefore, has a Huntington disease–like result of hyperkinesia.

Tourette syndrome is characterized by involuntary tics and sometimes brief vocalizations. It has a strong genetic component, but its exact cause is unknown. Some studies have indicated a reduction in the size of the caudate associated with Tourette syndrome. There is also an unknown causal link association between Tourette syndrome and obsessive-compulsive disorder.

THE CEREBELLUM: COORDINATOR OF MOVEMENT SEQUENCES

The cerebellum is one of the least understood areas of the brain. It is thought to contain over 50 billion neurons, a count on the order of half of the total neurons in the entire brain! It

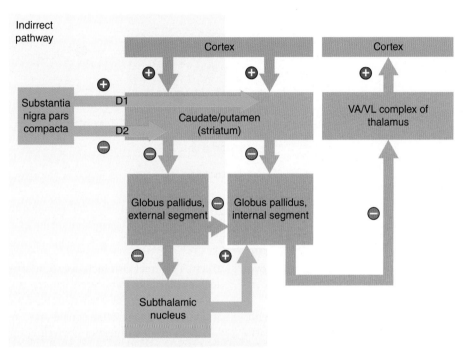

A Normal configuration of basal ganglia connections

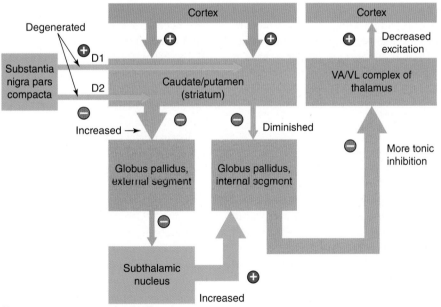

B Parkinson disease (hypokinetic)

FIGURE 17–9 A comparison of basal ganglia circuit activity in normal subjects (**A**) and those with Parkinson disease (**B**) and Huntington disease (**C**). Parkinson disease is characterized by reduced dopamine-mediated output from the substantia nigra, resulting in excessive inhibition in the projection from globus pallidus internal segment (GPi) to thalamus. Huntington disease is associated with reduced striatal activity and output and insufficient inhibition in the GPi-to-thalamus pathway. VA, ventroanterior; VL, ventrolateral. (Reproduced with permission from Ropper AH, Samuels MA, Klein JP: *Adams and Victor's Principles of Neurology*, 11th ed. New York, NY: McGraw Hill; 2019.)

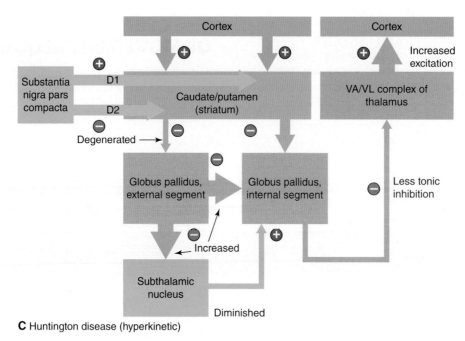

C Huntington disease (hyperkinetic)

FIGURE 17–9   *(Continued)*

has also expanded considerably in primate and hominid evolution, but this is rarely mentioned in deference to the expansion of the prefrontal neocortex.

What does the cerebellum do, and what can't you do without it? The cerebellum is a crucial structure in motor learning and coordination. Given this function, it is not surprising that cerebellar injury is associated with difficulties in making coordinated movements. Patients with cerebellar injuries walk with a slow, staggering, wide gait and are unable to make rapid alternating hand movements or reach to a target and stop before hitting it. These symptoms are similar to what is checked in a traffic stop sobriety test because the cerebellum is one of the first areas of the brain to be affected by alcohol.

Structure & Inputs & Outputs of the Cerebellum

The cerebellum extends from the posterior brainstem opposite the pons, where much of it is tucked underneath the occipital lobe (Figure 17–10A). Its surface is highly convoluted, derived from the architecture of generating a large surface area within a small volume, in a manner similar to that of the neocortex. It has 10 major lobules, numbered I through X.

Figure 17–11 shows some features of the input/output connections of the cerebellum, made through fiber tracts called peduncles. There are 3 peduncles on each side of the brainstem, called superior, middle, and inferior. The cutaway view in Figure 17–11A shows these tracts at the junction between the posterior brainstem and the cerebellum. Figure 17–11B shows details of some of the tracts within the superior peduncle, the main output tract of the cerebellum, via the cerebellorubral, fastigioreticular, and dentatothalamic

tracts. This tract also includes some afferents, such as the tectocerebellar and spinocerebellar tracts. The superior peduncular tracts enter the brainstem beneath the inferior colliculi in the midbrain.

Important connections traveling in the superior, middle, and inferior cerebellar peduncles are shown in Figure 17–12. The middle cerebellar peduncle is primarily an afferent tract from the pons to the cerebellum conveying vestibular and proprioceptive sensory information to the spinocerebellum (spinocerebellar, cuneocerebellar, olivocerebellar, and trigeminocerebellar tracts) and vestibulocerebellum (vestibulocerebellar tract). Minority efferent fibers in the middle cerebellar peduncle include cerebellar Purkinje cell output to vestibular nuclei in the brainstem. The inferior peduncle receives afferents from the Clarke nucleus in the spinal cord and several midbrain nuclei including the inferior olive and the trigeminal and arcuate nuclei. A major efferent of the inferior peduncle is to the vestibular nucleus.

Gross Organization of the Cerebellum

The cerebellum has a complex anatomic organization, with 10 cerebellar lobules (Figure 17–10) and divisions between anterior, medial, and lateral areas (Figure 17–13). Functionally, the cerebellum has 3 main divisions: the vestibulocerebellum, spinocerebellum, and cerebrocerebellum.

The vestibulocerebellum (also called the archicerebellum) is the phylogenetically oldest region of this structure. It consists anatomically of the ventral nodulus of the vermis and the flocculus. This part of the cerebellum receives inputs from the vestibular system and visual input driven by motion-sensitive retinal ganglion cells and mediates balance, equilibrium, and

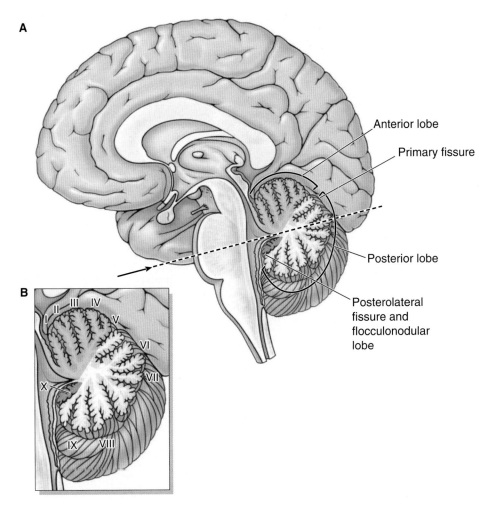

FIGURE 17–10 **A.** Midsagittal view of the cerebellum in relation to the entire brain. **B.** Details of the cerebellar lobules. The vermis is the midline (medial) region of the cerebellum. (Reproduced with permission from Martin JH. *Neuroanatomy: Text and Atlas*, 4th ed. New York, NY: McGraw Hill; 2012.)

coordinated eye movements such as the maintenance of fixation by eye movement compensation for head and body movement (vestibulo-ocular reflex; VOR).

Anatomically, the spinocerebellum is the medial region of the cerebellum consisting of the vermis and areas slightly lateral to the vermis called paravermis (see Figure 17–12). This cerebellar region mediates coordinated limb movement, including participating in the learning of complex movements. It receives proprioceptive and kinesthetic inputs from the spinal cord (spinocerebellar tract), inputs from the head and face via the trigeminal nerve, and auditory and visual input. Typical of cerebellar circuits, external sensory inputs synapse on cells in the cerebellar cortex, and these relay to deep cerebellar nuclei. The proprioceptive output of the spinocerebellum is to frontal cortical areas via the thalamus, whereas the vestibular output projects to several midbrain nuclei that in turn may project to the frontal lobe. The spinocerebellum mediates feedforward motor control that involves an internal model of the results of motor actions, such as reaching for a glass of water and stopping the hand in the proper grasping position.

The lateral regions of the cerebellum comprise the cerebrocerebellum (also called the neocerebellum). This part of the cerebellum, which has expanded greatly in primates and humans, mediates high-level planning and motor behavior evaluation. It is also involved in cognition. For example, the cerebrocerebellum is active while imagining the movement of pieces when playing chess and is thus important in anticipatory planning. Inputs to the cerebrocerebellum come mostly from proprioceptive areas of the parietal lobe via several pontine nuclei. The output of the cerebrocerebellum is to the frontal lobe (primarily to M1) via the VL thalamus and to the red nucleus in the brainstem, both of which modulate motor sequence production. The red nucleus projects to the inferior olive, which sends a reciprocal signal back to the cerebellum.

Neural Circuits, Physiology, & Learning in the Cerebellum

The cerebellum has a unique, highly repeated cellular architecture involving 5 major cell types: Purkinje, granule, stellate, basket, and Golgi cells, shown in Figure 17–14A. Input axons to the

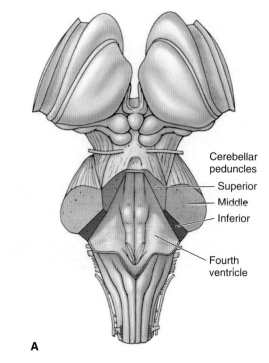

A

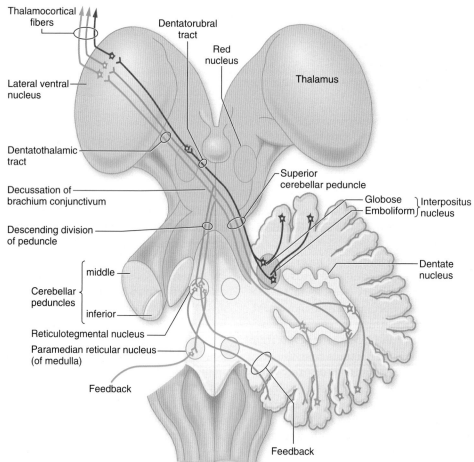

B

FIGURE 17–11 **A.** Cutaway view of the superior, middle, and inferior cerebellar peduncles (fiber tracts). **B.** Some constituents of the superior peduncular fiber tract. Afferent axons from the reticulotegmental nucleus are shown in light blue. Efferent axons projecting to thalamus are shown in green, blue, and purple. (Part A, reproduced with permission from Martin JH. *Neuroanatomy: Text and Atlas*, 4th ed. New York, NY: McGraw Hill; 2012; part B, reproduced with permission from Ropper AH, Samuels MA, Klein JP: *Adams and Victor's Principles of Neurology*, 10th ed. New York, NY: McGraw Hill; 2014.)

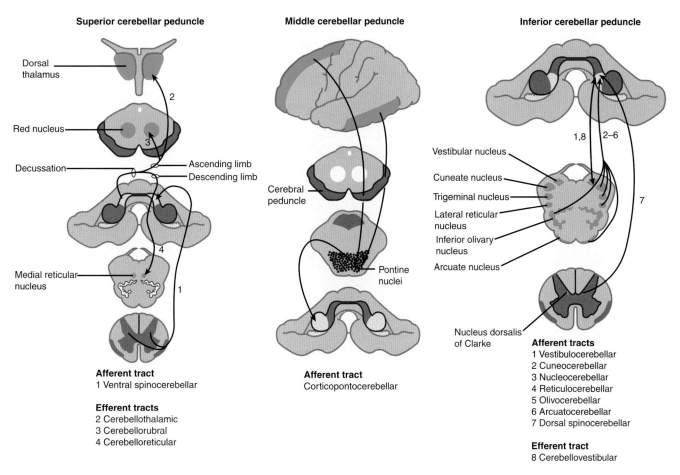

FIGURE 17-12 Connections of the superior, middle, and inferior cerebellar peduncles. (Reproduced with permission from Aminoff MJ, Greenberg DA, Simon RP: *Clinical Neurology*. 9th ed. New York, NY: McGraw Hill; 2015.)

cerebellum enter via the peduncles as mossy and climbing fibers. The axons of granule cells within the granule cell layer generate the parallel fibers of the molecular layer. Cerebellar computations are done in the outer layers (cortex) and are then projected to deep cerebellar nuclei that provide most of the output.

Outside the deep nuclei are 3 major layers in the cerebellar cortex: molecular, Purkinje, and granule (see Figure 17-14A). The molecular layer is composed of the flat, fan-shaped Purkinje cell dendritic trees with the parallel fibers running through them perpendicular to their major extent, where they make excitatory synaptic contacts with Purkinje cell dendrites. The major interneurons in this layer are GABAergic stellate and basket cells that make inhibitory synapses onto the Purkinje cell dendrites.

Below the molecular layer is the Purkinje cell layer where the Purkinje cell bodies and the soma of glial cells are located. Below that is the granule cell layer with the numerous small granule cell bodies that constitute a majority of the neurons in the cerebellum. Also in this layer are the cell bodies of Golgi cells and several other classes of cells.

Mossy Fibers

The mossy fiber input originates in brainstem pontine, vestibular, and reticular nuclei and spinocerebellar tracts. There

are approximately 200 million mossy fiber axons, making this tract comparable in size to the massive corpus callosum that connects the 2 cerebral hemispheres. Each mossy fiber arborizes to make approximately 500 excitatory synapses onto many granule cells, as well as projecting directly to deep cerebellar nuclei (see Figure 17-11B). The granule cell axons are the parallel fibers that contact Purkinje cells, whose axons also project to the deep cerebellar nuclei.

Climbing Fibers

Climbing fibers originate from the contralateral superior olive, which in turn receives input from the spinal cord, brainstem nuclei, and proprioceptive areas of the parietal lobe. Like the mossy fibers, these axons also send collaterals to deep cerebellar nuclei. The synaptic output of the climbing fibers is very specific, with each axon giving off approximately 10 axon terminals, each of which contacts 1 and only 1 Purkinje cell in a characteristic "wrapping" morphology (see Figure 17-14B). This single climbing fiber axon terminal makes several hundred contacts onto the Purkinje cell, such that a single climbing fiber action potential reliably produces a complex Purkinje cell action potential, called a complex spike. This unique complex spike is an important,

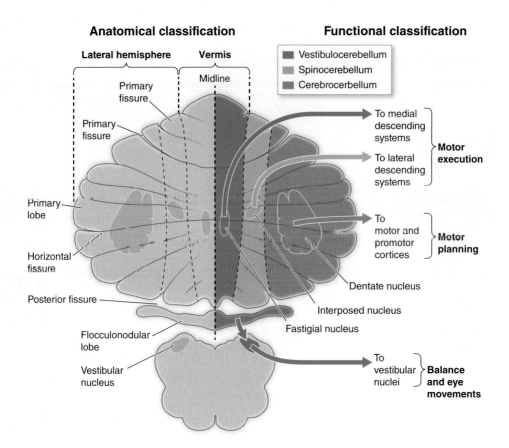

FIGURE 17–13 Anatomic divisions of the cerebellum with outputs and functions shown.

although not well-understood, essential mechanism in cerebellar output and learning.

The Cerebellum & Learning

The cerebellum controls subtle changes in motor performance that occur when a task is repeated or practiced. Tasks that are completely novel depend primarily on working memory in the prefrontal cortex. As tasks are practiced, sensory feedback from the parietal cortex and learning signals from the cerebellum shift control to the premotor cortex (see Chapter 16) and then, ultimately, to the supplementary motor area. The learning mechanism involves the interplay between mossy and climbing fiber inputs to Purkinje cells. Individual Purkinje cells receive inputs from many mossy fibers from an extended region of body sensors but are activated by only 1 climbing fiber. The complex spike induced by the climbing fiber, when it occurs, produces long-term changes in the efficacy of mossy fiber inputs, changing the timing modulation produced by different Purkinje cells. The stacking of the fan-shaped Purkinje cell dendritic trees one on top of another represents a timing layout for programming the sequence of motor activations in performing a complex task.

Cerebellar Output

Virtually all cerebellar output is from the deep nuclei except for the flocculonodular lobe in the vestibulocerebellum that projects to the vestibular nuclei. Neurons in the deep nuclei receive inhibitory inputs from Purkinje cells in the cerebellar cortex and collaterals from mossy and climbing fibers. Figure 17–11B shows 3 of the 4 major deep nuclei: the 2 interpositus nuclei (globose and emboliform) and the dentate nucleus. The fastigial nucleus on each side (not shown) is immediately medial and superior to the globose nucleus. The dentate and interpositus nuclei are part of the spinocerebellum, whereas the dentate nucleus receives almost exclusive input from the cerebrocerebellum.

The cerebellum is unique among brain structures in being associated with the ipsilateral side of the body. This occurs because sensory inputs cross before entering the cerebellum, and modulatory outputs from the deep nuclei cross again as efferents. The majority of deep nuclear cerebellar output is to the VL thalamus and the red nucleus via glutamatergic axons, although a few projection cells to the inferior olive are GABAergic.

Dysfunctions & Diseases Affecting the Cerebellum

Cerebellar damage or genetic abnormalities in the cerebellum are exhibited as various kinds of ataxia, or movement difficulties. These include slowness, inability to reach to an object and stop at the right time, oscillations (tremor) during reaching,

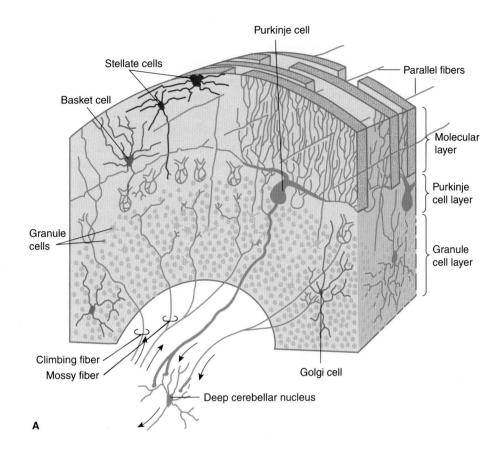

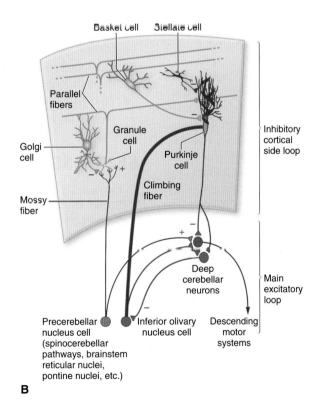

FIGURE 17–14 **A.** Schematic section of the cerebellar cortex showing the molecular, Purkinje, and granule layers and location of constituent cell types and fiber tracts. **B.** Detailed view of the canonical cerebellar circuit involving the external mossy and climbing fiber inputs to the Purkinje cell, and the granule cell parallel fiber projection. (Part A, reproduced with permission from Waxman SG. *Clinical Neuroanatomy*, 28th ed. New York, NY: McGraw Hill; 2017; part B, reproduced with permission from Raymond JL, Lisberger SG, Mauk MD: The cerebellum: a neuronal learning machine? *Science.* 1996 May 24;272(5265):1126-1131.)

balance problems, a wide-based unsteady gait, and slurred speech. Patients with cerebellum damage also characteristically have difficulty coordinating multijoint movements smoothly. They tend to produce a sequence of joint rotations rather than a single smooth movement of all joints simultaneously, called movement decomposition. Deficiencies in the compensatory eye movement during head movement to retain fixation vestibulo-ocular-reflex (VOR) are also characteristic of cerebellar damage, as is the failure to demonstrate classical (Pavlovian) conditioning, wherein a tone, predicting an air puff to the eye, does not yield by learning the conditioned response to blink.

CONCLUSION

Extrapyramidal motor systems are the components of motor control outside the corticospinal direct upper motor neuron to lower motor neuron pathway. These systems include the basal ganglia, thalamus, frontal and prefrontal lobe system, and cerebellum. The basal ganglia are a phylogenetically old motor control system for initiating movement and modifying ongoing movement sequences to meet environmental challenges, such as obstacles. Although many of the details of numerous motor sequences are represented in the frontal lobes, the specific motor sequence path from the overall goal to which muscles are activated in what order is mediated by the connections with the basal ganglia operating as a feedforward controller. That is, given the current motor state and environmental feedback, they choose the next motor component in the sequence. Two well-known diseases of the basal ganglia, Parkinson and Huntington disease, are characterized by inability to initiate or modify movement sequences, respectively.

The cerebellum also coordinates motion sequences by learning the precise timing and motor gain for various tasks. Within the cerebellum are 3 major subsystems: the vestibulocerebellum, spinocerebellum, and cerebrocerebellum. The vestibulocerebellum deals with balance and equilibrium via vestibular and visual motion-sensitive inputs. The spinocerebellum coordinates limb movements, whereas the cerebrocerebellum deals with higher order planning and goal implementation, including activity in cognitive tasks that involve motion imagery. The cerebellum is also a feedforward controller that builds a model of the motor system allowing accurate ballistic sequences, such as smoothly reaching out and extending one's arm to grasp to a cup of water and stopping with the hand open at exactly the right position. Damage to the cerebellum resembles a drunken state with characteristics such as slurred speech, uncoordinated movement, and inability to execute accurate ballistic movements. The cerebellum is, in fact, one of the first brain structures affected by alcohol consumption.

SUMMARY

- Extrapyramidal motor systems are the components of motor control outside the corticospinal direct upper motor neuron to lower motor neuron pathway.

- Extrapyramidal motor systems include the basal ganglia, thalamus, frontal and prefrontal lobe system, and cerebellum.
- The basal ganglia are a phylogenetically old motor control system for initiating movement and modifying ongoing movement sequences to meet environmental challenges, such as obstacles.
- The basal ganglia initiate and sequence movement via their projections to the thalamus.
- The inputs to the basal ganglia are via the caudate and putamen, which together are called the striatum.
- The globus pallidus, divided into internal and external segments, is the main processing area of the basal ganglia.
- Two midbrain areas, the SN and STN, are extensively connected with the basal ganglia and often considered part of the basal ganglia complex.
- Most of the output of the basal ganglia is from the globus pallidus internal segment to the thalamus, with most of this output being primarily inhibitory, with excitation only to the chosen motor sequence subset and inhibition of all other alternatives.
- Parkinson disease is caused by degeneration of dopaminergic neurons in the basal ganglia.
- The cerebellum coordinates motor sequences through learning.
- The neocerebellum, or lateral cerebellum, coordinates motor sequences through connections to premotor cortical areas.
- The spinocerebellum coordinates motor sequences through connections to brainstem and spinal neurons.
- The vestibulocerebellum coordinates balance and posture during movement.

SELF-ASSESSMENT QUESTIONS

1. A 46-year-old woman receives a diagnosis of having a movement disorder associated with disturbances of the basal ganglia. In particular, she presents with writhing, uncoordinated movements at rest of her left arm and leg. A magnetic resonance imaging scan reveals the presence of a tumor affecting mainly the right caudate nucleus and putamen. Which of the following best explains why the dysfunction is expressed on the side of the body contralateral to the region of the basal ganglia directly affected by the stroke?

   A. Fibers from the basal ganglia to the spinal cord are crossed.
   B. Fibers from the basal ganglia project to motor nuclei of the brainstem, whose axons then project to the contralateral spinal cord.
   C. Fibers from the basal ganglia project to the ipsilateral motor cortex.
   D. Axons from the basal ganglia project to the cerebellum, whose outputs are known to modulate the contralateral side of the body.
   E. Fibers from the basal ganglia project directly to the contralateral motor cortex.

2. A 43-year-old man who began to display marked involuntary movements at times of rest is seen by a neurologist, who concludes that he is suffering from Huntington disease. Which of the following neurotransmitters is lost or reduced in this individual?

A. Dopamine in the neostriatum

B. Substance P in the substantia nigra

C. Acetylcholine (ACh) and γ-aminobutyric acid (GABA) in intrastriatal and cortical neurons

D. Serotonin in the neostriatum

E. Histamine in subthalamic nucleus

3. Two 18-year-old men were experimenting with designer drugs, and after they took the drugs, each of the men presents with a movement disorder associated with basal ganglia dysfunction. The drug is later identified as the neurotoxin 1-methyl-4-phenyl-l,2,3,6-tetrahydropyridine (MPTP), which has recently been applied experimentally with considerable success as a model for the study of which of the following diseases?

A. Huntington disease

B. Hemiballismus

C. Parkinson disease

D. Tardive dyskinesia

E. Dystonia

4. A 25-year-old man, who began to have difficulty in walking, is examined by a neurologist and neurosurgeon. They conclude that a tumor is pressing on the lateral aspect of his spinal cord, affecting primarily the spinocerebellar tracts. Which of the following structures is the principal region within the cerebellum that receives these fibers?

A. Anterior lobe

B. Posterior lobe

C. Flocculonodular lobe

D. Fastigial nucleus

E. Dentate nucleus

5. A 23-year-old woman is exposed to a neurotoxin that selectively destroyed the Purkinje cell layer of the cerebellum, resulting in loss of balance and coordination. Which of the following structures or regions is most directly affected by the loss of Purkinje cells?

A. Red nucleus

B. Deep cerebellar nuclei

C. Reticular formation

D. Ventrolateral nucleus (thalamus)

E. Spinal cord

Autonomic Nervous System: Sympathetic, Parasympathetic, & Enteric

Franklin R. Amthor

Franklin R. Amthor

OBJECTIVES

After studying this chapter, the student should be able to:

- Understand the differences between the central, peripheral, autonomic, and enteric nervous systems (ENS).
- Understand the antagonism between the sympathetic and parasympathetic divisions of the autonomic nervous systems.
- See how the neurotransmitters acetylcholine (ACh) and norepinephrine mediate autonomic nervous system control.
- Understand the organization and projections of the cephalic portion of the autonomic nervous system.
- See how the sympathetic and parasympathetic divisions of the autonomic nervous system operate at the spinal cord level.
- Understand the role of the brainstem in autonomic nervous system processing.
- See the crucial roles of the hypothalamus and pituitary gland in autonomic control.
- Understand the organs controlled by the autonomic nervous system and notable disorders associated with autonomic nervous system dysfunction.

OVERVIEW

The nervous system consists of the central, peripheral, autonomic, and enteric systems. This chapter will discuss the autonomic and enteric nervous systems (ENS). The autonomic nervous system receives inputs from receptors in glands and cardiac and smooth muscle and sends motor commands to those areas. The enteric nervous system is the nervous system of digestion. Previously, the ENS was considered part of the autonomic nervous system, but it is now generally treated separately, occasionally being referred to as the "second brain."

The autonomic nervous system consists of sympathetic and parasympathetic branches that generally have opposite effects on organs such as the heart and lungs. The sympathetic system activates the fight-or-flight response, whereas parasympathetic activity promotes homeostatic functions such as digestion and the immune system. A major output of the autonomic nervous system is the hypothalamus via the reticular formation.

OUTSIDE THE CENTRAL NERVOUS SYSTEM: THE ENTERIC & AUTONOMIC NERVOUS SYSTEMS

The brain is the locus of consciousness and consciously controlled behavior. The brain also interacts with an extended nervous system outside the brain that controls body metabolic processes such as respiration, heart rate, temperature, and digestion. This control is mediated by neural clusters in various parts of the body called ganglia, which exist even in invertebrates. Vertebrate ganglia are the control centers for the autonomic and enteric nervous systems. These systems interact with the central nervous system (CNS) in the brainstem and hypothalamus.

The Enteric Nervous System

Life requires the consumption of nutrients and water and the removal of waste products of digestion. The ENS mediates homeostasis by controlling digestion and influencing hunger and satiety. This control requires interaction with the autonomic nervous system and CNS. The more central systems set priorities for digestion versus other body functions. **Figure 18–1** shows a block diagram of the neural control of digestion that illustrates the location of the ENS in the control scheme and the means and loci of interaction with other parts of the nervous system. Digestive control includes both neural projections and neurohumoral regulatory mechanisms.

Overview of the Autonomic Nervous System

The autonomic nervous system is composed of 2 opposing divisions, called the sympathetic and parasympathetic branches. These 2 branches have well-defined neurotransmitters and projection pathways in both the head and spinal cord. **Figure 18–2** shows a comparison between the projection system for somatic voluntary motor control versus that for the

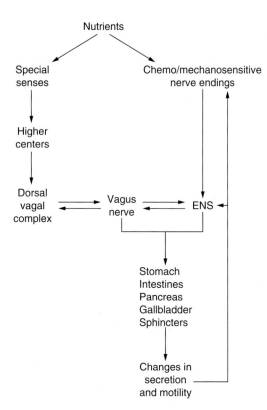

FIGURE 18–1 Neural control of the gastrointestinal system. Receptors in the digestive system have direct connections to the enteric nervous system (ENS) and indirect connections via the autonomic nervous system. The output of the ENS controls digestive system sphincters and modulates secretion and motility. (Reproduced with permission from Barrett KE. *Gastrointestinal Physiology*, 2nd ed. New York, NY: McGraw Hill; 2014.)

sympathetic and autonomic nervous systems. In the somatic motor nervous system (Figure 18–2, top), cholinergic neurons project from a CNS nucleus or ventral spinal cord root to a muscle.

The sympathetic and parasympathetic systems share a similar first stage in which a cholinergic (acetylcholine-releasing) neuron in the CNS (brain and spinal cord) projects toward an organ outside the CNS. In the parasympathetic nervous system, the CNS cholinergic neuron projects directly to a ganglion (concentration of neurons) at the effector organ. These neurons are also typically cholinergic (Figure 18–2, middle).

CNS cholinergic neurons of the sympathetic nervous system, however, project to a set of ganglia just outside the CNS. The output of these ganglia are neurons that release norepinephrine (NE) at the target effector organ (Figure 18–2, bottom). Acetylcholine (ACh) from the parasympathetic system and NE from the sympathetic system typically have opposite effects on the target organ. Parasympathetic ACh slows the heart, for example, whereas NE increases heart rate. The bottom of Figure 18–2 also shows the sympathetic projection to the outer portion of the adrenal gland (adrenal medulla). The adrenal medulla participates in neurohumoral control via the release of several neurotransmitters into the bloodstream, particularly epinephrine but also NE and dopamine. The adrenal medulla also releases neuroactive peptides into the bloodstream.

A simplified overall view of the organization of the autonomic projections from the spinal cord can be seen in **Figure 18–3**. Cholinergic CNS neurons in the parasympathetic system project directly to ganglia associated with peripheral organs, such as shown for brainstem cephalic neurons at the top of the figure. Cholinergic sympathetic neurons project to sympathetic ganglia just outside the spinal cord, illustrated in the middle of the figure. Norepinephrine neurons in these ganglia project to the target organs. Below that, the figure illustrates the sympathetic projection to the adrenal medulla. At the bottom of the figure is shown a typical voluntary somatic motor projection to a skeletal muscle, as in the top of Figure 18–2.

OVERALL ORGANIZATION OF THE AUTONOMIC NERVOUS SYSTEM

The organization of the autonomic nervous system is somewhat different depending on whether the CNS control of it emanates from the brain or spinal cord. **Figure 18–4** shows a more detailed schematic diagram of connections between the CNS and autonomic nervous system that illustrates some differences between the connection schemes of the brain versus those of the spinal cord. Parasympathetic control by the brain of various peripheral targets such as glands and involuntary muscles in the head is mediated by cranial nerves, particularly cranial nerves III, VII, and IX. Cranial nerve X projects to body organs such as the heart and lungs (right side of Figure 18–4).

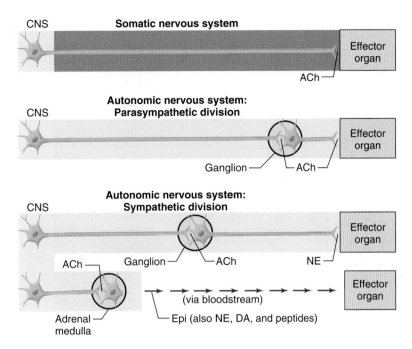

FIGURE 18–2 Cellular circuits of the somatic nervous system and parasympathetic and sympathetic divisions of the autonomic nervous system. In the somatic nervous system (*top*), cholinergic neurons project from a central nervous system (CNS) nucleus or ventral spinal cord root to a muscle. In the parasympathetic division of the autonomic nervous system, the CNS cholinergic neuron projects directly to a ganglion (concentration of neurons) at the effector organ. The neurons of the ganglion are also typically cholinergic (*middle*). Cholinergic CNS neurons of the sympathetic division of the autonomic nervous system, however, project to a set of ganglia just outside the CNS. The output of these ganglia are neurons that release norepinephrine at the target effector organ (*bottom*). The sympathetic division of the autonomic nervous system also projects to the outer portion of the adrenal gland (adrenal medulla). The adrenal medulla participates in neurohumoral control via the release of several neurotransmitters into the bloodstream, particularly epinephrine (Epi), but also norepinephrine (NE), dopamine (DA), and peptides (*bottom*). ACh, acetylcholine. (Reproduced with permission from Widmaier EP, Raff H, Strang KT. *Vander's Human Physiology*, 11th ed. New York, NY: McGraw Hill; 2008.)

Note that the only parasympathetic output from the spinal cord is via sacral segments (Figure 18–4, bottom right) that innervate colon, kidney, bladder, and sex organs.

Some of the sympathetic output from the spinal cord is shown on the left side of Figure 18–4. Several thoracic segments project upward to the superior sympathetic ganglion, which projects sympathetic control to organs in the head such as the pupil and various glands, generally opposing parasympathetic innervation of those same targets. Thoracic and lumbar spinal segments project to the spinal sympathetic ganglia system, from which NE neurons project to target organs in the body.

Organization of the Cephalic Portion of the Sympathetic & Parasympathetic Systems

The cranial portion of the autonomic nervous system is mediated by cranial nerves III, VII, and IX. Highlights of its layout are shown in Figure 18–5, with parasympathetic projections shown as solid blue lines and sympathetic axons as dashed blue lines. At the top of the figure, parasympathetic neurons in the Edinger-Westphal nucleus project via the inferior branch of the oculomotor nerve (cranial nerve III) to the ciliary ganglion. Cholinergic nerves there control pupil dilation.

Below this system in the figure is illustrated the projection of cranial nerve VII to the geniculate and sphenopalatine ganglia that innervate the lacrimal gland and nasal and palatine mucous membranes. A portion of cranial nerve VII projects in the chorda tympani nerve to the sublingual and submaxillary glands. Second from bottom in the figure, cranial nerve IX projects to the otic ganglion of the auditory system. At the bottom of the figure are sympathetic projections from thoracic spinal cord segments that ascend to the superior cervical sympathetic ganglion and project to the submaxillary ganglion and submaxillary gland. Some sensory afferents are shown in the figure (dotted blue lines) that run in the same nerves with autonomic axons.

Sympathetic & Parasympathetic Organization of the Spinal Cord

Figure 18–6 shows the overall organization of the sympathetic projections from the spinal cord with respect to the major organs innervated by the sympathetic ganglion. The majority of sympathetic projections are from cholinergic neurons in the thoracic and upper lumbar spinal cord segments. The dominance of sympathetic over parasympathetic innervation is a switch from emphasis on homeostatic processes such as digestion to voluntary action-oriented processes in which homeostasis is suppressed and metabolic resources are allocated to

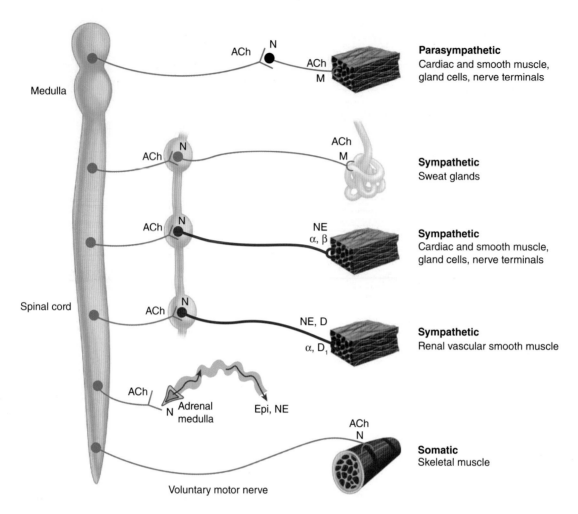

FIGURE 18-3 Overview of the general structure of the autonomic projections from the brain and spinal cord. Cephalic parasympathetic cholinergic neurons project to nicotinic acetylcholine (ACh) receptor neurons at target organs that are also cholinergic. These project to muscarinic receptors in the target organ. Spinal cholinergic neurons of the sympathetic division project to sympathetic neurons outside the spinal cord. Neurons in these ganglia project to the target organs and release norepinephrine (NE). The sympathetic projection to the adrenal medulla is also shown (*second from bottom*). The *bottom* of the figure shows the schematic organization of α motor neuron projection to voluntary skeletal muscle. ACh, acetylcholine; D, dopamine, D1, dopamine1 receptors; Epi, epinephrine; M, muscarinic; N, nicotinic; NE, norepinephrine. (Reproduced with permission from Katzung BG: *Basic and Clinical Pharmacology*, 14th ed. New York, NY: McGraw Hill; 2018.)

energetic fight-or-flight activity. The penalty of sympathetic dominance is the disruption of parasympathetic metabolic processing such as immune function, digestion, and organ repair and maintenance. These activities are postponed for the sake of short-term survival. It does no good to continue digesting your food properly if you are threatened to become food for a leopard.

The far right of Figure 18–6 shows the direction of the effect of sympathetic innervation on the target organs. Heart rate and contraction force increase, as does salivary gland secretion. Note that different receptor types for NE mediate different effects in different parts of the same target organ. For example, α_1 receptors in the pancreas decrease insulin secretion, but β_2 receptors there increase it. Similar opposing effects occur in other organs and in the vascular system. Sympathetic activation shunts blood toward voluntary muscles and away from areas of organs that mediate homeostatic processes.

An additional sympathetic target is the adrenal medulla (see Figures 18–2 and 18–3 and Figure 18–7), from which postsynaptic neurons release epinephrine and NE into the bloodstream. The release of NE produces rapid effects.

Neurons of the parasympathetic division of the autonomic nervous system have cell bodies in the brainstem and sacral spinal cord. These, like the CNS neurons of the sympathetic division, use the neurotransmitter ACh. Parasympathetic neural axons project all the way to the target organs, such as the heart, rather than relaying through extra-CNS ganglia, as is the case for the sympathetic division. Generally, parasympathetic neurons synapse on ganglia at target organs. In some cases, there are secondary neurons in those ganglia. These ganglionic neurons also typically use ACh as a neurotransmitter. The parasympathetic target organ cholinergic receptors are almost exclusively muscarinic, in contrast with those of muscles in the

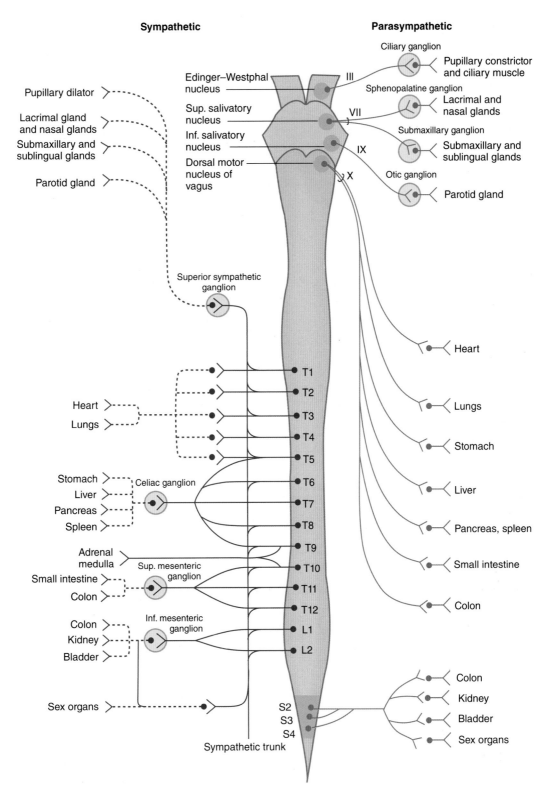

FIGURE 18–4 Overview of some differences between the cephalic versus spinal cord portions of the autonomic nervous system. Parasympathetic control by the brain of various peripheral targets such as glands and involuntary muscles in the head are mediated by cranial nerves III, VII, and IX. Cranial nerve X descends and projects to body organs such as the heart and lungs (*right side*). Parasympathetic projections in the spinal cord occur only from sacral segments (*bottom right*), which innervate colon, kidney, bladder, and sex organs. The *top left* of the figure shows that several thoracic segments project upward to the superior sympathetic ganglion that mediates sympathetic control of organs in the head such as the pupil and various glands, generally opposing parasympathetic innervation of those same targets. Below that is the sympathetic output from the spinal cord, shown on the *left*. Thoracic and lumbar spinal segments project to the spinal sympathetic ganglia system instead of the superior cervical ganglion. The neurons in the superior cervical ganglion and sympathetic spinal ganglia are norepinephrine releasing at target organs in the body. (Reproduced with permission from Waxman SG. *Clinical Neuroanatomy*, 28th ed. New York, NY: McGraw Hill; 2017.)

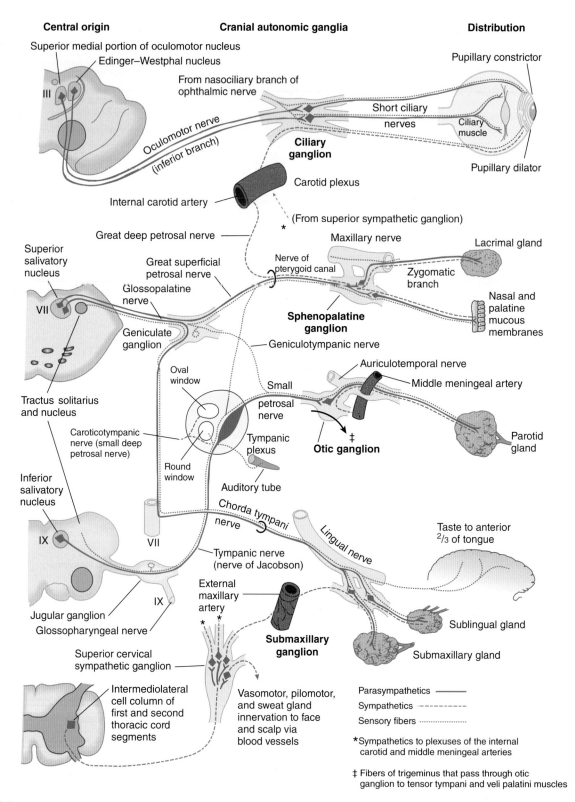

FIGURE 18–5 Cranial autonomic ganglia of the parasympathetic and sympathetic divisions of the autonomic nervous system. Parasympathetic projections are shown by *solid blue lines*; sympathetic axons are shown by *dashed blue lines*. Some sensory afferents are shown (*dotted blue lines*) that are in the same or nearby nerves with autonomic axons. At the top of the figure are projections from the Edinger-Westphal nucleus via the inferior branch of the oculomotor nerve (cranial nerve [CN] III) to the ciliary ganglia from which emanate ciliary nerves that control pupil dilation. Below that is the projection of CN VII to the geniculate and sphenopalatine ganglia that innervate the lacrimal gland and nasal and palatine mucous membranes. A portion of CN VII projects in the chorda tympani nerve to the sublingual and submaxillary glands. Second from bottom, CN IX projects to the otic ganglion of the auditory system. At the bottom are projections from thoracic spinal cord segments that ascend to the superior cervical sympathetic ganglion that has sympathetic projections to several targets, of which the submaxillary ganglion and submaxillary gland are shown. (Reproduced with permission from Waxman SG. *Clinical Neuroanatomy*, 28th ed. New York, NY: McGraw Hill; 2017.)

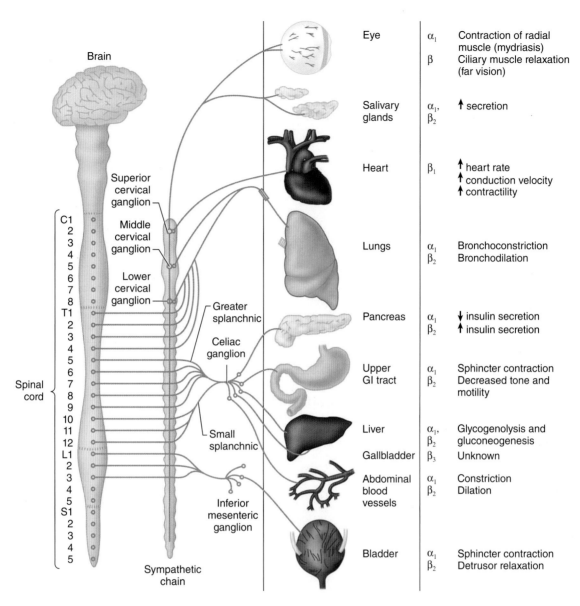

FIGURE 18−6 Sympathetic innervation of major organs. Cholinergic axons from the spinal cord synapse on the sympathetic ganglia chain outside it. Norepinephrine neurons project from these ganglia to the target organs. The effects on the target organs vary with the receptor types (α vs β). For example, in the case of blood vessels, flow is decreased to those involved in digestion, but increased to those serving voluntary musculature. (Reproduced with permission from Butterworth JF, Mackey DC, Wasnick JD: *Morgan & Mikhail's Clinical Anesthesiology*, 6th ed. New York, NY. McGraw Hill, 2018.)

somatic system that have nicotinic cholinergic receptors. Figure 18–7 illustrates somatic versus parasympathetic and sympathetic autonomic neurotransmitters and projection schemes.

Sensory Input to the Autonomic Nervous System

Sensory receptors in organs innervated by the autonomic nervous system project information into the system, in some cases in feedback arrangements in spinal cord circuits whose organization is similar to that of the stretch reflex for the somatic motor system. Autonomic receptors report

information about blood pressure, temperature, and carbon dioxide levels used to maintain homeostasis of those parameters. For example, the carotid artery neck has baroreceptors for blood pressure. These receptors project via the vagus nerve to the nucleus of the solitary tract (NST) of the medulla in the brainstem. The NST projects to the nucleus ambiguus and vagal nucleus. These ganglia are part of the parasympathetic division and release ACh to reduce heart rate. Thermoreceptors in the skin send temperature signals to autonomic motor neurons that control sweating and shivering. There are also thermoreceptors in the hypothalamus that regulate temperature. The hypothalamus is a major control center for the autonomic nervous system.

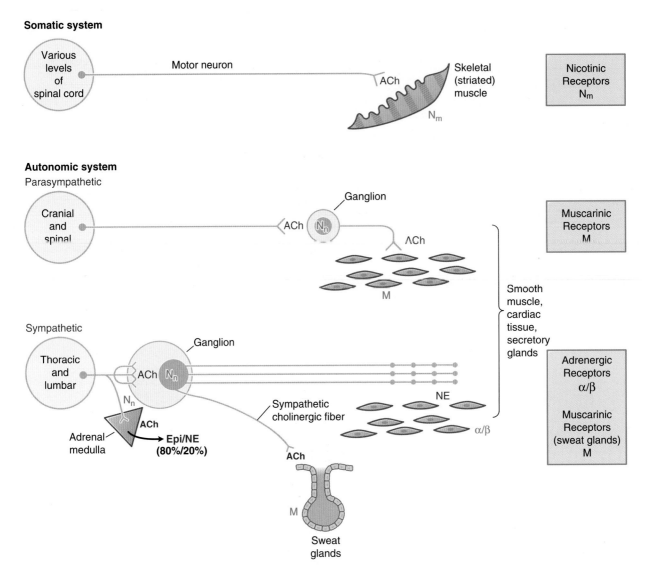

FIGURE 18–7 Comparison of the neurotransmitters and receptors of the somatic motor, parasympathetic, and sympathetic autonomic systems. In the somatic motor system, cholinergic spinal neurons project out the ventral root to nicotinic receptors on muscle cells. In the parasympathetic system, cranial and spinal cholinergic neurons project to ganglia at the target organs onto muscarinic synapses. In the sympathetic system, cholinergic neurons in thoracic and lumbar spinal cord segments project to sympathetic ganglia. From there, norepinephrine (NE)-releasing neurons project to target organs at α- or β-adrenergic synapses or muscarinic receptors on sweat glands. The sympathetic system also projects to the adrenal medulla, which releases both epinephrine (Epi) and NE. ACh, acetylcholine. (Reproduced with permission from Brunton LL, Hilal-Dandan R, Knollmann BC: *Goodman & Gilman's: The Pharmacological Basis of Therapeutics*, 13th ed. McGraw Hill; 2018.)

CONTROL OF THE AUTONOMIC NERVOUS SYSTEM

The autonomic nervous system mediates control of involuntary functions in a dynamic balance between fight-or-flight responses versus those of body homeostasis, maintenance, and immune response functions. This dual, balanced control includes heart rate, respiration, and reproductive behaviors, among many others. Although there is considerable, reflex-like low-level control of autonomic function at the spinal level, there is also a CNS hierarchy of control that includes brainstem nuclei and the hypothalamus. The switch of organ function from feeding to fleeing, for example, depends on CNS sensory input from vision, audition, and olfaction and the brain's evaluation of that input that a threat is approaching.

Brainstem Nuclei

Autonomic nuclei of the medulla in the brainstem exercise control of cardiac and respiratory function, vasoconstriction and dilation, and reflexes such as swallowing, coughing, sneezing, and vomiting. Different brainstem nuclei tend to be associated with sympathetic versus parasympathetic output. Sympathetic control is mediated by the caudal and rostral ventrolateral medulla, the mesencephalic locus ceruleus, and the Raphe nuclei of the pons and medulla. Neurons in the Raphe nuclei are serotonergic, whereas those of the locus ceruleus use NE. The locus ceruleus, one of the main producers of norepinephrine in the brain, has reciprocal connections with the hypothalamus.

Some CNS control of the parasympathetic output also comes from the Raphe nuclei. Other parasympathetic control is mediated by projections from the dorsal vagus motor nucleus, the amygdala, the parabrachial nucleus, the nucleus ambiguous, and the periaqueductal gray. Limbic structures, including the hippocampus, rhinal cortex, insula, cingulate

cortex, and orbitofrontal cortex, influence the autonomic output balance via brainstem nuclei and the hypothalamus.

The Hypothalamus

The hypothalamus, which is part of the diencephalon, consists of a cluster of autonomic nuclei that lie below the thalamus. Figure 18–8 shows the location of a number of these nuclei, with the table below indicating some of their functions. The autonomic nervous system projects to the hypothalamus via

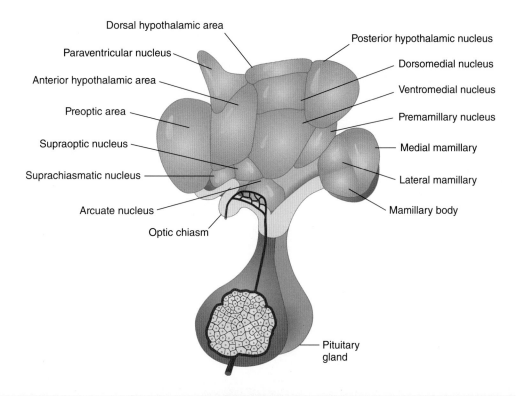

Function of the Hypothalamus	Area of the Hypothalamus
Secretion of hormonal release factors controlling the pituitary gland	Arcuate and paraventricular nuclei; periventricular area
Activation of sympathetic nervous system	Dorsal and posterior areas
Eating behavior	Ventromedial and arcuate nuclei; lateral area
Drinking behavior and thirst	Lateral area
Water and electrolyte balance	Supraoptic and paraventricular nuclei
Body temperature regulation	Preoptic area
Sexual behavior	Preoptic and anterior area
Circadiam rhythms	Suprachiasmatic nucleus

FIGURE 18–8 Anatomy of the hypothalamic nuclei and their involvement in some homeostasis functions. *Top*, hypothalamic nuclei and the spatial relationship between the hypothalamus and pituitary gland. *Bottom*, functions of some hypothalamic nuclei. (Reproduced with permission from Kibble JD, Halsey CR. *Medical Physiology: The Big Picture*. New York, NY: McGraw Hill; 2009.)

the brainstem reticular formation. The hypothalamus is typically divided into anterior, medial, and posterior nuclei. Anterior nuclei include the anterior nucleus and suprachiasmatic nucleus. The latter receives input from the retina and is the central governor of circadian rhythms. Medial nuclei include the ventromedial and dorsomedial nuclei. The mammillary body and posterior nucleus are in the posterior region. Sensory input from the heart and stomach reaches the hypothalamus via projections from the ventrolateral medulla. Feeding behavior is controlled by inputs from the NST in the medulla that communicates taste and visceral inputs associated with feeding.

An important hypothalamic nucleus that mediates control of the autonomic nervous system is the paraventricular nucleus. Neural cell bodies there are divided into magnocellular and parvocellular cells. Magnocellular cells are found in the paraventricular and supraoptic nuclei. Magnocellular cells cause the release of either vasopressin or oxytocin in the posterior pituitary. The parvocellular neurons include a class that projects to the median eminence of the pituitary using the neurotransmitter NE. Other parvocellular cells release thyrotropin-releasing hormone, which also regulates prolactin in conjunction with oxytocin; corticotropin-releasing hormone (CRH), which controls adrenocorticotropic hormone (ACTH) levels in conjunction with the secondary regulator vasopressin; and neurotensin, which controls luteinizing hormone and prolactin levels.

The limbic system also projects to the hypothalamus from above, thus connecting spinal autonomic neural circuitry with that of the limbic system. Brain areas that project to the hypothalamus include the amygdala, septum, olfactory bulb, and ventral tegmental area. The hippocampus projects to the hypothalamus via the mammillary body. A portion of this system is shown in Figure 18–9, including some of the major neurotransmitter systems involved. The hypothalamus

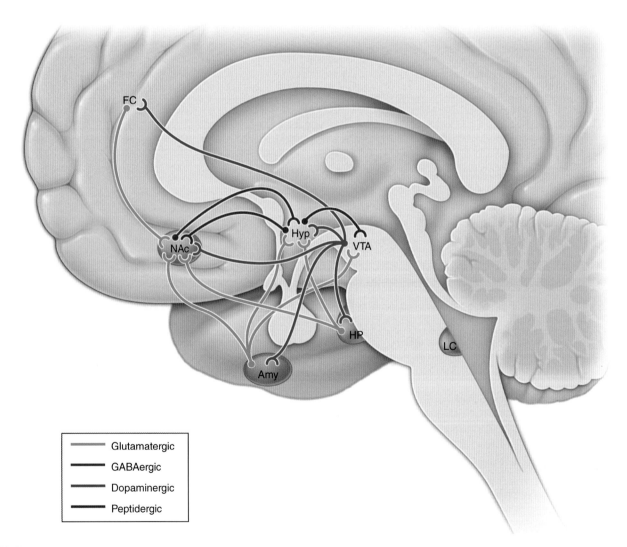

FIGURE 18–9 Relationship between the hypothalamus (Hyp) and limbic system areas known to be important for reward and addiction behaviors. Amy, amygdala; FC, frontal cortex; HP, hippocampus; LC, locus ceruleus; NAc, nucleus accumbens; VTA, ventral tegmental area. (Reproduced with permission from Jameson JL, Fauci AS, Kasper DL, et al: *Harrison's Principles of Internal Medicine*, 20th ed. New York, NY: McGraw Hill; 2018.)

integrates autonomic sensory input with the priorities set by the limbic system.

There are numerous types of inputs to the hypothalamus from the CNS. Recently, it has been shown that a special class of intrinsically photoreceptive retinal ganglion cells project to the suprachiasmatic nucleus to mediate circadian rhythms. These ganglion cells have their own photopigment-controlled ion channels and can respond to light directly, without being driven by rods and cones. There is also input to the hypothalamus from the olfactory system and hormonal input mediated by steroid hormones and feeding/satiety hormones such as ghrelin, leptin, and angiotensin. Hypothalamic neurons respond to circulating glucose, blood osmolarity, and body (blood) temperature.

Much of the output of the hypothalamus goes to the pituitary gland just below it, as shown in Figure 18–8. The hypothalamus controls the endocrine system via the neural and neurohumoral projections to the pituitary gland to control temperature, thirst, hunger, fatigue, and circadian rhythms.

The Pituitary & Control of the Endocrine System

The hypothalamus projects to the pituitary gland below it to control the endocrine system. The projection system includes hypothalamic neurons that project to sinuses or blood vessels in the pituitary (Figure 18–10). The anterior portion of the pituitary, called the adenohypophysis, contains a dense capillary bed of the portal hypophyseal system. Hypothalamic axons cause the release of neurotransmitters and neurohumoral agents into these capillaries at a structure called the median eminence. The projections of several hypothalamic nuclei to the pituitary are shown in Figure 18–10, such as the projection from the hypothalamic tuberal nuclei via the tuberoinfundibular tract to the median eminence. Somatostatin peptides released by the anterior pituitary reduce smooth muscle contractions in the intestine and suppress the release of pancreatic, thyroid-stimulating, and growth hormones.

The posterior pituitary, called the neurohypophysis, receives inputs from the supraoptic and paraventricular hypothalamic nuclei. These axonal projections release CRH, oxytocin, vasopressin, and antidiuretic hormone (ADH). Vasopressin is a peptide hormone that, among other functions, controls water uptake in the kidneys. Oxytocin produces distension of the cervix during birth and stimulates lactation (its synthetic version, Pitocin, is sometimes administered during labor). Circulating oxytocin also affects maternal behaviors such as pair bonding and social interaction. It has been experimentally administered to autistic people via nasal spray to determine whether it stimulates social interaction.

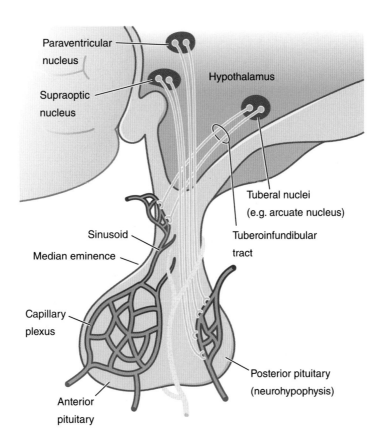

FIGURE 18–10 Projections from several hypothalamic nuclei (paraventricular, supraoptic, and tuberal) and the pituitary gland. (Reproduced with permission from Brunton LL, Chabner B, Knollmann BC: *Goodman & Gilman's the Pharmacological Basis of Therapeutics*, 12th ed. New York, NY: McGraw Hill; 2011.)

The hypothalamus, pituitary, and adrenal cortex complex within the endocrine system is often called the hypothalamic-pituitary-adrenal (HPA) axis. This system not only regulates the body in favor of either homeostasis (parasympathetic) versus voluntary motor (sympathetic) states, but it also controls mood, sexuality, and related emotions. The general circuit for the HPA axis involves the paraventricular nucleus of the hypothalamus, the anterior pituitary, and the adrenal cortex. Vasopressin and CRH are the 2 most important peptides released by the paraventricular nucleus to the pituitary. These induce the pituitary to secrete ACTH, which stimulates the adrenal cortex to produce glucocorticoid hormones such as cortisol (from cholesterol). There is a negative feedback pathway in this HPA circuit by which glucocorticoids secreted by the adrenal cortex suppress release of CRH and ACTH in the hypothalamus/ pituitary system.

Visceral Motor Reflex Functions: Cardiovascular, Bladder, & Sexual Functions

The autonomic system control of smooth and cardiac muscles and glands is called the visceral motor system, which is controlled by the hypothalamus, brainstem, and spinal cord. An example of the complex system controlling cardiac output (heart rate and contractile force) is shown in Figure 18–11. The system is comprised of a number of different sensor types distributed throughout the vasculature that maintain homeostasis for the parasympathetic branch, or fight-or-flight capability in the sympathetic system.

Figure 18–12 shows how the somatic, voluntary motor system interacts with the autonomic system to control urination from the bladder. Voluntary control is mediated by upper motor neurons in the medial area of primary motor cortex. Autonomic control is mediated by lower level spinal circuits, with lumbar spinal segments mediating sympathetic control and sacral segments mediating parasympathetic control (see Figures 18–4 and 18–6). An overall view of autonomic innervation of the female pelvic region is shown in Figure 18–13.

DISORDERS OF THE AUTONOMIC NERVOUS SYSTEM

Sympathetic activation changes body function priorities to enable rapid action in fight-or-flight situations. However, continuous or excessive sympathetic activation comes with a price, which is the disruption of necessary homeostatic

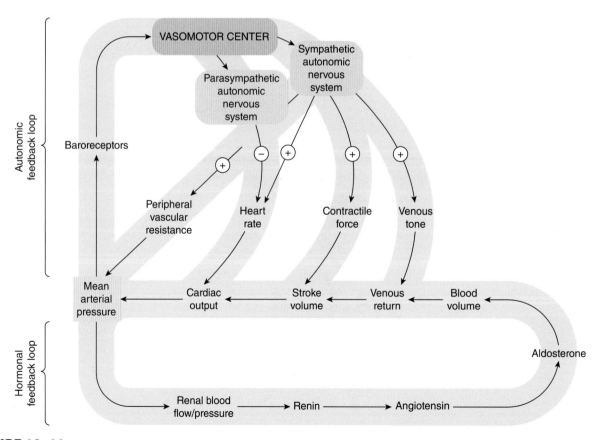

FIGURE 18–11 Autonomic cardiac control scheme showing autonomic and hormonal feedback loops. (Reproduced with permission from Katzung BG: *Basic and Clinical Pharmacology*, 14th ed. New York, NY: McGraw Hill; 2018.)

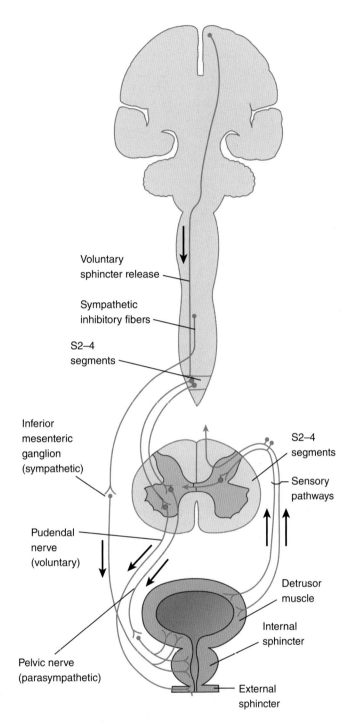

FIGURE 18-12 Descending pathways that innervate the bladder. Voluntary control comes from upper motor neurons in primary motor cortex. Autonomic control is mediated by lumbar sympathetic and sacral parasympathetic outputs. (Reproduced with permission from Waxman SG. *Clinical Neuroanatomy*, 28th ed. New York, NY: McGraw Hill; 2017.)

processes ranging from digestion to immune system function. Chronic stress can occur without a real threat, such as from excessive noise or light or social subordination. Chronic stress is typically associated with elevated release of cortisol by the adrenal cortex into the bloodstream. Cortisol acts on 2 main types of receptors in the brain, glucocorticoid and mineralocorticoid receptors.

Symptoms of chronic stress include sleep problems and memory dysfunction. In children, chronic stress can reduce growth due to the suppression of growth hormones. Behavioral signs of chronic stress include depression and ulcers. Women undergoing chronic stress tend to deposit fat around the waist; men may experience erectile dysfunction and increased risk of alcoholism.

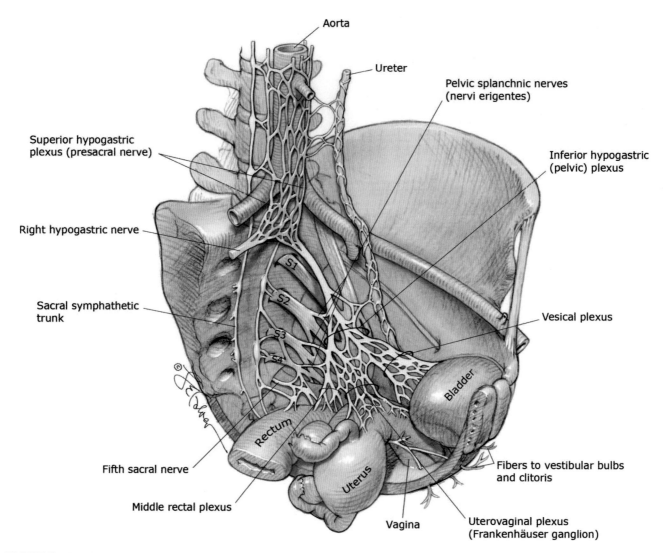

FIGURE 18–13 Pelvic autonomic nerves and organs innervated. (Reproduced with permission from Hoffman BL, Schorge JO, Bradshaw KD, et al: *Williams Gynecology*. 3rd ed. New York, NY: McGraw Hill; 2016.)

Obesity

There is increasing evidence that stress is partly responsible for the recent epidemic of obesity in the United States. The type of stress that appears to be the culprit is psychosocial stress, the reaction to assessment of threat to social status, esteem, group acceptance, and status. Diet quality deterioration appears to be an important mechanism by which psychosocial stress mediates its effects. Chronic stress is clearly correlated with weight gain and associated with dietary preferences for foods high in fat and sugar. People who tend to be heavier than normal, but not previously obese, seem to be at higher risk for stress-induced obesity.

Horner Syndrome

Damage to the superior sympathetic ganglion (see Figures 18–4 and 18–6) produces a constellation of symptoms known as Horner syndrome ipsilateral to the damage site. Visible symptoms include ptosis (droopy eyelid), miosis (constricted pupil), and enophthalmos (posterior retraction of the eyeball into the orbit). There is also decreased ability to sweat on the affected side.

SUMMARY

- The nervous system consists of the central, peripheral, autonomic, and enteric systems.
- The autonomic nervous system receives inputs from receptors in glands and cardiac and smooth muscle and sends control commands to those areas.
- Autonomic receptors report information about blood pressure, temperature, and carbon dioxide levels used to maintain homeostasis of those parameters.
- The autonomic nervous system projects to the hypothalamus via the brainstem reticular formation.
- The ENS is the nervous system of digestion.

- The autonomic nervous system is composed of 2 opposing divisions, called the sympathetic and parasympathetic branches.
- The sympathetic and parasympathetic systems share a similar first stage in which a cholinergic (acetylcholine-releasing) neuron projects from the CNS.
- Sympathetic nervous system axons project to a set of ganglia just outside the CNS from which neurons that release the neurotransmitter NE project to the target organ.
- Parasympathetic neurons project directly to the target organ without relaying in an intervening ganglion.
- Thus, at target organs such as the heart, generally opposing actions occur from the sympathetic division releasing NE versus the parasympathetic division releasing ACh.
- Sympathetic axons arise from the cervical, thoracic, and lumbar segments of the spinal cord, whereas parasympathetic axons arise above and below these segments, namely from the brainstem and sacral spinal cord segments.
- Sympathetic and parasympathetic autonomic nervous system control above the spinal cord is integrated and transmitted by a number of brainstem nuclei, particularly in the medulla.
- The hypothalamus projects to the pituitary gland below it to control the endocrine system.

SELF-ASSESSMENT QUESTIONS

1. A 58-year-old woman is suffering from hypertension, and the drugs available to her seem to be of little help. Recently, a new drug was approved for distribution, and the patient's physician recommended that she try it. The specific feature of this drug is that it selectively blocks synaptic transmission in autonomic ganglia in order to control blood pressure. Which of the following best characterizes this drug?

   A. Cholinergic antagonist
   B. Noradrenergic antagonist
   C. Serotonergic antagonist
   D. γ-Aminobutyric acid (GABA)-ergic antagonist
   E. Peptidergic antagonist

2. A patient is diagnosed with a hypothalamic tumor that results in significant alteration of autonomic functions, including loss of regulation of blood pressure and heart rate. Such effects upon autonomic functions can be understood in terms of the functional connections of the hypothalamus with a brainstem or spinal cord structure. Which of the following structures normally receives such inputs?

   A. Ventrolateral nucleus of the thalamus
   B. Nucleus accumbens
   C. Solitary nucleus
   D. Red nucleus
   E. Ventral horn cells at the level of C8 to T12 of the spinal cord

3. A patient is brought to the emergency department of a local hospital after he experienced orthostatic hypotension following a rapid response to a postural change. Magnetic resonance imaging (MRI) suggests that this change in blood pressure was caused by a tumor. At which of the following locations could a tumor most likely account for such a deficit?

   A. Lateral thalamus
   B. Premotor cortex
   C. Posterior fossa
   D. Midline region of basilar pons
   E. Collicular region of midbrain

4. An elderly patient experiences orthostatic hypotension. Which of the following could logically account for this disorder?

   A. Lesion of the dorsal motor nucleus of the medulla
   B. Lesion of sacral spinal cord autonomic neurons
   C. Reduction in release of ACh for preganglionic parasympathetic neurons
   D. Failure of damaged nerve terminals to synthesize and release NE
   E. Lesions involving serotonergic neurons in the pons

SECTION IV Cognitive Neuroscience

Consciousness

Franklin R. Amthor

- See how biologists believe consciousness evolved on earth from preceding species.
- Understand the brain structures that support consciousness.
- Understand the overall function of various cortical areas and their relationship with subcortical structures.
- See the crucial role of the thalamus in consciousness.
- Be familiar with the idea of association cortex and the origin of this idea in behaviorist/associationist concepts of perception and knowledge.
- Be aware of the crucial role of the prefrontal cortex in consciousness and its expansion in humans compared to other mammals and primates.
- Understand the different functions of lateral prefrontal, ventromedial prefrontal, and anterior cingulate (AC) cortices.
- Be aware of evidence about consciousness from laterality and split-brain studies.
- Understand what brain states such as sleep stages and phenomena such as blind sight and neglect indicate about consciousness.
- Be familiar with theories of consciousness based on mechanisms such as synchronous firing and global brain oscillations.
- Learn about recent quantum theories of consciousness.
- Learn about the debate about consciousness and the existence of free will.

A fundamental goal of neuroscience is to understand how consciousness arises in the human brain and how brain damage alters or destroys it. However, studying consciousness is difficult. Consciousness is a subjective inner experience whose content is not measurable using scientific instruments. What can be measured are what are called "correlates" of consciousness—brain activities or activity patterns that occur when consciousness is present compared to the brain activity when consciousness is lost, such as during coma or sleep. If consciousness is defined as an introspective, linguistic-based, inner thought stream that exists only in humans but not in any other animal, then it can only be studied in humans. This ethically precludes virtually all invasive neurophysiologic recording and manipulation techniques except for notable exceptions such as invasive physiologic recordings carried out during epilepsy surgery.

Neuroscientists and philosophers do not all agree with the materialistic idea that consciousness is created by brain activity. Alternative explanations for consciousness range from quantum mechanics to dualistic religious traditions that hold that a nonmaterial soul is the real seat of conscious. In this chapter, we examine aspects of consciousness that we understand depend on neural activity in the brain, such as differences between highly conscious states like normal wakefulness versus sleep or coma, and alterations in consciousness resulting from brain damage.

HOW DID CONSCIOUSNESS ARISE ON EARTH?

Life began on earth about a billion years after its formation 4.5 billion years ago. This life consisted of unicellular prokaryotes such as bacteria. Roughly a billion and a half years later, eukaryotes arose, cells with nuclei. About a billion and a half years after that, complex animals arose during the Cambrian explosion 500 million years ago, giving rise in a few million years to primitive vertebrates. Mammals arose about 200 million years ago, and primates about 60 million years ago, after the Cretaceous dinosaur extinction. Several hominid lines arose in the last 5 million years, with humans, *Homo sapiens*, showing up a few hundred thousand years ago.

Brain size and, in particular, brain size in relation to body size have increased significantly in some vertebrates over the eons. Invertebrates such as insects and mollusks have concentrations of neurons called ganglia containing a few thousand neurons. These ganglia differ greatly from each other and bear little resemblance to the brains of vertebrates. The most primitive vertebrate brains, however, such as those of amphibians (eg, frogs) or reptiles (eg, lizards and turtles), have structures very similar to those in mammalian, primate, and human brains, except that nonmammalian vertebrate brains have little or no neocortex, a largely mammalian invention. Mammalian brains are similar to each other in overall structure, cell types, and circuits, being distinguished mostly by the amount and distribution of neocortex. Primates have even more neocortex than most mammals, and humans more than most primates. Somewhere along this evolutionary path, consciousness evolved, and most neuroscientists think it has something to do with the evolution and growth of the neocortex.

BRAIN STRUCTURES MEDIATING CONSCIOUSNESS

Although consciousness and high general intelligence clearly are associated with the neocortex, the existence of these mental abilities clearly still depends on lower brain structures such as the brainstem and thalamus, whose function is necessary but not sufficient for consciousness. In particular, an intact reticular formation is necessary for basic awareness in all vertebrates.

The Reticular Formation

The central nervous system consists of the brain, spinal cord, and cephalic sensory ganglia such as the retina. The earliest vertebrates possessed a complex spinal cord and cephalic sensory ganglia before their brains became very large. The spinal cord is not just a fiber tract; it is also a distributed microcontroller that receives sensory information from the muscles, tendons, joints, and skin and produces complex coordinated motor output for various types of locomotion, ranging from swimming to walking, running, and climbing. The spinal cord also transmits sensory information from sensors in the viscera of the autonomic nervous system that mediate control of

respiration, heart rate, digestion, and blood oxygenation. This information projects upward to the phylogenetically oldest part of the vertebrate brain, the brainstem.

The brainstem also receives vestibular, visual, and other information necessary for balance and complex aspects of locomotion. A crucial central organizer of this information is the cerebellum, whose input/output tracts emanate from the pontine region of the brainstem. Half of all neurons in the brain may reside in the cerebellum. The reticular formation is a distributed brainstem neural network that integrates and executes information from both the autonomic nervous system and central nervous system. This distributed network of nuclei and tracts extends throughout the brainstem (medulla, pons, and midbrains) and upward to the diencephalon. The reticular formation regulates states of arousal and consciousness through both ascending axon tracts that modulate a large number of neurons in the brain and descending tracts that influence spinal reflexes and processing. Although the reticular formation is small relative to the rest of the brain, its function is crucial in controlling brain state and homeostasis. Damage to the reticular formation often produces death through loss of respiratory or cardiac control or results in coma due to loss of the ability to maintain an awake brain state. In contrast, it takes damage to much larger areas of neocortex to produce sustained complete loss of consciousness (**Figure 19–1**).

If we define (for vertebrates, at least) *awareness* as the brain state that permits active movement and response to the environment (as opposed to sleep) and *consciousness* as a state of awareness possessed only by humans, then the reticular formation is necessary for awareness, which itself is necessary, but not sufficient, for consciousness.

Overview of Cortical Structure

Above the brainstem is the diencephalon, consisting of the thalamus and hypothalamus. The reticular formation projects to the thalamus and modulates its function, whereas the thalamus reciprocally projects to the cortex, forming an even higher order brain system. The hypothalamus is a controller of the autonomic system, receiving projections from viscera sensors via spinal cord tracts and the reticular formation. The integration of autonomic brain states related to hunger, thirst, and reproductive goals with the brain's motor control hierarchy is through a neural network called the limbic system.

A well-known theory about the evolution of the hierarchical organization of brain structure is the triune theory of MacLean. Although not correct in some details, it still provides a framework for linking the evolution of the brain with the function of major subsystems within it. The 3 components of the MacLean triune system are, in order of evolution, (1) the reptilian complex, (2) the limbic system, and (3) the neocortical system. The reptilian complex is composed of the spinal cord and brainstem, including the cerebellum. This is the dominant brain system in fish and reptilian vertebrates. Next in evolution came the limbic system. This system enables sensory discrimination and motor behavior to be more complex and have more dependence on learning. **Figure 19–2A**

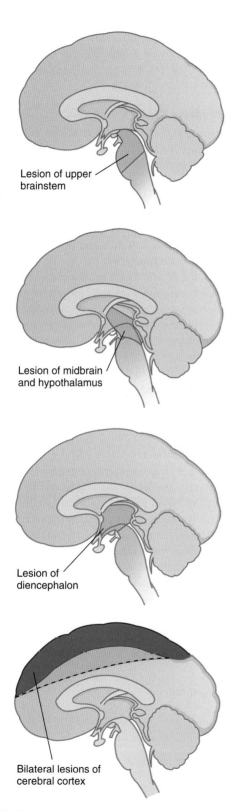

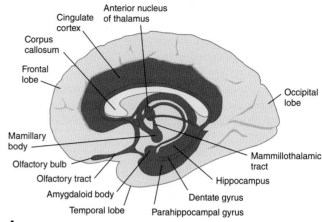

A

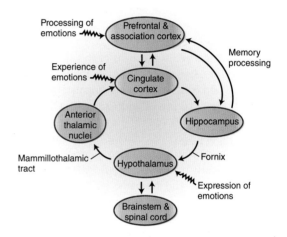

B

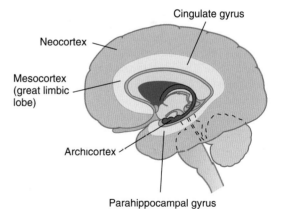

C

FIGURE 19–1 Brain lesions that cause loss of consciousness (sagittal sections). *Top:* Upper brainstem. *Second from top:* Midbrain and hypothalamus. *Second from bottom:* Diencephalon, particularly the thalamus. *Bottom:* Large bilateral lesions of neocortex. (Reproduced with permission from Waxman SG. *Clinical Neuroanatomy*, 28th ed. New York, NY: McGraw Hill; 2017.)

FIGURE 19–2 The limbic system. **A.** Sagittal view of classic limbic system structures (the limbic lobe), including the mesocortical cingulate gyrus, hippocampal gyrus, amygdala, olfactory bulb, and associated tracts. **B.** Limbic circuits and their general role in emotional processing. **C.** The main components of the limbic system emphasizing its concentric organization. (Parts A and B, reproduced with permission from Kibble JD, Halsey CR. *Medical Physiology: The Big Picture*. New York, NY: McGraw Hill; 2009; part C, reproduced with permission from Waxman SG. *Clinical Neuroanatomy*, 28th ed. New York, NY: McGraw Hill; 2017.)

shows a sagittal view of the limbic system with a number of its main structures. Notably, structures such as the amygdala and hippocampus mediate the formation of memories that control future behavioral contingencies based on experience. Many neuroscientists today object to calling the hippocampus limbic because, among other reasons, the hippocampus connects extensively to neocortex, part of the third, neocortical system. Connections between several limbic structures and neocortex are shown in Figure 19–2B.

The neocortical system is the third and phylogenetically newest part of the brain. It composes the largest part of most mammalian brains but is small or minimal in nonmammalian vertebrates such as amphibians, reptiles, and birds. The neocortex is distinguished from 2 older types of cortex, the allocortex and mesocortex (Figure 19–2C), which are associated with the limbic system, by its structure and location. The phylogenetically oldest allocortex (itself composed of archicortex, paleocortex, and periallocortex) is associated with the hippocampus and related structures and some areas of the olfactory system. Allocortex has 3 or 4 layers, versus 6 in neocortex. Mesocortex has 3 to 6 layers and consists of (1) the cingulate cortex immediately above the huge corpus callosum fiber tract that connects the 2 cerebral hemispheres and (2) the parahippocampal gyrus that organizes input projections into the hippocampus.

The neocortex, which composed a small percentage of the total brain in early mammals, became the dominant brain structure in primates and humans. Its 6-layered structure has similar cell types and functional organization throughout the brain. Current theory for mammalian brain function generally postulates that mammalian ancestors prior to the Cretaceous extinction were primarily olfactory animals that used a small primitive neocortex to differentiate and learn complex smells. After the dinosaurs disappeared, mammals radiated into the now unoccupied niches by expanding neocortex for complex processing in visual, auditory, and other domains. An important consequence of adapting a similar neural processing structure for almost all brain processing was that information could then be easily transmitted across the entire brain based on a common underlying neural circuit representation. This intrinsically integrated brain function permitted a high level of unified awareness that then permitted (with other factors) consciousness to arise in humans, as the theory goes.

Functions of Major Neocortical Lobes

The 4 major lobes of the neocortex are shown in Figure 19–3. All mammals have a similar neocortical organization. Mammals considered highly intelligent, such as primates, have more neocortex than other mammals, much of which involves enlargement of the frontal lobes. Apes in general and humans in particular not only have larger brains than other mammals, but also have a larger prefrontal (anterior) area of the frontal lobes. The prefrontal area is where working memory and abstract planning are represented.

In general, the occipital lobe processes vision; the temporal lobe processes audition and visual form information and is important for memory; the parietal lobe processes somatosensory, visually guided movement and auditory location information; and the frontal lobe generates movement. The output of the frontal lobe is primarily via the primary motor cortex at its posterior extent. Posterior to the central sulcus and across from primary motor cortex is the somatosensory area of the parietal lobe.

Control by Thalamus

Buried underneath the neocortex are the thalamic nuclei. Virtually all sensory input projects to primary cortical areas via so-called relay nuclei in the thalamus. Motor control signals from the basal ganglia and modulation of motor commands via the cerebellum and tendon and joint receptors project through the thalamus. Neocortical areas that receive inputs from the thalamus tend to project back to those and other thalamic areas. Thalamic nuclei and the mesocortical cingulate gyrus are like the hub of a wagon wheel and interact with and control the entire neocortex. Damage to these areas has severe impacts on consciousness. Brain imaging studies also show that conscious brain activity always consists of activity in 1 or more sensory

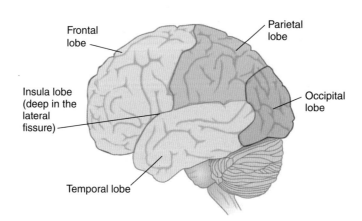

FIGURE 19–3 The 4 major lobes of the neocortex: frontal (blue), parietal (green), occipital (orange), and temporal (beige). (Reproduced with permission from Kibble JD, Halsey CR. *Medical Physiology: The Big Picture.* New York, NY: McGraw Hill; 2009.)

neocortical areas, the thalamus, and the prefrontal cortex simultaneously. This organization has been called the "vital triangle" by Cotterill.

The Association Cortices

Vertebrates have the largest brains and appear to be the most intelligent animals, mammals are the most intelligent vertebrates, primates are the most intelligent mammals, and humans are the most intelligent and only conscious primates. The neural basis of this chain is the enlargement of the brain, enlargement of neocortex, enlargement of the frontal lobe, and enlargement of prefrontal cortex. Human and chimpanzee DNA have about 99% overlap. Human brains are a little over twice the size of chimpanzee brains, with much of the added increase in the prefrontal cortex. What is this extra prefrontal neocortex doing that enables consciousness?

Is There Such a Thing as Association Cortex?

Early in the 20th century, tract-tracing histologic studies showed that particular areas of the occipital, parietal, and temporal cortices received direct thalamic input from visual, somatosensory, and auditory areas, whereas lower motor neurons in the spinal cord received direct projections from upper motor neurons in primary motor cortex in the frontal lobe. These came to be called "primary" cortical areas. The size of these areas generally follows the number of sensory receptors in the periphery for sensory areas or the number of lower motor neurons for motor areas. The cortical area sizes correspond to the acuity needed in the ecological niche occupied by various species. For example, moles that dig with their noses have enormous parietal representations of tactile receptors around their mouth and nose.

Beyond the relative cortical allocation based on ecological niche, mammals differ greatly in how much neocortex is not primary, that is, not directly connected to a sensory input or motor output. Early 20th-century behaviorist/associationist ideas about the brain supposed that it was a general, nondifferentiated learning apparatus, the details of whose specific circuit organization outside primary areas was of little consequence in understanding behavior. Nonprimary areas of neocortex were called "association" cortex. The idea was that although it was undifferentiated, the more you had of it, the better for learning and intelligence, and since humans had the most of it, that explained their superior intelligence.

Specific Features of the Association Cortices

At a late 20th-century brain meeting, Jon Kaas famously said that primate association cortex was rapidly shrinking. What he meant was best illustrated in the visual system. Visual thalamus, the lateral geniculate nucleus, projects to the pole of the occipital cortex, called primary visual cortex (V1; also striate cortex and Brodmann area 17). V1 projects to V2 (area 18), which is also visual, and V2 projects to V3, V4, V5, and so on, all with different visual response properties. The retina and visual thalamus respond to light and dark things of certain sizes, V1 responds to oriented edges, V4 to specific color patterns, and V5 to specific motion directions. These are all visual areas, not general association learning tissue.

The same is true in other sensory systems. High-level (as in more synapses away from primary) sensory areas tend to have neurons that respond to more "abstract," less receptor-response sensory attributes. These higher order areas tend to remain sensory modality specific until very high-level multimodal areas are reached, such as in the parietal lobe, where neurons that are influenced by visual, auditory, or somatosensory input from particular areas of space are found. Neurons in primary motor cortex tend to drive specific muscles in a topologically oriented map of the body. Anterior to primary motor cortex are areas such as premotor cortex and the supplementary motor area whose activation drives groups of related muscles.

The one place in the brain where many neurons are found whose firing (as far as we currently know) has no obvious topologic relation to body location or location on a sensory receptor sheet is the prefrontal cortex. Rather, many neurons in the prefrontal cortex are thought to mediate working memory, forming a transient firing group that can represent any arbitrary constellation of features that exist in the environment that needs to be remembered as a contingency for future action. If we are to differentiate the conscious human brain from the very similar but nonconscious chimpanzee brain, prefrontal cortex is an obvious place to consider.

THE FRONTAL & PREFRONTAL LOBES

Figure 19–4 shows sagittal views of the 3 principle regions of prefrontal cortex and some of their subcortical connections. On the left is the anterior cingulate (AC), which is older mesocortex. The AC is a master control area that allocates processing resources among various neocortical areas. The center view in Figure 19–4 shows the orbitofrontal cortex (OFC), also called ventromedial prefrontal cortex, which occupies the ventral and medial portion of prefrontal cortex. This cortical area receives low-level sensory input in pathways that parallel the main sensory projections to the thalamus. The OFC interacts with the amygdala, and this system is a kind of emotional working memory that can represent a sensory constellation (eg, the appearance of a snake in the grass) to be associated with an emotionally salient response (escape). On the right of Figure 19–4 is the dorsolateral prefrontal cortex (DLPFC). This large brain area instantiates a working memory for representing sensory constellations arising from either external actual events or imagined, internally generated imagery. This leads to the question of how an increase in DLPFC and, therefore, working memory capacity is associated with consciousness.

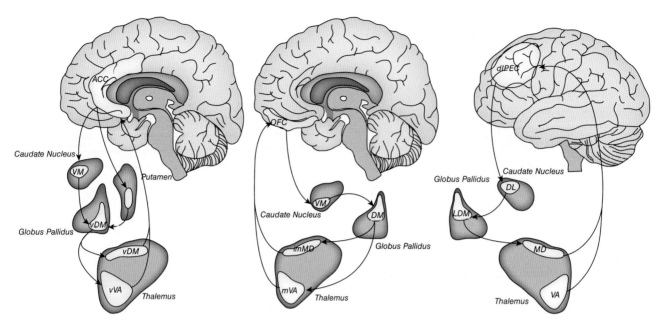

FIGURE 19–4 The 3 main prefrontal lobe areas and associated subcortical interaction areas. *Left:* The anterior cingulate cortex, which interacts with the basal ganglia caudate and putamen (striatum) areas, and the thalamus. *Center:* The orbitofrontal cortex (OFC), also called the ventromedial prefrontal cortex, which interacts with different zones of the striatum and thalamus, and the amygdala (not shown). *Right:* The dorsolateral prefrontal cortex (DLPFC) and interaction zones in the striatum and thalamus. (Adapted with permission from Perez DL, Catenaccio E, Epstein J: Confusion, Hyperactive Delirium, and Secondary Mania in Right Hemispheric Strokes: A Focused Review of Neuroanatomical Correlates. *J Neurol Neurophysiol.* Sept 2011:S1.)

Dorsolateral Prefrontal Cortex & Working Memory

Working memory is a concept that replaced the older concept of short-term memory, the ability to remember a list of several items such as phone number digits spoken or presented visually. Short-term memory lasts for only a few seconds without rehearsal, which begins the transference to long-term memory. Rehearsal depends on language, a fundamental component of human intelligence. Working memory extends the concept of short-term memory to include, among other things, the transference of information from long-term memory into a mental "scratchpad" by which this information can be quickly accessed. For example, if you were asked a series of questions about the first car you ever owned, you would bring into this scratchpad long-term memory information about the car's make, color, and so forth. This would permit answering further questions about the car more quickly.

The DLPFC is the major site for the operation of working memory. DLPFC interacts with the hippocampus and other appropriate area of neocortex to store, activate, and maintain mental memory images. One idea about how a larger DLPFC might support a qualitative increase in intelligence underlying consciousness comes from a memory model postulated by Lisman and colleagues. Their model was motivated by the observation that 2 prominent brain oscillations, gamma and theta, typically occur in a ratio of about 7:1. In their model, each gamma oscillation is like a pointer that enables a particular constellation of neural firing that represents 1 memory item. The Miller limit of 7 memory items occurs because the

theta cycle maintains the total memory representation, and only 7 gamma cycles that generate the neural code for 7 distinct items can be loaded or read out each theta cycle.

There are several implications of this model for intelligence and consciousness. Human gamma frequencies range from approximately 40 to 100 Hz, whereas the theta range is 4 to 8 Hz. The gamma/theta ratio varies somewhat in a particular person and between people. Evidence links better working memory to intelligence and indicates a correlation between the gamma/theta ratio and working memory capacity.

There is another, more speculative conjecture that can be made from this theory that suggests a function for a larger DLPFC. This has to do with what is called "chunking." The human memory limit is about 7 items (plus or minus 2). However, the sets of items can be quite different things. One can remember approximately 7 individual letters. However, one can also remember approximately 7 words, which obviously contain more than 7 letters. Under favorable circumstances, one can remember approximately 7 short sentences. The items in the 7-item memory limit can be complex things as long as they are familiar and can be represented as a unit or "chunk." What is a chunk, and how complex can it be?

In terms of number of items, human memory capacity is not significantly greater than that of many animals. Many studies have suggested that birds, with brains less than 1/100th the size of human brains, can remember up to 5 or 6 items. It is conceivable that some fundamental aspect of brain architecture, such as the gamma/theta ratio, limits the number of chunks that can be held in working memory for any vertebrate brain, but the complexity of the chunks increases with brain size, particularly the size of the DLPFC. The most complex chunks are enabled by language and linguistic categories.

The Orbitofrontal Cortex & Emotional Memory

The ventral part of the prefrontal cortex is called the orbitofrontal cortex (OFC) or ventromedial prefrontal cortex. Whereas the DLPFC is extensively connected to the hippocampus, the OFC has a similar relationship to the amygdala, which is instrumental in learning about situations of high "limbic" significance, such as those involving physical or social danger. Although most mammals may have in inbred fear of spiders and snakes, one must learn to be wary when encountering flashing red lights or particular facial expressions of one's boss.

The output of the OFC is also qualitatively different from that of the DLPFC. DLPFC working memory is highly consciousness and language dependent, requiring attention, and is often associated with linguistic maintenance via subvocal rehearsal. The OFC, in contrast, signals the "sense" of danger or inappropriateness by what are colloquially called "gut feelings" of unease, termed by Damasio as *somatic markers*. Intuitive gut feeling are generated by a fast, subcortical system termed the *low road* by LeDoux whose output may begin generating avoidance behavior before conscious awareness of the source of the feeling. To paraphrase the famous William James quote: "I see a bear, I run, and then I am afraid."

The OFC system exists in all mammals, but it is particularly highly developed in social mammals such as primates, presumably to deal with complex aspects of social rank in primate species. Enlargement of the OFC in humans, compared to other primates, increases the sophistication and differentiation of environmental cues associated with threat or risk. Driving a car is an example of a situation of constant, largely unconscious management of responses to a host of environmental cue threats ranging from the behavior of other cars to road signals. These threats are obeyed below the level of conscious awareness, with the sophistication of threat assessment and response enabled by expansion of the OFC.

The Anterior Cingulate Cortex

The cingulate cortex, although phylogenetically older mesocortex, remains an important controller of neocortical processing. This is particularly true of the AC. This structure receives inputs from most of the neocortex and the thalamus. Its most important output is to the entorhinal cortex, part of the hippocampal formation. The AC compares goals, set largely by the DLPFC, to current progress toward those goals, as relayed by sensory information controlled by the thalamus. Cells in the AC are activated by task difficulty and errors. The AC is also instrumental in the perception of pain and the anticipation of pain. Lesions of this area reduce pain perception.

LANGUAGE, LATERALITY, & CONSCIOUSNESS

There are numerous difficulties associated with the scientific study of consciousness. The most discussed of these, of course, is the fact that consciousness is a personal experience not directly accessible to instrumental measurement. The best neuroscience can do at present is to look at the various borderlines between neural states or systems that have it, versus those that do not. This includes, primarily, differences between conscious humans and near relatives that are not conscious, and between conscious and unconscious states in humans.

Language & Consciousness

The biggest problem in determining the substrate of consciousness based on species differences is that there is only 1 species, humans, that is generally agreed to have full consciousness. Of all the differences between conscious humans and all other nonconscious species, the 1 difference that stands out is language. As Helen Keller said, "Before my teacher came to me, I did not know that I am. I lived in a world that was a no-world. I cannot hope to describe adequately that unconscious, yet conscious time of nothingness. I did not know that I knew aught, or that I lived or acted or desired. I had neither will nor intellect. I was carried along to objects and acts by a certain blind natural impetus. I had a mind which caused me to feel anger, satisfaction, desire."

Consciousness is highly impaired without language, which all typically developing humans acquire purely by exposure with little explicit instruction. Some nonhuman primates can learn hundreds of words and even generate novel word pairs, but none have mastered the grammar of any language, even with extensive instruction. It is hard to argue against the proposition that human consciousness is derived from language.

One thing that language might contribute to consciousness is the ability to have episodic memory. Episodic memory is distinguished from semantic memory in that episodic memory and learning can arise from single events, whereas semantic memories are typically associated with the world knowledge semantic system in the brain established mostly through repetition and association. Episodic memory allows single-trial learning and learning by observation and verbal instruction. It must depend significantly on the ability to categorize experience through language and generate rules from categorized experience that help to make predictions about future outcomes. Many neuroscientists would argue that no animals other than humans have episodic memory. In this scheme, language-enabled episodic memory is a significant element of human consciousness. The planning ability it supports has obvious survival utility. Evolution has not produced any nonconscious human zombies lacking language; all normally developing humans have language, episodic memory, and consciousness.

Left & Right Brains

To the extent that human consciousness depends on language, it must also depend on the distinct capability of the left versus the right side of the brain (where most control of language resides in virtually all right-handers and a majority of left-handers). Yet, no significant functional differences are known to exist between the right and left hemispheres in overall structure, cell types, or neural circuit architecture. In fact, the right hemisphere competently develops normal language in some left-handers and in many cases of left hemisphere damage in infancy.

Elegant studies of the difference in language competence between the right and left hemispheres were done by Sperry, Gazzaniga, and colleagues in so-called "split-brain" patients. These were people in whom the large fiber tract connecting the 2 hemispheres (the corpus callosum) was transected to prevent the spread of epileptic seizures between the 2 hemispheres. Visual stimuli were presented to either the left or the right visual field for intervals too short for any eye movements to occur, which isolated these stimuli to the right or left side of the brain, respectively. These patients could not make verbal reports about stimuli isolated to the right side of the brain. Moreover, the ability (intelligence) of the right side of the brain to integrate aspects of visually presented stimuli into a coherent whole was very deficient compared to that of the left hemisphere.

Gazzaniga concluded from these studies that the isolated (by callosal transection) left hemisphere, which is about the same size as a chimpanzee brain, has normal language competence and consciousness. The isolated right hemisphere was deficient in language and in any many aspects of consciousness. Therefore, brain size alone cannot be the cause of the consciousness difference between humans and similar species such as chimpanzees. Some developmental process that occurs universally in humans, but only in humans, enables the left side of the brain to produce language and consciousness.

Sleep

Sleep is the daily transition between consciousness and unconsciousness that virtually all humans experience daily. Sleep itself is complex, composed of rapid eye movement (REM) and non-REM categories. Non-REM sleep is further divided into 4 different stages that differ in electroencephalogram (EEG) brain waves and physiologic attributes such as muscle tone. Most dreams occur during REM sleep, during which brain waves resemble those during wakefulness, including activity in motor cortex, although actual movement is suppressed via the parabrachial pathway.

Sleep and sleep cycles are controlled by the brainstem reticular formation (particularly the pons parabrachial area), several nuclei in the basal forebrain, and the hypothalamus, via the neurotransmitters acetylcholine (ACh), norepinephrine, and serotonin. The release of ACh, which occurs during REM sleep, increases EEG amplitudes but decreases EEG synchronous activity. The neurotransmitters norepinephrine and serotonin are also involved in the control of sleep. Norepinephrine is released by neurons in the brainstem locus coeruleus nucleus whose axons project widely (but diffusely) throughout the brain. Norepinephrine release increases cortical activation and EEG enhancement but, unlike ACh, does not induce REM sleep. Serotonin is released from axons whose somas are in the Raphe nucleus in the brainstem. Like norepinephrine, serotonin is important for the maintenance of the stages of non-REM sleep.

REM sleep EEG activity is so similar to that of normal waking consciousness that REM sleep is sometimes called paradoxical sleep. The thalamus and other subcortical structures control the progression of neural activity across the brain during sleep, but with brain activity generated more by internal sources than sensory input, which is highly attenuated during all stages of sleep. Sleep, particularly REM sleep has been hypothesized to have restorative and memory consolidation functions. REM sleep appears to be particularly important for the consolidation of memory because REM sleep deprivation has negative effects on learning. After moderate sleep deprivation, the proportion of REM to non-REM sleep increases. Prolonged sleep deprivation can produce psychosis, a disturbance of normal consciousness.

NEUROLOGIC DEFICITS & CONSCIOUSNESS

Another way of investigating the neural basis of consciousness is to examine how brain damage affects particular aspects of consciousness. Several disorders of visual consciousness give some interesting clues about the neural circuitry that supports it.

Blindsight

There are many things humans see, in the sense of processing information from visual input, of which we have no awareness. We are not aware of the blind spot in each eye where there are no photoreceptors at the optic nerve head. We are not aware of the letter configuration at the locations to which our eyes saccade during reading, despite the fact that these saccades are optimally accurate. Conscious vision is mediated by retinal projections to the thalamus, whereas the retinal projections to the superior colliculus and other retinal recipient zones process information in an unconscious manner.

A particularly interesting dissociation of conscious from unconscious visual processing is that of so-called "blindsight," studied by Weiskrantz. Patients who have extensive loss of primary visual cortex in the occipital lobe (V1, or striate cortex) report no awareness of stimuli presented in the corresponding visual field. However, when forced to guess whether an object was presented there or move their eyes to the object location, they perform far better than chance. Thus, behaviorally, they can use visual information presented in their blind hemi-field despite having no conscious awareness of any stimuli presented there.

It is interesting that humans alone are especially dependent on the thalamus–occipital lobe pathway for vision. Other primates with similar lesions in the V1 occipital cortex exhibit far less visual dysfunction than humans, with a loss of some visual acuity and form discrimination but less symptoms of actual blindness.

Neglect

Neglect is another type of loss of visual consciousness, usually due to damage to the right parietal lobe (which receives input from the left visual hemi-field). Patients with neglect tend to ignore objects on their left side, shaving only the right side of their face, for example. This is despite the fact they can freely move their eyes to place objects in the nonneglected right visual hemi-field. When asked to describe from memory a familiar place from a particular point of view, patients with neglect may also fail to describe any objects that would be seen on their left side. However, when asked to describe the scene from the opposite point of view, they neglect objects they described previously that now would appear in their left hemi-field.

THEORIES OF CONSCIOUSNESS

There are nearly as many theories about consciousness are there are neuroscientists and philosophers. The following discussion samples a few ideas that have recently received considerable attention or that can be related to psychophysical or physiologic data. The section on the quantum brain discusses some consciousness theories at the intersection of neuroscience and physics.

Priming & the Unconscious Brain

Most people have some idea of the existence of priming from the phenomenon of subliminal advertising. The most well-known example is of the insertion of 1 frame out of every 24 frames per second in a movie that says, "buy popcorn." The briefness of the presentation (<50 milliseconds) is such that people are not consciously aware of its existence. Nevertheless, in carefully controlled psychophysical experiments, it has been shown that such presentations have small but statistically significant influence on subsequent choices or the speed of processing of prime-related versus unrelated stimuli.

One of the most interesting aspects of this type of experiment is that because the prime image is a short text phrase, it must have been processed through the language system to generate semantic meaning, even though the subject is not conscious at all of its existence. Priming is just one example of data that indicate that most human brain processing is unconscious. Which of all the underlying unconscious brain activity rises to consciousness depends on both top-down and bottom-up attention mechanisms. These mechanisms must maintain neural activity for at least about half a second in the

vital triangle of the thalamus, sensory cortex, and frontal cortex as a prerequisite of conscious awareness.

Illusory Conjunctions & Working Memory

Ann Treisman and colleagues performed a number of experiments whose basic format is as follows. A set of 3 letters each of a different color, such as a red X, blue S, and green T, are flashed briefly on a projection screen. The stimulus duration is adjusted to obtain a criterion level of correct reports by the subjects. The experiment is then changed by the addition of a "mask" or noise figure immediately after the set of letters. The mask appears to "erase" the early visual system eidetic representation of the stimulus. A type of error now occurs that did not occur in the first experiment, which is that subjects now sometimes report letters correctly that were in the display, but with the wrong color (that of a different letter). This switching of the colors in the report between letters in the display is called an illusory conjunction.

Illusory conjunctions of this type are interesting because we know that the visual system processes some aspects of form and color with different neurons in different brain areas. That is, there are visual neurons in cortex that respond well to particular colors but are agnostic about shape, and visual neurons that respond to shape independent of the color of the shape. Thus, in this experiment, the stimulus activated color neurons that respond to red, blue, and green and shape neurons that respond to the X, S, and T shapes. The DLPFC maintains some "neural image" of this activity after the stimulus flash. How does the brain know which activated color neurons go with which activated letter neurons in order to report it correctly after the mask? This has been called the "binding problem": how activity in different areas of the brain associated with multiple objects can be sorted or bound so that encoded properties of each object are associated with that object and no others. This ability clearly depends on conscious working memory. One mechanism proposed for mediating this type of working memory is synchronous firing.

Synchronous Firing & Brain Oscillations

Most of the discussion in this chapter has been about the location of brain substrates that support consciousness. However, few neuroscientists believe that consciousness is located in any specific part of the brain or is dependent on any particular type of neuron. Consciousness is a process for which some particular brain areas appear to be necessary, but not sufficient. Considerable brain activity can persist under the influence of many anesthetics, but the pattern of activity no longer supports consciousness.

Sensory neurons produce trains of action potentials whose pattern is modulated by the presentation of some stimulus. It is well known that such patterns are noisy; that is, repeated presentations of the same stimulus produce slightly different spike patterns with each presentation. This suggests that the spike response of sensory neurons consists of a stimulus-associated component that is perturbed by random noise that varies for each specific presentation. The implication of this is that the information in neural spike trains must be in the average overall rate of firing that corresponds to the stimulus-generated component, with the exact spike pattern conveying little information because, if the spike pattern is not the same for repetitions of the same stimulus, it is unlikely to enable distinguishing between different similar stimuli.

This view of spike pattern irrelevance changed with the finding from dual- and multi-electrode recordings that, depending on the stimulus and attention state of the nervous system, sometimes neurons fire synchronously despite the noise. Synchronous firing means that the spikes in one neuron occur at about the same time as those in another neuron more often than chance would predict due to the overall mutual firing rates. Synchronous firing could solve the binding problem if, during different cycles of an ongoing brain EEG rhythm such as the gamma rhythm, the constellation of neurons that encoded properties of 1 object fired synchronously on 1 particular cycle, or cycle phase, whereas those associated with other objects fired synchronously on different cycles or phases. Attention and consciousness could then be mediated by control of neural synchronous firing across large areas of the brain with readout neurons being sensitive to spikes from multiple inputs occurring synchronously. The existence of stimulus-dependent and attention-dependent neural synchrony is beyond dispute, but the idea that synchrony mediates attention or consciousness is controversial. Some neuroscientists have suggested that firing epochs called bursts, characterized by very high firing rates for tens of milliseconds, mediate attention and conscious control effects, with synchrony being a by-product of burst firing.

The Quantum Brain

There has been considerable theorizing in the past 2 decades about the relationship between consciousness and the outcome of some quantum mechanics experiments. The fact that decisions made by conscious observers determines the outcome of quantum experiments has led to the suggestion that consciousness itself creates reality and is not reducible to, or identical with, the neural firing patterns going on in the brain.

The argument is best illustrated with the double-slit experiment, as pointed out by Feynman. Light can behave as a wave. If light passes through 2 closely spaced slits, an interference pattern will exist on some detector after the slits that is predictable from the wavelength of light and slit widths and spacing. However, if the intensity of the light is reduced until only 1 photon at a time is sent toward the slits, the pattern of hits on the detector after multiple single-photon transits is still an interference pattern. Did each single photon go through both slits and interfere with itself? According to current quantum physics, a probability function, described by the Schrödinger wave equation, passes through both slits, and the photon exists in a superposition of all allowed states until observation collapses the wave function into a particular outcome. The observation occurs in the system that consists of the mechanical detector and the human observer. The question is, where in this system does the collapse occur? Is it when the wave function interacts with the detector, or when the result of this interaction is consciously observed?

The difficulty is embodied in the Schrödinger's cat paradox. A cat is placed in a sealed box with a quantum device that has a probability of one-half of releasing a poison gas and killing the cat in the next hour. After the hour has passed, is the cat dead or alive before the box is opened? The mainstream so-called Copenhagen (Bohr) interpretation of this situation is that the cat exists in a live/dead superposition until the box is opened and the state of the cat is observed by a conscious human.

Physicists attempted to resolve the single photon passing through 2 slits paradox by using another detector, such as a polarizer, to tell which slit the single photon went through. The existence of the which-slit detector, however, eliminates the interference pattern at the photon detector screen. If a measurement can be made of which slit the photon passed through, the impact pattern is what would be expected if the slit that the photon did not pass through were not present. An experiment can be set up in which a which-slit measurement is made after the photon has passed through the slits, and this measurement still destroys interference pattern. The observation by a human of some quantum properties of a quantum system can alter the state of the system everywhere, including in its past. In so-called entangled systems, a consciously observed measurement in 1 place on 1 particle can change the state of an entangled particle at the far end of the universe instantaneously.

Given that the measurement collapses the wave function, the debate in physics is over where the collapse occurs. Most physicists believe that the detector causes the wave function collapse by a process called decoherence. However, because the various parts of the detector apparatus must obey the laws of quantum mechanics, it is a problem to decide where in the detector apparatus the decoherence occurs, and a significant number of physicists place this point in human consciousness. Theories about how this might occur in brains, such as in neural microtubules, are too complex to discuss within the space available in this treatment. Almost no one understands or is happy about this situation. As Feynman supposedly said, "Anyone who says that they understand quantum mechanics does not understand quantum mechanics."

Consciousness & Free Will

Two of the most fundamental questions in all of science are as follows: (1) Is consciousness causal or merely an epiphenomenal by-product of mechanistic brain operation? (2) Does free will really exist? The implications of the answers to these questions extend far beyond science into religion, ethics, law, and societal governance. These questions are intimately related because, if consciousness is not causal but an epiphenomenon, it is hard to see how there could be such a thing as free will. Until the late 20th century, these topics were almost taboo for most neuroscientists, who preferred to work on problems that were directly approachable or related to human mental and neurologic health. However, now that neuroscientists think they have a basic understanding of the principles of brain operation, the debate has ensued about whether the brain is just a "machine made of meat" whose operational principles are generally understood and whose behavior should be as predictable as that of any machine.

Deterministic arguments that deny the existence of causal consciousness and free will are generally motivated at least partly by a reaction against the Western dualistic ideas of the existence of a soul that inhabits and controls a mechanistic body. In Western religious traditions, the soul is the possessor of free will, while the body is an organic machine in humans that is similar to that in animals, except they lack a soul. If one does not believe in a soul, what is left is a machine. The feeling of free will has been postulated to be an evolutionary trick that motivates us to feel good about some decisions (completely determined by the machine) that promote survival value and bad about decisions that do not promote survival.

Those who argue against consciousness being causal also tend to view the principles of the operation of the brain to be grounded in Newtonian, pre-quantum physics, which views the universe as being filled with particles and forces whose future unfolding proceeds entirely according to a set of physical laws. The state of any physical system should be, at least in theory, entirely predictable from knowledge of its current state and physical laws that govern its evolution from the current state. In this scenario, there can be no free will or any causal role for consciousness. However, ironically, modern quantum physics does not actually view the universe this way, and as discussed earlier, some quantum physicists assign consciousness to a primary role in the creation of reality.

Another objection to deterministic theories of brain function that exclude free will and causal consciousness is that they are based on ideas of linear causation that are appropriate for describing simple systems but not complex dynamic systems characterized by extensive feedback and self-modification from experience. Much of the nervous system consists of loops in which firing of cell A drives cell B, which drives cell C, which feeds back to cell A. Of course, if these connections were all excitatory, this system would blow up, as in epilepsy. However, operating under normal homeostatic control, the locus of causality in this loop is difficult to assign. Feedback systems generated by completely deterministic rules can also operate in a chaotic manner such that tiny differences in the initial conditions can produce large differences in subsequent behavior.

Some neuroscientists advocate a middle ground in which the brain is regarded as a meat machine operating according to physical laws, but something like free will exists as an emergent phenomenon enabled by consciousness. Consciousness has causal efficacy via its enabling of decision making using categorization, episodic memory, and the ability to calculate future outcomes explicitly, which are all enabled by language. The brain constructs, through experience and previous decisions, its own architecture for using information to predict the future and make decisions based on that information. Conscious introspection is a significant part of this architecture.

The essence of science is the ability to make accurate predictions from data. No one doubts that biology depends on chemistry, and chemistry depends on physics. However, in the search for the DNA mutation that causes some neurologic disorder, neuroscientists typically do not look for the answer to physics, or even chemistry. DNA is part of an information processing system whose operation is best understood in terms of information coding rather than its chemistry (although the mutation may have been a result of chemistry, such as a teratogen). Brains that possess consciousness act on information itself. You choose the lumber size for the support posts for your deck based on a calculation of loads and tensile strengths. You do not know the result of the calculation before you do it. Perhaps your action was determined from the beginning of the universe at the big bang, but believing this does not seem to be of any use in guiding decisions you actually make.

The informed decision point of view of consciousness being causal does not depend on postulating the existence of a nonphysical soul. The human agent who acts is a biologic mechanism that obeys the laws of chemistry and physics. Choice is certainly constrained by the biologic hardware that executes decisions because drives and motivations are built into the hardware by biology and personal and species evolution. However, choices also depend on information stored in the brain and its use for the evaluation of likely outcomes. Failing to use information to consciously make decisions results in poorer decisions. Failing to understand the role of conscious introspection in human behavior reduces the scientific ability to predict human in it.

Choice is not the exclusive domain of humans. A dog can be trained to do and not do certain things. Dogs appear to experience conflict in situations where their basic instincts and their training conflict. They hesitate in those situations before making choices. The difference is that when a dog chooses, it is not aware of the explicit outcomes of the choice or the factors that went into the choice, other than an association between one possible behavior and reward or punishment, whereas humans are aware of episodic history and can foresee the future.

The idea of free will as the conscious introspective processing of information is admittedly a functional and operational definition of it. The issue for most neuroscientists is not whether there exists an unconstrained freedom to make any choice whatsoever but, rather, whether it is of predictive power to consider the chooser's conscious calculations in understanding what choice is made (behavior). One could imagine making 100 identical robots with a variety of goals embedded in their programming but whose programming was modifiable by experience. If these robots were turned out to roam the world, one could imagine at some particular time some particular choice would be made by half of them, and the opposite choice by the other half, because of the differences in their history. If they had language modules, we would find it more instructive, in terms of predicting their future behavior, to ask them why they made the choice they did, than to record their entire experience to reconstruct the changes in the operation of their neural net programming. Presumably, the robots would use the results of their decisions to make better future decisions based on their "belief" in their own consciousness and free will. Free will may be an illusion, but it is one that can have considerable explanatory and predictive power.

The moral principles related to values, conscience, and societal norms are called ethics. Belief in the brain as a deterministic machine has implications for ethics because, obviously, if there is no free will it is difficult to see how to make people responsible for their choices. With or without free will, if a human is demonstrably a threat, such as by committing a number of murders, there will be little controversy about society acting to remove the threat via imprisonment, although the harshness of the punishment may depend on the assessment of the mental state and mental competence of the killer. Killings may be attributed to a free-willed decision to kill for some gain (during a robbery), or the killer may be a psychopath unable to control killing. The psychopathy may have been inborn (genetics), the result of acquired brain dysfunction (a tumor in the amygdala), or psychologically acquired (parental abuse).

Difficult ethical questions arise related to neuroscience and physiologic psychology in the case of risky behavior. It is not illegal, per se, to be intoxicated. Fifty years ago, arguments were sometimes made in court that someone should be less harshly punished for a traffic accident because they "had one too many" and were not really responsible for their subsequent actions. Now, the opposite view is the norm. Driving while intoxicated is itself a crime punishable by loss of one's driving license (removal) and, in some cases, incarceration (punishment).

Do lower grade risky behaviors that are habitual reduce the ability to exercise free will and justify legal action? Does playing violent video games lead to violent behavior? Is smoking marijuana the gateway to more dangerous drugs? Does watching pornography lead to the commission of rape? There are neuroscientific components to all of these questions concerning whether any habit leads to any subsequent unacceptable behavior, and if so, in which people and under what other circumstances. Should bad habits that are associated with subsequent unacceptable behavior be legally sanctioned? Choices people make are caused not only by the hardware of their brain, but also by the hardware configuration modified by education, experience, knowledge of law and societal norms, and anticipated future consequences. Although the brain is a machine that operates on principles of chemistry and physics, the existence of ethics depends on the assumption that choices can be and should be made at the level of conscious knowledge. This knowledge includes the ethical norms of the society

about making choices. Most neuroscientists would say that the phrase "free will" is a construct that is useful for explaining and predicting behavior. How free one's will is in any particular situation depends on parameters that are at least partly amenable to neuroscientific investigation.

SUMMARY

- Brain activity is highly correlated with consciousness, but philosophers and religious traditions disagree about the causal relationship between the two.
- Intelligence appears to be generally correlated with the ratio of brain size to body weight.
- Although conscious capabilities appear to reside mostly in the neocortex, the integrity and operation of subcortical structures such as the reticular formation are necessary to sustain consciousness.
- A common evolutionary scenario thought to underlie the rise of consciousness is the triune theory in which nonmammalian vertebrates evolved the brainstem "reptilian complex," mammals added the limbic system and rudimentary neocortex, and primates evolved a significantly larger neocortex with particularly enlarged frontal lobes.
- Current research suggests that previous labeling of large neocortical areas such as the "association cortex" is misleading because much of this area is now known to be sensory or motor.
- The closest approximation to the role of association cortex in the brain is the prefrontal area of the frontal lobe.
- The DLPFC is crucial for the instantiation of working memory, a necessary component of consciousness.
- Ventromedial prefrontal cortex underlies representation and learning of social and emotionally salient contingencies whose valence and intensity produce "gut feelings" rather than rational verbal narratives.
- Given that *Homo sapiens* is the only species on earth thought to have true consciousness and the only species to have true language, most neuroscientists believe these facilities are strongly linked.
- The 2 brain hemispheres differ significantly in their capabilities, with the left being predominant in most individuals for language and the right being superior at spatial processing.
- Different stages of consciousness, or its lack, range from deep sleep to hypervigilance, controlled by brainstem mechanisms.
- Some specific neurologic and psychiatric disorders can be related to dysfunction in specific brain areas.
- Theories for the existence of consciousness range from brain size to synchronous neural firing to quantum

mechanical wave functions, with none being universally accepted.

- By their nature, different theories for the origin of consciousness also differ regarding the existence and causality of free will.

SELF-ASSESSMENT QUESTIONS

1. A patient is diagnosed as having a brain infarct and presents primarily with contralateral hemiparesis and dysarthria. Which of the following regions is affected by the infarct?

   A. Medial thalamic nuclei
   B. Lateral thalamic nuclei
   C. Dorsomedial thalamus
   D. Ventromedial thalamus
   E. Medial hypothalamus

2. A middle-aged woman, who is suffering from a rare autosomal recessive condition that results in calcification and degeneration of specific regions of the forebrain, is seen by a psychiatrist. The patient is given a battery of tests and is found to be unable to recognize fear in pictures presented to her. Nor is she able to draw a picture depicting fear; however, she is capable of drawing pictures depicting other emotions. A magnetic resonance imaging (MRI) scan indicates significant atrophy of tissue in a specific region of the brain. Which of the regions indicated below is the most likely target of this rare autosomal recessive condition?

   A. Mammillary bodies
   B. Septal area
   C. Amygdala
   D. Cingulate gyrus
   E. Lateral hypothalamus

3. A 65-year-old man suddenly finds himself unable to recognize the speech of individuals and the sounds of animals, whistles, or bells, but is still able to discriminate tones and hear sounds. On an MRI, a lesion was detected in which of the following regions?

   A. Inferior parietal cortex
   B. Superior parietal cortex
   C. Inferior temporal cortex
   D. Superior temporal cortex
   E. Medial geniculate nucleus

4. A patient is described as being socially disinhibited and displaying severe impairments in judgment, foresight, and insight. An MRI reveals the presence of a brain lesion. Where is the likely locus of this lesion?

   A. Premotor cortex
   B. Superior parietal lobule
   C. Prefrontal cortex
   D. Hippocampal formation
   E. Amygdala

20

Learning & Memory

Cristin F. Gavin & Anne B. Theibert

O B J E C T I V E S

After studying this chapter, the student should be able to:

- Define the 3 components of memory: encoding, storage, and retrieval.
- Distinguish and describe the temporal phases of memory: sensory, short-term/working, and long-term memory.
- Diagram the working memory model and its components, and identify the underlying brain mechanism of short-term working memory.
- Define the 2 information processing systems—declarative/explicit and nondeclarative/implicit memory—and describe their subsystems.
- Identify the brain regions involved in the information processing subsystems.
- Explain synaptic and systems consolidation and the role of sleep in memory consolidation.

OVERVIEW OF MEMORY & MEMORY SYSTEMS

One of the essential cognitive functions, memory involves the mental processes by which information is encoded, stored, and retrieved. Memory is thought to involve physical changes in the brain, called engrams or memory traces. In cognitive neuroscience, memory is defined not only by encoding and storing of the engram, but also through expression, which refers to the retrieval of stored information that leads to modification of behavior or conscious thought. Memory allows us to accomplish everyday physical and living activities and is critical for other key cognitive processes including language, planning, reasoning, and problem solving; it is also a fundamental component of our personality and consciousness.

Memory is the basis for the amassment of knowledge, the importance of which is exemplified by Francis Bacon's quote "Knowledge itself is power." Diminished learning and memory occur in normal aging and are common features of intellectual disability, traumatic brain injury, schizophrenia, Parkinson disease, and Alzheimer disease. Based on its central role in human behavior and disruption in many brain disorders, memory has been studied extensively in the fields of psychology, neuroscience, and clinical medicine. In this chapter, the various memory systems will be elaborated. Complementing this chapter is Chapter 10, "Synaptic Plasticity," in which

synaptic plasticity mechanisms implicated in encoding of memory are described.

In the broadest sense, memory can be categorized into collective memory and individual memory. Collective memory is a shared pool of knowledge by members of a social group, usually requiring symbolic representation such as language, and often studied in the discipline of sociology. The modern concept of human individual memory (hereafter memory) involves characteristic features. First, memory encompasses at least 4 components: acquisition, consolidation, storage, and retrieval, also called recall. Consolidation involves processes that stabilize a memory trace after its initial acquisition; learning consists of acquisition and consolidation and is also called encoding. Learning is a graded phenomenon, and most forms of memory can be either short lasting or long lasting. Second, memory involves multiple memory systems that depend on the specific type of information processed. Consequently, memory can be classified according to 2 features: the time course of learning and storage and the nature of the information learned and stored.

Focusing first on the time course, human memory involves informational processing systems with distinct temporal components. The idea that there are temporal forms of memory was expressed by William James and others in 1890, who distinguished between primary and secondary memory. The "modal" or "multistore" model of memory, published

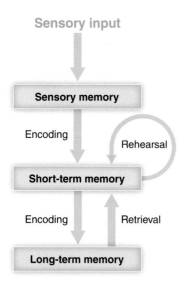

FIGURE 20–1 The modal/multistore model of memory. Proposed by Richard Atkinson and Richard Shiffrin in 1968, this structural model proposes that memory consists of three separate stores, each with its own characteristics. Information is processed and passed from store to store in a linear way.

in 1968 by Atkinson and Shiffrin, proposes a structure of memory composed of sensory memory (also called a sensory register) and a dual memory store that includes short-term memory and long-term memory (Figure 20–1).

Sensory memory involves initial sensing and processing of chemical and physical stimuli from the outside world, has a relatively high capacity, and is very short lived, on the order of a few hundreds of milliseconds to seconds. Short-term memory is defined as a short-term store of pertinent or goal-directed information; it depends on attention, the cognitive process that involves selectively concentrating on 1 aspect of the environment while ignoring other aspects. Short-term memory has a limited capacity and a lifetime of a few tens of seconds to minutes. In 1974, Baddeley and Hitch proposed a revision to the short-term memory model, transitioning to the concept of working memory. Working memory encompasses short-term memory and serves as both an encoding and retrieval processor, with an active maintenance of information in short-term memory storage and processes to manipulate information in the store. Long-term memory is the permanent store where information is retained for extended periods, from months to years to decades.

Focusing next on the nature of the information encoded, long-term memory is typically divided into declarative and nondeclarative types, also known as explicit and implicit memory, respectively, with several subtypes in each category (Table 20–1). Declarative memory includes semantic memory and episodic memory. Semantic memory includes memory of facts and information that is encoded with specific meaning. Episodic memory refers to experience and events that are encoded along spatial and temporal dimensions. Declarative memory usually involves conscious encoding and conscious recall and is also called explicit memory because it consists

TABLE 20–1 Forms of long-term memory.

Form	Examples
Declarative, or explicit	Facts, information, events
Nondeclarative, or implicit	Procedures, skills, conditioning

of information that is explicitly stored and retrieved. Nondeclarative memory includes memory for procedures, tasks, and skills, as well as emotional and conditioned responses. Nondeclarative memory is also called implicit memory and can be consciously or unconsciously encoded but is usually unconsciously recalled. These different memory systems can operate independently and in parallel, which allows conscious and unconscious memory systems to operate simultaneously and maximize memory throughput of the brain.

Different functional areas in the brain are involved in encoding and storing different types of information (Figure 20–2). Sensory memory involves primary, secondary, and association sensory cortices for each modality. Short-term memory and working memory are thought to involve predominantly the prefrontal cortex (PFC), but also include functions of the parietal and medial temporal lobes (MTLs) and basal ganglia. For long-term memory encoding, the majority of neuroanatomic regions that are associated with specific memory systems have been identified using clinical approaches. The hippocampus is involved in declarative and spatial learning, whereas the amygdala is involved in emotional memory. The basal ganglia and cerebellum are involved in procedural learning. Much less is known about the neuroanatomy of memory storage. In general, memories are thought to be stored in distributed neocortical circuits.

SENSORY MEMORY

Defined as the first component of the modal model, sensory memory involves the acquisition of sensory information obtained by sensory receptors and processed within the sensory cortices in the brain. Sensory memory, also called the sensory register, provides a moment-to-moment snapshot of an individual's overall sensory experience. Sensory information is stored for only a few hundreds of milliseconds to seconds, allowing a brief but high-resolution impression of the sensation, just long enough for pertinent information to be conveyed to short-term memory. Sensory memory is specific for each of the senses, of which humans have 5: vision, hearing, smell, touch, and taste; the sensory stimuli are called sensory modalities.

Common features have been identified for all forms of sensory memory studied. First, information stored in sensory memory is modality specific. The visual sensory store is called iconic memory; the auditory store is echoic memory; and the somatosensory store is haptic memory. Olfactory memory and gustatory memory have also been identified but are not as well characterized. Second, the formation of a sensory trace

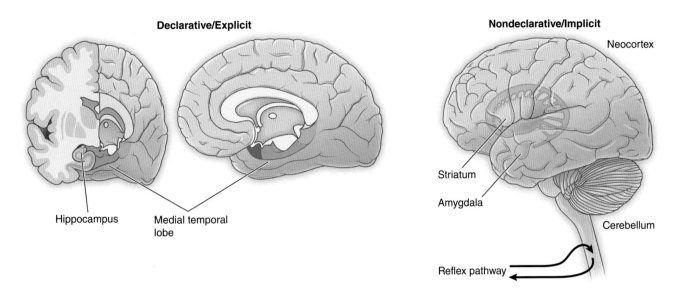

FIGURE 20-2 Long-term memory encoding systems involve different brain regions. Declarative/explicit memory requires the hippocampus and nearby structures in the medial temporal lobe. For non-declarative/implicit memory, procedural memory involves the basal ganglia and cerebellum, emotional memory involves the amygdala, priming involves the cerebral cortex, and classical conditioning involves the cerebellum, brainstem, and spinal cord.

is only weakly dependent on attention to the stimulus, and the duration and capacity of sensory memory are outside of cognitive control. Third, the sensory stores are very brief in duration, on the order of about 0.2 to 2 seconds, depending on the modality. Fourth, the sensory stores have a relatively large capacity, facilitating details that provide high resolution.

The sensory memory engram or trace is thought to involve the transient activation of sensory circuits underlying that modality, which occur within the primary, secondary, and association sensory cortices for that modality. A subset of information can be transferred from the rapidly decaying sensory memory into short-term memory via the process of attention. This filters sensory stimuli such that only relevant information at any given time will be transferred into short-term memory. Thus, the function of sensory memory is to provide a detailed representation of our sensory experience, from which specific relevant or goal-oriented information is extracted into short-term memory and processed.

SHORT-TERM & WORKING MEMORY

Short-term memory maintains current representations of goal-relevant information in a temporary store. In the modal model, movement of information from sensory memory into short-term memory requires attention, which can be either bottom up, stimulus driven, or top down, goal oriented. Short-term memory has a limited capacity of about 4 to 7 pieces, depending on the nature of the information stored, and a limited duration, on the order of tens of seconds to minutes. The capacity and duration of short-term memory can be enhanced. Chunking, the process of organizing material into meaningful

groups, can increase the capacity of short-term memory. Rehearsal, the ongoing repetition of the information held in short-term storage, can extend the duration. Thus, in its original conception, short-term memory is the capacity for holding, but not manipulating, limited amounts of information in the mind in an accessible store for short periods of time.

The term *working memory* was coined by Miller, Galanter, and Pribram in the 1960s in the context of the mind operating like a computer, but it was not until the 1970s and 1980s that Baddley and Hitch proposed a model that defines working memory in its current structure (Figure 20–3). In their scheme, information in the short-term memory store can

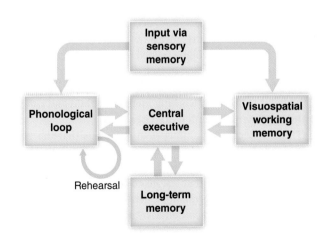

FIGURE 20-3 Working memory model. Proposed by Alan Baddeley and Graham Hitch in 1974, this model organizes short term memory into sub-components and defines working memory. A fourth component, the episodic buffer (not shown) was added later.

be dynamically organized and manipulated; addition of this functional role is a key feature of working memory. Working memory handles information that enters not only from sensory memory but also from recently recalled long-term stores. Hence, working memory is bidirectional, serving as both an input and output device, for the holding and processing of new and already stored information, for the purpose of cognitive tasks.

Another feature of working memory is that it contains at least 2 storage subsystems—one for visual and spatial information, called the visuospatial sketchpad, and another for verbal information, called the phonological loop. These subsystems are under the control of a component called the central executive. The central executive enables working memory systems to selectively attend to some stimuli and ignore others and coordinate cognitive processes especially when more than 1 task is simultaneously performed. In 2000, Baddeley extended the model by adding another component, the episodic buffer, which holds representations that integrate phonologic, visual, and spatial information, and possibly information not covered by those subsystems, such as semantic and musical information. The episodic buffer also provides the link between working memory and long-term memory.

Many cognitive scientists and psychologists today use the concept of working memory to replace or include the previous scheme of short-term memory, emphasizing the functional role of working memory in manipulating and using information in the store, compared with the storage role of short-term memory. For simplicity, hereafter the term *short-term working memory* will be used to refer to both the temporary storage and manipulation of information in the store. Short-term working memory has received substantial attention over the past few decades. Impairment of short-term working memory is observed in several brain disorders, including attention-deficit/hyperactivity disorder, Parkinson disease, and Alzheimer disease. In normal cognition, short-term working memory, together with attention, plays a major role in the processes of thinking. Short-term working memory facilitates planning, comprehension, reasoning, decision making, and problem solving. Consequently, measures of short-term working memory capacity are strongly related to performance in other complex cognitive tasks, and in fact, working memory is a better predictor of academic success than is intelligence quotient (IQ). Finally, short-term working memory is fluid and can be enhanced by mental training exercises.

There is consensus among neuroscientists that the PFC plays a substantial role in short-term working memory (Figure 20–4). Research on monkeys in the 1930s by Jacobsen and Fulton showed that lesions to the PFC impaired spatial short-term working memory performance. In the 1970s, Fuster and colleagues recorded activation of PFC neurons in monkeys while they performed short-term working memory tasks. Functional imaging studies over the past 2 decades confirmed activation of the PFC in humans during short-term working memory tasks. Functional magnetic resonance imaging and transcranial magnetic lesion studies have revealed

potential additional roles for the parietal lobe, MTL, and basal ganglia in short-term working memory. This is not entirely surprising given the roles of the parietal lobe in attention and computation of sensory information and the roles of the MTL and basal ganglia in encoding long-term memories.

Research by Goldman-Rakic and others in the 1990s demonstrated that networks of PFC excitatory pyramidal neurons continue to fire during, and are required for, short-term working memory. These and other studies led to a model stipulating that the encoding of short-term working memory involves increased and persistent firing of PFC neurons in recurrent networks. In the models, persistent activity is induced by sensory input (and presumably via input from long-term memory), which persists even after the input disappears, and different PFC subregions contribute to different components of the working memory system. More recently, researchers have hypothesized that working memory mechanisms involve activity-dependent (Hebbian) short-term synaptic plasticity (defined in Chapter 10, "Synaptic Plasticity"). Both short-term potentiation and short-term depression have been implicated in short-term working memory. In fact, potentiation has been proposed as a candidate mechanism that underlies the enhanced persistent firing model. Short-term potentiation involves enhanced neurotransmitter release by increasing presynaptic calcium ion (Ca^{2+}) levels or duration and/or enhanced release mechanisms. Short-term depression is thought to involve depletion of neurotransmitter stores. These synaptic changes could function as short-term working memory traces. The memory trace would decay over time as the release activities and neurotransmitter levels are restored to their prestimulus levels. Other non-Hebbian synaptic and neuronal plasticity mechanisms may act in parallel with synaptic plasticity in short-term working memory mechanisms.

LONG-TERM MEMORY

Long-term memory is the second stage of the dual memory store model where large amounts of information can be stored for prolonged periods of time, from years to decades. In the model, long-term memory depends on short-term working memory for its input and is accessed by the process of recall, also known as retrieval, in which information is located and then brought back to short-term working memory (Figure 20–5). Long-term memory encompasses the concept of multiple memory systems, which are defined based on the types of information being learned and stored. The 2 main types of memory are declarative, also called explicit memory, and nondeclarative, also called implicit memory. Declarative memory encodes and stores semantic, episodic, and spatial information; is consciously learned and recalled; and depends specifically on the hippocampus for encoding. Nondeclarative memory includes procedural and motor memory and nonassociative and classical associative learning; is unconsciously learned; and can be unconsciously or consciously recalled. Each of the nondeclarative subsystems requires specific brain

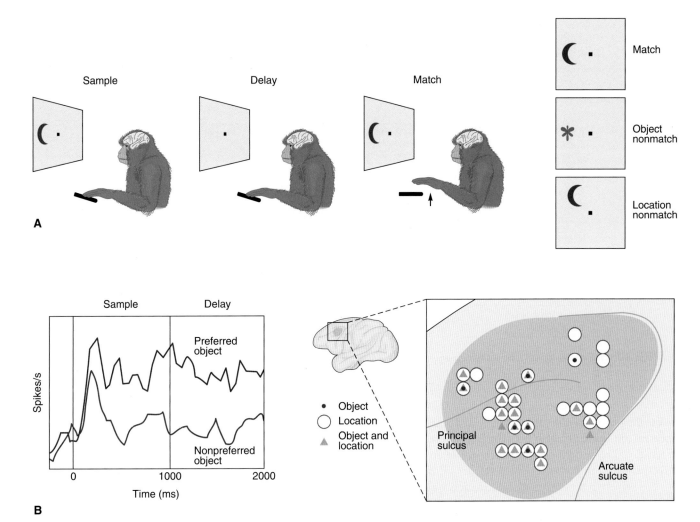

FIGURE 20–4 The prefrontal cortex is involved in short-term working memory. **A.** Neuronal activity is assessed in monkeys during the delayed-match-to-sample (DMS) task. A trial begins when the monkey grabs a response lever and fixates a small target at the center of a computer screen. An initial stimulus (Sample) is briefly presented and must be held in working memory until the next stimulus (Match) appears. The monkey was required to remember the sample and its location and release the lever only in response to stimuli that "matched" on both dimensions. **B.** Neuronal firing rates in the lateral prefrontal cortex during the delay period in the task are often above baseline and represent responses to the type of stimulus, the location, and the integration of the two. Left is activity of a prefrontal neuron to preferred objects (to which the neuron responds robustly) and to nonpreferred objects (to which the neuron responds minimally) during the task. Activity is robust when the monkey encounters the preferred object (sample) and during the delay. At right the symbols represent recording sites where neurons that maintained each type of information (what, where, and what and where) were found.

regions, such as the basal ganglia, cerebellum, or amygdala, for encoding of information in long-term memory.

It is well accepted that the formation of long-term memories progresses as a time-dependent process and that, as time advances, memories become stronger and less susceptible to interference. Before the memory is stabilized, long-term memory is subject to fading through the normal processes of forgetting. There are numerous hypotheses about forgetting, including mechanisms of passive and active forgetting. The 3 main passive forgetting models are (1) the loss of context cues that hinder retrieval, (2) interference from other similar memories that hinder retrieval, and (3) the natural decay of memory traces, called trace decay theory. Four forms of active forgetting have also been postulated. In interference-based

forgetting, other competing information or activities accelerate the decay of memory traces. In motivated forgetting, cognitive mechanisms are voluntarily engaged to weaken a memory trace, often for unpleasant memories. In retrieval-induced forgetting, some aspects of a memory are recalled that suppress the recall of other aspects related to the recalled memory. In intrinsic forgetting, activity of forgetting cells and intrinsic biochemical and molecular pathways degrade the previously encoded memory traces. It seems likely that, depending on the region or type of information affected, different mechanisms may be employed for forgetting.

Repetition or rehearsal is often required to encode and preserve a long-term memory. For most declarative and procedural memory, items stored in short-term working memory

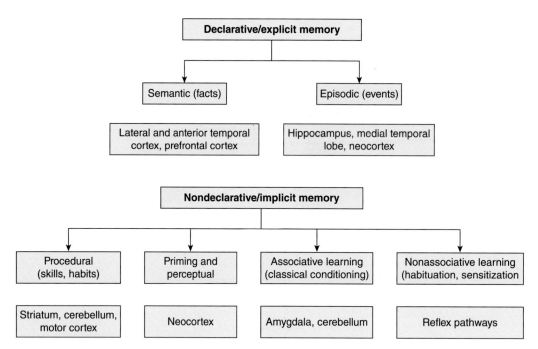

FIGURE 20–5 Subdivisions of long-term memory.

move to long-term memory through repeated practice and use. Rehearsal can occur through behavior, reflection, or deliberate recall, called recapitulation, which are often dependent on the perceived importance, called valence, of the information. For some types of memory, information with extremely high valence, for example, fear, may transition rapidly into long-term memory with just 1 learning experience. Memory research has shown that learning is subject to interference. In contrast, once a memory has been stored in a long-term memory store, it no longer requires rehearsal and becomes immune to interference. However, after long-term memories are recalled and undergo reconsolidation, memories can become labile and malleable.

It is well established that human long-term memory can store a massive number of items, which has been well studied in visual memory, where subjects can recall details about thousands of images after viewing. Because it is thought that the engram involves biochemical and physical changes in synapses and neurons, it is expected there must be a physical limit to how many memories we can store. Although the size of the memory store has not been measured, it has been estimated. If each neuron participated in the storage of a single memory, the limit of the store would be 86 billion (nearly 10^{11}) pieces of information. Because 1 neuron can receive thousands of synaptic inputs and each neuron probably participates in multiple memories, this exponentially increases the brain's memory storage capacity, with current estimates of the store at around a petabyte (a million gigabytes or 10^{15} units of information).

Learning involves acquisition and encoding of information, leading to the formation and stabilization of the memory trace, which for long-term memory involves processes called memory consolidation, of which there are 2 types, termed synaptic consolidation and systems consolidation. These types of memory consolidation occur with different but overlapping time courses, mechanisms, and brain areas. Synaptic consolidation represents the first phase, beginning within the first minutes after acquisition and lasting for several hours. During synaptic consolidation, the memory trace is encoded as changes in synapses that involve synaptic plasticity mechanisms, molecular changes that alter synaptic transmission, and morphology. Synaptic consolidation is thought to occur through modification of synapses in small groups of neurons in a specific brain region required for learning, for example the hippocampus for semantic information. Candidate mechanisms underlying synaptic consolidation are detailed in Chapter 10, "Synaptic Plasticity." Some investigators now refer to this phase as synaptic and cellular consolidation because additional neuronal activities such as gene expression and global modulation of excitability may be involved.

During systems consolidation, which begins within hours but takes weeks to months to years to be accomplished, memory traces that were first encoded by synaptic consolidation are then distributed to other areas of the brain and are stored as stable alterations of neuronal circuits. One hypothesis is that the memory trace is gradually consolidated within a population of engram neurons in the region where the memory is stored. Recurrent activation, or "training," of the engram neurons in the storage circuit by neurons in the learning circuit may be involved. In addition, changes in gene expression in the neurons of the consolidated memory circuit have also been demonstrated.

There is consensus that long-term memories are stored in widely distributed neuronal circuits throughout the cerebral cortex. Numerous intriguing ideas have been proposed about memory storage. Specific aspects of memories may be encoded within individual neural networks by specific patterns of synaptic connections. The memory of all the aspects of an object, fact, event, location, skill, or response likely involves several different groups of neurons in different parts of the brain. Memories may be stored as connections between groups of neurons that are primed to fire together in the same pattern that created the original experience. Each component of a memory may be stored in the brain area that initiated it. Long-term memories may be accessed independently, by visual, verbal, or other sensory clues. Memories may be encoded redundantly in various regions of the cortex, such that if 1 memory trace is lost, the duplicated engram or alternative route allows the memory to still be recalled. These compelling ideas await support by experimental data. Studies have demonstrated that sleep is an important factor in establishing long-term memories, because processes that occur during sleep play key roles in system consolidation.

The recall of memory refers to the process of retrieval of information from long-term memory stores. The 2-stage theory proposes that recall begins with a search and retrieval process and then progresses to a decision or recognition process where the correct information is chosen from what has been retrieved. Once a previously consolidated memory has been recalled, it can be actively reconsolidated. It has been proposed that reconsolidation serves to maintain, strengthen, and modify memories that had already been stored in long-term memory. During reconsolidation, memories become labile and malleable. Importantly, reconsolidation may provide the opportunity for significant memories to become updated, incorporating new information into the long-term memory store. Many important questions about long-term memory are currently under investigation in basic neuroscience research. For example, what are the mechanisms whereby previously stored memories remain stable but accessible and malleable. Another key question is: How does the brain maintain previously learned memories while it continues to learn new information that becomes incorporated into the networks of preexisting long-term memories?

DECLARATIVE/EXPLICIT MEMORY

One of the 2 main types of human long-term memory, declarative/explicit memory, is a memory system for factual knowledge, concepts, experiences, and spatial information. Four common features define declarative/explicit memory. It is consciously learned and consciously recalled (hence, the term *explicit*); after recall, it can be described or articulated (hence, the term *declarative*). Declarative/explicit memory is extremely flexible; numerous pieces of information can be associated under different situations. Anatomically, declarative/explicit memory requires the MTL, including the hippocampus and surrounding entorhinal, perirhinal, and parahippocampal cortices, for learning (Figure 20–6).

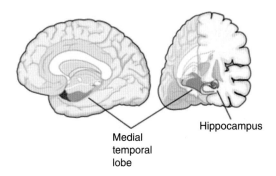

FIGURE 20–6 The medial temporal lobe contains the hippocampus and surrounding entorhinal cortex and perirhinal cortex involved in encoding long-term declarative/explicit memory. (Reproduced with permission from Kandel ER, Schwartz JH, Jessell TM, et al: *Principles of Neural Science*, 5th ed. New York, NY: McGraw Hill; 2013.)

The 2 main subcategories of declarative memory are semantic memory and episodic memory. Semantic memory reflects factual information, meaning ideas and concepts; it includes vocabulary, verbal symbols, object knowledge and function, social customs, geography, understanding of math, and all the factual knowledge acquired over a lifetime. Episodic memory involves observational information attached to specific life experiences and events. These can be memories about what happens to a person directly or events that occur in situations around a person. Episodic memory involves the encoding and recall of events and experiences that include a location context and time component.

Two additional subcategories of declarative/explicit memory, termed autobiographical and spatial memory, have been defined. Autobiographical memory consists of episodic memory about personal experiences combined with semantic knowledge associated with those experiences and information about oneself. These include our personal experiences, such as likes, dislikes, and opinions that contribute to our sense of identity and form part of the "self-memory system" proposed by Conway and Pleydell-Pearce in 2000. Spatial memory is involved in recording and recalling information about one's environment and spatial orientation. Spatial memory provides essential components for episodic memory but is also key for representation of location, spatial orientation, and goal directed spatial navigation and thus has earned its own subcategory in declarative/explicit memory.

Evidence for the role of the MTL in long-term memory was first discovered in the 1950s from the study of patients who had undergone surgery for epilepsy or suffered damage to the MTL. The first, most famous, and most thoroughly studied patient was H.M. By age 27, H.M. had suffered for over 10 years from intractable temporal lobe epilepsy, caused by brain damage following a bicycle accident. Recurrent uncontrolled seizures were debilitating and rendered him unable to live a normal life. Experimental surgery was performed to reduce the seizures that involved a bilateral MTL resection, including removal of the hippocampal formation, amygdala, and parts of the multimodal association area of the temporal cortex. Although the surgery resulted in better control of his seizures, H.M. was left with a devastating memory deficit. He suffered from anterograde amnesia and was unable to form new semantic or episodic long-term memories. Consequently, H.M. lived minute to minute for the next 50 years of his life.

H.M.'s memory deficit was remarkably specific. His short-term working memory was largely intact. His prior memories were mostly intact for his lifetime up to several years before the surgery; he experienced some retrograde amnesia for information acquired in the several years before his operation. H.M. retained the command of language, including his vocabulary, indicating that semantic memory was preserved; his IQ remained the same. His ability to learn new procedural and motor skills and classical and operant conditioning appeared normal. What H.M. lacked after the surgery was the ability to transfer new information about people, places, and objects he had encountered or other daily experiences from short-term working memory into long-term memory. Other patients who have experienced bilateral lesions of the hippocampus or MTL, from surgery or as a result of disease, have shown comparable long-term memory deficits.

These clinical studies, together with a multitude of studies using animal models and human functional brain imaging, support the conclusion that the hippocampus and adjacent entorhinal cortex, the main input area from the cerebral cortex to the hippocampus, play essential roles in forming new declarative/explicit memories, and other structures in the MTL contribute important functions as well. In addition, these studies demonstrate that the MTL is not essential for short-term working memory, nondeclarative/implicit memory, or storage and retrieval of the majority of declarative/explicit memory (although a role for the MTL in recall of some autobiographical memory has been shown). After his death, H.M.'s name was revealed; the field of neuroscience owes a large debt of gratitude to Henry Molaison and other patients, whose participation in experimental studies catapulted the understanding of human long-term memory.

Regions in the MTL are also involved in perception and spatial representation, which in addition to providing input for memory, may perform additional cognitive functions. For example, the perirhinal cortex has been implicated in object recognition. Neurons have been identified in the rodent hippocampus, called "place cells," that fire bursts of action potentials when the animal passes through a particular location in its environment. Other hippocampal neurons called "head direction cells" respond when the animal's head points in a specific direction; "boundary cells" respond to the presence of an environmental boundary. Specific neurons in the entorhinal cortex act as "grid cells," which respond when the animal traverses a set of small regions, and "speed cells," which respond to the speed of the animal's running. Together these MTL cells are thought to form a network that provides a neural representation of the animal's specific location and movement in space, acting as a cognitive map and contributing to spatial memory as well.

What are the mechanisms involved in the formation of long-term declarative/explicit memory? As described in Section 4, it has been proposed that long-term memory involves consolidation. In a popular model, changes in synapses and neuronal gene expression within hippocampal neurons in the first few hours of learning underlie synaptic and cellular consolidation for declarative/explicit memory. These involve synaptic plasticity mechanisms, in particular long-term potentiation (LTP) and long-term depression (LTD). Described in Chapter 10, "Synaptic Plasticity," LTP and LTD are activity-dependent persistent changes in synaptic transmission, which encompass signaling cascades that produce biochemical and morphologic changes in synapses, as well as signaling to the nucleus that leads to changes in neuronal gene expression. In systems consolidation, information is actively transferred as the hippocampus teaches the cortex more and more about the information it has acquired. The standard model of systems consolidation proposes that soon after learning, the same hippocampal and cortical neurons that encode memory are reactivated during retrieval; in the early stages, the hippocampus guides the reactivation of neocortical circuits during retrieval of memory. However, as time progresses, neocortical circuits are reactivated during memory retrieval and no longer require input from the hippocampus. Studies demonstrate that neocortical plasticity is required for memory consolidation, with many of the signaling cascades and genes identified in hippocampal LTP and LTD implicated in systems consolidation.

It is well documented that sleep plays an important role in formation of declarative/explicit memory. One model contends that, during slow wave sleep (SWS), reactivation of newly learned hippocampal memory representations transfers information to neocortical networks, where it is integrated into long-term representations through systems consolidation. Research suggests the sleep spindles, a sleep wave generated in the thalamus, play an additional role in boosting consolidation of declarative memories and/or incorporating new information into existing knowledge. Rapid eye movement (REM) sleep has also been implicated in declarative memory. Sleep may play an active role in producing specific brain waves or other processes that facilitate memory consolidation processes, or a passive role to protect from interference or provide ideal conditions for memory consolidation. In an active role model, specific brain waves or other processes that occur during SWS may contribute to the regulation of gene expression that controls proteins required for synaptic plasticity. It has been suggested that systems consolidation occurs during sleep, because this is a period when the necessary retrieval of memory required for consolidation occurs and would not interfere with daily cognitive functions.

NONDECLARATIVE/ IMPLICIT MEMORY

Nondeclarative/implicit memory is the other major category of long-term human memory. Nondeclarative memory is reflected in automatic changes in behavior, tasks, responses, or performance that do not require conscious thought or conceptual recollection. It allows people to do things by rote without thinking about them. It allows us to perform many tasks effortlessly, but it is often difficult to explain exactly how we do them, hence the term *nondeclarative*. The 4 main subcategories of nondeclarative/implicit memory are (1) procedural, which includes motor and perceptual skills, tasks, and habit formation; (2) priming; (3) simple, classical and associative conditioning; and (4) nonassociative learning.

These subtypes of nondeclarative/implicit memory share several features in common. They are all types of unconscious memory that is evident in the performance of a task, behavior, or response. They are inflexible (ie, insensitive to surface perceptual changes). They are tightly connected to the original context under which the learning occurred. However, although similar in their characteristics, each of these subcategories involves different, but sometimes overlapping, brain regions for their functions. Similar to declarative/explicit memory, nondeclarative/implicit learning involves changes in the effectiveness of the synaptic pathways that underlie those memory systems, which is further described in Chapter 10, "Synaptic Plasticity." Indeed, many of the signaling pathways and mechanisms involved in synaptic plasticity underlying memory were first discovered in nondeclarative/implicit systems.

One of the most well-recognized forms of nondeclarative/implicit memory is procedural memory, which enables people to perform certain tasks, skills, and habits automatically, without being consciously aware or remembering how to perform the actions (Figure 20–7). It is the "how to" knowledge and constitutes a large majority of nondeclarative/implicit memory. In everyday life, people rely on procedural memory for physical actions such as tying a shoe, driving a car, washing dishes, and turning on a smart phone, without conscious awareness or thinking. Even behaviors that we consider innate, such as walking, require components of procedural memory. Procedural memory also involves learning motor sequences that are inherent in more complex skill learning, such as playing a musical instrument or hitting a tennis ball. Many procedural memory tasks are unconsciously learned, but components can also involve conscious learning as well. Improving procedural skills involves repetition and practice. Studies of human clinical disorders provided the first clues as to the brain regions involved in procedural memory, which is now known to involve the basal ganglia and cerebellum. Parkinson disease pathology is largely limited to the basal ganglia, and patients with this disorder have deficits in the acquisition of new motor skills. Within the basal ganglia, the striatum contains the main neuronal cell nuclei linked to procedural memory. Damage to the cerebellum can affect learning of motor and procedural skills. The cerebellum

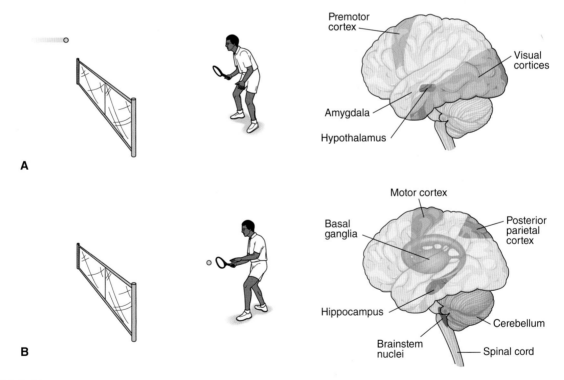

FIGURE 20–7 Procedural memory involves the basal ganglia and cerebellum. **A.** A tennis player uses the visual cortex to perceive the size, direction, and velocity of the ball. The premotor cortex develops a motor program to return the ball. **B.** The basal ganglia becomes involved in initiating motor patterns. To execute the shot the motor cortex sends signals to the spinal cord that control muscles in the arms and legs. The basal ganglia and cerebellum are also involved in learning/encoding movements in the racket swing, and those memories are recalled to hit the ball properly. The posterior parietal cortex sends feedback sensory information and the cerebellum also adjust movements. The hippocampus is not involved in hitting the ball but is involved in storing the memory of the shot so the player can describe it later. (Reproduced with permission from Kandel ER, Schwartz JH, Jessell TM, et al: *Principles of Neural Science*, 5th ed. New York, NY: McGraw Hill; 2013.)

functions in correcting movement and fine tuning the motor agility found in complex procedural skills such as painting, instrument playing, and accuracy sports.

Priming is a subcategory of nondeclarative/implicit memory concerned with perceptual identification of words, objects, and other stimuli. Priming produces an improved facility for detecting or processing a perceptual object based on recent experience; exposure to 1 stimulus using pictures, words, or music influences the response to a subsequent stimulus. A typical example of priming is when a person reads or hears a word, and for some period of time afterward, the person is more likely to use that word in conversation or in a word completion experiment. Priming not only improves the ability to identify stimuli but also alters judgments and preferences that involve the same stimuli. For example, priming leads to the illusion-of-truth effect, which suggests that subjects are more likely to believe or rate as true those statements that they have already heard, regardless of the truth of the statement. Studies on stroke patients indicate that priming involves the occipital and prefrontal cortices.

Associative memory is a subcategory of nondeclarative/implicit memory where an animal learns the predictive value of one stimulus for another. Essential for survival and generally reliable, associative memory is the neural correlate of cause and effect. Two types of associative learning, called classical conditioning and operant conditioning, were defined through extensive experimental studies used throughout the 20th century, which still form the core of associative memory research today. Classical conditioning involves associating 2 environmental stimuli, such that a response is conditioned to an unrelated stimulus, and involves unconscious reflexive responses and skeletal musculature. Operant conditioning involves associating a specific behavior with a reinforcing environmental event and involves the execution of a voluntary motor response.

Classical conditioning was first studied in detail by Ivan Pavlov, through his seminal experiments with dog behavior. Subsequently, other experimental paradigms were developed, including conditioned fear response, classical eye blink response, and odor and taste aversion. Pavlovian classical conditioning involves a specific paradigm. Before conditioning occurs, a stimulus, called the unconditioned stimulus (US), produces a natural unlearned response, called the unconditioned response (UR). The US needs to be biologically potent and can be pleasant and even rewarding or unpleasant and even painful. The UR is an involuntary, automatic, or reflexive response. In Pavlov's experiments, prior to conditioning, presentation of food was the US, and it produced salivation, the UR. The experiment involves another stimulus, called the neutral stimulus (NS), which has no effect on an animal before learning. The NS could be a person, object, place, noise, smell, or some other stimulus. For Pavlov, the NS was the sound of a metronome.

Conditioning begins when the NS is paired with the US. As soon as the pairing begins, the NS becomes what is called the conditioned stimulus (CS), and it becomes associated with the pleasant/unpleasant and rewarding/painful qualities of the US. After pairing is repeated, the animal exhibits a conditioned

response (CR) to the CS when the CS is presented alone. The CR is usually similar to the UR, although there may be some differences. Consequently, with successful pairing, the CS is able to produce a CR that is reminiscent of the UR to the US. For Pavlov, the sound of the metronome elicited a salivation response in the dogs, before and even without the presentation of food.

In the conditioned fear response, an aversive stimulus, such as a foot shock, becomes associated with a specific environmental context or stimulus sound, resulting in the expression of a fear response, such as freezing. Fear conditioning involves the amygdala and, depending on the type of US, can also involve the hippocampus (for contextual fear conditioning) (Figure 20–8). In eye blink conditioning, before learning, a mild puff of air or shock to the cornea, the US, produces a reflexive eye blink response, the UR. During conditioning, the pairing of an auditory or visual stimulus (initially a NS, which becomes the CS) together with the US (air puff) leads to the CR, the eye blink. Studies have shown that eye blink conditioning involves the cerebellum. In olfactory conditioning, pairing of an odor with an aversive stimulus results in the animal's aversion to that particular odor and involves the olfactory bulb. Conditioned taste aversion occurs when an animal associates the taste of a certain food with symptoms caused by a toxic, spoiled, or poisonous substance that produce nausea, sickness, or vomiting. The nucleus tractus solitarius in the brainstem has been implicated in conditioned taste aversion.

Many human behaviors can be modified through positive and negative reinforcement, so behavior can be controlled by predicted consequences. Operant conditioning is a type of learning in which the strength of a behavior is modified by the behavior's consequences, such as reward or punishment. In operant conditioning, an individual makes an association between a particular behavior and a consequence, and the stimuli present when a behavior is rewarded or punished can also become associated. Throughout humanity, behaviors that lead to a successful outcome are often retained, whereas those that are unsuccessful or produce adverse effects are usually discarded. Moreover, operant conditioning has likely been used by parents in teaching children for tens of thousands of years.

Famously studied first by Edward Thorndike in the late 19th century and then B.F. Skinner in the mid-20th century, operant conditioning experiments can involve positive or negative reinforcement or punishment. Positive reinforcement occurs when a behavior or response is itself rewarding or the behavior is followed by another stimulus that is rewarding. Negative reinforcement occurs when a response or behavior is followed by the removal of an adverse stimulus. Positive punishment occurs when a behavior or response is followed by an aversive stimulus. Negative punishment occurs when a behavior or response is followed by the removal of a positive stimulus. The goal in both types of reinforcement is for the behavior to increase, whereas the goal in both types of punishment is for a behavior to decrease. Evidence suggests that both acetylcholine (produced by neurons in the basal nuclei)

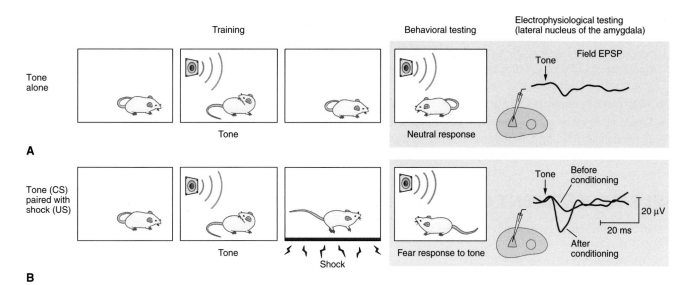

FIGURE 20–8 Fear conditioning (learned fear). **A.** An animal ordinarily ignores a neutral tone, which produces a small field excitatory postsynaptic potential (EPSP) recorded in the amygdala. **B.** When the tone is presented immediately before a foot shock, called the unconditioned stimulus (US), the animal learns to associate the tone, called the conditioned stimulus (CS) with the shock. Subsequently the tone alone causes the mouse to freeze, an instinctive fear response. After fear conditioning the electrophysiological response in the lateral nucleus of the amygdala to the tone is greater than the response prior to conditioning.

and dopamine (produced by neurons in the midbrain) are involved in operant conditioning.

Regarded as one of the simplest forms of implicit learning in animals, nonassociative learning is considered a fundamental form of learning that can be observed across all animal phyla and most sensory modalities. Nonassociative memory involves a change in the strength of a response to a single stimulus, resulting from repeated exposure to that stimulus, but does not require the formation of an association between one environmental stimulus and another. It automatically classifies the valence of a sensory input based on its temporal pattern without the need for concomitant or feedback signals. Nonassociative learning can be divided into habituation and sensitization. Habituation occurs when an animal learns, after repeated exposure, to ignore a stimulus that is neither beneficial nor harmful in its environment. In habituation, the strength or probability of a response, which is usually a reflex response, decreases when the stimulus and its response are repeated. Sensitization is the progressive increase of a response following repeated administrations of a stimulus. Well studied in invertebrates, nonassociative memory in humans is best characterized in adaptation in reflex responses involving sensory stimuli.

SUMMARY

- Memory involves information encoding, storage, and retrieval.
- Memory is organized according to temporal components called sensory memory, short-term/working memory, and long-term memory.

- Sensory memory involves sensing and initial processing of sensory stimuli.
- Short-term memory is defined as a short-term store of goal-directed information; it depends on attention and involves reverberating circuits in the prefrontal cortex.
- Working memory encompasses an active short-term memory store that can be accessed to process and manipulate information; in addition to the prefrontal cortex, it involves other areas of the frontal lobe and parietal cortex.
- Long-term memory is the permanent store where information is retained for extended periods, from years to decades; the long-term memory engram or trace involves biochemical and physical changes in the brain.
- Memory is also organized along informational components, called declarative/explicit and nondeclarative/implicit memory.
- Declarative/explicit memory includes semantic memory, which is memory of facts and information encoded with specific meaning, episodic memory of experiences and events, and spatial memory about one's environment and spatial orientation.
- Nondeclarative/implicit memory includes memory for procedures, tasks, and skills, as well as emotional and conditioned responses.
- Encoding of long-term memory involves different brain regions: Declarative/explicit memories require the hippocampus and other temporal lobe structures, whereas nondeclarative/implicit memory requires the basal ganglia, cerebellum, amygdala, and/or reflex circuits.

■ Encoding of long-term memory involves synaptic consolidation, which involves synaptic plasticity mechanisms and systems consolidation, where memory traces are distributed to other areas of the brain and stored as stable alterations of neuronal circuits.

■ Sleep plays an important role in memory consolidation.

■ Different memory systems operate independently and in parallel, which allows simultaneous and maximal memory throughput of the brain.

SELF-ASSESSMENT QUESTIONS

1. Short-term working memory mainly involves which brain region(s)?
    A. Only the prefrontal cortex (PFC)
    B. Only the posterior parietal cortex and temporal cortex
    C. Only the hippocampus
    D. The PFC, posterior parietal cortex, and temporal cortex
    E. All regions of the frontal, parietal, and temporal lobes

2. The hippocampus is required for the formation of new _____ memories.
    A. semantic, episodic, and spatial
    B. explicit and implicit
    C. declarative and nondeclarative
    D. procedural and spatial
    E. short-term working

3. The majority of long-term explicit memories are thought to be stored in many
    A. structures of the medial temporal lobe (MTL).
    B. regions of the hippocampus.
    C. parts of the basal ganglia.
    D. domains of the cerebellum.
    E. areas of the cerebral cortex.

4. Long-term potentiation (LTP) is thought to be a neuronal mechanism involved in
    A. sensory memory.
    B. short-term working memory.
    C. long-term memory.
    D. only hippocampal-dependent memory.
    E. all types of memory: sensory, short-term, and long-term.

5. Sleep has been proposed as an ideal period for system consolidation because during sleep there is _____ the transmission or transfer of information from hippocampus to neocortex.
    A. little use of adenosine triphosphate (ATP) by other regions of the brain, so more ATP will be available for
    B. no incoming sensory activity; hence, there is no interference with
    C. detoxification of free radicals and toxic proteins that improves
    D. a decrease in rogue brain waves that might complicate and confound
    E. an increase in a specific brain wave that enhances

Language

Daniel Mirman

- Describe the representation of concepts and identify the semantic hub(s).
- Describe and diagram the speech perception and production systems.
- Identify the white matter tracts most relevant to language processing.
- Identify the neural system for reading and describe how it changes during reading development.

CLASSIC MODEL

The classic model of the neural basis of language emerged from the work of 19th-century cognitive neurologists Paul Broca, Carl Wernicke, and Ludwig Lichtheim. Broca described patients with relatively preserved ability to understand speech but profound deficits in producing speech: slow, labored, telegraphic speech, often with speech errors or distortions of speech sounds and omission of function words (eg, articles and prepositions) and inflections (eg, –s for plurals, –ed for past tense). This disorder came to be known as Broca aphasia or expressive aphasia and to be associated with damage to the left inferior frontal gyrus (Broca area) and the underlying white matter. In contrast, Wernicke described patients with profound comprehension deficits but relatively fluent speech production. Although relatively rapid and well-articulated, the speech production in Wernicke aphasia (also called receptive aphasia) tends to have limited meaningful content due to use of a small set of high-frequency words and made-up words (also called "nonwords" or "abstruse neologisms"). Wernicke aphasia was thought to be associated with damage to Wernicke area, the posterior portion of the left superior temporal gyrus.

Lichtheim developed an integrated description of the language system and its instantiation in the cortical regions around the left hemisphere's Sylvian fissure. This distinction between nonfluent expressive aphasia and fluent receptive aphasia and the role of peri-Sylvian regions in language remained largely unchanged into the late 20th century and remains deeply influential despite being challenged by 3 kinds of observations. First, many individuals with aphasia do not fit the classic aphasia subtypes; rather, they exhibit "mixed" or "unclassifiable" clusters of language deficits. Second, the symptoms are functional/behavioral and may be caused by a variety of very different underlying cognitive and neurologic deficits. For example, the telegraphic speech typical of Broca aphasia can be caused by a deficit in syntax (grammar) and sentence planning, a deficit in word retrieval and selection, or a deficit in articulatory motor planning and execution. Third, focal damage to the Broca area does not tend to produce Broca aphasia, and focal damage to the Wernicke area does not tend to produce Wernicke aphasia. Rather, those syndromes are caused by broader damage that includes the traditionally associated regions as well as other regions.

Partly motivated by these challenges, an alternative has emerged that focuses on the "primary systems"—the cognitive and neural systems that support language processing. These systems are as follows: (1) a distributed semantic system for representation of conceptual knowledge, with particularly important integrative hubs in the anterior temporal lobe and temporoparietal cortex (angular gyrus and posterior superior temporal gyrus) and related white matter tracts (particularly the inferior frontal-occipital fasciculus and the uncinate fasciculus); (2) a speech recognition system for recognizing and distinguishing speech sounds and spoken words, which builds on higher level auditory processing and primarily involves the superior temporal lobe; (3) a speech production system in which (i) segment-level or syllable-level articulatory planning and motor control rely on inferior parietal regions including somatosensory representations of the articulators in the inferior postcentral gyrus and extend into inferior precentral gyrus motor representations of the articulators; and (ii) sentence-level or utterance-level planning and execution (ie, grammatically structuring multiword utterances) rely on inferior and middle frontal gyri and underlying white matter (aslant tract); and (4) a ventral visual object recognition system for reading, particularly a region within the left fusiform gyrus known as the visual word form area.

MEANING

Semantic Representation

Language is ultimately about the communication of meaning, so semantic or conceptual representations are the keystone of the language system. When we encounter and interact with objects in the world, the primary perceptual and motor representations converge to more abstract conceptual representations of those objects. When we recall and think about object and action concepts, such as "hammer" and "kick," we reactivate those perceptual, motor, and emotional experiences of the objects or events. For example, the representation of the concept "hammer" is based on the visual experiences of seeing hammers, the motor-action experiences of pounding nails, the auditory experiences of hearing hammering, and so on. This is called grounded or embodied semantics or perceptual symbol systems; that is, the conceptual representations are grounded in our bodily experiences. The neural consequence is that semantic knowledge draws on a distributed system that includes lateral occipital cortex representations of object shape, middle temporal/medial superior temporal representations of object motion, secondary auditory cortex representations of meaningful sounds, posterior temporal and inferior parietal representations of object-related action, and other perceptual, motor, and limbic regions.

Damage to individual components of this distributed system can cause specific semantic deficits associated with individual components. For example, atrophy of the auditory association cortex produces a specific deficit for processing words that refer to concepts with strong auditory elements (eg, thunder) compared to concepts with strong visual elements (eg, pyramid) or manipulation elements (eg, scissors). Damage to inferior temporal regions in the later stages of the ventral visual stream tends to produce deficits for concepts that are primarily distinguished by visual features, such as animals. In contrast, damage to inferior parietal cortex regions in the later stages of the dorsal visual stream tends to produce deficits for concepts that are primarily distinguished by action or manipulation features, such as tools.

This distributed system of modality-specific representations is integrated in 2 cross-modal "hubs": 1 in the anterior temporal lobes (ATLs) and 1 in temporoparietal cortex (TPC). Figure 21–1 shows a schematic depiction of the distributed semantic system with hubs in the ATL and TPC. The ATL hub is particularly important for object identification and categorization. Frontotemporal lobar degeneration that particularly affects the ATL produces a deficit of semantic knowledge: the semantic variant of primary progressive aphasia (sPPA, also called semantic dementia). Individuals with sPPA have profound semantic deficits, while other aspects of perception and

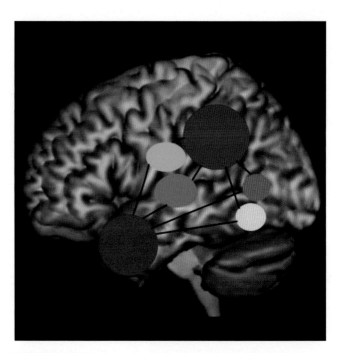

FIGURE 21–1 Schematic depiction of the distributed semantic system with integrative "hubs" in the anterior temporal lobe (red) and temporoparietal cortex (purple). The "spokes" of the system connect the hubs with modality-specific areas for processing auditory features (ie, auditory association cortex; blue), color features (ie, V4; yellow), motion features (ie, middle temporal; orange), and action (frontoparietal action system; green).

cognition are largely intact. In sPPA, errors in picture naming are almost exclusively more common or more typical category members (eagle → duck) or superordinate category labels (eagle → bird). Similar errors are made by patients with ATL damage due to focal epileptogenic lesions or stroke lesions (which typically extend beyond ATL). The semantic deficit in sPPA extends beyond just verbal tasks: In nonverbal tasks such as delayed copying and object decision, individuals with sPPA also make category typicality errors. For example, they may choose the elephant with small ears instead of large ears or draw a camel with no hump or a duck with 4 legs—all cases where the patient produced a response that is typical for the category (animals) but fails to reflect object-specific properties. That is, degeneration of the ATLs produces gradual blurring of object-specific within-category distinctions, while broader between-category distinctions are comparatively spared.

The TPC hub is particularly important for event or scenario representations, such as relationships between objects that are not members of the same category and do not share features but frequently co-occur together (also called thematic relations), for example, object–instrument relations (eg, dog – leash) or object–location relations (eg, zebra – savannah). TPC stroke damage tends to increase the production of thematically related semantic errors in picture naming (eg, cow → milk), and these relations are spared relative to perceptual features in patients with sPPA, which tends to affect the ATL hub more than the TPC hub.

Both cerebral hemispheres are involved in semantic processing, with a substantial degree of redundancy between the hemispheres, but also some hemispheric specialization. The profound semantic deficit in sPPA tends to arise from bilateral deterioration of the ATL. Unilateral damage to the semantic system tends to produce more limited semantic deficits, indicating that the spared contralesional hemisphere is able to largely compensate. Unilateral left ATL damage tends to affect verbal semantic tasks more strongly (eg, picture naming and word matching), whereas unilateral right ATL damage tends to affect visual semantic tasks more strongly (eg, picture matching). Presumably, this is due to the left ATL being more strongly connected to the (typically) left-lateralized language system.

White Matter

There is one notable exception to the pattern that unilateral damage produces modality-specific semantic deficits: Broad semantic deficits can arise after unilateral stroke damage to a "white matter bottleneck" medial to the insula and lateral to the basal ganglia. The inferior fronto-occipital fasciculus (IFOF), uncinate fasciculus, and anterior thalamic radiations converge in this region, so the diverse semantic deficits arise because a small amount of bottleneck damage can cause widespread dysfunction throughout the semantic system

(key white matter tracts involved in language processing are shown in Figure 21–2). The IFOF is particularly important for linking visual processing in the occipital and ventral temporal cortex with the semantic hub in the ATL. The role of the uncinate fasciculus is somewhat more controversial, with alternative accounts focusing on its role in semantics of valence and social semantics (due to connecting the ATL with the orbitofrontal cortex) or in semantic control (due to connecting the ATL with the inferior frontal regions). There may also be a posterior white matter bottleneck in the vicinity of the TPC, but its anatomy and function are less well documented.

Semantic Access

Deficits such as sPPA and category-specific impairments (eg, impaired semantics of animals but not tools) suggest damage to the neural system that stores or represents semantic knowledge, such that part of that knowledge is lost. In these deficits, impaired performance is fairly consistent across repeated testing, different tasks, and different testing conditions. There is also a very different kind of semantic deficit in which semantic knowledge appears to be intact but *access* to that knowledge is ineffective, inefficient, or inconsistent. Patients with semantic access deficits (1) are sensitive to cueing (picture naming is facilitated by hearing the start of the target word), (2) perform better when test trials are separated by a long delay than

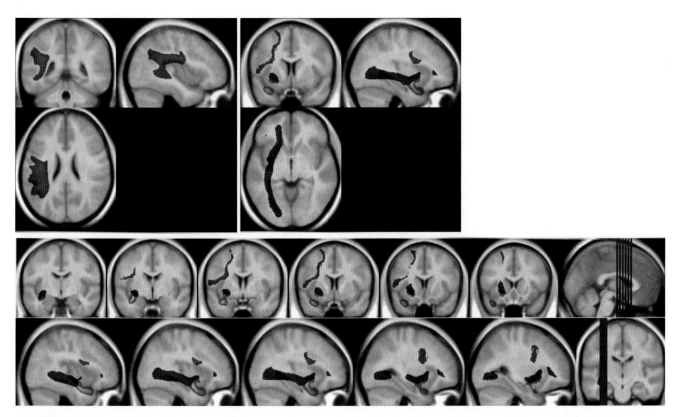

FIGURE 21–2 White matter tracts particularly critical for language processing. *Top left:* Arcuate fasciculus (largely overlapping with the superior longitudinal fasciculus). *Top right and bottom:* Inferior fronto-occipital fasciculus (blue), uncincate fasciculus (green), and frontal aslant tract (red).

by a moderate delay, (3) perform inconsistently on multiple tests of the same stimulus (ie, sometimes can name a picture and sometimes cannot name that same picture, usually with declining performance over repeated presentations), (4) perform worse in the presence of semantically related distractors, and (5) tend to have a correlation between their semantic deficit and executive function deficits. Each of these phenomena stands in stark contrast to the semantic deficit in sPPA, which exhibits none of them. Observation of these deficits—and their striking difference from the semantic deficit in sPPA—indicates that semantic cognition requires key components or mechanisms: storage of semantic knowledge and access to or control over that knowledge. However, there is not yet agreement about the computational basis of the access/control component or its neural basis, although the frontal cortex and the underlying white matter likely play an important role.

RECOGNITION & PRODUCTION OF SPEECH SOUNDS

The sound structure of language is called phonology, and the speech sound units are called phonemes. Phonemes are typically defined by "minimal pairs": The difference in the initial sound between "tape" and "cape" produces a different word; therefore, the initial sounds in those 2 words are different phonemes. In contrast, the initial sound in "tape" will be acoustically different between "Christmas tape" and "Spanish tape," but it will be heard as the same word in both cases, so that acoustic difference is not phonemic.

Speech Recognition: Ventral Stream

Recognition of phonemes is the major higher level auditory function of the auditory association cortex in the posterior portion of the superior temporal gyrus. Early spectrotemporal analysis of speech input is bilateral, with left hemisphere auditory cortex specialized for temporal analysis of rapid acoustic changes and right hemisphere auditory cortex specialized for fine-grained spectral frequency analysis. This division of labor is driven by a fundamental signal-processing limitation: a trade-off between temporal resolution and spectral resolution known as the Gabor limit. Asymmetric temporal sampling allows the auditory system to overcome this limitation with higher temporal resolution and lower spectral resolution in the left hemisphere and higher spectral resolution and lower temporal resolution in the right hemisphere.

One consequence of asymmetric temporal sampling is the relative dominance of the right hemisphere for auditory functions that are more reliant on spectral resolution than on temporal resolution. Such functions include music processing, recognition of emotion in speech, and speaker identification and recognition. Auditory agnosias—deficits of auditory recognition that are not attributable to hearing or cognitive deficits—tend follow this lateralization pattern. Impaired recognition of environmental sounds and music (amusia) generally results from right hemisphere damage, whereas deficits of speech sound recognition (verbal auditory agnosia, or word deafness) generally result from left hemisphere damage.

After initial spectrotemporal processing, subsequent stages of speech recognition are generally left-lateralized and rely on progressively more anterior portions of the superior temporal lobe. Recognition of phonemes and syllables engages the middle portion of the superior temporal gyrus; recognition of words and phrases engages the anterior portion, making contact with the semantic hub in ATL. This posterior-to-anterior progression in the superior temporal lobe is known as the ventral speech stream (Figure 21–3) and is the speech analog of the ventral visual processing stream for object recognition.

Speech Production: Dorsal Stream

Speech production requires very precise motor control of the articulatory apparatus—the lips, jaw, tongue, vocal folds, and velum (which controls whether air is allowed through the nasal passage, distinguishing sounds such as /m/ and /n/ from /b/ and /d/). This relies on core motor control systems of the basal ganglia, cerebellum, and motor cortex and can be disrupted by stroke and other disorders of the motor system such as Parkinson disease. Such motor-based disorders of speech production are called dysarthria. Stuttering is also thought to be due to dysfunction in the basal ganglia–thalamocortical motor circuits that impairs timing cues for the initiation of speech.

In addition to low-level motor control of the articulators, speech production requires articulatory action planning. The articulatory action planning system relies on a frontoparietal circuit that includes the precentral gyrus, insula, postcentral gyrus, and inferior parietal lobule. This system is known as the dorsal speech stream (see Figure 21–3) and is the speech analog of the dorsal visual processing stream for visually guided action. Damage to the dorsal speech stream tends to impair production of speech sounds with relatively spared lower level motor control of the articulatory apparatus and higher level aspects of language processing.

One such disorder is apraxia of speech, in which speech sounds can be distorted with abnormal rhythm, stress, or prosody, and patients struggle to initiate words or "grope" for the right arrangement of articulators to produce the correct speech sound. Patients may also make frank speech sound substitution errors, producing well-articulated nonwords that are similar to the target word (eg, ghost → "goath"). Although subtly different and possibly having somewhat different underlying causes, speech sound distortions and substitution errors tend to be fairly highly correlated and to be caused by very similar patterns of neurologic damage to the precentral and postcentral gyri, insula, and inferior parietal lobule.

The analogy between the dorsal visually guided action system and the dorsal speech production system also helps to understand the computational architecture of speech production. Limb actions are guided by visual perception of object location and size and by somatosensory feedback of limb position. However, the neural transmission and processing of these

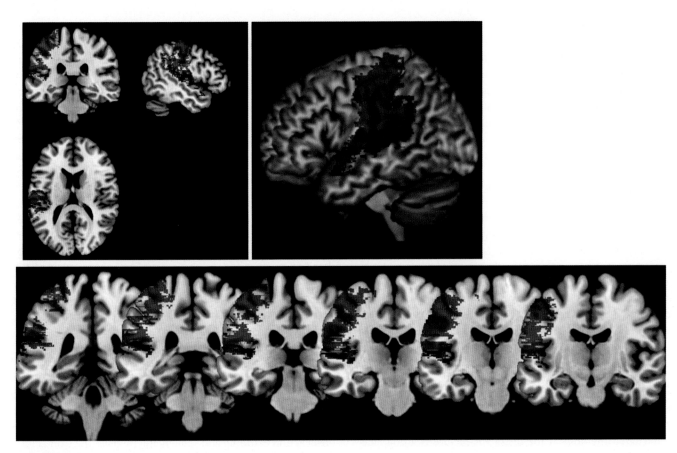

FIGURE 21–3 Ventral speech recognition stream (blue) and dorsal speech production stream (red).

sensory feedback signals is too slow for efficient correction; by the time the feedback signal was processed and a correction signal sent, the position of the limb would have changed substantially and the correction signal would be wrong. To overcome this problem, motor control systems use an internal forward model, which makes online predictions regarding the state of the effector and the sensory feedback. This internal forward model allows the system to predict errors and send correction signals before the errors occur (and before sensory feedback is sent), so the correction signal can arrive in time for efficient, online error correction. The internal forward model is tuned by actual sensory feedback, so its predictions can (gradually) adjust to changes in the environment or effector properties. The computational forward model principles apply to both limb and articulatory motor control.

The targets of speech production are both motor and acoustic. That is, the target is an articulatory action sequence that produces a particular acoustic signal. The auditory system provides feedback about the outcome of the articulatory actions (like the visual system does for limb actions). The somatosensory system provides online feedback about the configuration of the articulators (as it does for limb actions). Internal forward models make predictions about the somatosensory and acoustic/auditory consequences of the articulatory motor actions, which are compared against the targets to allow online correction. Immediate error corrections are

a simple example of the prediction-based correction mechanism in action; for example, utterances such as "v-horizontal," where the production of "vertical" is corrected to "horizontal" within 150 milliseconds. This is far less than the approximately 400-millisecond minimum that would be required to recognize that an incorrect speech sound was produced and execute a new articulatory command. More generally, a substantial proportion of error corrections happen too fast for an external feedback system, indicating the involvement of an internal prediction-based error detection and correction system.

Because the formats of motor and sensory representations are different, these correction signals require sensory-motor transformation in order to make the forward model prediction and to compute the correction signal. The precise neural implementation of these sensory-motor transformations is still being debated, although the cerebellum and the planum temporale (or the parietotemporal boundary at the posterior end of the Sylvian fissure) have been proposed as promising candidates.

SENTENCE PROCESSING

Sentences unfold gradually over time but have a hierarchical or propositional underlying structure. That is, even simple sentences such as, "John loves Mary" or "Bill gave the book to Susan," are expressions of relationships between constituents that are distributed throughout the sentence. Sentence comprehension requires assembling those constituents into the correct relational structure, and sentence production requires unfolding that structure into an appropriate sequence of words. Thus, temporal sequencing, working memory, planning, and cognitive control are key elements of sentence processing.

From the earliest days of neurolinguistics, the neural basis of syntax has been a central question. The syntax or grammar of a language is the set of rules or patters that govern how sentence constituents can be assembled. That is how we know that "The boy chased the dog" means roughly the same thing as "The dog was chased by the boy," but that "The dog chased the boy" describes a very different event. Much of this research has focused on so-called agrammatism, a disorder thought to be specific to syntactic or grammatical processing. Despite these efforts, it has proven virtually impossible to disentangle syntactic processing from closely related cognitive functions such as sequence processing, working memory, and cognitive control. Therefore, although a neural basis for syntax remains elusive and controversial, there is substantial agreement about the neural systems that support sentence processing.

Sentence Comprehension

Sentence comprehension can be measured by asking participants to find the picture that matches a sentence such as, "The boy chased the dog." If the distractor picture is a dog chasing a boy, then it can be correctly rejected only after correct comprehension of the full sentence. Comprehension of such "reversible" sentences can be compared against a "lexical" case where just recognizing the individual constituents is sufficient; for example, a distractor picture of a boy chasing a girl. Impaired comprehension of reversible sentences with spared lexical sentence comprehension is associated with damage to the inferior parietal cortex (angular gyrus and supramarginal gyrus), extending into the posterior superior temporal gyrus. The role of this region in sentence comprehension may be related to the event semantic hub in TPC; sentences describe events, so sentence comprehension is a form of event comprehension. It may also be related to the role of the parietal cortex in working memory because sentence comprehension requires active memory for word sequences.

Multiword Utterances

Following the general pattern that language production is more difficult than language comprehension, deficits of sentence production are more readily apparent than deficits of sentence comprehension. Agrammatism is typically defined in terms of impaired sentence production, such as omission of grammatical morphemes (eg, function words such as articles and prepositions and suffixes such as –s for plural and –ed for past tense) and making word order errors. In both progressive aphasia (agrammatic variant of primary progressive aphasia) and nonprogressive aphasia (stroke), these deficits tend to co-occur with other aspects of nonfluent language production

such as slow, effortful speech, short utterances, and production of speech sound errors (discussed earlier). They are, perhaps surprisingly, *not* strongly associated with impaired sentence comprehension; many so-called agrammatic patients perform relatively well on sentence comprehension tasks that require syntactic analysis, which is one reason to doubt the existence of a central syntactic processing mechanism.

Effective sentence production requires articulatory control and word retrieval. As discussed in previous sections, speech production depends on a dorsal system of inferior parietal regions and frontal motor control regions, and the left ATL plays a particularly important role in semantically driven production of individual words. Broader speech rate measures (eg, words per minute) tend to also reflect integrity of the dorsal speech production system. When syntactic errors are isolated from other factors, the critical regions are substantially more anterior: the inferior and middle frontal gyri, possibly extending into the frontal aslant tract, a white matter tract that connects inferior frontal regions with the anterior cingulate and presupplementary motor area.

The neural systems supporting speech and sentence production bear a striking resemblance to the neural systems supporting limb action production and planning. Disorders of object-related actions (limb apraxia) are primarily associated with inferior parietal damage, extending into frontal motor regions, much like disorders of speech production. Higher level action planning and sequencing involves the frontal lobe in a hierarchical posterior-to-anterior progression: Posterior frontal cortex (ie, motor and premotor areas) is responsible for simple motor acts such as picking up a milk carton or pouring milk into coffee, more anterior regions represent larger action "chunks" or subgoals such as adding milk to coffee (which requires picking up the milk, pouring it, and putting it down), and even more anterior regions represent even larger action plans such as making a cup of coffee. Speech and sentence production can similarly be understood in terms of simple actions (articulating an individual speech sound or syllable), small action chunks (articulating a word or common word sequence), larger action chunks (planning and articulating a complete sentence), and overall action goals (telling a story). As with limb actions, there is a nested, hierarchical structure of goals and subgoals that requires maintenance and updating, and it is supported by a frontal-parietal cortical neural system.

READING

Basics & Mechanics

Spoken language appears to have emerged spontaneously a fairly long time ago and is learned by (almost) all children without formal instruction. In contrast, written language is a relatively recent invention (at least in evolutionary terms)—approximately 6000 years ago—and learning to read and write requires formal instruction. Thus, the reading system is based on some of the same neural systems as spoken language, with additional reliance on particular kinds of visual processing.

Writing systems differ substantially across languages, but they have some consistent elements: Most characters are drawn with 1 to 4 strokes, and character shapes tend to be as distinct as possible. At the initial input stage, reading is constrained by the anatomy of the retina and oculomotor dynamics. Text needs to be fixated (foveated) in order to extract enough high spatial frequency detail for character recognition. Text that appears in the parafovea provides partial information and allows a parafoveal preview of the next word. Eye movements during reading are typically short saccades, covering about 7 letters or 2 degrees, and moving from word to word. About 30% of words are skipped; these are typically short, very common words (eg, "the") that can be processed without a dedicated fixation (ie, based on parafoveal preview and context). About 10% to 15% of saccades are regressions—refixations of an earlier word. Regressions are important for reading comprehension, especially for correcting initial comprehension failures: Comprehension accuracy decreases if regressions are prevented, especially for "garden path" sentences that have misleading structures.

Average fixation time during reading is approximately 250 milliseconds, but this varies widely. Fixation duration is primarily determined by linguistic and cognitive factors such as word familiarity and predictability, rather than visual factors such as word length. Even if a word disappears after 60 milliseconds, the fixation duration is largely unaffected: Visual perception of the word happens very quickly; the fixation time is the time required to comprehend the word, integrate it into the sentence representation, and plan the next saccade. Fixation times are widely used to study reading processes because they provide such a precise, natural, and minimally invasive measure of the cognitive demands of reading.

Reading a single word requires connecting 3 components of the language system: visual recognition of the characters (orthography), production (and recognition) of speech sounds (phonology), and word meaning (semantics). These 3 components are bidirectionally interconnected for the purpose of typical language tasks (eg, word recognition, word production, word reading) and are commonly called the "triangle model." In alphabetic orthographies such as English, Spanish, and Hebrew, there is a systematic relationship between the visual characters and the sound of the word. In these cases, the orthography-phonology part of the triangle can directly decode (ie, read aloud) a word based on those grapheme-phoneme correspondences. This works well for words such as mint, lint, and hint, and for pseudo-words such as deest and beest. However, this system will have more difficulty with words that deviate from the pattern, such as pint. Decoding such "irregular" or "inconsistent" words is additionally supported by the semantic route of the triangle, and patients with semantic deficits (eg, sPPA) often have difficulty reading these kinds of words (discussed more later in the section on dyslexias). The triangle model also identifies the 3 main neural components of the reading system: inferior/basal temporal-occipital cortex for visual orthographic processing,

peri-Sylvian regions for phonological processing, and anterior temporal cortex for semantic processing.

Ventral Stream & Visual Word Form Area

Like other kinds of object recognition, letter recognition is based on the ventral visual stream, including V1 and V2 edge and contour detectors (letter features), and ventral occipito-temporal representations of letter-like shapes and 2-letter combinations (bigrams). This pathway culminates with the visual word form area (VWFA), a region of the left fusiform gyrus near the lateral occipitotemporal sulcus, which is reliably activated more strongly when processing real words than nonword letter strings or mirror-reversed words. The VWFA response to real words increases as people learn to read in both their first language and in a second language. This is an experience-dependent process and not just developmental maturation. Adult illiterates who learn to read show increased VWFA activation specifically for real words. Among adult native English speakers, those who can also read Hebrew show greater VWFA response to Hebrew words than those who cannot read Hebrew (both groups show equal VWFA response to English words). VWFA lesions produce pure alexia, which is characterized by letter-by-letter reading, indicative of intact low-level visual processing (letter recognition) but impaired holistic word recognition.

Recall that reading is a recent invention (and widespread literacy is even more recent)—too recent for human genome evolution to have produced an innate neural word recognition module. VWFA is properly understood as an emergent property of the visual object recognition system, a system that is co-opted (or "recycled") for reading and that itself influenced the form of writing systems. As a visual object recognition task, word recognition is paralleled by face recognition, which is similar in 3 key respects: (1) it is highly practiced, (2) it requires fine-grained visual discrimination of high spatial frequency information, and (3) it requires holistic object recognition. The VWFA is homologous to the fusiform face area (FFA), a portion of the right fusiform gyrus that responds selectively to faces in a way that is similar to the VWFA response to visual words. In young (preliterate) children, the FFA is bilateral; the right-lateralization of the FFA emerges as children learn to read, and this portion of the left fusiform gyrus becomes specialized for visual word recognition rather than face recognition (ie, becomes the VWFA), presumably because spoken language is left-lateralized.

Dyslexias

Acquired Dyslexia

Acquired dyslexia is a disorder of reading in previously literate individuals as a result of brain damage that spares (most) other perceptual and cognitive functions. Acquired dyslexia has 3 main forms. Pure alexia (also called alexia without agraphia or pure word blindness) is typically due to damage to the VWFA and is primarily characterized by slow reading aloud with abnormally large (linear) effects of number of letters. Damage to the white matter fibers that connect the VWFA to the posterior occipital cortex areas (ie, inferior longitudinal fasciculus) also plays an important role in chronic pure alexia, suggesting that VWFA is a contact point between visual processing and language processing. For patients with pure alexia, the reading deficit is paralleled by impaired performance for matching unfamiliar visual symbols (eg, Kanji), consistent with a deficit of holistic visual discrimination of high spatial frequency information.

Phonological dyslexia is a relatively selective deficit of reading (and writing/spelling) nonwords relative to real words, often involving lexicalization errors (eg, gat → "cat"). This pattern reflects increased reliance on semantics during reading due to impaired direct connections between orthography and phonology. Patients with phonological dyslexia often also exhibit phonological deficits in spoken language processing, suggesting a more general phonological processing deficit (although a few notable exceptions to this pattern have been documented). Phonological dyslexia is generally associated with damage to peri-Sylvian speech processing regions (discussed earlier), including the superior temporal lobe, angular and supramarginal gyri, inferior frontal cortex, frontal operculum, and insula.

Surface dyslexia is characterized by impaired reading (and writing/spelling) of irregular words, especially low-frequency irregular words such as pint, with comparatively spared reading of regular words (eg, mint, lint, hint) and nonwords (sint). Spared ability to sound out nonwords and regular words indicates that the system for mapping orthography to phonology remains intact. Intact grapheme-phoneme mapping is reflected by the errors for irregular words, which are typically regularizations (eg, reading pint to rhyme with mint). Surface dyslexia is strongly associated with semantic deficits in nonreading tasks, commonly arising in neurodegenerative diseases (especially sPPA) and rarely due to focal lesions (eg, stroke). Thus, the impairment appears to be specific to a semantically mediated system for reading irregular words, while leaving the direct orthography-to-phonology mapping system intact.

In addition to these main types of acquired dyslexia, reading deficits can also arise as a result of damage to related peripheral (ie, visual) systems. One example of a peripheral dyslexia is neglect dyslexia, in which patients fail to identify the initial portion of a letter string and which tends to occur in patients with left-sided spatial neglect. Deep dyslexia is an intriguing and complex syndrome in which patients produce semantic (eg, castle → "knight") and visual (eg, skate → "scale") errors in reading, tend to lexicalize nonwords (as in phonological dyslexia), and perform better when reading concrete nouns (eg, table, chicken) than abstract words or modifiers such as adjectives and adverbs (eg, envy, swiftly). Deep dyslexia may be a particularly severe form of phonological dyslexia, possibly with some additional semantic deficit (although some patients appear to have intact comprehension, arguing against a semantic deficit). Another possibility is that deep dyslexia is a consequence of (not very effective) reading using the right hemisphere. The ability of the right hemisphere to take over language functions in response to left hemisphere damage and whether such compensation is adaptive or maladaptive are active areas of current research.

Developmental Dyslexia

Developmental dyslexia is characterized by difficulties with word recognition and by poor spelling and decoding abilities, in the absence of frank deficits of other perceptual or cognitive abilities and despite the provision of effective classroom instruction. These difficulties typically result from a deficit in phonological processing, although secondary consequences may include problems in reading comprehension and reduced reading experience. The phonological deficits in developmental dyslexia are frequently framed in terms of phonological awareness, the ability to intentionally manipulate phoneme-level aspects of spoken language; for example, a phoneme deletion task such as saying the word "split" without the /p/ sound. Phonological awareness skills in children are early predictors of reading ability, and dyslexic deficits in phonological awareness tend to persist into adulthood. Interventions that strengthen phonological awareness skills are effective strategies for improving decoding in children with dyslexia. Speeded word production (eg, rapid naming of letters, numbers, or colors) and verbal short-term memory are also often impaired in developmental dyslexia.

Dyslexia is highly heritable, with a 30% to 50% chance of being passed from parent to child. Several genes in the DYX2 (dyslexia susceptibility-2) locus on chromosome 6p22 have been associated with dyslexia, including *KIAA0319*, *TTRAP*, and *DCDC2*. Magnetic resonance spectroscopy has revealed *N*-acetyl-aspartate, choline, and glutamate abnormalities in developmental dyslexia. Neuroanatomic studies have found reduced gray matter volume in the left planum temporale and bilateral posterior superior temporal lobe and inferior parietal lobe, as well as reduced white matter volume in temporoparietal regions, particularly the arcuate fasciculus (superior longitudinal fasciculus) and corona radiata.

Functional neuroimaging studies reveal that, relative to control participants, dyslexics exhibit less activation in posterior portions of the reading system, particularly the inferior occipitotemporal cortex (ie, VWFA), but also the posterior superior temporal gyrus and inferior parietal cortex (angular and supramarginal gyri). In contrast, dyslexics exhibit greater activation of frontal language areas, such as left inferior frontal and precentral gyri. These findings align with the broader set of results showing that reading development is associated an anterior-to-posterior shift: Early (novice) readers show more activity in frontal language areas; as reading skill and automaticity increase, frontal activation decreases and activation of the posterior temporoparietal areas increases. This shift appears to be delayed in dyslexia, either due to (possibly genetic) neuroanatomic abnormalities in those posterior regions or due to cognitive deficits in phonological processing that engages those areas.

CONCLUSION

The neural system supporting human language is centered on the left peri-Sylvian cortex. Building on higher level auditory processing, the superior temporal cortex is responsible for speech perception and spoken language comprehension. The posterior-to-anterior progression of speech sound representations to word and phrase representations is called the ventral speech stream. Inferior frontoparietal cortical regions are responsible for articulatory planning and execution, and this speech production system is closely related to neural systems involved in limb action planning and execution. This dorsal speech stream also follows a posterior-to-anterior progression from speech sound and syllable production (parietal and frontal motor/premotor regions) to sentence planning and production (inferior and middle frontal gyri). Semantic knowledge relies on a distributed system of modality-specific representations of perceptual, motor, and other experiences integrated in "hubs" in the ATLs and TPC. Reading is relatively recent development that requires explicit training and builds on existing systems for spoken language, semantic knowledge, and expert visual object recognition. The visual word form area in the left fusiform gyrus is a critical connection between the visual system and the language system that is particularly important for efficient word reading.

SUMMARY

- In the traditional model, the neural language system is primarily in the left hemisphere, and composed of a posterior superior temporal region (Wernicke area) and an inferior frontal region (Broca area). This model has been substantially extended and revised, largely due to contemporary neuroimaging methods.
- Semantic processing depends on anterior temporal and temporoparietal hubs that integrate information from a distributed system of cortical regions.
- Recognition of speech sounds and spoken words builds on bilateral cortical auditory processing and primarily involves the ventral speech stream in the left superior temporal lobe.
- Production of speech sounds and syllables begins with motor control systems in the cerebellum, basal ganglia, and motor cortex.
- Phonological aspects of speech production rely on the dorsal speech stream inferior parietal regions: angular and supramarginal gyri, somatosensory representations of the articulators in the inferior postcentral gyrus, and

inferior precentral gyrus motor representations of the articulators.
- Sentence planning and production (grammatically structuring multiword utterances) relies on inferior and middle frontal gyri.
- The primary white matter tracts involved in language processing are the arcuate fasciculus (superior longitudinal fasciculus), IFOF, uncinate fasciculus, and aslant tract.
- Reading builds on the spoken language system, adding a visual word recognition component primarily in the left fusiform gyrus to the phonological and semantic systems of spoken language.

SELF-ASSESSMENT QUESTIONS

1. A 64-year-old woman presents with a reduction in fluency of speech with a serious deficiency in naming of objects and repetition of words when requested to do so. The patient's writing is poor, and she also displays a hemiparesis. Comprehension of speech appears to be preserved. A magnetic resonance imaging (MRI) scan and overall neurologic examination reveal that the patient has a lesion. Which of the following regions is likely to contain the lesion?
   A. Medial convexity of the premotor cortex
   B. Frontal operculum and convexity
   C. Supramarginal gyrus
   D. Angular gyrus
   E. Inferior parietal lobule

2. A 67-year-old woman is brought to a local hospital following complaints by her family because of recent difficulties that the patient has experienced in communicating with others. In particular, the patient has great difficulty in comprehending words and understanding simple commands. A neurologic examination confirms that the patient experiences difficulties in language comprehension, and an MRI reveals a cortical lesion. Which of the following regions was observed to be the locus of the lesion?
   A. Medial convexity of the premotor cortex
   B. Frontal operculum and convexity
   C. Medial aspect of occipital cortex
   D. Posterior aspect of superior temporal lobe
   E. Superior (posterior) parietal lobule

3. A 75-year-old man, who is right handed, was told in the past by his internist that he has an irregular heartbeat. The patient decides that he does not wish to learn anything further about this condition, so he does not return to this physician, and it remains untreated. One morning, he awakes to find that his face droops on the right side and that he cannot move his right arm or right leg. When he tries to call an ambulance for help, he has a great deal of difficulty communicating with the operator because his speech is slurred, nonfluent, and missing some pronouns. The call is traced by the police; an ambulance arrives at his house and takes him to an emergency room. A neurologist is called to see the patient in the emergency room. When he listens to the patient's heart, he detects an irregular heartbeat.

It is very difficult to understand his speech because it is halting, with a tendency to repeat the same phrases over and over. He has difficulty repeating specific sentences given to him by the neurologist, but he is able to follow simple commands such as, "Touch your right ear with your left hand." His mouth droops on the right when he attempts to smile, but his forehead remains symmetric when he wrinkles it. He cannot move his right arm at all, but he is able to wiggle his right leg a little bit. Which of the following language problems does this patient have?

A. Dysarthria
B. Wernicke aphasia
C. Broca aphasia
D. Alexia
E. Pure word deafness

CHAPTER

22

Emotion

Franklin R. Amthor

OBJECTIVES

After studying this chapter, the student should be able to:

- Know how emotion is defined and manipulated for study.
- Understand the usefulness of emotion in guiding behavior.
- Know more about the limbic system and other brain areas important for generating emotion.
- Recount recent evidence about the crucial role of the amygdala in emotional processing and learning.
- Understand the role of the ventromedial prefrontal cortex in high-level emotional intelligence.
- Understand the physiologic changes associated with emotional states and the role of the autonomic nervous system.
- Understand the brain mechanisms thought to underlie some emotional disorders such as sociopathy and autism.

OVERVIEW

Emotions are the feelings generated by basic instincts and drives and by the assessment of progress or frustration of those drives. Emotions depend on the limbic system. The limbic system, in turn, interacts with the autonomic nervous system to control whether the body should be in the sympathetic fight/flight body state or oriented toward homeostasis. The limbic system also interacts with sensory organs that assess the state of the environment and with the neocortex, which modulates behavior based on contextual memories. A particularly important part of the brain related to emotion and limbic function is the amygdala–ventromedial frontal lobe system that is responsible for assessing emotionally salient risks, such as those associated with living in social groups.

DEFINING EMOTION

Basic instincts and drives make their presence felt by generating emotions that motivate the organism toward some action. Emotional drive is both generated by and produced from the state of the autonomic nervous system. Emotional drives are typically based on immediate survival needs such as thirst, hunger, reproductive activity, and social rank maintenance.

Note that some of these are internally generated, such as thirst and hunger, whereas others are externally triggered, such as the appearance, sound, or smell of a potential mate or predator. External emotion-generating inputs are transmitted from cephalic sensory organs. The behaviors triggered by external sensory input often depend on learned associations from previous experience.

Emotions can be described as existing along dimensions such as approach/withdrawal and intensity. Fear and disgust are emotions that are associated with withdrawal behavior, whereas happiness promotes approach. Each type of emotion has an associated intensity that is also experienced. Emotions are associated with body states mediated by different relative levels of sympathetic versus parasympathetic neurotransmitters as well as other neurotransmitters and neuromodulators. According to the James-Lange theory of emotion, emotional responses are processed initially at limbic brain levels and the autonomic nervous system, with cognitive responses occurring later along a slower pathway involving higher brain areas. By this theory, the initial emotional reaction to sensory input should be similar in humans to that of primates and other mammals because we share similar, phylogenetically older limbic brain structures. The cognitive human overlay would be unique because of unique human consciousness and language.

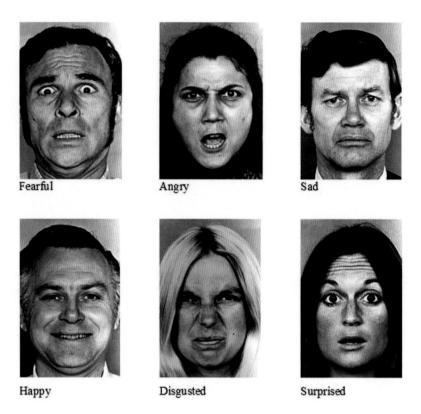

FIGURE 22–1 Faces exhibiting the 6 major emotions universally expressed by humans in all cultures. (Reproduced with permission from National Institute of Mental Health, Washington, DC. Photography by Paul Ekman and Wallace V. Friesen.)

It is also clearly the case, however, that cognitive processes, such as imagination, can generate emotions in a top-down manner.

The Uses of Emotion

Emotions bring about behaviors that satisfy basic needs necessary for survival, such as eating and fleeing predation. At this level, emotions exist in virtually all mammals and probably all vertebrates. Seeking pleasure (food, mates) and avoiding pain (predation, heights) are associated with a similar constellation of behaviors in all vertebrates. In non-mammalian, so-called cold-blooded vertebrates, many of the triggers for emotion have evolved to be inborn, such as fear of snakes and spiders and attraction toward the opposite sex. These inborn emotions are likely to be universal across many vertebrates because they are tied to the basic operation of the autonomic nervous system and the limbic system that controls it.

In mammals, there is more emotionally driven generation of risks and rewards based on learned associations from previous experience. This is particularly true in mammalian social hierarchies where every single individual has a unique rank, sometimes across multiple rank dimensions, and all interactions between individuals must follow socially defined rank protocols. In many mammals, emotion is communicated by body posture, facial expressions, and vocalizations.

Emotional Expression

Social mammals communicate more complex emotional repertoires than nonsocial mammals or nonmammalian vertebrates. Darwin, in his book *The Expression of the Emotions in Man and Animals*, argued that emotional communication is selected for because it aids survival in social groups. Given the similarity in hierarchical structures in primate social groups, it is not surprising that some emotional facial expressions are nearly universal. Figure 22–1 shows 6 faces displaying what are thought to be the 6 universal human facially displayed emotions of fear, anger, sadness, happiness, disgust, and surprise, from the work of Ekman and colleagues.

ANATOMIC AREAS MEDIATING EMOTION

The limbic system in nonmammalian vertebrates is the top of the hierarchy of autonomic control. The limbic system processes and integrates sensory information from internal sensors of body state such as blood pressure, sugar level, and temperature with external sensory input from smell, vision, audition, taste, and skin senses. In its interaction with the ventromedial prefrontal cortex, the limbic system evaluates this sensory input in light of learned associations from experience. The cingulate cortex, which is mesocortex, is an executive area at the top of the limbic system. Two memory areas, the

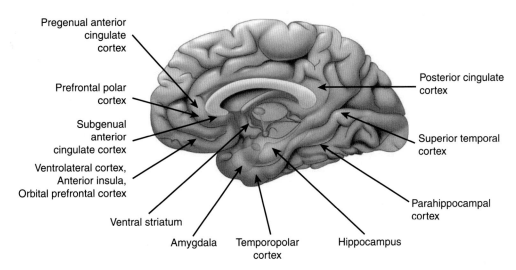

FIGURE 22–2 Major structures of the limbic system. The top of the limbic control hierarchy is the cingulate cortex. Ventromedial prefrontal cortex interacts with the amygdala for the learning of high salient survival contingencies, such as the fear reaction one has when running a red light. The insula, hippocampus, and some areas of the temporal lobe are also heavily connected with other limbic structures. (Reproduced with permission from Nestler EJ, Hyman SE, Holtzman DM, et al: *Molecular Neuropharmacology: A Foundation for Clinical Neuroscience*, 3rd ed. New York, NY: McGraw Hill; 2015.)

hippocampus and amygdala, are associated with the creation and use of memory by the limbic system. The hippocampus has both limbic and nonlimbic connections for creating and learning the context associated with an event to be remembered. The amygdala processes inputs from the brainstem and autonomic nervous system and interacts reciprocally with the ventromedial (also called orbitofrontal) cortex and the basal ganglia.

The Limbic System

The main limbic areas involved in mood and emotion are shown in Figure 22–2. Executive areas include the cingulate cortex above the corpus callosum and the ventromedial prefrontal cortex in the prefrontal lobe area below the dorsolateral prefrontal cortex. Several temporal lobe cortical areas also interact extensively with limbic areas. The amygdala is a memory area whose

relationship to the ventromedial prefrontal cortex is similar to that of the hippocampus with the rest of neocortex. The hippocampus was originally included as an area of the limbic system by Maclean. Although there are connections between the hippocampus and the limbic system, the hippocampus is extensively connected to other, nonlimbic areas of neocortex.

Another major brain area associated with the limbic system is the insula, located medial to the temporal lobe. Some of the main connections between the limbic system and several cortical areas are shown in Figure 22–3. There are also connections between limbic structures and the dorsolateral prefrontal cortex, the seat of working memory.

The overall connection scheme of cortical and subcortical limbic connections is shown in a block diagram format in Figure 22–4. The bold lines indicate the original Papez circuit of the limbic system, which includes the projection of several

Cortico-Limbic Connectivity

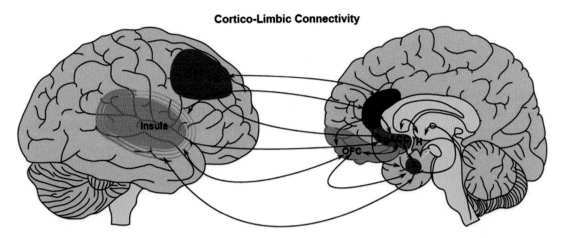

FIGURE 22–3 Corticolimbic connectivity. Low-level structures such as the amygdala (A) and hippocampus (H) interact with the cingulate cortex, dorsolateral prefrontal cortex (dlPFC), and ventromedial prefrontal cortex. OFC, orbital frontal cortex; pACC, perigenual anterior cingulate cortex; sgACC, subgenual anterior cingulate cortex. (Reproduced with permission from Perez DL, Barsky AJ, Daffner K, et al. Motor and somatosensory conversion disorder: a functional unawareness syndrome? *J Neuropsychiatry Clin Neurosci*. 2012 Spring;24(2):141-151.)

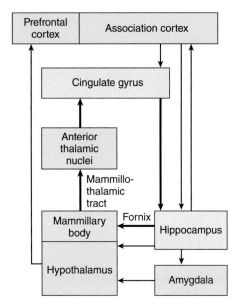

FIGURE 22–4 Block diagram of the limbic system with emphasis (bold lines) on the internal Papez circuit, which includes the anterior thalamic nuclei, cingulate gyrus, and fornix output of the hippocampus. (Reproduced with permission from Kandel ER, Schwartz JH, Jessell TM, et al: *Principles of Neural Science*, 5th ed. New York, NY: McGraw Hill; 2013.)

anterior thalamic nuclei to the cingulate cortex. The input to these thalamic nuclei comes chiefly from the hippocampus via its output tract, the fornix, via the mammillary body. The thin lines in Figure 22–4 show limbic projections mostly discovered more recently that are not part of the original Papez circuit, although the amygdala has long been known to be limbic.

The Amygdala

The amygdala on each side of the brain sits just anterior to the hippocampus. It has 3 main divisions: the basolateral, central, and cortical nuclei, shown in Figure 22–5. The basolateral nucleus receives significant input from the hippocampal formation and projects to medial prefrontal, orbito- (ventromedial) prefrontal, and cingulate cortical areas. The central nuclei receive ascending input from the brainstem and project to the hypothalamus. The cortical nuclei receive inputs from the olfactory bulb and also project to the hippocampus.

The amygdala interacts with the ventromedial prefrontal cortex in a manner somewhat similar to the interaction between the hippocampus and dorsolateral prefrontal cortex. Much of the prefrontal cortex instantiates a working memory of the configuration of the environment associated with a situation about which learning needs to occur. Activated neurons in the prefrontal cortex project to and activate coincidence detectors in the hippocampus and amygdala where synaptic weight changes, typically associated with *N*-methyl-D-aspartate (NMDA) receptors, allow the reactivation of the prefrontal neurons that activated neurons in the hippocampus and amygdala by reciprocal connections.

How the amygdala encodes situation context for learning is illustrated schematically in Figure 22–6. Neurons in the amygdala receive inputs from different neurons in multiple cortical areas, the hippocampus, and the limbic system. For any given contextual situation, a few neurons in the amygdala "grid" will receive inputs from the arbitrary set of activated neurons associated with that situation. The activated synaptic weights will be increased. Because the connections are reciprocal, similar situations that activate those amygdala neurons will activate the situation-coding neurons that constituted the representation of that situation.

The hippocampus is associated with learning nearly any context, such as navigational routes. The amygdala–ventromedial prefrontal cortex system, on the other hand, is involved in learning about risk and reward situations, particularly situations that are followed by negative consequences. This system creates memories that can engender fear of things such as guns pointed at someone or aggressive facial expressions. Damage to the amygdala does not eliminate fear of intrinsically fearful things such as snakes, heights, or leopards. However, it reduces the appropriate fear reactions to fear that must be learned, such as the sudden appearance of brake lights on the car ahead.

Ventromedial Prefrontal Cortex

The ventromedial or orbitofrontal cortex is shown in the sagittal section on the right in Figure 22–3 (some treatments consider the orbitofrontal cortex to be restricted to only the most ventral part of the ventromedial cortex, with the latter comprising a larger area). Ventromedial prefrontal neocortex is reciprocally connected to the amygdala and is essential for the assessment of risk and the associated emotional response of fear. In addition to the amygdala, inputs to the ventromedial prefrontal cortex come from the dorsolateral thalamus, olfactory bulb, and temporal lobe. Outputs from the ventromedial prefrontal cortex go reciprocally to the amygdala, as well as to the hypothalamus, hippocampus, cingulate cortex, and temporal lobe.

Ventromedial prefrontal cortex damage results in an inability to inhibit inappropriate behavior, particularly learned, socially inappropriate behavior. Humans with ventromedial prefrontal cortex damage often cannot avoid risky behavior because of the lack of a gut feeling of fear associated with the risks. Thus, they are poor at avoiding high reward but high loss activities such as gambling. Humans with ventromedial prefrontal damage are also poor at detecting and avoiding behavior that is socially unacceptable, such as speech laced with pointless profanity.

Another hallmark of ventromedial or orbitofrontal damage is what is called "utilization behavior." A patient with damage to this part of the brain may, when left in a room with paint cans and brushes, begin painting the wall. The sight of objects triggers their use, even when inappropriate, because the gut feeling normal people get about socially inappropriate behavior is missing. Extreme damage to ventromedial prefrontal cortex is associated with the inability to experience empathy, and some patients with this damage become sociopaths.

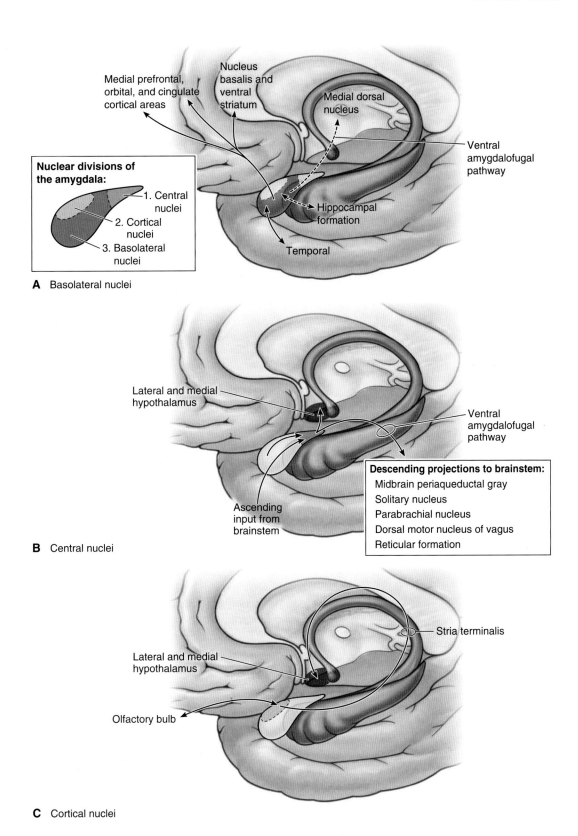

Nuclear divisions of the amygdala:
1. Central nuclei
2. Cortical nuclei
3. Basolateral nuclei

A Basolateral nuclei

Medial prefrontal, orbital, and cingulate cortical areas

Nucleus basalis and ventral striatum

Medial dorsal nucleus

Ventral amygdalofugal pathway

Hippocampal formation

Temporal

B Central nuclei

Lateral and medial hypothalamus

Ventral amygdalofugal pathway

Ascending input from brainstem

Descending projections to brainstem:
Midbrain periaqueductal gray
Solitary nucleus
Parabrachial nucleus
Dorsal motor nucleus of vagus
Reticular formation

C Cortical nuclei

Lateral and medial hypothalamus

Stria terminalis

Olfactory bulb

FIGURE 22–5 The amygdala on each side of the brain sits just anterior to the hippocampus. It has 3 main divisions: the basolateral, central, and cortical nuclei. The basolateral nucleus receives significant input from the hippocampal formation and projects to medial prefrontal, orbito- (ventromedial) prefrontal, and cingulate cortical areas. The central nuclei receive ascending input from the brainstem and project to the hypothalamus. The cortical nuclei receive input from the olfactory bulb and also project to the hippocampus. (Reproduced with permission from Martin JH. *Neuroanatomy: Text and Atlas*, 4th ed. New York, NY: McGraw Hill; 2012.)

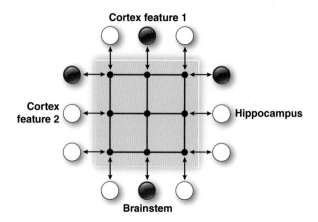

FIGURE 22–6 Neurons in the amygdala receive inputs from different neurons in multiple cortical areas, the hippocampus, and the limbic system. For any given contextual situation, a few neurons in the amygdala "grid" will receive inputs from the arbitrary set of activated neurons associated with that situation. The activated synaptic weights will be increased. Because the connections are reciprocal, similar situations that activate those amygdala neurons will activate the situation-coding neurons that constituted the representation of that situation.

There are notable lateralization differences in the prefrontal cortex, including the ventromedial prefrontal cortex. Activity in the left prefrontal cortex is biased toward approach on an approach/withdrawal axis, while activity in the right prefrontal area is associated with withdrawal. Damage to the left prefrontal cortex is thought to tip the approach/withdrawal balance toward right-dominated withdrawal and depression. Damage to the right prefrontal cortex, in contrast, shifts the balance to the left and is associated with manic behavior. These laterality effects are stronger in the ventromedial than dorsolateral prefrontal cortex.

Although the limbic system is phylogenetically old, the ventromedial prefrontal cortex has expanded in primates and humans with the rest of the cortex to mediate more complex emotional processing. It has often been supposed that emotion is the opposite of reason. Emotions, however, are the product of a complex neural processing system that is experience and case based, rather than rule based. The fact that the output of this system is via a low-dimensional feeling matrix rather that a high-dimensional language-based cognitive matrix does not imply that the calculations performed by this system are primitive. The autonomic/limbic/ventromedial prefrontal system acts rapidly before complex conscious processing and awareness, as is necessary for survival. Some aspect of how the car in front of you is being driven causes you to back away without your being aware of doing so or being able to say why, but it saves your life.

PHYSIOLOGIC CHANGES ASSOCIATED WITH EMOTION

Emotions are the "language" by which the limbic and autonomic nervous systems communicate with the rest of the brain. The fact that this language of is low dimensionality compared to conscious, verbal language used by other parts of the brain does not mean that the calculations done by this system are primitive and low dimensional. The guidance given by emotion for appropriate behavior in complex social situations may be based on complex, unconsciously processed cues and nondeclarative memories, including body language, tone of voice, facial expressions, and previous experiences with these elements. Humans experience strong "gut feelings" when their behavior in social groups is deemed unacceptable and may even experience such feelings in anticipation of unacceptable behavior, such as fear of making a mistake in public speaking. We are constantly unconsciously processing facial expressions, body postures, and tones of voice of those around us. Even the contemplation of particular dangerous moves in a cerebral exercise such as playing chess can evoke such feelings.

The output of the emotion-processing system tends to be mostly describable along the approach/withdrawal and intensity axes, which can be partly mapped onto the autonomic nervous system sympathetic/parasympathetic polarities and intensities for each division.

High & Low Road Inputs

The American neuroscientist Joseph LeDoux has proposed a low and high road theory for sensory processing. In this scheme, information that is sent by cephalic sensors to the thalamus for transmission along the slow high road to the neocortex is also sent in parallel on the fast low road to the amygdala for more immediate action. Olfactory input, for example, which is dominated by emotional approach/withdrawal motivation, projects directly to the amygdala–ventromedial prefrontal system, which can trigger avoidance behavior before conscious awareness of the identity of the smell, which is based on slower high road cortical processing. The block diagram of olfactory bulb projections in Figure 22–7 shows the direct projection from the olfactory bulb to the amygdala versus the more complex olfactory projection system that involves prefrontal and frontal cortex.

A similar situation exists for other senses in which a high road projection to thalamus and neocortex is paralleled by a low road projection to the limbic system. The low road system activates both the autonomic nervous system and initiates behavior before conscious processing informs us of the identity of the stimulus. Danger in both physical and social situations activates the amygdala–ventromedial system.

Autonomic Responses

LeDoux's term for the output of the amygdala–ventromedial system is *somatic markers*, what we usually call "gut feelings." These have a strong autonomic component, often switching the body from homeostasis (parasympathetic) to fight/flight sympathetic activation. Sympathetic activation increases activity in the hypothalamus-pituitary-adrenal (HPA) axis, leading to internal changes such as increased heart rate, sweating, and pupil dilation. A general term for activators of the HPA axis

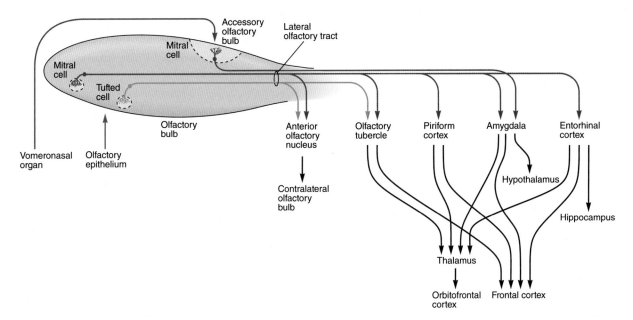

FIGURE 22–7 Projections of the olfactory bulb. Note the direct projection to the amygdala and the more complex paths involving projections to the cortex. The amygdala has a direct output to the hypothalamus that activates the hypothalamus-pituitary-adrenal axis. (Reproduced with permission from Kandel ER, Schwartz JH, Jessell TM, et al: *Principles of Neural Science*, 5th ed. New York, NY: McGraw Hill; 2013.)

is *stress*, as shown in Figure 22–8. An important transmitter in this system is cortisol. Cortisol levels increase during stress, which acts as a negative feedback signal to reduce adrenal activation. However, chronic stress associated with continuously elevated cortisol levels that is not effective in reducing sympathetic activation has negative effects on the body, such as impairment of immune function, heart disease, and impairment of learning and memory.

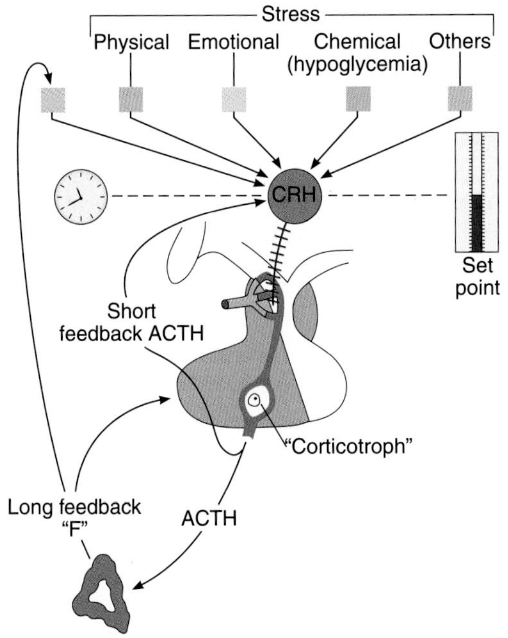

AFFECTIVE DISORDERS

Patients with damage to ventromedial prefrontal cortex lack normal aversion to risky behavior, such as gambling, but are cognitively aware that the behavior may be detrimental. This type of damage is also characterized by utilization behavior. In contrast, the hallmark of amygdala damage is an extreme loss of any fear.

Sociopathy

There is considerable overlap between psychopathy and sociopathy, with the consensus being that sociopathy is a weak form of psychopathy. A unifying scheme for defining psychopathy is that it is characterized by a lack of gut feelings of remorse or empathy. It may occur in individuals who are often otherwise above average in intelligence. Overlapping sociopathic traits include lack of emotional attachment and manipulativeness. Given the considerable evidence that damage to the amygdala–ventromedial system produces such traits, it seems highly likely that unknown damage to this system underlies most sociopathic behavior. Such damage may be organic, from, for example a tumor or head blow, or possibly secondary to environmental effects such as child abuse.

Autism

Autism is a spectrum disorder, probably originating from mutations at more than 10 gene loci and arising from multiple other causes. As a spectrum, it ranges in severity from

FIGURE 22–8 Inputs to the hypothalamus-pituitary-adrenal (HPA) axis, the feedback loops with cortisol (F) and adrenocorticotropic hormone (ACTH). CRH, corticotropin-releasing hormone. (Reproduced with permission from Gwinup G, Johnson B: Clinical testing of the hypothalamic-pituitary-adrenocortical system in states of hypo- and hypercortisolism, *Metabolism*. 1975 Jun;24(6):777-791.)

extremely mild (the absent-minded college professor) to profound mental retardation. Unifying concepts for autism include Simon Baron-Cohen's idea of an autistic lack of theory of mind, the ability to comprehend and react to another's point of view and intentions. This is exhibited as antisocial behavior that, although once was interpreted as maliciousness, is now seen as an inability to comprehend that others have feelings that can be hurt. Autistic people are thought to be socially withdrawn and inept because of an inability to act in a socially appropriate manner, due to an underlying perceptual deficit.

Baron-Cohen has extended the theory of mind idea of autism to the idea of autism as an ultra-male brain. Females, on average, score much higher than males on tests of empathy, while males score higher on tests of systemizing, such as spatial manipulations and mechanical knowledge. An essential point of this idea is that both males and females exist on a spectrum of male versus female "brains," with some females having more male-type brains, and some males with more female-type brains. His theory then is that autistics, whether male or female, have brains at the extreme male end, with very poor empathy, but sometimes savant abilities in calculation or art. Some data have suggested that prenatal exposure to high testosterone tends to produce male brain types and associated autistic traits in humans and laboratory animals. These effects may be mediated by underdevelopment of the ventromedial prefrontal system that underlies social intelligence. As such, autism would be viewed as a deficiency in emotional intelligence or perception, not a lack of emotional experience.

CONCLUSION

The autonomic and limbic systems evolved to control the balance between homeostasis and species-typical action behaviors such as fight, flight, and reproduction. Highly social mammals, such as primates, have extensive autonomic reaction to risks and dangers associated with social interactions and signals, many of which are learned. The amygdala–ventromedial system and the anterior cingulate cortex are high-resolution executives that reciprocally interact with limbic and lower structures to mediate complex social and emotional intelligence. Although the outputs of these systems are embedded in low-dimensional matrices such as gut feelings, their unconscious computations are high dimensional, complex, and necessary for existence in a complex social environment.

SUMMARY

- Emotions are feelings generated by drives and instincts and by assessment of progress toward those drives.
- Emotion depends on the limbic system, the middle component of the proposed evolutionary triune structure of the brain.
- Emotional reactions can be characterized along the dimensions of valence and intensity.

- According to the James-Lange theory of emotion, emotional reactions precede cognitive appraisal.
- In mammals, emotions are particularly evoked by social hierarchy situations.
- Approximately 6 basic human emotions are thought to be universal.
- Emotional expression involves activation of the limbic and autonomic nervous systems.
- The amygdala is crucial for emotional learning via its interaction with ventromedial prefrontal cortex.
- According to LeDoux's "low road" theory, emotions are processed by a rapid path from the thalamus to other subcortical structures such as the amygdala, independently from a slower, but more accurate "high road" path involving the projection from thalamus to neocortex.
- Affective disorders are characterized by disturbances in emotional cognition and behavior.

SELF-ASSESSMENT QUESTIONS

1. A car accident victim continues to exhibit a normal lack of fear of intrinsically fearful entities such as snakes and leopards but has lost fear for images that one learns are dangerous, such as guns and fearful facial expressions. Normal semantic and episodic memories of non–fear-associated items remain intact and continue to be learned. The lesion is likely to be located where?

   A. Hippocampus
   B. Amygdala
   C. Insula
   D. Ventromedial prefrontal cortex
   E. Dorsolateral prefrontal cortex

2. After a stroke, a 57-year-old man suddenly develops a gambling addiction and loses most of his savings at a casino. He also exhibits what is called utilization behavior, the tendency to use objects that do not belong to him, such as grabbing coins from someone else's pile at the casino and inserting them in the slot machine. Where is the lesion likely to be?

   A. Hippocampus
   B. Amygdala
   C. Thalamus
   D. Ventromedial prefrontal cortex
   E. Dorsolateral prefrontal cortex

3. Two patients present at a neurology clinic with mirror image brain lesions. One patient has become high risk taking and manic, while the other is lethargic and depressed. The manic/depressed mirror lesions are where?

   A. Left/right ventromedial prefrontal cortex
   B. Right/left ventromedial prefrontal cortex
   C. Left/right dorsolateral prefrontal cortex
   D. Right/left dorsolateral prefrontal cortex
   E. Left/right amygdala

Circadian Rhythms & Sleep

Christopher M. Ciarleglio, Rachel C. Besing, & Karen L. Gamble

OBJECTIVES

After studying this chapter, the student should be able to:

- Understand how circadian rhythms are ubiquitous throughout all life and in virtually all cells in most species.
- Know how circadian rhythms are derived from intrinsic clock mechanisms.
- Understand how light sensed by some cells within an organism synchronizes the circadian rhythms of the entire organism.
- Understand the difference between synchronization and entrainment of circadian clocks.
- Understand how circadian rhythms work in terms of sleep/activity epochs.
- Understand the molecular basis of intrinsic circadian rhythms and its robustness with respect to temperature and other perturbations.
- Recount the role of the suprachiasmatic nucleus (SCN) and retinal output in circadian rhythms.
- Be aware of the importance of vasoactive intestinal polypeptide (VIP) in circadian rhythms.
- Understand how the SCN influences the rest of the body's circadian rhythms.
- Understand dysfunctions in circadian rhythms such as seasonal affective disorder and sleep problems.

INTRODUCTION

The result of billions of years of evolution, the innate biological clock is a nearly ubiquitous feature of life on Earth. The conservation of its basic function—the maintenance of a stable relationship between the organism's internal physiologic processes and the environmental light cycle—across such a wide swath of species speaks volumes about its importance. This timekeeping mechanism is not simply a response to changing light, but rather an innate clock that responds slowly and predictably to changes in the architecture of daily light cycles. Behaviorally, this clock allows organisms to predict daily changes in the environment and to react accordingly. Physiologically, the clock serves as a master regulator of many processes, providing a temporal pattern for internal organization and output. In humans and other mammals, the master circadian clock is located in the suprachiasmatic nuclei of the hypothalamus—a pair of densely packed nuclei receiving direct light input from specialized cells in the retina and other indirect timing and physiologic information from a slew of other areas in the nervous system and body. In this chapter, we will explore the basic properties of circadian and seasonal rhythms, the more complex molecular constituents of the clock, and finally, their impact on human health.

EVOLUTIONARY ORIGINS

At the formation of the solar system, the planetary nursery in the accretion disk had a natural motion, orbiting our nascent Sun and serving as the birthplace of dozens of planetoids colliding with each other like a game of cosmic pinball. These planetoids had a natural rotation parallel with the orbit of the accretion disk, but these planetary rotations tended to vary

VOCABULARY

Actigraphy: A type of activity monitoring that uses accelerometry to record amount of activity (usually wrist movement) over time and plots it on an **actigraph** (or **actogram**). Algorithms can be applied to determine the amount and quality of sleep.

Activity bout (α): The segmented time of day at which an organism is active.

Aftereffect: A transient reorganization of the circadian rhythm evident in constant conditions, particularly after a stimulus or perturbation.

Chronotherapy: Therapeutic strategy in which knowledge of the internal circadian clock is used to treat patients with strategies aimed at realigning circadian rhythms or giving medication at a particular time of day to improve treatment response.

Chronotype: The time of day at which a person prefers to sleep and/or be awake in reference to the outside environment. Early types are sometimes referred to as "early birds," and late types are sometimes referred to as "night owls."

Circadian: Of or about a day in length; in biology, a circadian rhythm is a self-sustaining physiologic rhythm of nearly 24 hours in length that continues to oscillate in the absence of external factors or stimuli.

Circadian time (CT): All the temporal phases of a circadian rhythm that occur in 1 cycle under constant conditions. That cycle is arbitrarily divided into 24 circadian hours regardless of local time, where CT 0 is the onset of activity in diurnal animals and CT 12 is the onset of behavioral activity in nocturnal animals. Any use of CT in vitro is based on an extrapolation from a measurable behavior.

Constant darkness: A photoperiod in which light is completely absent and organisms are allowed to free-run based on their individual circadian properties.

Cyanobacteria: An ancient photosynthetic bacterial phylum that exhibits robust circadian rhythms in culture.

Desynchronization: Process by which an oscillatory network with many coupled subcomponents becomes uncoupled due to inconsistent changes in the time interval between the subcomponents so that the phase relationships among components are lost.

Diurnal: Of or due to the partitioning of an organism's main bout of behavioral activity to the daytime.

Entrain: To achieve entrainment; the act of an environmental zeitgeber setting the phase of the clock.

Entrainment: The state of a circadian clock in which the rhythm is at a stable phase angle with the environment and is due to an entraining stimulus from that environment, called a *zeitgeber*.

Free-running period (FRP or τ or period): The temporal length of a single rhythmic waveform. Circadian rhythms generally have a τ around but not exactly equal to 24 hours.

Light therapy: A type of antidepressant and/or circadian (chrono-)therapy using daily white or blue (488-nm) light to artificially entrain the clock. See **chronotherapy**.

Nocturnal: Of or due to the partitioning of an organism's main bout of behavioral activity to the nighttime.

Periodicity: A rhythm, especially with relatively stable characteristics from 1 cycle to the next.

Phase (Φ or φ): A specific temporal point in a rhythm. The phase of an environmental rhythm (the zeitgeber) is denoted as Φ, whereas the phase of a circadian rhythm is denoted as φ.

Phase advance (+Δφ): The amount of time that the phase of a rhythm happens earlier than was predicted by that rhythm's free-running period (τ). If light is the zeitgeber, a phase advance is usually achieved when the light pulse is given in the late subjective night. Also, the act of achieving an earlier phase than predicted.

Phase angle (ψ): The stable temporal relationship between a point in a circadian rhythm and an environmental stimulus (zeitgeber). This is arguably the most important evolutionary characteristic of a circadian clock.

Phase delay (−Δφ): The amount of time that the phase of a rhythm happens later than was predicted by that rhythm's free-running period (τ). If light is the zeitgeber, a phase delay is usually achieved when the light pulse is given in the early subjective night. Also, the act of achieving a later phase than predicted.

Phase response curve: A type of graph that illustrates magnitude of phase shifts (y-axis; phase advances are positive, whereas phase delays are negative) to pulses of light as a function of circadian time (x-axis). This type of graph is useful in determining how capable an organism is of entraining to the varying length of daylight.

Photoperiod: The proportion of time within each day that is allotted to either day or night, usually leading to the expression of seasonal or photoperiodic traits in living organisms.

Photoperiodic: Of or having any physiologic change due to the environmental photoperiod; having the condition of **photoperiodism**; a more exaggerated form of **seasonality**.

Rapid eye movement sleep: A phase of sleep wherein the brain is highly active and the body is in a deeply relaxed state (sleep paralysis).

Seasonality: Condition in which animals experience behavioral changes in response to environmental season but which does not wholly constitute **photoperiodism**.

Subjective day/night: The time of day according to the circadian clock regardless of the external local time.

(*Continued*)

VOCABULARY (*CONTINUED*)

Suprachiasmatic nucleus (SCN): A pair of nuclei (paradoxically referred to in the field as a single nucleus) in the anteroventral hypothalamus, just dorsal to the optic chiasm. These nuclei house the central mammalian circadian pacemaker with some 20,000 densely packed and generally GABAergic neurons, although many produce an array of other neuropeptides.

T-cycle: Any photoperiod whose light and dark portions add up to a day length other than 24 hours.

Zeitgeber: German meaning "time giver"; a phase-setting environmental stimulus (for circadian rhythms, usually light)

that serves to align the environmental rhythm to the biological clock.

Zeitgeber time (ZT): All the temporal phases of a rhythm that occur in 1 cycle under the influence of a rhythmic zeitgeber. Assuming that the length of that cycle is 24 hours (a non–24-hour environmental cycle is called a "T-cycle"), it is divided into hours where ZT 0 is defined as the onset of activity in diurnal animals, and ZT 12 is defined as the onset of behavioral activity in nocturnal animals.

---

wildly as their axes wobbled in space or they slowed until they were tidally locked with their star. For Earth, the planet's rotation was cemented and stabilized approximately 4.4 billion years ago when a Mars-sized planetoid named Theia crashed into it and formed our moon. The Moon stabilized Earth's axis, slightly off perpendicular to the planet's orbit around the Sun. The Moon also gave us tides once the planet had cooled enough from the impact that liquid water oceans could form. It is through geologic evidence of these powerful tides—when first formed, the Moon was 6 to 10 times closer than present—that we know that the early Earth spun at the absolutely blistering pace of 4 hours per day. Over time, as the radius of the Moon's orbit drifted outward to its current position, the drag of the lunar tide slowed Earth's rotation to the 24 hours we now know. Because **circadian** clocks can be found in life-forms as ancient as **cyanobacteria** and in most living things today, including humans, one cannot help but appreciate that they must have given early life an advantage. In fact, a TimeTree of Life analysis would indicate that the most recent common ancestor of cyanobacteria and humans lived some 4.1 billion years ago (with estimates as early as approximately 4.3 billion years ago), when we know that the Earth's rotation was still much accelerated. Along with the extraordinary discovery of 4.1 billion-year-old organic carbon in 2015, this evidence suggests that the earliest life on Earth not only had to deal with its harsh and downright inhospitable environs, but also had to be able to synch their daily cycle with a period of only several hours. Yet, genes used by animals to control parts of their clocks are exaptations of older, more ancient genes that can be found in bacteria and are being used for such processes as DNA repair.

As such, the day–night cycle is a critical environmental factor shaping the evolution of life on Earth. In Earth's tumultuous history, extraterrestrial impacts such as the Moon-forming event, along with geologic upheaval and vulcanism, were not uncommon. Although early life evolved in the water, these factors wreaked havoc on the ability of the Sun's light to reach the oceans, at times darkening the planet for many years. In at least 3 extreme instances in the planet's history, the entire globe was covered with a sheet of white ice that was miles thick in some places—the so-called "Snowball Earth." The last of these deep ice ages lasted millions of years 800 to 600 million years ago, bouncing most of the Sun's light back into space and trapping early life in a dark ocean. *Yet we find in the present that the endogenous circadian clock is an almost ubiquitous feature of life on Earth, suggesting that it would have offered some increased fitness, even then.* How did circadian rhythms become the rule rather than the exception? It is thought that the ability to anticipate day/night transitions and coordinate internal metabolic processes was advantageous for the earliest life on the planet. The evolution of photosynthesis led to large amounts of oxygen in the atmosphere and an ozone to filter damaging solar radiation. Before that time, it is thought that organisms used their circadian clocks to judge surface safety by sinking to deeper water during the day and surface feeding at night—the so-called "escape from light" hypothesis proposed by Colin Pittendrigh, who was a founding father of the chronobiology field. By tracking light–dark transitions, later photosynthetic organisms could capture the Sun's light and fix carbon on a regular schedule. Organisms that fed on these photosynthesizers shared the ancestral characteristic and used their own clocks to time their feeding behavior. Regardless of the predator and prey relationship, an endogenous circadian rhythm allowed an organism to maintain a fairly consistent relationship (or **phase angle**) with the external day–night cycle, despite changes in the primary time cues (or **zeitgebers**). Circadian clocks could be **entrained**, rather than purely driven or synchronized, allowing the organismal clock to generally keep time despite irregularities in weather and seasons and/or the absence of light, such as due to volcanic ash, asteroid impact, or even Snowball Earth. This stable phase angle provided a mechanism for adaptive flexibility to the ever-changing geophysical day: the ability to predict time of day persistently, even in periods of bad weather, geologic upheaval, or severe climate change. Thus, **entrainment** offered some fitness that allowed feeding or photosynthesis to occur on a generally regular schedule. This last point explains why completely divergent species such as cyanobacteria and humans evolved the ability to produce circadian rhythms, despite the fact that their last common ancestor lived some 4.1 billion years ago when the length of the day was far shorter than 24 hours. Either circadian rhythms were so important to early evolving life that they persist in most species today, or circadian rhythms have become so important that convergent evolution has made them a general property of life on Earth.

Seminal work by Carl Johnson and colleagues elegantly demonstrated in cyanobacteria that circadian clocks do offer competitive fitness when the endogenous rhythm is resonant with the external environment. In mammals, where such direct competition experiments are difficult, Pat DeCoursey made a fortuitous observation in captive ground squirrels that having a functional circadian clock did indeed decrease mortality rates: While the squirrels could not get out of a pen, a predatory weasel somehow got in and disproportionately picked off clock-lesioned squirrels while at the same time providing invaluable evidence for the importance of a behavioral circadian rhythm in mammals. This incident inspired DeCoursey and her team to monitor the behavior of wild-type and clock-lesioned ground squirrels using Global Positioning System tags in the wild, further bolstering the initial results. In addition to compromised survival due to predator–prey relationships, the circadian clock can also offer fitness due to overall health of the organism. Recent work in rodent species shows that certain genetic mutations can change the speed of the clock. For example, mice with a mutation that causes a faster clock with a shorter period (ie, 22-hour cycle) die from heart and kidney failure at earlier ages when housed in conditions that provide a standard, 24-hour, light:dark (LD) 12:12 **photoperiod**. Remarkably, these mutant mice appear to age and live normally when housed in a 22-hour **T-cycle** with an LD 11:11 photoperiod.

Thus, the mammalian biological circadian clock, located in the hypothalamus of the brain (see later section on the suprachiasmatic nucleus), is an indispensable component of life in the wild. It would follow, then, that understanding how mutations in circadian genes disrupt the function of behavioral and physiologic rhythmicity is important not only on the merits of scientific interest, but also for its implications to human health.

PROPERTIES OF CIRCADIAN RHYTHMS

By definition, circadian rhythms are the physiologic processes whereby an organism regulates its activity and coordinates other physiologic processes on a self-sustained, daily cycle. The word *circadian* comes from the Latin words *circa*, which means "about," and *diem*, which means "day." Behavioral rhythms govern several characteristics in animals: feeding/fasting, drinking, waking/sleeping, attention, cognitive performance, torpor, and body temperature, among others. Physiologic circadian rhythms can be found in hormone release, immune system function, and even cell division. Presently, a circadian rhythm has 3 fundamental properties: (1) the rhythm is self-sustained and approximately 24 hours in length; (2) the rhythm is temperature compensated; and (3) the rhythm is entrained by external factors such as light.

The first property of circadian clocks was initially observed by a French scientist named Jean-Jacques d'Ortous de Mairan, who was fascinated with the daily leaf movements of the heliotropic plant, *Mimosa pudica*, and so he examined whether his observations were simply a direct response to the sunlight or something more ingrained in the plant. After placing the plant in a dark cabinet, he observed that daily leaf movement persisted, thus illustrating the first characteristic of a circadian clock: persistence of the rhythm in constant conditions (generally light and temperature) at a near 24-hour period. In rodent models, this endogenous period is most often assessed by behavioral monitoring—such as activity recorded by wheel running (Figure 23–1, *left*), infrared motion detection (Figure 23–1, *right*), laser beam break, or water drinking—in constant darkness. Mice, for example, are the **nocturnal** species that exhibit activity during the dark of night. If placed in a monitored cage in **constant darkness**, mice will generally exhibit a **free-running period** (**FRP** or τ) of slightly less than 24 hours and continue to

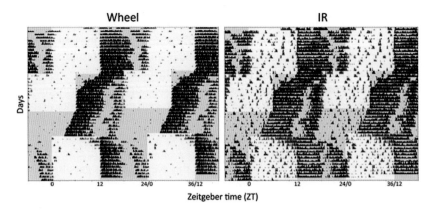

FIGURE 23–1 Representative double-plotted actograms illustrate mouse behavioral circadian characteristics in response to changing lighting conditions. *Left*, actogram of wheel-running activity; *right*, actogram of the same mouse (*left*) as monitored by infrared (IR) motion detection. *Black* ticks represent activity in 5-minute bins; yellow background denotes lights on; gray background denotes lights off.

run only during what they perceive as "night." The same form of activity monitoring (known as **actigraphy**) may be used to assess behavioral rhythms of humans, but the FRP of **diurnal** humans tends to run slightly longer than 24 hours. Even in humans, wakefulness occurs during what they perceive as "day" in the absence of photic or social cues in constant routine conditions in which people are kept awake with a constant posture in continual dim ambient light, with hourly meals. The imperfect, non–24-hour clock timing found across the animal kingdom has a purpose: The closer an animal's FRP is to 24 hours, the more difficult it is to entrain to the 24-hour, light–dark cycle.

The second property of circadian rhythms is rather remarkable: Unlike other basic biochemical reactions that increase their reactivity as the temperature increases—usually 2- to 3-fold for every 10°C increase—biological clocks are seemingly unaffected by temperature. In other words, the clock continues to run at a normal **periodicity** regardless of ambient environmental temperature. How the clock manages to accomplish this feat is rather a mystery, but it may have something to do with redundancy built into the molecular feedback loop (see later section titled "Molecular Architecture of the Circadian Clock"). Regardless, as discussed on the topic of clock evolution, the clock must be able to maintain its innate circadian rhythm at or near its native period and be able to process incoming signals from the environment. That latter property is the third and final characteristic of a circadian rhythm.

The light–dark cycle created by the Earth's rotation is a natural, robust, and reliable oscillation. In the modern world, each day is exactly 24 hours. In a seminal series of papers on mammalian rhythms by Colin Pittendrigh and Serge Daan, the fourth paper suggests that conservation of the phase relationship between the master oscillator (Earth's rotation—Φ) and its slave oscillator (the circadian biological clock—ϕ) is the essence of entrainment. This relationship is called **phase angle** (ψ) and is arguably the most important aspect of a circadian rhythm. A **zeitgeber** (German for "time giver") is an external cue that sets or aligns the internal biological clock to the external 24-hour light–dark cycle. The most ancient and influential of all zeitgebers is light, which readily adjusts the **phase** of the biological clock such that the internal circadian rhythm is synchronized to the environmental stimulus. In humans, entrainment manifests as a behavioral period equal to the period of the 24-hour entraining stimulus with a stable phase relationship (ie, phase angle) between the circadian rhythm and the environment. There are 2 proposed models of entrainment: the continuous (parametric) model and the discrete (nonparametric) model. Both models have been championed by founders of the field, and both have merits and drawbacks. In the continuous model, Jurgen Aschoff suggested that the intensity of light proportionally changed the speed of the biological clock in a phase-dependent manner, thus squeezing or stretching the internal circadian clock period to fit into the actual environmental day. In contrast, Colin Pittendrigh suggested that a discrete model could explain entrainment of the circadian clock by simply shifting the phase ($\Delta\phi$) or timing

of each cycle by a specific amount. This model used a **phase response curve** (**PRC**) to explain phase-dependent shifts to discrete pulses of light that, alone or in combination, added up to the period of the environmental day (Figure 23–2). Thus, in a 24-hour light–dark cycle, the internal circadian period (τ) is equal to the external 24-hour cycle of light and darkness (**T**).

In Pittendrigh's discrete model, a zeitgeber adjusts clock phase by an amount of time that corrects for the difference between the period of the master oscillator and the internal circadian clock. Light phase shifts a particular rhythm (eg, hormone levels, neuronal activity, behavioral activity levels) by an amount that depends on when the light is presented with respect to the animal's **subjective** time, as defined by the animal's internal circadian clock. With regard to light, the largest **phase delays** occur when presented during the early subjective night, and the largest **phase advances** occur when light is presented during the late subjective night, just before dawn. The functional result of a phase delay is that the rhythm peaks later than it would have if there had been no stimulus given. When a phase advance occurs, the rhythm peaks earlier than it would have if there had been no light stimulus given. The relationship between when a light pulse is given during the animal's subjective day or night and the resulting phase shift can be plotted using a PRC, in which the time of the light presentation (with respect to the internal circadian day) is on the x-axis and the size of the phase shift is plotted on the y-axis (see Figure 23–2).

The ability to entrain to the geophysical day with a constant phase angle is of paramount importance, especially when considering that the amount of time between dawn and dusk changes with the seasons. These changes in **photoperiod**, or the amount of daytime relative to nighttime over a 24-hour period, may perturb the phase relationship between the master and slave oscillators. Further work on mammalian entrainment by Pittendrigh and Daan sought to address how phase angle is conserved across changes in photoperiod due to season (see later section titled "Seasonality"). They proposed that the circadian clock consists of 2 coupled oscillators—a morning and an evening oscillator. They suggested that each oscillator is entrained to a light–dark transition (either dawn or dusk) and that the relationship between these oscillators accounts for photoperiodic encoding. For diurnal species such as humans, where the majority of activity is relegated to the daytime, dawn is referred to as **zeitgeber time** 0, or ZT 0, regardless of the local time at which dawn occurs. Likewise, the onset of activity in diurnal animals is referred to as **circadian time** 0, or CT 0, when the individuals are left to free-run in constant conditions. Rather confusingly, dusk is referred to as ZT 12 regardless of what the local time is for primarily nocturnal species, whose activity is generally isolated to nighttime. The onset of activity for nocturnal species is therefore referred to as CT 12 when the animal is left to free-run in constant conditions (constant darkness).

These distinctions between how we refer to the passage of time on a circadian scale relative to the local time are difficult but important to understand. For example, consider 2

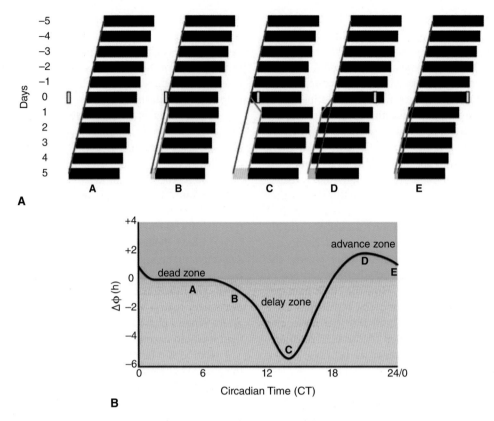

FIGURE 23–2 Phase shifts to discrete pulses of light and the phase response curve (PRC) of wild-type mice (*Mus musculus*). **A.** Idealized constant darkness (DD) actograms showing that a 30-minute pulse of light (*yellow*) on day 0 shifts the phase of activity onset (*black bars* are activity) on subsequent days in a phase-dependent manner. *Red line* is activity onset based on free-running period; *green line* is the new activity onset after the light pulse; *gold bar* represents the total phase delay; and *blue bar* represents the total phase advance. **B.** Idealized PRC (*black line*) tracing the phase shifts (in hours) from the top figure over circadian time. *Gold area* of the graph represents the phase delay zone, and *blue area* of the graph represents the phase advance zone. Letters A to E in the top figure represent the shift responsible for the point in the PRC (bottom) represented by the same letters.

nocturnal mice with different internal circadian periods and therefore different onsets of activity relative to the local time. If a person in Bangor, Maine, were to check on the behavior of these 2 mice at local sunset on the first day of summer (ie, 8:25 pm Eastern Daylight Time [EDT] or 20:25 EDT), that would correspond to ZT 15:35 for that person, but the internal time for the 2 mice could be very different, depending on their native period and how long they have been in the dark (eg, CT 3 or CT 16). In other words, it's complicated. The further away from the equator one goes, the bigger is the photoperiodic disparity between seasons: In the continental United States, its northernmost city of Lynden, Washington, has a summer photoperiod of LD 16.2:7.8 but only goes through a period of astronomical twilight rather than "night," whereas the southernmost incorporated place in the United States, Key West, Florida, has a summer photoperiod of only LD 13.7:10.3 with full night and day. It is difficult enough to keep track of the nuances of seasonally changing and latitude-dependent photoperiods to even consider how the circadian clock actually processes the information. How seasonality and photoperiodism are encoded in mammals will be discussed in the later section titled "Seasonality," along with the rules outlined by Pittendrigh and others concerning

how entrainment and the conservation of phase angle persist at a tissue or cellular level.

SUPRACHIASMATIC NUCLEUS: THE CENTRAL MAMMALIAN PACEMAKER

In the latter half of the 20th century, the nascent field of chronobiology picked up speed on the mammalian front with the publication of classic and brilliant works by the field's founding fathers. Colin Pittendrigh and Serge Daan published a masterpiece on the properties of rodent behavioral rhythms. Jurgen Aschoff furthered our understanding of human rhythms and the effects of light on the speed of the clock, postulating what Pittendrigh would later call Aschoff's Rules, and Franz Halberg was finding rhythms in all types of organisms. What eluded these investigators, however, was the specific location of the mammalian biological clock. In 1967, Curt Richter published a study suggesting that ablation of the hypothalamus led to circadian behavioral arrhythmicity. Exactly who should receive credit for the subsequent discovery of the central pacemaker is still hotly debated, but in 1972, 2 groups independently identified the **suprachiasmatic nucleus (SCN)** of the hypothalamus as the biological clock in mammals. Robert Moore and Nicholas Lenn identified the retinohypothalamic tract projecting from the retina—long thought to be the primary sensor of circadian light in mammals—to the SCN. Simultaneously, Friedrich Stephan and Irving Zucker followed Richter's lead and concluded that the SCN was the pacemaker by electrolytic lesioning of specific nuclei in the hypothalamus. Only lesioning of the SCN produced behavioral **arrhythmicity**. Progress in the field quickened as the SCN was found to exhibit rhythmicity of neuronal firing rates in vivo and in vitro. The SCN was firmly established as the master circadian pacemaker in mammals by transplant studies that rescued behavioral rhythmicity in SCN-lesioned animals and even conveyed upon the transplant recipient the donor's circadian period.

The SCN is medially located in the anterior hypothalamus, dorsal to the optic chiasm and inferolateral to the third ventricle in mice (Figure 23–3A). Each nucleus is approximately 200-μm wide at its widest point on the coronal plane, 200 to 250 μm dorsoventrally, and approximately 500 to 600 μm from the rostral to caudal extremes. It is densely packed with about 10,000 small (approximately 10-μm wide) neurons, most of which are γ-aminobutyric acid (GABA)-ergic. Due to their density, these SCN neurons are readily identifiable in a coronal mouse brain section as translucent bulbs above a darker optic chiasm (Figure 23–3B). These neurons increase their spike frequency during the circadian day and upregulate nighttime firing rate in response to phase-shifting light pulses.

SCN cells have several characteristics that make them unique from other cells. One distinguishing feature is that SCN cells receive photic information directly from the retina, allowing them to remain entrained to the 24-hour light–dark cycle. The SCN sends efferent projections to other hypothalamic nuclei, ultimately influencing pineal gland function and melatonin release. Second, SCN cells have network properties that allow them to synchronize their activity with one another due to neuronal firing, chemical synapses, and gap junctions. Third, these small compact neurons are capable of regeneratively firing action potentials (eg, pacemaking). The frequency of these electrical events exhibits a 24-hour rhythm at the population and single-cell level, even when neurons are maintained in a low-density culture that minimizes synaptic communication.

The SCN Is Innervated by the Retina & Is Characterized by Anatomically Localized Neuropeptides

As mentioned earlier, the mammalian circadian clock is entrained to the external environment primarily by light through **phase delays** in the early night and **phase advances** in the late night. This phase-shifting process begins with photic activation of conventional photoreceptors and specialized melanopsin ganglion cells within the retina. These intrinsically photosensitive ganglion cells then signal photic information directly to the SCN via glutamatergic innervation by the retinohypothalamic tract. Glutamate and pituitary adenylate cyclase–activating peptide (PACAP) released from retinal terminals activate postsynaptic N-methyl-D-aspartate (NMDA) receptors (as well as $VPAC_1$, $VPAC_2$, and PAC_1 receptors), resulting in an influx of calcium, membrane depolarization, and an increase in spontaneous action potential firing. Early work suggested that these retinorecipient neurons are located in the ventrolateral core of the SCN (see Figure 23–3B). However, more recent studies suggest that projections from melanopsin ganglion cells actually innervate the entire nucleus more extensively than previously thought. There are slight species-specific differences in the pattern of innervation, but most rodent models follow a general layout. Studies on light-induced expression of the immediate-early gene c-Fos suggest that many retinorecipient cells express vasoactive intestinal polypeptide (VIP) and gastrin-releasing peptide (GRP).

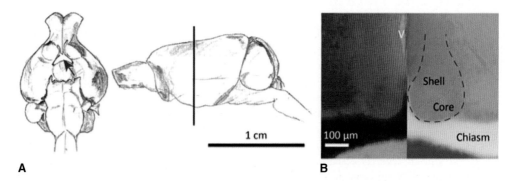

FIGURE 23–3 Murine suprachiasmatic nucleus (SCN) of the hypothalamus. **A.** *Left*, in this ventral sketch of the mouse brain, the SCN is located in the hypothalamus, just dorsal to the caudal extreme of the optic chiasm (*red arrow*). *Right*, in this sagittal view of the mouse brain, coronal SCN slice cultures are typically made on the *vertical black line*. *Horizontal scale bar* represents 1 cm. **B.** Dim red backlighting of a coronal hypothalamic slice culture (*left*); the *right half* of the image is inverted and grayscale to view detail as seen under regular illumination. The general shape of the nucleus is outlined in *red* with core/shell demarcated by *blue*. The ventrolateral core containing retinorecipient cells synapsing with intrinsically photosensitive retinal ganglion cells is labeled. The dorsomedial shell is also labeled, along with the chiasm. V, third ventricle. *Horizontal scale bar* represents 100 μm. (Part A, reproduced with permission from Ciarleglio CM, Resuehr HE, McMahon DG. Interactions of the serotonin and circadian systems: nature and nurture in rhythms and blues, *Neuroscience.* 2011 Dec 1;197:8-16.)

A conserved anatomic pattern of neuropeptide expression exists in the SCN from multiple rodent models. In addition to the retinorecipient core, the SCN is also characterized by a dorsomedial shell that produces arginine vasopressin, met-enkephalin, and angiotensin II. Core neurons innervate not only each other, but also the shell of the same nucleus. There are also internuclear connections between the 2 cores and the 2 shells.

VIP Plays a Key Role in Circadian Entrainment & Behavior

Prepro-VIP is the precursor from which VIP and peptide histidine isoleucine are derived, and both are structurally similar to PACAP. VIP is a secreted peptide in the glucagon family that is expressed rhythmically in the core cells of the SCN, with a peak during the night in 12:12 LD conditions, but not in constant lighting conditions (constant darkness [DD] and constant light [LL]). All 3 share binding affinity for 3 receptor types in the brain—$VPAC_1$, $VPAC_2$, and PAC_1—but VIP has a higher specificity for the VPAC receptor subtypes. $VPAC_2$ (gene name *Vipr2*) is a G-protein–coupled receptor that is highly expressed in the mammalian SCN, and its mRNA shows a biphasic pattern of expression in LD and DD. Signaling through this receptor activates adenylyl cyclase to increase the concentration of cyclic adenosine monophosphate (cAMP), and it has been shown that rhythms in firing activity in the SCN are responsive to the phase-dependent phase-shifting effects of VIP and $VPAC_2$ agonists via protein kinase A and mitogen-activated protein kinase (MAPK) in vitro. Exposure to constant light has been shown to significantly depress VIP concentrations in the rat SCN in a light dose–dependent manner. This result is supported by in vitro data suggesting that NMDA phase-delays neuronal firing activity in rats and causes a drop in the VIP content of core cells. These same cells respond to pulses of light during the dark period by upregulating transcription of the core circadian clock genes (*Per1* and *Per2*; see later section titled "Molecular Architecture of the Circadian Clock"), producing a phase shift. Previous studies have shown that VIP is sufficient to phase-advance and alter electrical activity when applied alone at CT 20 to 24 in vivo and moderately sufficient to phase-delay when applied alone at CT 12 to 14 in hamsters. Altogether, these results strongly suggest a key role for VIP in photic entrainment and for $VPAC_2$ as the essential VIP receptor in the mammalian circadian clock.

In addition to VIP, GRP and GABA also contribute to SCN coupling. For example, mice lacking VIP receptors ($Vipr2^{-/-}$) and VIP ($VIP^{-/-}$) have arrhythmic SCN electrical activity, along with arrhythmic or severely disrupted wheel running activity. Furthermore, daily application of a $VPAC_2$ agonist restores molecular rhythmicity and synchrony of firing rate rhythms to $VIP^{-/-}$ SCN neurons, indicating that VIP is mediating SCN coupling and behavioral rhythms. When GRP is applied to SCN cultures from $Vipr2^{-/-}$ mice, SCN synchronization is also restored, suggesting that other neuropeptides are important in this network. Finally, daily GABA application to 2 dissociated neurons from the same

culture results in resynchronization of firing rate, indicating that GABA is sufficient for SCN coupling. However, in the intact SCN network, $GABA_A$ receptor activation slows resynchronization after SCN organotypic cultures are forced into a state in which 2 populations in a single nucleus are uncoupled. Ironically, decoupling induced by $VPAC_2$ antagonists can be reversed by blockade of $GABA_A$ receptors, suggesting that GABA signaling also mediates VIP-induced synchronization.

The Mammalian Circadian Clock Can Be Set by Nonphotic Stimuli

In addition to light, nonphotic zeitgebers or stimuli are also able to entrain the circadian clock. Such nonphotic stimuli include arousal-producing stimuli and exercise such as sleep deprivation, novel wheel running activity, saline injection, and intermittent shaking of cages. When these stimuli are presented during the subjective day, rodents will advance the onset of their activity on following days. The presence of a nonphotic stimulus is conveyed to the SCN through the following 2 main pathways: (1) a geniculohypothalamic tract (GHT) and (2) the median raphe nuclei pathway. The GHT originates from the thalamic intergeniculate leaflet (IGL) and uses neuropeptide Y (NPY), GABA, and endorphins as neurotransmitters, whereas the dorsal and median raphe nuclei pathway, which projects to the IGL, is primarily serotonergic and projects to the SCN either directly (median raphe) or indirectly (dorsal raphe) via the IGL.

The large phase shifts that occur during the subjective day when animals are presented with nonphotic stimuli are mediated, at least in part, by NPY release into the SCN from the IGL. During the subjective day, NPY itself can produce large phase advances in vivo when injected into the SCN region or applied in vitro directly to SCN slices. Furthermore, confining hamsters to a small box could not block the phase advances that were caused by NPY injections into the SCN during the subjective day, demonstrating that activity or exercise is not needed to induce a phase advance when the SCN is injected with NPY. In a second experiment within the same study, hamsters were also exposed to a novel wheel for 3 hours, with the experimental group being injected with NPY antiserum into the SCN and the control group being injected with normal rabbit serum into the SCN. Hamsters injected with normal serum exhibited phase advances similar to those of the unoperated hamsters, suggesting that NPY conveys nonphotic information to the SCN, whereas the hamsters injected with the antiserum to NPY shifted their activity by <15 minutes.

Early studies showed that VIPergic neurons are under the influence of serotonergic innervation and that treatment with the serotonin-depleting reagents para-chlorophenylalanine or 5,6-dihydroxytryptamine causes a marked decrease in VIP immunoreactivity—an effect that can be reversed with a 5-hydroxytryptamine (5-HT) receptor 1B agonist. This depletion initiates the rhythmic property of VIP mRNA expression in DD and suggests that serotonin works antagonistically to light. The increase of available serotonin by treatment with monoamine oxidase (MAO) inhibitors or by knocking out the *MAOA* gene increases VIP expression in rats and mice, respectively. 5-HT$_{1B}$ receptors are localized to the retinohypothalamic tract, suggesting an indirect effect on VIP expression by modulation of glutamate release. Similarly, 5-HT$_{1A}$ or 5-HT$_7$ receptors are located on the core neurons of the SCN and allow serotonin to directly modulate VIP release and neuronal activity. Because serotonin plays a role in nonphotic entrainment and modulates the SCN directly, mice with VIP signaling deficiency—and thus lacking robust responses to photic stimuli—may have enhanced responses to nonphotic stimuli.

The Efferent Projections of the Mammalian Circadian Clock Include Both Paracrine & Synaptic Signals

As mentioned earlier, the SCN is both necessary and sufficient for driving 24-hour rhythms in physiology and behavior, including rhythms in sleep–wake activity, energy homeostasis, heart rate/blood pressure, body temperature, and hormone release. Thus, it is not surprising that the SCN projects to a wide array of brain regions and impacts the entire brain through both direct and indirect neural pathways. A classic study showed that blocking the SCN output signal (ie, sodium-dependent action potentials) with tetrodotoxin (TTX) will dissociate the "hands" of the clock, while the "gears" keep on turning. Specifically, hamsters received chronic delivery of TTX to the SCN for several weeks while housed in running wheels in DD. During the TTX delivery, 24-hour locomotor rhythms were eliminated; however, they were reinstated after TTX was discontinued. Remarkably, the phase of the reinstated locomotor rhythm was predicted by the pre-TTX phase, indicating that the internal clock had been running all along, even though the outward manifestation of the clock was disrupted.

Numerous brain regions receive direct synaptic connections from the SCN, including the median preoptic area, the bed nucleus of the stria terminalis, the IGL, the paraventricular nucleus of the hypothalamus, the dorsal medial nucleus of the hypothalamus, and the arcuate nucleus. A primary direct efferent pathway from the SCN is the subparaventricular zone, which is also a putative "switch" for diurnality. Indirect pathways to the pineal gland and pituitary are critical for 24-hour rhythmic release of hormones such as melatonin and corticosterones, respectively. The pathway from the paraventricular nucleus is important for 24-hour control of the autonomic nervous system. Altogether, this system produces 24-hour rhythms in nutrients (eg, glucose, fatty acids) and hormones (eg, insulin, glucagon, leptin, adiponectin, ghrelin).

Hormones, regulation of body temperature, and feeding behavior have all been implicated as possible mediators of the efferent resetting signal from the SCN to downstream neural and peripheral targets. Humoral output of the SCN may also be a mediator of peripheral tissue synchronization. A classic study lesioned the SCN in hamsters and then restored locomotor rhythms by transplanting fetal SCN "micropunches" into the ventricles of arrhythmic animals. Furthermore, to determine whether restoration of rhythmicity was dependent upon neural outgrowth or humoral signaling, the SCN tissue was contained within a semi-permeable capsule before transplantation, and the same result was observed. However, it is important to note that not all circadian rhythms are restored by SCN fetal transplants; specifically, rhythmic release of glucocorticoids, melatonin, and luteinizing hormone fails to recover. Taken together, these results indicate that both humoral and neuronal signals are important for synchronization of peripheral clocks. Several candidate releasable factors proposed are transforming growth factor-α, prokineticin 2 (PK2), and cardiotrophin-like cytokine. For example, PK2 expression peaks during the subjective day in the SCN, and injection of PK2 to the SCN region suppresses locomotor activity in rats at night but results in an increase in activity during the day.

CIRCADIAN MULTIOSCILLATOR SYSTEM

So far, we have introduced the circadian system as relying on a single, primary master oscillator. However, research over the past 2 decades has revealed a much more complex system in which individual cells and tissues, both neural and peripheral, have the ability to generate 24-hour rhythms in isolation from the SCN. Rhythmicity of these secondary oscillators frequently damps out after several cycles due to reduction of both cellular clock gene expression amplitude and tissue-level amplitude, due to the individual cellular oscillators drifting out of phase with one another. Thus, the SCN provide an important daily resetting signal to the secondary pacemakers in the brain as well as in tissues throughout the body such as the lung, liver, heart, and spleen. The hierarchical structure of the circadian system is also evident during resynchronization following a large shift in the light–dark cycle—simulating jet lag. Using a bioluminescent reporter of clock gene activity (see later section titled "Molecular Architecture of the Circadian Clock"), researchers have been able to track ex vivo rhythms of various tissue clocks in real time. Explants of numerous peripheral and neural tissues have been cultured following a 6-hour phase advance of the light–dark cycle at 1, 3, and 6 days following the shift. Several studies have now shown that the SCN rather quickly reentrains to the new light–dark cycle, whereas other tissues take much longer. Locomotor behavior generally takes 1 day for each hour of jet lag to adjust, so a 6-hour phase shift would take at least 6 days for full reentrainment. These ex vivo clock gene reporter studies show that for some tissues, such as the liver, 6 days is not sufficient for reentrainment.

The first autonomous neural oscillator outside of the SCN to be discovered was the retina. The retinal clock is critical for adaptation to changes in environmental lighting, including dark adaptation (via melatonin) and light adaptation (via dopamine). Not surprisingly, these neurotransmitters can also

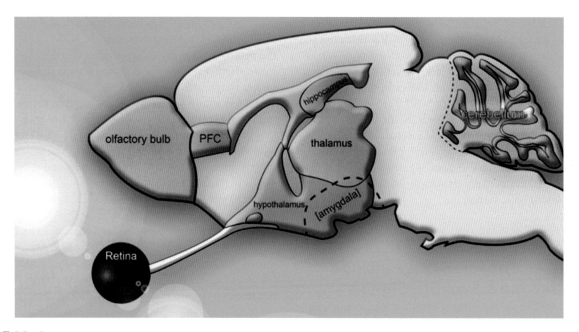

FIGURE 23–4 Multiple oscillators in the rodent brain contribute to circadian behavioral output and physiology. Medial parasagittal view; major loci are indicated by color and label. The amygdala is more lateral than can be viewed in this section and is denoted by the *dashed line*. PFC, prefrontal cortex. (Adapted with permission from Ciarleglio CM, Resuehr HE, McMahon DG. Interactions of the serotonin and circadian systems: nature and nurture in rhythms and blues, *Neuroscience*. 2011 Dec 1;197:8-16.)

directly regulate retinal circadian phase. Since then, other extra-SCN brain regions have been identified as having daily oscillations in clock gene expression. These include nuclei in the thalamus, hypothalamus, amygdala, olfactory bulb, cerebellum, hippocampus, and many others (Figure 23–4). Outside of the SCN, the olfactory bulb has been shown to maintain the most robust rhythms ex vivo in clock gene expression reported using bioluminescence. In situ hybridization studies of the rat brain have reported rhythmic clock gene expression in numerous regions of the forebrain (prefrontal cortex, rostral agranular insula, paraventricular nucleus, amygdala, and hippocampus). The majority of the extra-SCN oscillators have circadian phases that are delayed by 4 to 12 hours from the SCN.

Among the forebrain regions mentioned earlier, the hippocampal clock has been a primary focus of research in the past few decades because of documented 24-hour rhythmicity in neurogenesis, long-term potentiation, and signaling cascades that are important for memory formation (eg, MAPK and cAMP). Rhythms in these processes contribute to day–night differences in several hippocampal-dependent tasks including acquisition, recall, and extinction. For example, spatial working memory and novel location memory are augmented during the awake phase (night for nocturnal rodents), and these day–night differences persist when mice are housed under DD (and, thus, are under circadian clock control). The molecular clock in the forebrain appears to be necessary for these rhythms in memory since knocking out the positive limb of the molecular clock (see next section) results in poor memory at both times of day. The local clock in the hippocampus

is entrained by the light–dark cycle (via the SCN) as well by other external factors. For example, food availability is critical for resetting the phase of the hippocampal clock, and synchronization of the feeding–fasting cycle with the light–dark cycle is necessary for memory and long-term potentiation. Mice that are fed during the day (rest phase) show a shifted rhythm of clock gene expression in the hippocampus as well as poor performance in novel object recognition and reduced long-term potentiation. Like the hippocampus, it is likely that the local circadian clocks in other extra-SCN oscillators also play important roles in neural function and behavior.

MOLECULAR ARCHITECTURE OF THE CIRCADIAN CLOCK

The Transcription/Translation Feedback Loop

Several clock genes take part in an interlocking transcriptional and translational feedback loop to activate and repress each other in a manner that results in an approximate 24-hour rhythm of gene expression (Figure 23–5). The key circadian genes in mammals include the activators *Bmal1* and *Clock* (or also *Npas2*), which activate the E-box promoter for the *Period* genes *Per1* and *Per2* and the repressor *Cryptochrome* genes *Cry1* and *Cry2*. In mammals, *Clock* is constitutively expressed, and *Bmal1* peaks in expression during the subjective circadian night, or "lights off." The transcription factor RORa serves to activate *Bmal1* transcription and, in addition, competes with

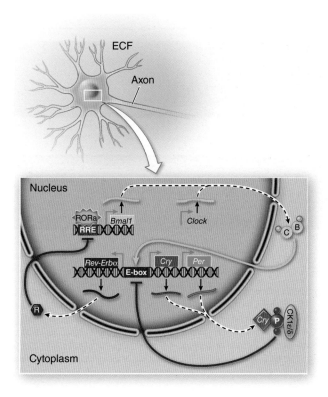

FIGURE 23-5 Genetic mechanisms of the circadian neuron. Mammalian neuronal circadian rhythms are governed by an intricate gene–protein feedback loop known as the transcription/translation feedback loop (TTFL). *Black dashed arrows* represent movement of transcripts out of the nucleus for translation. *Green arrows* represent the positive loop where the resultant proteins activate transcription of *Per*, *Cry*, and *Rev-Erba*. *Red lines* represent the negative loop where the resultant proteins inhibit their own transcription, in the case of PER and CRY, or inactivate *Bmal1* transcription by competing with RORa, as in the case with REV-ERBα. ECF, extracellular fluid.

Rev-Erbα for binding to the promoter of *Bmal1*. CLOCK and BMAL1 dimerize in the cytoplasm after translation, are phosphorylated by casein kinase (CK)-2α, and then translocate back into the nucleus to bind to E-boxes that upregulate *Per*, *Cry*, and *Rev-Erbα* expression, forming the "positive arm" of the negative feedback loop.

After translation, either PER1 and CRY1 or PER2 and CRY2 dimerize and then are phosphorylated by CK-1ε/δ. This serves to either degrade the proteins or to repress their own transcription in the "negative arm" of the feedback loop by translocating back into the nucleus and inhibiting their own promoter's activation by BMAL1/CLOCK. Concurrently, Rev-Erbα inhibits *Bmal1* transcription by competing with RORa for promoter binding in a second negative feedback loop. Because the *Per* genes are highly transcribed during the circadian day, they are a useful measure of circadian period ex vivo (**Figure 23-6**).

Altogether, both positive and negative arms of the feedback loop result in rhythmic expression, with PER and CRY expression levels being highest during the late day and lowest during the middle of the night within the SCN. In particular, posttranslational modification has been shown to play a major role in determining period and phase. Phosphorylation is the main posttranslational modification being considered. In addition to CK2-α, CK1-ε, and CK1-δ, other kinases such

as CK2-β and glycogen synthase kinase 3 (GSK3)-β have been shown to phosphorylate BMAL1, CRY1, CRY2, PER1, and PER2, which either allows the transcription factors to enter the nucleus or to be degraded by the proteasome.

Nearly every cell in the body (and many brain cells) rhythmically expresses these core circadian clock genes. The molecular clock drives transcription of a plethora of other clock-controlled genes (43% of all protein-coding genes in humans); however, which genes are rhythmically transcribed depends on the cell or tissue type. One important resource for exploring and comparing clock-controlled genes among rhythmic tissue is CircaDB (http://circadb.hogeneschlab.org). This website reports >3000 cycling genes from cell lines as well as peripheral and neural (brainstem, cerebellum, hypothalamus, and SCN) tissues. The relationship between the central clock in the SCN and the local molecular clocks in peripheral tissues is somewhat complex. One way to study this relationship is to disrupt the molecular clock throughout the body and then restore the clock only in the brain (restoring SCN output). Several years ago, the Hogenesch laboratory followed this approach and found that restoration of the molecular clock in the brains (only) of *ClockΔ19*-mutant mice rescued behavioral arrhythmicity and clock gene rhythmicity in the liver. These results suggest that SCN output is sufficient to drive the local clock in peripheral organs. However, clock-controlled genes

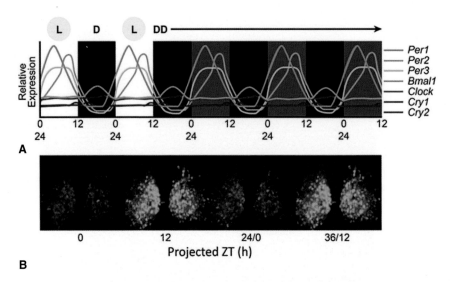

FIGURE 23–6 Circadian gene expression in mammals. **A.** Gene expression profiles of 7 key circadian genes over 4.5 days, demonstrating the self-sustaining oscillations of molecular rhythms in the presence and absence of a zeitgeber (light). Genes are denoted by colored lines (see key to *right*). **B.** Representative example of the circadian expression of *Per1*::GFP in suprachiasmatic nucleus (SCN) neurons over 36 hours ex vivo in projected zeitgeber time (ZT). A single brain slice from a mouse carrying the *mPer1*::GFP was cultured and the gene expression dynamics of the SCN were assayed via time-lapse confocal microscopy. D, dark; DD, constant darkness; GFP, green fluorescent protein; L, light. (Part B, reproduced with permission from Ciarleglio CM, Resuehr HE, McMahon DG. Interactions of the serotonin and circadian systems: nature and nurture in rhythms and blues, *Neuroscience*. 2011 Dec 1;197:8-16.)

specific to the liver were reduced in number and had lower amplitude rhythms. Thus, the local clock in peripheral tissues is important for functions specific to that cell type. This approach has yet to be applied to SCN–extra-SCN relationships. The results of such a study would reveal the importance of the SCN signal versus the local molecular clock in secondary oscillators in the brain.

SEASONALITY

After the Moon-forming impact, the new Earth was left spinning on an axis slightly off perpendicular to the planet's orbit around the Sun. While this is not thought to be unusual, planets that lack a proportionally large moon either proceed with a floating axis or will right their axis to perpendicular (with respect to its orbit around a star) with time. The gravitational influence of the nascent Moon served to stabilize this off-kilter axis, creating reliable seasons. The amount of seasonal daily light, or **photoperiod**, varies from the most light on the first day of summer to the least light on the first day of winter. The range of light per day depends on latitude, with the most extreme latitudes (the poles) receiving the most extreme photoperiods. As life flourished on the planet, strategies for thriving with seasonal changes in photoperiod developed and are maintained today. The ability to predict oncoming hardship in the winter or abundance in the summer is thought to increase fitness in plants and animals alike. For plants such as trees, the shorter daytime indicates a decrease of higher energy short-wavelength light and the coming colder temperatures. The trees lose their foliage at this time of year and go relatively dormant. As daytime length increases, photoperiod signals

the oncoming warmth and a transition to photosynthesis, and an increase in foliage and gamete production occurs.

In animals, change in photoperiod indicates a necessity for behavioral change. For nocturnal animals, summer photoperiod means that all activity has to be squeezed into a shorter night, and with the abundance of growing plant life, it is the prime time of year to breed, and thus, some male animals experience gonadal growth while females become receptive to mating. As winter approaches, the photoperiod indicates a time for hibernation and/or pelage change—lighter color and thicker coat to prepare for winter cold.

Not all animals experience these physiologic changes, but those that do are said to be **photoperiodic**. Laboratory mice (*Mus musculus*) are thought not to be photoperiodic, but they do experience a behavioral reorganization called **seasonality** following changes in photoperiod. In their seminal paper on entrainment, Pittendrigh and Daan demonstrated that rodents compress their main **activity bout (α)** in long photoperiods. In addition, this compression of activity length results in an **aftereffect**, or transient reorganization of the circadian rhythm that is evident in constant conditions. Specifically, the compression or shortening of the primary activity bout that is evident in long photoperiods correlates with a decreased FRP in mice—a faster clock.

The reorganization of the clock and how this accounts for behavioral changes had remained a mystery until recently, with the development of in vivo electrophysiologic and ex vivo circadian gene reporter techniques. In situ hybridization experiments showed that gene expression in response to a light pulse is different in animals taken from short (LD 8:16) and long (LD 16:8) photoperiods, specifically the immediate early gene *c-Fos* and pineal *N*-acetyltransferase, the enzyme used to produce the neurohormone melatonin. In fact, the tissue-level architecture of in vivo electrical activity of mouse SCN is dramatically different between photoperiods, initially suggesting that seasonality is encoded in the SCN by changes in the phase distribution of individual neuronal clocks.

It turns out that how seasonality is encoded in the SCN is a bit more complicated, but in an interesting way: How the SCN encodes season is not just dependent on the photoperiod that the organism inhabits presently, but also on what photoperiod they had been exposed to early in perinatal development. Several different labs demonstrated that for animals reared in an equinox photoperiod (LD 12:12), the phase relationship of neurons relative to each other is the major factor behind how the SCN encodes season and, therefore, how an animal subsequently behaves. In other words, if one were to record the circadian rhythm from a single neuron using something like the *Period* gene reporter in Figure 23–6B, one would find that the rhythms from many neurons in the SCN would line up (synchronize) in phase if they were recorded from an animal that had just experienced a short, winter photoperiod (LD 8:16) before the experiment. Contrarily, one would find that the rhythms from neurons derived from an animal that had just experienced a long, summer photoperiod (LD 16:8) would be much more asynchronous, peaking across the circadian "daytime." Reasonably, SCNs harvested from equinox photoperiod demonstrate an intermediate phenotype. Therefore, in equinox-developed animals, season is encoded by neuronal circadian phase relationships. But this is only part of the story.

How the SCN encodes season, it turns out, depends on what photoperiod the animal experienced around birth. Although the phase distribution of neurons within the SCN is due to proximal photoperiod, the resultant tissue-level integration in response to seasonal change is profoundly different based on one's season of development. Summer-developed mice exhibit remarkably stable molecular clock rhythms regarding the phase at which SCN neurons peak in *Per1* expression, very close to dusk (ψ). Winter-developed mouse SCN, in contrast, varies phase angle widely, depending on the proximal season, with *Per1* expression peaking more than an hour after dusk in animals harvested from LD 8:16 or peaking 2 hours before dusk in animals harvested from LD 16:8. Equinox-developed animals display an intermediate phenotype. The ethologic implications alone are stunning: If the peak of *Per1* expression correlated with time of activity onset, imagine how this result might impact Dr. DeCoursey's study involving ground squirrels discussed earlier! Furthermore, the tissue-level dynamics are not just a result of changing neuronal phase distributions, as mentioned in the previous paragraph, but also altered neuronal rhythms themselves, with the shape of the distribution changing drastically by broadening or narrowing between summer and winter photoperiods, but *only if the animal was developed in a short, winter photoperiod*. In addition, neuronal period decreases in long photoperiod, but only if the animal was developed in a long photoperiod.

Taken together, it is fairly clear that seasonal encoding in the SCN occurs not only at the tissue level, but also at the neuronal level, and because the environment has such a profound and lasting effect on the animal's physiology, seasonal encoding may be an example of an epigenetic modification.

These fascinating results on what should otherwise be a mundane topic are underscored by further work on the behavioral ramifications of seasonal birth, seasonality, and photoperiodism. A series of studies on seasonally developed hamsters and mice have demonstrated correlates of anxiety and depression dependent not only on the proximal photoperiod (ie, a tendency to be sadder in short photoperiod), but also on developmental photoperiod (ie, long photoperiod–developed mice are generally more anxious, and short photoperiod–developed mice are generally more "depressed"). With that in mind, one is forced to wonder what effect seasonality and seasonal birth have on humans. *Homo sapiens* are, in nature, seasonal breeders, with most births happening in the summer to early fall. In an industrialized society, we lose that natural behavior because we can provide for infants year-round, so an understanding of the seasonal effects of light is critical in explaining aberrations in human health.

Changes in seasonal photoperiod have been associated with mood disorders and mental disease in humans. Seasonal affective disorder, for example, is a mood disorder that affects between 0.4% and 2.7% of the US population every year and is treated with bright light therapy or selective serotonin reuptake inhibitors. A 5% to 8% winter-spring excess of births has been reported for both schizophrenia and mania/bipolar disorder. There is a spring and summer excess of births for autism and a winter-spring excess of births for neurosis. Winter-born humans have been reported to show both stronger morning preference than the other seasons on the Morningness-Eveningness Questionnaire and significantly lower (sadder) Global Seasonality scores than individuals born in the summer. Many of these disorders revolve around the serotonergic system, and for good reason: A recent study in mice reported that photoperiod at birth programs the intrinsic electrical and receptive properties of neurons in the dorsal raphe nuclei—the midbrain region that is responsible for serotonergic signaling to higher order areas of the brain. These studies suggest that birth season—or perhaps the seasonality of late gestation—imprints the organization of the brain systems that control cognition, emotion, and/or circadian rhythmicity.

In all, seasonality is an important aspect of circadian rhythmicity on a planet with changing light cycles. Its impact on human health is profound, but it is important to reiterate 1 particular aspect of seasonal physiology, and that is on sleep properties. In humans, summer sleep is very different from winter sleep. Summer sleep is usually consolidated into a single bout and compressed into a shorter night than other times of year. Winter sleep, on the other hand, is wholly different: It is decompressed, spread over a much longer night, and usually occurs in 2 or more bouts. This compression and decompression of sleep, which correlates with duration of melatonin release, can contribute to the aforementioned disorders of human health, especially in those who may be prone to the disorders because of seasonal birth.

HUMAN SLEEP

Sleep Architecture

An in-depth discussion of sleep is covered in Chapter 34, but a brief description is included here to describe the interrelationship between sleep and circadian systems. During waking, electroencephalogram (EEG) recordings show 2 different types of brainwave activity: alpha activity (at 8 to 12 Hz) and beta activity (at 13 to 30 Hz). Alpha activity occurs when a person is resting quietly and not engaging in any strenuous activity. Beta activity has a lower amplitude because many different neural circuits are being activated at once.

Sleep has been divided into 2 main types: rapid eye movement (REM) and non–rapid eye movement (NREM). The original scoring guidelines include 4 stages of NREM sleep and 1 stage of REM sleep. The new system developed by the American Academy of Sleep Medicine identifies 3 stages of NREM sleep (NREM stages 1, 2, and 3) and 1 REM sleep stage. Once an individual falls asleep, he or she will progress through stages 1 to 3 of NREM sleep (with stage 3 being the deepest level of sleep) and then ascend back up through the stages until the REM sleep stage is reached. One cycles lasts approximately 70 to 90 minutes. A person experiences approximately 4 or 5 of these cycles per night (Figure 23–7).

Stage 1 represents the transition from wakefulness to sleep and consists of theta activity (3.5 to 7.5 Hz), indicating neuronal firing is becoming more synchronized. At this point, a person may experience hypnic jerks, which are sleep twitches caused by muscle contractions followed immediately by relaxation. This may also be experienced as a falling sensation. Upon entering stage 2 sleep, EEG activity is characterized by sleep spindles and K complexes (Chapter 34). A sleep spindle is a burst of waves (12 to 14 Hz) that lasts about half a second. K complexes are sharp waves that

are associated with inhibition of neuronal firing. Stage 3 EEG activity is then characterized by synchronized, high-amplitude, delta waves (<3.5 Hz). Heart rate, breathing rate, and brain activity also decrease at this stage, which is also known as slow-wave sleep.

After stage 3, EEG activity during REM sleep is characterized by irregular, low-voltage, fast waves that mimic those during stage 1 sleep. Using this criterion, REM sleep is very light. Eyes also begin to move rapidly back and forth while eyelids remain closed. At this point, postural muscles become very relaxed. This is referred to as sleep paralysis. Using this criterion, REM sleep is deep. This is why REM sleep is sometimes known as paradoxical sleep. Heart rate, blood pressure, and breathing also tend to vary more in REM sleep than in stages 2 to 3. People who are woken up out of REM sleep also tend to report that they had been dreaming, whereas someone woken up out of slow-wave sleep would deny that they had been dreaming.

Two-Process Model of Sleep

Sleep is regulated by 2 different processes: the circadian clock (process C) and the sleep homeostatic process (process S) (Figure 23–8). Homeostatic sleep builds up exponentially during time awake and declines exponentially during sleep. At the same time, the circadian clock drives a rhythm in attention and arousal that is independent of the duration of prior wakefulness. The distance between the 2 processes adds up to account for total sleep pressure. During a 24-hour period of sleep deprivation, many people feel a "second wind" on the following morning as process C kicks back in, overcoming the continual increase in process S.

The 2-process model of sleep can also help explain dips in performance often experienced as an afternoon slump after lunch or as an early morning fog. Process C drives a 24-hour rhythm in performance that peaks in the evening for most people. Process S results in peak performance in the morning after recovering from the initial wake-up period (approximately

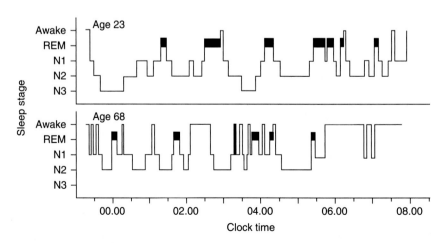

FIGURE 23–7 Sleep hypnogram demonstrating changes in sleep architecture due to age (23 years vs 68 years). REM, rapid eye movement.

(Reproduced with permission from Jameson JL, Fauci AS, Kasper DL, et al: *Harrison's Principles of Internal Medicine*, 20th ed. New York, NY: McGraw Hill; 2018.)

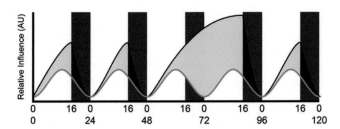

FIGURE 23–8 Two-process model of sleep. Schematic demonstrating how sleep timing is controlled by 2 different processes that together contribute to overall sleep pressure. Process C (*green line*) is driven by the internal circadian clock and persists as a 24-hour rhythm of arousal in constant conditions, even under 40 hours of wakefulness (shown between 48 and 88 hours). Process S (*black line*) demonstrates the sleep homeostat that builds exponentially with increased wakefulness and decreases exponentially during sleep, resetting the homeostat. The difference between the 2 lines is the total sleep pressure. Night is represented by *gray bars*, and day is represented by *white bars*. The upper row of numbers represents zeitgeber time (ZT), whereas the lower row of numbers represents the number of consecutive hours displayed. AU, arbitrary units.

1 to 4 hours), referred to as sleep inertia. After that, performance driven by process S slowly declines throughout the day, but overall performance results from a combination of both process C and process S. Thus, performance is fairly high during the early part of the day due to process S and fairly high during the evening hours due to process C. That leaves the afternoon as a time when process S is declining but process C has yet to reach a full peak, causing a reduction in performance at this time of day. Of course, during the overnight hours, performance is low due to reductions in both processes. As a result, jobs that require workers to be awake and alert in the middle of the night often struggle with balancing productivity, performance, and worker safety.

Functions of Sleep

For millennia, people and scientists have wondered about the purpose of sleep—even Aristotle recognized its importance for preservation of life because sleep allows the body's organs to rest and recover. A related hypothesis states that the purpose of sleep is to conserve energy. During sleep, energy is conserved due to decreased body temperature. As a result, animals increase sleep duration when food is in short supply, thus reducing energy expenditure. Sleep improves memory. In humans, task learning improves following a night of sleep. REM sleep specifically aids in consolidation of nondeclarative (procedural) memory, whereas NREM sleep aids in consolidation of declarative memories. Similarly, natural immune response is modified by partial sleep deprivation. After just 1 night of sleep deprivation, the activity of natural killer cells, a type of white blood cell, is reduced by 28%. Sleep loss can also result in a reduction of circulating immune complexes, secondary antibody responses, and antigen uptake. Finally, recent research has highlighted the importance of sleep for proper function of the glymphatic

system, in which glial cells regulate the flow of cerebrospinal fluid by shrinking and swelling. The results showed that the flow of fluid slows and the space between cells decreases during waking and increases during sleep by as much as 60%! This mechanism of sleep is very important for removing toxins from the brain, including β-amyloid, a protein implicated in Alzheimer disease.

CLINICAL CORRELATES

As described earlier, circadian rhythms impact a variety of physiologic functions. Therefore, it is no surprise that circadian disruption can impair memory, reduce mental and physical reaction times, and exacerbate or increase the risk of human disease such as depression, insomnia, diabetes, obesity, immune dysfunction and cancer. In the laboratory, mice are often used to model the impact of circadian disruption on human disease since they exhibit many of the same circadian characteristics as humans, including 24-hour rhythms in temperature, melatonin, cortisol, attention, and activity. Like mice, the SCN serves as the central circadian pacemaker and is entrained by photic and nonphotic input. One notable difference is temporal niche, such that humans are **diurnal** and active in the daytime, whereas mice are **nocturnal** and active at night. Despite this major behavioral difference, clock genes are also expressed in a circadian rhythm in human tissues including white blood cells and buccal cells. As with all genes, circadian genes are prone to heritable mutations over time. These conserved variants have been identified in many of the circadian genes, with significant phenotypic consequences that have driven the field of circadian geneticists to create mouse models of the genetic change and further our understanding of circadian protein roles, function, and dysfunction.

Much effort has been made to identify genetic causes for circadian sleep disorders, which have been defined by the International Classification of Sleep Disorders (ICSD) as "a persistent or recurrent pattern of sleep disturbance due primarily to alterations in the circadian timekeeping system or a misalignment between the endogenous circadian rhythm and exogenous factors that affect the timing or duration of sleep." Six disorders have been recognized as true circadian rhythm sleep disorder by the ICSD; these include advanced sleep phase syndrome (or familial advanced sleep phase syndrome [FASPS]), delayed sleep phase syndrome (DSPS), non–24-hour sleep–wake disorder (N-24; also known as free-running disorder), irregular sleep–wake rhythm/phase (ISWR), jet lag, and shift work.

To date, FASPS has been the only circadian disorder found to display true Mendelian inheritance. This disorder is characterized by an approximate 4-hour advanced phase angle of sleep onset every day. These people wake up in the very early morning (1 to 4 am) and fall asleep very early as well (6 to 7 pm), even in the presence of social pressure to stay awake. Although this disorder is likely to have many genetic sources, 2 such sources have been identified as either of 2 complementary mutations: a S662G mutation in the *hPer2* phosphorylation site or a T44A mutation in the phosphate transfer domain of CK1-δ.

The etiology of DSPS has not been as straightforward. DSPS is the most common of the CRSDs and is characterized by extremely late bedtimes (2 to 6 am) and midday wake times (10 am to 2 pm). Although there is 1 reported case of inherited DSPS where the genetic defect is unknown, a length polymorphism located in exon 18 of the *Per3* gene has shown the most promising association with the phenotype. A single nucleotide polymorphism in the *Clock* gene (3111 T>C) has also been a promising genetic lead, with people carrying the C/C genotype exhibiting strong evening preference, although not DSPS per se. Like FASPS, however, there are likely many genetic causes for the phenotype that have yet to be identified. Numerous clinical trials have attempted to treat delayed circadian phase with **light therapy**. Even delayed sleep phase associated with mental illness such as attention-deficit/hyperactivity disorder (ADHD) was successfully treated in 1 pilot study using early morning light therapy. Moreover, the reduction in ADHD symptoms was correlated with the size of the phase advance induced by light therapy.

N-24 is common in blind people and is a result of a lack of perception of photic entraining stimuli, which then leads to the person free-running through the geophysical days. N-24, therefore, does not necessarily have a primary genetic component. ISWR is characterized by the absence of circadian sleep–wake, and its cause is unknown. Jet lag is the unpleasant physiologic and psychological aftereffects of traveling across multiple time zones, and its severity is proportional to the number of time zones crossed, direction of travel (west to east is considered more severe for humans), sleep deprivation, presence of zeitgebers at the destination, and individual tolerance. While the cause of jetlag is known to be the misalignment of circadian phase with the geophysical phase at the destination (or disruption/misalignment of multiple internal endogenous oscillators), much work has been done to alleviate the symptoms and elucidate their root causes. To date, no major genetic studies have been undertaken in humans regarding N-24, ISWR, or jet lag.

The final recognized circadian rhythm sleep disorder, shift work disorder, is caused by circumstances similar to jet lag, in that misalignment of circadian phase with the zeitgebers (light, social pressure, stimulants) during the work shift causes unpleasant aftereffects or sleepiness, especially in people on a rotating schedule. Studies in individuals involved in shift work (estimated at 1 in 5 American workers) have discovered how genetic polymorphisms in circadian genes associate with shift work tolerance, sleep strategy, and other CRSDs. For example, multilocus models of polymorphisms in several clock genes are associated with alcohol or caffeine consumption and sleepiness of hospital shift work nurses. One contributing factor to sleepiness and adaptation to shift work is the decision of when to sleep on days off. For example, many shift workers switch back to sleeping at night on days off. Different sleep strategies are used by hospital shift work nurses, who frequently work several 12-hour night shifts in a row followed by several days off. The most maladaptive strategies are ones in which nurses take long, daily naps on or stay awake for >24 hours on at least 1 day per week. Nurses using these strategies reported greater sleep disturbance, an earlier **chronotype**, and more cardiovascular problems.

Characteristics of human mental health display an intriguing association with circadian rhythms. The symptoms of jet lag and shift work briefly described earlier offer evidence that disruption of circadian phase angle can lead not only to side effects, but also the possibility of more serious conditions. Patients with mood disorders often exhibit altered circadian phase in body temperature, cortisol, and even melatonin. It has been suggested that the connection between mood disorders and circadian rhythms may involve the literal connection between the serotonergic raphe nuclei of the brainstem and the SCN, both directly and indirectly via the IGL of the thalamus. Numerous 5-HT receptor subtypes are expressed in the SCN, and the interplay between the circadian system and the serotonergic system is thought to be extensive at both the molecular and tissue levels. In combination with the extant data on the role of clock genes in normal and abnormal human circadian rhythmicity, these data suggest not only that circadian genes could play a potentially huge role in mental health, but also that human circadian neural organization is an appropriate starting point for research into novel treatments for mental disorders. For example, some medications may have improved efficacy or reduced side effects when taken at a particular time of day. This approach is often referred to as **chronotherapy**.

CONCLUSION

Circadian rhythms are 24-hour oscillations in behavior and physiology that arose out of necessity to survive in a world with regularly occurring light and dark periods. In mammals, these rhythms are controlled by a primary clock located in the SCN of the hypothalamus that orchestrates secondary clocks throughout the rest of the brain and body. The SCN is necessary and sufficient for driving 24-hour rhythms in sleep/wake, locomotor activity, feeding/fasting, hormone release, heart rate/blood pressure, and so on. SCN neurons and nearly every cell in the body can generate 24-hour rhythms in transcription due to a molecular clock composed of interlocking feedback loops. However, SCN neurons have an additional feature of being able to couple into a network that allows animals to shift their clock phase to match the environmental cycle of light and dark, food availability, and even the presence of predators. This network also allows adaptation to changes in the length of the light period as the seasons change across an annual cycle. The core features of an internal clock—persistence in constant conditions, entrainment to the environment, and temperature compensation—are evident in nearly all life on Earth, including humans. The circadian clock is important for human health, and disruption of circadian rhythms (as in jet lag and shift work) can exacerbate and/or increase the risk of disease. Translation of the findings from animal models and human laboratory studies may lead to novel chronotherapeutic treatments for disease.

SUMMARY

- Circadian rhythms are 24-hour oscillations in behavior and physiology that arose out of necessity to survive in a world with regularly occurring light and dark periods.

- Mammalian circadian rhythms are controlled by a primary clock located in SCN of the hypothalamus that orchestrates secondary clocks throughout the rest of the brain and body.

- Nearly every cell in the body can generate 24-hour rhythms in transcription due to a molecular clock composed of interlocking feedback loops.

- The SCN is necessary and sufficient for driving 24-hour rhythms in, for example, sleep/wake, locomotor activity, feeding/fasting, hormone release, heart rate, and blood pressure, and SCN neurons form a coupled network that allows animals to shift their clock phase to match the environmental cycle of light and dark, food availability, and even the presence of predators.

- The circadian network allows adaptation to changes in the length of the light period as the seasons change across an annual cycle.

- The core features of an internal clock—persistence in constant conditions, entrainment to the environment, and temperature compensation—are evident in nearly all life on Earth, including humans.

- The circadian clock is important for human health, and disruption of circadian rhythms (as in jet lag and shift work) can exacerbate and/or increase the risk of disease.

- Translation of the findings from animal models and human laboratory studies may lead to novel chronotherapeutic treatments for disease.

SELF-ASSESSMENT QUESTIONS

1. When did circadian rhythms originate?
   A. Soon after the origin of life
   B. After the dinosaur extinction at the end of the Cretaceous
   C. After the Permian extinction 250 million years ago
   D. At the onset of the Cambrian explosion about 530 million years ago
   E. At the transition from prokaryotes to eukaryotes

2. How does entrainment differ from synchronization?
   A. Entrainment works by always setting the circadian clock when the amount of light exceeds a certain threshold.
   B. Entrainment works by always setting the circadian clock when the amount of light falls below a certain threshold.
   C. Entrainment allows continuity in clock phase to be robust with respect to temporary changes in light levels, such as from cloud cover or volcanoes.
   D. Synchronization allows continuity in clock phase to be robust with respect to temporary changes in light levels, such as from cloud cover or volcanoes.
   E. Entrainment and synchronization are 2 names for the same thing.

3. What is the primary, central pacemaker brain area in mammals?
   A. The striatum
   B. The SCN of the hypothalamus
   C. The nucleus interpositus of the cerebellum
   D. The lateral geniculate nucleus of the thalamus
   E. The superior colliculus deep layers

4. What is the retinal output to the SCN?
   A. Magnocellular retinal ganglion cells
   B. Kinocellular retinal ganglion cells
   C. Motion-selective retinal ganglion cells
   D. Intrinsically photoreceptive retinal ganglion cells
   E. Starburst amacrine cells

5. Which gene is involved in circadian clocks?
   A. *Per2*
   B. *Clock2*
   C. *Sync1*
   D. *Sync2*
   E. *Per-cyc1*

6. Which of the following is a common circadian rhythm disorder?
   A. Seasonal affective disorder
   B. Metabolic asynchronicity
   C. Overactive immune responses
   D. Sleep problems
   E. Poor night vision

7. The retinal projection to the suprachiasmatic nucleus that mediates circadian rhythms is mediated by what types of retinal neurons?
   A. Magnocellular cells.
   B. Parvocellular cells.
   C. A special class of amacrine cells.
   D. Intrinsically photosentive melanopsin ganglion cells.
   E. Photoreceptors with axons that project to the brain.

PART II
NERVOUS SYSTEM DISORDERS & THERAPEUTICS

SECTION V

Neurologic & Neurosurgical Disorders

Stroke & Neurovascular Disorders

Michael Lyerly

PREVALENCE & BURDEN

Cerebrovascular diseases represent a heterogeneous class of disorders affecting the central nervous system including ischemic and hemorrhagic strokes, cerebral venous thrombosis, aneurysms, and vascular malformations. These disorders are frequently associated with high morbidity and mortality. Fortunately, advances in diagnostic and therapeutic options for cerebrovascular diseases have led to improved clinical outcomes for many of these conditions.

Cerebrovascular diseases now represent the fifth leading cause of death in the United States. Approximately 3% of adults have experienced a clinical stroke; however, the incidence of subclinical or "silent" strokes is likely much higher. Nearly 795,000 strokes occur annually in the United States, of which approximately 610,000 are first-time strokes and 185,000 are recurrent attacks. It is estimated that someone has a stroke every 40 seconds. The highest incidence and mortality rates are seen in the southeastern states (termed the "Stroke Belt") and among racial and ethnic minorities. As the population ages, it is expected that the number of incident strokes will more than double in the coming decades, especially among patients age ≥75 years. Despite the declining incidence and mortality of stroke, the global burden of stroke is increasing, particularly in low- and middle-income countries.

CEREBROVASCULAR LOCALIZATION

Clinical localization is perhaps no better demonstrated than in cerebrovascular diseases. Medical students frequently encounter their first opportunity to "localize a lesion" when evaluating a stroke patient. In addition to determining what level of the neuroaxis or which lobes of the brain are affected, symptoms of cerebrovascular disease can frequently be localized by vascular territories. For example, in a patient with right hemiparesis and hemianesthesia affecting the face and arm, coupled with aphasia, one can say that the frontal, parietal, and temporal lobes are affected in the left hemisphere. Knowledge of the homunculus will further localize the motor and sensory deficits to the lateral aspect of the hemisphere. Taken together, it becomes apparent that all of the affected areas fall within the left middle cerebral artery (MCA) territory. When a cerebrovascular disorder appears on the differential diagnosis for a patient, it is important to consider not only the anatomic localization but also the vascular localization for the symptoms.

ISCHEMIC STROKE

Among all strokes, approximately 80% to 85% are categorized as ischemic strokes. Ischemic strokes occur when a blood vessel becomes blocked, depriving a region of the brain of oxygen

VOCABULARY

Embolism: Blockage of a blood vessel by something that has been carried in the bloodstream. Can be a clot (thromboembolism), bacteria from endocarditis (septic embolism), fat (fat embolism, as with trauma), or gas (air embolism).

Epidural hemorrhage: Bleeding into the space between the dura mater and skull, commonly due to trauma.

Hemorrhagic stroke or intracerebral hemorrhage: A neurologic syndrome attributable to blood vessel rupture or leakage.

Intraparenchymal hemorrhage: Bleeding within the brain tissue, commonly due to hypertension, cerebral amyloid angiopathy, trauma, or vascular malformations.

Ischemic stroke: A neurologic syndrome attributable to blockage of blood supply to a region of the brain. Common mechanisms of ischemia include large-vessel **thrombosis, lacunar infarction, embolism,** and hypoperfusion.

Large-vessel stroke: Ischemic stroke due to blockage of 1 or more of the brain's arteries, often named vessels such as the middle cerebral artery, usually due to thrombosis or embolism.

Penumbra: Area of ischemic, but still viable, brain tissue surrounding an ischemic core that is necrotic and not salvageable.

Small-vessel stroke: Ischemic stroke due to thrombosis of the penetrating arteries/arterioles. Also known as lacunar stroke.

Subarachnoid hemorrhage: Bleeding into the space between brain/pia and arachnoid, commonly due to ruptured aneurysms or trauma.

Subdural hemorrhage: Bleeding into the space between arachnoid and dura mater, commonly due to trauma.

Thrombosis: Local coagulation/clotting of the blood.

and glucose. Fortunately, reperfusion options are available for some ischemic stroke patients that have the potential to reverse stroke symptoms and improve functional outcomes.

Pathophysiology

Cellular Changes in Ischemia

Although the brain represents <5% of total body weight, it is responsible for 20% to 25% of energy consumption. Approximately 20% of total cardiac output is directed to the brain. Since the brain has essentially no intrinsic energy stores, even brief disruptions in cerebral blood flow (CBF) can have devastating consequences.

Normal CBF in an adult is approximately 50 mL/100 g/min. As CBF falls, protein synthesis fails and cells shift toward anaerobic glycolysis. Below 20 mL/100 g/min, neuronal electrical

activity starts to fail, which usually correlates with the onset of neurologic symptoms. With further decline in CBF, cellular membranes cannot maintain their gradient and cell death ensues unless reperfusion is quickly restored. Electrical failure leads to activation of a variety of cellular cascades (eg, release of excitatory amino acids, depletion of adenosine triphosphate, activation of proteolytic processes) that ultimately result in cell death via both necrotic and apoptotic pathways. Cell survival is determined by the severity and duration of CBF reduction. Because of collateral blood flow, variable degrees of ischemia exist within an infarct. While the central core of an ischemic stroke may have irreversible cellular injury, the surrounding tissue (termed the penumbra) may have higher CBF, which is potentially salvageable if perfusion is restored.

In the days following irreversible tissue injury, infarcted tissue will become edematous with eosinophilic, pyknotic neurons ("red dead neurons"; Figure 24–1). In the ensuing days, an inflammatory response develops, initially marked by an influx of mononuclear cells that phagocytize dying cells. Subsequently, macrophages predominate after the first 24 to 48 hours, and astrocytes start to proliferate, laying down a network of glial fibers. Ultimately, liquefactive necrosis develops, and the region of the infarct is left as a cavity with a surrounding glial scar.

Cerebral Perfusion & Autoregulation

Cerebral perfusion pressure (CPP) is defined as the mean arterial pressure (MAP) minus the intracranial pressure (ICP). Because the brain is highly sensitive to fluctuations in CBF, there are mechanisms in place to protect it from variations in systemic MAP. This is principally achieved through modulation in vascular resistance, which occurs by varying the diameter of cerebral blood vessels, primarily arterioles. Because CBF is proportional to CPP but varies inversely to cerebral vascular resistance (CVR), the brain is able to maintain a fairly

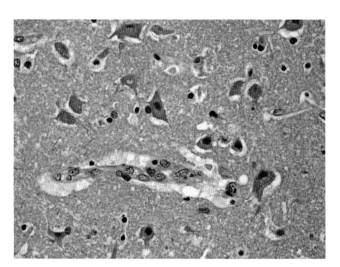

FIGURE 24–1 This photomicrograph demonstrates several eosinophilic, pyknotic neurons. (Reproduced with permission from Reisner H. *Pathology: A Modern Case Study*, 2nd ed. New York, NY: McGraw Hill; 2020.)

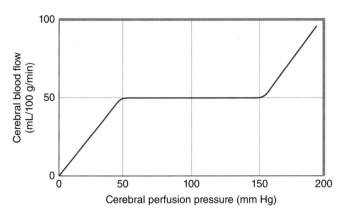

FIGURE 24–2 This curve shows normal cerebral autoregulation. Over a wide range of cerebral perfusion pressure, cerebral blood flow is able to remain fairly constant. (Reproduced with permission from Hall JB, Schmidt GA, Kress JP: *Principles of Critical Care.* 4th ed. New York, NY: McGraw Hill; 2015.)

constant CBF despite fluctuations in perfusion pressure. This protective mechanism is known as autoregulation.

$$CPP = MAP - ICP$$
$$CBF = CPP/CVR$$

Under physiologic conditions, autoregulation allows the brain to maintain stable blood flow over a wide range of perfusion pressure (Figure 24–2). In patients who are chronically hypertensive, this curve shifts to the right. It may not be safe to acutely lower their blood pressure because they may drop below the lower threshold of autoregulation and have a drop in their CBF. Because many stroke patients have chronic hypertension, physicians have to be extremely careful about acutely lowering patients' blood pressure and causing further ischemic damage by worsening cerebral perfusion.

Mechanisms of Ischemia

Cerebral ischemia can typically be broken down into 3 primary pathophysiologic mechanisms: thrombosis, embolism, and hypoperfusion. The goal of acute stroke evaluation is to determine this mechanism to guide appropriate long-term treatment strategies.

Thrombosis

Thrombosis refers to the occlusion of a vessel as a consequence of a local vascular process. Formation of a local thrombus may cause cerebral ischemia by reducing blood flow distal to the thrombotic plaque or fragmentation of the plaque causing an artery-to-artery embolism. Acute occlusion may also occur when platelets adhere to an ulcerated plaque, locally occluding the vessel lumen. Thrombotic mechanisms are commonly divided into large- and small-vessel subtypes.

Large-vessel disease may affect the major precerebral vessels (carotid and vertebral arteries) or the vessel comprising and emanating from the circle of Willis. The most common cause of large-vessel pathology is atherosclerosis. Atherosclerotic

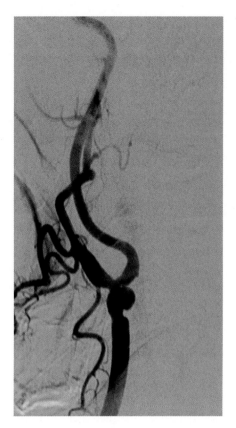

FIGURE 24–3 A digital subtraction angiogram showing a large carotid plaque with ulceration at the carotid bifurcation. (Reproduced with permission from Papadakis MA, McPhee SJ, Rabow MW: *Current Medical Diagnosis & Treatment 2019.* New York, NY: McGraw Hill; 2019.)

plaques typically develop in regions of turbulent blood flow, particularly in close proximity to vascular bifurcations, such as the origin of the internal carotid artery (Figure 24–3). Less common large-vessel pathologies include arterial dissections, vasculitides, vasospasm/vasoconstriction, and arteriopathies such as fibromuscular dysplasia or moyamoya syndrome. Patients may present with 1 or more infarcts confined within a specific vascular territory. Knowledge of clinical syndromes attributable to each vascular bed is useful to diagnose a large-vessel infarct (eg, a dominant MCA territory infarct will cause motor and sensory deficits of the contralateral arm and leg, contralateral visual field impairment, and aphasia). Depending on hemodynamic fluctuation relative to the stenosis, patients may have stroke symptoms that progress with a stuttering time course that may evolve over minutes to hours.

Small-vessel infarcts (commonly referred to as lacunar strokes or "lacunes") are <1.5 cm in diameter and occur in the basal ganglia, thalamus, brainstem, or cerebellum. These regions of the brain are supplied by small, penetrating blood vessels that arise from large parent vessels such as the MCA. Hypertension and diabetes mellitus are particularly strong risk factors for this stroke subtype. Through a pathologic process called lipohyalinosis, these small vessels develop vascular wall thickening and endothelial dysfunction, which results in a reduction of the luminal diameter. A less common mechanism

TABLE 24–1 Lacunar stroke syndromes.

Lacunar Stroke Syndrome	Localization	Clinical Symptoms
Pure motor stroke	Internal capsule or corona radiata	Contralateral face, arm, and leg weakness
Pure sensory stroke	Thalamus	Contralateral face, arm, and leg numbness
Ataxia hemiparesis	Pons, internal capsule, or corona radiata	Unilateral weakness (particularly leg) and limb ataxia
Mixed sensorimotor stroke	Thalamus and internal capsule	Weakness and numbness of the face, arm, and leg
Dysarthria–clumsy hand	Pons, corona radiata	Dysarthria with limb ataxia (particularly arm)

for the development of small-vessel occlusion is when a microatheroma in the parent vessel grows over the origin of the small vessel, causing proximal occlusion. Despite their small size, lacunar strokes can present with significant neurologic deficits due to the fact that they occur in regions of the brain densely populated by motor and sensory pathways. Several characteristic clinical syndromes that may assist in the diagnosis of a lacunar stroke have been described (Table 24–1). Patients typically present with symptoms that evolve over minutes to hours, and worsening of symptoms after initial presentation is not uncommon.

Embolism

Embolic strokes occur when a clot (or other material) formed in another part of the body travels to the brain and occludes a vessel. Emboli frequently arise from cardiac sources. A common embolic etiology is atrial fibrillation, which may cause clots to form in the left atrium or left atrial appendage. Valvular disease, ventricular mural thrombus following myocardial infarction, atrial myxoma, and endocarditis are additional cardiac sources of emboli. In patients with a patent foramen ovale or other cardiac wall defects, systemic emboli may shunt from the right to the left heart, bypass the lungs, and pass into the cerebral circulation. Other systemic sources of emboli include fat (long bone fractures), air (typically iatrogenic), and amniotic fluid. Clinically, embolic strokes may be small or large depending on the size of vascular bed occluded. Unlike thrombotic strokes, emboli may shower to several blood vessels, causing infarcts in multiple vascular territories simultaneously. Neurologic deficits from embolic strokes reach maximum intensity relatively abruptly, as opposed to the stuttering course that may be seen with thrombotic stroke mechanisms.

Hypoperfusion

Like other end organs, the brain is vulnerable to systemic hypoperfusion. This may occur in the setting of blood loss, systemic hypotension (eg, sepsis), or reduced cardiac output

from acute heart failure or pulmonary embolism. Neurologic deficits tend to be more diffuse but preferentially affect the arterial border zone (watershed) regions of the brain, which are the boundaries between major vascular territories. Clinically, this may produce symptoms such as cortical blindness and proximal limb weakness (the arterial border zone corresponds to these areas on the homunculus). In addition to neurologic deficits, patient typically have other systemic signs of hemodynamic dysfunction.

Other Ischemic Stroke Mechanisms

Less common ischemic stroke mechanisms include hypercoagulable states and genetic conditions. Coagulation disorders more commonly cause venous thrombosis, although some conditions such as antiphospholipid syndrome may be associated with arterial events. Sickle cell disease, essential thrombocytosis, and polycythemia vera are other examples of hematologic conditions associated with ischemic stroke. Pregnancy, malignancy, and systemic inflammatory conditions such as human immunodeficiency virus (HIV) and ulcerative colitis may induce a prothrombotic state. Stroke may be seen as a late effect in genetic conditions such as Down syndrome but can also be a defining feature in genetic diseases such as CADASIL (cerebral autosomal dominant arteriopathy with subcortical infarcts and leukoencephalopathy). Clinicians should consider hypercoagulable or genetic conditions in stroke patients who are under the age of 55 years, patients without vascular risk factors, and patients with a strong family history of stroke or thrombotic events.

Cryptogenic Stroke

Despite thorough diagnostic evaluations, a defined etiology is not determined in 20% to 40% of ischemic stroke patients. These patients are termed *cryptogenic*. This represents a heterogeneous class of patients, although many have an embolic pattern on neuroimaging. As new diagnostic tools emerge and sensitivity of existing modalities improves, it is likely that many of these patients will be able to have a stroke etiology determined. For example, the increased utilization of prolonged cardiac monitoring (>30 days) has identified paroxysmal atrial fibrillation as a common and important mechanism in cryptogenic stroke patients.

Ischemic Stroke Risk Factors

Risk factors are patient attributes and medical conditions that increase an individual's risk of having an ischemic stroke. It is important to differentiate stroke risk factors from stroke mechanisms (described in the previous section), which are the pathophysiologic processes that result in impairment of CBF. Risk factors can be classified as modifiable and nonmodifiable.

Age is a significant nonmodifiable risk factor for stroke, with the risk of stroke doubling for each decade beyond the age of 55. As the population ages, it is expected that the proportion of stroke patients >75 years old is going to double by the year 2050. Men are at higher risk of stroke compared to women, although this difference is less pronounced in young patients. Race and ethnicity are also important nonmodifiable risk factors, with African Americans being at higher risk than whites. Finally, a family history of stroke, particularly among first-degree relatives, increases stroke risk. There are likely many additional genetic factors that shape an individual's risk of stroke that remain poorly understood.

Numerous modifiable risk factors for stroke have been identified, although their relative contribution may differ among the ischemic stroke subtypes. Identification of these risk factors is imperative in the determination of an appropriate long-term treatment strategy for each patient. By far, hypertension is the most significant modifiable risk factor and is present in nearly 80% of ischemic stroke patients. Diabetes, dyslipidemia, cardiac disease (coronary artery disease, atrial fibrillation, congestive heart failure), and obstructive sleep apnea are also commonly encountered and contribute to stroke risk. Migraine, particularly among those who experience aura, has been shown to be associated with increased stroke risk, although the exact mechanism remains unclear. Several lifestyle risk factors, including tobacco abuse, excessive alcohol consumption, illicit drug use, diet, and physical inactivity, should also be addressed with each stroke patient and factored into their treatment plan.

Clinical Presentation of Ischemic Stroke

Ischemic stroke typically presents with the acute onset of focal neurologic deficits. Depending on the stroke subtype, symptoms may evolve over minutes to a few hours. Neurologic deficits frequently occur without warning or prodromal symptoms. Common symptoms include focal weakness, focal numbness, visual field defects, aphasia, dysarthria, and coordination deficits. Although some patients may present with 1 of these symptoms in isolation, more commonly patients have a combination of several neurologic deficits. Alterations in level of consciousness are not common with solitary infarcts within the cerebral hemispheres but may be seen with bihemispheric or brainstem strokes. Headache may also be reported but is more common with intracerebral hemorrhages than ischemic strokes.

As arterial anatomy does not vary substantially between patients, infarcts of vascular territories have characteristic constellations of symptoms that can be useful in clinical localization. Anterior cerebral artery territory infarctions cause weakness and numbness of the contralateral lower extremity and may also be accompanied by gait apraxia, mutism, reduced motivation, and urinary incontinence. MCA territory infarcts cause contralateral face and arm weakness and numbness, gaze deviation toward the side of the stroke (from impairment of the frontal eye fields), and contralateral visual field defects (from impairment of the optic radiations). Patients with dominant MCA infarcts may also have varying degrees of aphasia, whereas those with nondominant MCA infarcts may have hemineglect. Infarctions of the posterior cerebral artery (PCA) produce contralateral

visual field defects. Because the thalamus also receives blood supply from perforators of the PCA, contralateral sensory deficits may be found on examination. Strokes involving the posterior circulation tend to be less stereotyped but commonly involve motor and sensory deficits as well as cranial nerve impairments. Cerebellar symptoms may also be seen with posterior circulation infarctions.

Acute Diagnosis & Management

After initial stabilization, a focused history should be performed with emphasis on determining the definitive time of symptom onset. In some cases, this time cannot be determined, and the "last known normal" time should be established. Symptom progression, presence of seizure symptoms, current medications (particularly antithrombotics), and known vascular risk factors should also be collected in the history. In many cases, it is necessary to gather information from family members or bystanders. Acutely, it is generally not possible to do a full general examination, although attention should be given to cardiovascular exam to assess for arrhythmias, bruits, or murmurs. The neurologic exam is also abbreviated acutely to allow for determination of significant neurologic deficits without causing delays in acute treatment decisions. Scales such as the National Institutes of Health Stroke Scale (NIHSS) are commonly used to guide a standardized, rapid neurologic assessment and facilitate communication of stroke severity between healthcare providers.

Given the potential for hypoglycemia to mimic a stroke, it is important to check a serum glucose level on any patient with stroke symptoms. Serum electrolytes, blood cell count, cardiac enzymes, and a coagulation profile should also be ordered. The preferred initial neuroimaging study in the acute setting is a noncontrasted computed tomography (CT) scan of the head. CT has a high sensitivity for intracerebral hemorrhage, which is necessary to exclude as the cause of the patient's symptoms when considering acute reperfusion therapies. Radiographic evidence of ischemia may not be apparent on CT for several hours. The earliest findings may be blurring of the gray-white junction, local edema leading to sulcal effacement, and hypodensity of the infarcted brain tissue (Figure 24–4). Although cerebral blood vessels are generally not visible on a noncontrasted CT, occasionally an acutely thrombosed vessel will appear bright (hyperdense vessel sign) and signifies a large-vessel occlusion. Increasing emphasis is being placed on obtaining vascular imaging during the acute evaluation of ischemic stroke to help identify patients with large-vessel occlusion who may be amenable to endovascular thrombectomy.

Once the patient has been stabilized and the initial evaluation is complete, the patient can be evaluated for acute reperfusion therapies. Currently, intravenous (IV) tissue plasminogen activator (tPA; alteplase) is the only US Food and Drug Administration–approved medical treatment for acute ischemic stroke. This drug catalyzes the conversion of plasminogen to plasmin, which promotes fibrinolysis. It is administered as a

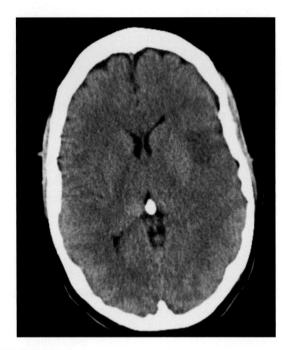

FIGURE 24–4 This noncontrasted head computed tomography shows hypodensity within the left middle cerebral artery territory (right side of the image, with radiologic orientation). Loss of the gray-white junction and sulcal effacement are also present. (Reproduced with permission from Maitin IB, Cruz E: *Current Diagnosis & Treatment Physical Medicine & Rehabilitation*. New York, NY: McGraw Hill; 2015.)

weight-based dose with 10% given as an IV bolus followed by a slow infusion of the remainder over the course of an hour. Many inclusion and exclusion criteria must be considered, however. The primary inclusion criteria include clinical diagnosis of ischemic stroke resulting in disabling neurologic deficits. Patients with any hemorrhage on their CT scan should not receive IV-tPA. Other major contraindications include history of bleeding disorders or coagulopathy; recent surgery or trauma; uncontrolled blood pressure; active bleeding; thrombocytopenia; elevated prothrombin time (PT), partial thromboplastin time (PTT), or international normalized ratio (INR); or significant ischemic changes on the initial CT scan. IV-tPA is a time-sensitive medication and must be administered within 3 hours from onset of symptoms (up to 4.5 hours in select patients, although this is considered off-label). Patients who receive IV-tPA are significantly more likely to have minimal or no neurologic deficit at 3 months compared to patients who receive placebo, but are at a higher risk of symptomatic intracerebral hemorrhage. Unfortunately, despite increases in public awareness, many patients do not arrive at a hospital within the treatment window, and nationwide, IV-tPA treatment rates are <10%.

Recently, several randomized trials demonstrated benefit for endovascular thrombectomy in acute ischemic stroke patients with large-vessel occlusion. Although endovascular procedures have been investigated since the late 1990s, older interventional devices have not been shown to be more

---

CASE 24–1

A 69-year-old man presents to the emergency department after he experienced right hand weakness and slurred speech at home. His wife says these symptoms progressed to complete right arm paralysis with right facial droop and inability to speak over the course of 15 minutes. She immediately called 9-1-1 and had him brought to the emergency department. On examination, you note that he is mildly tachycardic with a blood pressure of 203/108 mm Hg. He has near global aphasia and right facial weakness sparing the forehead, and he is unable to lift his right arm off the bed. His glucose returns at 110 mg/dL, and you escort him to have a computed tomography (CT) scan.

His noncontrasted head CT demonstrates no evidence of hemorrhage or evolving ischemia, but he does have a linear hyperdensity in the region of the left middle cerebral artery (MCA) suggesting a thrombosed vessel. When you return with the patient to the emergency department and notify his wife that you are concerned that he may be having a stroke, she breaks down crying, stating that she has been worried about him having a stroke because of his poorly controlled hypertension and diabetes. He also smokes 1 pack of cigarettes each day. His wife confirms that his symptom started approximately 1.5 hours previously. She verbally consents to the patient receiving intravenous (IV) tissue plasminogen activator (tPA) after you review the inclusion and exclusion criteria with her. Before you can administer this medication, you must lower his blood pressure

to a safe threshold (<185/110 mm Hg) using labetalol. His blood pressure is brought down to a safe range, and he receives IV-tPA without complication.

Because of the size of the clot suggested on the CT scan, you are concerned that IV-tPA will not be enough to allow for full recanalization. The interventional team is activated, and he undergoes mechanical thrombectomy approximately 3 hours from his symptom onset. During the procedure, angiography confirms complete occlusion of the left MCA. No stenosis is otherwise seen in the intra- or extracranial vasculature. The procedure is successful, and the next morning, he is starting to regain some of his speech and motor function. The MRI shows a subcortical MCA territory infarction, likely significantly smaller than the infarct that would have occurred had he not received any reperfusion therapy. As part of his hospital workup, his telemetry monitoring demonstrates paroxysmal atrial fibrillation.

Although he is initially placed on aspirin during the early course of the hospitalization, this is transitioned to apixaban on hospital day 5 because of his presumed cardioembolic mechanism from atrial fibrillation. He is also placed on high-dose statin therapy and several antihypertensives. A diabetic educator works with him during the hospitalization on glycemic control, and he also receives tobacco cessation counseling. After 7 days in the hospital, he is discharged to inpatient rehabilitation where he continues to show neurologic improvement.

efficacious than IV-tPA alone. The latest classes of mechanical thrombectomy devices have been shown to produce higher recanalization rates and better clinical outcomes compared to IV-tPA alone. It should be noted that these interventions should be viewed as adjunctive therapies to IV-tPA rather than substitutes. Current guidelines recommend consideration of endovascular thrombectomy in patients with evidence of large-vessel occlusion who can be treated within symptom onset. Recently, several clinical trials have shown that multimodal imaging such as CT perfusion studies can be used to select patients up to 24 hours from last known normal. Like IV-tPA, intracerebral hemorrhage remains the biggest safety concern.

Diagnostic Studies to Determine Stroke Mechanism

After initial evaluation, stroke patients are admitted to the hospital for further diagnostic studies to determine their stroke mechanism. Each patient should be screened for vascular risk factors including testing for diabetes and lipid profiles. Each patient should then undergo brain parenchymal imaging and vascular imaging. Unless contraindicated, magnetic resonance imaging (MRI) is the preferred parenchymal imaging modality because it clearly defines the size and extent of the infarct (Figure 24–5). CT or magnetic resonance angiography provides imaging of the intra- and extracranial vessels to identify

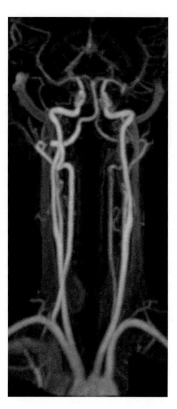

FIGURE 24–6 This magnetic resonance angiogram of the neck provides visualization of the carotid and vertebral systems as well as the intracranial circulation. (Reproduced with permission from Ropper AH, Samuels MA, Klein JP: *Adams and Victor's Principles of Neurology*. 10th ed. New York, NY: McGraw Hill; 2014.)

sites of occlusion or stenosis as well as other patterns of vascular irregularity such as fibromuscular dysplasia or vasculitis (Figure 24–6). Ultrasonography is another noninvasive imaging modality commonly used to assess the extracranial carotid artery. Although catheter cerebral angiography is viewed as the "gold standard" vascular imaging test, it is reserved for patients needing better definition of vascular anatomy given the potential risks of the procedure. Finally, each patient should undergo a cardiac evaluation including cardiac rhythm monitoring and cardiac enzyme assessment. Although not required for all patients, most should have an echocardiogram to assess for intracardiac thrombi, wall motion abnormalities, and valvular disease. In patients in whom an occult arrhythmia is suspected, prolonged outpatient cardiac monitoring can be pursued. Hypercoagulability assays should be considered in patients with otherwise negative evaluations, particularly young patients without vascular risk factors. Taken together, these tests will allow the clinician to develop an understanding of the likely pathophysiologic mechanism that will guide selection of secondary stroke prevention strategies.

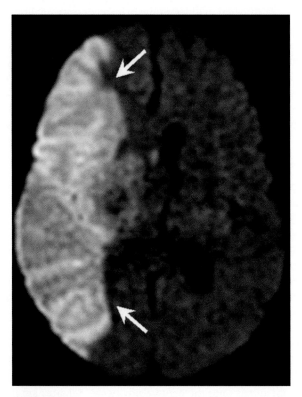

FIGURE 24–5 An example of the diffusion-weighted imaging series of a magnetic resonance imaging scan demonstrating an acute ischemic infarction within the right MCA territory (*arrows*). (Reproduced with permission from Chen MYM, Pope TL, Ott DJ. *Basic Radiology*. 2nd ed. New York, NY: McGraw Hill; 2011.)

Secondary Stroke Prevention

Long-term prevention of recurrent ischemic stroke generally consists of antithrombotic agents, statin therapy, and risk factor modification. For most pathophysiologic mechanisms of ischemic stroke, antiplatelet agents, such as aspirin or clopidogrel, are preferred over anticoagulation. The exception to this is ischemic stroke secondary to atrial fibrillation where oral anticoagulants have been demonstrated to be superior to antiplatelet therapy. Unless medically contraindicated, ischemic stroke patients should also be placed on high-dose statin therapy. The benefits of statins likely result from numerous properties beyond the lipid-lowering effects, such as plaque stabilization and anti-inflammatory properties. Effective treatment strategies should be developed to modify each individual's vascular risk factors including promoting healthy lifestyle choices. Finally, for patients with carotid artery stenosis >50%, revascularization procedures should be considered such as endarterectomy or stenting. No benefit has been seen with revascularization of major vessels other than the extracranial carotid artery.

INTRACEREBRAL HEMORRHAGE

Intracerebral hemorrhages are the second most common type of stroke, accounting for about 15% to 20% of all strokes. They are associated with higher morbidity and mortality compared to ischemic strokes. These hemorrhages can be classified based on their location within the cranium, each with different underlying pathophysiology and treatment strategies.

Classification & Pathophysiology

Classification of Intracranial Hemorrhage

Hemorrhages within the cranium can be classified according to the anatomic space that they occupy. Epidural hemorrhages occur between the calvarium and the dura matter and most commonly result from traumatic injury to the middle meningeal artery. Subdural hemorrhages occur between the dura and arachnoid meningeal layers and are typically related to rupture of bridging veins. Hemorrhages within the subarachnoid space may be caused from trauma or aneurysmal rupture. Finally, intraparenchymal hemorrhages occur within the brain tissue itself and have a multitude of etiologies. The discussion within this chapter will focus on intraparenchymal and nontraumatic subarachnoid hemorrhages. Further details on epidural, subdural, and traumatic subarachnoid hemorrhage can be found in Chapter 33 (Neurotrauma).

Etiology & Pathophysiology of Intraparenchymal Hemorrhage

Intraparenchymal hemorrhage secondary to chronic hypertension is the most common etiology of spontaneous intraparenchymal hemorrhage. These hemorrhages occur from rupture of the same small penetrating blood vessels that are affected in lacunar ischemic stroke and are found in deep brain nuclei and the brainstem (Figure 24–7). Chronic hypertension leads to disruption in the vascular layers, which predisposes the vessel to rupture. Another common etiology is cerebral amyloid angiopathy, which leads to deposition of amyloid protein into the vessel wall, resulting in focal areas of fragility, hemorrhages,

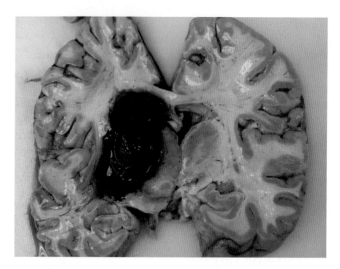

FIGURE 24–7 This gross specimen of the brain shows an intracerebral hemorrhage originating from the basal ganglia, characteristic of a hypertensive hemorrhage. (Reproduced with permission from Kemp WL, Burns DK, Travis Brown TG. *Pathology: The Big Picture.* New York, NY: McGraw Hill; 2008.)

and cognitive impairment. Unlike hypertensive hemorrhage, cerebral amyloid angiopathy tends to cause more superficial (termed *lobar*) hemorrhage. Less common causes of intraparenchymal hemorrhage include vascular malformations (discussed in the next section), vasculitis, sympathomimetic drug abuse, and coagulopathies. Some primary intracranial tumors and metastases have a tendency to hemorrhage and may be initially mistaken as a primary intraparenchymal hemorrhage. Central nervous system infections such as herpes simplex virus and *Aspergillus* may cause hemorrhage and should be considered in immunocompromised patients. Finally, hemorrhages can occur within infarcted brain tissue following reperfusion injuries and infarcts secondary to venous sinus thrombosis.

Clinical Presentation

Patients with spontaneous intraparenchymal hemorrhages have onset of neurologic deficits that evolve over minutes to hours. Symptoms tend to be less abrupt at onset and evolve as the hematoma expands. Because intraparenchymal hematomas are adding volume into the intracranial compartment, symptoms of increased ICP typically accompany the focal neurologic symptoms. Early in the course, this may include headache, nausea, and diplopia. As the pressure increases, symptoms may progress to lethargy, respiratory irregularity, and ultimately coma or death if not treated. Papilledema may be an accompanying exam finding with increased ICP. A dilated, unreactive pupil is a particularly ominous finding and may suggest mass effect causing herniation of the temporal lobe uncus onto the oculomotor nerve. Seizures are more common in the early phase of intraparenchymal hemorrhage compared to ischemic stroke. In a hemorrhage patient with fluctuating levels of consciousness, there should be a high index of suspicion for nonconvulsive status epilepticus.

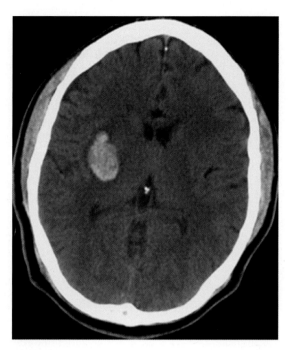

FIGURE 24-8 A noncontrasted head computed tomography scan shows an intraparenchymal hemorrhage within the right basal ganglia.

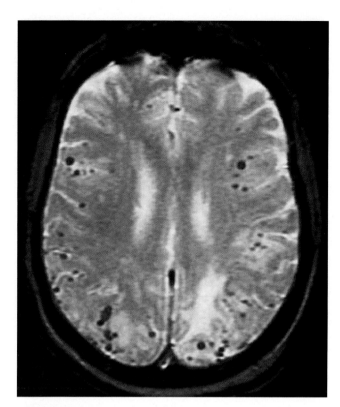

FIGURE 24-9 This magnetic resonance image with susceptibility-weighted imaging shows scattered microhemorrhages throughout the cerebral hemispheres consistent with cerebral amyloid angiopathy. (Reproduced with permission from Ropper AH, Samuels MA, Klein JP: *Adams and Victor's Principles of Neurology.* 10th ed. New York, NY: McGraw Hill; 2014.)

Diagnosis

The noncontrasted head CT is the initial radiographic study of choice for a patient presenting with the acute onset of neurologic deficits. Acutely, hemorrhage will appear bright (hyperdense) on a head CT (Figure 24–8). This scan will provide anatomic localization and hematoma volume and can show the presence of intraventricular extension and mass effect. Coagulation studies and toxicology profiles should routinely be performed on any patient with an intraparenchymal hematoma. Beyond the acute phase, neuroimaging is frequently repeated in the first 24 hours given the risk for hematoma expansion. In patients with poorly controlled hypertension and a hematoma in a location typical for hypertensive hemorrhages deep in the brain, further diagnostic workup is frequently not needed. For more peripherally located (lobar) hemorrhages, MRI is useful to identify cerebral microhemorrhages characteristic of amyloid angiopathy (Figure 24–9). An MRI may also aid in the diagnosis of underlying structural lesions such as neoplasms. Vascular imaging is necessary to investigate potential vascular malformations or vasculitis. Diagnostic catheter angiography may be necessary to fully visualize these lesions if less invasive imaging studies are inconclusive.

Management of Intraparenchymal Hemorrhage

Many patients with acute intraparenchymal hemorrhage initially present with impaired consciousness and potential respiratory collapse. As with other medical emergencies, the initial steps are focused on hemodynamic stability and securing the

airway. Once the diagnosis of an intraparenchymal hemorrhage has been made, the patient should be placed with the head of bed up, and frequent blood pressure monitoring should be initiated. Whereas acute lowering of blood pressure is avoided with ischemic strokes, this has been shown to be safe in patients with intraparenchymal hemorrhage. Although current data are conflicting regarding the initial target blood pressure for these patients, lowering systolic blood pressure to at least 160 mm Hg is recommended. This is best achieved by IV antihypertensives such as labetalol or nicardipine. Invasive blood pressure monitoring techniques may be necessary to ensure appropriate titration of these medications. Antithrombotic medications should be discontinued, and if the patient is on therapeutic anticoagulation, these medications should be reversed. Hemorrhage patients are generally admitted to an intensive care setting where they can be closely monitored for neurologic deterioration and medical complications such as infections and deep venous thromboses.

If the patient has evidence of increased ICP, invasive pressure monitoring should be considered. The patient should be provided with adequate sedation and analgesia. Although steroids should be avoided, other measures to treat elevated ICP such as hyperosmolar therapies are reasonable. The role for surgery to evacuate the hematoma is limited and is typically only undertaken for lobar hemorrhages that extend to the cortex or those with cerebellar hemorrhages and evidence of brainstem compression. If there is evidence of obstructive hydrocephalus, particularly in those with intraventricular hematoma extension, an external ventricular drain may be placed to relieve the pressure within the ventricular system. Despite advances in understanding the pathophysiology and treatment options for intraparenchymal hemorrhages, prognosis is poor for many patients. Up to half of patients will die within 30 days of the hemorrhage, and only about a quarter will regain functional independence.

VASCULAR MALFORMATIONS

Cerebral Aneurysms

Cerebral aneurysms are saccular-appearing outpouchings from the vascular wall that result from a focal weakening of the layers of the blood vessel due to absence or disruption of the tunica media or internal elastic lamina. Hypertension, tobacco abuse, and alcohol abuse are major risk factors, although aneurysms are also commonly seen in some connective tissue diseases (eg, Ehlers-Danlos) and genetic conditions (eg, autosomal dominant polycystic kidney disease). It is estimated that approximately 3% of the population has a cerebral aneurysm, although rupture is relatively uncommon. Risk of rupture is directly related to the diameter of the aneurysm. Aneurysms <7 mm in diameter pose the lowest risk and can frequently just be monitored.

In patients who do have aneurysmal rupture, blood will rapidly accumulate in the subarachnoid space (aneurysmal subarachnoid hemorrhage [SAH]). Sudden, severe headache ("worst headache of my life") is the hallmark presenting symptom. Patients will frequently also have nausea, vomiting, meningismus, and ultimately decreased level of arousal. Because of the rapid progression of symptoms, 10% of patients die before arriving at a hospital. Diagnosis can usually be made with a noncontrasted head CT scan (Figure 24–10). In rare circumstances, a lumbar puncture may be necessary to demonstrate red blood cells in the CSF in patients with a strong clinical suspicion for SAH with normal neuroimaging. After initial stabilization, vascular imaging should be undertaken to identify the location of the aneurysm. Surgical clipping and endovascular coiling are commonly used techniques to stabilize and secure the aneurysm to prevent rebleeding. Complications following SAH include hydrocephalus, ischemic injury from vasospasm, and hyponatremia from syndrome of inappropriate antidiuretic hormone (SIADH). Increased ICP is common, and an external ventricular drain may be needed to alleviate hydrocephalus. Nimodipine has been shown to improve neurologic outcomes; however, the exact mechanism of action for this effect is not well understood. Unfortunately, even with prompt treatment, the 30-day mortality for aneurysmal SAH is nearly 50%, and many who survive are left with severe neurologic deficits.

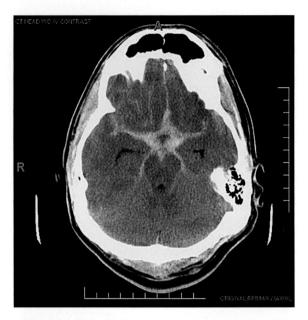

FIGURE 24–10   A noncontrasted head computed tomography scan demonstrating a subarachnoid hemorrhage. Note the extension of the hemorrhage anteriorly in the interhemispheric fissure, laterally into the Sylvian fissure, and posteriorly around the midbrain ("star sign"). (Reproduced with permission from Doherty GM: *CURRENT Diagnosis & Treatment Surgery*, 14th ed. New York, NY: McGraw Hill; 2015.)

Arteriovenous Malformations

Cerebral arteriovenous malformations (AVMs) are uncommon congenital malformations within the brain parenchyma consisting of direct artery to venous connections without the normal intervening capillary bed. Intraparenchymal hemorrhage is the presenting symptom for most of these patients, although headache and seizures are also frequently reported. Unlike hypertensive hemorrhages and cerebral amyloid angiopathy, hemorrhages from AVMs tend to occur in patients younger than age 40. Although CT and MRI may confirm the diagnosis, catheter angiography is frequently employed to fully define the anatomy of the lesion and to investigate for cerebral aneurysms, which may coexist with AVMs and be the source of the hemorrhage (Figure 24–11). AVMs may be treated with open surgery, radiosurgery, and/or endovascular embolectomy, although many patients with asymptomatic, unruptured AVMs can be managed conservatively with observation.

Other Vascular Malformations

Developmental venous anomalies (DVAs), cavernous malformations, and capillary telangiectasias are other forms of cerebral vascular malformations. DVAs are compositions of small medullary veins draining into a large central vein. They are typically benign and rarely result in hemorrhage. Cavernous malformations are tufts of thin, dilated capillaries that are sometimes detected as incidental findings on MRIs obtained for other indications and occasionally cause intraparenchymal hemorrhages. In most cases, these are simply observed, although surgical treatment may be

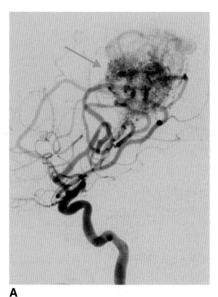

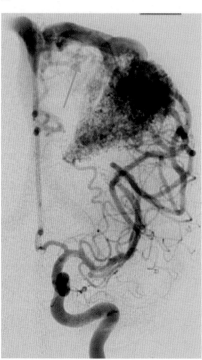

FIGURE 24–11 **A.** This digital subtraction angiogram shows a cerebral arteriovenous malformation with feeding arteries entering the nidus of the vascular malformation (*blue arrow*). **B.** The venous phase of the angiogram demonstrates early drainage into a cortical vein (*blue arrow*). (Reproduced with permission from Elsayes KM, Oldham SA: *Introduction to Diagnostic Radiology.* New York, NY: McGraw Hill; 2014.)

considered in those with recurrent hemorrhage, seizures, or neurologic impairment. Capillary telangiectasias are small, dilated capillaries within the brain that are benign and do not warrant treatment. They may be seen in some systemic conditions such as hereditary hemorrhagic telangiectasia (Osler-Weber-Rendu disease).

VENOUS SINUS THROMBOSIS

Cerebral venous sinus thrombosis (CVST) is an uncommon cause of ischemic stroke and intracerebral hemorrhage but warrants discussion due to its pathophysiology and tendency to affect unique patient populations. These patients tend to be young adults with either genetic or acquired procoagulable states such as pregnancy, the puerperium, malignancies, inflammatory conditions, and oral contraceptive use. Thrombosis of the draining venous system of the brain can produce injury through 2 primary pathophysiologic mechanisms. If venous blood is unable to drain from a region of the brain, edema can develop which can ultimately lead to tissue infarction and/or hemorrhage. If the major venous sinuses (eg, the superior sagittal sinus) are occluded, cerebrospinal fluid cannot be reabsorbed through the arachnoid granulations, leading to hydrocephalus and increased ICP. In many cases, both of these mechanisms occur simultaneously.

Because the venous drainage of the brain is more variable than its arterial system, venous thrombosis syndromes are less well defined than those affecting the arterial tree. Headache is a nearly universal presenting complaint. Focal neurologic deficits may also be seen depending on the region of the brain affected. Signs and symptoms of increased ICP may also be seen. Seizures are more common with CVST than with arterial ischemic strokes. Although CVST may be detected on a non-contrasted head CT, the diagnosis is typically made with MRI of the parenchyma coupled with either magnetic resonance or CT venography demonstrating occlusion of a dural sinus or cortical draining vein (Figure 24–12). CVST should be

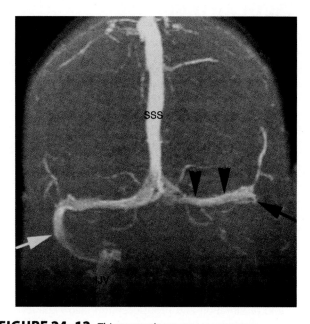

FIGURE 24–12 This magnetic resonance venogram demonstrates normal venous anatomy on the left side (*white arrow*). The superior sagittal sinus (SSS) and internal jugular vein (IJV) are labeled. The right transverse sinuses (*double arrow*) abruptly terminates (*black arrow*), indicating a venous thrombosis. (Reproduced with permission from Lalwani AK: *CURRENT Diagnosis & Treatment in Otolaryngology—Head & Neck Surgery*, 4th ed. New York, NY: McGraw Hill; 2020.)

considered in a patient with an ischemic stroke that does not conform to an arterial territory on imaging. Hypercoagulable studies and malignancy screens are valuable tools in patients in whom the etiology of the CVST is not clear.

Patients with CVST should be treated with therapeutic anticoagulation using either unfractionated heparin or low-molecular-weight heparin (LMWH) to prevent further propagation of the thrombus. Even in cases where there is associated intraparenchymal hemorrhage, anticoagulation can still be used because the risk of hematoma expansion is low in comparison to the benefits of preventing further venous infarction. For patients with neurologic worsening despite anticoagulation, endovascular thrombectomy may be considered. After the initial period, the patient can be transitioned to oral anticoagulation (typically with warfarin) with a total duration of anticoagulation treatment of 3 to 12 months. Because vitamin K antagonists are contraindicated in pregnancy, LMWH is typically used and continued for 6 weeks postpartum. Anticoagulation should be considered for future pregnancies, particularly in the third trimester. For patients with a known hypercoagulable disorder or those with recurrent venous thrombotic events, indefinite anticoagulation may be warranted. In general, prognosis for patients with CVST is relatively good, with the majority of patients experiencing a full recovery. Less than 15% of patients will have significant residual neurologic deficits, and <5% will experience a recurrent cerebral venous thrombosis.

SPINAL CORD VASCULAR DISEASES

Although the spinal cord can be affected by a number of vascular disorders, this discussion will focus on spinal cord infarctions and spinal dural arteriovenous fistulas because of their unique clinical presentations.

Spinal Cord Infarction

Infarction of the spinal cord most commonly involves the anterior spinal artery (ASA). The ASA territory includes the ascending spinothalamic pathway and descending corticospinal pathway, sparing the dorsal columns (Figure 24–13). This syndrome typically affects both sides of the cord and presents with weakness and sensory loss to pain and temperature below the level of the lesion as well as back pain but no loss of vibration or proprioception. Bowel and bladder symptoms may also be present in three-quarters of patients. The posterior spinal artery syndrome is less common and typically involves isolated loss of vibration and proprioception below the level of the lesion. Spinal cord ischemia most commonly affects the mid and lower thoracic cord. This region of the cord receives a significant radicular artery, the artery of Adamkiewicz, which can lead to spinal cord ischemia when occluded.

Spinal cord infarcts frequently do not have an identifiable cause. Common mechanisms that have been implicated

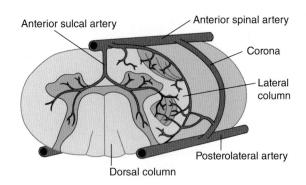

FIGURE 24–13 Spinal cord vascular anatomy. (Reproduced with permission from Waxman SG. *Clinical Neuroanatomy*, 28th ed. New York, NY: McGraw Hill; 2017.)

include mechanical compression of supplying vessels, systemic embolism or hypotension, atherosclerotic disease of the aorta, and fibrocartilaginous emboli from rupture of an intervertebral disk. Iatrogenic causes are frequently reported as part of surgical or endovascular procedures involving the abdominal aorta. Diagnosis is most frequently made by MRI with diffusion-weighted imaging. Additional vascular imaging is necessary to evaluate for aortic disease and patency of the radicular arteries supplying the spinal cord.

Data on effective treatment strategies for spinal cord infarction are limited. In the majority of patients, the diagnosis of spinal cord infarction is made beyond the window for treatment with thrombolytics. In cases where infarction is secondary to aortic surgery, many authors advocate for augmenting MAP with vasopressors and lumbar drainage. Steroids have not been shown to be of benefit. Patients with high thoracic or cervical cord lesions should be monitored closely because they are at risk for spinal shock, autonomic dysreflexia, and respiratory failure. Prognosis is highly variable and is dependent on the location and severity of the spinal cord infarction.

Spinal Dural Arteriovenous Fistula

Although there are several spinal vascular malformations, dural arteriovenous fistulas are by far the most common. They most commonly come to clinical attention between the ages of 30 and 70 years and have a significant male predominance (male-to-female ratio of 9:1). They occur when a radiculomeningeal artery connects directly to a radicular vein without an intervening capillary bed. They typically occur in the thoracic or lumbar regions. Presenting symptoms include back pain, weakness, and sensory deficits that may develop acutely or more insidiously. Later in the course, bowel and bladder symptoms and gait impairment may occur.

Although MRI is frequently obtained as an initial imaging study, definitive diagnosis typically requires selective spinal catheter angiography, which can identify the full anatomy of the vascular malformation. The MRI may show cord edema in the area of the malformation (Figure 24–14). Treatment may consist of open surgical resection or endovascular

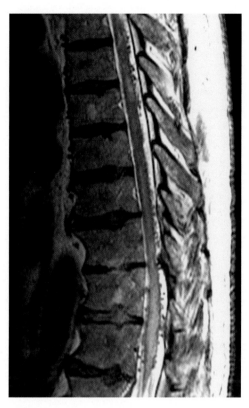

FIGURE 24–14 A T2-weighted magnetic resonance image of the spinal cord showing cord edema and flow voids along the dorsum of the cord consistent with a spinal dural AV fistula. (Reproduced with permission from Ropper AH, Samuels MA, Klein JP, et al: *Adams and Victor's Principles of Neurology*. 11th ed. New York, NY: McGraw Hill; 2019.)

embolization, although a combination of these 2 approaches may be necessary for some patients.

HYPERTENSIVE ENCEPHALOPATHY

Sudden and drastic increases in blood pressure can lead to cerebral edema and neurologic deficits. In some cases, it may be difficult to distinguish hypertensive encephalopathy from other central nervous system insults on clinical grounds alone. Most patients have headache, confusion, agitation, and,

in more advanced cases, lethargy, seizures, and coma. Neuroimaging may show evidence of cerebral edema but does not show discrete ischemic lesions. The diagnosis is confirmed by the resolution of neurologic deficits after lowering of the patient's blood pressure. Edema on neuroimaging also typically resolves.

SELF-ASSESSMENT QUESTIONS

1. A 64-year-old patient presents with the sudden onset of impaired vision. On examination, you find a right homonymous hemianopia without any other neurologic deficits. What is the most likely vascular territory involved?

    A. Left middle cerebral artery (MCA)
    B. Right MCA
    C. Left posterior cerebral artery (PCA)
    D. Right PCA

2. The patient in Question 1 is noted to have an irregularly irregular rhythm on cardiac auscultation. Based on this finding, what is the most likely mechanism for the stroke?

    A. Occlusion of a small, perforating vessel in the thalamus
    B. Embolism of a clot from the left atrium of the heart
    C. Symmetric hypoperfusion of both hemispheres
    D. Intracerebral hemorrhage from thrombosis of the superior sagittal sinus

3. A 48-year-old man is brought to the emergency department after collapsing at home with left hemiparesis. Computed tomography reveals an intraparenchymal hemorrhage in the right basal ganglia with intraventricular extension. What is the most likely etiology for his hemorrhage?

    A. Hypertensive hemorrhage
    B. Amyloid angiopathy
    C. Superior sagittal sinus thrombosis
    D. Herpes simplex virus encephalitis

4. A 24-year-old woman presents with 3 days of headache and blurred vision to the emergency department. She has papilledema on examination, and magnetic resonance venography demonstrates a parietal infarction with loss of flow in the superior sagittal sinus. What is the best acute therapy for this condition?

    A. Start oral aspirin daily
    B. Start a therapeutic heparin drip and transition to warfarin
    C. Start dexamethasone, scheduled 4 times per day
    D. Administer intravenous tissue plasminogen activator (tPA)

Neurooncology

Paula Warren

OBJECTIVES

After studying this chapter, the student should be able to:

- Understand the overall incidence and impact of nervous system tumors.
- Identify common primary brain tumors in both the adult and pediatric populations.
- Be able to describe common clinical presentations of primary brain tumors and recognize classic diagnostic features.
- Identify common peripheral nervous system tumors.
- Recognize tumors that commonly metastasize to the brain.
- Recognize and describe common paraneoplastic syndromes.
- Recognize common cancer-predisposing syndromes and familial tumor syndromes.

Nervous system tumors are a large and diverse group that can involve the brain, the meninges, the spinal cord, nerve roots, or peripheral nerves. In addition, there can be either primary nervous system tumors or metastatic spread of other primary cancers to involve the nervous system. In general, primary brain tumors and other nervous system cancers are relatively rare when compared to other cancers such as lung or breast cancer. However, despite their relative rarity, they are an important source of morbidity and mortality for patients. This chapter is not meant to be an all-inclusive review of nervous system tumors but rather will highlight key tumors and syndromes and will review common clinical presentations and basic diagnostic and treatment strategies.

PREVALENCE & BURDEN

Overall, brain tumors are uncommon, and according to the 2015 Central Brain Tumor Registry of the United States, they account for only 2% of all cancers. Meningiomas are the most common primary brain tumors (36.1%), followed by Glial cell tumors (25.8%), and pituitary tumors (15.1%) (**Figure 25–1**). The incidence of brain tumors varies by age, sex, and race, and there is an overall higher rate of nervous system cancers in individuals with certain predisposing genetic syndromes. Over the past 3 decades, the incidence

and mortality of brain tumors have increased dramatically, especially in patients >75 years of age. Reasons for this may include improved diagnostic imaging, increased access to medical care, improved care for elderly patients, and/or changes in causal factors. Ultimately, more research is required to understand this observation.

A considerable amount of research has been devoted to identifying risk factors for nervous system cancers in order to understand why they occur and to discover better treatment options. Unfortunately, however, most brain tumors have no known cause. High-dose therapeutic ionizing radiation to the head has been associated with an increased risk for both meningiomas and glioblastomas (GBMs). In addition, there are certain hereditary genetic conditions that are established risk factors. These include, but are not limited to, Li-Fraumeni syndrome, neurofibromatosis types 1 and 2 (NF1 and NF2), and von Hippel-Lindau (VHL) syndrome. There has also been considerable interest over the question of whether cell phones cause brain tumors, and as of yet, there is no conclusive evidence of an association between cell phone use and the development of brain tumors. Other potential etiologies that have been examined are infections, head trauma, diet, tobacco, alcohol, allergies, and environmental factors. There have been some associations between these factors and the development of brain tumors, but no formal causations have been identified.

VOCABULARY

- **Extra-axial:** External to the brain parenchyma, arising from the skull, meninges, cranial nerves, etc.

- **GBM (glioblastoma):** It is the most common malignant primary brain tumor in adults.

- **Glioma:** Tumor originating from glial cells, including astrocytomas, oligodendrogliomas, and ependymomas.

- **Infratentorial:** Below the tentorium cerebelli, also called the posterior fossa.

- **Intra-axial:** Within the brain parenchyma.

- **Primary brain tumor:** Tumor originating from brain cells, as opposed to brain metastases that originate from cells outside the brain

- **Supratentorial:** Above the tentorium cerebelli, ie, in the cerebrum.

- **WHO grade:** Histological tumor grading scheme from the World Health Organization.

GLIOMAS

Glioma is a general term that is used to refer to all glial tumors in the central nervous system (CNS). These tumors are classified based on their histologic similarity to glial cells: astrocytes (astrocytoma), oligodendrocytes (oligodendroglioma), or ependymal cells (ependymoma). The World Health Organization (WHO) grading system is based on histologic criteria that

are used to classify tumors as 1 of 4 grades, with grade I being the least malignant and grade IV being the most malignant. WHO grade I tumors are described as well circumscribed with benign cytologic features. WHO grade II tumors have some degree of cytologic atypia. WHO grade III tumors have anaplasia and increased mitotic activity, and WHO grade IV tumors demonstrate grade III features in addition to having either microvascular proliferation or necrosis. Although this is primarily a histologic classification system, molecular markers are increasingly being used to provide information on diagnosis, prognosis, and potential responsiveness to therapeutics, and their significance will likely continue to increase.

In general, *low-grade glioma* (LGG) refers to WHO grade I and II tumors, and *high-grade glioma* (HGG) refers to WHO grade III and IV tumors. LGGs tend to be more slow-growing tumors that are associated with a better prognosis, whereas HGGs tend to be more aggressive and can be rapidly fatal. We will discuss these 2 groups of tumors in the following sections.

Low-Grade Gliomas

LGGs are WHO grade I and II tumors and have a biphasic age distribution, with the first peak in childhood at around 6 to 12 years and a second peak in adulthood around 30 to 50 years. There is an increased incidence of LGGs in males as compared to females. Grade I tumors are more common in younger patients, and a common example is juvenile pilocytic astrocytoma, which is discussed further in the section on pediatric brain tumors. In adults, most LGGs are WHO grade II (diffuse infiltrating) astrocytomas but can also be WHO grade II oligodendrogliomas. We will discuss key features of oligodendrogliomas separately later in this chapter.

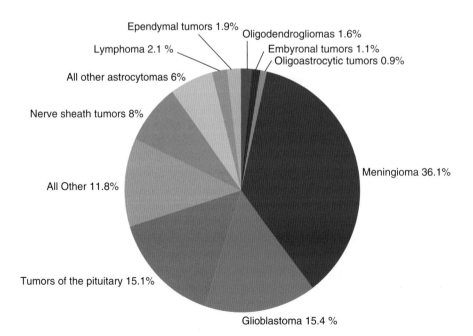

FIGURE 25-1 Distribution of all primary brain and central nervous system tumors by histology, Central Brain Tumor Registry of the United States (CBTRUS) 2007 to 2011 (N = 343,175). (Reproduced with permission from Ostrom QT, Gittleman H, Liao P, et al. CBTRUS statistical report: primary brain and central nervous system tumors diagnosed in the United States in 2007-2011. *Neuro Oncol.* 2014 Oct;16 Suppl 4:iv1-63.)

In terms of clinical presentation, most patients with LGGs have seizures, and in most cases, seizures are the presenting symptom of the tumor. Interestingly, most patients with LGGs do not have focal neurologic deficits such as aphasia or hemiparesis. Magnetic resonance imaging (MRI) is the preferred diagnostic imaging method, and generally, LGGs do not enhance with contrast, which can be used as a diagnostic clue (Figure 25–2). Management of these patients can be very challenging; sometimes, a "watch and wait" approach is taken with frequent imaging studies to monitor tumor growth, and at other times, the decision is made for earlier treatment with surgical intervention (biopsy vs resection, as possible). The role of chemotherapy and radiotherapy in the treatment of LGGs is a contentious area, and the intricacies of this treatment are beyond the scope of this chapter. However, it is important to consider that most LGGs will ultimately transform into higher grade gliomas, and decisions regarding up-front treatment may ultimately affect treatment choices later on and may affect patient quality of life, especially as related to the cognitive effects of radiotherapy.

High-Grade Gliomas

HGGs are malignant tumors that include the WHO grade III anaplastic astrocytomas, the WHO grade III anaplastic oligodendrogliomas, and the WHO grade IV GBMs. Of these

high-grade tumors, GBMs are most common and represent about 60% of all HGGs. Most HGGs occur in the adult population, although they can occur in children. The median age at diagnosis is 64 years for GBM, 51 years for anaplastic astrocytoma, and 48 years for anaplastic oligodendroglioma, and in general, HGGs occur at slightly older ages than LGGs. There is an increased incidence of GBM in men compared to women, and they also seem to occur more frequently in whites compared to other ethnic groups.

HGGs are very aggressive, and the median overall survival with treatment is as follows: 14 to 16 months for GBM, 3 to 5 years for anaplastic astrocytoma, and 15 years for anaplastic oligodendroglioma. Clinical presentation for these tumors varies with tumor location, tumor growth rate, and associated tumor-related edema and can include focal neurologic deficits, seizures, headaches, and other symptoms of increased intracranial pressure such as nausea and vomiting. Again, MRI is the preferred imaging method and generally shows an infiltrative lesion that enhances with contrast and has associated peritumoral edema. In addition, there can be solitary or multifocal lesions. In cases of GBM, the tumors often have necrotic cores and hemorrhagic components that are seen on MRI (Figure 25–3). When a GBM crosses the corpus callosum on imaging, it may be described as a "butterfly" GBM (Figure 25–4). The histologic criteria for diagnosis were discussed earlier, but key histologic findings of GBMs are areas of pseudo-palisading necrosis where the hypercellular tumor nuclei appear to line up around areas of tumor necrosis (Figure 25–5).

There are 3 main treatment modalities for HGGs: surgical resection, radiation therapy, and chemotherapy. Standard treatment for GBM has been established by randomized,

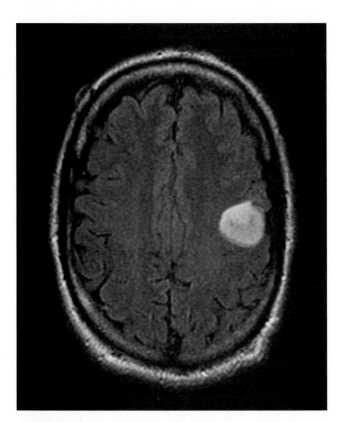

FIGURE 25–2 Fluid-attenuated inversion recovery (FLAIR) magnetic resonance image of a left frontal low-grade astrocytoma. This lesion did not enhance. (Reproduced with permission from Jameson J, Fauci AS, Kasper DL, et al: *Harrison's Principles of Internal Medicine*, 20th ed. New York, NY: McGraw Hill; 2018.)

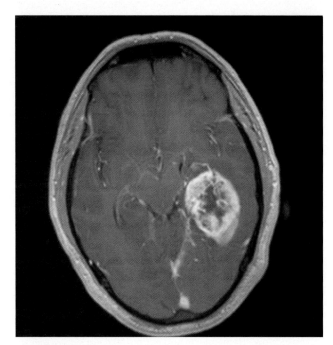

FIGURE 25–3 Glioblastoma. (Reproduced with permission from Kantarjian HM, Wolff RA: *The MD Anderson Manual of Medical Oncology*, 3rd ed. New York, NY: McGraw Hill; 2016.)

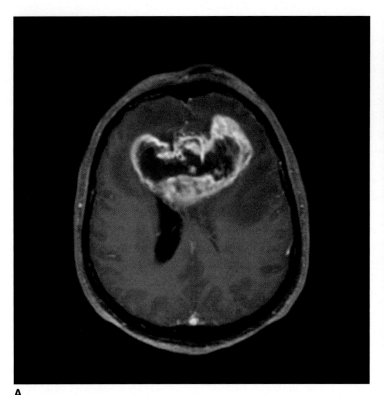

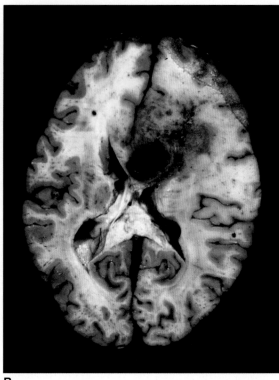

A   **B**

FIGURE 25–4 Glioblastoma. **A.** Magnetic resonance imaging reveals that this glioblastoma crosses the corpus callosum and involves both hemispheres ("butterfly glioma"). **B.** Postmortem specimen shows the necrosis and hemorrhage typical of these high-grade gliomas. (Reproduced with permission from Reisner H. *Pathology a Modern Case Study*, 2nd ed. New York, NY: McGraw Hill; 2020.)

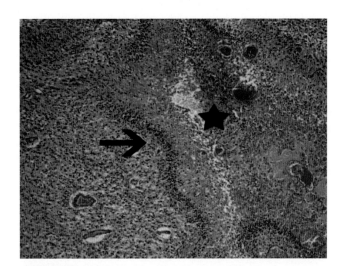

FIGURE 25–5 The distinction between the various grades of infiltrating astrocytic neoplasms is based on 4 histologic features: nuclear pleomorphism, mitotic figures, microvascular proliferation, and necrosis. Glioblastomas (GBMs), by definition, contain at least 3 of these 4 histologic features. In this section, the necrosis is apparent (*star*). As is characteristic for GBMs, this tumor has palisading of neoplastic cells at the edge of the necrosis (*arrow*). Hematoxylin and eosin, 100×. (Reproduced with permission from Kemp WL, Burns DK, Brow TG: *Pathology: The Big Picture.* New York, NY: McGraw Hill; 2008.)

phase III clinical trials and includes maximal safe surgical resection followed by concurrent radiation therapy and chemotherapy followed by adjuvant chemotherapy. This same approach is often used for anaplastic astrocytomas. Current research is investigating the optimal treatment for anaplastic oligodendrogliomas. In general, patients who are younger, who have a complete surgical resection, and who have limited neurologic disability are thought to have a better prognosis. There are also molecular features of tumors, such as tumor methylation status and *IDH* gene mutation status, that are increasingly being used to prognosticate and to guide treatment decisions. When HGGs progress or recur, treatment options are limited and are often dictated by the availability of clinical trials.

Oligodendrogliomas

We have already discussed oligodendrogliomas in the sections on LGGs and HGGs, but they have some characteristic features that warrant individual discussion. Oligodendrogliomas are relatively uncommon and account for only about 5% to 6% of gliomas. As compared to astrocytomas, these tumors are more likely to occur in the cerebral hemispheres and are therefore even more likely to be associated with seizures. Histopathologically, these tumors also have some distinguishing features. Microscopically, they demonstrate calcifications;

CASE 25–1

A 47-year-old white male with past medical history significant for mild hypertension presents with a 2-month history of gait difficulty. In particular, the patient notes that he is dragging the left foot and is having difficulty climbing stairs. During this same time frame, he reports mild headaches that are minimally responsive to over-the-counter medications. He underwent magnetic resonance imaging (MRI), which revealed a right temporal ring-enhancing mass with central necrosis and surrounding edema. He underwent a craniotomy with resection; pathology demonstrated brisk mitotic activity, necrosis, and microvascular proliferation. The patient had improvement in his symptoms after surgery and was able to walk without any gait abnormality or assistive devices. The patient was referred to neuro-oncology for further treatment recommendations.

Discussion

This patient has a glioblastoma (GBM), a World Health Organization grade IV astrocytoma, which is the most common malignant brain tumor in adults. There are 2 types of GBMs: primary, meaning a de novo lesion that develops without evidence of a less malignant precursor lesion, and secondary, meaning that the GBM arose from a lower-grade astrocytoma that transformed. In general, primary GBMs develop rapidly in older patients, are more aggressive, and have a worse prognosis. The patient in this case has a primary GBM. The patient underwent first-line therapy with complete surgical resection and, unless he is eligible for or chooses to participate in a clinical trial, will likely receive standard of care, which will include concurrent radiation and chemotherapy (temozolomide) followed by maintenance chemotherapy (temozolomide). The patient will have regular MRI scans during and after maintenance chemotherapy in order to monitor for tumor progression. When these tumors recur, patients' treatment options may include repeat surgery, additional radiation therapy, and/or additional chemotherapy agents. In addition, patients may or may not be eligible for clinical trials.

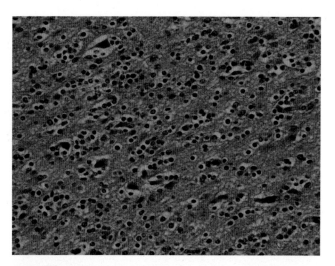

FIGURE 25–6 This medium-power photomicrograph illustrates the histologic features of an oligodendroglioma. Note the "fried egg" appearance (ie, prominent clearing around the cells) and the comparatively uniform round nuclei characteristic of this neoplasm. Hematoxylin and eosin, 200×. (Used with permission from Dr. Stephen Cohle, Spectrum Health-Blodgett Campus, Grand Rapids, MI.)

Ependymomas

Ependymomas are another type of glial tumor. They primarily occur in children and are therefore discussed later in the section on pediatric brain tumors.

MENINGIOMAS

Meningiomas are generally benign, slow-growing neoplasms that arise from the arachnoid cap cells. They are the most common primary brain tumor in adults, accounting for >30% of all CNS tumors. The incidence of meningiomas appears to increase with age, and they occur more frequently in women, with a 2:1 female-to-male ratio. The only established environmental risk factor for meningioma is ionizing radiation, especially among those exposed in childhood. There are genetic syndromes that increase the risk of meningioma, and these will be discussed later in the chapter.

Meningiomas are classified by the WHO into 3 grades based on local invasiveness and cellular features of atypia. Grade I meningiomas are referred to as benign meningiomas and have a low mitotic rate and do not demonstrate brain invasion. Grade II meningiomas, or atypical meningiomas, demonstrate any of the following: higher mitotic rate, brain invasion, or specific histologic features. Grade III meningiomas, or anaplastic meningiomas, have a very high mitotic rate or have a specific histology, either papillary or rhabdoid meningioma. There are specific subtypes within each of the grades. Meningiomas may also be characterized microscopically by the presence of spindle cells concentrically arranged in a whorled pattern and psammoma bodies.

Meningiomas are frequently detected incidentally as part of the workup for other problems, such as headaches.

perinuclear halos, which have a "fried egg" appearance; and a delicate capillary network, which is often described as looking like "chicken wire" (Figure 25–6). The perinuclear halos are artifact and are due to fixation of the tissue specimens. Molecularly, oligodendrogliomas may have allelic losses on 1p and 19q, either separately or combined, with the combined loss being most common. The 1p/19q codeletion is a favorable prognostic sign, and these patients have improved responses to chemotherapy and longer survival.

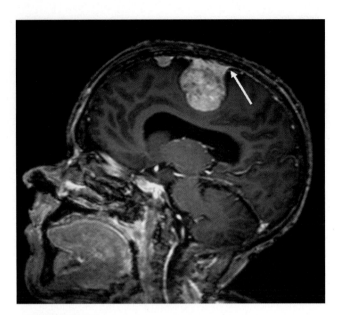

FIGURE 25–7 Sagittal magnetic resonance image demonstrating a contrast enhancing dural-based lesion (*arrow*) proven to be a meningioma at time of resection. (Reproduced with permission from Doherty GM: *CURRENT Diagnosis & Treatment Surgery*, 14th ed. New York, NY: McGraw Hill; 2015.)

However, some patients can experience focal neurologic deficits, seizures, increased intracranial pressure, and/or neurocognitive deficits, which are likely related to the anatomic location and size of the tumor. Most meningiomas can be diagnosed with imaging studies including MRI and computed tomography (CT). They are extra-axial tumors (meaning external to the brain parenchyma). They are typically contrast enhancing and often have a "dural tail," which is a thickening of the dura mater at the periphery of the tumor (Figure 25–7). CT scans often demonstrate calcification within the tumor and can also help to identify bony involvement.

Not all meningiomas require treatment, and the decision to treat is often based on the age of the patient and whether or not the patient is experiencing side effects related to the tumor. Incidental, asymptomatic meningiomas can often be safely monitored with imaging studies. If treatment is required, surgical intervention is often first-line treatment. Factors that affect whether or not patients undergo surgery include, but are not limited to, the age of the patient, the patient's performance status and current neurologic condition, the patient's comorbidities, and tumor factors, such as size and location. Complete surgical removal is the goal, but in approximately 1/3 of cases, this is not possible. In those cases, radiation therapy is often given after surgery. In addition, more aggressive or recurrent tumors may require repeat surgeries, multiple rounds of radiotherapy, or even chemotherapy.

HEMANGIOBLASTOMAS

Hemangioblastomas are benign (WHO grade I) vascular tumors that can occur anywhere in the body but are especially common in the brainstem, cerebellum, and spinal cord.

They predominately occur in young adults and seem to occur more frequently in men than women. Hemangioblastomas can occur sporadically (70% of cases) or in association with VHL disease (30% of cases; see separate section on VHL). Patients with hemangioblastomas in association with VHL typically present at younger ages than patients with sporadic tumors. Clinical presentation varies with tumor location, but common symptoms include headaches, hydrocephalus, or cerebellar symptoms. Pain is commonly noted with spinal hemangioblastomas. Hemangioblastomas can produce erythropoietin, which can cause secondary polycythemia in approximately 5% of patients. The characteristic MRI finding is a fluid-filled cyst with an enhancing mural nodule. Hemangioblastomas also tend to have "flow voids" present on MRI, which correspond to enlarged vasculature. Histopathologically, they demonstrate tightly packed, thin-walled vessels with neoplastic stromal cells. Treatment for hemangioblastomas can involve surgical resection or radiation therapy or both. The highly vascular nature of the tumor and the anatomic location can make surgical resection difficult or impossible. In these cases, radiation therapy would be more likely. In addition, antiangiogenic agents are being investigated as potential therapies for this type of tumor.

PEDIATRIC PRIMARY BRAIN TUMORS

Pediatric brain tumors differ from adult brain tumors and therefore require individual discussion. Although the incidence rates of brain tumors in children are less than those in adults, pediatric brain tumors are the leading cause of cancer-related morbidity and mortality in children. It is also important to recognize that one of the major differences between primary brain tumors in adults versus children is location, with most adult primary brain tumors being supratentorial and most of those in children being infratentorial in location. There are many different types of childhood primary brain tumors, and we focus on the most common in this chapter.

Pilocytic Astrocytomas

Pilocytic astrocytomas are low-grade (WHO grade I) astrocytomas that are found predominately in the pediatric age group, most commonly occurring around 9 to 10 years of age. Although they can be located throughout the brain, in children, they are most often found in the posterior fossa, specifically in the cerebellum. If these tumors occur in the adult population, they are more likely to be located in the cerebrum. In general, these tumors tend to arise from midline structures, such as the cerebellum, optic nerves/optic chiasm, hypothalamus, and brainstem.

Patients often present with signs of increased intracranial pressure and cerebellar symptoms, especially if their tumor is located in the posterior fossa. Radiographically, these tumors are well circumscribed and classically have a large cystic

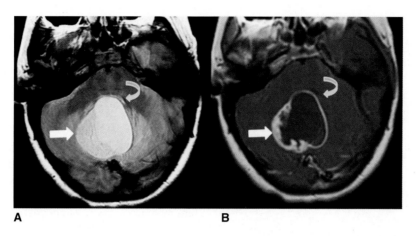

A   B

FIGURE 25–8 Pilocytic astrocytoma. Axial T2-weighted (**A**) and T1-weighted (**B**) post-contrast images show a cystic lesion with peripheral enhancement and an enhancing solid component located in the posterior fossa (*arrows*). These findings are suggestive of a pilocytic astrocytoma. Note that the lesion exerts mass effect on the fourth ventricle, which is compressed (*curved arrows*). (Reproduced with permission from Jameson J, Fauci AS, Kasper DL, et al: *Harrison's Principles of Internal Medicine*, 20th ed. New York, NY: McGraw Hill; 2018.)

component with a brightly enhancing solid mural nodule (Figure 25–8).

Histologically, they are sparsely cellular without anaplasia or mitoses. These tumors often contain Rosenthal fibers, which are corkscrew-shaped, eosinophilic intracytoplasmic inclusions (Figure 25–9), and eosinophilic granular bodies, which are globular aggregates within astrocytic processes. Neither Rosenthal fibers nor eosinophilic granular bodies are specific for pilocytic astrocytomas, and both may be seen in other neoplasms and disease processes. In general, pilocytic astrocytomas are slow-growing tumors with a relatively good prognosis (5-year survival >90%), and they rarely progress to a higher grade neoplasm. Surgical resection is first-line therapy and is usually curative if a complete resection is achieved.

Medulloblastomas

Medulloblastoma is the most common malignant brain tumor of childhood, accounting for 25% of all pediatric brain tumors. These tumors occur most commonly in the first decade of life and have a bimodal peak in incidence between 3 and 4 years old and then again between 7 and 10 years old. Medulloblastomas occur in the posterior fossa, predominately in the region of the fourth ventricle. As a result of this location, they often lead to hydrocephalus, because of obstruction of cerebrospinal fluid (CSF) flow, and patients present with symptoms of increased intracranial pressure, such as headache, lethargy, and vomiting. Tumors also often involve the cerebellum and can cause cerebellar signs such as truncal or limb ataxia and nystagmus.

Medulloblastoma is an aggressive embryonal tumor and is classified as a CNS primitive neuroectodermal tumor (WHO grade IV). Histologically, these tumors are extremely cellular and are composed of small, round blue cells with hyperchromatic nuclei (Figure 25–10) and Homer-Wright rosettes. The most updated WHO classification also classifies medulloblastomas according to molecular characteristics; however, the details of this are beyond the scope of this chapter. On MRI, medulloblastomas are generally contrast enhancing and show effacement of the fourth ventricle (Figure 25–11). All patients with medulloblastoma should have entire neuraxis imaging to assess extent of disease dissemination and for spinal drop metastases and CSF cytology to assess for CSF involvement because these tumors have a high propensity for spread within the CNS. Surgery is first-line therapy for these tumors. Postsurgically, patients are divided into standard-risk and high-risk groups based on age, degree of surgical resection, and presence of metastasis. In general, the standard-risk group receives postsurgical radiotherapy alone, and the high-risk group receives postsurgical

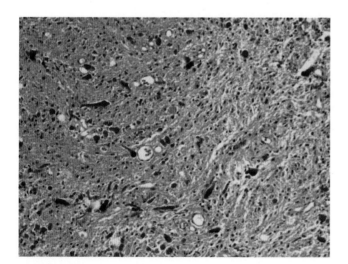

FIGURE 25–9 Rosenthal fibers. The thick, irregular, eosinophilic structures scattered throughout this image are Rosenthal fibers. Rosenthal fibers are associated with pilocytic astrocytomas and a number of other indolent central nervous system neoplasms but can also be seen at the edge of chronic nonneoplastic processes. In this regard, Rosenthal fibers indicate slow growth, which is consistent with pilocytic astrocytomas. Hematoxylin and eosin, 200×. (Reproduced with permission from Kemp WL, Burns DK, Brow TG: *Pathology: The Big Picture*. New York, NY: McGraw Hill; 2008.)

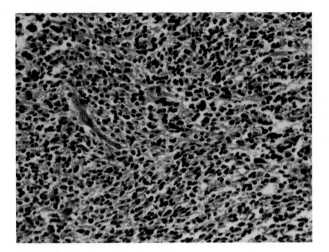

FIGURE 25–10 Medulloblastoma. One of the small round cell tumors of childhood, medulloblastomas originate in the cerebellum. Hematoxylin and eosin, 200×. (Reproduced with permission from Kemp WL, Burns DK, Brow TG: *Pathology: The Big Picture.* New York, NY: McGraw Hill; 2008.)

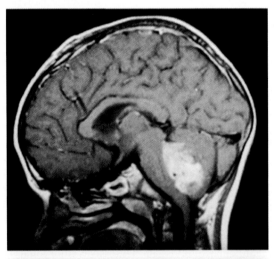

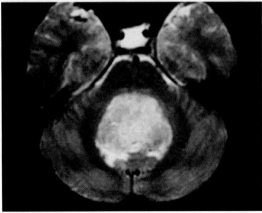

FIGURE 25–11 Medulloblastoma. Magnetic resonance imaging in the sagittal (*above*) and axial (*below*) planes, illustrating involvement of the cerebellar vermis and neoplastic obliteration of the fourth ventricle. (Reproduced with permission from Ropper AH, Samuels MA, Klein JP: *Adams and Victor's Principles of Neurology*, 11th ed. New York, NY: McGraw Hill; 2019.)

radiotherapy plus chemotherapy. Five-year survival rates for the standard-risk and high-risk groups are 70% and 40%, respectively. Long-term survivors of medulloblastoma often have neurologic disabilities, including significant learning disabilities.

Ependymomas

Ependymoma is the third most common CNS tumor of childhood and is especially prevalent among children younger than 3 years old. There is an increased incidence in males (1.7:1 male-to-female ratio). The WHO classification system includes 3 grades of ependymomas: grades I, II, and III. Ependymomas can occur anywhere throughout the CNS, but infratentorial tumors are most common. Infratentorial ependymomas are also commonly located intraventricularly, especially in the fourth ventricle. Ependymomas can also occur in the spinal cord, and patients who have only intraspinal lesions but not intracranial lesions are often found to have NF2. Patients with infratentorial lesions commonly present with signs of increased intracranial pressure due to hydrocephalus. Ependymomas may have calcifications that are visible on CT scans, and they are typically well-circumscribed masses with varying degrees of enhancement on MRI. Histologically, these tumors have characteristic perivascular pseudorosettes, which are formed when ependymal cells form rings around vessels. Ciliary basal bodies (blepharoplasts) can be demonstrated on electron microscopy. Surgical resection is first-line therapy in these tumors, and the extent of resection is the most significant prognostic factor for patients with ependymoma. In most cases, local irradiation is given after surgical resection. Chemotherapy appears to have a limited role in the treatment of these patients.

Craniopharyngiomas

Craniopharyngioma is the most common supratentorial tumor in childhood; however, it is a rare tumor overall. This tumor has a bimodal age distribution with 1 peak in children between ages 5 and 10 years and another peak in adults between ages 50 and 60 years. Craniopharyngiomas are slow-growing, benign (WHO grade I) tumors that are derived from remnants of the Rathke pouch. There are 2 subtypes of craniopharyngiomas that are histologically and molecularly distinct. The classic adamantinomatous subtype is more common and occurs more frequently in children. The papillary subtype occurs predominantly in adults. Craniopharyngiomas are usually located in the suprasellar region of the brain. Common clinical presentations for these tumors include hypopituitarism, visual changes (diplopia or bitemporal hemianopsia), and/or hydrocephalus. Craniopharyngiomas contain both solid and cystic areas. The cystic areas contain dark fluid that is composed of cholesterol crystals and necrotic debris. This cystic fluid has a dark brown or black color and is often described as "motor oil." Calcification is common in these tumors, and they often appear as a calcified mass in the parasellar region on head CT. On MRI,

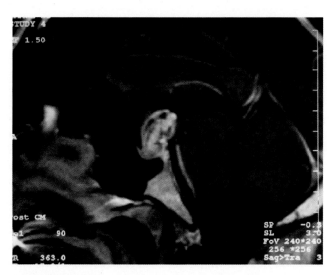

FIGURE 25–12 Sagittal magnetic resonance imaging showing contrast-enhanced suprasellar craniopharyngioma. (Reproduced with permission from Riordan-Eva, P, Augsburger JJ: *Vaughan & Asbury's General Ophthalmology*, 19th ed. New York, NY: McGraw Hill; 2018.)

these are usually intensely enhancing lesions (Figure 25–12). Craniopharyngiomas are most commonly treated with complete resection or subtotal resection followed by radiotherapy. Like the pituitary tumors, craniopharyngiomas can produce significant endocrine abnormalities, and patients should be managed by a multidisciplinary team that includes neurosurgeons, radiation oncologists, and endocrinologists.

PITUITARY TUMORS

Pituitary tumors are the third most common intracranial neoplasm. Recent studies suggest that the incidence of pituitary tumors is actually higher but is underestimated because many tumors are asymptomatic and therefore go undiagnosed. Pituitary tumors are uncommon in pediatric populations, and their incidence increases with age. Some pituitary tumors may be associated with genetic syndromes, such as multiple endocrine neoplasia type 1 (MEN1), multiple endocrine neoplasia type 4 (MEN4), McCune-Albright syndrome, or Carney complex.

Before discussing pituitary tumors, it is important to review the pituitary gland, which plays a key role in regulating the body's hormones and the hormones it secretes. The pituitary gland is divided into 2 parts: the adenohypophysis (the anterior lobe) and the neurohypophysis (the posterior lobe). The adenohypophysis, or anterior pituitary, contains 5 types of endocrine cells, which are defined by the hormones they secrete: corticotrophs (adrenocorticotropic hormone), thyrotrophs (thyroid-stimulating hormone), gonadotrophs (follicle-stimulating hormone and luteinizing hormone), somatotrophs (growth hormone), and lactotrophs (prolactin). The neurohypophysis, or posterior pituitary, is responsible for the secretion of oxytocin and vasopressin. Pituitary tumors result from hyperplasia of the previously listed endocrine

cells, and most pituitary tumors arise from the anterior pituitary gland.

Pituitary adenomas are the most common pituitary tumor, and are generally benign tumors that do not spread outside the skull. For a pituitary tumor to be classified as a pituitary carcinoma, there has to be metastasis, which is rare. Pituitary adenomas are typically classified according to size: pituitary microadenomas, which are <10 mm, and pituitary macroadenomas, which are ≥10 mm. In general, pituitary macroadenomas are approximately twice as common as pituitary microadenomas. Although these tumors are considered "benign," they can have a significant impact on health because of the symptoms they produce. Most pituitary adenomas present clinically because of inappropriate hormone secretion or because of compression of adjacent structures. The optic chiasm is most often compressed (Figure 25–13), which results in bitemporal hemianopsia. In addition, headaches and/or hydrocephalus may result from compression or disruptions in CSF flow.

Pituitary adenomas are also classified by whether or not they make excessive hormone ("functional" adenoma vs a "nonfunctional" adenoma, respectively). Most pituitary adenomas that come to clinical attention are functional, and these tumors are named for the hormones they produce. For example, a prolactin-producing adenoma is called a prolactinoma. The prolactinoma is the most common functional pituitary adenoma, and common signs and symptoms associated with it are galactorrhea, amenorrhea, hypogonadism, and sexual dysfunction. The second most common functional pituitary adenoma is a growth hormone–secreting adenoma, and affected individuals may experience acromegaly. The type of hormone secreted by the adenoma dictates the signs and symptoms the patient may experience, diagnostic testing choices, and treatment options. In most cases, neurosurgical intervention is

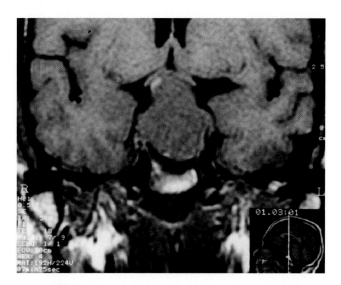

FIGURE 25–13 Coronal magnetic resonance imaging showing large pituitary adenoma elevating and distorting the optic chiasm. (Reproduced with permission from Riordan-Eva, P, Augsburger JJ: *Vaughan & Asbury's General Ophthalmology*, 19th ed. New York, NY: McGraw Hill; 2018.)

first-line therapy for these tumors. However, some cases can be treated with medical management, such as bromocriptine, a dopamine agonist, for prolactinoma. In some cases, radiation therapy or chemotherapy may be necessary. In all cases, patients will require long-term follow-up to assess disease status and close monitoring by endocrinology for management of hormonal abnormalities.

PINEAL REGION TUMORS

Pineal tumors are rare, accounting for <1% of all primary brain tumors. They are a very heterogenous group made up of benign pineal region tumors, glial tumors, pineal parenchymal tumors, and germ cell tumors. Each of these categories of tumors has distinct histopathologic features as well as differences in disease course, treatment modalities, and prognosis. Clinical presentation among these different tumors is similar, however, and commonly includes hydrocephalus, manifested by lethargy, nausea, headache, and/or Parinaud syndrome, which is characterized by absent upgaze, lid retraction, near-light dissociation (better pupillary reaction to accommodation than to light), and convergence nystagmus and is caused by compression of the midbrain tectum. In addition, adolescent males may experience precocious puberty due to β-human chorionic gonadotropin production. Most pineal tumors require at least a biopsy for tissue diagnosis, but some can be diagnosed by detection of secreted hormones in CSF or serum. Treatment usually involves surgical resection with or without additional radiation therapy. Chemotherapy is also used in certain situations.

PRIMARY CNS LYMPHOMA

Primary CNS lymphoma (PCNSL) is rare and represents only approximately 3% of all primary brain tumors. PCNSL mainly occurs in older individuals, with a median age at diagnosis of 59 years. According to the Surveillance, Epidemiology, and End Results (SEER) database, the incidence of PCNSL appears to be increasing among patients age 65 years and older, with the highest incidence in patients age 75 years or older. PCNSL occurs in both immunocompetent and immunocompromised patients, but at a higher frequency among the latter group. The most significant risk factor for CNS involvement of lymphoma is an immunocompromised state, either acquired, such as acquired immunodeficiency syndrome (AIDS) or after transplantation, or congenital, such as Wiskott-Aldrich syndrome or severe combined or common variable immunodeficiency. PCNSL in AIDS patients and in posttransplant patients is almost exclusively associated with Epstein-Barr virus infection. PCNSLs are unique in that they are confined to the CNS, but they do not arise from neural tissue. Instead, they are extranodal, malignant non-Hodgkin lymphomas of primarily B-cell origin. PCNSL can involve the brain, the eyes, the leptomeninges, or the spinal cord.

PCNSL can present in a variety of ways, but cerebral symptoms including personality/cognitive changes, hemiparesis, aphasia, or headache are most common. MRI is the preferred imaging modality for diagnosis and typically demonstrates a highly infiltrative tumor with an intense, homogenous enhancement pattern. In patients with AIDS-related PCNSL, brain lesions are often ring enhancing and may be associated with hemorrhage or necrosis. Stereotactic brain biopsy is most commonly used for diagnosis of PCNSL. In addition, cytologic and/or flow cytometric analysis of lymphoma cells isolated from CSF or via vitreous biopsy may result in the diagnosis.

Surgical resection has a very limited role in PCNSL and is generally not associated with improved survival and may actually result in worsened neurologic status of patients. Current mainstays of treatment include steroids, chemotherapeutics primarily involving high-dose intravenous methotrexate with or without additional agents, rituximab (a monoclonal CD20 antibody), and radiotherapy. In general, whole-brain radiation therapy is delayed as long as possible, especially among elderly patients, due to associated neurotoxicity. Untreated PCNSL is rapidly fatal, and patients typically die within 1.5 months from time of diagnosis. With treatment, 5-year survival rate in immunocompetent adults is approximately 30%. Poor prognosis is associated with age >60 years old, poor functional status, elevated serum lactate dehydrogenase, elevated CSF protein concentration, and involvement of deep regions of the brain (ie, periventricular regions, basal ganglia, brainstem, and/or cerebellum). Even patients who have an initial good response to treatment will likely have disease recurrence at some point, and treatment options at recurrence include additional chemotherapy, radiation therapy, or palliative care.

PERIPHERAL NERVE TUMORS

Schwannomas

Schwannomas are the most common peripheral nerve tumor. They are benign (WHO grade I) nerve sheath tumors that arise from Schwann cells, which produce the myelin sheath around nerve fibers. Most schwannomas occur extracranially in the peripheral nerves of the skin and subcutaneous tissues. They can arise from spinal nerve roots and can cause radicular symptoms and signs of nerve root or spinal cord compression. When schwannomas occur intracranially, they have a strong predilection for cranial nerve VIII in the cerebellopontine angle and are referred to as vestibular schwannomas or acoustic neuromas. Vestibular schwannomas can cause tinnitus, hearing loss, and/or dizziness. Approximately 90% of schwannomas occur as solitary, spontaneous tumors, and approximately 4% of schwannomas arise in the setting of NF2 (see later section on NF2). MRI is the preferred diagnostic imaging modality and often shows a well-circumscribed mass with intense contrast enhancement (Figure 25–14). Schwannomas are encapsulated and do not infiltrate into the nerve fibers, but rather displace them. Pathologically, these

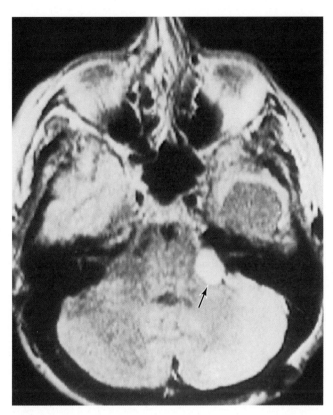

FIGURE 25–14 Magnetic resonance image of a horizontal section through the head at the level of the lower pons and internal auditory meatus. A left acoustic nerve schwannoma with its high intensity is shown in the left cerebellopontine angle (*arrow*). (Reproduced with permission from Waxman SG. *Clinical Neuroanatomy*, 28th ed. New York, NY: McGraw Hill; 2017.)

tumors consist of alternating highly cellular regions (Antoni A regions) that have areas of nuclear palisading (Verocay bodies) and loosely arranged hypocellular regions (Antoni B regions). Most schwannomas strongly express the S100 protein (Figure 25–15). Surgical resection is most often used to treat these slow-growing tumors, and there is a low risk of recurrence or malignant transformation.

Neurofibromas

These are also benign (WHO grade I) nerve sheath tumors that typically occur as solitary and sporadic tumors. There is, however, a strong association with multiple neurofibromas and NF1. Neurofibromas are composed of Schwann cells and fibroblasts. These tumors, unlike schwannomas, are not encapsulated, and they infiltrate between nerve fascicles of the parent nerve. MRI often demonstrates fusiform lesions that enhance with contrast. Surgery is often used to treat these tumors, but unlike schwannomas, it is difficult to resect these tumors completely without sacrificing the entire nerve that is involved. In neurofibromas associated with NF1, surgery is less often used because there are typically multiple lesions. In addition, recurrence and malignant transformation are more common in neurofibromas associated with NF1.

NERVOUS SYSTEM METASTASES

Systemic cancers can metastasize to various parts of the nervous system, including the brain parenchyma, the leptomeninges, the dura, and the spinal cord and are associated with significant morbidity and mortality. Parenchymal brain metastases are the most common type of brain tumor and occur in 10% to 15% of people with cancer. The overall incidence of brain metastases appears to be increasing, and this is likely related to improved overall survival times of cancer patients, increased awareness of brain metastases, and improved diagnostic techniques. The frequency with which systemic cancers metastasize to the brain varies according to the type of primary cancer. Common cancers that spread to the brain are lung, breast, melanoma, renal, and colorectal cancers, in decreasing order of frequency. Although some cancers are more likely to metastasize to the brain, any primary cancer can spread to the brain, and therefore, metastasis should always be considered as part of the differential diagnosis in cancer patients who also have brain lesions. Brain metastases can produce a significant amount of peritumoral edema, which, in turn, can produce clinical symptoms such as headache, seizures, and/or focal neurologic deficits.

Pathologically, most brain metastases are spheroid and appear to be well demarcated from surrounding brain tissue on gross examination. In addition, the majority of brain metastases are multiple lesions, and they are often located at the junction of the gray and white matter (Figure 25–16). The cerebrum is the site of 80% to 85% of brain metastases, whereas the cerebellum is the site of 10% to 15% and the brainstem is the site of only 3% to 5%. Some brain metastases are more likely to hemorrhage, and these include melanoma, renal cell carcinoma, thyroid cancer, and choriocarcinoma. The gold standard for diagnostic imaging is MRI with contrast, which is more sensitive that CT in determining the location and number of metastases. Often, the diagnosis of brain metastasis can be assumed, especially in the setting of a known primary cancer and multiple typical-appearing lesions, and other times, tissue must be obtained for diagnosis, especially in the setting of no known primary cancer and a solitary brain lesion.

There are several treatment options for patients with brain metastases, including whole-brain radiotherapy, stereotactic radiosurgery, conventional surgical resection, and use of systemic therapies. Decisions regarding which therapy to use are made based on such factors as the number, size, and location of the lesions; the overall and neurologic condition of the patient; the status of the primary cancer; and the goal of therapy (ie, to provide palliation or symptom management or to extend survival).

PARANEOPLASTIC SYNDROMES

Paraneoplastic syndromes are a group of rare disorders that are associated with cancer but are not directly attributable to cancer cells. Instead, these syndromes are either due to substances secreted by the tumor or due to immune

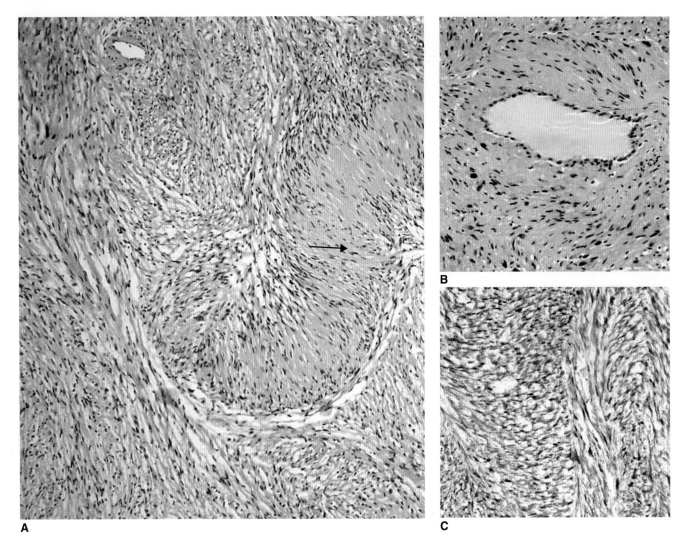

FIGURE 25–15   Schwannoma. **A.** Spindle cell neoplasm demonstrating a hypercellular pattern of growth (Antoni A pattern) and a characteristic Verocay body consisting of 2 palisading columns of nuclei separating an amorphous area of fibrillary cell processes (*arrow*). **B.** Characteristic hyalinized vessel within tumor. **C.** S100 immunostaining characteristic of Schwann cells. (Reproduced with permission from Reisner H. *Pathology a Modern Case Study*, 2nd ed. New York, NY: McGraw Hill; 2020.)

cross-reactivity between tumor and normal host tissues. Paraneoplastic syndromes were first recognized more than a century ago, and since that time, the understanding of paraneoplastic syndrome pathogenesis has increased significantly. It is estimated that up to 8% of patients with cancer will be affected by a paraneoplastic syndrome, and this number will likely increase as patients with cancer continue to live longer and diagnostic techniques for these syndromes continue to improve.

Paraneoplastic syndromes can represent the first manifestation of cancer, even in a patient without a known primary malignancy. Therefore, if a patient with an unknown primary cancer presents with a common paraneoplastic syndrome, then a diagnostic workup for malignancy must be done. Paraneoplastic syndromes can affect many organ systems, with the nervous system often being severely affected. Commonly associated malignancies include small-cell lung cancer, breast cancer, gynecologic tumors, and hematologic malignancies. Diagnosis of a paraneoplastic syndrome is based on clinical presentation, exclusion of other causes, performance of autoantibody and other diagnostic testing such as imaging studies, and workup for relevant cancers. Treatment of paraneoplastic disorders can involve immunotherapy and identification and treatment of the underlying malignancy.

Paraneoplastic syndromes of the peripheral nervous system can include paraneoplastic sensory neuropathy or Lambert-Eaton myasthenic syndrome (LEMS). LEMS is characterized by muscle weakness and is often associated with dry mouth, constipation, and sexual dysfunction. LEMS is clinically similar to myasthenia gravis (MG), with the main difference being that patients with LEMS get temporarily stronger with exertion unlike patients with MG, who get weaker with exertion. LEMS is seen in approximately 1% to 3% of patients

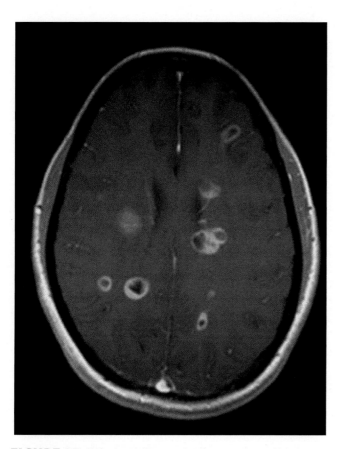

FIGURE 25-16 Multiple brain metastases, breast. (Reproduced with permission from Kantarjian HM, Wolff RA: *The MD Anderson Manual of Medical Oncology*, 3rd ed. New York, NY: McGraw Hill; 2016.)

with small-cell lung cancer and is caused by autoantibodies directed against the presynaptic P/Q-type voltage-gated calcium channels, which leads to a decrease in acetylcholine release. Paraneoplastic disorders that affect the CNS can include limbic encephalitis, paraneoplastic encephalomyelitis, and paraneoplastic cerebellar degeneration. See Table 25–1 for a list of common paraneoplastic disorders and their associated autoantibodies.

FAMILIAL TUMOR SYNDROMES/ CANCER-PREDISPOSING SYNDROMES

Most nervous system tumors occur sporadically. However, there are some syndromes that predispose affected individuals to cancers of both the nervous and other systems. We will review some of the more well-known syndromes in this chapter.

Neurofibromatosis Type 1

Neurofibromatosis type 1 (NF1), also known as von Recklinghausen syndrome, is a relatively common syndrome, affecting approximately 1 in 3000 people. NF1 is autosomal dominant but can also occur as the result of a spontaneous mutation. NF1 is due to a germline mutation of the *NF1* tumor suppressor gene (neurofibromin) on chromosome 17q11.2. Neurofibromin is a major negative regulator of Ras, which is a key protein involved in signaling for cell growth and division. NF1 affects multiple organ systems, with the central and peripheral nervous systems, the skin, the eyes, and the bones being most frequently involved. NF1 is commonly characterized by cutaneous findings of café-au-lait spots, axillary and inguinal freckling, optic gliomas, osseous lesions, and pigmented iris hamartomas (Lisch nodules) (Figure 25–17). Patients with NF1 are at increased risk of tumors including benign neurofibromas and intracranial tumors such as optic gliomas and meningiomas. The most common primary CNS tumors seen in NF1 are optic gliomas, and bilateral optic gliomas are considered to be virtually pathognomonic for NF1. Patients with NF1 are also at increased risk for other malignancies such as pheochromocytomas, malignant peripheral nerve sheath tumors, thyroid carcinomas, and leukemias. Most patients with NF1 are monitored closely with neurologic and ophthalmologic examinations, and any treatment is directed at specific complications.

Neurofibromatosis Type 2

Neurofibromatosis type 2 (NF2) is less common than NF1. It is an AD disorder, but spontaneous mutations do occur. NF2 is caused by germline mutations in the *NF2* gene on chromosome 22. *NF2* encodes for the tumor suppressor protein merlin (also called schwannomin) that plays an important role in the interaction of cytoskeletal components with proteins in the cell membrane. Clinically, NF2 primarily affects the nervous system, and one of the hallmark features of this disease is bilateral vestibular schwannomas, classically located at the bilateral cerebellopontine angles. Vestibular schwannomas can cause significant hearing loss, and management often involves surgical resection and/or radiation therapy. Other findings include cutaneous manifestations, such as café-au-lait spots and subcutaneous schwannomas, cataracts, gliomas, meningiomas, and spinal intramedullary ependymomas.

Tuberous Sclerosis

Tuberous sclerosis (TS) is a rare, multisystem autosomal dominant disorder that is characterized by hamartomas involving the nervous system, skin, and other organs such as the kidneys, heart, and lungs. Clinically, the nervous system is most often affected, and clinical manifestations can include seizures, developmental delay, intellectual disability, and behavioral problems. Other common clinical manifestations include cutaneous abnormalities, including facial angiofibromas, hypopigmented ash leaf spots, subungual fibromas, fibrous forehead plaques, and shagreen patches; cardiac rhabdomyomas; mitral regurgitation; and

TABLE 25–1 The main paraneoplastic disorders and their associated autoantibodies.

Neurologic Disorder	Clinical Features	Predominant Autoantibody	Tumor
Cerebellar degeneration	Ataxia, subacute	Anti-Yo (anti-Purkinje cell)	Ovary, fallopian tube, lung, Hodgkin disease (anti-Tr)
Encephalomyelitis including limbic and brainstem encephalitis	Subacute confusion, brainstem signs, myelitis	Anti-Hu (ANNA 1)	Small cell lung, neuroblastoma, prostate, breast, Hodgkin, testicular (Ma)
	Anti-Ma, Anti-CRMP-5, Anti-Caspr2		Psychosis, seizures, hypersympathetic state
Anti-NMDA, Anti-mGluR5	Ovarian (and other site) teratoma	Opsoclonus–myoclonus–ataxia	Ocular movement disorder, gait ataxia
Anti-Ri (ANNA 2)	Breast, fallopian tube, small cell lung	Retinal degeneration	Scotomas, blindness, disc swelling
Antirecoverin (Anti-CAR)	Small cell lung, thymoma, renal cell, melanoma	Subacute sensory neuropathy and neuronopathy	Distal or proximal sensory loss
Anti-Hu (ANNA-1)	Small cell lung, Hodgkin, other lymphomas	Lambert-Eaton myasthenic syndrome	Proximal fatiguing weakness, autonomic symptoms (dry mouth)
Anti-voltage-gated (VGCG) calcium channel	Small cell lung, Hodgkin, other lymphomas	Stiff person syndrome and neuromyotonia	Muscle spasms and rigidity
Antiamphiphysin, Anti-Caspr2, Anti-GAD	Breast, lung	Chorea	Bilateral choreoathetosis
Anti-Hu, Anti-CRMP-5	Lung, Hodgkin, others	Optic neuropathy	Blindness

In many cases, a particular autoantibody is associated with a specific tumor type rather than with the clinical syndrome (e.g., small cell lung cancer and polyneuropathy with ANNA 1, breast cancer with anti-Purkinje cell antibody, testicular tumors with anti-Ma). Clinical syndromes similar to each of these may occur with non–small cell lung cancer and lymphoma, most often in the absence of detectable antibodies.

Reproduced with permission from Ropper AH, Samuels MA, Klein JP: *Adams and Victor's Principles of Neurology*, 11th ed. New York, NY: McGraw Hill; 2019.

renal angiomyolipomas. Possible brain lesions include subependymal giant-cell astrocytomas (SEGAs) and cortical tubers, so called because these nodules become calcified and hard and resemble potatoes. SEGAs generally form in the ventricles of the brain and can lead to disruption in CSF flow, which can result in hydrocephalus that may clinically manifest as headaches and blurred vision. Individuals with tuberous sclerosis have germline mutations in either *TSC1* (chromosome 9q34), which encodes the protein hamartin, or *TSC2* (chromosome 16p13.3), which encodes the protein tuberin. Treatment of patients with tuberous sclerosis is primarily symptomatic and involves seizure control and tumor surveillance.

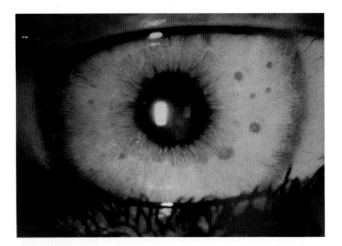

FIGURE 25–17 Hamartomas of the iris (Lisch nodules), typical of neurofibromatosis type 1. (Reproduced with permission from Spalton DJ, Hitchings RA, Hunter PA: *Atlas of Clinical Ophthalmology*, 3rd ed. Oxford, United Kingdom: Mosby Elsevier; 2005.)

Von Hippel-Lindau Disease

Von Hippel-Lindau (VHL) disease is a rare, AD condition that is characterized by hemangioblastomas of the retina and the CNS (particularly involving the brainstem, cerebellum, and spine), renal cell carcinomas, pheochromocytomas, and epididymal cysts. Hemangioblastomas are slow-growing, benign tumors that are highly vascular and have hyperchromatic nuclei. Hemangioblastomas are seen in approximately 75% of patients with VHL; however, only approximately 30% of patients with hemangioblastomas will have VHL. Regardless, patients who have a hemangioblastoma should also have a thorough workup that includes a funduscopic exam, a renal ultrasound, and consideration of imaging of the entire spine in order to exclude other lesions. VHL results from germline mutations in the *VHL* gene on chromosome 3q25. Patient with VHL require lifelong monitoring for associated tumors, and treatment of any tumors typically involves surgical resection.

Li-Fraumeni Syndrome

Li-Fraumeni syndrome (LFS) is an autosomal dominant cancer predisposition syndrome. It is linked to germline mutations of the *p53* tumor suppressor gene, which plays an important role in regulating cell cycles. Individuals with LFS are at increased risk for multiple malignancies including sarcomas, premenopausal breast cancers, leukemias, CNS neoplasms, and adrenal cortical carcinomas. Approximately 12% of the malignancies seen in LFS involve the CNS and can include astrocytomas, medulloblastomas, primitive neuroectodermal tumors, choroid plexus carcinomas, and ependymomas. As a result of the increased lifetime risk of cancer, individuals with LFS must be followed indefinitely.

Sturge-Weber Syndrome

Sturge-Weber syndrome (also known as encephalotrigeminal angiomatosis) is a congenital, noninherited disorder that is characterized by a port-wine nevus affecting the skin in the ophthalmic (V1) or maxillary (V2) distributions of the trigeminal nerve, leptomeningeal angiomas on the side of the brain ipsilateral to the port-wine stain (usually occipital), glaucoma, seizures, stroke, and intellectual disability. It is caused by a somatic activating mutation in the *GNAQ* gene, which plays a role in vascular development. There are several classical imaging findings associated with this syndrome, including gyral calcifications seen on head CT and "tram-track" calcifications, due to leptomeningeal vascular malformations, seen over the occipital or parietal regions on head CT or skull radiographs. Sturge-Weber syndrome is not associated with the development of either central or peripheral nervous system tumors.

CONCLUSION

Nervous system tumors are a large and varied group that can present diagnostic and treatment challenges. It is important to recognize the impact that these types of tumors can have on patients' lives and productivity and the significant morbidity and mortality associated with them. Treatment options largely consist of surgery, radiation therapy, and chemotherapy, and management often involves a multidisciplinary team of physicians.

SELF-ASSESSMENT QUESTIONS

1. A 50-year-old man is diagnosed with a malignant brain tumor. Which of the following is the most likely cause of malignant brain tumors in this age group?
   A. Malignant meningioma
   B. Glioblastoma
   C. Oligodendroglioma
   D. Anaplastic astrocytoma
   E. Pilocytic astrocytoma

2. A 9-year-old girl presents with headache and is found by imaging to have a cystic lesion with a protruding nodule in the cerebellum. On biopsy, the tumor is glial in origin, does not have brisk mitotic activity, and has eosinophilic granular droplets. What type of tumor is this?
   A. Craniopharyngioma
   B. Pilocytic astrocytoma
   C. Medulloblastoma
   D. Germinoma
   E. Oligodendroglioma

3. Which of the following finding is one of the features used to distinguish glioblastoma (GBM) from lower-grade astrocytomas?
   A. Mitoses
   B. Cellular density
   C. Necrosis
   D. Marked anaplasia

4. A patient presents with a tumor in the cerebellopontine angle. On biopsy, the pathology shows Verocay bodies, and the cells stain positive for S100. What type of tumor is this?
   A. Craniopharyngioma
   B. Germinoma
   C. Astrocytoma
   D. Neurofibroma
   E. Schwannoma

Headache Disorders & Neurologic Pain Syndromes

Cristina Wohlgehagen

OBJECTIVES

After studying this chapter, the student should be able to:

- Recognize and indicate treatment for the main primary headache disorders, including migraine with and without aura, tension-type headache, and trigeminal autonomic cephalgias.

- Recognize and indicate treatment for the main secondary headache disorders, including medication overuse headache, medication/caffeine withdrawal headache, idiopathic intracranial hypertension (pseudotumor cerebri), and spontaneous intracranial hypotension.

- Recognize the diagnostic "red flags" that warrant imaging and further workup.

- Identify the major neurologic pain syndromes, including fibromyalgia, complex regional pain syndrome, postherpetic neuralgia, trigeminal neuralgia, phantom limb pain, and central pain syndrome.

PREVALENCE & BURDEN

Headache is perhaps the most common neurologic syndrome. About half the world's population experiences headache at least once each year, and up to three-quarters of people will have a headache at some point in their lives. The most common type of headache is tension-type headache, followed by migraine. The 1-year prevalence of migraine in the United States is 12%, with a female predominance. Migraine prevalence is highest during some of the peak productive years of life (age 30 to 39 years), and 1 of every 4 migraineurs misses at least 1 day of work every 3 months. Migraine is among the top 10 causes of disability worldwide and accounts for the most years lived with disability of any neurologic disorder.

EVALUATION OF HEADACHE DISORDERS

The workup of a headache is guided by several factors in the history and exam (Figure 26–1). The more common primary headache disorders, namely migraine and tension-type headache, are diagnosed based on a thorough history and physical exam. Neuroimaging is not required unless the patient has an abnormal neurologic exam or the history is concerning. However, secondary headaches could masquerade as trigeminal autonomic cephalgias and some of the headaches classified under other primary headache disorders; therefore, further workup is often warranted. There are a number of potential "red flags" in the history that may suggest the need for further workup (Table 26–1).

PRIMARY HEADACHE SYNDROMES

Migraine

Migraine can present in childhood, but generally begins around puberty during adolescence or young adulthood. The pathophysiology of migraine is likely secondary to genetic predisposition and environmental factors leading to the phenotypic presentation of migraine. Three genetic mutations have been identified in familial hemiplegic migraine. These are the *CACNA1A* gene on chromosome 19, which encodes a P/Q type calcium channel subunit and increases presynaptic calcium; the *SCN1A* gene on chromosome 2, which encodes a sodium channel subunit and causes persistent sodium influx; and the *ATP1A2* gene on chromosome 1, which encodes a subunit of the sodium-potassium ATPase and decreases potassium and glutamate clearance. Mutations in the *PRRT2* gene, which is not an ion channel gene but encodes for synaptosomal-associated protein 25 (SNAP25), may also cause hemiplegic migraine. The genetics behind the more common

VOCABULARY

Abortive treatment: Treatments given at the onset of symptoms to reduce the severity of a headache.

Aura: Sensation that typically occurs shortly before a migraine headache begins. Auras are most commonly visual but can involve motor or other sensory changes as well.

Cephalgia: Synonym for headache.

Neuromediators: Also known as neuromodulators, chemical substances released in the central nervous system or in the periphery that can regulate a broad population of neurons.

Phonophobia: Discomfort associated with sensitivity to sound/noise.

Photophobia: Discomfort associated with light sensitivity.

Preventative treatment: Treatments used on a daily basis to reduce the frequency of headaches.

Primary headaches: Those in which headache is the primary problem, such as tension or migraine headaches.

Secondary headaches: Those due to another condition, such as sinusitis or intracerebral hemorrhage.

Trigger: A stimulus that can set off a migraine, for example, stress or a particular food.

types of migraine are likely multifactorial and still under study. It is thought that patients with migraine have cortical neuronal hyperexcitability and likely abnormal brainstem function.

The initiating mechanism of a migraine headache is thought to be secondary to cortical spreading depression (Figure 26–2). This is a wave of increased cortical neuronal activity, followed by neuronal suppression. Cortical spreading depression propagates at a velocity of 2 to 3 mm per minute. The aura spreads at a similar speed, and therefore, it has been attributed to cortical spreading depression. When the cortical spreading depression initiates in the occipital lobes, a visual aura ensues. Migraine without aura may result from cortical spreading depression in a clinically silent area of cortex. Cortical spreading depression (via an unknown mechanism) is thought to activate the trigeminal vascular system and release of substances involved in pain pathways including calcitonin gene-related peptide and glutamate. The trigeminal vascular system and neuromediators cause the headache and likely lead to neurogenic inflammation and peripheral sensitization. If the headache persists, central sensitization and allodynia can occur in a pattern similar to that which arises with chronic pain in other parts of the body (Figure 26–3).

A migraine attack can be divided into 4 phases: (1) the premonitory phase, which occurs hours to days before the onset of head pain and includes various symptoms ranging from euphoria to fatigue; (2) the aura phase, when neurologic symptoms occur just before or during the headache onset; (3) the headache phase, which includes the associated migrainous

symptoms; and (4) the postdrome. Migraine is a recurrent headache disorder that is diagnosed clinically based on diagnostic criteria. Neuroimaging is not indicated unless historical warning signs (see Table 26–1) are present or the neurologic exam is abnormal, but may reveal small subcortical hyperintensities that are not periventricular or in the corpus callosum.

Migraine headache can be episodic or chronic, and chronic migraine is defined as a headache on at least 15 days per month with a minimum of 8 days meeting criteria for migraine. Migraine can be further characterized as migraine with or without aura. Based on diagnostic criteria, an untreated migraine attack lasts 4 to 72 hours in adults but can be of shorter duration in children. It has at least 2 of the following 4 characteristics: (1) unilateral location (Figure 26–4), (2) pulsating quality, (3) moderate to severe pain intensity, and (4) aggravation by or causing avoidance of routine physical activity. During the headache, the patient must have 1 of the following features: (1) nausea and/or vomiting or (2) phonophobia and photophobia.

Migraine aura has ≥1 visual, sensory, speech and/or language, motor, brainstem, or retinal symptoms that are fully reversible, with at least 2 of the following 4 characteristics: (1) aura spreads gradually over >5 minutes and/or symptoms occur in succession; (2) each individual aura symptom lasts 5 to 60 minutes; (3) at least 1 aura symptom is unilateral; or (4) the aura is accompanied or followed within 60 minutes by headache. Each individual aura can last up to 1 hour, so if a patient has multiple aura symptoms in succession, the total aura time will be longer than 60 minutes.

Migraine with aura has several different variants; these include migraine with typical aura, migraine with brainstem aura, hemiplegic migraine, and retinal migraine. In migraine with typical aura, the aura consists of visual, sensory, and/or speech and language symptoms. However, it excludes motor, brainstem, and retinal symptoms. The typical visual aura is described as a scintillating scotoma with a zig-zag "fortification spectra," which slowly enlarges at a speed similar to that of cortical spreading depression (Figure 26–5). Migraine with brainstem aura requires at least 2 of the following brainstem symptoms: (1) dysarthria, (2) vertigo, (3) tinnitus, (4) hypoacusis (hearing impairment), (5) diplopia, (6) ataxia, and (7) decreased level of consciousness. Hemiplegic migraine is a subtype of migraine with aura in which the aura is a syndrome of fully reversible motor weakness and fully reversible visual, sensory, and/or speech or language symptoms. Retinal aura is distinguished from the typical visual aura because it is a monocular positive or negative visual phenomenon. This is confirmed by clinical visual examination during an attack or the patient's drawing of a monocular field defect.

Migraine Treatment: Preventive

The treatment of migraine headaches hinges on both preventive and abortive therapies. All patients who suffer from migraine headaches should be counseled on lifestyle modifications, such as regular sleep and meals, healthy diet and exercise, and avoidance of triggers, as part of their preventive therapy.

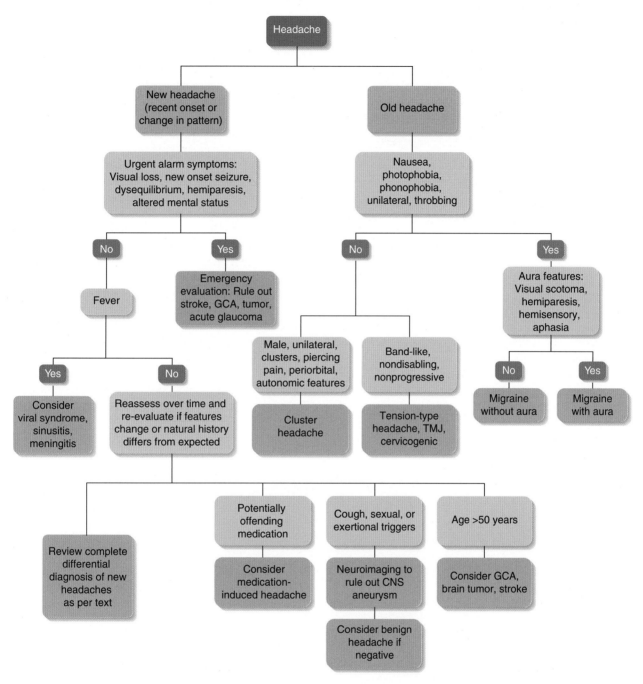

FIGURE 26–1 Headache algorithm. It is important to understand new-onset versus chronic headache and then tease out warning signs for potential secondary headache from a patient's history and physical exam. CNS, central nervous system; GCA, giant-cell arteritis; TMJ, temporomandibular joint. (Reproduced with permission from Henderson MC, Tierney LM, Smetana GW: *The Patient History: Evidence-Based Approach to Differential Diagnosis.* 2nd ed. New York, NY: McGraw Hill; 2012.)

Common triggers for migraine headache include stress, hormonal changes, skipping meals, weather changes, sleep disturbances, strong odors (eg, perfume, gasoline, smoke), lights, alcohol, food (eg, tyramine in aged meat/cheese and ripe bananas, aspartame), and heat. Some migraine triggers cannot be avoided. Migraine patients should be offered prescription preventive migraine therapy if they have >3 migraine days *without* disability per month or >2 migraine days *with* disability per month.

For optimal prevention of migraine headaches, it is important to involve patients in their care. Consider comorbidities, and when possible, choose a single medication to treat multiple diseases. With women of childbearing age, discuss contraception and the potential risk of medication use during pregnancy. Each preventive medication should be started at a low dose and slowly titrated up. It is important to give each preventive medication an adequate trial. Generally, once at a therapeutic dose, a preventive medication should be

TABLE 26–1 Warning signs in the history that raise concern.

- Change or progression in pattern (increasing frequency or severity)
- The first and/or worst headache of a person's life
- New headache in an individual >40 years old
- New headache in a patient with cancer, immunosuppression, or pregnancy
- Sudden and abrupt onset of attacks (thunderclap), including awakenings from sleep
- Headaches triggered by exertion, sexual activity, or Valsalva maneuvers (bearing down, coughing, or sneezing)
- Neurologic symptoms lasting >1 hour
- Associated alteration of consciousness
- Indications of systemic illness (fever, rash, weight loss, meningismus)
- History of head trauma

continued for at least 6 weeks before reevaluating. The use of headache calendars before and after initiation of migraine preventive therapy can give objective data on the efficacy of the drug in that patient.

Medications with established efficacy (level A evidence) for the prevention of migraine include antiepileptic agents (divalproex sodium, topiramate) and β-blockers (metoprolol, propranolol). Divalproex sodium should be considered in someone with concomitant mood disorders and requires monitoring for weight gain, hyponatremia, and hepatitis. Topiramate might be helpful in an overweight patient, as it can cause weight loss. It is contraindicated in patients with renal calculi and glaucoma. Patients need to be monitored for cognitive complaints and should be warned about tingling and changes in taste (carbonated drinks taste "flat"), which are common side effects. Other antiepileptics that can be beneficial in the treatment of headaches include gabapentin, levetiracetam, zonisamide, and lacosamide. Propranolol should be considered in someone with concomitant hypertension or anxiety. It should be avoided in individuals with asthma or diabetes. Patients on an antihypertensive need to be monitored for signs and symptoms of hypotension and bradycardia. Other antihypertensives that can be considered in the preventive treatment of migraine are verapamil and candesartan.

Medications that are probably effective (level B evidence) for the prophylaxis of migraine headaches include antidepressants (amitriptyline, venlafaxine). Amitriptyline should be considered in someone with insomnia or mild depression. It should be used with caution in patients with cardiovascular disease because it can lead to arrhythmia, and an electrocardiogram is warranted prior to initiation in this population of patients. The main side effect is sedation, although it has the potential

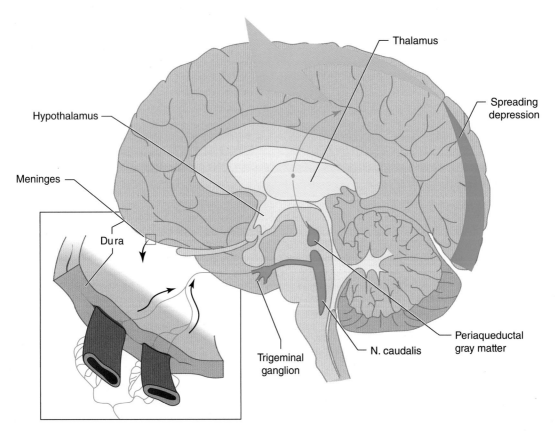

FIGURE 26–2 Cortical spreading depression. Cortical spreading depression is a wave of increased cortical neuronal activity, followed by neuronal suppression that propagates at a velocity of 2 to 3 mm per minute. It is thought to be the initiating mechanism in migraine. (Reproduced with permission from Simon RP, Aminoff MJ, Greemberg DA: *Clinical Neurology*, 10th ed. New York, NY: McGraw Hill; 2018.)

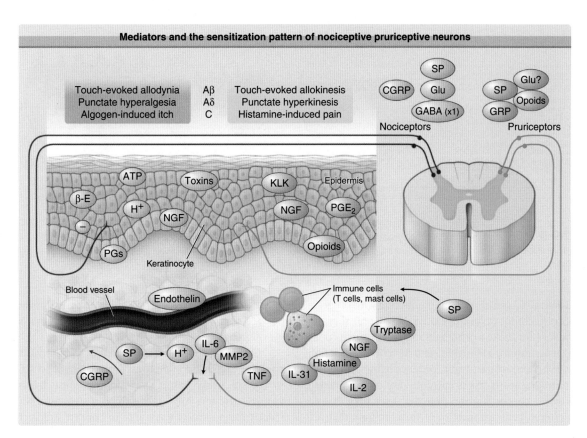

FIGURE 26–3 Allodynia. Central sensitization and allodynia can occur in patients with refractory headache. It is similar to other types of chronic pain. This phenomenon is thought to be mediated by neuromodulators such as calcitonin gene-related peptide (CGRP) and glutamate (Glu). ATP, adenosine triphosphate; GABA, γ-aminobutyric acid; GRP, gastrin-releasing peptide; IL, interleukin; KLK, kallikrein; MMP, matrix metalloprotease; NGF, nerve growth factor; PGs, prostaglandins; PGE_2, prostaglandin E_2; SP, substance P; TNF, tumor necrosis factor. (Reproduced with permission from Goldsmith LA, Katz SI, Gilchrest BA, et al: *Fitzpatrick's Dermatology in General Medicine*, 8th ed. New York, NY: McGraw Hill; 2012.)

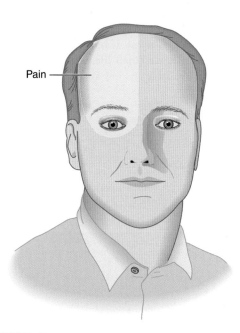

FIGURE 26–4 Migraine. The pain pattern in migraine is most often severe unilateral frontal and/or temporal throbbing that can radiate to involve the retro- or supraorbital region. (Reproduced with permission from Simon RP, Aminoff MJ, Greemberg DA: *Clinical Neurology*, 10th ed. New York, NY: McGraw Hill; 2018.)

to cause other anticholinergic side effects including xerostomia, dizziness, blurred vision, constipation, and urinary retention (especially in the elderly). Patients should also be monitored for suicidal ideation. Alternative tricyclic antidepressants that can be used for the prevention of migraine include nortriptyline and protriptyline. Venlafaxine might be useful in a migraine patient who suffers from moderate depression. It requires routine laboratory monitoring of renal function and lipids. Patients should also be monitored for hypertension and, as with many of the antidepressants, suicidal ideation.

If medications in the anticonvulsant, antihypertensive, and antidepressant categories are ineffective or contraindicated, memantine (category B in pregnancy) should be considered in the prevention of migraine headaches. Supraorbital nerve stimulation has also been shown to be an effective preventive therapy. In addition, in a patient who meets criteria for chronic migraine, injection of botulinum toxin in the face, occiput, neck, and shoulders following the chronic migraine paradigm is effective at decreasing the intensity and frequency of migraine attacks. The calcitonin gene-related peptide (CGRP) receptor antagonists are a newer class of preventive treatments made specifically for migraine. CGRP antagonists appear to have good efficacy with a low side effect profile, though their long term effects are unknown.

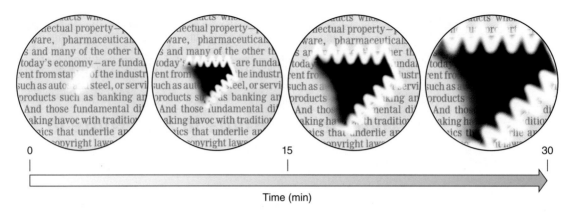

Time (min)

FIGURE 26–5 Visual aura in migraine. The typical visual aura associated with migraine headache is described as a scintillating scotoma, which spreads at about 2 to 3 mm per minute. (Reproduced with permission from Simon RP, Aminoff MJ, Greemberg DA: *Clinical Neurology*, 10th ed. New York, NY: McGraw Hill; 2018.)

These treatments can be used in conjunction with progressive relaxation techniques and cognitive behavioral therapy. There is evidence for the use of herbal supplements such coenzyme Q10, magnesium, riboflavin, and feverfew. Although *Petasites hybridus* extract has strong evidence in the preventive treatment of migraine, its use is currently not recommended because of safety concerns given potential liver toxicity and carcinogenic/teratogenic properties of formulations that are not free of pyrrolizine alkaloids. Trigeminal and occipital distribution nerve and sphenopalatine ganglion blocks, as well as trigger point injections using local anesthetic, may also be beneficial as adjunctive therapy for both the prophylaxis and acute treatment of migraine.

If a patient has predictable migraine headaches during menses, she may qualify for a "mini-prophylaxis." Instead of taking a daily preventive medication, she would use therapy the week of her expected migraine headache, which can be calculated fairly accurately in someone with regular menstrual cycles. Although the traditional preventive migraine medications can be used during the week of prophylaxis, using frovatriptan has been found to be effective (level A evidence) for this purpose. Aside from this setting, medications in the triptan category are traditionally used for migraine abortive treatment, especially because of their potential to cause medication overuse headache.

Migraine Treatment: Abortive

As an adjunct strategy to preventive therapies in the treatment of migraine, patients should be offered abortive agents. Migraine-specific medications include ergot derivatives and triptans. These medications act as serotonin (5-HT) receptor agonists. Triptans are more selective 5-HT receptor agonists than ergotamine and dihydroergotamine, acting on 5-HT 1B/1D receptors. Triptans are the abortive treatment of choice in migraine headache (level A evidence). Contraindications to triptans include untreated arterial hypertension, coronary artery disease, history of ischemic stroke, administration of an ergot compound within 24 hours of triptan use, severe renal or

hepatic disease, peripheral vascular disease, Raynaud disease, age >65 years, and migraine with brainstem aura or hemiplegic migraine.

Originally, migraine was thought to be a vascular disorder, and brainstem symptoms were thought to be secondary to basilar artery vasoconstriction. Because triptans induce vasoconstriction, migraine with brainstem aura was excluded from triptan clinical trials due to concerns of increasing the risk of brain infarction and is thus not a formal indication for triptan therapy. However, it is now clearer that aura is primarily a neuronal process related to cortical spreading depression, and more recent literature suggests that treating these patients with triptans may actually be beneficial without increased risk for ischemic vascular events.

A variety of triptans are approved for migraine treatment (**Figure 26–6**). Sumatriptan was the first triptan introduced for acute migraine treatment. It has the fastest time to peak levels but also the shortest half-life. Sumatriptan and zolmitriptan are both available in oral and nonoral formulations.

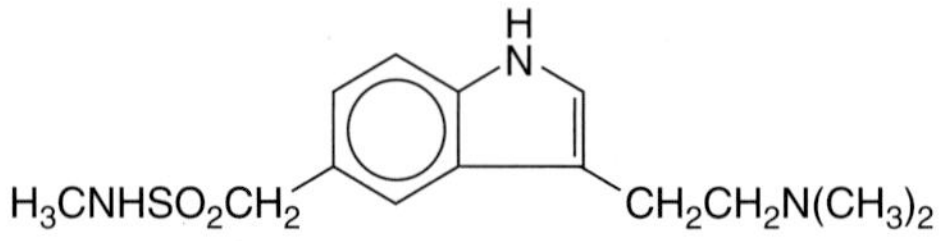

H$_3$CNHSO$_2$CH$_2$ — CH$_2$CH$_2$N(CH$_3$)$_2$

Sumatriptan

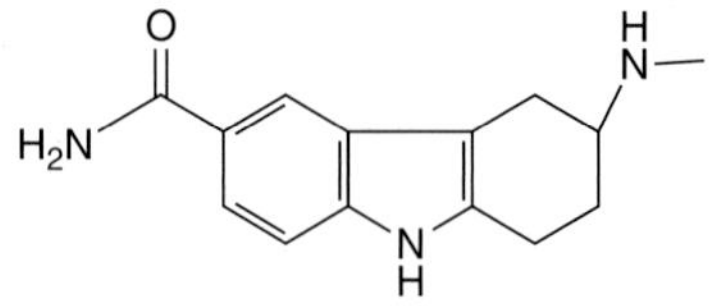

H$_2$N — **Frovatriptan**

FIGURE 26–6 The chemical structure of triptans. Sumatriptan was the first triptan introduced for acute migraine treatment. It has the fastest time to peak levels, but also the fastest half-life. Because of a variation in chemical structure, frovatriptan has a slower onset and lower potency, but also the longest half-life of this class of medications.

Rizatriptan is available in an oral tablet, as well as an oral disintegrating tablet. Almotriptan, eletriptan, frovatriptan, and naratriptan are only available in an oral tablet formulation. Frovatriptan and naratriptan have a slower onset and lower potency but also a lower headache reoccurrence rate because they are longer lasting. Frovatriptan has the longest half-life of the triptans.

When choosing a triptan, it is important to consider how quickly the headache climaxes, as well as associated symptoms of nausea and vomiting. Gastroparesis is common during migraine. Although a patient might be able to tolerate oral medications without symptoms of nausea, vomiting, or bloating, the absorption of medications may be delayed. Therefore, nonoral triptans should be considered early, especially if gastrointestinal symptoms are present. Unlike preventive therapy where one would "start low and go slow," symptomatic therapy should be prescribed at the dose most likely to be effective within the prescribing range. If a lower dose formulation is partially effective, the patient should be instructed to redose, and the practitioner should prescribe the equivalent higher dose formulation in the future.

In patients who cannot take triptans, longer acting nonsteroidal anti-inflammatory drugs (NSAIDs) such as diclofenac and naproxen can be used as abortive therapy (level A evidence). These have less of a potential for medication overuse headache. If triptans and NSAIDs cannot be used, then combination medications with isometheptene can be considered. Cyclobenzaprine has a similar chemical structure to amitriptyline and can also be used as an adjunct for symptomatic headache therapy. It is unlikely to cause medication overuse headache. Adding antiemetics, especially in the setting of gastrointestinal symptoms, may also be beneficial. In patients with migraine with aura, transcranial magnetic stimulation at the occipitalis is another option.

The patient should also be counseled on how to use symptomatic medication effectively, using migraine-specific medications when possible at headache onset. Waiting until the headache has built up in intensity may render the symptomatic medication less effective. The goal is to stop the headache, not just to decrease the intensity. The patient should limit all pain medications to 9 days or less per month to avoid medication overuse headache. Note that it is the number of days, not the total number of times during a day, that puts the patient at risk. Therefore, if within prescribing range, the patient should redose or use multiple medications from different categories in an effort to completely abort the headache.

Medication overuse headache only occurs in patients with primary headache disorders. It is defined as a headache occurring ≥15 days per month, with regular overuse for >3 months of ≥1 medication that can be taken for symptomatic relief of headache. The top 3 offenders are caffeine, butalbital, and opioids. However, any symptomatic pain medication or decongestant, whether used for headache or another condition, has the potential to cause medication overuse headache in a patient with a primary headache disorder. Therefore, patients should avoid, if possible: (1) opioids (including butorphanol nasal spray); (2) combination medications containing

CASE 26–1

A 33-year-old obese woman presents with headaches that started around puberty. The headaches have become more frequent and more intense over the years but have not changed in character. They begin with visual distortion that is described as a scintillating scotoma that slowly enlarges over 10 minutes to involve the right hemifield and then dissipates over 30 minutes. This is accompanied by a dull ache and followed by severe hemicranial pain that builds up over an hour and is pounding in character. Associated symptoms include severe photophobia and phonophobia but no nausea or vomiting. Movement makes the headaches worse. The patient can sometimes have nasal congestion, but there are no unilateral autonomic symptoms. The headaches are not positional and not worsened by Valsalva. The headaches are disabling and last for about a day. They occur 3 times per month. Triggers include work-related stress, sleep deprivation, and red wine. She is on oral contraceptive pills and takes ibuprofen (which only minimally decreases the intensity) for her headaches 3 days per month. The patient's neurologic examination, which includes funduscopy, is normal.

The diagnosis is episodic migraine with aura. The patient should be counseled on lifestyle modifications and trigger avoidance and offered a preventive treatment. She is obese and on birth control, so topiramate might be a good option for her in the absence of a history of renal calculi or glaucoma. The patient has migraine with aura and should be counseled on progesterone only or other non-hormonal forms of birth control given small increase in risk for stroke in this patient population. She is a good candidate for oral sumatriptan for abortive therapy because she can tolerate oral medications during a headache and her migraine builds up relatively slowly. She should be counseled to take the sumatriptan at headache onset and limit symptomatic medications to ≤9 days per month.

butalbital, tramadol, or caffeine; and (3) short-acting NSAIDs (eg, ibuprofen). In addition, because many symptomatic medications are available over the counter, it is important to ask patients about nonprescription medication use (type and number of days per week). This is especially important because in the setting of medication overuse headache, preventive and abortive medications are less efficacious.

Tension-Type Headache

The prevalence of episodic tension-type headache is high, as it is the most common primary headache disorder in the population. It affects women slightly more than men, with an onset between the second and third decades of life and the highest prevalence between the third and fourth decades of life. Much like migraine, there is a decline in the prevalence of tension-type headache later in life. Because the severity of tension-type headache remains mild to moderate, patients are less likely to seek medical attention unless the headache becomes more frequent and meets criteria for the frequent episodic or chronic tension-type headache subtypes. The pathophysiology of tension-type headache is under investigation. It is thought that peripheral pain mechanisms are involved in episodic tension-type headache, whereas central pain mechanisms are more significant in chronic tension-type headache.

Tension-type headache is further subdivided into the following subtypes: infrequent episodic (once per month; <12 days per year), frequent episodic (<15 days per month; >12 days but <180 days per year), and chronic (>15 days per month; >180 days per year). The headache can last 30 minutes to 7 days in the episodic subtype and hours to days if not unremitting in the chronic tension-type subtype. It requires 2 of the following 4 characteristics: (1) bilateral location (Figure 26–7), (2) pressing or tightening (nonpulsating) quality, (3) mild or moderate intensity, and (4) not aggravated by routine physical activity. Tension-type headache requires no more than 1 symptom of photophobia, phonophobia, or mild nausea and neither of the symptoms of moderate or severe nausea or vomiting.

Episodic infrequent tension-type headache can be treated with over-the-counter analgesics including acetaminophen, aspirin, and ibuprofen. There is always the potential for medication overuse headache, and the patient should be instructed to take symptomatic medications 9 days or less per month, or about twice per week. Episodic frequent and chronic tension-type headaches can cause moderate to severe disability and are treated with a treatment strategy similar to migraine headache. Amitriptyline has been shown to be efficacious in the preventive treatment (level I evidence) of tension-type headache; however, given the overlap between migraine and tension-type headache, other migraine prophylactic agents can also be used.

Trigeminal Autonomic Cephalgias

The trigeminal autonomic cephalgias are a group of headache disorders characterized by unilateral headache associated with ipsilateral autonomic features. These include cluster headache, paroxysmal hemicrania, short-lasting unilateral neuralgiform headache attacks (with 2 forms: short-lasting unilateral neuralgiform headache attacks with conjunctival injection and short-lasting unilateral neuralgiform headache attacks with cranial autonomic symptoms), and hemicrania continua.

Cluster headaches are very severe headaches that occur in bouts, typically every 6 to 24 months. During a bout, patients have a number of cluster attacks (headaches), usually 0.5 to 8 per day when the disorder is active. Although not part of the diagnostic criteria, circadian periodicity is a hallmark of cluster headaches, and the times of attacks are often predictable, frequently occurring at night. The syndrome is relatively rare and male predominant.

Cluster headaches attacks cause unilateral orbital, supraorbital, and/or temporal pain lasting 15 to 180 minutes (Figure 26–8). These headaches are very intense and are often referred to as "suicide headaches" because they pain is

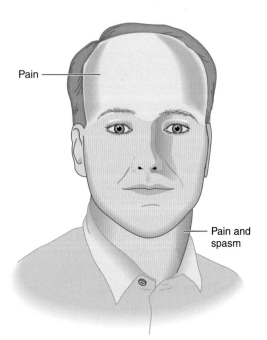

FIGURE 26–7 Tension-type headache. The pain pattern in tension-type headache is most often bilateral and frontal pressure or aching that is mild to moderate in intensity. (Reproduced with permission from Simon RP, Aminoff MJ, Greemberg DA: *Clinical Neurology*, 10th ed. New York, NY: McGraw Hill; 2018.)

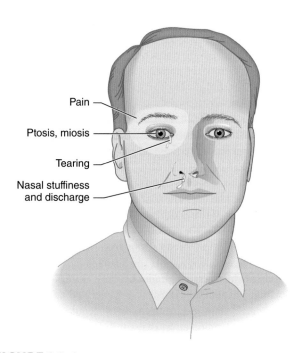

FIGURE 26–8 Autonomic symptoms in a patient with cluster headache. This patient has severe right-sided headache, mainly involving his eye, that is associated with right-sided ptosis. It is difficult to appreciate other autonomic symptoms such as miosis, flushing, and rhinorrhea that may also be present in this picture. (Reproduced with permission from Simon RP, Aminoff MJ, Greemberg DA: *Clinical Neurology*, 10th ed. New York, NY: McGraw Hill; 2018.)

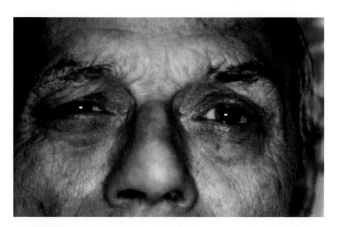

FIGURE 26-9 Cluster headache. The pain pattern in cluster headache is most commonly abrupt, excruciating orbital or periorbital pain associated with autonomic symptoms. These include unilateral conjunctival injection, lacrimation, eyelid edema, ptosis, miosis, nasal congestion/rhinorrhea, sweating, and/or flushing on the same side as the headache. (Reproduced with permission from Simon RP, Aminoff MJ, Greemberg DA: *Clinical Neurology*, 10th ed. New York, NY: McGraw Hill; 2018.)

so severe it can lead to suicidal ideation or attempt during an attack. Cluster headaches must have either or both of the following: (1) at least 1 ipsilateral autonomic symptom including conjunctival injection, lacrimation, eyelid edema, ptosis, miosis, nasal congestion and/or rhinorrhea, forehead and facial sweating and/or flushing, and/or a sensation of fullness in the ear (Figure 26–9), or (2) a sense of restlessness or agitation during an attack. Unlike migraine patients who prefer to be still during an attack, patients with cluster headache tend to pace and move around during a cluster episode.

Prior to diagnosis, secondary disorders that can present like cluster headache, including pituitary tumors, need to be ruled out. Therefore, this patient population needs neuroimaging with magnetic resonance imaging (MRI) of the brain at presentation. If the history is suspicious for vascular etiology, then further vascular imaging of the head and neck may be warranted to look for arterial dissection, aneurysm, or arteriovenous malformations, among other causes. Management of cluster attacks involves counseling against alcohol use during the cluster bout and discussing the use of preventive and abortive therapies.

The drug treatment of choice for a cluster attack is subcutaneous sumatriptan. When available, continuous inhalation of 100% oxygen at 7 to 12 L/min via a non-rebreathing facial mask for 15 to 20 minutes can completely abort a cluster attack. However, a quarter of patients find that oxygen only delays an attack. Preventive medications are used to speed up the time to remission and to decrease the frequency and intensity of cluster attacks during a bout. Except in patients with chronic cluster headache, there is no evidence that continuing prophylactic medications beyond the cluster bout is beneficial. Preventive treatments that can be used include lithium, verapamil, gabapentin, topiramate, valproic acid, corticosteroids, and high-dose melatonin. Greater occipital nerve and

sphenopalatine ganglion blocks using local anesthetic in combination with steroid can also be effective.

Hemicrania continua is more common in women and generally presents in adulthood. It is a unilateral, mild to moderate continuous headache with exacerbations of moderate to severe intensity that often has both autonomic and migrainous associated symptoms. The diagnostic criteria require either or both of the following: (1) at least 1 ipsilateral autonomic symptom and/or (2) a sense of restlessness or agitation or aggravation of pain by movement. Hemicrania continua is an indomethacin-responsive headache. The treatment and diagnosis rest on the response to indomethacin, and the dose should be up titrated to at least 50 mg 3 times per day before efficacy is determined. If needed, it can be increased to 75 mg 3 times per day as tolerated. In patients who cannot tolerate indomethacin, *Boswellia serrata* extract is an herbal supplement with a similar chemical structure that may be beneficial.

Other Primary Headache Disorders

The other primary headache disorders include primary cough headache, primary exercise headache, primary headache associated with sexual activity, primary thunderclap headache, cold-stimulus headache, external-pressure headache, hypnic headache, primary stabbing headache, new daily persistent headache, and nummular headache.

Hypnic headache mainly occurs in the elderly (age >40 to 50 years) and is more common in women. It presents as frequent headaches that are only present during sleep and usually occur around the same time each night. The diagnostic criteria require that the recurrent headache attacks (1) develop only during sleep and cause awakenings; (2) occur on ≥10 days a month; (3) last from 15 minutes to 4 hours after awakening; and (4) have no autonomic symptoms or a sense of restlessness. Other causes of secondary headache that can lead to nocturnal awakenings such as sleep apnea, nocturnal hypertension, subdural hematomas, communicating hydrocephalus, vascular lesions, temporal arteritis, pheochromocytomas, subacute angle-closure glaucoma, and medication overuse or withdrawal headache need to be excluded. Scheduled bedtime caffeine, melatonin, indomethacin, and lithium have been found to be effective in the treatment of hypnic headache.

Primary stabbing headache often occurs in migraine patients and can coexist in those with other primary headache disorders. Among other descriptions, it has been referred to as "jabs and jolts syndrome" and "ice pick headache." It is characterized by brief and localized stabs of pain that occur in the absence of pathologic damage to underlying structures or cranial nerves. The diagnostic criteria require head pain occurring spontaneously as a single stab or a series of stabs where (1) each stab lasts for up to a few seconds; (2) stabs recur with irregular frequency, from 1 to many per day; and (3) there are no cranial autonomic symptoms. Other causes for similar pain such as meningioma and pituitary tumors, cerebrovascular diseases, cranial or ocular trauma, and herpes zoster need to be ruled out prior to diagnosis. This is usually an indomethacin-responsive headache at total daily doses of 25 to 150 mg. However, if a patient is unable to tolerate indomethacin, success has been reported with high-dose melatonin or the use of gabapentin.

New daily persistent headache is described as development of a daily and unremitting headache in a patient who does not have history of major life stressor, trauma, or illness prior to the onset of headaches. There usually is no history of prior headaches; however, if such history is present, then the patient does not report a crescendo in headache frequency and/or intensity over the time preceding onset of daily headaches. If present, this pattern might suggest medication overuse headache or other types of secondary headache. A patient with new daily persistent headache is able to give a definitive date of when the headache started. The diagnostic criteria necessitate a distinct and clearly remembered onset, with pain becoming continuous and unremitting within 24 hours. Since the diagnosis of new daily persistent headache is one of exclusion, it requires normal neuroimaging, lumbar puncture, and blood work. Preventive medications used for other headache disorders are often tried in new daily persistent headache with variable efficacy.

Nummular headache has a female predominance with a mean age of onset in the fourth decade of life. The root of the word means "resembling a coin," and the pain usually affects a small, coin-shaped area of the scalp. The character of the pain can differ from one patient to the next and has been described as pressure-like, sharp, achy, throbbing, burning, or itching. There can also be exacerbations in the intensity of pain. The diagnostic criteria require continuous or intermittent head pain felt exclusively in the scalp with the following 4 characteristics: (1) sharply contoured, (2) fixed in size and shape, (3) round or elliptical, and (4) 1 to 6 cm in diameter. Gabapentin, tricyclic antidepressants, and injections of botulinum toxin at the headache site have been found to be effective in the treatment of nummular headache.

SECONDARY HEADACHE SYNDROMES

It is important to know the warning signs that need to be worked up in order to distinguish primary from secondary headache disorders. Historical "red flags" or an abnormal neurologic exam needs to be expeditiously investigated. Despite being aware of these warning signs, some secondary headaches can be missed if the practitioner does not have a high level of suspicion, and these include medication overuse headaches and medication or caffeine withdrawal headaches. Further, the presence of these headaches can have a great impact on the efficacy of preventive and abortive headache treatments. **Medication overuse headache** was described earlier in the migraine section to emphasize the most common offending agents and stress the importance of limiting symptomatic migraine therapy to ≤9 days per month.

Medication withdrawal headache requires daily intake of a substance for >3 months that has been interrupted. Evidence

of causation is demonstrated by both of the following: (1) the headache has developed in close temporal relation to withdrawal from the substance, and (2) the headache has resolved within 3 months after total withdrawal from the substance. Caffeine withdrawal headache requires caffeine consumption of >200 mg/d (~2 cups of coffee) for >2 weeks, which has been interrupted or delayed. There is also evidence of causation demonstrated by development of the headache within 24 hours of last caffeine intake and either headache relief within 1 hour of taking 100 mg of caffeine or resolution within 7 days of total caffeine withdrawal.

Medication overuse and withdrawal are probably the most common causes of intractability in migraine patients. These causes can be missed by a practitioner because patients often do not include over-the-counter analgesics, decongestants, and herbal supplements in their medication list. In addition, caffeine intake is generally not part of a routine social history and can be overlooked. Some patients are also embarrassed about medication misuse, and therefore, it is essential to take a detailed medication history focusing on both prescription and over-the-counter medications, including vitamins, herbs, and natural products. Excessive use of symptomatic agents and caffeine overuse (on average more than once a day) can cause intractable migraine, and vitamin A or D overuse may lead to headaches. When stopping or tapering the offending agent, the patient may have an initial worsening of the headache before there is improvement. This worsening can be bridged with relaxation therapy and outpatient pharmacologic treatment using long-acting NSAIDs, muscle relaxers, or steroids, but may require inpatient admission for detoxification from an offending agent if the patient has daily use of potent opioids and/or barbiturates or has failed outpatient attempts.

High- and low-pressure headaches can also be tricky to diagnose. The historical warning signs (see Table 26–1) and neurologic exam can raise the clinician's level of suspicion, but it can sometimes be difficult to distinguish between the 2 conditions.

Idiopathic Intracranial Hypertension

Idiopathic intracranial hypertension, also known as pseudotumor cerebri, most commonly occurs in obese women of childbearing age. The disease is most prevalent in the second and third decades of life. The majority of patients present with headache that is worse with lying down and Valsalva maneuvers. It is accompanied by symptoms of increased intracranial pressure including transient episodes of visual loss and visual obscurations, pulse-synchronous tinnitus, diplopia due to cranial nerve VI palsy, and papilledema (**Figure 26–10**), which is the hallmark of idiopathic intracranial hypertension, with associated visual loss.

Idiopathic intracranial hypertension is characterized by increased cerebrospinal fluid opening pressure (>250 mm H$_2$O) without evidence of ventriculomegaly. It is thought to be secondary to decreased absorption of cerebrospinal fluid, although increased production may also play a role. Neurodiagnostic

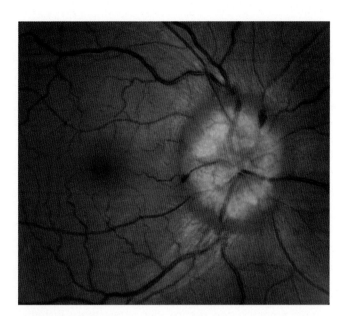

FIGURE 26–10 Papilledema. Optic disk swelling caused by raised intracranial pressure. (Reproduced with permission from Kasper D, Fauci A, Hauser S, et al: *Harrison's Principles of Internal Medicine*, 19th ed. New York, NY: McGraw Hill; 2015.)

studies reveal no ventricular obstruction, abnormal enhancement, or intracranial lesion to explain the increased pressure. MRI of the brain can show signs of increased intracranial pressure including flattening of the posterior sclera and a partial empty sella turcica. Potential intracranial lesions include scarring secondary to previous inflammation (eg, meningitis, subarachnoid hemorrhage) leading to decreased flow through the arachnoid granulations and venous sinus thrombosis causing obstruction of venous flow. Arteriovenous malformations and dural shunts are also associated with intracranial hypertension. Other potential secondary causes of intracranial hypertension include corticosteroid withdrawal, increased vitamin A, and the use of isotretinoin and tetracycline. The differential also includes obstructive sleep apnea and orthostatic edema (abnormal systemic retention of sodium and/or water).

Most patients with idiopathic intracranial hypertension and papilledema have visual loss, and perimetry to assess visual field defects is the main measure used to determine the course of therapy. The management of idiopathic intracranial hypertension is divided into symptomatic treatment of headaches and treatment of increased intracranial pressure. Medications used in prophylaxis of migraine can be effective in symptomatic treatment of headaches; however, agents that cause weight gain should be avoided or monitored closely. Topiramate can be used for the treatment of headache, but it is a weak carbonic anhydrase inhibitor, and therefore, it should not be used alone to decrease intracranial hypertension.

Patients should be counseled on weight loss (about 10% of the patient's body weight) as an effective treatment of intracranial hypertension. A low-sodium diet and avoiding excessive fluid intake can also help in the management of idiopathic intracranial hypertension. Acetazolamide is effective at

lowering intracranial pressure because it is a carbonic anhydrase inhibitor that reduces production of cerebrospinal fluid. It can cause changes in taste, paresthesias, and drowsiness. Furosemide is a second-line agent that is efficacious in the treatment of idiopathic intracranial hypertension either alone or in combination with acetazolamide. It is thought to work both by decreasing sodium transport to the brain and increasing urine production. However, potassium supplementation is required. If the patient is refractory to medical treatment and has progressive visual loss, optic nerve sheath fenestration is indicated. Ultimately, if other therapies have failed and vision loss continues, lumboperitoneal or ventriculoperitoneal shunting should be considered. Surgical procedures should not be used if refractory headache is the only symptom.

Spontaneous Intracranial Hypotension

The presentation of spontaneous intracranial hypotension is analogous to that caused iatrogenically in post–lumbar puncture headache. Spontaneous intracranial hypotension is often preceded by trivial trauma (eg, lifting boxes, falls, coughing, roller coaster rides, exercise). Patients who are hyperflexible or have a history of connective tissue disorders seem to be predisposed to developing spontaneous intracranial hypotension. It is thought to be caused by cryptogenic cerebrospinal fluid leaks via dural fistulas adjacent to the spinal roots. Tears in the arachnoid and dural layers can also lead to chronic cerebrospinal fluid leaks. The majority of the leaks in this condition are in the thoracic spine or near the cervicothoracic junction. Cranial nerve abnormalities are thought to be secondary to downward traction caused by decreased pressure.

Spontaneous intracranial hypotension presents as a postural headache that is worse when upright and better lying down, and it tends to be worse toward the end of the day. The character and location of headaches in spontaneous intracranial hypotension can be variable, but most often, they are either holocephalic or in the bilateral frontal, occipital, or occipitofrontal regions. Neck stiffness or pain, nausea, and tinnitus tend to be more common, and other associated symptoms of interscapular pain, upper extremity radicular pain, vomiting, auditory muffling, dizziness, diplopia, or visual blurring may also be present. In extreme cases, intracranial hypotension can cause alterations in consciousness. Physical exam can be normal, but often the patient's headache improves or resolves after being placed in the Trendelenburg position for about 5 minutes.

Neuroimaging can show pachymeningeal gadolinium enhancement (Figure 26–11) and cerebellar tonsillar descent. Sometimes, subdural hematomas can be present, although in roughly 25% of cases, MRI of the brain with contrast is normal. On lumbar puncture, opening pressure is low or unobtainable; otherwise, cerebrospinal fluid studies are normal. Patients can improve with caffeine and hydration; however, often treatment with an epidural blood patch is warranted. In this procedure, approximately 20 mL of the patient's blood is drawn and then injected into the epidural space, and clotting factors in the blood help seal the leak. Computed tomography and MRI

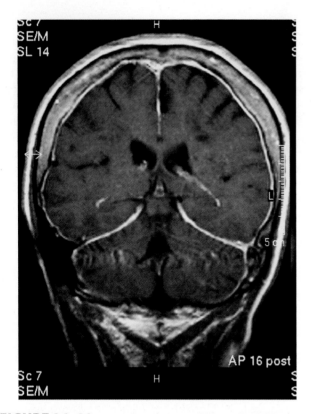

FIGURE 26–11 Pachymeningeal gadolinium enhancement on magnetic resonance imaging of the brain with contrast can be seen in patients with spontaneous intracranial hypotension, as is demonstrated on this coronal cut. Another clue to this diagnosis is cerebellar tonsillar descent (not shown); however, 25% of imaging in patient suffering from this condition can also be normal. (Reproduced with permission from Ropper AH, Samuels MA, Klein JP: *Adams and Victor's Principles of Neurology*, 11th ed. New York, NY: McGraw Hill; 2019.)

myelography may be necessary to confirm and locate the leak for directed high-volume epidural blood patching or fibrin glue, among other options if initial treatments fail.

NEUROLOGIC PAIN SYNDROMES

Fibromyalgia

Fibromyalgia is often a comorbid condition in patients with chronic headaches. It is more common in women, with a prevalence of 2% to 3% worldwide that is similar across different socioeconomic classes. It manifests as chronic widespread musculoskeletal pain and tenderness. The pathophysiology is likely multifactorial, and associated genes are linked to pathways controlling pain sensitivity and the stress response. There are theories that chronic fibromyalgia can elicit the same central sensitization that is seen in chronic migraine, likely through similar neuropeptide cascades (eg, calcitonin gene-related peptide and substance P). The term *fibromyalgia* is something of a misnomer, and there is no evidence of inflammation or lesions of the fibrous tissues of the muscles, fascia, and aponeuroses.

The diagnosis is based on clinical symptoms of widespread pain and neuropsychological symptoms. Tenderness to palpation (4 kg of digital pressure) of predefined sites in the occiput, trapezius, supraspinatus, gluteal region, greater trochanter, low cervical region, second rib, lateral epicondyle, and knee bilaterally on exam can help with diagnosis (Figure 26–12). Management of patients with fibromyalgia revolves around counseling on improvement of quality of life rather than abolition of pain. Physical therapy, relaxation techniques, and cognitive behavioral therapies are used in conjunction with pharmacologic treatments such as antidepressants (amitriptyline, duloxetine, milnacipran) and anticonvulsants (gabapentin, pregabalin).

Complex Regional Pain Syndrome

Complex regional pain syndrome is a neurogenic pain syndrome. Complex regional pain syndrome type I develops spontaneously and was formerly known as reflex sympathetic dystrophy. Complex regional pain syndrome type II is more common and occurs after nerve injury including trauma or immobilization of a limb and was formerly known as causalgia. The pathophysiology underlying complex regional pain syndrome is under investigation. It was initially postulated that the pain was related to short-circuiting of impulses; however, it is now thought that the abnormal cross-excitation is chemical (secondary to neurotransmitters) rather than electrical. Studies are underway to define the molecular changes that occur in the nervous system with this type of chronic pain.

In both types of complex regional pain syndrome, there is persistent disabling regional neuropathic pain in the absence of recognizable pathology to adjacent nerves. There is also associated regional autonomic dysfunction, and patients can present with limb edema, skin discoloration, altered temperature/sweating, allodynia, and hyperalgesia. Medications used to treat neuropathic pain disorders that are similar to those used as preventive therapy in migraine should be used. Early mobilization of the limb also helps. Overall, current treatment options are unsatisfactory.

Postherpetic Neuralgia

Herpes zoster, commonly known as shingles, is a relatively common condition affecting older individuals and those who are immunocompromised. The herpes virus primarily lies dormant in the spinal ganglia, especially in the unilateral thoracic or lumbar segments. In a significant minority of patients, the cranial ganglia, especially the ophthalmic division of the trigeminal ganglion, can be involved (Figure 26–13). When the virus reactivates, neuralgic pain or dysesthesia is the presenting symptom. This is followed in about 4 days by cutaneous erythema and vesicular eruption in the area supplied by the affected roots. The vesicular eruption scabs over in about 10 to 14 days. Postherpetic neuralgia can persist for ≥3 months in a significant minority of patients. Diagnosis is based on history and clinical exam; however, if necessary, the vesicular fluid can be cultured for varicella-zoster virus.

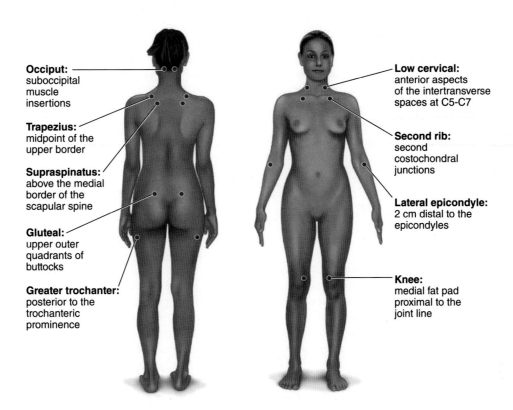

FIGURE 26–12 Tender points in fibromyalgia. Shown are the predetermined tender points in the body that are associated with a diagnosis of fibromyalgia. There are 18 total points, 9 on each side. (Data from Wolfe F, Clauw DJ, Fitzcharles MA, et al: The American College of Rheumatology preliminary diagnostic criteria for fibromyalgia and measurement of symptom severity, *Arthritis Care Res* (Hoboken). 2010 May;62(5):600-610.)

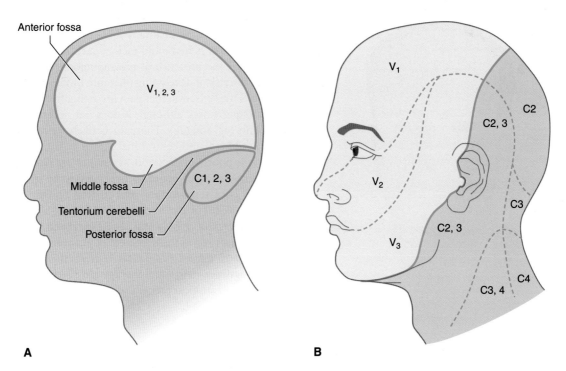

FIGURE 26–13 Divisions of the trigeminal nerve. There are 3 division of the trigeminal nerve. V1 is the ophthalmic division, V2 is the maxillary division, and V3 is the mandibular division. In a minority of patients, the herpes virus can lie dormant in the cranial ganglia. If this happens, the ophthalmic division of the trigeminal ganglion is most commonly involved. (Reproduced with permission from Simon RP, Aminoff MJ, Greemberg DA: *Clinical Neurology*, 10th ed. New York, NY: McGraw Hill; 2018.)

The zoster vaccine is recommended as preventive treatment in all patients age 60 or older. Antiviral therapy with acyclovir is the treatment of choice for acute herpes zoster, but valacyclovir and famciclovir can also be used and may be more successful at decreasing healing time and the duration of postherpetic neuralgia. The prompt administration of antivirals within the first 72 hours of varicella-zoster virus reactivation may decrease the duration of postherpetic neuralgia. Amitriptyline and other tricyclic antidepressants, as well as antiepileptic medications including carbamazepine, gabapentin, and phenytoin, can be effective, although postherpetic neuralgia is often refractory to medical treatments.

Trigeminal Neuralgia

Trigeminal neuralgia is also known as *tic douloureux* and is the most common of all neuralgias. Idiopathic trigeminal neuralgia presents in middle age and later in life. It is characterized by severe, paroxysmal, sharp and stabbing facial pain without numbness or objective findings in the distribution of the fifth cranial nerve. The second and third divisions of the trigeminal nerve are more commonly affected (**Figure 26–14**). The cause of trigeminal neuralgia is unknown. Theories based on patients' response to treatments suggest that it may be related to excessive firing within the fifth cranial nerve nucleus with concomitant peripheral excitation and abnormal neuronal chemical discharges. The diagnostic criteria require attacks of unilateral facial pain in 1 or more divisions of the trigeminal nerve (without radiation outside of the nerve) with at least 3 of the following 4 characteristics: (1) recurring in paroxysmal attacks lasting from a fraction of a second to 2 minutes; (2) severe intensity; (3) electric shock–like, shooting, stabbing, or sharp pain; and (4) precipitated by innocuous stimuli to the affected side of the face. Although some attacks can be spontaneous, patients report minimal stimulation provoked by chewing, facial movements, touch, or temperature (even a breeze) can trigger an attack.

Trigeminal neuralgia can be symptomatic due to underlying neurologic lesions and therefore is a diagnosis of exclusion that requires imaging of the brain and arterial vasculature to look for compression of the trigeminal nerve, basilar artery aneurysm, tumor in the cerebellopontine angle, or multiple sclerosis among the potential causes. Trigeminal neuralgia in a young female, especially if bilateral, should raise the suspicion for multiple sclerosis. The most effective treatment for trigeminal neuralgia is carbamazepine, which can cause drowsiness, dizziness, and ataxia. Blood work should be monitored for renal toxicity, hepatotoxicity, pancytopenia, and hyponatremia. Other antiepileptic medications such as phenytoin, valproic acid, gabapentin, and pregabalin can help as well. Baclofen is also effective, especially as adjunctive therapy to an anticonvulsant. If the pain is refractory, the patient may be a candidate for botulinum toxin injections to the affected trigeminal division or surgical procedures including microvascular decompression, radiofrequency ablation, chemical gangliolysis, and rhizotomy.

Phantom Limb Pain

The incidence of phantom limb pain in patients requiring amputations is high, and factors such as the site of amputation and the presence of preamputation pain are associated with the risk of developing phantom limb pain. Phantom limb pain is the sensation that pain is coming from a body part that no longer exists, although it does not necessarily need to be a limb (eg, tongue). The pain is likely generated secondary to peripheral and central mechanisms. Although the mechanism is poorly understood, symptoms are likely secondary to a combination of neuroma hypersensitivity in the periphery, spinal cord sensitization, and cortical reorganization. Tricyclic antidepressants; anticonvulsants such as carbamazepine, oxcarbazepine, gabapentin, and pregabalin; and memantine are agents used in the treatment of phantom limb pain. Transcutaneous nerve stimulation, mirror therapy, biofeedback, and cognitive-behavioral therapy can also be beneficial. Nerve blocks and surgical procedures can be considered if conservative therapies fail.

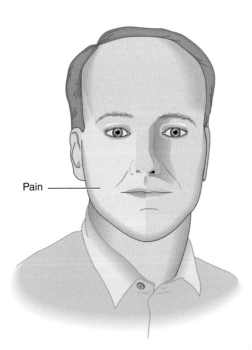

Pain

FIGURE 26–14   Trigeminal neuralgia. The second (maxillary) and third (mandibular) divisions of the trigeminal nerve are most commonly affected in trigeminal neuralgia. These patients have severe, paroxysmal, sharp or stabbing pain in this distribution of the face. (Reproduced with permission from Simon RP, Aminoff MJ, Greemberg DA: *Clinical Neurology*, 10th ed. New York, NY: McGraw Hill; 2018.)

Central Pain Syndrome

Central pain syndrome is also known as thalamic pain syndrome and Dejerine-Roussy syndrome. Patients with this syndrome have continuous moderate to severe pain (with variable characterization: tingling, aching, stabbing, burning, pressure-like) secondary to a lesion in the central nervous system (brain, brainstem, and spinal cord) that can be exacerbated by trivial cold or hot stimuli, emotional disturbances, and loud noises. Despite this, the patient has a higher pain threshold to objective testing in the affected hemibody. The syndrome was first described secondary to stroke in the ventral posteromedial and ventral posterolateral nuclei of the thalamus (posterior cerebral artery–penetrating branches). Classically, there is initial hemisensory loss that is followed by hemibody pain. In this instance, the pain is thought to be secondary to partial recovery of the thalamus. Acute but incomplete lesions (eg, vascular insult, multiple sclerosis, tumors, epilepsy) affecting the central nervous system can also produce central pain syndrome. Lesions causing central pain syndrome have been reported in the thalamus, parietal lobe, medial lemniscus, and posterior columns of the spinal cord. Stress reduction in conjunction with tricyclic antidepressants or anticonvulsants, including gabapentin, can help in the treatment of central pain syndrome.

SELF-ASSESSMENT QUESTIONS

1. A 34-year-old obese woman presents to her neurologist for disabling headaches that occur 4 times per month. The headaches started when she was 19 and have not changed in character. She has severe unilateral throbbing that is accompanied by nausea and vomiting. She does not have phonophobia or photophobia, and the headaches are not preceded by neurologic symptoms. The headaches are worse with movement. She has a history of asthma, which is well controlled, but otherwise, her history is unremarkable. Her neurologic exam, which includes funduscopic exam, is normal. What would be the best preventive medication in this patient?

   A. Topiramate
   B. Acetazolamide
   C. Propranolol
   D. Sumatriptan
   E. Amitriptyline

2. A 23-year-old woman presents with headaches that occur once every other month. Prior to the onset of headache, she sees flashing lights for about 15 minutes. The headache starts as a pressure pain and climaxes over 45 minutes to become throbbing and severe over the right or left frontotemporal region. She prefers to lay down in a dark and quiet room. She has no nausea or vomiting. A diagnosis of migraine with aura is made, and she is started on sumatriptan. The medication is effective at aborting her headaches because it works at which by which of the following mechanisms?

   A. Agonism of serotonin (5-HT) 2B/2D receptors
   B. Antagonism of 5-HT 2B/2D receptors
   C. Agonism of 5-HT 1B/1D receptors
   D. Antagonism of 5-HT 1B/1D receptors
   E. Antagonism of 5-HT 2A/2C receptors

3. A 44-year-old man presents with severe pain that wakes him up in the middle of the night, around 11:00 pm and again at 1:00 am. The pain is in the right periorbital region and comes on abruptly. The pain is severe and associated with ipsilateral tearing and a sense of restlessness. The episodes last 30 minutes and have occurred every day for the past 2 weeks. He is pain free between attacks. He has mild hypertension that is well controlled on verapamil but otherwise does not take other medications and has no other medical conditions. His neurologic exam is normal. What is the best next step in management?

   A. Increase verapamil
   B. Trial of sumatriptan
   C. Schedule caffeine nightly
   D. Order a sleep study
   E. Order neuroimaging studies

Epilepsy

Ashley Thomas

A seizure is a transient occurrence of signs and/or symptoms due to abnormal, excessive, or synchronous neuronal activity in the brain. Seizures can be caused by a wide variety of provoking insults, including electrolyte disturbances, brain injury/insult, and fevers in children, or can occur completely unprovoked (Table 27–1). After a single unprovoked seizure, only about 30% of patients will go on to have another seizure. After 2 seizures have occurred, the recurrence risk for additional seizures is approximately 75%.

Epilepsy is a disorder of the brain characterized by a predisposition to generate recurrent unprovoked epileptic seizures. It is defined by any of the following conditions: (1) at least 2 unprovoked seizures occurring >24 hours apart; (2) 1 unprovoked seizure and a high probability of further seizures occurring over the next 10 years because of an underlying predisposing condition; or (3) diagnosis of an epilepsy syndrome.

PREVALENCE & BURDEN

Approximately 2 million Americans and >65 million people worldwide have epilepsy. The prevalence of epilepsy in the general population is about 1%. Each year, approximately 300,000 people have their first seizure and 150,000 new cases of epilepsy are diagnosed. The incidence of epilepsy is highest in young children and older adults. Risk factors for developing epilepsy include intellectual or developmental delay, family history of seizures, cerebral palsy, autism, hypoxia, stroke, head trauma, central nervous system infection, intracranial hemorrhage, dementia, brain tumors, and tubers or other brain malformations.

Risk of death is up to 3 times higher in patients with epilepsy than the general population. Causes of death in epilepsy include injury, drowning, suicide, status epilepticus, and sudden unexpected death in epilepsy (SUDEP). SUDEP is defined as a sudden, unexpected, nontraumatic, nondrowning, witnessed or unwitnessed death while in a reasonable state of health in a person who has epilepsy and no other obvious or structural cause. SUDEP is the leading cause of epilepsy-related death, with >1 out of 1000 people with epilepsy dying each year. The main risk factors for SUDEP include the presence of generalized convulsive seizures and frequent or uncontrolled seizures of any kind. Other risk factors include long duration of epilepsy, epilepsy beginning at a young age, medication nonadherence, stopping or changing medications suddenly, intellectual disability, young adult age, and diffuse generalized suppression noted on electroencephalogram (EEG) immediately following a seizure. The exact cause of SUDEP is unknown at this time.

SEIZURE CLASSIFICATION (GENERALIZED TONIC-CLONIC, PARTIAL, & ABSENCE)

Seizures are classified according to the scheme proposed by the International League Against Epilepsy (Figure 27–1). This classification scheme divides seizures into partial onset and generalized based on the origin of the seizures, with partial-onset seizures arising from 1 focal area in the brain and generalized seizures arising from epileptic networks that affect the entire brain at the same time. *Partial-onset seizures* can be further divided into *simple partial seizures*, which are focal

VOCABULARY

Hypsarrhythmia: An abnormal encephalogram that is characterized by slow waves of high voltage and a disorganized arrangement of spikes.

Ictal: Referring to what occurs during a seizure event.

Interictal: Referring to what occurs between seizure events.

Opisthotonos: Spasm of the muscles causing backward arching of the head, neck, and spine

Postictal: Referring to what occurs after a seizure event.

seizures with preserved consciousness, and *complex partial seizures*, which are focal seizures with loss of consciousness. Partial-onset seizures can arise from any cortical region, and the clinical manifestations of the seizure correspond to that location. For example, partial-onset seizures arising from the occipital region manifest with visual phenomena. Generalized seizures can be further divided into types of seizures based on

TABLE 27–1 Common causes of new-onset seizures.

Primary neurologic disorders
Benign febrile convulsions of childhood
Idiopathic/cryptogenic seizures
Cerebral dysgenesis
Symptomatic epilepsy
Head trauma
Stroke or vascular malformations
Mass lesions
CNS infections
Encephalitis
Meningitis
Cysticercosis
HIV encephalopathy
Systemic disorders
Hypoglycemia
Hyponatremia
Hyperosmolar states
Hypocalcemia
Uremia
Hepatic encephalopathy
Porphyria
Drug toxicity
Drug withdrawal
Global cerebral ischemia
Hypertensive encephalopathy
Eclampsia
Hyperthermia

Reproduced with permission from Simon RP, Aminoff MJ, Greemberg DA: *Clinical Neurology*, 10th ed. New York, NY: McGraw Hill; 2018.

their clinical manifestations: tonic-clonic, tonic, clonic, atonic, myoclonic, and absence.

Tonic-clonic seizures have an initial tonic phase whereby there is continuous contraction of the muscles of the limbs, initially in a flexed position, followed by extension. There may also be contraction of the respiratory muscles, which can result in a vocalization called an "ictal cry." Contraction of the masticatory muscles can lead to tongue biting and other oral trauma. The tonic phase is followed by a clonic phase where there is symmetric, rhythmic jerking of the limbs. The jerking is initially of lower amplitude and faster frequency, and as this phase progresses, the jerking becomes larger in amplitude and slower in frequency. As the seizure subsides, respiratory effort returns and can result in deep gasping and/or snoring sounds.

Tonic seizures consist only of continuous contraction of the limb, respiratory, and masticatory muscles without the subsequent clonic phase.

Clonic seizures consist only of symmetric, rhythmic jerking of the limbs, without the initial tonic phase.

Atonic seizures are also called "drop attacks" and result in a loss of muscular tone. This seizure type has a strong association with injury and is frequently seen in patients with Lennox-Gastaut syndrome.

Myoclonic seizures consist of brief, shock-like muscle contractions. They can occur in 1 or both hemispheres simultaneously and involve small or large muscle groups. Typically, they occur in the arms but can involve the legs or have a more generalized distribution. This seizure type is frequently seen in patients with juvenile myoclonic epilepsy.

Absence seizures consist primarily of staring with loss of consciousness and without a significant postictal period. Minor eye and mouth movements can be seen, but more complex automatic behaviors are uncommon.

Etiologies of epilepsy can be classified as genetic, structural/metabolic, or unknown. Genetic epilepsies are the result of a known or presumed genetic defect. Structural causes can include stroke, trauma, or tumors. When they are not genetic and no structural or metabolic cause is found, they are unknown.

EPILEPSY SYNDROMES

In addition to the descriptive terms used to classify epilepsy, there are a number of recognizable epilepsy syndromes. These are diagnosed because of the presence of a constellation of consistent clinical and electrical features (Figure 27–2). Recognizing epilepsy syndromes can help to guide treatment and predict outcome. Some of the most common seizure syndromes are listed here. For additional details, please see Chapter 35, "Pediatric Neurology."

West syndrome is characterized by the triad of infantile spasms, hypsarrhythmia on EEG, and developmental regression. West syndrome is most often caused by tuberous sclerosis but can also be seen in patients with focal cortical dysplasias, malformations of cortical development, perinatal hypoxia, and various metabolic syndromes. Many of these

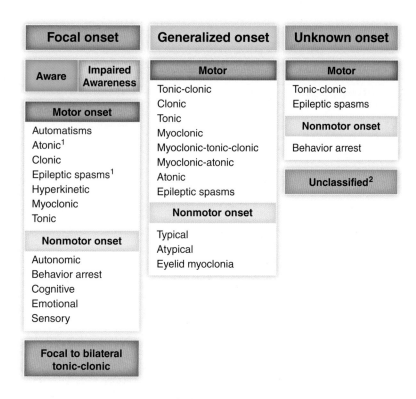

FIGURE 27-1 International League Against Epilepsy (ILAE) 2017 classification of seizure types. [1]Degree of awareness usually is not specified. [2]Due to inadequate information or inability to place in other categories. (Reproduced with permission from Fisher RS, Cross JH, D'Souza C, et al: Instruction manual for the ILAE 2017 operational classification of seizure types, *Epilepsia*. 2017 Apr;58(4):531-542.)

patients evolve to develop Lennox-Gastaut syndrome or other generalized epilepsies.

Dravet syndrome usually begins in infancy with febrile and afebrile generalized and unilateral clonic or tonic-clonic seizures. Up to 80% of patients will have a mutation in the sodium channel α1 subunit (*SCN1A*) gene.

Childhood absence epilepsy (CAE) begins in children age 3 to 8 years old. Seizures consist mainly of staring off with loss of consciousness and a minimal postictal period. Typically, they occur multiple times per day and are provoked by hyperventilation. Minor eye or mouth movements can be seen, but more complex automatic behavior is uncommon. The EEG is typically normal interictally except for generalized spike and wave discharges that occur at 3 Hz. During a seizure, the EEG shows prolonged bursts of 3-Hz generalized spike and wave discharges that can last up to 10 to 20 seconds. Absence seizures resolve by the teenage years in >90% of patients, and those who continue to have seizures often evolve to have juvenile myoclonic epilepsy (Figure 27–3).

Lennox-Gastaut syndrome begins in children age 3 to 8 years old and is preceded by West syndrome in 20% of patients. Lennox-Gastaut syndrome is defined by a triad of mixed seizure types, abnormal EEG, and encephalopathy. The most common seizure type is the "drop attack" or atonic seizure, followed by tonic and atypical absence seizures. Generalized tonic-clonic and focal seizures can also occur. The EEG pattern shows diffuse background slowing as well as interictal slow spike and wave discharges at <2.5 Hz and generalized paroxysmal fast activity noted during sleep. Seizures are frequently medically refractory, and intellectual prognosis is poor.

Benign epilepsy with centrotemporal spikes is the most common form of epilepsy in childhood, with onset between 3 and 13 years of age. Seizures are mostly nocturnal and consist of focal sensory and motor seizures, particularly beginning in the face. These seizures infrequently progress to generalized tonic-clonic seizures. The interictal EEG shows single and repetitive unilateral or bilateral independent spike and wave discharges in the centrotemporal region. Rarely is medical treatment needed, and seizures generally remit within several years of onset.

Febrile seizures occur between 6 months and 6 years of age and typically affect 2% to 5% of children. They usually occur during the first 24 hours of a febrile illness. Simple febrile seizures consist of brief, generalized convulsions that lack focal features. Approximately two-thirds of children with simple febrile seizures have a single seizure, and <10% of children have >3 febrile seizures. Complex febrile seizures can be prolonged, have focal features, or occur with multiple seizures during the first 24 hours. These features increase the likelihood of subsequently developing epilepsy, which occurs in 2% to 6% of children with febrile seizures. *Febrile seizures plus* is an epilepsy syndrome that begins with febrile seizures in infancy or childhood. Patients then go on to develop other seizure types that are not necessarily associated with fever. This is a genetic syndrome with multiple gene mutations identified,

Electroclinical syndromes

One example of how syndromes can be organized: Arranged by typical age at onset*

Neonatal period
- Benign neonatal seizures^
- Benign familial neonatal epilepsy (BFNE)
- Ohtahara syndrome
- Early myoclonic encephalopathy (EME)

Infancy
- Febrile seizures^, Febrile seizures plus (FS+)
- Benign infantile epilepsy
- Benign familial infantile epilepsy (BFIE)
- West syndrome
- Dravet syndrome
- Myoclonic epilepsy in infancy (MEI)
- Myoclonic encephalopathy in nonprogressive disorders
- Epilepsy of infancy with migrating focal seizures

Childhood
- Febrile seizures^, Febrile seizures plus (FS+)
- Early onset childhood occipital epilepsy (Panayiotopoulos syndrome)
- Epilepsy with myoclonic atonic (previously astatic) seizures
- Childhood absence epilepsy (CAE)
- Benign epilepsy with centrotemporal spikes (BECTS)
- Autosomal dominant nocturnal frontal lobe epilepsy (ADNFLE)
- Late onset childhood occipital epilepsy (Gastaut type)
- Epilepsy with myoclonic absences
- Lennox-Gastaut syndrome (LGS)
- Epileptic encephalopathy with continuous spike-and-wave during sleep (CSWS)+
- Landau-Kleffner syndrome (LKS)

Adolescence - Adult
- Juvenile absence epilepsy (JAE)
- Juvenile myoclonic epilepsy (JME)
- Epilepsy with generalized tonic-clonic seizures alone
- Autosomal dominant epilepsy with auditory features (ADEAF)
- Other familial temporal lobe epilepsies

Variable age at onset
- Familial focal epilepsy with variable foci (childhood to adult)
- Progressive myoclonus epilepsies (PME)
- Reflex epilepsies

Distinctive constellations/surgical syndromes

Distinctive constellations/surgical syndromes
- Mesial temporal lobe epilepsy with hippocampal sclerosis (MTLE with HS)
- Rasmussen syndrome
- Gelastic seizures with hypothalamic hamartoma
- Hemiconvulsion-hemiplegia-epilepsy

Nonsyndromic epilepsies**

Epilepsies attributed to and organized by structural-metabolic causes
- Malformations of cortical development (hemimegalencephaly, heterotopias, etc.)
- Neurocutaneous syndromes (tuberous sclerosis complex, Sturge-Weber, etc.)
- Tumor, infection, trauma, angioma, antenatal and perinatal insults, stroke, etc.

Epilepsies of unknown cause

* The arrangement of electroclinical syndromes does not reflect etiology.
^ Not traditionally diagnosed as epilepsy.
+ Sometimes referred to as Electrical Status Epilepticus during Slow Sleep (ESES).
** Forms of epilepsies not meeting criteria for specific syndromes or constellations.

FIGURE 27–2 International League Against Epilepsy (ILAE) Proposal for Revised Terminology for Organization of Seizures and Epilepsies 2010. Electroclinical syndromes and other epilepsies are grouped by specificity of diagnosis. (Data from Berg AT, Berkovic SF, Brodie MJ, et al: Revised terminology and concepts for organization of seizures and epilepsies: report of the ILAE Commission on Classification and Terminology, 2005-2009, *Epilepsia*. 2010 Apr;51(4):676-685.)

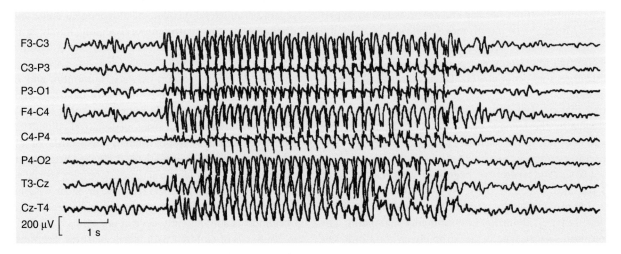

FIGURE 27–3 Electroencephalogram of a patient with typical absence (petit mal) seizures, showing a burst of generalized 3-Hz spike-wave activity (center of record) that is bilaterally symmetric and bisynchronous. Odd-numbered leads indicate electrode placements over the left side of the head; even numbers indicate electrode placements over the right side. (Reproduced with permission from Simon RP, Aminoff MJ, Greemberg DA: *Clinical Neurology*, 10th ed. New York, NY: McGraw Hill; 2018.)

A 17-year old girl presented to the emergency department (ED) after having a witnessed generalized convulsive seizure. She was evaluated in the ED, and her bloodwork and MRI were normal. She reported that over the past year she has been having episodes where she drops things, particularly in the morning. These episodes occur 3 to 4 days per week and are worse if she is sleep deprived. Her parents have also noticed some episodes where she is "spacing out." An EEG was obtained, and it showed generalized 4-Hz spike and wave and polyspike and wave discharges. The clinical history and EEG findings are consistent with juvenile myoclonic epilepsy. She was started on lamotrigine and is currently doing well.

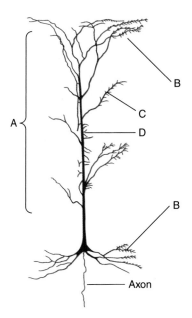

FIGURE 27–4 Neocortical pyramidal cell, showing the distribution of neurons that terminate on it. *A* denotes nonspecific afferents from the reticular formation and the thalamus; *B* denotes recurrent collaterals of pyramidal cell axons; *C* denotes commissural fibers from mirror image sites in the contralateral hemisphere; *D* denotes specific afferents from thalamic sensory relay nuclei.

such as those affecting *SCN1A* and type A γ-aminobutyric acid (GABA) receptor.

Juvenile absence epilepsy (JAE) begins at age 8 to 12 years old and consists of absence seizures and rare generalized tonic-clonic seizures. The absence seizures in JAE are less frequent than those in CAE. The interictal EEG is similar to that in CAE, consisting of 3-Hz generalized spike and wave discharges. Seizure remission occurs in >80% of patients with JAE by the end of the teenage years.

Juvenile myoclonic epilepsy is the second most common epilepsy syndrome across all age groups and accounts for approximately one-sixth of adult epilepsies. Seizures usually begin between age 12 and 18 years and may follow CAE or JAE. The hallmark of this syndrome is frequent myoclonic jerks, particularly upon awakening, in addition to generalized tonic-clonic seizures. Approximately one-third of patients also have absence seizures. The interictal EEG consists of 4- to 6-Hz generalized spike/polyspike and wave discharges. Seizures typically respond well to medication, with prolonged seizure-free intervals easily attainable, but seizures will recur upon medication withdrawal.

DIAGNOSIS

Origins of EEG

The EEG is recorded from wires placed on the surface of the head and represents electrical activity in the brain transmitted through the skull and skin. Pyramidal cells are the primary output neurons of the cerebral cortex. They are glutamatergic and compose approximately 80% of the neurons of the cortex. Their cell bodies are triangular shaped and have a single apical dendrite that is oriented toward the pial surface, multiple basal dendrites, and a single axon (Figure 27–4). Pyramidal cells are grouped closely together and organized in the same orientation. The EEG signal is derived from the summation

of excitatory postsynaptic potentials and inhibitory postsynaptic potentials of the apical dendrites of pyramidal cells. The activity of a single cell is too small to detect, but when pyramidal cell activity becomes synchronized over a large number of cells, then the electrical activity can be detected (Figure 27–5). EEG is recorded from highly conductive silver or gold cup electrodes placed on the surface of the scalp. The electrodes are placed at regular intervals and labeled according to the International 10–20 System (Figure 27–6). The electrical signal must travel through many layers before reaching the recording electrode, including pia mater, subarachnoid space, arachnoid mater, dura mater, skull, subcutaneous tissues, and scalp. All of these layers degrade the electrical signal to a degree, such that there is temporal and spatial dispersion, as well as decreased amplitude. Because pyramidal cells are oriented perpendicular to the cortical surface, EEG best measures electrical activity from the gyri close to the skull and does not accurately measure electrical activity from the sulci. The paroxysmal depolarization shift (PDS) is the pathophysiologic cellular phenomenon that underlies all types of epileptic seizures and interictal epileptiform activity. The PDS occurs when rapidly repetitive action potentials are not followed by the usual refractory period, which causes a prolonged membrane depolarization. An interictal epileptiform discharge occurs when a large number of neurons generate a synchronous PDS (Figure 27–7). An epileptic seizure occurs when a large number of neurons repeatedly generate synchronous PDSs.

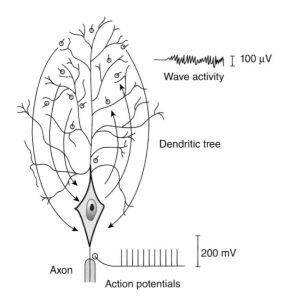

FIGURE 27–5 Diagrammatic comparison of the electrical responses of the axon and the dendrites of a large cortical neuron. Current flow to and from active synaptic knobs on the dendrites produces wave activity, while all-or-none action potentials are transmitted along the axon. When the sum of the dendritic activity is negative relative to the cell body, the neuron is depolarized; when it is positive, the neuron is hyperpolarized. The electroencephalogram recorded from the scalp is a measure of the summation of dendritic postsynaptic potentials rather than action potentials. (Reproduced with permission from Barrett KE, Barman SM, Brooks HL, et al: *Ganong's Review of Medical Physiology*, 26th ed. New York, NY: McGraw Hill; 2019.)

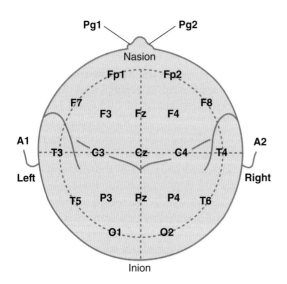

FIGURE 27–6 A single-plane projection of the head, showing all standard positions of electrode placement and the locations of the central sulcus (fissure of Rolando) and the lateral cerebral fissure (fissure of Sylvius). The outer circle is drawn at the level of the nasion and inion; the inner circle represents the temporal line of electrodes. This diagram provides a useful guide for electrode placement in routine recording. A, ear; C, central; Cz, central at zero, or midline; F, frontal; Fp, frontal pole; Fz, frontal at zero, or midline; O, occipital; P, parietal; Pg, nasopharyngeal; Pz, parietal at zero, or midline; T, temporal. (Reproduced with permission from Grass Technologies, An Astro Med, Inc. Produce Group, West Warwick, RI.)

Importance of EEG

EEG is the main diagnostic tool used for epilepsy; however, a normal EEG does not exclude the diagnosis of epilepsy. The EEG has a sensitivity of approximately 50% to 60% and a specificity of approximately 70% to 90% in predicting seizure recurrence. Interictal epileptiform discharges are detected in approximately 30% to 55% of patients with seizures on their initial EEG and are associated with a 2-fold increased risk of seizure recurrence. Several methods can further increase the diagnostic value of the EEG. If the EEG is obtained within 24 hours of the seizure episode, the sensitivity is increased by 15%. If the EEG is obtained during sleep, the sensitivity is increased by 25%. If no abnormalities are noted on the initial EEG, then repeated testing increases the likelihood by 15% to 20% that interictal epileptiform discharges will be seen, up to 90% by the fourth EEG obtained. Different types of EEG studies can be performed based on the clinical situation and needs of the patient.

A *routine EEG* is performed in the EEG laboratory and records approximately 20 minutes of cerebral activity. Prolonged EEG recordings of an hour or more can be performed at the physician's discretion. Additional time for EEG recording increases the probability that interictal epileptiform discharges will be seen during the test.

A *sleep-deprived EEG* is performed in the EEG laboratory after a night of voluntary sleep deprivation. Because EEG during sleep improves sensitivity, this test is ordered to improve the likelihood that the patient will fall asleep during the test.

A *continuous video EEG* is performed while the patient is hospitalized. It can be performed on comatose patients or those who need a definitive diagnosis or characterization of their events. The video is beneficial because it can be correlated with EEG to improve diagnostic accuracy. Subtle changes on the EEG can be mistaken for epileptic patterns where video would confirm that such changes are simply due to artifact. Continuous EEG is performed on patients while admitted to the hospital where medical staff are available for close monitoring. During the hospitalization, medications are withdrawn and other provocative measures are performed to try to induce seizures, which puts patients at high risk for status epilepticus. An epilepsy monitoring unit (EMU) is a designated area in the hospital where several patients can undergo continuous video EEG monitoring at the same time. The EMU is designed to evaluate, diagnose, and treat seizures of all kinds, as well as perform medication adjustments and evaluate for potential surgical and other therapies.

An *ambulatory EEG* is performed for 1 to 3 days while the patient is going about his or her daily routine, after an initial placement of electrodes in the EEG laboratory. This study allows for prolonged recording of cerebral activity and can capture clinical events. It is beneficial because the patient is allowed to remain in his or her usual environment where stress and activity levels are more typical. Unfortunately, because simultaneous EEG and video cannot usually be obtained, it is difficult to use this type of EEG to obtain a definitive diagnosis of epilepsy. In addition, because this is not performed in the

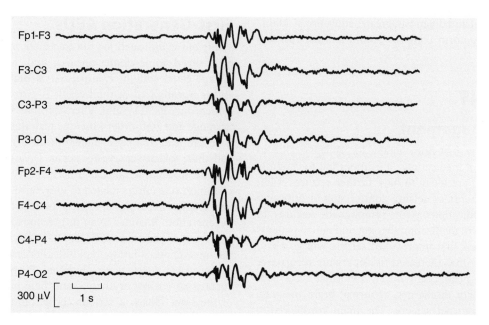

FIGURE 27-7 Electroencephalogram of a patient with idiopathic (primary generalized) epilepsy. A burst of generalized epileptiform activity (center) is seen on a relatively normal background. These findings, obtained at a time when the patient was not experiencing seizures, support the clinical diagnosis of epilepsy. Odd-numbered leads indicate electrode placements over the left side of the head; even numbers indicate electrode placements over the right side. (Reproduced with permission from Simon RP, Aminoff MJ, Greemberg DA: *Clinical Neurology*, 10th ed. New York, NY: McGraw Hill; 2018.)

hospital, medication withdrawal cannot be performed due to a high risk of status epilepticus.

DIFFERENTIAL DIAGNOSIS

The diagnosis of epilepsy is essential to initiate treatment and reduce morbidity and mortality. The principal steps toward making a proper diagnosis are obtaining a thorough history, performing a complete physical exam, and conducting appropriate testing.

A surprising number of patients referred for evaluation of epilepsy turn out to have other disorders. Events that mimic epileptic seizures typically fall into 1 of 2 categories: physiologic events or psychiatric events. Physiologic events can include syncope, migraine, transient ischemic attack, transient global amnesia, vertigo, sleep disorders, delirium, and intermittent movement disorders. Psychiatric events can include panic attack, conversion disorder, dissociative state, acute psychosis, and malingering. By far, the most common mimic for epileptic seizures is conversion disorder, which manifests as psychogenic nonepileptic spells (PNESs).

Psychogenic Nonepileptic Spells

PNESs consist of paroxysmal changes in movements, responsiveness, or behaviors that resemble epileptic seizures. These events can be distinguished from epileptic seizures by the absence of ictal EEG epileptiform abnormalities and typical clinical features. Typical clinical features of PNES include asynchronous limb movements, pelvic thrusting, side-to-side head movements, dystonic posturing including opisthotonos,

out-of-phase clonic activity, and waxing and waning movements. Although these clinical features are often seen in PNES, none are pathognomonic for the disorder. Simultaneous video and EEG recordings are required to confirm the diagnosis of PNES.

PNES is common, composing 5% to 10% of outpatients in epilepsy clinics and 20% to 40% of inpatients in EMUs. It can occur at any age, but peak incidence is in young adulthood, and it is up to 3 times more common in women than men. It can also coexist in up to 5% of patients with a diagnosis of epilepsy. Predisposing factors for developing PNES include female sex; history of prior trauma including sexual abuse, physical abuse, or neglect; traumatic brain injury; and psychiatric comorbidities. These are factors that make someone susceptible to developing PNES. Precipitating factors include injury, death of a loved one, rape, surgical procedures, giving birth, natural disasters, family/relationship difficulties, and impending legal action. These factors can trigger a patient to begin having PNES. Perpetuating factors include anxiety, depression, misdiagnosis, and inappropriate treatment. These factors may worsen the severity of PNES and make it harder for patients to recover.

Treatment for PNES lies in formal psychological assessment and treatment with psychotherapy, such as cognitive-behavioral therapy. Psychopharmacology can also be helpful in certain circumstances where perpetuating factors are playing a large role. Once a diagnosis of PNES is confirmed, antiepileptic drugs (AEDs) should be tapered off because they do not treat conversion disorder. Unfortunately, even with proper psychotherapeutic treatments, many patients continue to have PNES. Factors associated with improved outcomes include younger age at onset and diagnosis, greater educational attainments, fewer somatoform complaints, and attacks with less dramatic features.

TREATMENT

Medical Management

Medications are the first-line therapy for epilepsy. Due to the potential risks of medications, it is important to carefully select patients who are likely to have further seizures if left untreated. The benefits of seizure control should outweigh the risks of the medications. Acute symptomatic seizures do not require long-term medication therapy, and not all patients presenting with their first unprovoked seizure will go on to have additional seizures. Increased risk of seizure recurrence is associated with prior brain insult, abnormal EEG with interictal epileptiform discharges, abnormal brain imaging, and history of nocturnal seizure. The main consideration in AED selection is one based on the seizure types that the patient experiences. Approximately two-thirds of patients will become seizure-free on the first or second AED used. It is also important to consider possible side effects in choosing AEDs. Adverse events occur in 10% to 30% of patients and are usually mild and reversible. Finally, drug interactions and patient comorbidities may also play a role in the decision-making process. For example, certain AEDs such as valproic acid should be avoided in patients with comorbid liver disease. Comparative effectiveness studies on initial monotherapy and adjunctive therapy for partial-onset seizures and generalized seizures have failed to demonstrate that one AED is clearly superior to any other AEDs. Therefore, practice guidelines recommend considering unique patient characteristics to guide AED selection, such as patient age, concomitant medications, and AED tolerability, safety, and efficacy. Some of the most commonly used AEDs are described in the following sections.

CASE 27–2

A 42-year-old man presented to clinic for evaluation of episodes of confusion and altered speech. He is unaware that he is having episodes and is unable to give any description of the events. His wife described that his episodes begin with staring off and unresponsiveness, followed by garbled speech. Upon further questioning, she stated that at the beginning of episodes he will repeatedly lick his lips and rub his thighs. The episodes last for 2 to 3 minutes and occur 1 to 2 times per week. He has been evaluated by another physician who found that his bloodwork and brain MRI were normal. He underwent an EEG and was found to have left temporal interictal epileptiform discharges. Based on his EEG, he was diagnosed with left temporal lobe epilepsy and was started on carbamazepine.

First-Generation AEDs

Phenytoin is indicated for the treatment of partial-onset and generalized tonic-clonic seizures and works by blocking voltage-gated sodium channels. It is highly protein bound and is metabolized in the liver. It is a strong inducer of the cytochrome P450 system. Phenytoin has a narrow therapeutic range and zero-order kinetics, such that a small change in dose can lead to a large change in the serum concentration, and thus, toxicity can easily occur. Dose-related side effects include nystagmus, ataxia, dysarthria, and encephalopathy. Common side effects related to long-term use include hirsutism, gingival hyperplasia, reduced bone density, and cerebellar degeneration. It comes in an intravenous formulation for the treatment of status epilepticus. Due to the alkaline nature of the intravenous solution, rapid infusion can lead to a complication called *purple glove syndrome*. Purple glove syndrome consists of edema, erythema, and blue-purple discoloration of the skin. This is a serious complication that can lead to necrosis and subsequent amputation if left unrecognized. When rapid infusion of phenytoin is necessary, it is best to use fosphenytoin, a water-soluble prodrug of phenytoin, which can be infused at a high rate more safely. Rapid infusion of phenytoin or fosphenytoin can cause severe hypotension and cardiac arrhythmias, so careful monitoring is required.

Carbamazepine is also indicated for the treatment of partial-onset and generalized tonic-clonic seizures and works by blocking voltage-gated sodium channels. It can exacerbate absence and myoclonic seizures and therefore is contraindicated in these patients. Carbamazepine is metabolized in the liver and induces the cytochrome P450 system. It also induces its own metabolism, called autoinduction, whereby increased dose may not lead to a significant increase in plasma concentration. Common dose-related side effects include hyponatremia, drowsiness, ataxia, diplopia, vertigo, and blurred vision. Serious side effects include skin rash, bone marrow suppression, and hepatic failure.

Valproic acid is indicated for the treatment of partial-onset and absence seizures that occur in isolation or in combination with other seizure types. It is a first-line treatment for juvenile myoclonic epilepsy. Valproic acid enhances GABA activity and may block voltage-gated sodium channels. It is highly protein bound and metabolized in the liver. It inhibits uridine diphosphate–glucuronosyltransferase (UGT) and the cytochrome P450 system. Common side effects include drowsiness, nausea, gastrointestinal disturbances, tremor, weight gain, and hair loss. Serious side effects include hyperammonemia, encephalopathy, hepatotoxicity, and pancreatitis. Valproic acid has a high incidence of birth defects, particularly neural tube defects, and should be used with caution in women of childbearing age.

Ethosuximide is indicated for the treatment of absence seizures and blocks low-threshold, "transient" (T-type) calcium channels in thalamic neurons. It is not effective against partial-onset or generalized seizures. It is primarily renally excreted but does undergo some hepatic metabolism. Common side effects include nausea, abdominal discomfort, drowsiness, anorexia, and headache.

Second-Generation AEDs

Topiramate is indicated for the treatment of partial-onset seizures, generalized tonic-clonic seizures, and seizures associated with Lennox-Gastaut syndrome. It blocks voltage-gated sodium channels, inhibits carbonic anhydrase, and increases the frequency at which GABA opens chloride channels. It is metabolized in the liver and is a weak inducer of the cytochrome P450 system, particularly at higher doses. Common dose-related side effects include somnolence, paresthesias, weight loss, and naming difficulties. Serious side effects include nephrolithiasis and acute open-angle glaucoma. It is also associated with hypohidrosis, which can lead to overheating.

Lamotrigine is also indicated for the treatment of partial-onset seizures, generalized tonic-clonic seizures, and seizures associated with Lennox-Gastaut syndrome. There are some reports of efficacy against absence seizures. It should be used with caution in patients with myoclonus because there are some reports of myoclonus exacerbation. Lamotrigine primarily blocks voltage-gated sodium channels and is metabolized in the liver through the UGT system. Due to UGT metabolism, lamotrigine has substantially increased clearance during pregnancy, and lamotrigine levels should be checked regularly with concomitant dose increases. Common dose-related side effects include vertigo, diplopia, blurred vision, ataxia, headache, and insomnia. Serious side effects include Stevens-Johnson syndrome and toxic epidermal necrolysis.

Levetiracetam is indicated for the treatment of partial-onset and generalized tonic-clonic seizures and binds to a synaptic vesicle protein known as SV2A, which is important in vesicle exocytosis. It is mainly excreted unchanged in urine. Common dose-related side effects include somnolence, dizziness, and headache. Uncommon side effects include behavior change, irritability, depression, and psychosis.

With the use of antiepileptic medications, approximately 70% of patients can have their seizures controlled or substantially improved. The remaining 30% of patients have medically refractory epilepsy. When trials of 2 different medications at therapeutic doses fail to achieve seizure freedom, <10% of patients will respond to a third medication. Moreover, patients who initially respond to a medication may become unresponsive after a period of time. Uncontrolled seizures have a 0.5% risk of death per year due to SUDEP. In addition, uncontrolled seizures can lead to cognitive decline over time and decreased quality of life. Therefore, it is reasonable to consider surgical interventions to treat seizures in medication-refractory patients.

Dietary Therapy

Modified diets have been proven safe and effective for treating many different intractable epilepsy syndromes and seizure types. All of these diets mimic the physiology of fasting. During periods of decreased glucose availability, fats are metabolized into ketone bodies—acetone, β-hydroxybutyrate, and acetoacetate. As ketone body levels rise and blood glucose levels fall, ketones become the primary source of fuel for the brain. At the cerebral level, ketones act to suppress seizures, but the exact mechanism is unknown. Possible mechanisms include: (1) decreased membrane excitability, (2) decreased synaptic excitation, (3) enhancement of synaptic inhibition, and (4) improved mitochondrial function. The classic ketogenic diet is the most well-known diet and uses a ratio of 4:1 grams of fat to carbohydrates plus protein. All food must be weighed on a scale and carefully monitored. This diet is typically initiated in the hospital due to potential complications, such as hypoglycemia and acidosis. Other complications include nephrolithiasis, hyperlipidemia, and gastrointestinal distress. Serious side effects such as hepatic failure, pancreatitis, and cardiomyopathy have also been reported. Approximately 50% of patients on the classic ketogenic diet achieve >50% reduction in seizures, and up to 30% of patients achieve >90% seizure reduction.

Alternative ketogenic diets are less restrictive than the classic ketogenic diet and may produce similar anticonvulsant efficacy. The main benefit for these diets is their dietary flexibility. Alternative diets include the medium-chain triglyceride (MCT) diet, modified Atkins diet, and low glycemic index treatment. The MCT diet uses MCT oils, which are very ketogenic, as the main fat source and allows a higher amount of protein and carbohydrate than the classic ketogenic diet. The modified Atkins diet uses 60% daily calories from fat and also allows more carbohydrates than the classic ketogenic diet. The low glycemic index treatment uses only carbohydrates with a low glycemic index and allows for more carbohydrates than any of the other dietary therapies for epilepsy.

Surgical Treatment

Medication remains the first-line treatment for epilepsy; however, patients with refractory epilepsy are unlikely to respond to additional medication trials. Patients with disabling complex partial seizures who have failed first-line AEDs should be considered for epilepsy surgery. A patient is considered medically refractory once there is failure of ≥2 appropriate AEDs to control seizures. When a person has a lesion causing epilepsy, a surgical resection of the lesion (and possibly surrounding tissue) is often required to improve seizure outcomes.

Resective surgery involves removing the epileptogenic area of the brain with the intent of reducing seizure frequency without injuring vital cortical functions, such as language, motor, or sensory functions. This can only be done safely after careful investigation of the seizure focus as well as the surrounding brain tissue. Investigation of the seizure focus includes ictal and interictal video EEG, magnetic resonance imaging (MRI) of the brain, positron emission tomography scan, and psychological and neuropsychological assessments. Additional testing can be performed as needed, such as magnetoencephalography, ictal single-photon emission computed tomography, functional MRI, or intracarotid amobarbital test (Wada test). If surface EEG yields inconclusive results, then further localization is required with intracranial electrodes. Subdural grid and strip electrodes and intraparenchymal depth electrodes can be placed to more accurately localize the seizure onset zone. Functional mapping can also be performed to localize eloquent cortex.

Once the seizure focus is clearly defined, then a more detailed surgical plan can be formed. Ideally, the entire epileptogenic zone will be resected without disrupting eloquent cortex. For patients with lesions causing epilepsy, often the surrounding brain tissue becomes irritated and generates seizures. In this case, it is important that this tissue does not remain since it is generating seizures and there may be little or no change to seizure frequency. For patients with temporal lobe epilepsy, there is a standard resection protocol that consists of resection of the anterior temporal lobe and mesial structures. The middle and inferior temporal gyri and the hippocampus and amygdala are removed, while the superior temporal gyrus often remains. The resection goes posteriorly from the temporal pole approximately 5.5 cm on the nondominant hemisphere and 4.5 cm on the dominant hemisphere (to reduce the likelihood of producing language deficits). In patients who have an epileptogenic lesion noted on MRI, such as a tumor, cavernoma, or hippocampal sclerosis, there is an approximately 70% chance of seizure freedom from surgery. In nonlesional epilepsy, the success rate drops to approximately 50%.

Vagus nerve stimulation (VNS) should be considered when patients are refractory to medications and resective brain surgery is not a good option. VNS therapy leads to a 50% reduction in seizure frequency in 25% to 50% of patients, and this reduction improves over time and is sustained at long-term follow-up. VNS consists of a generator, which is implanted in the subcutaneous tissues of the left chest wall, and a bipolar helical lead that is attached to the cervical portion of the left vagus nerve. The generator delivers a biphasic current in an open-loop fashion, such that the generator cycles between on and off periods at predetermined time intervals. The stimulus intensity, frequency, and duration can all be programed by the physician, and interrogation and device programming are carried out via an external programming wand connected to a handheld computer. A handheld magnet is provided to the patient for the purpose of on-demand stimulation, whereby the patient can swipe the magnet across the generator and initiate a stimulation. On-demand stimulation performed at the onset of a seizure can modulate the intensity or even abort or terminate the seizure. The precise mechanism through which VNS works is poorly understood. Previous research has shown that VNS therapy alters cerebral electrical activity and blood flow by activation of neuronal networks via the vagus nerve's connections in the ventroposterior and

intralaminar regions of the thalamus and thalamocortical pathways. Voice alteration and throat pain are the most common side effects, followed by cough, paresthesias, worsened obstructive sleep apnea, nausea, and chest pain. Transient arrhythmias have been rarely reported, and no serious cardiac dysfunction has been noted. In addition, the generator must be replaced approximately every 10 years, which requires outpatient surgery. The major benefits to VNS are that it does not interact with other medications, has no known systemic neurotoxic effects (eg, somnolence, vertigo, fatigue, cognitive impairment), does not cause bone marrow suppression, does not lead to liver or renal impairment, can improve mood, and is considered safe during pregnancy.

Responsive neurostimulation (RNS) uses implanted electrodes to record EEG activity, recognize epileptiform activity, and provide electric stimulation to suppress or disrupt seizures. This is a closed-loop system whereby the generator only delivers stimulation in response to epileptiform abnormalities recognized on the intracranial EEG. The device requires the seizure-onset zone to be in a localized area and precisely identified, since the implanted electrodes only record EEG activity and perform stimulations over a small area of cortex. Complex algorithms are used to detect possible seizure activity very early on, in order to provide a stimulation before the seizure activity has spread. The generator is placed in a partial-thickness cavity in the skull (under the scalp). The generator is interrogated and programmed by an external wand that is connected to a computer. The patient is also given a wand and computer for use at home to download recordings performed by the device. Patients are asked to perform frequent downloads initially, and these can be spaced out after longer periods of time. Prospective clinical trials have demonstrated median seizure frequency reductions of 44% at 1 year and 53% at 2 years and seizure reductions ranging from 60% to 66% 3 to 6 years after implant. The main benefit of RNS is that very precisely localized stimulation is delivered only when seizure activity is detected and that stimulation can be given in multiple locations or over eloquent cortex. In addition, there are no systemic effects of the device, and it does not interact with other medications. The main risks associated with RNS occur at the time of electrode and device implantation and include bleeding and infection. In addition, the device must be replaced every 2 to 3 years in outpatient surgery.

STATUS EPILEPTICUS

Status epilepticus is a neurologic emergency. Untreated, it is usually fatal, and even with best therapy, it has a mortality rate of approximately 20%. It is commonly defined as continuous seizure activity lasting for ≥30 minutes or repetitive seizures without returning to neurologic baseline between seizures. Continuous seizures of this duration produce irreversible brain damage, primarily through the release of excitotoxic levels of glutamate. Thus, rapid treatment is essential. Practically speaking, any seizure lasting >5 minutes is unlikely to resolve on its own and should be treated as status epilepticus.

Status epilepticus can be classified using the partial-onset or generalized dichotomy and whether or not the patient has convulsive activity present. The main types of convulsive status epilepticus include generalized convulsive, focal motor, and myoclonic, and the main types of nonconvulsive status epilepticus include subtle generalized, complex partial, and absence. Nonconvulsive status epilepticus can be difficult to detect, so continuous video EEG monitoring should be used in any patient with suspected nonconvulsive status epilepticus to confirm the diagnosis. Approximately 40% of patients with status epilepticus report a prior history of epilepsy. In fact, 15% of epilepsy patients will experience an episode of status epilepticus in their lifetime, and 12% of the time, status epilepticus is the first manifestation of epilepsy. Often, the cause for status epilepticus in patients with epilepsy is related to low levels of their antiepileptic medications or changes in their medication regimen. Additional causes of status epilepticus include acute stroke, various metabolic causes, alcohol, hypoxia, infection, tumor, and trauma. The etiology of status epilepticus is important to determine because this may affect treatment and predicts prognosis. Predictors of poor outcome after status epilepticus include hypoxia, prolonged seizure, advanced age, low initial Glasgow Coma Scale score, and other complications.

Treatment of status epilepticus is most effective when initiated early. Immediately after the diagnosis of status epilepticus, basic life support measures should be taken including evaluating airway, breathing, and circulation. Additionally, blood should be obtained to evaluate for metabolic abnormalities, toxicology screen, and AED levels. Initial pharmacotherapy is initiated with intravenous thiamine 100 mg followed by 50 mL of D50 dextrose solution. Intravenous lorazepam is given in 2-mg increments every 2 minutes as long as seizures persist up to a maximum dose of 0.1 mg/kg. If venous access has not been obtained, intramuscular midazolam and rectal diazepam are options, given at 10 mg and 20 mg, respectively. Next, intravenous fosphenytoin should be administered as a loading dose of 20 mg/kg with a rapid infusion rate of 150 mg/min. Continuous blood pressure and cardiac monitoring should be performed throughout the infusion, because fosphenytoin can cause hypotension and cardiac arrhythmias. If seizure activity persists, then continuous intravenous infusion is required, along with intubation, central venous access, and continuous blood pressure and cardiac monitoring. Midazolam, pentobarbital, and propofol are options for continuous intravenous infusion. Continuous EEG monitoring is necessary during continuous infusion because these medications are titrated to burst suppression pattern seen on the EEG. Supplemental seizure medications can be used to aid in long-term seizure control. Examples of these medications include levetiracetam, phenobarbital, valproate, and lacosamide. The goal for treatment with continuous infusions is to maintain burst suppression and seizure control for at least 24 hours. After this point, the continuous infusion can be slowly weaned. If seizures recur during the continuous infusion taper, then the continuous infusion should be increased back to achieve burst suppression, and a supplemental seizure medication should be added. After another 24 hours of seizure freedom, the weaning process can be tried again. Continuous EEG monitoring should be maintained for at least 24 hours after the continuous infusion is discontinued to monitor for seizure recurrence.

CONCLUSION

Epilepsy is diagnosed when a person has the propensity for recurrent unprovoked seizures. EEG is the primary diagnostic tool, and the presence of interictal epileptiform discharges is associated with a 2-fold increased risk of seizure recurrence. Proper diagnosis is important so that appropriate treatment can be initiated. Mortality is higher in people with epilepsy than in the general population, particularly due to SUDEP. Medical management is the primary treatment for epilepsy. There is similar efficacy between AEDs chosen for the particular seizure type, so patient factors should guide the medication choice. Up to one-third of people with seizures will be refractory to medications and should consider surgical options. Status epilepticus is a state of continuous seizure activity and is considered a neurologic emergency. It is associated with high morbidity and mortality and should be recognized early and treated aggressively for the best overall outcome.

SELF-ASSESSMENT QUESTIONS

1. A 6-year-old boy is brought to clinic by his mom because she was told by his first-grade teacher that he is daydreaming in class. His mom has also noticed over the past few months that he does not always follow directions at home. She reports that previously her son was very eager to please and would always follow instructions. She is worried that he may have attention-deficit disorder (ADD). Because you are a thorough neurologist, you decide to check a routine electroencephalogram (EEG), which shows 2- to 3-second bursts of generalized spike and wave discharges at 3 Hz. What is the boy's diagnosis, and what can you tell his mom about his prognosis?

   A. He has ADD and will need lifelong medication.

   B. He has absence seizures and will need lifelong medication.

   C. He has ADD and should try harder at school.

   D. He has absence seizures and will need medication now but will likely outgrow his epilepsy by adulthood.

2. A 32-year-old woman with complex partial epilepsy is seen in the emergency department for a breakthrough seizure. Her phenytoin dose is increased from 300 mg/d to 400 mg/d. A few days later, she comes to your office complaining of constant ataxia, nystagmus, and confusion. What is the most likely cause of her new symptoms?

   A. She continues to have frequent complex partial seizures.

   B. She has developed cerebellar ataxia.

   C. She has phenytoin toxicity.

   D. She has opioid intoxication.

3. A 42-year-old woman with depression and anxiety has been having seizure-like events for the past 6 months. Her general physician has tried her on levetiracetam and lamotrigine, but she continues to have episodes 4 to 5 times per week, which is unchanged since starting medication. Her bloodwork, brain magnetic resonance imaging, and routine EEG are unremarkable. What is your next step?

A. Increase the doses of her medications since she has not responded to the current doses of medications yet.

B. Check a sleep-deprived EEG to evaluate for epileptiform abnormalities.

C. Refer her to a psychologist because you diagnose her with psychogenic nonepileptic spells (PNES) since she has failed to respond to antiepileptic drugs (AEDs) and her EEG was normal.

D. Refer her for epilepsy surgery since she has failed trials of 2 medications.

Movement Disorders

Victor W. Sung

- Understand the various pathologies underlying movement disorders.
- Identify and distinguish the clinical features of the various movement disorders and correlate these with basal ganglia anatomy.
- Identify the various medical and surgical treatments for movement disorders.

PREVALENCE & BURDEN

Given the breadth of pathologies responsible for the various movement disorders, there is great variation in disease prevalence. More will be discussed later for each of the diseases, but in general, movement disorders are relatively common neurologic problems. The most prevalent movement disorder is essential tremor, with a prevalence of roughly 400 per 100,000. While essential tremor is common, many of the cases are mild, and often these patients do not seek treatment. The most common movement disorder encountered in clinical practice is Parkinson disease, a serious and debilitating disorder affecting approximately 200 people per 100,000 population and >1 million people in the United State and 10 million people worldwide. Combined direct and indirect cost of care of US patients with Parkinson disease is estimated at $25 billion per year. Huntington disease is rare, with a prevalence in the 7 per 100,000 range.

LOCALIZATION

The entire motor system is quite extensive, spanning from motor cortex to muscle. For simplicity, however, disorders of the motor system are divided anatomically. Disorders involving the corticospinal tract (pyramidal) extending out to the peripheral muscle are classified as neuromuscular disorders (see Chapter 31). Disorders of the basal ganglia and cerebellum (extrapyramidal) are grouped into the field of movement disorders and will be discussed here. Pathways through the basal ganglia moderate and adjust voluntary movement (Figure 28–1). The direct pathway primarily facilitates movement ("go"), whereas the indirect pathway primarily inhibits movement ("no go").

DISORDERS

We will discuss each of the main movement disorders, but to establish a framework, most movement disorders are classified as either predominately hypokinetic (too little movement) or hyperkinetic (too much movement). The prototypical hypokinetic movement disorder is Parkinson disease, whereas the prototypical hyperkinetic movement disorder is Huntington disease.

HYPOKINETIC MOVEMENT DISORDERS

Parkinsonism is the umbrella term for a tetrad of symptoms: rigidity, resting tremor, bradykinesia, and postural instability. Together, these are the cardinal signs of parkinsonism. **Rigidity** is a velocity-independent muscular stiffness. This means that with the patient's limb relaxed, there is still resistance to passive range of motion, and the amount of resistance is the same whether the limb is moved quickly or slowly. This is often described in the context of parkinsonism as "lead pipe rigidity," meaning that moving the limb passively feels like trying to bend a lead pipe. This is in contrast to spasticity, which is a velocity-dependent increase in muscular tone, usually with more resistance when the limb is moved quickly and less when moved slowly. Spasticity is often described as being like a "clasp knife" (like opening a pocket knife) and is seen in motor disorders where the corticospinal (pyramidal) tract has been disrupted. **Resting tremor** is present when the body part is at rest and diminishes with action. The presence of resting tremor can help distinguish idiopathic Parkinson disease from other forms of parkinsonism, as will be described later. **Bradykinesia** is a slowness of movement that can

VOCABULARY

Movement disorders can be defined as neurologic syndromes in which there is either an excess or paucity of voluntary or involuntary movements unrelated to weakness or spasticity. Movement disorder diagnosis starts with the classification of a patient's predominant abnormal movements. Therefore, proper definition of each of the types of abnormal movements is critical for the understanding of movement disorders. The 5 major categories of abnormal movements are tremor, chorea, dystonia, myoclonus, and tics. These are defined as follows:

- **Tremor:** Involuntary rhythmic oscillating movement
  - **Resting tremor:** Tremor occurring with the body part at rest (eg, hand tremor occurring with arm rested in patient's lap)
  - **Postural tremor:** Tremor occurring with sustained posture (eg, with arms outstretched)
  - **Action tremor:** Tremor occurring with active movement (eg, with finger-to-nose task)
    - **Intention tremor:** Subtype of action tremor where tremor worsens as the limb approaches the target
- **Chorea:** Brief, semi-directed, nonrhythmic, dance-like movements
  - **Athetosis:** Slow, involuntary, writhing movement that is a slower variant of chorea
  - **Ballismus:** Flailing, ballistic, involuntary movement that is a larger amplitude variant of chorea
- **Dystonia:** Sustained or repetitive movements that result in twisting or other abnormal postures of the body
- **Myoclonus:** Rapid, lightning-like twitch of a muscle group or groups that results in a brief jerk
- **Tics:** Sudden, repetitive, nonrhythmic movement or vocalization involving discrete muscle groups

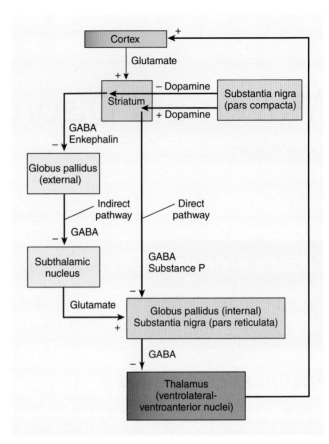

FIGURE 28–1 Functional circuitry between the cerebral cortex, basal ganglia, and thalamus. The major neurotransmitters and their excitatory (+) or inhibitory (−) effects are indicated. In Parkinson disease, there is degeneration of the pars compacta of the substantia nigra, leading to overactivity in the indirect pathway (*red*) and increased glutamatergic output from the subthalamic nucleus. GABA, γ-aminobutyric acid. (Reproduced with permission from Katzung BG: *Basic and Clinical Pharmacology*, 14th ed. New York, NY: McGraw Hill; 2018.)

manifest as decreased facial expression, decreased blink rate, impaired fine movements of the hands, and an overall statue-like appearance. **Postural instability** refers specifically to a tendency to fall and is associated with the classic stooping of posture, shortening of stride length, and shuffling of gait seen in Parkinson disease.

Parkinson Disease: Pathology & Diagnosis

The most common cause of parkinsonism is **idiopathic Parkinson disease** (PD). PD is a degenerative disorder that results from loss of dopaminergic neurons in the substantia nigra pars compacta (Figure 28–2A). These neurons normally project to the putamen and provide dopaminergic input

to *both* the direct and indirect pathways. Therefore, death of these cells leads to loss of stimulation in the *direct* pathway (less "go") as well as loss of inhibition in the indirect pathway (increase in "no go"). These changes in output from the putamen are, at a basic level, an explanation for the bradykinesia and overall loss of movement seen in PD. Affected dopamine (DA) neurons develop intracellular protein accumulations called **Lewy bodies** (Figure 28–2B), and the abnormal protein that composes Lewy bodies is known as **α-synuclein**.

The diagnosis of PD is purely clinical and based on presence of at least 2 of the 4 cardinal parkinsonian symptoms, which were described earlier. The average age of onset of PD is 65 years, and the average time from diagnosis to severe disability or death is 15 to 20 years. At the time of diagnosis, idiopathic PD patients usually have parkinsonian symptoms that are more severe on 1 side of the body than the other. This reflects asymmetric degeneration of DA neurons in the substantia nigra, a feature that is characteristic of the disease. The classic resting tremor of PD is a 4- to 6-Hz tremor that tends to begin distally in 1 hand. Because it involves the fingers, in early

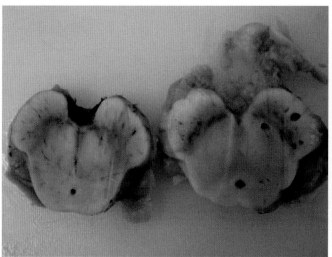
A

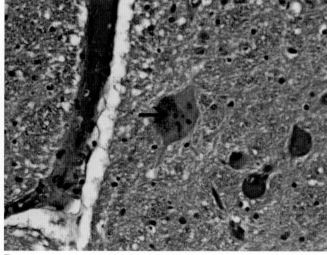
B

FIGURE 28-2 Idiopathic Parkinson disease (PD). **A.** The brainstem on the left side of the image has a pale substantia nigra compared to the age-matched control on the right side of the image. A grossly pale substantia nigra is characteristic of PD and is caused by a selective loss of pigmented dopamine-secreting neurons in this nucleus. The well-circumscribed defects near the substantia nigra in the brainstem on the right side are artifacts, due to early decomposition and gas formation. **B.** The neuron in the center of the image has several Lewy bodies, visible in this section as basophilic homogeneous cytoplasmic inclusions surrounded by a clear halo (*arrow*). Lewy bodies are the hallmark of PD and are rich in a protein known as α-synuclein. Hematoxylin and eosin, 400×. (Reproduced with permission from Kemp WL, Burns DK, Brow TG: *Pathology: The Big Picture.* New York, NY: McGraw Hill; 2008.)

stages, it often has the appearance of rolling pills between the thumb and index finger and thus is described as "pill rolling." The bradykinesia of idiopathic PD may present as decreased facial expression (masked facies) or slowness in the fingers (causing micrographia, which is very small handwriting). The rigidity of PD is often described as cogwheeling, and this is simply tremor superimposed on rigidity in that limb, which gives a cogwheeling or ratcheting type of feel when the limb is moved passively. The postural instability of PD tends to occur later in the disease and is the least responsive of the cardinal symptoms to DA replacement therapy.

Other common motor features of PD can be grouped as follows. From a posture and gait standpoint, stooping forward and having decreased arm swing on the more affected hemibody are common early symptoms. As the gait problem progresses, patients develop shorter stride length, which leads to shuffling of the feet and difficulty with turning (described as "en bloc" turns, a French term that refers to the body turning as if it were a rigid block). Speech and swallowing problems are common and related to rigidity and bradykinesia of the oropharynx. The decrease in involuntary swallowing can lead to drooling (overflow of pooled saliva). Decreased speech volume (hypophonia) and mild dysphagia are common as well.

Nonmotor symptoms are also common in PD. Anosmia (impaired sense of smell) is an early feature. Autonomic symptoms such as constipation and orthostatic hypotension can be seen. Rapid eye movement sleep behavior disorder, depression, and dementia can all be seen, although dementia is usually not seen until later in the disease. Psychosis (usually in the form of visual hallucinations) can be seen and is often associated with dopaminergic therapy being used to treat motor symptoms.

Other Hypokinetic Movement Disorders: The Parkinson-Plus Syndromes

In addition to idiopathic PD, there are 4 other main causes of parkinsonism that are collectively called the Parkinson-plus syndromes, or atypical parkinsonism. The term *Parkinson-plus syndromes* is particularly helpful because all of the disorders in the group are characterized by parkinsonism *plus* other symptoms that are either completely atypical for idiopathic PD or in greater proportion than would be seen in PD. The 4 Parkinson-plus syndromes that will be discussed here are dementia with Lewy bodies, multiple system atrophy, progressive supranuclear palsy, and corticobasal syndrome. In general, the parkinsonism seen in these 4 disorders is more symmetric at onset than PD, and they generally have less tremor but more rigidity and bradykinesia. None of the 4 have specific pharmacologic treatments and, in general, are treated symptomatically with antiparkinsonian medications. All 4 disorders have a much poorer response to dopaminergic therapy and thus a worse prognosis than idiopathic PD.

Dementia with Lewy bodies (DLB) is sometimes referred to simply as Lewy body disease and is characterized pathologically by the same α-synuclein inclusions and Lewy bodies as idiopathic PD. The difference between the 2 conditions is the distribution, as the pattern of Lewy body accumulation within the brain is much more diffuse in DLB but more concentrated in the basal ganglia in PD. Clinically, patients with DLB have parkinsonism and dementia within the first year of symptom onset. This differs from PD, where only 30% to 40% of patients develop dementia, and if it occurs, the onset of the dementia is usually 10 years after the onset of motor symptoms. Other common features of DLB include visual hallucinations, prominent clinical fluctuations, and neuroleptic sensitivity. Notably, the visual hallucinations occur even without exposure to dopaminergic therapy (unlike in PD, where this is primarily seen as a side effect of dopaminergic therapy). The fluctuations are in the cognitive status and can be dramatic, even within the same day, where the patient at times seems cognitively normal and at other times is completely demented. Likewise, the neuroleptic sensitivity refers to a cognitive, delirious/agitated response to neuroleptic treatment (which is usually initiated to treat the hallucinations). Recent work has emphasized that DLB and PD are likely part of a spectrum with shared pathophysiology, and patients with mixed features or who are intermediate between the 2 extremes will be encountered. See Chapter 29 for more information on the cognitive deficits in DLB.

Multiple system atrophy (MSA) is also characterized pathologically by α-synuclein inclusions, but these are found in glia (glial cytoplasmic inclusions) as opposed to the intraneuronal inclusions that are Lewy bodies. However, because the primary abnormal protein accumulation is α-synuclein, it is still organized with PD and DLB as 1 of the synucleinopathies. The prevalence of MSA is less than that of PD, at approximately 4 cases per 100,000 population. As the name alludes, MSA is a multisystem neurodegenerative disorder that is characterized by cerebellar and pyramidal tract signs and autonomic dysfunction in addition to parkinsonism. The cerebellar signs include intention tremor when reaching for objects, slurred speech, and an uncoordinated, ataxic gait. Autonomic symptoms are nonmotor features such as orthostatic hypotension, urinary retention, constipation, and abnormal heat or cold intolerance. There are 2 clinical variants distinguished based on the predominant presenting symptoms. If parkinsonism is the dominant feature, it is called MSA-P, and if cerebellar ataxia is the dominant feature, it is called MSA-C. Both variants have the preponderance of autonomic dysfunction. Although autonomic dysfunction can be seen in idiopathic PD, it occurs earlier and to a more severe degree in MSA than in PD.

Progressive supranuclear palsy (PSP) is pathologically different from the previously discussed causes of parkinsonism because there is abnormal accumulation of the protein tau instead of α-synuclein. Aggregates of tau, particularly in glial cells, are the pathologic hallmark of PSP. The prevalence of PSP in the United States is significantly less than that of PD, approximately 6 cases per 100,000 population. In addition to parkinsonism, the most striking clinical feature is the supranuclear gaze palsy referenced by the disease name. The patient has difficulty volitionally initiating gaze in a certain direction, but when performing the oculocephalic maneuver, the patient's extraocular muscles can physically still make the appropriate movements. Therefore, the problem localizes above the level of the brainstem nuclei that control eye movements, hence the term *supranuclear* gaze palsy. This is most commonly seen early with vertical eye movements, which present as difficulty with reading or frequent stumbling over

impediments due to inability to look down. As it progresses to a complete gaze palsy in all directions, the patient may move his or her entire head in order to look around the room. The gaze issue combined with parkinsonism leads to early gait problems and frequent falls. Speech and swallowing are significantly affected, and the speech of PSP patients can have a characteristic growling quality. As PSP progresses, patients can develop disproportionate atrophy of the dorsal midbrain, which can sometimes be seen on magnetic resonance imaging (MRI), as noted in Figure 28–3.

Corticobasal syndrome (CBS) is another Parkinson-plus syndrome that is often marked pathologically by abnormal accumulation of tau in a form called corticobasal degeneration (CBD). (CBS refers to the clinical syndrome while CBD refers to the specific neuropathological findings that are often associated.) Because both PSP and CBD have accumulation of tau isoforms containing four microtubule-binding repeats, they are considered related and sometimes referred to as "4R tauopathies." Although there are no formal studies on the prevalence of CBS, estimates are that it is roughly half as common as PSP. Unlike PSP, however, CBS tends to present asymmetrically with parkinsonism plus prominent apraxia of 1 hand. The patient may report progressive loss of use of that hand. On testing, apraxia manifests as intact motor strength but difficulty performing complex voluntary tasks, such as brushing teeth or giving a thumbs-up signal. When the

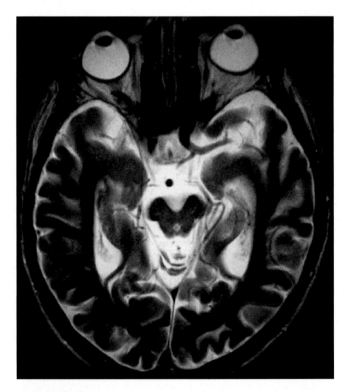

FIGURE 28–3 Progressive supranuclear palsy. T2-weighted axial magnetic resonance image showing the atrophic dorsal midbrain that gives rise to the "mouse ears" (also "Mickey mouse") appearance. (Reproduced with permission from Ropper AH, Samuels MA, Klein JP: *Adams and Victor's Principles of Neurology*, 11th ed. New York, NY: McGraw Hill; 2019.)

apraxia becomes severe, the patient has little voluntary control of the limb, and it may move on its own. This is known as the "alien limb phenomenon." Ultimately, the disease progresses to involve the other side of the body, and the cortical reference in the disease name means that patients will ultimately develop dementia as well.

One additional cause of parkinsonism is **drug-induced parkinsonism** from medications being taken for other conditions. The clinical key is that unlike idiopathic PD, the parkinsonism is symmetric at onset and begins after introducing 1 or more agents that interfere with central nervous system (CNS) DA. Medications known to cause drug-induced parkinsonism are DA antagonists (antipsychotics, certain antiemetics such as metoclopramide), DA depleters (reserpine, tetrabenazine), and chemotherapeutic agents (fluorouracil, doxorubicin, cyclophosphamide). All of these causes are reversible, meaning that removal of the offending agent should lead to resolution of parkinsonism over weeks to months, depending on exposure. Certain toxins can poison and damage the basal ganglia, causing irreversible parkinsonism. These include the compound 1-methyl-4-phenyl-1,2,3,6-tetrahydropyridin (MPTP; a byproduct of synthetic opioid manufacturing that caused a spate of drug-induced parkinsonism in the 1980s), organophosphates (pesticides), carbon monoxide, cyanide, and methanol.

Parkinson Disease: Pharmacology & Other Treatments

Currently available treatments are mostly *symptomatic* and do not alter the underlying degenerative process. Symptomatic treatments are useful and can restore function and quality of life for many years, but ultimately, the progression of the disease leads to increasing difficulty in managing the symptoms.

Most of the pharmacologic interventions currently used in PD are aimed at restoring DA levels in the brain. In general, medications used in the management of PD can be divided into DA precursors, DA receptor agonists, and inhibitors of DA degradation. There is a smaller but still useful role for existing nondopaminergic therapies, such as anticholinergic agents that modify the function of striatal interneurons.

Dopamine Precursors

DA itself is not useful for therapy because it cannot cross the blood–brain barrier (BBB). However, DA's immediate precursor, **levodopa**, is readily transported across the BBB, and once in the CNS, levodopa is converted to DA by the enzyme aromatic L-amino acid decarboxylase (AADC). Orally administered levodopa is readily converted into DA by AADC in the gastrointestinal tract, which both diminishes the amount of levodopa that can reach the CNS and increases the peripheral DA-related adverse effects (predominantly nausea, due to binding of this DA to receptors in the area postrema). When levodopa is administered alone, only 1% to 3% of the administered dose reaches the CNS unchanged (**Figure 28–4**). To boost the levels of levodopa available to the brain and reduce the adverse effects of peripheral levodopa metabolism,

levodopa is almost always administered in combination with carbidopa, which inhibits peripheral AADC without affecting central AADC. Carbidopa increases the fraction of orally administered levodopa available in the CNS from 1% to 3% (without carbidopa) to 10% (with carbidopa), allowing a significant reduction in the dose of levodopa and reducing the incidence of peripheral adverse effects. The combination of carbidopa/levodopa (trade name Sinemet, from the Latin for "without emesis") is still considered the gold standard of therapy for PD. By increasing CNS DA levels, carbidopa/levodopa effectively treats all 4 cardinal symptoms of PD, although gait instability tends to be slightly less responsive.

In later stage PD, use of high doses of carbidopa/levodopa can cause hyperkinetic choreiform movements at peak doses. This phenomenon is known as levodopa-induced dyskinesia and is thought to be due to temporary DA excess in the direct and indirect pathways causing chorea. Other adverse effects of levodopa therapy include hypotension, vivid dreams, and visual hallucinations. It is an important distinction that levodopa-related hallucinations are usually visual and not auditory, because auditory hallucinations are almost always due to a primary psychiatric disorder. The classic levodopa-related visual hallucinations are miniature-sized people or animals, sometimes referred to as "Lilliputian figures."

DA Receptor Agonists

Another strategy for enhancing dopaminergic neurotransmission is to target the postsynaptic DA receptor directly using DA receptor agonists. The earliest therapies in this class were the ergot derivatives bromocriptine (D_2 agonist) and pergolide (D_1 and D_2), but these have been found to induce long-term side effects such as cardiac valve fibrosis and have fallen out of favor. The newer nonergot agonists are pramipexole, ropinirole, and rotigotine (all $D_3 > D_2$). All DA agonists are nonpeptide molecules and do not compete with levodopa for transport across the BBB. Furthermore, because they do not require enzymatic conversion by AADC, they remain effective late in the course of PD. All of the DA receptor agonists in current use have half-lives longer than that of levodopa, which allows for less frequent dosing and a more uniform response to the medications.

The major limitation on the use of the DA receptor agonists is their tendency to induce unwanted adverse effects, which may include nausea, peripheral edema, and hypotension. All of the DA agonists may also produce a variety of adverse cognitive effects, including excessive sedation, vivid dreams, and hallucinations, particularly in elderly patients. A rare but problematic side effect is **DA dysregulation syndrome**, in which patients develop problems with impulse control. Common manifestations include pathologic gambling, overspending, compulsive eating, and hypersexuality. These behaviors may be socially destructive and require discontinuation of the medications.

Inhibitors of DA Metabolism

Another strategy to treat PD involves the inhibition of DA breakdown. Inhibitors of both monoamine oxidase type B

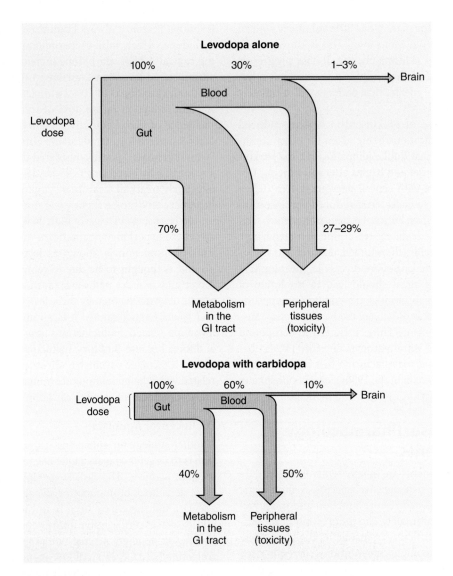

FIGURE 28-4 Fate of orally administered levodopa and the effect of carbidopa, estimated from animal data. The width of each pathway indicates the absolute amount of the drug at each site, whereas the percentages shown denote the relative proportion of the administered dose. The benefits of coadministration of carbidopa include reduction of the amount of levodopa required for benefit and of the absolute amount diverted to peripheral tissues and an increase in the fraction of the dose that reaches the brain. GI, gastrointestinal. (Data from Nutt JG, Fellman JH: Pharmacokinetics of levodopa, *Clin Neuropharmacol.* 1984;7(1):35-49.)

(MAO-B; the isoform of monoamine oxidase [MAO] that predominates in the striatum) and catechol-*O*-methyltransferase (COMT) have been used as adjuvants to levodopa in clinical practice. **Selegiline** is an MAO inhibitor that is selective for MAO-B at low doses. One potential problem with selegiline is that it has an amphetamine metabolite, which can cause sleeplessness and confusion, especially in the elderly. **Rasagiline** is a newer MAO-B inhibitor that does not form amphetamine metabolites and is more specific for MAO-B than selegiline. The specificity for MAO-B over MAO-A allows these drugs to avoid the tyramine effect associated with nonselective MAO blockade. Both rasagiline and selegiline improve motor function in PD when used alone, and both can augment the effectiveness of levodopa therapy.

Tolcapone and **entacapone** inhibit COMT and thereby inhibit the degradation of levodopa as well as DA. Tolcapone is a highly lipid-soluble agent that can cross the BBB, whereas entacapone distributes only to the periphery. Both drugs decrease the peripheral metabolism of levodopa and thereby make more levodopa available to the CNS. There have been reports of fatal hepatic toxicity associated with tolcapone, and thus in practice, entacapone is the most widely used COMT inhibitor.

Nondopaminergic Pharmacology in PD

Amantadine was developed primarily as an antiviral that reduces the length and severity of influenza A infections. In patients with PD, however, amantadine can have mild benefits on the cardinal motor symptoms but also can treat levodopa-induced dyskinesias. Although the exact mechanism of action for amantadine in PD is unknown, the mechanism for reducing dyskinesia is thought to involve blockade of excitatory *N*-methyl-D-aspartate receptors. **Trihexyphenidyl** and **benztropine** are muscarinic receptor antagonists that reduce cholinergic tone in the CNS. They reduce tremor more than bradykinesia and are therefore more effective in treating patients for whom tremor is the major clinical manifestation of PD. These anticholinergic drugs are thought to act by modifying the actions of striatal cholinergic interneurons, which regulate the interactions of direct and indirect pathway neurons. They also cause a range of anticholinergic adverse effects, which may include dry mouth, urinary retention, and importantly, impairment of memory and cognition.

Surgical Therapy for PD

Deep brain stimulation (DBS) therapy is approved by US Food and Drug Administration (FDA) for the treatment of medically refractory PD. DBS involves surgical placement of an electrode into the basal ganglia, either in the subthalamic nucleus or the globus pallidus internal segment. The electrode wire is tunneled under the skin and connected to a subcutaneous pacemaker-type pulse generator that controls electrical stimulation to the implanted basal ganglia site. High-frequency stimulation is applied through the electrode and has an ablative effect on cells in these nuclei and results in decreased output from the indirect pathway (less "no go") and alleviation of PD motor symptoms. Although DBS provides powerful suppression of PD motor symptoms and can be adjusted over time to address symptom progression, on its own, it does not alter progression of the disease. Risks of the procedure are infection related to the implanted hardware and hemorrhage during intracranial placement of the electrode. Most patients receiving DBS therapy can reduce their antiparkinsonian medications, but the ability to completely replace oral medications is rarer. Candidates for DBS must have proven response (at some point in the disease course) to levodopa, because DBS only benefits symptoms that are responsive to levodopa. Thus, DBS has no effect on the nonmotor symptoms of PD. The most common PD patients to receive DBS therapy are those who have advanced disease requiring such high doses of oral medications that they frequently alternate between adverse effects and insufficient benefit when the medications wear off.

HYPERKINETIC MOVEMENT DISORDERS

Essential Tremor

As mentioned previously, the most prevalent of all movement disorders is **essential tremor (ET)**. The exact pathologic mechanism of ET is not known, but degeneration of the cerebellum and its outflow tracts is most commonly implicated. ET is characterized by a bilateral postural and action tremor most commonly involving the arms. Head and voice tremor are also very common, whereas leg tremor is less common. ET is a pure tremor disorder because there are no other major clinical features other than the tremor. This distinguishes it from PD, but the tremor itself is also different because PD tremor is present at rest but abates with posture and action while the tremor of ET is present with posture and action but absent at rest. Patients with ET frequently have a positive family history of a similar tremor, indicating a genetic component of ET, although no single gene has been identified. ET is thought to be polygenic, not unlike hair color. Although ET is most common in the elderly, it can occur at younger ages when there is a strong family history of earlier onset tremor. The tremor itself is slowly progressive with age, but in later stages, the amplitude of the tremor can become quite large, to the extent that it impairs activities of daily living due to impaired use of the hands. Pharmacologic treatments for ET include propranolol and primidone. Propranolol is a nonselective β-blocker, can cross the BBB, and has a sedative effect on the tremor. Primidone is a prodrug for phenobarbital and thus exerts a γ-aminobutyric acid (GABA)-ergic effect to reduce the tremor. Both are symptomatic and do not prevent worsening of the tremor with time. DBS is also an FDA-approved therapy for ET. The target for electrode placement is the ventral intermediate nucleus of the thalamus. Thalamic DBS is highly effective at treating ET and is considered by most to be superior to either propranolol or primidone in suppressing tremor. As in PD, DBS remains a symptomatic therapy for ET.

Dystonia

Dystonia is defined as involuntary, sustained contraction of muscles around a joint that often results in (often painful) twisting postures and/or repetitive movements. The exact pathophysiology of dystonia is poorly understood, although the origin of the aberrant signal for the muscle contraction is central (coming from the basal ganglia) and not peripheral (ie, originating in the peripheral nerves or muscles). There are increasing numbers of genetic mutations identified that cause dystonia as 1 of the primary clinical manifestations, and the current nomenclature for these genes is *DYT1*, *DYT2*, and so on. Dystonia is most commonly categorized as being either focal or generalized based on the part of body involved. The most common focal dystonia is cervical dystonia, which involves the neck (cervical) region. Depending on the direction that the neck is twisted or pulled due to the abnormal muscle contractions, cervical dystonia is subdivided further. Torticollis is a cervical dystonia that primarily causes twisting of the neck and turning of the head (**Figure 28–5**). Anterocollis is when the head and neck are pulled forward, laterocollis is when they are pulled to the side, and retrocollis is when they are pulled backward. Another common focal dystonia is blepharospasm, which involves the orbicularis oculi, thus causing eye blinking or eye closure. Writer's cramp, which is often provoked by the hand posture required to write with a pen on paper, primarily involves wrist and

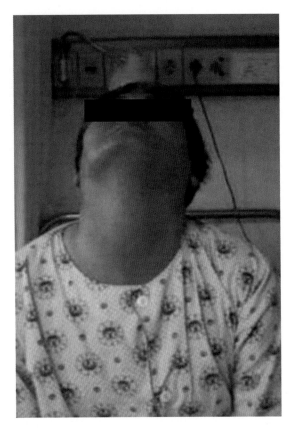

FIGURE 28–5 Retrocollis. (Reproduced with permission from Jeong SG, Lee MK, Kang JY, et al: Pallidal deep brain stimulation in primary cervical dystonia with phasic type: clinical outcome and postoperative course, *J Korean Neurosurg Soc.* 2009 Oct; 46(4):346-350.)

finger flexors. The treatment of choice for all focal dystonias is botulinum toxin injections into the affected muscles. Although botulinum toxin does not address the aberrant brain signal generating the movement, it does effectively abort the muscle contraction itself. Botulinum toxin works by preventing presynaptic release of acetylcholine into the neuromuscular junction. On average, 1 set of botulinum toxin injections can relieve a focal dystonia for up to 3 to 6 months. Oral medications such as antiparkinsonian medications (eg, carbidopa/levodopa or trihexyphenidyl) or muscle relaxants/benzodiazepines are sometimes used for generalized dystonias but are rarely effective for focal dystonias.

One unique genetic dystonia is **dopa-responsive dystonia**, which is usually caused by a mutation in the gene for guanosine triphosphate (GTP) cyclohydrolase 1. Both autosomal dominant and autosomal recessive mutations have been described. GTP cyclohydrolase is a critical enzyme in the pathway to synthesize tetrahydrobiopterin, which is a cofactor needed for the generation of DA. This disorder is extremely rare, with a prevalence of 1 in 2,000,000. Dopa-responsive dystonia causes childhood-onset dystonia and parkinsonism. The dystonia is worse in the legs than the arms and tends to worsen in the evenings. The dystonia and parkinsonism are highly responsive to very-low-dose levodopa, although patients require lifelong therapy. The dramatic responsiveness

to treatment makes it one of the most easily treatable of all dystonias, and therefore, many advocate for an empiric trial of carbidopa/levodopa in all patients who present with a dystonia, regardless of age.

There are also secondary dystonias that are not felt to be idiopathic. Most common are symptomatic dystonia and Wilson disease (which are discussed later in this chapter). Symptomatic dystonia is due to basal ganglia damage by stroke or trauma. Treatment for the secondary dystonias is similar to that of the primary dystonias.

Chorea

Chorea is an abnormal hyperkinetic movement consisting of nonrhythmic, irregular muscle contractions appearing to flow from 1 muscle group to the next. The word *chorea* is derived from the Greek word for dance, describing the dance-like quality of the movement. It is felt to be on the spectrum with athetosis, which has a more writhing quality, and ballismus, which has a more thrashing, large-amplitude quality. Causes of chorea can be divided into genetic causes and acquired causes.

Huntington Disease

The most well-known genetic cause of chorea is **Huntington disease (HD)**. HD is the prototypical pure genetic neurodegenerative disorder. The HD gene (*HTT*) on chromosome 4 encodes the protein huntingtin and contains a trinucleotide (CAG) repeat. HD was 1 of the first **trinucleotide repeat disorders** to be discovered, and the *HTT* gene was 1 of the first human genes to be completely sequenced. In an affected patient, the mutated allele will usually have ≥40 repeats, whereas there are normally only 15 to 20 repeats. CAG repeat expansions in the elevated range of 36 to 39 may lead to the disease, but there is reduced penetrance in this range. Expansions of >40 repeats are considered to be fully penetrant. As with all trinucleotide repeat disorders, HD can exhibit anticipation (an earlier age of onset in each generation, reflecting instability and expansion of the repeat), but interestingly, anticipation is primarily with paternal inheritance in HD. Patients who are homozygous for the mutation have been reported but are rare. There is a direct correlation between the CAG repeat length and disease onset and severity. The average age of symptom onset is 40 years, but larger repeat expansions (ie, CAG repeats >55) can have juvenile onset, whereas a CAG repeat of exactly 40 can result in symptom onset in the 70s. The exact function of the huntingtin protein is unknown, but it is thought to be a toxic gain of function. Pathologically, mutant huntingtin causes neuronal loss diffusely in the brain but most selectively in the medium spiny neurons of the striatum (caudate and putamen). Disproportionate caudate atrophy can often be seen on brain imaging in an HD patient (Figure 28–6).

Phenotypically, HD has a classic triad of motor, cognitive, and behavioral symptoms. The most common motor symptom is chorea, and 90% of patients with HD will develop chorea at some point in their disease course. Other hyperkinetic movements such as dystonia, myoclonus, and tics can

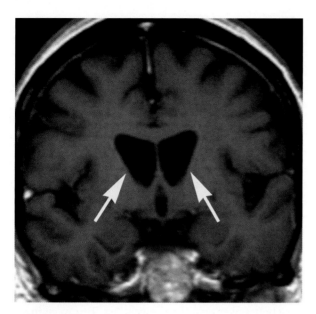

FIGURE 28-6 Image demonstrates enlarged frontal horns with flattened edge due to caudate atrophy (*arrows*) with abnormal configuration. (Reproduced with permission from Jameson J, Fauci AS, Kasper DL, et al: *Harrison's Principles of Internal Medicine*, 20th ed. New York, NY: McGraw Hill; 2018.)

be seen in HD but are less common. It should be noted that juvenile-onset HD is much different phenotypically in that it actually presents with parkinsonism instead of chorea. Cognitive symptoms can range from mild executive dysfunction to dementia. Behavioral symptoms can range from

---

CASE 28-1

A 60-year-old man presents for evaluation of abnormal movements. He has had at least 6 months of progressive nonpatterned involuntary movements of all 4 extremities. He has a past medical history of hypertension but denies any history of psychiatric illness. He has never had exposure to antipsychotics or antiemetics. On examination, he has moderate-amplitude chorea of the trunk and extremities. He has mildly impaired tandem gait. He denies any family history of similar abnormal movements. His mother died at age 85 years of natural causes, and his father died at age 52 years of a myocardial infarction.

Despite the lack of family history, it is still most likely that this patient has Huntington disease (HD). His father died relatively young and may have been the affected parent who gave him the mutation. He should have genetic testing to confirm this. Adults of any age who present with chorea should have HD and tardive dyskinesia as the top conditions on the differential diagnosis list. The absence of exposure to any known dopamine antagonists makes tardive dyskinesia unlikely, although sometimes patients are not aware of or may forget to report prior treatment with these medications.

---

mild depression or anxiety to severe agitation or psychosis. Diagnosis is confirmed by genetic testing after clinical suspicion is raised, usually with chorea and a positive family history. Genetic testing is available for at-risk presymptomatic patients as well, although there are significant ethical considerations, and thus, genetic testing should always be done with the involvement of a genetic counselor. At present, there are no curative treatments available, although gene silencing clinical trials are underway. The only approved symptomatic treatment is **tetrabenazine**, which treats the chorea only. Tetrabenazine is an irreversible vesicular monoamine transmitter (VMAT) type 2 inhibitor that depletes presynaptic DA. As might be expected with this mechanism, tetrabenazine can cause the adverse effect of parkinsonism at high doses. Like its fellow DA depleter, reserpine, tetrabenazine also carries a risk of worsening depression. DA-blocking agents such as typical and atypical antipsychotics can also suppress the chorea of HD and may also treat psychosis if present.

Acquired Causes of Chorea

Other important acquired causes of chorea include cerebrovascular disease, Sydenham chorea, and tardive dyskinesia. When cerebral ischemia involves the basal ganglia, the irritation may result in chorea or ballismus. Given the focality of strokes, the clinical result is usually a hemichorea or hemiballismus contralateral to the side of the infarct or ischemia. The classic presentation of **hemiballismus** is the result of a lacunar infarct to the subthalamic nucleus. The treatment for hemiballismus is a short course of a DA antagonist (neuroleptic) or DA depleter.

Sydenham chorea is a complication of childhood infection with group A β-hemolytic *Streptococcus*. It occurs in 20% of children and adolescents with rheumatic fever, although this incidence is decreasing due to better and earlier treatment of streptococcal infection. Sydenham chorea primarily affects the face, feet, and hands. No treatment is necessary because the chorea usually remits within a few months.

Tardive dyskinesia is a chorea that develops after chronic exposure to DA-blocking agents such as antipsychotics and certain antiemetics (eg, metoclopramide). Development of tardive dyskinesia usually requires years of daily exposure to the DA-blocking agent, although it has been seen with much shorter exposure periods. It is thought that downregulation of DA receptors over time plays a role in the pathogenesis. The classic presentation of tardive dyskinesia is with repetitive lip-smacking/tongue-protruding movements, but the chorea can involve any part of the body. Treatment of tardive dyskinesia involves withdrawal of the offending agent, and 50% of patients will have resolution of the chorea within 6 months. However, if persistent, the chorea can be suppressed by DA depleters (which do not tend to cause tardive dyskinesia).

Tics

Tics are sudden, repetitive, nonrhythmic movements that tend to be stereotyped. If involving the face or body, they are classified as motor tics, but if involving an utterance or sound, they are classified as vocal tics. Tics may also be simple or complex. If the tics become persistent, it is classified as a disorder, and all tic disorders are felt to be on the spectrum with obsessive-compulsive disorder (OCD). Most patients describe a premonitory urge to make the tic prior to the initiation of the tic itself. The tic can also usually be suppressed temporarily, but the longer it is suppressed, the more uncomfortable this becomes and the larger the cluster of tics to relieve the urge.

Tourette syndrome is defined as the combination of both motor and vocal tics that have been persistent for >1 year. Average age of onset is 8 to 12 years old, and symptoms tend to improve into adulthood. Patients with Tourette syndrome may have obscene vocal tics (coprolalia) as a feature, but this occurs in only 15% of patients and tends to develop later in the course of the disease. Comorbid psychiatric symptoms such as attention-deficit/hyperactivity disorder (ADHD) and OCD are common. These should be treated aggressively because they are felt to be more debilitating than the tics themselves. Treatments to suppress the tics include clonidine, topiramate, DA depleters, and DA antagonists (antipsychotics).

Myoclonus

Myoclonus is a rapid lightning-like involuntary twitch and has numerous causes. Hiccups are an example of a myoclonic jerk of the diaphragm muscle. Physiologic (benign) myoclonus includes examples such as sleep starts or sleep myoclonus of infancy. Myoclonus can also be a feature of certain myoclonic epilepsies, all of which have epileptiform discharges on electroencephalography that correlate with myoclonus. These include myoclonic epilepsy with ragged red fibers and Lafora progressive myoclonic epilepsy. Both are genetic diseases that affect multiple organ systems and are progressive and ultimately fatal at a young age. Myoclonus is commonly seen in hospitalized patients due to severe metabolic derangements such as uremia or cerebral anoxia. Spinal cord injury can cause myoclonus, and it can also be associated with advanced neurodegenerative disorders such as Alzheimer disease, subacute sclerosing panencephalitis, and Creutzfeldt-Jakob disease. Certain drugs such as lithium, bismuth, meperidine, and cyclosporine can also cause myoclonus. Definitive treatment for myoclonus depends on the etiology. Symptomatic suppression of myoclonus can be attempted with clonazepam or a variety of other antiepileptic drugs (eg, levetiracetam, valproate).

Other Atypical Movement Disorders
Neuroleptic Malignant Syndrome

Neuroleptic malignant syndrome (NMS) is a rare and life-threatening adverse reaction to DA antagonists. The most common drugs to precipitate NMS are the typical antipsychotics, although NMS has been reported from atypical antipsychotics, usually the ones with the highest D_2 antagonism. NMS has been reported with DA depleters such as reserpine and tetrabenazine, as well as potent DA-blocking antiemetics such as metoclopramide. NMS can also be seen with abrupt withdrawal of prodopaminergic drugs, such as carbidopa/levodopa. This is clinically relevant for PD patients who become hospitalized for other reasons and have their antiparkinsonian agents stopped during the inpatient stay, which can precipitate NMS.

NMS typically consists of parkinsonism (primarily rigidity), fever, and autonomic instability. Although encephalopathy and elevated serum creatine kinase levels are commonly seen, these are not required to make the diagnosis of NMS. Fever is thought to be due to hypothalamic DA receptor blockade. The most significant risk factor for the development of NMS is the titration schedule, because rapid titration of high-potency DA-blocking agents carries the highest risk for NMS. Other risk factors include dehydration, exhaustion, and agitation. The incidence of NMS has been reported at 1 in 500 but is decreasing due to increased physician awareness and resultant changes in management as well as increased use of atypical antipsychotics over typical antipsychotics. Treatment involves removal of the DA antagonist as a first step. Prodopaminergic agents such as the DA precursors and DA agonists can be used as treatment, although the most commonly used treatment is dantrolene. Intensive care unit care with aggressive rehydration, temperature regulation, and correction of electrolytes is also critical for survival. Finally, if the NMS was precipitated by withdrawal of prodopaminergic agents, then these should be reinitiated as soon as possible.

Wilson Disease

Another important mixed movement disorder is Wilson disease, which is an autosomal recessive disorder of copper metabolism. Mutations in the *ATP7B* gene lead to abnormal copper accumulation, which leads to organ dysfunction. Although prevalence of mutation carriers is 1 in 100, prevalence of the actual disease is much rarer, at 2 per 100,000. The primary sites of copper accumulation are in the liver and brain, and those with more accumulation in the liver (60%) present with hepatic dysfunction and jaundice as children or teenagers. Patients with more brain accumulation (40%) present with neuropsychiatric symptoms in their 20s or 30s. The most common neurologic symptoms of the disease are parkinsonism, an unusual postural/action tremor that is often described as "wing-beating tremor," dysarthria, sialorrhea, dystonia, and ataxia. Psychiatric symptoms can include personality change, depression, anxiety, and psychosis. Wilson disease is treatable if caught early but can be fatal if it is missed. When neurologic or psychiatric symptoms are present, this should correlate with basal ganglia hyperintensities on brain MRI and copper deposition in the irises of the eyes, known as Kayser-Fleischer rings (Figure 28–7). Diagnosis is confirmed by lab test results, which include low ceruloplasmin levels, elevated 24-hour urine for copper, and/or high copper content on liver biopsy. Treatment of Wilson disease involves chelation therapy with agents such as penicillamine or liver transplant if disease is severe.

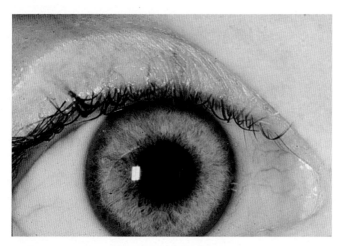

FIGURE 28–7 Kayser-Fleischer ring in Wilson disease. This corneal ring is brown and located at the outer edge of the gray-blue iris. Its darkness increases as the outer border (limbus) of the cornea is approached. (Reproduced with permission from Usatine RP, Smith MA, Mayeaux EJ, Chumley HS: *The Color Atlas and Synopsis of Family Medicine*, 3rd ed. New York, NY: McGraw Hill; 2019. Photo contributor: Marc Solioz, University of Berne.)

SELF-ASSESSMENT QUESTIONS

1. A 60-year-old man is brought in by his family for a dementia evaluation. The patient is no longer able to feed himself without assistance. On examination, he demonstrates bradykinesia, left-sided rigidity, postural instability, and apraxia. The patient frequently raises his left arm into the air but appears unaware of this action. A brain MRI shows cortical atrophy that is greater on the right than the left. Which of the following is the most likely diagnosis?

    A. Frontotemporal dementia
    B. Dementia with Lewy bodies (DLB)
    C. Progressive supranuclear palsy
    D. Parkinson disease with dementia
    E. Corticobasal syndrome

2. A 55-year-old woman presents with 4 months of tremor that affects both upper extremities and is present "most of the time." She has a 15-year history of type 2 diabetes and hypertension. Medications are insulin, lisinopril, hydrochlorothiazide, and metoclopramide. On exam, her speech and mental status are normal. She has a paucity of facial expression, slow movements, and mild bilateral upper and lower extremity rigidity. Motor strength is normal, but sensory exam reveals distal pinprick loss. There is a 4-Hz resting tremor in both upper extremities that disappears with voluntary movement. Which of the following is the most likely diagnosis?

    A. DLB
    B. Drug-induced parkinsonism
    C. Multiple system atrophy
    D. Parkinson disease (PD)
    E. Vascular parkinsonism

3. A 65-year-old man initially developed a left upper extremity resting tremor with mild left upper extremity rigidity and was diagnosed with PD. He returns for follow-up, and his wife reports that although his tremor is improved, he has been spending hours each day on the computer playing online poker. He has spent thousands of dollars, and this is creating significant stress for the family. Which of the following medications is the most likely culprit for causing this problem?

    A. Carbidopa/levodopa
    B. Donepezil
    C. Selegiline
    D. Pramipexole
    E. Amantadine

4. A 20-year-old woman presents for evaluation of a problem with gait. She reports that she has walked with a limp since at least 9 or 10 years old. She occasionally feels that her calves are cramping, and she is noted to have a dystonic inversion of her right foot when she walks. She feels the symptoms usually worsen over the course of the day. She has some parkinsonism manifested as mild rigidity in her legs with mild bradykinesia of rapid toe tapping. Eye movements and all exams of the upper extremities are normal. She has no family history of any such condition. What should be done next to confirm the diagnosis in this patient?

    A. Empiric trial of carbidopa/levodopa
    B. Magnetic resonance imaging of the brain
    C. Routine electroencephalogram
    D. Genetic testing for Huntington disease (HD)
    E. Electromyography of the gastrocnemius muscle

Age-Associated Cognitive Disorders & Dementia

Marissa C. Natelson Love & Rabia Jamy

OBJECTIVES

After studying this chapter, the student should be able to:

- Define the terms *dementia* and *mild cognitive impairment* (MCI).
- Understand how patients are screened and diagnosed by history, physical exam, and standardized tests.
- Identify different types of dementia based on clinical presentations, neuropathology, and pathogenesis.
- Explain pharmacologic and nonpharmacologic management of cognitive disorders.

PREVALENCE & BURDEN

One of the most striking demographic trends over the past century has been a dramatic extension of life expectancy, which has almost doubled from 44 years in 1890 to >80 years today. An unfortunate accompaniment of this change is an increase in age-related cognitive change, perhaps the most common and feared result of aging. Age-related cognitive change includes both "normal" cognitive aging and several neurodegenerative diseases causing dementia.

Among the neurodegenerative diseases, Alzheimer disease (AD) is the most common, affecting >5 million people in the United States. Interestingly, the incidence (rate of new cases per unit of population) of dementia seems to be declining worldwide, with improvement in control of vascular risk factors and other public health improvements. However, the prevalence (overall number of cases) of dementia is still growing at an alarming rate. The risk of developing dementia due to AD doubles every 5 years after age 65 years, and with the growth of the aged population, AD prevalence is expected to continue increasing dramatically.

NEUROANATOMY

One of the reasons it is important to define which cognitive domains are involved in a patient's cognitive decline is the fact that each domain has a particular anatomy. Thus, identifying an impaired domain is the primary mode of localization in behavioral neurology. Episodic memory localizes to the medial temporal lobe, including the hippocampus (Chapter 20).

Language is generally localized to the left hemisphere and can be more precisely localized based on the type of aphasia (Chapter 21). Visuospatial function is generally localized more to the right hemisphere and occipital, and executive function is primarily frontal.

SCREENING & DIAGNOSIS

History

The history is the most important part of the workup in diagnosing cognitive disorders. A collateral informant is usually helpful because the patient's deficits may prohibit the patient from providing a reliable history. An important goal is to identify the initial symptoms, which enables inferring the initial cognitive domain involved and in turn defining the initial neuroanatomy, a key factor in differential diagnosis. Later in the course of neurodegenerative diseases, multiple brain regions invariably become involved, and thus multiple domains are affected. Elucidating the initial symptoms can suggest where in the brain the pathologic process might have started. It is important to remember that patients may use the term "memory" to refer to other cognitive domains. For example, "I can't remember words" is likely to reflect language impairment, and "I forget how to get to the grocery store" is likely to reflect visuospatial impairment. Asking for anecdotes or specific examples of cognitive functions that the patient can no longer perform is most informative.

Other important details include the time course of the onset and progression of the cognitive changes (eg, acute,

VOCABULARY

Clinical diagnosis: Diagnosis based on clinical criteria, such as symptoms, exam findings, neuroimaging, and other clinical tests.

Cognitive aging: Normal, but highly variable, decline in cognition that occurs with aging, apart from any disease.

Cognitive domains: The individual components of cognition, such as memory, language, complex attention, visuospatial, and executive function. Most of these are self-explanatory, with the possible exception of **executive function**, which is a set of processes related to cognitive control and self-regulation, including ability to plan, organize, multitask, shift attention purposefully, inhibit undesirable behavior, initiate tasks, and generate ideas.

Delirium: An acute confusional state of cognitive change with disturbance of consciousness. Delirium is commonly caused by metabolic, infectious, or other medical conditions and must be excluded to diagnose the neurodegenerative diseases discussed in this chapter.

Dementia: A syndrome with cognitive decline sufficient to impair daily functioning. Dementia can be staged as mild, moderate, or severe. Mild dementia is characterized by difficulties with **instrumental activities of daily living**, which are activities generally necessary for independent living, such as doing housework, preparing meals, or managing money. Patients with moderate dementia have further difficulties with basic **activities of daily living**, such as bathing and dressing. Patients with severe dementia are generally fully dependent and unable to participate in most aspects of their own care.

Major neurocognitive disorder: Although the term *dementia* is generally used by neurologists, psychiatry introduced new terminology in *Diagnostic and Statistical Manual of Mental Disorders*, fifth edition (DSM-V), replacing *dementia* with this diagnosis (Table 29–1).

Mild cognitive impairment (MCI): Cognitive change more than normal for age or education but not enough to impair daily functions (ie, more than normal cognitive aging but less than dementia). Note that the terms *MCI* and *dementia* are syndromic, describing a degree of cognitive decline but not referring to a specific disease. One can have MCI (or dementia) due to Alzheimer disease, due to another neurodegenerative disease, due to vascular disease, or due to head trauma or chronic alcoholism, among many other possible causes. This chapter is focused on the neurodegenerative diseases causing dementia.

Minor neurocognitive disorder: DSM-V diagnosis congruous with mild cognitive impairment.

Pathologic diagnosis: Diagnosis based on neuropathologic examination of the brain at autopsy. Compare with earlier definition of **clinical diagnosis**. Most of the disorders discussed in this chapter have separate clinical and pathologic diagnostic criteria. Clinical criteria are used by clinicians to make diagnoses, provide prognosis, and guide treatment plans for patients under their care, whereas pathologic criteria come into play only after death. The degree to which the clinical diagnosis predicts neuropathologic findings varies. For example, a clinical diagnosis of Alzheimer disease carries a fairly high (but certainly not 100%) likelihood of finding the plaque-and-tangle neuropathology that makes a pathologic diagnosis of Alzheimer disease. In other conditions, such as frontotemporal dementia, the clinical syndrome can have several different possible neuropathologic causes, so the pathologic diagnosis is hard to predict based on the clinical diagnosis.

TABLE 29–1 DSM-V diagnostic criteria for major neurocognitive disorder.

A. There is insidious onset and gradual progression of impairment in at least 2 cognitive domains.
   1. Complex attention
   2. Executive function
   3. Learning and memory
   4. Language
   5. Perceptual-motor (visuospatial)
   6. Social cognition
B. Interfering with independence in everyday activities
C. Not exclusively with delirium, psychiatric disorders

DSM-V, *Diagnostic and Statistical Manual of Mental Disorders*, fifth edition.

Data from American Psychiatric Association: *Diagnostic and Statistical Manual of Mental Disorders*, 5th ed. Arlington, VA, American Psychiatric Association, 2013.

subacute, intermittent, or chronic). A cognitive review of systems may include asking specifically for any history of change in gait, the presence of a tremor, language dysfunction, visuospatial deficits, or sleep changes. The patient should be screened for symptoms of depression, anxiety, psychosis, or other behavior change.

Cognitive Examination

A brief bedside cognitive screening exam can be performed. The Mini Mental State Exam (MMSE) is widely used. Somewhat more challenging tests that are more sensitive for detecting milder deficits include the Montreal Cognitive Assessment (MoCA) and the Saint Louis University Mental Status (SLUMS) exam. Full neuropsychological evaluation requires up to a full day of testing, but provides standardized scores normed to age and education across a range of cognitive domains and may be helpful in subtler or atypical cases of impairment.

To assess learning and memory, the patient is typically asked to repeat and remember 3 unrelated words. Normal performance is to learn and repeat all 3 words. After generally 5 or more minutes of other mental state testing, the patient should be asked to recall the words. Remote memory can be checked by asking the patient to describe his or her medical, family, and social history; however, a knowledgeable informant must be available to confirm the information.

The evaluation should also include orientation testing. Disorientation to self occurs only in advanced dementia. Its presence in the context of mild or moderate cognitive disability suggests delirium or a primary psychiatric disturbance.

Assessment of language includes naming, sentence repetition, fluency (effortfulness of speech), comprehension, reading, and writing. This can be tested with everyday objects available to the examiner, such as a jacket, shoe, or pen. Parts of objects are more difficult to name than whole objects. Therefore, in addition to a jacket as a whole, the patient might be asked to name the collar, lapel, sleeve, pocket, and cuff.

A brief sequence of commands can further assess language comprehension, praxis, and left–right orientation. The patient should be asked to show how he or she would perform actions with each hand (eg, using a hammer to hit a nail or a key to open a lock). A subsequent 2-handed task, such as slicing bread or opening a jar, tests the patient's ability to integrate the actions of both hemispheres in a single task. These can be followed with commands that require the patient to correctly identify right and left, both in reference to his or her own body (eg, "Touch your right thumb to your left ear") and the examiner's body (eg, "Point to my left hand with your left hand").

Visuospatial or perceptual-motor function can be tested by asking the patient to copy a drawing of a cube or other simple 3-dimensional figure. Normal performance is to accurately depict 3 sides and 3 dimensions. The integration of motor behavior in space can be further tested with a drawing task. The clock drawing test assesses multiple realms of cognition, including executive function (planning), spatial relationships, and semantic knowledge. Normal performance requires placing all numbers and the hands in the correct position.

Executive functions can be evaluated in different ways. Category (also called semantic) fluency tests the patient's ability to name as many words as possible belonging to a category set, such as animals or fruits. Patients who name <15 animals in 1 minute have a high likelihood of cognitive impairment. Attention, concentration, and working memory can be tested by asking the patient to add the value of a penny, a dime, a nickel, and a quarter. For this task, it is important that the names of the coins be used, because the working memory system is engaged throughout the process of translating the names to numerical values, performing addition, and reporting the answer in a unit different than what was provided. This pocket change addition task is useful as a cognitive screening tool because it can assess calculation simultaneously with working memory. The patient who answers "36 cents" can add numbers, but has failed to include all 4 coins. Other tests of working memory or related aspects of attention can be used if pocket change addition is inappropriate (eg, for someone unfamiliar with the common names of US coins). Alternatives include asking the patient to state the months of the year or days of the week in reverse order. Digit span is a common test of primary memory that also depends on attention. In this task, the patient is asked to repeat a string of random digits in the order that he or she heard them. Normal performance is to repeat strings of 5 or more correctly. Deficits may be more pronounced when patients are asked to repeat digits in reverse order. Normal performance in this task is to reach a span at least 2 digits less than the forward span.

Physical Examination

A general physical and neurologic examination should be completed. These are often normal in AD and other dementias. Parkinsonism can develop in several disorders and can be helpful in narrowing a differential diagnosis. Focal neurologic finding can suggest the presence of a structural or vascular lesion.

Ancillary Testing

The American Academy of Neurology evidence-based practice parameter for the diagnosis of dementia recommends blood tests to exclude systemic illnesses as the cause of dementia (Table 29–2). General metabolic and hematologic states, as well thyroid function and vitamin B_{12} levels, should be tested. Syphilis serology tests are no longer considered part of the routine screening.

Imaging is also recommended as part of the routine assessment of patients with dementia symptoms. Computed tomography (CT) is useful to exclude structural lesions that may contribute to the dementia such as cerebral infarctions, neoplasm, extra-axial fluid collections, and hydrocephalus. However, magnetic resonance imaging (MRI) is preferred due

TABLE 29–2 Recommended testing for the patient presenting with possible dementia.

Screen for depression
Blood tests
■ Comprehensive chemistry panel, including hepatic and renal function
■ Complete blood count
■ Thyroid function tests
■ Vitamin B_{12} level
Cerebral imaging
■ Computed tomography is generally sufficient for screening, but magnetic resonance imaging provides much more information

Data from Knopman DS, DeKosky ST, Cummings JL, et al: Practice parameter: diagnosis of dementia (an evidence-based review). Report of the Quality Standards Subcommittee of the American Academy of Neurology, *Neurology*. 2001 May 8;56(9):1143-1153.

to its greater resolution and the additional information provided. Medial temporal atrophy on MRI strongly supports the likelihood of AD when appropriate clinical features are present (Figure 29–1). Fluorodeoxyglucose (FDG) positron emission tomography (PET) scans reveal temporoparietal hypometabolism in patients with AD and frontotemporal hypometabolism in frontotemporal dementia. The presence or absence of amyloid plaques can be determined by amyloid PET.

Cerebrospinal fluid (CSF) examination by lumbar puncture is not a routine part of the dementia evaluation. Standard CSF tests (cell count, protein, glucose) have a low likelihood of influencing diagnosis in most people with dementia. CSF examination is more useful in cases with serologic evidence of past syphilis, as well as in patients with immunosuppression or atypical dementia symptom patterns, such as young age at onset or very rapid progression. CSF assays for soluble amyloid-beta (Aβ) and tau are commercially available. The finding of abnormal CSF Aβ and tau increases the probability that cognitive impairment is due to AD but is not highly specific.

Electroencephalography (EEG) is also not recommended as part of the routine evaluation of dementia. EEG findings are nonspecific. They are frequently normal in early stages and evolve toward generalized slowing.

COGNITIVE AGING

Cognitive aging is a decline in cognition that is considered to be generally inevitable with age, although the degree of cognitive change is highly variable, and some individuals age with very little cognitive decline. It is a common feature of aging across species. Declines associated with cognitive aging begin as early as the 40s. Some cognitive domains are more susceptible than others. Processing speed commonly declines with aging, and difficulty remembering names, especially proper names, is also typical. Overall, the degree of change is milder compared to the neurodegenerative diseases, although it can limit abilities to perform technical or highly demanding tasks.

Cognitive aging is not a disease, and the biological basis is still under study. Generally, neuronal death is not involved, as in the neurodegenerative dementias. Some brain "pathology," such as development of neurofibrillary tangles in the medial temporal lobe and brain atrophy on imaging, is considered a nearly universal accompaniment of aging, but the relationship of these changes to cognitive aging is not clear.

ALZHEIMER DISEASE

AD is by far the most common cause of dementia and thus is almost always a consideration in the workup of cognitive change. Its hallmark is early change in episodic memory, although formal diagnostic criteria also require change in a second cognitive domain, such as language, visuospatial processing, or executive function. Social graces remain intact early. Noncognitive symptoms, including apathy and unawareness, are important contributors to the impact of disease. The general neurologic exam is usually normal.

Clinical Manifestations

Memory dysfunction is usually the first symptom recognized in AD. Recent memories are impaired because new information cannot be adequately stored for later recall. This leads to the characteristic rapid forgetting of people with AD. Declarative memory is most impaired in AD and is impaired early in the disease. This fact-oriented memory system allows us to store and recall specific information and experiences.

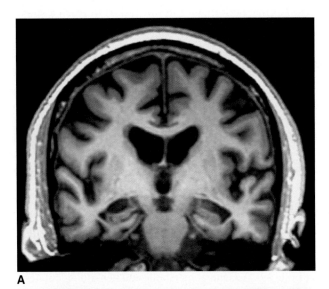

A

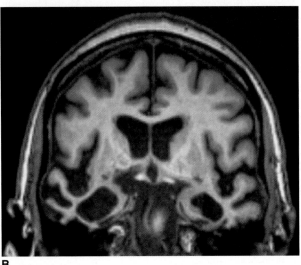

B

FIGURE 29–1 **A.** Coronal T1-weighted magnetic resonance image (MRI) of a 74-year-old man with moderate Alzheimer-type dementia. Diffuse cerebral and hippocampal atrophy with ex vacuo ventricular and cortical sulcal dilation is noted. **B.** Coronal T1-weighted MRI of a 70-year-old woman with behavioral variant frontotemporal lobar dementia. Atrophy of the right greater than left temporal lobes is out of proportion to atrophy of the frontal and parietal lobes. (Reproduced with permission from Ropper AH, Samuels MA, Klein JP: *Adams and Victor's Principles of Neurology,* 11th ed. New York, NY: McGraw Hill; 2019.)

Procedural memory (eg, knowing the steps to perform a task) is often better preserved, which contributes to the appearance of normalcy to a casual observer in mild AD. Emotionally charged memories are often better maintained. Orientation to time is often affected in early AD, and as the illness progresses, orientation to place becomes more disrupted. This may result in becoming lost in familiar settings.

Language impairments are prominent in AD. They usually begin as word-finding difficulty in spontaneous speech, which may later become severe enough to interrupt the flow of speech. The language of AD patients becomes progressively vaguer as semantic memories are lost. Their verbal output frequently lacks specifics. Prosody, the normal rhythm, melody, and emotional intonation of speech, is affected in many AD patients, particularly in more severe stages. Reading skills and verbal comprehension worsen as AD progresses. In late stages, global aphasia is common.

Disorders of higher visual processing and visual impairment are also common in AD. The dysfunction is evident at the level of basic visual processing, including impaired sensitivity to movement and visual contrast. Deficits in depth perception are also observed.

Executive dysfunction, including problems with judgment, problem solving, planning, and abstract thought, affects the majority of AD patients. Executive function behaviors require selecting tasks appropriately, sequencing their execution, and monitoring performance to ensure successful completion. Intact executive function also requires the suppression of inappropriate responses to the environment. Failures in this area of cognition are manifested as failure to manage more complicated tasks such as family finances or meal preparation. Socially inappropriate behavior, disinhibition, and poor task persistence may also emerge. The presence of executive dysfunction predicts the transition from more benign age-related cognitive changes to early dementia.

Noncognitive or behavioral symptoms are also important, especially as the disease evolves. Personality changes involving passivity and apathy are frequent in the early phases of the illness. Apathy is separable from depression and represents an organic loss of motivation. It occurs in 25% to 50% of AD patients. Another common noncognitive problem in AD is unawareness of illness (called anosognosia or lack of insight), which occurs in >50% of patients. Unawareness of illness is a major impediment to early diagnosis and may reduce the effective implementation of management strategies. Psychosis and agitation tend to occur later in the disease course. Delusions are often paranoid in character and may lead to accusations of theft, infidelity, and persecution. The delusion that caregivers or family members are impostors or that one's home is not his or her real home is a common trigger for wandering or aggression. Anxiety and depression can lead to catastrophic reactions, an intense emotional outburst of short duration. They are characterized by the abrupt onset of tearfulness, aggressive verbalizations or actions, and contrary behaviors. Sundowning is commonly used to describe predictable increases in confusion and behavioral symptoms in the afternoon and evening hours. It is reported in up to 25% of AD patients.

AD follows a relentlessly progressive course, although there may be periods of relative symptom stability. Symptoms tend to progress less rapidly in both early and late disease, with more rapid losses, especially in activities of daily living, in moderate disease. It is a fatal disease, with an average survival of 8 to 12 years following diagnosis. Approximately half of AD patients die from complications of global neurologic dysfunction such as immobility and malnutrition; the other half of deaths are attributed to other factors, typically other age-related diseases such as stroke and cancer. Life expectancy is reduced by about 50%.

Diagnosis

The symptoms of AD begin insidiously and progress gradually. Most patients are initially diagnosed when their symptoms are still not functionally limiting, so the clinical diagnosis is mild cognitive impairment (MCI) due to AD. With time, as the disease progresses and activities of daily living become impaired, the diagnosis becomes dementia due to AD.

Pathologic diagnosis of AD, of course, requires autopsy. On gross examination, the AD brain is atrophic with enlarged ventricles and sulci (Figure 29–2), and on microscopic examination, there is neuronal loss and gliosis. The basis for a pathologic diagnosis of AD, though, is the presence of 2 hallmark findings on microscopic examination: amyloid plaques and neurofibrillary tangles. Amyloid plaques (Figure 29–3), also known as neuritic or senile plaques, are extracellular aggregates composed primarily of Aβ peptide, 39- to 43–amino acid fragments derived from cleavage of amyloid precursor protein (APP). Neurofibrillary tangles (Figure 29–4) are intracellular accumulations of tau, a microtubule-associated protein that is normally found in cells but becomes hyperphosphorylated and aggregates in AD.

The diagnoses of MCI and dementia, as described under "Vocabulary," are based on the severity of cognitive impairment and do not themselves indicate etiology. MCI is diagnosed when the symptoms are more than expected with normal cognitive aging but do not have a significant impact on daily function, and dementia is diagnosed when the line of functional impairment is crossed. A patient can have MCI (or dementia) due to any of a multitude of causes. The determination that a patient's MCI or dementia is due to AD has traditionally been based on purely clinical characteristics, especially the memory predominance of the cognitive symptoms.

More recently, biomarkers that help to identify AD pathophysiology have begun to be used in clinical diagnosis. The primary clinical biomarkers for AD are designed to detect changes related to the pathologic findings of AD, specifically Aβ, tau, and neurodegeneration, either by neuroimaging or CSF analysis. Aβ plaque deposition can be detected with a PET scan using amyloid tracers (Figure 29–5). In CSF, Aβ levels decrease in AD, which is somewhat paradoxical since overall Aβ levels are higher in brain due to accumulation in plaques;

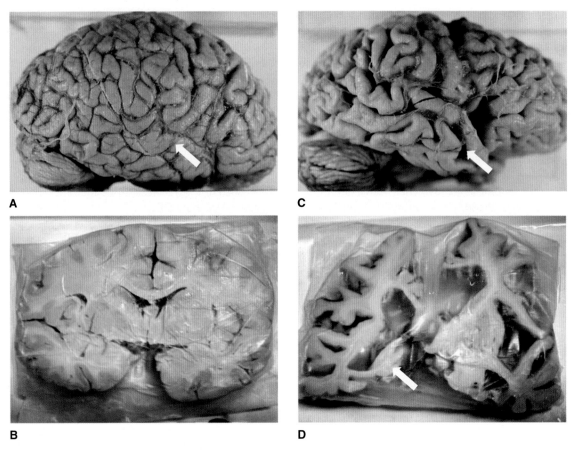

FIGURE 29–2 Neuroanatomical comparison of normal brain and Alzheimer disease brain. **A/B,** Normal brain. **C/D,** Alzheimer disease brain. **A/C,** Lateral views show prominent neocortical atrophy in AD (arrows). **B/D,** Coronal sections show enlargement of the ventricles and hippocampal atrophy (arrow). (Reproduced with permission from Zerr I: *Alzheimer's Disease: Challenges for the Future.* London: IntechOpen Limited; 2015.)

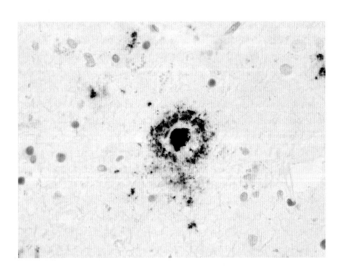

FIGURE 29–3 Senile plaque. A brown-staining senile plaque with a central core of β-amyloid protein is seen in the cerebral cortex of a patient with Alzheimer disease. (Reproduced with permission from Reisner H. *Pathology: A Modern Case Study*, 2nd ed. New York, NY: McGraw Hill; 2020.)

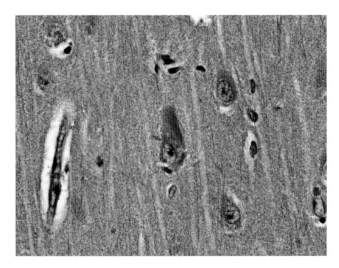

FIGURE 29–4 Neurofibrillary tangle (NFT). A bright red, elongated NFT partially fills the cell body of a large neuron (center of field) in the cerebral cortex of a patient with Alzheimer disease. (Reproduced with permission from Reisner H. *Pathology: A Modern Case Study*, 2nd ed. New York, NY: McGraw Hill; 2020.)

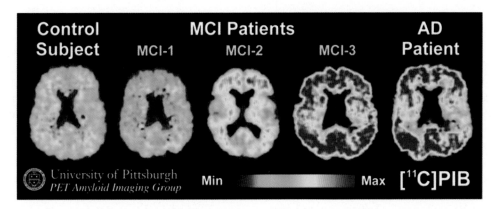

FIGURE 29–5 Positron emission tomography (PET) images obtained with the amyloid-imaging agent Pittsburgh Compound-B ([¹¹C] PIB) in a normal control (*left*); 3 different patients with mild cognitive impairment (MCI; center); and a patient with mild Alzheimer disease (AD; *right*). Some MCI patients have control-like levels of amyloid, some have AD-like levels of amyloid, and some have intermediate levels. (Used with permission from William Klunk and Chester Mathis, University of Pittsburgh.)

presumably the shift toward plaque deposition lowers Aβ concentrations in the interstitial fluid. Levels of both total and phosphorylated tau increase in CSF, so the ratio of CSF Aβ to tau is a sensitive measure (since the numerator decreases and denominator increases). Neurodegeneration can be detected by either structural imaging showing atrophy, particularly in the hippocampus, or by functional imaging with FDG-PET scans, which show decreased metabolic activity in areas with neurodegeneration.

The growing use of AD biomarkers has revealed that many changes begin well before symptoms emerge. For example, amyloid plaque deposition begins about 15 years before clinical symptoms develop, and typical AD changes in CSF Aβ and tau are also detected in a similar time frame. Thus, many older individuals with completely normal memory and no symptoms have evidence of AD pathophysiology on testing, which is known as preclinical AD. Although preclinical AD is a research concept, not a clinical diagnosis, the fact that people with AD pathophysiology can be identified even before they are symptomatic raises the hope of applying future AD therapies and arresting disease in a presymptomatic (ie, asymptomatic) stage.

Pathophysiology

Merely identifying certain brain changes in a disease state is not sufficient evidence that those changes play a causal role in the disease, of course. Genetics provides some of the strongest evidence for causality, and although the vast majority of AD cases are sporadic, there are rare families in which an early-onset form of AD is inherited in an autosomal dominant pattern. These families have mutations in 1 of 3 genes: *APP*, presenilin 1 (*PSEN1*), or presenilin 2 (*PSEN2*). All 3 genes are involved in the production of Aβ peptides, which are generated when presenilin, a component of the γ-secretase protease, cleaves APP. Aβ tends to aggregate and can form both small oligomers, which have toxic effects on synapses, and larger aggregates that form amyloid plaques. The idea that Aβ plays a

central role in AD pathogenesis is based largely on this genetic evidence and is known as the amyloid hypothesis of AD.

The exact mechanism by which neuronal dysfunction and death occur in AD is unknown. APP or its normal derivatives might play a role in maintaining synaptic function and neuronal health. Aβ also is an activating trigger for microglial cells, leading them to produce several inflammatory cytokines with cytotoxic properties, including tumor necrosis factor-α. Activation of microglia may contribute to a self-propagating cycle of local inflammation and neuronal dysfunction. Although most models of AD pathophysiology place Aβ in a causative role, other approaches suggest oxidative stress or bioenergetic failure as triggering factors in the amyloid cascade. It is possible that AD is a disorder with heterogeneous origins, with different primary mechanisms resulting in similar patterns of neuronal failure and pathologic expression in different individuals.

Treatment

There are several US Food and Drug Administration (FDA)-approved drugs for AD. First-line treatment is usually a cholinesterase inhibitor, such as donepezil, rivastigmine, or galantamine. These drugs inhibit the enzyme that degrades acetylcholine in the cleft of cholinergic synapses and thus serve to boost cholinergic transmission. The rationale for using cholinesterase inhibitors in AD stems from early observations of cholinergic cell loss in AD and the known role of cholinergic transmission in memory. Because cholinesterase inhibitors do not halt the pathophysiologic processes that kill cholinergic neurons, they are considered a symptomatic, not disease-modifying, treatment. Their effect is modest; most patients do not experience actual improvement in symptoms but do benefit from slowing or arresting symptom progression for 6 to 12 months. The most common side effects are gastrointestinal, which can be avoided to some extent with the transdermal preparation of rivastigmine. Because these drugs are procholinergic, muscle cramps and bradycardia can also occur.

The other FDA-approved AD treatment is memantine, which blocks overstimulation of *N*-methyl-D-aspartate (NMDA)-subtype glutamate receptors. NMDA receptor activity is critical for normal learning and memory, but excessive activation results in excitotoxicity due to abnormal calcium influx. Memantine is a use-dependent blocker designed to allow physiologic NMDA receptor stimulation but prevent excitotoxicity. It is indicated for the moderate and severe dementia stages of AD and so is generally added to a cholinesterase inhibitor later in the disease. Memantine, like the cholinesterase inhibitors, provides a modest benefit by temporarily slowing progression of impairment.

Other drugs can be used to treat the behavioral and psychiatric symptoms that can occur in AD. Selective serotonin re-uptake inhibitors (SSRI) or serotonin-norepinephrine reuptake inhibitors should be considered, with side effect profiles guiding the choice of agent. Citalopram has shown efficacy in reducing agitation. Antipsychotics can be used to treat agitation or psychosis in patients with dementia, but because of the FDA Black Box warning for increased mortality when used in these patients, antipsychotics should be reserved for cases when nonpharmacologic intervention and other treatments fail. Atypical antipsychotics may be better tolerated compared with traditional agents.

Nonpharmacologic strategies are generally more effective and better tolerated approaches for treating behavioral and psychiatric symptoms in dementia. These include scheduled toileting and prompted toileting for incontinence, offering graded assistance (as little help as possible to perform activities of daily living [ADLs]), role modeling, cueing, positive reinforcement to increase independence, and avoiding adversarial debates by using redirection instead. Caregivers should be advised to maintain a calm demeanor and use the services of caregiver support groups. In addition, a systems-based approach to treatment might decrease caregiver burden. Home health services or assisted living facilities where multiple healthcare disciplines can become involved in the care of the person with dementia are likely to prevent caregiver burnout and subsequent skilled nursing facility placement. Sleep hygiene should be addressed, and if necessary, pharmacologic sleep aides with the least cognitively slowing effects can be used. Antihistaminic and anticholinergic agents are relatively contraindicated.

CASE 29–1

A 75-year-old woman presents to her physician accompanied by her daughter who is concerned about her memory. The daughter reports that for the past 9 months, her mother has been repetitive and forgets plans that they have made. Furthermore, the mother seems more withdrawn from social activities. She is able to do all of her previous activities of daily living, still drives without problems, and cooks for herself. Past medical history is significant for hypertension and hyperlipidemia. Family history is positive for dementia in the patient's mother with onset at age 85 years. The patient is widowed and denies using tobacco, alcohol, or drugs. Medications include several antihypertensives, a statin, and diphenhydramine as needed for insomnia. On exam, she is alert; pleasant; and oriented to person, place, and situation but not to time. On a cognitive screening test, she scores 22/30, missing 3/3 points on recall, 2/5 on serial calculations, and 3/4 on orientation to time. No apraxia is noted in either upper extremity, and speech is fluent. The remainder of her neurologic exam is normal.

Because her cognitive problems are clearly more than just normal aging but are not impairing her day-to-day functioning, the appropriate diagnosis is mild cognitive impairment. The etiology of her mild cognitive impairment would require further study to determine, but Alzheimer disease is the most common and most likely etiology, and her history is typical, with her symptoms primarily in the domain of episodic memory. Vascular disease is another consideration. Management would likely begin with a cholinesterase inhibitor, recommendation to minimize her anticholinergic sleep aid, and counseling about the importance of exercise and blood pressure control.

FRONTOTEMPORAL DEMENTIA

Clinical Manifestations

Frontotemporal dementia (FTD) is a progressive, degenerative disorder characterized by behavioral changes that have some clinical similarities to bipolar disorder and psychoses, such as social withdrawal, apathy, disinhibition, and compulsive behavior. It has an earlier onset than AD, with a median age of onset of 58 years, and unlike AD, memory is typically not particularly impaired in early stages of disease.

The earliest signs of disease in FTD are frequently subtle personality and behavioral changes, which become increasingly pronounced as time progresses. Patients typically do not have insight into their problems, so the history is usually provided by a family member. Other symptoms may include impaired social behavior, reduced emotional reactivity, and changes in personality or beliefs, including compulsive behavior and poor judgment. Examples of problems include childish behavior, rudeness, inappropriate sexual remarks or jokes, impatience, careless driving, excessive spending or hoarding of certain items, perseverative routines, compulsive pacing, insistence of certain foods or excessive food intake, neglect of personal hygiene, and disinterest in the immediate family. The patient's cognitive abilities may remain intact for some time after the onset of behavior changes. Survival from time of symptom onset ranges from 6 to 11 years.

In addition to referring to this specific clinical syndrome, the term FTD can also refer to a family of disorders including 2 others that have similar underlying pathology. In the context of this broader use of the term FTD, the specific disorder discussed here is called behavioral variant FTD (bvFTD), and the other 2 clinical syndromes are semantic variant primary progressive aphasia (PPA) and nonfluent variant PPA. Semantic variant PPA is a fluent aphasia (meaning that the rate and ease of spoken language is not affected) in which patients lose their knowledge about what things are called and, later, what those things do or are used for. Thus, the speech of semantic variant PPA patients is often rather vague and lacks the use of specific nouns. Nonfluent variant PPA patients have progressive difficulties speaking, with effortful and fragmented speech lacking normal grammatical structure.

Diagnosis

Diagnosis of FTD is based on these clinical symptoms and is supported by evidence of frontal and temporal atrophy on structural neuroimaging or frontal and temporal hypometabolism on functional neuroimaging, such as PET scans with the radiolabeled glucose tracer FDG. As one would expect, the exact location of the imaging abnormalities varies with the clinical syndrome. In bvFTD, it is often worse on the right side, and in the PPAs, it is usually on the left.

Pathophysiology

The pathology of FTD, including bvFTD and the semantic and nonfluent variants of PPA, is referred to as frontotemporal lobar degeneration (FTLD). Unlike AD, there is not 1 single pathology for FTD. Most patients have accumulation of either transactive response DNA-binding protein 43 kDa (TDP-43) or tau (the same microtubule-associated protein found in neurofibrillary tangles in AD). When TDP-43 is present, the pathologic diagnosis is FTLD-TDP, which occurs in about half of cases. In most other cases, tau pathology is present, and the pathologic diagnosis is FTLD-tau, which has several subtypes. One subtype of FTLD-tau is Pick disease, which is manifested by Pick bodies in neurons. Other subtypes are progressive supranuclear palsy and corticobasal degeneration, which are discussed in Chapter 28.

The heterogeneity of pathology in FTD and overlap with other conditions emphasize that FTD is part of a spectrum of related disorders. In addition to the conditions already mentioned (bvFTD, semantic variant PPA, nonfluent variant PPA, progressive supranuclear palsy, and corticobasal degeneration), the other major neurodegenerative disease that is part of the FTD spectrum is amyotrophic lateral sclerosis (ALS), which is discussed in Chapter 31. In fact, FTD patients often develop features of ALS, and ALS patients often develop features of FTD, and the 2 disorders can develop similar pathology (particularly FTLD-TDP) and be driven by similar genetic mutations.

Genetic causes are much more common in FTD than in AD, with autosomal dominant mutations in up to 25%. The most common gene for both FTD and ALS is a hexanucleotide expansion in *C9ORF72* on chromosome 9. Other common genes involved in FTD (but less so in ALS) are *MAPT*, the gene for tau, and progranulin (*GRN*).

Treatment

There are no FDA-approved therapies for FTD. The drugs used for AD are generally not effective and can actually exacerbate some FTD symptoms. SSRIs and atypical antipsychotics are often used to help control behavioral symptoms.

DEMENTIA WITH LEWY BODIES

Dementia with Lewy bodies (DLB) causes a decline in cognition, usually with parkinsonism. Three cardinal features that distinguish DLB from other degenerative dementias are marked fluctuations in cognitive function or level of alertness, visual hallucinations, and rapid eye movement (REM) sleep behavior disorder. DLB is closely related to Parkinson disease dementia (PDD), and the 2 disorders are called the Lewy body dementias because both have these microscopic inclusions composed of α-synuclein. In fact, the main difference between DLB and PDD is the timing of symptoms: In DLB, the cognitive symptoms begin before or <1 year after the onset of motor symptoms, whereas in PDD, the motor symptoms precede the cognitive symptoms by at least a year.

Clinical Manifestations

Cognitive decline in DLB starts with deficits in attention, executive function, and visuospatial skills, unlike AD, in which memory is affected first. Parkinsonian symptoms such as bradykinesia and rigidity also develop, but they are usually milder and more likely to be symmetric than in Parkinson disease, and tremor, a cardinal feature of Parkinson disease, is less commonly seen. Autonomic dysfunction is also common, and patients may have repeated falls and fainting spells secondary to orthostatic hypotension.

There are several distinguishing features of DLB. Fluctuating cognition is present in almost 80% of the cases. However, it can be subtle, and caregivers and patients may have to be directly asked about changes in the level of alertness over the course of a day. Visual hallucinations most commonly involve seeing animals or well-formed people. Finally, DLB patients often seem to act out their dreams, a condition known as REM sleep behavior disorder, in which the atonia that normally suppresses dream enactment during REM sleep does not occur.

DLB is a progressive and debilitating disease. Survival from the time of diagnosis is variable and is often worsened due to the patients' increased risk of falls, immobility, and aspiration pneumonia.

Diagnosis

Diagnosis of DLB is largely based on clinical history and physical exam findings. It is important to make a prompt and correct diagnosis because of the sensitivity of patients to antipsychotic medications. Reactions can be acute and severe. Symptoms can range from worsening of orthostatic hypotension, to irreversible parkinsonism, to death. MRI scans may reveal cortical atrophy. Single-photon emission CT (SPECT) and PET scans of patients with DLB have shown decreased perfusion in the occipital lobes, which in some studies has been shown to correlate with severity of visual hallucinations. In cases where clinical features are not clear cut, DaTscan (GE Healthcare; SPECT scanning using the dopamine transporter ligand ioflupane iodine-123) can be used to provide support for final diagnosis, which has a specificity of 90%.

Pathophysiology

DLB is a synucleinopathy, or disorder characterized by α-synuclein inclusions, like Parkinson disease and multiple system atrophy (discussed in Chapter 28). α-Synuclein is a normal component of the presynaptic terminal. In synucleinopathies, α-synuclein accumulates in the cytoplasm of neurons in inclusions known as Lewy bodies. These are the same type of inclusions that are found in Parkinson disease, although in DLB, they tend to be found more in cortical regions. Lewy bodies are also found in the substantia nigra and other brainstem nuclei. Patients have a loss of dopamine- and acetylcholine-producing neurons, similar to patients with Parkinson disease and AD, respectively, and as a result, they suffer from symptoms seen in both these diseases. DLB is usually sporadic, and there are no well-recognized autosomal dominant genes for DLB.

Treatment

The cholinesterase inhibitors used in AD are also effective in DLB. Visual hallucinations are perhaps the most responsive symptom to treatment. Sinemet and other anti-Parkinson treatments can be used and may help with the motor symptoms. It is important to avoid antipsychotics, particularly typical antipsychotics.

VASCULAR DEMENTIA

Unlike the dementing diseases discussed thus far, vascular dementia is not a primary neurodegenerative condition associated with proteinopathic inclusions, but rather, it is a disorder caused by chronic ischemia due to impaired cerebral perfusion. It can result either from the cumulative effect of discrete strokes, which is often called poststroke vascular dementia or multi-infarct dementia, or it can take a more insidious course, even without clinically apparent strokes, due to gradual accumulation of small-vessel ischemic disease. Cerebrovascular disease is also often a co-contributor to dementia syndromes, along with other pathology.

Clinical Manifestations

Vascular risk factors are present, and clinical history of stroke can be informative. The most commonly affected cognitive domain in vascular cognitive impairment is executive function, specifically processing speed. However, symptoms and cognitive deficits can vary depending on which areas suffer ischemia. Classically, vascular dementia progresses in a stepwise, rather than continuously progressive, manner, although with small-vessel disease, this is not always the case and progression can be gradual.

The physical exam often has residual neurologic deficits that localize to the area of the prior lesion (eg, aphasia, dysarthria, hemiparesis). Even without suggestive history or physical exam findings, vascular causes of cognitive impairment cannot be ruled out without neuroimaging, preferably MRI of the brain. Clinical judgment is required to determine whether the vascular lesion is responsible for the presenting cognitive impairment. Single lesions in strategic areas such as the left hemisphere perisylvian language areas, thalamus, midbrain, medial temporal lobe, and medial frontal lobe have been associated with causing cognitive impairment. These appear to be critical hubs in maintaining skills in language, memory, and attention.

Pathophysiology

Cerebrovascular disease has many different etiologies. Single or multiple large-vessel atherothromboembolic lesions can lead to impairment. Small-vessel disease can be from multiple lacunar infarcts, ischemic white matter damage, or microhemorrhages. Intracerebral hemorrhages and hypoperfusion injuries are also considered vascular causes of dementia.

Treatment

Although there is no specific treatment for vascular dementia once it develops, patients often respond to cholinesterase inhibitors, with effectiveness similar to that seen in AD patients. Vascular cognitive impairment is considered the most preventable form of dementia, and treatment tends to focus on secondary prevention by optimizing cerebrovascular health, minimizing cardiovascular risk factors, and instituting lifestyle modifications including diet and exercise.

NORMAL PRESSURE HYDROCEPHALUS

Normal pressure hydrocephalus (NPH) is a syndrome of acquired hydrocephalus in adulthood. Patients develop dilated cerebral ventricles leading to the classic triad of gait disorder, dementia, and urinary incontinence. The diagnosis should be suspected when these features are present in a patient with risk factors for hydrocephalus, such as prior intracerebral hemorrhage or infection. However, it is important to remember that impairments of gait, cognition, and urinary control are all common with aging, so not every patient with these symptoms has NPH.

Clinical Manifestations

The general neurologic exam is generally normal except for deficits in balance and gait. Findings include difficulty with moving from sitting to standing or the reverse; problems with initiating gait; and shuffling or poor foot clearance that leads to tripping, falling, or festination. The classic NPH gait is referred to as magnetic, since the feet seem difficult to lift off the floor. The cognitive deficits are explained by executive dysfunction such as slow processing and difficulty with problem solving. Memory deficits involve poor retrieval and relatively intact recognition memory, unlike that seen in AD. The urinary incontinence is usually urge incontinence, and patients are often aware of the need but unable to reach the restroom.

Diagnosis

When the diagnosis is suspected because of some or all of the classic features, neuroimaging is ordered to evaluate for hydrocephalus. It is important to distinguish between ventriculomegaly (enlarged ventricles) due to cerebral atrophy, which is called ex vacuo hydrocephalus, and ventriculomegaly due to hydrocephalus. Evidence of edema in the white matter surrounding the ventricles due to transependymal flow of CSF supports the diagnosis, although it can sometimes be difficult to distinguish this from ischemic changes in the white matter, which are also common.

If NPH is still suspected after imaging, a lumbar puncture is performed for large-volume drainage of CSF, with pre- and posttesting of gait. Documented improvement in walking speed after the procedure supports the diagnosis.

Pathophysiology

There are various models of the pathophysiology of idiopathic NPH. The end result is that the ventricles enlarge and neuronal and glial dysfunction occurs to produce the clinical features. The deficits presumably result from stretching of cortical fibers passing around the enlarged ventricles. Ventricular enlargement and subsequent dysfunction of the brain may be due to impaired CSF outflow resistance and increased intracranial pressure. Then, altered CSF dynamics and reduced subcortical blood flow and metabolism may give rise to ischemia that causes dysfunction, but not infarction in an anatomic distribution. The axons affected are periventricular and affect gait and cognition in the subcortical and frontal regions. Periventricular hyperintensities are typically seen on MRI in idiopathic NPH.

Treatment

The definitive treatment for NPH is neurosurgical insertion of a ventriculoperitoneal shunt that allows drainage of CSF from the lateral ventricle to the abdomen.

MANAGEMENT OF COGNITIVE DISORDERS

We have already discussed the specific treatments for each disorder. These are generally classed as symptomatic therapies and have not been demonstrated to alter the underlying pathologic process. Current clinical trials are evaluating putative disease-modifying treatments targeting the presumed pathophysiologic processes causing disease.

Most of these cognitive disorders are associated with the development of behavioral and psychiatric symptoms, such as agitation, depression, and anxiety. Treatment of emotional and behavioral symptoms is also symptomatically oriented, and no drugs have been specifically approved for these indications. However, because depression may cause acceleration of decline if untreated, treatment is highly recommended. Recreational programs and activity therapies have shown positive results. SSRIs or serotonin-norepinephrine reuptake inhibitors should be considered, with side effect profiles guiding the choice of agent.

Agitation may be in response to physical or emotional discomfort. Citalopram has shown efficacy in reducing agitation. Antipsychotics should be used to treat agitation or psychosis in patients with dementia where environmental manipulation fails. Atypical agents may be better tolerated compared with traditional agents.

Nonpharmacologic strategies for the prevention of agitation might include the following: use of scheduled toileting and prompted toileting for incontinence, offering graded assistance (as little help as possible to perform ADLs), role modeling, cueing, positive reinforcement to increase independence, and avoiding adversarial debates by using redirection instead. Caregivers should be advised to maintain a calm demeanor and use the services of caregiver support groups. In addition, a systems-based approach to treatment might decrease caregiver burden. Home health services or assisted living facilities where multiple healthcare disciplines can become involved in the care of the person with dementia are likely to prevent caregiver burnout and subsequent skilled nursing facility placement.

Almost as important as prescribing certain medicines is avoiding others. In particular, antihistaminic and anticholinergic agents are relatively contraindicated. This includes many over-the-counter and prescription drugs used for sleep, urinary incontinence, allergies, and other indications. Benzodiazepines are also generally to be avoided in the elderly, especially in those with cognitive impairment.

Finally, lifestyle modifications are an important aspect of preventing and treating these cognitive disorders. Physical exercise, especially aerobic exercise, has well-described beneficial effects. High levels of mental activity are associated with better outcomes. Certain diets, including the Mediterranean diet, have been associated with lower risk of cognitive impairment. In addition, reducing cardiovascular risk factors, particular hypertension, is also encouraged. These lifestyle factors probably have greater potential for positive effects than current pharmacologic treatments for the neurodegenerative dementias.

SELF-ASSESSMENT QUESTIONS

1. Which of the following reversible causes of cognitive impairment should you screen for in a patient with mild cognitive impairment?
   A. Depression
   B. Hypothyroidism
   C. Vitamin B$_{12}$ deficiency
   D. B and C
   E. All of the above

2. Which of the following medications is most likely to be associated with cognitive impairment?
   A. Carvedilol
   B. Hydrochlorothiazide
   C. Lisinopril
   D. Atorvastatin
   E. Diphenhydramine

3. Which of the following is the best choice for initial management of a patient with mild Alzheimer disease (AD)?
   A. N-methyl-D-aspartate (NMDA) receptor antagonist (eg, memantine)
   B. Peripherally acting cholinesterase inhibitor (eg, pyridostigmine)
   C. *Ginkgo biloba*
   D. Centrally acting cholinesterase inhibitor (eg, donepezil)
   E. Selective serotonin reuptake inhibitor (eg, fluoxetine)

4. Variations in the nucleotide sequence of which of the following genes is most closely associated with the development of late-onset AD?
   A. *LRRK2*
   B. Progranulin (*GRN*)
   C. Presenilin-1 (*PSEN1*)
   D. *APOE*
   E. Amyloid precursor protein (APP)

Neuroimmunology & Neuroinflammatory Disorders

William Meador

- Briefly discuss the epidemiologic aspects of neuroimmunologic diseases.
- Understand the basic premise of immunologic diseases involving the central and peripheral nervous systems.
- Understand prototypical diseases resulting from immune system damage to the nervous system.
- Briefly discuss treatment options available to patients with various neuroimmunologic diseases.

PREVALENCE & BURDEN

Although not described as common illnesses, neuroimmunologic diseases account for a significant proportion of disability in mid-to-late life in many developed countries. As a rule, these illnesses typically present with a progressive decline in neurologic function with superimposed flare-ups, resulting in significant neurologic deficits that can make basic functions of life quite difficult to perform. These illnesses are thought to collectively affect >500,000 people in the United States. Because the severity of illness within each disease can vary widely, studies looking at life expectancies can vary, but it is generally accepted that these illnesses result in a reduction of life expectancy that is commensurate with the severity of illness in each case.

OVERVIEW OF NEUROIMMUNOLOGIC ILLNESS

The immune system can cause protean manifestations of neurologic disease, and no single description can encompass all of them. To illustrate the range of disorders that the immune systems can cause, 2 classes of disorders will be discussed here in some detail: demyelinating disorders, which include multiple sclerosis (MS) and the related disorders neuromyelitis optica spectrum disorder and transverse myelitis (TM); and the neuromuscular disorders myasthenia gravis (MG) and Lambert-Eaton syndrome. Although this is far from a comprehensive review, these are common disorders and illustrate many of the principals of pathophysiology, diagnosis, and treatment.

MULTIPLE SCLEROSIS

Epidemiology

Almost all patients with MS are diagnosed between the ages of 20 and 49 years, with a mean age of diagnosis at 30 years. Approximately 5% of patients are diagnosed prior to age 20 years, and 9% are diagnosed after age 49 years. The disease has a female-to-male ratio of 3:1 and typically presents with acute onset of a neurologic symptom. The exact cause is still unknown. The illness has higher rates of prevalence in higher latitudes (farther distance from the equator), and many feel this may reflect an environmental component. Lack of sunlight exposure and low vitamin D have been proposed to contribute to the disease, but conclusive evidence for this is still lacking. It is generally accepted that there is also a genetic contribution to risk; >120 genes have been implicated as contributory to the development of MS, and almost all of these genes have direct or indirect effects on the immune system.

There are between 400,000 and 750,000 people living with MS in the United States and 2.3 million people with MS worldwide. This illness has a very high cost to society. The medications used to treat MS are typically very expensive, and monitoring of the disease is also quite expensive. Patients are often underemployed or disabled due to the illness, and lost productivity in mid-life can have a large impact on patients and their families. Depression is a common comorbidity in MS and further complicates patient care; in addition, it can increase patients' healthcare-related costs. Even when compared to other chronic illnesses, patients with MS have higher

VOCABULARY

Attack: Monophasic clinical episode of symptoms typical of MS, lasting ≥24h; aka exacerbation or relapse.

Clinically isolated syndrome (CIS): Initial attack in a patient not known to have MS.

Dissemination in Space (DIS): Occurrence in multiple locations within the CNS.

Dissemination in Time (DIT): Occurrence on different dates.

Juxtacortical: A lesion in the white matter directly abutting the cortex.

Lesion: Area of inflammatory damage in the brain; typically associated with a T2 hyperintense area ≥3mm on MRI.

Periventricular: A lesion in the white matter directly abutting the lateral ventricles.

Progressive: A time course with steadily worsening disease activity.

Relapsing: A time course with distinct attacks between periods of clinical stability.

Transverse myelitis: Acute inflammatory damage occurring in a defined segment of the spinal cord.

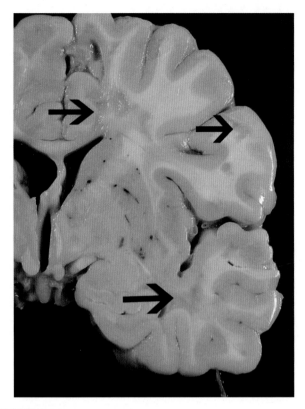

FIGURE 30–1 Autopsy examination of typical multiple sclerosis lesions. (Reproduced with permission from Kemp WL, Burns DK, Brow TG: *Pathology: The Big Picture.* New York, NY: McGraw Hill; 2008.)

rates of depression, and the rate of suicide is 7 times higher in MS patients than in age-matched controls.

Pathophysiology

MS damage to the CNS occurs primarily through demyelination of axons within the brain, optic nerves, and spinal cord (Figure 30–1). Some as-yet unrecognized trigger or process results in failure of tolerance of lymphocytes, leading to autoimmune destruction of central nervous system (CNS) tissue. As a result of cytokine and chemokine activation and production, the blood–brain barrier becomes more permeable, and activated T cells, B cells, macrophages, and other immune cells enter the CNS and cause autoimmune inflammation and destruction of nervous system tissue. Although T-cell lymphocytes have long been known to be a driving force in MS pathology, B-cell lymphocytes are becoming increasingly recognized in the pathophysiology of MS.

Examination of acute demyelinative plaques in the brain reveals denuded axons, dying oligodendrocytes, and "foamy macrophages," which are macrophages heavily laden with digested lipids from myelin breakdown. Microglia, the primary antigen-presenting cells within the CNS, are activated in the lesion and serve to further activate T cells through major histocompatibility complex (MHC) activation. Chronic lesions typically show demyelinated axons, astrocytic scarring, and little evidence of ongoing inflammatory cells or activity. They can also show evidence of decreased axon density and

remyelination, manifested as axons with thin myelination. Oligodendrocyte precursor cells can proliferate after CNS injury in MS, and it is suspected that these cells contribute to remyelination efforts.

Clinical Course

The clinical course of MS can be divided broadly into relapsing MS (RMS) and progressive MS. Most patients present initially with a relapsing-remitting picture; they experience a sudden attack of neurologic symptoms (blindness, weakness, or numbness are common) that gradually improve over weeks to months, only to be followed by another attack. Over time, the picture may become more progressive, with gradual worsening of neurologic symptoms and less and less recovery. Some patients may present with progressive, rather than relapsing, symptoms right from the start.

Relapsing MS

Most patients (85% to 90%) have a relapsing form of MS early in their course of disease (Figure 30–2). They typically present with an acute demyelinating event in their third or fourth decade of life. Typical events at onset include optic neuritis, TM, brainstem demyelinating events, and cerebral hemispheric syndromes. The most common presenting symptoms for MS are numbness and paresthesias, vision loss, motor weakness, ataxia, and polysymptomatic events.

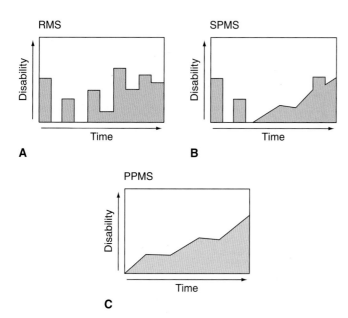

FIGURE 30–2 Clinical course of multiple sclerosis (MS).
A. Relapsing MS (RMS). **B.** Secondary progressive MS (SPMS).
C. Primary progressive MS (PPMS). (Reproduced with permission from
Jameson J, Fauci AS, Kasper DL, et al: *Harrison's Principles of Internal Medicine*, 20th ed.
New York, NY: McGraw Hill; 2018.)

Symptoms typically start abruptly, build in severity over hours to days, and then slowly resolve over several weeks. Patients often have very good recovery from these attacks early on, and many will improve to a point of being asymptomatic following the event. After the first attack, subsequent events are termed relapses. The typical MS patient has a relapse once every 13 to 15 months, and the symptoms that develop depend heavily on the location of the lesion within the CNS. Often, the symptoms of a relapse are quite different from the initial event, reflecting attack on a different part of the nervous system.

The disability produced by multiple relapses tends to accumulate over time. Most patients with MS will require ambulatory assistance 15 years from their initial diagnosis, but this can vary widely depending on the rate of disease progression and location of lesions. For example, one-fourth of patients will never require assistance with activities of daily living. However, it seems that a high level of disease activity in the first 5 years is strongly predictive of disability at 15 years from diagnosis. There are also early factors that portend a poorer outcome, and these include incomplete recovery from relapses, multiple relapses in the first year, spinal cord disease, male sex, African-American race, very active imaging studies, and early progressive course.

Fatigue is often cited as the most common cause of disability among patients with MS. It can manifest in different ways with patients, but typically they feel rested in the morning, but by late morning or early afternoon, they are too exhausted to carry on and have to rest before continuing with their daily activities. Although muscle fatigability is typically a significant problem for patients, it is mental and arousal fatigue that

is most limiting to most patients. Many patients have some form of cognitive decline during their illness, but this is often not their primary disabling manifestation. It tends to be mild and affect predominantly attention, concentration, working memory, and executive functioning, rather than being a true amnestic phenomenon. Very rarely, patients can have cognitive decline as their presenting manifestation of MS, but this is thought to occur in <5% of patients with MS.

Progressive MS

Approximately 10% of newly diagnosed patients with MS will be diagnosed with progressive MS. This illness presents quite differently from RMS and was historically known as primary progressive MS but now is simply referred to as progressive MS. Patients usually develop progressive MS later in life, with a median age of onset of 37 years, and have a very insidious initial course. Often, patients cannot clearly recall how long their symptoms have been ongoing. They typically present with a progressive myelopathic picture (ie, they have progressive weakness, ataxia and sensory loss that affects the legs more so than the arms). They typically have a slow progression with significant changes occurring over years and even decades for some. Disability usually develops from impairment in ambulation and bowel and bladder functioning and reduced dexterity.

Many patients who present initially with RMS will later develop a more progressive course. Classically, this was termed *secondary progressive MS* but is now considered to be progressive MS because it behaves clinically very much like progressive MS from the onset. In this state, relapses become rarer over time, and the frequency of relapses can diminish completely in many patients. Likewise, imaging studies will show little evidence of inflammatory changes over time. This transition is made strictly on clinical grounds when patients begin to report progressive accumulation of worsening symptoms or progressive changes on exam without intervening relapses.

Tumefactive MS

Rarely, patients with MS can present with large lesions that appear similar to a brain tumor. These lesions can be quite large with mass effects on surrounding structures; they may be associated with significant perilesion edema and they can have enhancement patterns suggestive of tumors. Patients can present with a clinical history and symptoms concerning for tumors, subacute infections, or strokes. Although the severity and type of symptoms encountered can vary dramatically, some patients can have minimal symptoms or exam changes despite extensive lesion sizes. Biopsy is often necessary to assess for true tumors versus demyelinating changes, and magnetic resonance spectroscopy is becoming more useful to help differentiate between the 2 conditions. Many patients will have a rapid and near-complete recovery, with many only having a single clinical event and not going on to develop MS in the future; however, limited data are available on this topic.

Pregnancy

Because MS affects predominantly women and is most active in mid-life, pregnancy is a common occurrence in patients with MS. Most of the treatments used to treat MS are considered risky in pregnancy, and generally it is recommended that patients forego treatment while pregnant and while breast-feeding to limit exposure to the fetus or infant. The annualized relapse rate (ARR) of patients with RMS decreases significantly during pregnancy, and in the third trimester, it is reduced by two-thirds. However, in the first 6 months after delivery, the ARR increases above a patient's baseline rate. When averaged over pregnancy and the first 6 months of postpartum life, the ARR for an MS patient remains at the normal rate. Therefore, there is no net benefit or harm for a patient with MS to become pregnant in regard to relapse occurrence.

Diagnostic Criteria

A diagnosis of MS is still based on the clinical assessment of a patient and has relied on 2 primary thresholds since the 1950s: dissemination in space (DIS) and dissemination in time (DIT). How DIS and DIT have been defined has changed significantly over the years, but these 2 basic principles remain the mainstay of diagnosing MS. In 2017, an international panel published the newest set of diagnostic criteria for MS, called the McDonald Criteria (Table 30–1). The McDonald Criteria are meant to be applied to patients who have a clinical event or a clinical history that is suggestive of MS. DIS can be fulfilled by having clinical evidence to support 2 areas of injury in the CNS, magnetic resonance imaging (MRI) showing lesions in 2 of 4 typical locations, or ancillary tests confirming two points in the CNS are affected. DIT can be fulfilled by a new clinical event, new lesions on follow-up imaging of any interval, an enhancing lesion at any time, or spinal fluid with evidence of CNS-specific production of immunoglobulin (such as oligoclonal bands or elevated IgG index). All diagnoses of MS are made in patients in whom there is no better alternative explanation.

Patients often present with a single demyelinating event (eg, optic neuritis or TM), and if the features of the event are suggestive of a demyelinating event in their history, exam findings, and ancillary testing, this is termed a *clinically isolated syndrome* (CIS). Basically, CIS refers to a patient who has had an event suggestive of MS but does not yet fulfill criteria for diagnosis of MS. Some patients with CIS may have evidence that puts them at high risk of MS and may warrant treatment initiation. Such evidence would include multiple brain lesions on MRI, abnormal spinal fluid, or a history suggestive of prior events without objective clinical evidence. In most cases, however, CIS alone is not enough to warrant starting long-term MS treatment.

If a patient has clear objective findings on exam to support 2 historical events typical of demyelinating disease, a diagnosis of RMS can be made at that time as long as alternative explanations are ruled out. No further testing is required for diagnosis in this scenario, but often MRIs will be obtained to assess for level of disease activity and to confirm the diagnosis. Moreover,

TABLE 30–1 The 2017 McDonald criteria for diagnosis of multiple sclerosis in patients with a typical attack at onset.

In a patient with a typical attack at onset...		
No. of Clinical Attacks	**No. of Lesions with Objective Clinical Evidence**	**Additional Evidence Needed to Diagnose MS**
≥2	≥2	None
≥2	1, with clear historical evidence of prior attack involving lesion in different location	None
≥2	1	DIS, demonstrated by an additional clinical attack implicating a different CNS site OR by MRI showing lesions in ≥2 typical MS locations
1	≥2	DIT, demonstrated by an additional clinical attack; an enhancing lesion typical of MS on MRI; new lesion on follow up MRI; OR demonstration of CSF-specific oligoclonal bands
1	1	DIS AND DIT, demonstrated by criteria above
In a patient with progressive worsening over 1 year typical of MS ...		
2 of these 3 criteria: ■ ≥1 T2 brain lesion typical of MS ■ ≥2 T2 spinal cord lesions typical of MS ■ CSF-specific oligoclonal bands		

DIS, Dissemination in Space; DIT, Dissemination in Time. In all cases, alternative explanations must be considered and ruled out.

Adapted with permission from Carroll WM: 2017 McDonald MS diagnostic criteria: Evidence-based revisions, *Mult Scler.* 2018 Feb;24(2):92-95.

if there are questions still unanswered after clinical assessment and imaging studies are performed, a spinal tap is often recommended to look for evidence of MS in the spinal fluid.

The diagnosis of progressive MS is somewhat different. According to the 2017 McDonald Criteria, patients must have 1 year of progressive disease activity plus 2 of the following 3 findings: 1 or more brain lesion(s) typical of MS, 2 or more spinal cord lesions typical of MS, CSF-specific oligoclonal bands (see Table 30–1). In diagnosing both RMS and progressive MS, an extensive evaluation for alternative explanations is warranted to rule out MS mimickers.

Ancillary Testing

The advent of MRI has been exceedingly beneficial in making the diagnosis of MS correctly, has enabled early diagnosis, and has completely changed our ability to track the disease course over time. MRI is irreplaceable in a clinical setting in which MS is suspected or diagnosed, and it is relied upon heavily for diagnosis discussions, treatment decisions, and prognosis. On MRI, lesions in the hemispheres tend to be oval in shape and oriented perpendicular to the ventricular surface. In contrast, lesions in the spinal cord tend to be 1 or 2 vertebral body heights and peripherally located. When the lesions are acute, often there is enhancement with MRI contrast agents. Several criteria have been proposed to support a diagnosis of MS on MRI. The most recent are the MAGNIMS criteria, which stipulate that for DIS, a patient should have 1 or more lesions in 2 of the following locations: periventricular, juxtacortical/cortical, infratentorial, optic nerve, or spinal cord. Although simplistic, when this rule is applied for diagnostic purposes, it has a sensitivity of 93% and specificity of 32%. When evaluating patients with CIS, the MRI is the best tool for predicting conversion to MS. Patients with CIS who have 1 or more lesions typical of MS are at much higher risk of developing MS over the next 15 years than patients without any identifiable brain lesions (72% vs 24% in isolated optic neuritis).

MRI is not only important in diagnosis, but is also very useful in prognosticating and in tracking disease activity over time. Patients who have multiple enhancing lesions or accumulate multiple new lesions rapidly in the early course of their illness are at higher risk of aggressive disease over time. In addition, patients with more spinal cord lesions on imaging tend to have a more aggressive course. Each T2 lesion visualized on MRI is thought to be related to scar tissue that developed from local inflammation and scarring due to MS disease activity. Many of these will occur in a clinically "silent" manner, whereby the patient will be unaware of their development. Therefore, it is recommended that patients who are being treated for MS have an MRI performed at least annually; in addition, they should have an MRI performed with any new symptoms concerning for a relapse.

Spinal fluid assessment is another useful tool in diagnosing MS and is abnormal in >90% of patients with MS. During the disease process, plasma cells take up residence inside the CNS and produce immunoglobulins at higher rates in the spinal fluid than in the serum. This results in unique immunoglobulin bands on protein electrophoresis, and these are classically referred to as oligoclonal bands. This is often associated with an elevated immunoglobulin G (IgG) index in the spinal fluid, which is present due to significant de novo synthesis of IgG in the spinal fluid. It is calculated as a ratio comparing the serum albumin and IgG to the cerebrospinal fluid (CSF) albumin and IgG. Patients with spinal fluid suggestive of MS will have either oligoclonal bands or an elevated IgG index (an elevated IgG synthesis rate is often found but is less specific). Therefore, spinal fluid assessment can help support a diagnosis of MS and, of equal importance, can help to rule out other causes of CNS dysfunction or disease.

Neurophysiologic testing can also be used to look for evidence of MS lesions and can be particularly useful when trying to assess patients for subtle evidence of CNS damage. Visual evoked potentials (EPs), brainstem auditory EPs,

and somatosensory EPs are used to assess the CNS for normal or abnormal function. An example of the utility of these tests would be a patient who has a history of unilateral blurry vision that is suggestive of optic neuritis but who has a completely normal exam. Obtaining visual EPs may show abnormal conduction speed in the optic nerve, helping to support the belief that the prior event of blurry vision was a result of optic neuritis.

CASE 30-1

A 25-year-old woman is evaluated in your clinic for a chief complaint of vision loss. She reports that a few days ago, she noticed that the vision in her right eye was slightly blurry, and she noticed a dull ache behind that same eye. She thought that her symptoms were related to a headache and did not seek medical evaluation. However, this morning she woke up with severe blurry vision in her right eye and a lot of pain behind her right eye when she moves her eyes. Currently, she reports she can make out people's shape, very large print, and large road signs but she cannot read or make out details on others' faces with the right eye. She denies any personal or family history of ocular disease.

This patient's presentation is highly suggestive of optic neuritis (ON). She has vision loss that is moderate in severity and developed over a period of a few days. It is associated with retrobulbar pain that is made worse with eye movement, a finding that occurs in >9 of 10 patients with ON. Pain in the setting of vision loss helps the provider rule out ischemic causes of vision loss, which are typically painless. Painful vision loss should always warrant consideration of acute angle-closure glaucoma, but this condition would be associated with a tense globe, scleral hypervascular appearance, and increased cupping of the optic disk along with increased intraocular pressure in the affected eye. Evaluation should begin with a thorough assessment of the visual system including visual acuity, visual fields, and fundoscopic exam combined with a detailed neurologic exam of the entire body. Magnetic resonance imaging (MRI) of the orbital structures (fat-suppressed) may be ordered to confirm the diagnosis of ON, but it should also include MRI of the brain, and both should be done with and without gadolinium contrast. This helps to risk-stratify the patient for the future development of multiple sclerosis. Other testing considerations include evoked potentials, formal visual field testing, testing for systemic autoimmune diseases, imaging of the spinal cord, and spinal fluid assessment, depending on the clinical scenario following a thorough bedside evaluation. Treatment with steroids is generally recommended, and typical agents would include intravenous methylprednisolone or oral prednisone. This has been shown to speed up the recovery of vision loss but does not seem to affect the ultimate outcome as it relates to visual acuity.

Treatment

Treatments for MS can be divided into treatments used in the acute setting of a relapse or rapid decline and those intended to modify the disease course chronically (disease-modifying therapy).

Corticosteroid treatment has long been the mainstay of acute relapse management. When patients present with new symptoms concerning for a relapse, a pseudorelapse is ruled out by assessing them for infectious causes, and then most patients are treated with a course of steroids. Both intravenous (IV) and oral steroids have been shown to improve the rate of recovery, but in general, they do not affect the overall outcome, and the extent of recovery is similar with or without treatment. There have been several studies comparing the efficacy of oral versus IV steroids; in general, they are similar, but IV steroids may reach their maximum improvement slightly faster. Short-term treatment with high-dose corticosteroids carries the risk of side effects including gastritis, insomnia, elevated blood sugars, and psychosis. Prolonged steroid therapy can result in osteoporosis, cataracts, diabetes, and adrenal failure. Injectable subcutaneous adrenocorticotropic hormone has been approved in the United States for MS patients who have suffered a relapse and who have failed treatment with steroids. It leads to endogenous production of steroid hormones that are thought to expedite recovery and has similar side effects as direct administration of synthetic steroids. Plasma exchange has also been shown to be beneficial for acute demyelinating events and MS relapses. This treatment entails placement of a large-bore central IV catheter; then, the plasma is removed from the bloodstream and replaced with sterile albumin in a method similar to dialysis. This treatment has been shown to be beneficial in MS patients with severe relapses, but it does carry risks such as severe blood pressure fluctuations, hemorrhage, catheter-associated clots and infections, and cardiac events.

The first therapies approved by the US Food and Drug Administration (FDA) and European Medicines Agency for MS were the interferon class of medications in the mid-1990s. This class of medication has been shown to reduce ARRs and reduce MRI activity and has well-established long-term benefit and safety data with very rare serious side effects. These medications are administered either subcutaneously or intramuscularly and at frequencies that vary from every other day to every 2 weeks, depending on the formulation. Common side effects of this class include injection site reactions and flu-like side effects, and monitoring for typically reversible transaminitis is important. Also around the mid-1990s, glatiramer acetate was also approved for MS. This is a subcutaneous medication given daily or 3 times weekly that has also been shown to reduce ARR and MRI disease activity. These injectable therapies are considered to be the most established and safest of the disease-modifying drugs.

Between the mid-2000s and 2014, several newer agents were approved for MS. These agents have higher efficacy than the injectable therapies previously available but carry rare but serious side effect risks that are unique to the agents. Natalizumab is an infusible therapy given every 28 days that has shown very high efficacy. It blocks α-4 integrin, which is a vesicle cellular adhesion molecule that, when bound, allows for lymphocyte egress into the nervous system. This medication works by blocking lymphocyte entry into the CNS but carries a risk of progressive multifocal leukoencephalopathy (PML). The first oral agent approved for MS was fingolimod, a capsule taken once daily that acts by blocking the S1P1 receptor on lymphocytes. Without signaling at this receptor, lymphocytes cannot egress out of lymph tissue, and the medication results in reduced lymphocytes in the bloodstream and significantly reduces disease activity and MRI progression of disease in MS. Serious side effects of this medication include prolonged lymphopenia, bradycardia, de novo hypertension, macular edema, and a slight increase in the risk of skin malignancies. Several cases of PML have also been documented with this medication, but they occur at a considerably lower frequency than in patients treated with natalizumab. Another oral agent, teriflunomide, is also a once-daily pill that reduces the production and activity of lymphocytes. It reduces ARR similarly to the injectable therapies and has some benefit on progressive disease, although it is not FDA approved for progressive MS. Side effects of this medication include hair loss, transaminitis, de novo hypertension, and gastrointestinal distress, and it is considered quite unsafe in both men and women who plan to have a child or become pregnant.

The mid-2010s brought even more treatment options for MS. Dimethyl fumarate was approved in 2013 by the FDA and is an oral therapy given twice daily. Dimethyl fumarate also reduces the production and activity of lymphocytes. It is a derivative of fumaric acid used to treat psoriasis for many years. It has shown significant efficacy in ARR reductions and reduction of MRI activity and is generally well tolerated. Side effects include gastrointestinal distress, flushing reaction, and lymphopenia, and rare cases of PML have also been reported. Alemtuzumab, a monoclonal antibody against CD52 on mature lymphocytes, is another infusible therapy approved by the FDA in 2014 and is given daily for 5 days followed 1 year later by daily infusions for 3 days. It requires prolonged bloodwork monitoring monthly for at least 48 months past the last infusion. Some of the concerning side effects include thyroid disease, secondary neoplasms, serious infusion reactions, immune thrombocytopenic purpura, and prolonged leukopenia. It is highly effective at controlling disease activity using relapse rate, MRI, and disability measures.

Ocrelizumab was approved in 2017 and is administered via infusion therapy every 6 months. This medication is a CD20 monoclonal antibody and kills circulating B cells. It is generally well tolerated and has shown very promising results in clinical trials for reduction in relapse rates and impressive reduction in MRI disease activity, and it is the first treatment approved for progressive MS (primary progressive MS). Side effects include infusion reactions, infections, and rare secondary malignancies.

In 2019, 2 medications were approved for adult-onset relapsing MS: cladribine and siponimod. Cladribine is an oral chemotherapeutic agent that exerts its effects through impairment of the production of both B and T cell lymphocytes. It is administered in two rounds, typically separated by a year, and carries side effects of increased infection rates, nausea, and reduced white blood cell counts. Siponimod is similar in its effects to fingolimod in acting as an S1P inhibitor. However, it binds more selectively to only two subunits of this receptor (instead of 4 by fingolimod) aiming to reduce the risk of side effects such as bradycardia. Hematopoietic stem cell transplantation is an area of great interest and research in the treatment of MS. It has been shown to reduce aggressive disease courses well but carries very serious risks. Ongoing studies will determine which patients may receive the best benefit from this aggressive therapeutic option.

NEUROMYELITIS OPTICA SPECTRUM DISORDER

Epidemiology

Neuromyelitis Optica Spectrum Disorder (NMOSD) is an autoimmune disease that affects the CNS predominantly by severe attacks of optic neuritis (ON) and TM. Although it was first described in the late 19th century, it was not until the late 20th century that it was recognized fully as an illness that is separate from MS. It is less common than MS, affecting approximately 2 in 100,000 people in the United States, but its attacks result in much greater disability with very poor recovery. The average age of patients at diagnosis of NMOSD (age 39 years) is almost a decade later than those developing MS.

Pathophysiology

The primary driving force in the pathology of NMOSD is the production of aquaporin-4 (AQP4) antibodies. This was first identified in 2004, and this discovery has led to a very useful diagnostic tool for NMOSD. These antibodies bind to a water channel (the AQP4 channel) and then activate both the innate and adaptive immune system, resulting in significant destruction of local tissue within the CNS. These antibodies have a predilection for the optic nerves, spinal cord, brainstem (especially near the fourth ventricle), hypothalamus, and thalamus. Therefore, the clinical manifestations are rooted in symptoms and signs connected to these regions of the CNS. Local examination of the lesions reveals activated complement cascades, thickened and hyalinized vessels, and necrosis that are quite different in appearance from lesions in MS. It is thought that some form of molecular memory brings about the production of these antibodies, but patients with NMOSD often have other measurable pathogenic antibodies such as Sjögren syndrome antibodies (SSa/b, anti-Ro/La), so it may be that they have an overactive plasma cell population in general.

Myelin Oligodendrocyte Glycoprotein (MOG) antibodies have also been described as another pathogenic marker of disease in NMOSD. In these patients, attacks tend to be less severe with better recovery than those attacks experienced by AQP4 antibody positive NMOSD. Although treatment for AQP4 positive NMOSD is typically very aggressive in approach, MOG associated NMOSD has more variable treatment approaches depending upon clinical behavior and some patients and providers elect to only treat relapses.

Clinical Course

Patients with NMOSD typically present after a severe event of ON and/or TM. ON in NMOSD frequently produces severe visual impairment, often to the point that little to no vision remains in the affected eye. It can also be bilateral, which would be very unusual for MS-related ON. Events of TM often result in severe weakness, sensory loss, and ataxia that often leave patients unable to walk. Patients accumulate disability rapidly as they have severe attacks with poor recovery. The initial event is TM or ON in 43% and 41% of patients, respectively, with 4% presenting with both. Unusual presentations can include persistent nausea and vomiting due to area postrema involvement, sleep or hormonal disorders due to hypothalamic involvement, or brainstem manifestations such as cranial nerve deficits. The disease activity occurs almost exclusively through relapses, and a progressive course is not thought to occur in this illness.

Diagnostic Criteria

Until 2015, patients had to suffer both an event of ON and TM to be formally diagnosed with NMOSD. However, updated diagnostic criteria published that year began to incorporate the AQP4 antibody into the diagnostic criteria. Currently, a patient presenting with ON or typical TM can be diagnosed with NMOSD after a single event if the patient tests positive for the AQP4 antibody. This helps to initiate treatment much faster and prevent significant disability from an additional attack. Table 30–2 contains the diagnostic criteria for NMOSD.

TABLE 30–2 Diagnostic criteria for neuromyelitis optica spectrum disorder (NMOSD).

NMOSD seropositive = any core syndrome plus presence of aquaporin-4 antibody	
NMOSD seronegative = 2 core syndromes, one of which is optic neuritis, transverse myelitis, or area postrema syndrome	
Core Syndromes	
Optic neuritis	Other brainstem syndrome
Transverse myelitis	Acute diencephalic syndrome
Area postrema syndrome	Symptomatic cerebral syndrome with abnormal magnetic resonance imaging

Data from Wingerchuk DM, Banwell B, Bennett JL, et al: International consensus diagnostic criteria for neuromyelitis optica spectrum disorders, *Neurology.* 2015 Jul 14; 85(2):177-189.

Ancillary Testing

Because patients often present with acute onset of vision loss or TM, MRIs are often obtained early in the disease course. Imaging can help to differentiate NMOSD from MS. In NMOSD, spinal lesions tend to be longitudinally extensive along the vertical course of the spinal cord and extend >3 vertebral body heights (Figure 30–3). Spinal cord lesions are more likely to involve the central cord in NMOSD than in MS and are more likely to be associated with significant cord edema and expansion. NMOSD spinal cord lesions often have a central area of enhancement with gadolinium but a T2 hyperintense signal that extends well beyond the central, enhancing portion of the lesion. In NMOSD, ON is often associated with edema of the optic nerve and enhancement. Contrary to MS, ON in NMOSD is more likely to have intracranial involvement along with involvement of the optic chiasm. In addition, in NMOSD, the length of the optic nerve affected on imaging tends to be much longer than that typically found in MS. Patients with

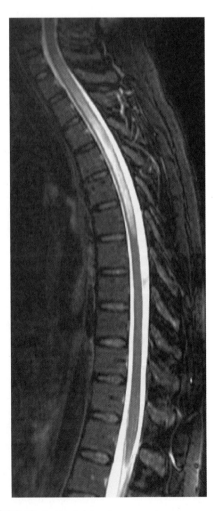

FIGURE 30–3 Sagittal thoracic magnetic resonance imaging with T2 hyperintense changes indicative of longitudinally extensive transverse myelitis (LETM) in neuromyelitis optica spectrum disorder. (Reproduced with permission from Ropper AH, Samuels MA, Klein JP: *Adams and Victor's Principles of Neurology*, 11th ed. New York, NY: McGraw Hill; 2019.)

NMOSD often have T2 hyperintense MRI findings affecting the hypothalamus and the floor of the fourth ventricle. True parenchymal brain lesions are not typical of NMOSD but can occur, and when present, they tend to be larger, more confluent lobar T2 hyperintense lesions and often resolve completely with treatment.

Because diagnosis is based in part on serum testing for AQP4 or MOG antibodies, performing the most sensitive form of this test is important. Labs that use cell-based assays with cells induced to overexpress AQP4 channels seem to have higher sensitivity for detecting AQP4 antibodies. Although reports of AQP4 positivity in the CSF and not in the serum exist, serum testing is typically sufficient because these antibodies are thought to be produced peripherally.

Treatment

Initiating treatment promptly is key in NMOSD because patients can accumulate disability rapidly with any new attacks. For acute attacks, NMOSD patients seem to be less responsive to steroids than MS patients, but some patients respond quite well to steroids. Plasma exchange is an increasingly used treatment for acute attacks of NMOSD and seems to be very beneficial for patients in small series. Broad immunosuppressive agents have been shown to be quite useful for chronic treatment with the goal of relapse reduction in medium-sized retrospective case series. Reductions in ARRs with treatment initiation with immunosuppressive agents can be >90% in retrospective case series. Agents that are typically used include azathioprine and mycophenolate mofetil. More targeted therapy affecting primarily B cells with CD20 monoclonal antibodies has also been very promising in this illness and seems to be well tolerated over the long term with impressive relapse rate reductions in retrospective series.

The first FDA-approved therapy for NMOSD was approved in 2019. This medication, eculizumab, is a complement inhibitor that reduced relapse rate by >90% and was generally well tolerated. Serious side effects include meningococcal meningitis and other serious infections. Because of this risk, patients must undergo a series of meningococcal vaccinations prior to initiation of the therapy. This medication is presently only approved for AQP4-positive NMOSD.

TRANSVERSE MYELITIS

Epidemiology

Although most cases of TM are associated with MS or other autoimmune diseases, some patients will develop what is determined to be idiopathic TM (ITM), meaning that the symptoms and demyelination are restricted to the spinal cord. Approximately 10,000 cases of TM occur in the United States every year, and up to one-third of these cases will remain idiopathic after thorough workup. Often there is an antecedent viral illness in the weeks preceding ITM, but a single infectious pathogen does not seem to be the culprit.

ITM has many clinical features that are often distinct from TM from other causes, and these differences will be reviewed in this section.

Pathophysiology

Early descriptions of ITM occurred in the late 19th century, and the first description of "acute transverse myelitis" was in 1948 by Suchett-Kaye. One leading hypothesis of this process is that of molecular mimicry. It is thought that an environmental exposure, such as a recent infection, promotes the development of an immune process that then attacks the spinal cord. Autopsy examination has shown chronic demyelination, and several infectious agents have been shown to have similar physical structure to factors directly embedded or instrumental to myelin structure, function, or development. There are also monocyte and lymphocyte infiltrates in the perivascular spaces, along with astrogliotic scarring with loss of axonal density in most lesions.

Clinical Course

Patients with ITM often develop progressively worsening symptoms that develop over 1 to 4 days with a mean of 3 days to peak clinical severity. Typically, patients will begin to have symptoms of numbness, weakness, imbalance, or bowel and bladder dysfunction that are mild in severity but worsen rapidly over hours or days. Roughly half of patients will have an antecedent illness in the preceding weeks. At their nadir, between half and two-thirds of patients will be unable to walk. Some form of autonomic dysfunction is almost universal, and up to 10% of patients with ITM will die from their illness or immediate complications. At initial evaluation, patients often have myelopathic findings on exam with hyperreflexia, sensory levels, weakness in the extremities, and ataxia. However, approximately one-third of patients will have a spinal shock presentation, where they have flaccid paralysis with absent reflexes and atonic bladder. Approximately 1 in 5 patients will have cervical cord sensory levels, and roughly two-thirds will have a thoracolumbar sensory level.

Clinical improvement occurs most rapidly in the first 3 months, with the majority of recovery complete between 6 months and 1 year. A general rule of prognosis is a rule of thirds: One-third of patients will have minimal to no disability, one-third will have moderate disability requiring assistance for some activities of daily living, and one-third will have severe disability. Most patients experience a single event without a recurrent event. However, up to one-fourth of patients will have recurrent ITM, with risk factors for recurrence being male sex, age >50 years, and severe motor and sphincter dysfunction.

Diagnostic Criteria

Formal diagnostic criteria were developed in 2002 by the Transverse Myelitis Consortium Working Group. These criteria are designed to eliminate common causes of TM such

TABLE 30–3 Transverse Myelitis Consortium Working Group diagnostic criteria for idiopathic transverse myelitis.

Inclusion Criteria	Exclusion Criteria
■ Deficits attributable to cord dysfunction ■ Bilateral signs/symptoms ■ Clearly defined sensory level ■ Exclusion of compressive lesion ■ Inflammation in the spinal cord ■ Progression to nadir between 4 hours and 21 days	■ Prior radiation to spine in past 10 years ■ Clear vascular distribution of deficits ■ Abnormal flow voids on imaging ■ Serologic or clinical evidence of connective tissue disease ■ Central nervous system manifestations of explanatory disease ■ History of clinically apparent optic neuritis

Data from Transverse Myelitis Consortium Working Group: Proposed diagnostic criteria and nosology of acute transverse myelitis, *Neurology*. 2002 Aug 27;59(4): 499-505.

as MS, ischemic TM, and connective tissue disease–related phenomena (Table 30–3).

Ancillary Testing

ITM usually presents with a longitudinally extensive spinal cord lesion (longitudinally extensive TM). These lesions are often several vertebral body heights in length and often involve the entire diameter of the spinal cord, unlike the partial, peripherally located, shorter lesions found in MS. Patients should have brain and entire spinal axis MRIs performed very early in the disease course, and those with brain lesions typical of MS have an 80% risk of developing MS over the ensuing few years. Workup for other causes of myelopathy should be conducted including testing for vitamin B_{12}, thyroid function, human immunodeficiency virus, vitamin E, copper, autoimmune disease markers, and AQP4 and MOG antibodies. CSF examination is recommended to rule out an infectious cause, such as cytomegalovirus- or Epstein-Barr virus–associated myelitis. Routine studies plus MS profiles should be ordered in addition to infectious studies to rule out MS as a cause. CSF studies often show a significant pleocytosis, and the differential diagnosis can vary, with more neutrophils found in infectious causes; eosinophil predominance should raise the possibility of parasitic or fungal infections. Nerve conduction studies may show a loss of F waves, raising the possibility of Guillain-Barré syndrome, but imaging should help to differentiate these processes. Seventeen percent of patients with ITM will have oligoclonal bands, but this also raises the possibility of MS as a cause and the possibility of paraneoplastic and infectious causes as well.

Treatment

The standard treatment for ITM, although not FDA approved, is high-dose steroids. In patients who do not respond rapidly to steroids, consideration should be given to IV immunoglobulin (IVIg) or plasma exchange. In patients with very severe deficits, it may be worth considering initiating plasma exchange early in the course, and the addition of cyclophosphamide to plasma exchange is more beneficial than plasma exchange alone. Close monitoring of respiratory function is warranted because some patients with cervical cord involvement may develop respiratory failure. In addition, physical therapy, occupational therapy, and monitoring for deep venous thrombosis and bed sores are essential. The remainder of treatments focus on symptom management such as addressing atonic bladders with catheterization, reducing spasticity with antispasmodics, and managing pain and tonic spasms with antiepileptics such as gabapentin or carbamazepine. Long-term follow-up to continually assess for etiology is warranted because some patients will lack evidence of systemic autoimmune processes initially but later develop more florid symptoms.

MYASTHENIA GRAVIS

Epidemiology

Myasthenia gravis was first described in 1672 and is thought to affect approximately 60,000 people in the United States. Prior to the age of 40 years, the female-to-male ratio is 3:1, but after age 40, more men develop MG than women. The incidence of MG has been increasing in the United States over the past few decades, and this is thought to be related to increasing longevity, and now more men than women are affected by MG. The classic presentation is fluctuating or fatigable weakness that affects the muscles controlling eye movements or the proximal musculature of the limbs. There are rare congenital myasthenic syndromes resulting from genetic defects in proteins at the neuromuscular junction; these are covered in Chapter 35.

Pathophysiology

The pathophysiology of MG was established in early 1970s. The disease develops when the immune system begins producing antibodies directed at postsynaptic acetylcholine (ACh) receptors at the neuromuscular junction (Figure 30–4). These antibodies have been described as 3 primary types based on their effects on the receptors: binding (most prevalent), blocking, and modulating antibodies. Electron microscopy has shown that the density of postsynaptic ACh receptors is significantly diminished in patients with MG and that the normal density of folds and pockets within the neuromuscular junction is also reduced, resulting in a flattened appearance of the junction relative to healthy controls. Once the antibodies are bound, complement-mediated destruction results in the decrease in postsynaptic ACh receptors. These antibodies are pathogenic; when transferred to a healthy recipient, symptoms of the disease will develop. Approximately 10% of MG patients will not have Ach receptor antibodies and instead will have muscle-specific tyrosine kinase (MuSK) antibodies. These patients tend to be less responsive to traditional therapies and have more bulbar symptoms than patients with ACh receptor antibodies. There seems to be a poorly understood link between genetics and the development of this disease because family members of patients have a risk as high as 1,000 times that of the general population and approximately 20% of a patient's first-degree relatives will show MG-related antibodies on serologic testing.

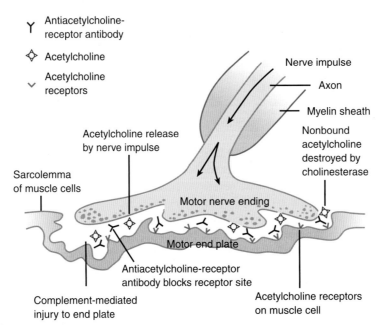

FIGURE 30–4 Neuromuscular junction changes found in myasthenia gravis. (Reproduced with permission from Chandrasoma P, Taylor CR: *Concise Pathology*. 3rd ed. Stamford, CT: Appleton & Lange; 1998.)

Clinical Course

Patients often present with muscle fatigability that predominantly affects the proximal musculature or the bulbar muscles. Most patients find that their symptoms are worse later in the day or when activities require them to use the involved musculature repeatedly. Approximately two-thirds of patients will present with diplopia or ptosis as their presenting symptom, and almost all patients will have both of these symptoms at 2 years from diagnosis. These are particularly noticeable late in the day when performing tasks that require significant eye movement and visual clarity, such as driving late in the day. Another classic presentation is that of systemic weakness. Patients report that late in the day or with significant physical exertion they notice their proximal muscles become weak, especially the shoulder and hip girdle musculature. Patients often present in mid-life, and their symptoms typically develop in a subacute or chronic manner. Approximately 10% to 15% of patients will have a disease course with weakness restricted to the oculomotor and bulbar muscles. Atrophy of the involved musculature is not a common presenting problem but can occur later in the illness or with particularly aggressive disease courses.

Diagnostic Criteria

A widely accepted, formal diagnostic set of criteria is not available for MG. Therefore, the diagnosis remains one based on clinical grounds and ancillary testing. The primary symptoms and signs that suggest a diagnosis of MG are fatigable weakness involving the proximal extremities and/or fluctuating and fatigable weakness of the bulbar musculature. When these symptoms are present, further workup that would support a diagnosis of MG are as follows: (1) serologic demonstration of ACh receptor or MuSK antibodies; (2) pharmacologic testing with edrophonium with rapid muscular recovery; and (3) repetitive nerve stimulation showing decrements or single-fiber electromyography (EMG) showing postsynaptic transmission deficits. Differential diagnosis considerations should include congenital myasthenic syndromes, Lambert-Eaton myasthenic syndrome (discussed later in this chapter), botulism poisoning, or organophosphate toxicity.

Ancillary Testing

Approximately 80% to 90% of patients with MS will have serologic testing that reveals ACh receptor or MuSK antibodies supporting the diagnosis. However, between 10% and 15% of patients will not have any serologic findings to confirm the diagnosis. One useful bedside test is to apply ice to the area affected to look for improvement in the symptom. This is best demonstrated with ptosis, and the ptosis can resolve within a few minutes of placing an ice pack over a patient's affected eye. The cold temperature inactivates acetylcholinesterase, which increases the amount of synaptic ACh. Moreover, fast acting acetylcholinesterase medications such

as edrophonium can be administered to quickly block the breakdown of ACh at the bedside. Caution should be used when performing this test; cardiac monitoring is required with atropine readily available in case of severe bradycardia or arrhythmia.

CASE 30-2

A 58-year-old man presents with a 4-month history of progressive fatigue. He reports that if he tries to do something physically strenuous, such as rake his yard or climb a few flights of stairs, his arms and legs begin to feel heavy. Initially, he attributed this to old age, but 2 weeks ago, he noticed some vision changes. He first noticed that when he was driving home from work late in the evening that the lines on the road would seem to split into double lines at times. This would last a few minutes and then spontaneously resolve. However, over the past 5 days, the frequency and severity of this double vision have worsened dramatically, and he has noticed that objects may appear side by side or one on top of the other. The events recently have been lasting 30 minutes or more and are only relieved with closing his eyes and resting. They also are occurring more frequently during the middle of the day. He reports that if he closes an eye when it happens that the double vision resolves completely.

This patient's presentation is suggestive of a problem with his skeletal and extraocular musculature. The fatigable weakness in his extremities may suggest a myopathic, myositis, or neuromuscular junction–related problem. His binocular diplopia (gets better with closing 1 eye) is highly suggestive of a neuromuscular junction disorder because it is brought on by fatigue, worse later in the day, and relieved with rest. In addition, there is no stereotypical orientation of the diplopia to suggest a specific cranial nerve is malfunctioning. Thus the presentation is highly suggestive of myasthenia gravis. Workup should begin with a thorough bedside evaluation looking for fatigable weakness in the proximal and distal extremities, thorough evaluation of all cranial nerves, and skin evaluation to look for rashes. The patient should next be evaluated using nerve conduction and electromyographic (EMG) testing to evaluate for a neuromuscular junction problem. This should include repetitive nerve stimulation and, if available, single-fiber EMG. In addition, bloodwork should be assessed for creatine kinase levels and for testing for acetylcholine receptor antibodies. A computed tomography scan of the chest should be performed to assess for thymoma, and even if no tumor is present, elective thymectomy could be considered. Treatment typically begins with acetylcholinesterase inhibitors such as pyridostigmine, and in severe cases, the addition of prednisone or other immunosuppressive agents may be warranted early on in the illness.

Nerve conduction and single-fiber EMG are useful tools in diagnosing MG. On nerve conduction testing, repetitive nerve stimulation is performed at 2, 5, and 10 Hz to look for a decrement in the compound motor action potential of >10%. This is a physiologic demonstration of the fatigability of muscles with a postsynaptic neuromuscular transmission deficit. Repetitive nerve stimulation has a sensitivity of approximately 60%. EMG is performed with a single-fiber technique to look for jitter, which is an abnormal firing interval between 2 adjacent motor units.

Treatment

All patients with recently diagnosed MG should undergo computed tomography of the chest to search for a thymic tumor. Thymomas are associated with MG, and if a thymoma is discovered, surgical resection can improve the clinical course of the affected patient. Although only approximately 10% of MG patients have a thymoma, up to 70% will have lymphoid follicular hyperplasia in the thymus on biopsy examination. A recent study has demonstrated a beneficial effect of thymic resection in patient under the age of 65 years and with a disease duration of ≤5 years.

As discussed previously, acute treatment of MG can involve short-acting acetylcholinesterase inhibitors, but these carry significant and potentially serious side effects. Although fast-acting agents such as edrophonium are used to aid in diagnosis, they are not typically used for disease management. Pyridostigmine and neostigmine have much longer half-lives and can be given 3 to 4 times per day for the management of MG. These are generally well tolerated, but some patients may experience severe abdominal cramping or diarrhea, which can be mitigated by adding oral glycopyrrolate with each dose. Acute treatment of a myasthenic crisis is usually managed with IVIg, plasma exchange, and ventilator support if needed. Close monitoring of respiratory status and clearance of secretion is paramount in any patient with a crisis or flare-up of their MG-related symptoms. Steroids have been shown to be quite helpful for long-term therapy, and these are typically paired with steroid-sparing immunosuppressive agents (eg, azathioprine or mycophenolate mofetil) early on with a planned transition to only the steroid-sparing agent over time. Other treatment modalities with probable efficacy include cyclosporine, cyclophosphamide, and rituximab.

LAMBERT-EATON MYASTHENIC SYNDROME

Lambert-Eaton myasthenic syndrome (LEMS) often has a clinical presentation similar to MG with fatigable weakness of the proximal extremities predominantly, but patients can have bulbar weakness. One clinical feature that helps to distinguish LEMS from MG is that patients with LEMS often have significant autonomic features such as dry mouth, constipation, and bladder dysfunction. Another distinguishing factor is that of facilitation: reflexes and strength may be diminished at rest, but after activation of the muscle repeatedly, the reflexes may return and strength may actually improve. Roughly have of LEMS patients will have a neoplasm as the root cause of their illness, with LEMS presenting in a paraneoplastic manner in those cases. The disorder is caused by antibodies targeted at the presynaptic voltage-gated calcium channels of the P/Q type. Once this diagnosis is made, extensive search for a neoplasm should be undertaken. Treatments for LEMS are similar to those for MG, with the exception that treatment of the underlying malignancy should also be initiated should a neoplasm be discovered during workup. See Chapter 31 for more details.

SYSTEMIC AUTOIMMUNE DISEASES

Systemic Lupus Erythematosus

Systemic lupus erythematosus (SLE) classically presents with a malar rash, arthritis, photosensitivity, serositis, and abnormal serologic testing and affects women 9 times more often than men. The American Academy of Rheumatology has developed diagnosis criteria based on the presence of 4 of 11 features, 1 of which is neurologic disease involvement, which speaks to the frequency of nervous system involvement in SLE. The clinical presentations of neurologic manifestations of SLE can vary greatly and can include acute inflammatory demyelinating polyneuropathy, mononeuropathy (single/multiplex), peripheral polyneuropathy, plexopathy, acute encephalitis or cognitive decline, strokes, myelopathy, seizures, and multiple psychiatric illnesses. The disparate possibilities make attributing neurologic involvement to SLE difficult unless the patient has known SLE prior to the development of neurologic symptoms. Treating the underlying illness of SLE will often cease any neurologic worsening, but many aspects may not improve or resolve, such as cognitive decline or peripheral polyneuropathy. There is a strong association between antiphospholipid antibodies and anticardiolipin antibodies and vascular events in the peripheral nervous system and CNS. The clinical course can be monophasic, polyphasic, or progressive and chronic.

Sjögren Syndrome

Sjögren syndrome (SS) is a chronic autoimmune disease typically related to SLE or rheumatoid arthritis but can develop singularly. Classically, it presents with sicca syndrome, which is severe xerostomia and keratoconjunctivitis sicca. Peripheral neuropathy is the most common neurologic manifestation of SS, but as in many other systemic autoimmune diseases, myelopathy, strokes, and cranial neuropathies can develop. Nerve biopsy may be warranted if mononeuritis multiplex is thought to be related to a vasculitis from SS. Treatment is only symptomatic from a neurologic standpoint because broad immunosuppressive medications should be used to treat the underlying systemic autoimmune process.

Sarcoidosis

Sarcoidosis is an idiopathic granulomatous inflammatory disease that primarily affects the lungs, but approximately 10% of patients will have nervous system involvement. Of those with neurosarcoidosis, half will present with neurologic symptoms as the initial manifestation of disease. Cranial neuropathies are the most common neurosarcoid manifestation, but patients can also develop hypothalamic dysfunction, myopathy, strokes, cognitive decline, ataxia, peripheral polyneuropathy, or myelopathy. CSF examination typically shows a lymphocytic pleocytosis with very low glucose levels, which can be helpful to differentiate sarcoid from MS, and CSF angiotensin-converting enzyme levels may be elevated but are an unreliable test for neurosarcoidosis. MRI often shows leptomeningeal enhancement, particularly along the basal meninges and in the posterior fossa. Broad-spectrum immunosuppression seems to be the best treatment using agents such as steroids, methotrexate, azathioprine, and infliximab, among others.

SELF-ASSESSMENT QUESTIONS

1. You are evaluating a 39-year-old woman in the hospital for a new event of transverse myelitis that has resulted in her inability to walk and severe bladder and bowel dysfunction. When reviewing her images, you note that her lesion extends through most of her thoracic spinal cord and into her lower cervical spinal cord with patchy enhancement in the central portion. The fact that this lesion is longitudinally extensive—defined as being longer than 3 vertebral body heights—makes which of the following diagnoses less likely?

    A. Multiple sclerosis

    B. Idiopathic transverse myelitis

    C. Neuromyelitis optica spectrum disorder

2. A patient presents to your clinic with a 2-year history of worsening gait trouble. He reports that he is not sure when it began but that he now has trouble walking short distances and has noticed increasing difficulty feeling where his feet are placed and controlling his bladder and bowel functioning. You suspect a diagnosis of progressive multiple sclerosis (MS). Which of the following findings would not help you fulfill the diagnostic criteria for progressive MS?

    A. Brain magnetic resonance imaging (MRI) with 1 or more lesions suggestive of demyelination

    B. Spinal fluid with elevated immunoglobulin G (IgG) index or oligoclonal bands

    C. Abnormal somatosensory evoked potentials of the lower extremities

    D. Spinal cord MRI showing 2 lesions typical of MS

3. Myasthenia gravis is a disorder of neuromuscular junction transmission resulting in weakness of the extremities and musculature of the head and neck. The primary pathogenesis of this illness is through which of the following mechanisms?

    A. Decreased production of acetylcholine

    B. Impaired release of acetylcholine from vesicles at the presynaptic membrane

    C. Antagonism of the postsynaptic acetylcholine receptors

    D. Increased activity of acetylcholinesterase, resulting in faster degradation of synaptic acetylcholine

Neuromuscular Disorders

Mohamed Kazamel

O B J E C T I V E S

After studying this chapter, the student should be able to:

- Provide an overview of the common neuromuscular disorders organized around their localization along the peripheral neural axis.
- Review the etiologies and pathophysiologic mechanisms involved in different neuromuscular disease processes.
- Discuss briefly the management of common neuromuscular disorders with a special focus on diagnostic testing and specific treatments.

Neuromuscular disorders are a diverse group of diseases that result from lesions in the nerve cells inside or close to the spinal cord, peripheral nerves, neuromuscular junction, or muscles. The cell bodies of the sensory nerves are located in the dorsal root ganglia just outside the intervertebral foramina (Figure 31–1), while the motor neuron cell bodies lie in the anterior horn of the spinal cord, within the gray matter. The motor unit is a functional entity that includes the anterior horn cell, its nerve axons, and the muscle fibers that are supplied by these axon terminals. Overall, neuromuscular disorders can be classified into disorders of the cell body (neuronopathy), nerve roots (radiculopathy), plexus, peripheral nerves, neuromuscular junction, or muscles.

PREVALENCE & BURDEN

The recent advances in diagnostic methods, specifically genetic testing and the development of consensus criteria for few neuromuscular disorders have led to some evolution in the epidemiologic data for these diseases. Compared to the 1991 first world survey of most inherited neuromuscular disorders, a 2015 comprehensive review of the available prevalence data of 30 neuromuscular diagnoses reported significant increases in some inherited neuromuscular disorders. Increases in prevalence rates were seen in myotonic dystrophy (7.1 to 26.5 per 100,000), Charcot-Marie-Tooth disease (3.1 to 82.3 per 100,000), facioscapulohumeral dystrophy (2.03 to 6.8 per 100,1000), and Becker muscular dystrophy (0.07 to 3.65 per 100,1000). In general, the prevalence rates of neuromuscular disorders were found to range from 0.1 per 100,000 population for oculopharyngeal muscular dystrophy

to 60 per 100,000 population for post-polio syndrome. Prevalence of neuromuscular disorders as a group was estimated to be at least similar to that of Parkinson disease worldwide (100 to 300 per 100,000). We still believe that this summed estimate for neuromuscular disorders as a group represents only the tip of the iceberg. Thus, although neuromuscular disorders are rare as individual disease entities, as a group they are not.

DISORDERS OF THE ANTERIOR HORN CELL

Poliomyelitis

Poliomyelitis is a paralytic disease that has historically been responsible for epidemics of weakness, disability, and death. The causative organism of poliomyelitis is the mRNA polio enterovirus that is transmitted by oral–fecal contamination. The virus has a strong predilection for the spinal cord, specifically the anterior horn cells. Infection leads to loss of the anterior horn cells and weakness of the associated motor unit. After the polio vaccine was introduced in 1955, the disease was eradicated from the United States. There are still a few countries in central Africa where new cases of poliomyelitis are seen. Most infected patients remain asymptomatic or present with mild gastrointestinal symptoms with no neurologic sequelae. However, neurologic manifestations of the more severe cases can be unilateral or asymmetric lower motor neuron limb weakness and atrophy. Rarely, the disease is extensive enough to involve the respiratory muscles. Survivors experience slow improvement in strength as time goes by due to

VOCABULARY

Mononeuropathy: Involvement of a single nerve by a localized pathology, as in median mononeuropathy in carpal tunnel syndrome or the ulnar mononeuropathy in cubital tunnel syndrome.

Muscular dystrophies: Genetically determined, progressive, degenerative disorders of the muscles.

Multiple mononeuropathies (or, more commonly, mononeuritis multiplex): A disorder of more than 1 nerve in the same limb.

Myopathy: A disorder of the skeletal muscles in general.

Neuronopathy: A disorder of the neuronal cell bodies, whether the anterior horn cells on the motor side or the dorsal root ganglia on the sensory side.

Neuropathy: A disorder of the peripheral nerves, usually with diffuse involvement (polyneuropathy) unless otherwise specified.

Polyradiculoneuropathy: A combined involvement of the roots and the nerves.

Radiculopathy: A disorder of the nerve root, which often combines motor and sensory involvement.

Radiculoplexus neuropathy: A combined disorder of the roots, plexus, and nerves.

reinnervation of the muscle fibers from the remaining healthy motor units. There is no specific treatment for the active phase of the disease other than supportive care, so prevention through vaccination is critical.

Patient with remote history of poliomyelitis can present with what is sometimes called *post-polio syndrome*. This happens when patients experience subacute deterioration of the old weakness or, rarely, new weakness in other regions that were not involved earlier by the disease. This phenomenon can be explained by premature aging of the motor units that are already supplying an increased number of muscle fibers

during the process of reinnervation. Treatment of post-polio syndrome is mainly supportive. The generally benign nature of post-polio syndrome should be explained to the patient after exclusion of any other superimposed new neurologic disorders.

Spinal Muscular Atrophy

Spinal muscular atrophies (SMAs) are a group of genetically determined autosomal recessive conditions that are caused by loss of the survival motor neuron gene (*SMN1*) on chromosome 5q13.2. The carrier frequency for these mutations is 1 in 50 in the United States. In general, SMAs are classified based on the age of onset, degree of disability, life expectancy, and the amount of genetic reserve.

The classical phenotypes are type I (Werdnig-Hoffman disease), type II (Dubowitz disease), type III (Kugelberg-Welander syndrome), and type IV, which is the adult form of the disorder. Types I, II, and III are infantile or childhood disorders that can be distinguished by different ages of onset and are often remembered using an aphorism: type I never sits, type II never walks, and type III never runs. Type IV patients have variable presentation and may even be able to play sports into their teenage years before weakness and muscle atrophy become manifest. In general, sensation is preserved in all of the types of SMA. Type I SMA manifests within the first 6 months of life. These patients are floppy infants who have poor feeding and recurrent respiratory infections. They are often alert with intact extraocular movements. The average survival is 2 years. Type II patients present between 6 and 12 months and can survive until the second decade of their lives. However, they are mostly wheelchair dependent. Restrictive lung disease and recurrent pneumonias are major sources of morbidity and mortality. Type III patients typically present after 18 months of life with limb weakness, proximal more than distal. This is associated with profound muscle atrophy and loss of deep tendon reflexes. Oropharyngeal weakness leads to a dysphagia and recurrent aspiration pneumonias, but patients can have normal life expectancy. Type IV patients do not present until adulthood.

Although the primary genetic defect in SMA is in the gene *SMN1*, there is an interesting interaction with a related gene,

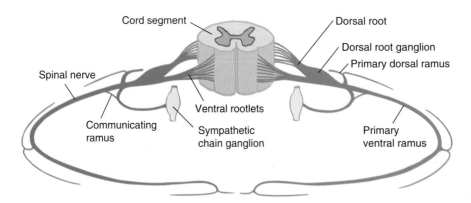

FIGURE 31-1 Schematic illustration of a cord segment with its roots, ganglia, spinal nerves, and rami. (Reproduced with permission from Waxman SG. *Clinical Neuroanatomy*, 28th ed. New York, NY: McGraw Hill; 2017.)

SMN2, also located on chromosome 5. The number of gene copies of *SMN2* in human being can range anywhere between 0 and 4. *SMN2* has the ability to partially compensate for loss of *SMN1*, so that a greater number of *SMN2* copies leads to a less severe form of disease. The diagnosis of SMA is confirmed by genetic testing. Genetic counseling should be considered in type III and type IV patients who are considering parenthood. Prenatal diagnosis is also available.

Motor Neuron Disease

Amyotrophic lateral sclerosis (ALS) is the most common type of motor neuron disease. The worldwide incidence is reported to be 4 to 8 per 100,000 population, and approximately 5000 cases are diagnosed every year in the United States. Ten to 15% of cases are familial, and the rest are sporadic. It is an aggressive disease, with a median survival of 3 years from onset. Diagnosis should be considered when there is history of asymmetric progressive motor weakness starting in 1 limb and later spreading to involve the other limbs. A mixture of upper and lower motor neuron findings is often seen in the limbs or the bulbar region. Upper motor neuron findings can be spasticity, hyperreflexia, positive Babinski sign, crossed adductor reflexes, Hoffman sign, hyperactive jaw jerk or gag reflex, pseudobulbar affect, or spastic tongue with spastic dysarthria. Lower motor neuron signs include hypotonia (flaccidity), muscle atrophy, diminished or lost reflexes, fasciculations, or flaccid dysarthria. Sensory exam is usually normal. One should always suspect the diagnosis when brisk reflexes are paradoxically elicited in an atrophic limb. Diagnosis should be confirmed with electromyography (EMG) where electrophysiologic signs of widespread active and chronic denervation are seen.

Several other variants of motor neuron disease are recognized. Primary muscular atrophy represents 10% of motor neuron disease cases. It is characterized by a lower motor neuron pattern of muscle weakness and atrophy similar to that seen in ALS, but with no upper motor neuron signs. The disease is usually limited to 1 limb. Primary lateral sclerosis (1% to 3% of cases) is an upper motor neuron variant of motor neuron disease and is caused by involvement of the corticospinal tracts. Hyperreflexia and spasticity are present, but without muscle atrophy. Some patients develop lower motor neuron signs later, and the diagnosis changes to ALS. This rarely happens after >5 years from disease onset. Progressive bulbar palsy (1% to 2%) is a variant of motor neuron disease that starts with bulbar involvement and symptoms of dysarthria and dysphagia due to preferential involvement of the lower cranial nerve nuclei.

Ideally, management of these patients should occur in an ALS multidisciplinary clinic where they are followed by healthcare providers from multiple specialties including neurology, physical therapy, occupational therapy, speech therapy, and respiratory therapy. A nutritionist and social worker should be a part of that team. Respiratory failure is the most common cause of death, and noninvasive ventilation (bilevel positive airway pressure) should be started when forced vital capacity decreases below 50% of what is predicted for patient age,

height, and weight. Malnutrition and loss of weight are universal, and percutaneous endoscopic gastrostomy tube insertion to maintain high protein and calorie intake has been proven to prolong survival. The majority of drug therapy is directed toward treating symptoms and complications such as muscle cramps, spasticity, drooling, depression, insomnia, and pseudobulbar affect. The first available treatment to be approved by US Food and Drug Administration specific for ALS was riluzole. The mechanism of action is through inhibiting the release of glutamate from presynaptic terminals. Riluzole was shown in 2 clinical trials to prolong tracheostomy-free survival by only 2 to 3 months. Side effects include gastrointestinal upset and hepatic impairment. Liver function tests should be checked at baseline before starting the medication and every 3 months as long as the patient continues treatment with riluzole. Edaravone was approved by the FDA in 2017 for treatment of ALS. The proposed mechanism of action is through its antioxidant properties. It was found to slow the clinical progression in ALS cases based on the ALS functional rating scale (ALS-FRS). Possible side effects include increased liability to skin contusions, gait instability, and headache.

DISORDERS OF THE DORSAL ROOT GANGLIA

Disorders of the dorsal root ganglia are relative uncommon but have distinctive clinical symptoms. The term *sensory neuronopathy* applies to conditions where the sensory neuron cell body in the dorsal root ganglia is preferentially affected. The clinical presentation can range from multifocal patchy sensory loss to a profound loss of proprioception and sensory ataxia. Differential diagnosis includes connective tissue disorders (Sjögren syndrome), paraneoplastic conditions (anti-Hu antibody syndrome in small-cell lung cancer), or toxicity as in vitamin B_6 and cisplatin toxicities, or it can be idiopathic.

DISORDERS OF THE NERVE ROOTS (RADICULOPATHIES)

Radiculopathies are one of the most common neuromuscular disorders. Degenerative spine disease is the culprit in the great majority of cases. However, infective, inflammatory, or neoplastic infiltrative processes can happen. Thus, radiculopathies are often seen in the more mobile and prone to wear and tear portions of the spine such as the cervical and lumbar spine rather than in the thoracic spine.

Radiculopathies often present with burning, electrical, or shock-like painful sensation and paresthesia radiating from the neck or the low back to the upper or lower limbs, respectively. Pain is often diffuse and not easily localized to the sensory territory of the involved dermatome. Weakness is less common and, if present, usually is associated with pain. Due to the intersection and branching that happens at the level of the brachial and lumbosacral plexuses, a single root lesion rarely presents with either dense sensory loss or marked weakness.

Spondylosis

Cervical spondylosis is a consequence of arthritis of the cervical vertebrae. Typical radiologic signs of cervical spondylosis (disk space narrowing and osteophytes) are seen in 50% of people older than age 50 years and 75% of people older than age 65 years. Limitation in neck rotational movement is the cardinal sign and can be associated with signs of radiculopathy or even myelopathy. Headache, felt mainly in the back of the head, may be present. Diagnosis is based on clinical presentation and magnetic resonance imaging (MRI). EMG is performed for accurate localization and prognostication when clinical suspicion of cervical radiculopathy exists. Treatment is often conservative, using muscle relaxants, physical therapy, and sometimes epidural steroid injections. Surgical intervention is indicated when clinical and radiologic evidence of compressive myelopathy exists. Overall, improvement is expected in the majority of cases (90%) with medical conservative treatment.

Lumbar spondylosis, from arthritic change in the lumbar vertebrae, usually presents with low back pain either with or without lumbar radiculopathic symptoms. Any of the lumbar or sacral roots may be affected as they exit the vertebral foramina. Symptoms may also arise from compression of multiple nerve roots in the spinal canal. The spinal cord usually ends at the level of the lower margin of the L1 vertebra. Caudal to this level, the subarachnoid space contains the lumbar and sacral nerve roots that are traveling downward to exit from their relevant intervertebral foramina. These nerve roots are termed the *cauda equina*. Severe lumbar spondylotic pathology can cause compression of these roots, leading to cauda equina syndrome. This syndrome is characterized by diminished sensation in the saddle area bilaterally and bowel or bladder control problems, as well as radicular pain in lumbar and sacral territories. EMG and MRI are still instrumental in the localization and diagnosis. Treatment is often conservative in this condition too. The classic indications for surgery include cauda equina syndrome with sphincteric disturbances, progressive weakness, and intractable pain despite medical treatment.

Herpes Zoster Infection

Herpes zoster, or shingles, is a disease of sensory nerves that leads to pain and blistering of the skin. The incidence of symptomatic herpes zoster is 480 per 100,000 population, and the age in the majority of patients ranges from 55 to 75 years. It is usually caused by reactivation of a latent prior infection with the varicella-zoster virus (VZV). Approximately 90% of the population are carriers of a VZV-latent infection, and one-third will experience reactivation. Reactivation most often occurs in the setting of compromised immunity due to another infection such as human immunodeficiency virus, immunosuppressive treatment, stress, surgery, delivery, or just old age. With reactivation, the virus starts to replicate and travels down the sensory nerves to cause the characteristic painful vesicular rash in the

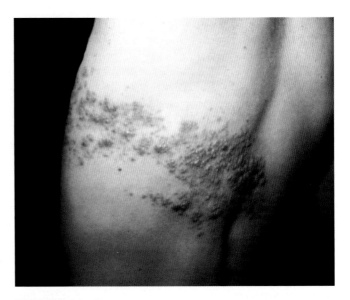

FIGURE 31–2 Zoster (shingles)—note vesicles along the dermatome of a thoracic nerve caused by varicella-zoster virus. (Reproduced with permission from Usatine RP, Smith MA, Chumley HS, et al: *The Color Atlas of Family Medicine*, 2nd ed. New York, NY: McGraw Hill; 2013. Photo contributor: Richard P. Usatine, MD.)

territories of the involved dermatome (shingles) (Figure 31–2). Treatment with oral acyclovir should be started as soon as the condition is recognized, ideally within 3 days from the onset of rash. Antiviral treatment decreases the duration of rash and sensory symptoms. In 25% of cases, patients have incapacitating residual local pain after resolution of the rash, a condition termed *postherpetic neuralgia*. Treatment of postherpetic neuralgic is mainly symptomatic with medications such as tricyclic antidepressants (amitriptyline or nortriptyline), gabapentin, or pregabalin. Lidocaine patches can be used in cases where oral treatment is contraindicated, but sometimes, the pain is refractory to all of these therapies. Earlier treatment with antiviral medication was not found to lower the probability of developing postherpetic neuralgia.

DISORDERS OF THE BRACHIAL PLEXUS

In general, plexopathies are characterized by multifocal limb weakness including the proximal and distal muscles. This is often associated with widespread patchy sensory loss. Proximal and distal deep tendon reflexes can be absent. The deficit is often unilateral, and if bilateral, it is almost always asymmetric.

The brachial plexus originates from the ventral rami of the lower 4 cervical nerves and the first thoracic ventral ramus (C5–T1). Its structural levels include trunks, divisions, and then cords. From the cords arise most of the major nerves of the upper limb. Above the clavicle, the C5–C6 rami unite to form the upper trunk, the C8–T1 rami join to form the lower trunk, and the C7 ramus becomes the middle trunk. Behind the clavicle, each of 3 trunks bifurcate into anterior and posterior divisions. The anterior divisions of the upper and middle trunks form the lateral cord that lies lateral to the axillary artery. The anterior division of the lower trunk descends at first behind and then medial to the axillary artery and forms the medial cord. The posterior divisions of all 3 trunks form the posterior cord that runs behind the axillary artery. An important branch of the lateral cord is the musculocutaneous nerve that supplies the flexor muscles of the elbow and gives sensation to the lateral surface of the arm. An important branch of the medial cord is the ulnar nerve. The axillary and radial nerves come out of the posterior cord. The median nerve originates from both the medial and lateral cords. Accurate localization is important, especially at the trunk level, since different pathologic processes have more or less specific predilections toward different portions of the plexus. Lesions affecting the upper trunk are usually traumatic or radiation induced, whereas those affecting the lower trunk may be caused by trauma, malignant infiltration, or thoracic outlet syndrome (TOS). Severe trauma can affect the whole plexus and cause concomitant multiple nerve root avulsions leading to an ominous prognosis.

Upper Trunk Brachial Plexopathy

Downward traction on an infant's arm during delivery (as in Erb-Duchenne palsy) or, in adults, a severe fall on the side of the head and shoulder, forcing the 2 apart (as frequently occurs in a motorcycle accident), may tear the upper trunk and cause C5–C6 root avulsion(s). This causes paralysis of the deltoid, periscapular, brachialis, and biceps muscles.

The last 2 are both elbow flexors, and the biceps is also a powerful supinator of the forearm. The arm therefore hangs adducted, with the forearm pronated and the palm facing backward, looking like a waiter hinting for a tip. There is sensory loss over the lateral aspect of the arm (the musculocutaneous and axillary nerve sensory territories).

Lower Trunk Brachial Plexopathy

Upward traction on the arm, such as in a forcible breech delivery (in Klumpke palsy), or malignant infiltration by an apical lung cancer (Pancoast tumor) may involve the lower trunk and its forming roots (C8–T1). These provide nerve supply to the intrinsic muscles of the hand. The hand assumes a clawed appearance (claw hand deformity) due to weakness of the interossei and lumbrical muscles. These muscle groups normally flex the metacarpophalangeal and extend the interphalangeal joints. Their weakness also leaves the action of the long extensors of the fingers, mainly innervated by the C7 root through the radial nerve, unopposed. There is sensory loss along the medial aspect of the forearm and often an associated Horner syndrome. The latter occurs as a result of traction on the superior cervical sympathetic ganglion.

Another example of lower trunk brachial plexopathies is the true neurogenic TOS. This is caused by gradual progressive entrapment of the lower trunk by a fibrous band that extends between the first thoracic rib and a rudimentary C7 rib or an elongated C7 vertebral transverse process. The presence of a cervical rib on its own is not synonymous with TOS because the incidence of the former is 20,000 to 80,000 times higher than that the rare true neurogenic TOS. Hence, careful clinical and EMG assessment is needed when there is a clinical suspicion of the condition. Often, patients present with mild aching and paresthesia in the medial aspect of the arm and forearm rather than the hand. This can be associated with a slowly progressive weakness of the forearm and hand intrinsic muscles. A pathognomonic sign of the disease is the preferential involvement of the T1 supplied thenar muscles rather than the hypothenar muscles (supplied by both C8 and T1 roots).

DISORDERS OF THE LUMBOSACRAL PLEXUS

The lumbosacral plexus originates from the ventral rami of the L1 through S4 nerve roots and is made up of 2 portions, the upper lumbar plexus and lower lumbosacral plexus. The upper lumbar plexus arises from the L1–L4 nerve roots. The lower lumbosacral plexus is derived from the L4–S4 nerve roots. The plexus is situated within the substance of the psoas major muscle and emerges at its lateral edge. The major branches from the upper lumbar plexus include the lateral femoral cutaneous nerve (L2–L3) transmitting sensation from the anterolateral aspect of the thigh; the femoral nerve (L2–L4) supplying the iliopsoas, pectineus, sartorius, and quadriceps muscles; and the obturator nerve (L2–L4) supplying the adductors of the thigh, gracilis, obturator externus, and a portion of the gluteus maximus. The major nerves originating from the lower portion of the plexus include the superior gluteal nerve (L4–S1) supplying the tensor fascia late, gluteus medius, and gluteus minimus muscles; the inferior gluteal nerve (L5–S2) supplying the main bulk of the gluteus maximus muscle; and the sciatic nerve (L4–S3) with its fibular (peroneal) and tibial nerve fibers.

Lumbosacral plexopathies can arise from a variety of pathologic processes, such as neoplastic; infective; inflammatory autoimmune; radiation induced; retroperitoneal hematoma; mechanical or stretch injury, especially after hip surgery; infiltrative (amyloid deposits); or interestingly idiopathic.

DISORDERS OF THE PERIPHERAL NERVES

In general, neuropathies can present with the following symptoms and signs:

- Motor deficit: Limb weakness and muscle atrophy with decreased or absent deep tendon reflexes.
- Sensory symptoms: Numbness, positive sensory phenomena (paresthesia, dysesthesia), and/or pain in a distal length-dependent (stock and glove) distribution (Figure 31–3).
- Variable involvement of the autonomic nervous system.

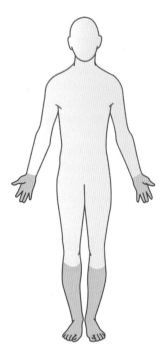

FIGURE 31–3 Distribution of sensory deficits in a patient with peripheral polyneuropathy. Notice the "stocking-and-glove" pattern of sensory loss. (Reproduced with permission from Waxman SG. *Clinical Neuroanatomy*, 28th ed. New York, NY: McGraw Hill; 2017.)

Nomenclature

A single nerve can be affected by a localized pathology as in median mononeuropathy in carpal tunnel syndrome or the ulnar mononeuropathy in cubital tunnel syndrome. The term *peripheral neuropathy* or *polyneuropathy* is used to describe diffuse symmetric involvement of the nerves in multiple limbs. The term *multiple mononeuropathies* (or more commonly *mononeuritis multiplex*) applies when ≥2 nerves in the same limb are affected. This pattern is usually encountered in inflammatory vasculitic neuropathies. Moreover, the pathologies that affect peripheral nerves may involve other portions of the peripheral nervous system such as the nerve roots (polyradiculoneuropathy) or roots and plexus (radiculoplexus neuropathy). This is more often seen in autoimmune or paraneoplastic processes.

There are different ways to classify peripheral neuropathies.

- Based on temporal course: In general, a neuropathy is considered acute when the time from its onset to the nadir is less than a month; subacute when this interval is 1 to 2 months; and chronic when the illness progresses over longer than 2 months or when the same neuropathy relapses.

- Based on the pathology: Peripheral neuropathies can be classified as demyelinating or axonal, with the latter often carrying a worse prognosis. Often, nerve conduction studies and EMG are able to make such differentiation and nerve biopsy is not needed for classification.

- Based on the etiology: Peripheral neuropathies can be classified as metabolic, endocrine, nutritional, toxic, genetic/hereditary, infectious, inflammatory, autoimmune, amyloid, neoplastic, or paraneoplastic. A large portion of patients are still labeled as having idiopathic peripheral neuropathy even after a thorough diagnostic workup.

Charcot-Marie-Tooth Disease

The eponym Charcot-Marie-Tooth disease (CMT) identifies a group of genetic or inherited neuropathies in which the peripheral neuropathy is either the sole or the predominant clinical component of the syndrome. CMT is considered the most common neuromuscular disease worldwide, with an estimated prevalence of 1 per 1214 population. CMT is subclassified based on the nature of pathology (demyelinating or axonal), mode of inheritance (autosomal dominant, recessive, or X linked), and specific genetic abnormality. CMT1A is the most common subtype and accounts for of 55% to 60% cases. It is due to duplication of the region containing the *PMP22* gene on chromosome 17p11.2. It is inherited in an autosomal dominant pattern. Normally, a nerve axon is surrounded by a single Schwann cell between the nodes of Ranvier. However, in CMT1A, when chronic progressive demyelination ensues, a reactive increase in the number of Schwann cells surrounding the intermodal axonal segments develops. These are classically known as onion bulbs.

The classic CMT phenotype features normal initial development followed by slowly progressive distal weakness and sensory loss manifesting within the first 2 decades of life, absent deep tendon reflexes, and skeletal deformities in the feet (pes cavus and hammertoes) (Figure 31–4). Affected children cannot keep up with their peers in running and have problems with activities that require balance (eg, biking or skating). Fine movements of the hands in activities such buttoning and zipping can be impaired, but the hands are rarely as affected as the feet. Most patients remain ambulatory throughout life and have a normal lifespan. Treatment is only supportive with physical and occupational therapy to prevent joint contractures. Ankle-foot orthotics are often needed for foot drop. Genetic counseling is imperative for the patient and the family.

Diabetic Neuropathy

The most common cause of neuropathy in the developed world is diabetes. The lifetime incidence of neuropathy is 59% and 45% in patients with type 1 and type 2 diabetes, respectively. The risk for developing peripheral neuropathy in a diabetic patient correlates with the degree of glycemic dyscontrol and the duration of diabetes. Diabetic neuropathy is commonly associated with other microvascular complications of diabetes such as nephropathy and retinopathy. The most common pattern is distal (length-dependent) symmetric sensory neuropathy. More than 25% of cases report deep aching foot pain with burning or electrical shooting quality. Significant

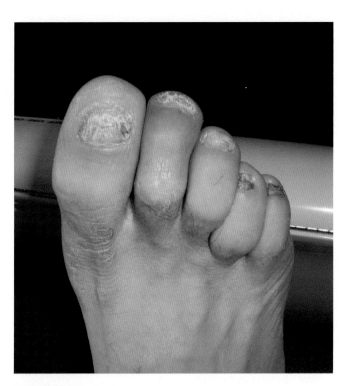

FIGURE 31–4 Hammer-toe deformity caused by Charcot-Marie-Tooth disease. (Reproduced with permission from Usatine RP, Smith MA, Mayeaux EJ, Chumley HS: *The Color Atlas and Synopsis of Family Medicine*, 3rd ed. New York, NY: McGraw Hill; 2019. Photo contributor: Richard P. Usatine, MD.)

weakness is uncommon. However, mild atrophy and weakness of the foot intrinsic muscles can be seen. Autonomic nervous system involvement (distal anhidrosis, gastroparesis, and erectile dysfunction) is commonly encountered. The mainstay of treatment is tight glycemic control. Symptomatic treatment of painful diabetic neuropathy can include pregabalin, gabapentin, tricyclic antidepressants, lidocaine patches for localized pain, and sometimes opioids such as tramadol.

Diabetic Amyotrophy

The site of pathology in this condition is more diffuse and may involve the nerves, lumbosacral plexus, and the nerve roots. Hence, the more anatomically descriptive term is *diabetic lumbosacral radiculoplexus neuropathy*. It more commonly affects older patients with type 2 diabetes. The condition is believed to be mediated through an immune-mediated attack on the vasa nervosa. The neuropathy starts with a unilateral severe pain involving the low back or hip and radiating down to the thigh and the leg. Within a few days or weeks, atrophy and weakness of the proximal and distal muscles of the affected lower limb become apparent. Patients also report sensory symptoms in the form of numbness, tingling, and contact allodynia. Interestingly, there is usually a considerable amount of weight loss that accompanies the disease onset. MRI of the lumbosacral plexus reveals signal hyperintensity and gadolinium enhancement of the lumbosacral roots and adjoining plexus. Nerve conduction studies and EMG show evidence of multifocal

axonal nerve damage that is often superimposed on the typical length-dependent pattern of diabetic sensory peripheral neuropathy. Cerebrospinal fluid (CSF) protein is elevated, whereas white blood cell count is normal. Early treatment with a short course of intravenous (IV) or oral glucocorticoids can shorten the duration of pain. However, it does not affect the long-term prognosis from the standpoint of motor deficits.

Acute Inflammatory Demyelinating Polyradiculoneuropathy (Guillain-Barré Syndrome)

Guillain-Barré syndrome can affect any age, with mean age of onset at 40 years and a worse prognosis in the elderly population. The reported annual incidence is 1.2 to 1.8 per 100,000 population. The first sign is usually weakness of the lower limbs, beginning distally, sometimes a few weeks after a preceding upper respiratory or gastrointestinal infection. Weakness progresses within a few hours or days, leading to gait impairment. Distal paresthesia and sensory disturbances are present in most patients. Deep tendon reflexes are absent and tone is flaccid. Although the weakness ascends rapidly, its ultimate extent is variable. It can go on to involve the upper limbs and cranial nerves, leading to dysphagia and bilateral facial palsy. The diaphragm and accessory muscles of respiration can be affected in severe cases, and life-threatening respiratory failure can develop rapidly, requiring prompt intubation and mechanical ventilation. Involvement of the autonomic nervous system can also occur resulting in life-threatening dysregulation of blood pressure control, cardiac rhythm, and central respiratory drive.

Guillain-Barré syndrome should always be clinically suspected in any rapidly progressing ascending flaccid paralysis that goes from onset to nadir over <4 weeks. Diagnostic workup should include CSF analysis and electrophysiologic evaluation with nerve conduction studies and EMG. There is often *albuminocytologic dissociation* in the CSF. This term refers to an elevation of the CSF protein concentration without any elevation of the white blood cell count. This is not usually seen until the second week from disease onset, and the CSF may be normal if tested early. Electrophysiologic studies usually reveal marked slowing of conduction velocities and conduction block, signs of a predominantly demyelinating pathology. Treatment with IV immunoglobulin (IVIg) or plasma exchange should be started as soon as possible with the goal of limiting severity and shortening the time to recovery. Both options were found to be equally efficacious. However, IVIg is often favored due to its ease of use and wide availability. The disease is usually a once in a lifetime event with no recurrence in 95% of cases.

The *Miller Fisher variant* of Guillain Barre syndrome is characterized by the acute onset of ataxia, ophthalmoplegia, and areflexia. Anti-GQ1b antibodies are present in the sera of 85% of patients. GQ1b is a ganglioside protein that is normally present in the oculomotor neurons, cerebellar cortex, and dorsal root ganglia. Management is the same as in Guillain-Barré syndrome.

Vitamin B₁₂ Deficiency

Vitamin B₁₂ deficiency is a common nutritional cause of neuropathy. A diet containing even a small amount of animal meat products provides sufficient vitamin B₁₂. Hence, vitamin B₁₂ deficiency due to poor intake occurs only in strict vegans. Vitamin B₁₂ deficiency can also be seen in malabsorption syndromes. An established etiology is pernicious anemia, where there is an antibody-mediated attack on the gastric parietal cells. These cells secret the intrinsic factor necessary for vitamin B₁₂ absorption in the ileum. Thus, vitamin B₁₂ deficiency may occur even with adequate oral intake, and it may be necessary to supplement the vitamin by injection.

Vitamin B₁₂ is essential for the demethylation of methyl tetrahydrofolate, which is important for DNA synthesis. The main neurologic pathology of vitamin B₁₂ deficiency is *subacute combined degeneration*, which involves the brain, spinal cord, and peripheral nerves (Figure 31–5). Patients often present with gait impairment due to spasticity and loss of proprioception along with simultaneous hand and feet paresthesias. On examination, patients show signs of combined upper and lower motor neuron dysfunction as well as

cognitive dysfunction. Megaloblastic anemia may be present due to defective DNA synthesis. The diagnosis of vitamin B₁₂ deficiency should be confirmed by testing serum vitamin B₁₂ and methylmalonic acid levels. The latter is a more accurate marker of cellular vitamin B₁₂ function and can be abnormal in the setting of borderline low vitamin B₁₂ levels (200 to 400 pg/mL). Vitamin B₁₂ supplementation should be administered parenterally since poor enteric absorption is usually the problem. Supplementation with vitamin B₁₂ typically halts progression of the disease but does not reverse it, since the major component of the disability is due to the unforgiving myelopathy.

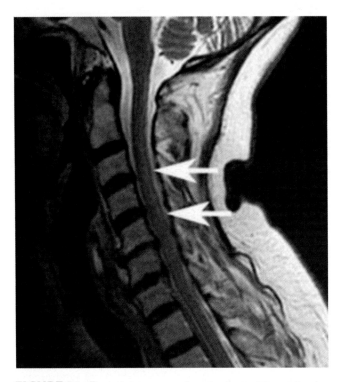

FIGURE 31–5 B₁₂ deficiency myelopathy. Sagittal T2-weighted MRI demonstrates high signal involving the posterior columns of the cervical spine (arrows). (Reproduced with permission from Jameson J, Fauci AS, Kasper DL, et al: *Harrison's Principles of Internal Medicine*, 20th ed. New York, NY: McGraw Hill; 2018.)

CASE 31–1

A 32-year-old woman developed bilaterally symmetric upper and lower limb weakness and numbness in feet and hands at the same time. She reported episodes of her legs "giving out" and dropping objects from both hands. She had been getting worse over the past 2 years before presentation. She did not have any neck or back pain. There were no changes in bowel or bladder function. She did not report any double vision, difficulty swallowing, or change in the character of her voice that she or others could notice.

On examination, she was alert and oriented to time, place, and person. Her speech was normal. Examination of the cranial nerves was grossly unremarkable. She had slight symmetric weakness of both lower limbs at both hip flexors and ankle extensors. She had loss of vibratory sense in the toes, ankles, and knees and loss of proprioception in the toes on both sides. Her reflexes were normal at the ankles and were brisk with crossed adductors at the knees. Romberg test was positive. Electrodiagnostic testing revealed a sensory neuropathy in the lower limbs. Magnetic resonance imaging (MRI) study of the brain was normal. MRI of the cervical spinal cord showed T2 signal hyperintensity in the dorsal column on both sides. On laboratory testing, she had a hemoglobin level of 10.5 g/dL (reference, 12 to 15.5 g/dL) with a mean corpuscular volume of 106 fL (reference, 81 to 98 fL). Her vitamin B₁₂ level was 100 pg/mL (reference, >200 pg/mL) and the methylmalonic acid level was 1600 nmol/L (reference, <318 nmol/L). Subsequent testing demonstrated a positive intrinsic factor antibody.

This patient has typical symptoms, neurologic examination, and laboratory findings for subacute combined degeneration secondary to vitamin B₁₂ deficiency. The preserved Achilles reflex and hyperreflexia throughout despite the neuropathy is evidence of a corticospinal tract lesion and myelopathy. Disruption of proprioception and vibration can result from large fiber sensory loss. Given the positive intrinsic factor antibody, the patient has pernicious anemia. She will likely need to be on intramuscular vitamin B₁₂ injections for life.

Vitamin B$_6$ (Pyridoxine)–Related Neuropathies

Pyridoxine is unique in the sense that it can cause neuropathy when it is deficient or in excess. Vitamin B$_6$ deficiency–related neuropathy can occur in the setting of isoniazid treatment for tuberculosis and can be avoided with concurrent supplementation with the vitamin while being on isoniazid. Vitamin B$_6$ toxicity can lead to sensory neuronopathy. This can be seen with megadose intake of vitamin B$_6$ (>2 g/d) and also with taking lower doses (50 mg/d) over long periods.

Vitamin B$_1$ (Thiamine) Deficiency

Thiamine deficiency–related neuropathy can occur with alcoholism or severe malnutrition. The classic severe form of vitamin B$_1$ deficiency is called *beriberi disease*. It is generally rare in developed countries, but recently, it has become more common in association with rising use of bariatric surgery. The neuropathy is progressive axonal and sensory more than motor. It can be associated with atrophic skin changes (dry beriberi) and/or congestive heart failure (wet beriberi). The latter is more common in nonalcoholic thiamine deficiency patients. Oral thiamine repletion is indicated unless the patient presents with Wernicke encephalopathy, in which case starting parenteral thiamine as soon as possible is required.

Alcoholism-Associated Neuropathy

Alcoholism is most commonly associated with the development of a progressive painful axonal sensorimotor polyneuropathy. It has been difficult to determine whether alcohol directly causes neuropathy or occurs due to alcoholism's association with chronic malnutrition and vitamin deficiencies. Moreover, underreporting of alcohol consumption is common. Thus, epidemiologic quantification of alcohol-associated neuropathy has been very challenging. Treatment of alcoholism-associated peripheral neuropathy requires abstinence and a well-balanced diet. This approach deals with both alcoholism and malnutrition. Indeed, given that alcohol was shown to be a neurotoxin, it is important to counsel any patient with an established diagnosis of peripheral neuropathy, regardless of its etiology, on moderation of alcohol intake.

Lead-Induced Neuropathy

The incidence of lead toxicity with peripheral neuropathy has substantially been lowered with the declining human exposure to the known environmental major sources, such as lead-based paint and lead addition to gasoline. Lead neurotoxicity can present as a combination of motor-predominant peripheral neuropathy (as seen when the radial nerve is involved, leading to wrist and finger drop) and encephalopathy. There is often concomitant constipation secondary to autonomic nerve involvement. Extraneural manifestations include microcytic hypochromic anemia and basophilic stippling of red blood cells. Measurement of lead level in a 24-hour urine collection

is done to screen for suspected cases. Chelation therapy with ethylenediamine tetraacetate (EDTA) is a treatment option.

Entrapment & Compression Mononeuropathies

Entrapment and compression mononeuropathies result from nerve compression by bony growth or fibrosis or external compression. The most common entrapment neuropathies in the upper limb affect the median nerve at the wrist level (carpal tunnel syndrome) and ulnar nerve at the level of elbow. The radial nerve can be compressed at the level of the humeral spiral groove (Saturday night palsy). In the leg, peroneal neuropathy across the head of the fibula may also occur. The pathology is focal demyelination and conduction block at the point of compression. Axonal degeneration can happen in chronic cases. Diagnosis depends on the clinical picture and the demonstration of slowing of nerve conduction velocity across the site of entrapment.

Carpal Tunnel Syndrome

Carpal tunnel syndrome is considerably more common in women and tends to develop around the time of the menopause. It usually affects the dominant hand, but it can affect both hands, with severity being greater on the dominant side. Factors that promote the development of carpal tunnel syndrome include hormonal changes (menopause, pregnancy), weight gain, hypothyroidism, and diabetes mellitus. Patients commonly experience pain and paresthesia that do not always follow the distribution of the median nerve in the hand. The sensory symptoms are worse at night, and patients usually wake up from sleep and shake their hands trying to get some relief. On examination, there is usually decreased sensation in the palmer aspect of the lateral 3½ fingers. A positive Tinel sign refers to paresthesia in the radial portion of the palm and the radial fingers induced by a tap on the transverse carpal ligament. Paresthesia in the fingers can sometimes be induced by sustained passive hyperflexion of the wrist (Phalen sign). Treatment should start with splinting the wrist at a neutral position for few months. If there is no improvement, patients should be referred to a surgeon for either open or endoscopic carpal release surgery via transecting the flexor retinaculum.

Ulnar Mononeuropathy at the Elbow (Cubital Tunnel Syndrome)

Ulnar nerve palsy is often traumatic in origin as the nerve is vulnerable to external compression at the level of medial epicondyle, the "funny bone." Clinical presentation includes a claw hand deformity that is similar to what was described in lower trunk brachial plexopathy. However, the sensory deficit is more often on the ulnar border of the hand rather than the forearm or arm. Conservative treatment with an elbow pad can be tried first, especially when sensory symptoms predominate. If there is no response, ulnar transposition surgery to transfer the nerve to the volar aspect of the elbow can be performed.

Radial Mononeuropathy at the Level of the Spiral Groove

The radial nerve is vulnerable to injury at the level of the humeral spiral groove as it lies directly on the bone at this location. This results in wrist and finger drop. Elbow extension is preserved as the branch that supplies the triceps comes out of the radial nerve proximal to the spiral groove. The sensory deficit is localized to the radial portion of the dorsum of the hand (anatomic snuff box).

Peroneal Mononeuropathy at the Level of the Fibular Head

This can be seen in patients who habitually sit with crossed legs, especially if they lose weight. Clinical presentation includes foot drop and steppage gait. Sensation is impaired on the dorsum of the foot and completely abolished in the first interosseous space. This is due to the fact that the compression often preferentially affects the nerve fibers of the deep branch of the common peroneal nerve. Treatment is mainly conservative by counseling patients to avoid crossing their legs. Physical therapy and ankle-foot orthosis may be needed.

DISORDERS OF NEUROMUSCULAR JUNCTION TRANSMISSION

Disorders of neuromuscular junction transmission can happen due to pathologic processes that involve either the postsynaptic end of the synaptic cleft, as in myasthenia gravis, or the presynaptic side, as in Lambert-Eaton myasthenic syndrome (LEMS) or botulism. Fatigable or fluctuating weakness is the hallmark of this entity of disorders. Deep tendon reflexes are usually preserved, with the exception of LEMS, in which they are typically lost. Sensation is preserved.

Myasthenia Gravis

Myasthenia gravis is an autoimmune disease that is caused by an antibody-mediated attack of the postsynaptic side of the neuromuscular junction. This leads to a decrease in the number of acetylcholine (ACh) receptors, loss of invaginations and simplification of the postsynaptic end, and widening of the synaptic cleft (Figure 31–6). Prevalence is approximately 20 per 100,000 in the US population. The reported female-to-male ratio is 3:2, and manifestations of the disease can start at any age. As many as 70% of myasthenia gravis patients have thymus hyperplasia, whereas 10% have thymoma. Other autoimmune diseases such as vitiligo and Hashimoto thyroiditis are common associations.

The clinical hallmark is symptomatic weakness that predominates in certain muscle groups and typically fluctuates in response to effort and rest. The disease manifestations become more overt over the course of the day and are worst in the evening. Patients often complain of binocular double vision and droopy eyelids. One-third of patients have dysphagia, which is more often to fluids than solids. Speech is usually nasal. Proximal limb and neck weakness occur from the onset in one-third of patients. Antibodies to ACh receptors are present to approximately 85% of generalized cases. Apart from antibody testing, establishing the diagnosis can be aided electrophysiologically by the presence of decrementing amplitudes of compound muscle action potential (CMAP) during repetitive nerve stimulation (RNS) testing.

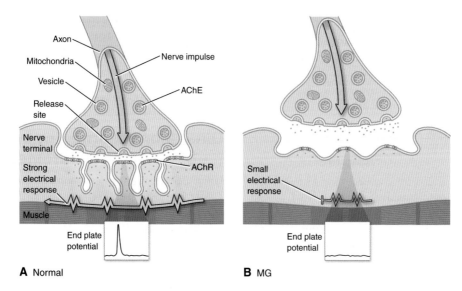

A Normal   **B** MG

FIGURE 31–6 Diagrams of (**A**) normal and (**B**) myasthenic neuromuscular junctions. The myasthenia gravis (MG) junction demonstrates a normal nerve terminal; a reduced number of acetylcholine receptors (AChRs); flattened, simplified postsynaptic folds; and a widened synaptic space. AChE, acetylcholinesterase.

Treatment should start with pyridostigmine. This medication delays the breakdown of ACh by inhibiting the enzyme acetylcholinesterase. This allows ACh to accumulate at the neuromuscular junction site for a longer time. Side effects may include increased bronchial secretions and bronchospasm and intestinal cramps. In the majority of cases, treatment with pyridostigmine is not sufficient and patients may need to take an immunosuppressive agent such as steroids, azathioprine, or mycophenolate. Rescue treatments with IVIg or plasma exchange are treatment options in myasthenic crisis. They can be also used regularly as maintenance treatment. Thymectomy was found to have long-term benefits on myasthenic symptoms and quality of life for at least 3 years. It should not be reserved for just those who have thymoma. See Chapter 30 for more information.

Lambert-Eaton Myasthenic Syndrome

The clinical manifestations of this disease are caused by antibodies targeting the voltage-gated calcium channels (VGCC) on the presynaptic side of the neuromuscular junction. Inactivation of these channels decreases the calcium influx induced by an incoming action potential and causes the release of inadequate amounts of ACh from the nerve terminal. The syndrome often has a paraneoplastic origin, and the underlying etiology in two-thirds of patients is a small-cell carcinoma of the lung. The disease often presents with fatigable weakness predominantly affecting the pelvic girdle and lower limbs. Ocular manifestations are often mild if present. Muscular strength transiently increases, at first, with exercise. Deep tendon reflexes are often absent. Many patients complain of dry mouth or other autonomic manifestations (orthostatic hypotension and impotence). Electrophysiologically, the disease is characterized by presence of incrementing CMAP amplitudes during RNS testing. Treatment follows the same lines of management that apply to myasthenia gravis. 3,4-Diaminopyridine is a voltage-gated potassium channel blocker that prolongs depolarization and facilitates ACh release, improving muscle power and fatigue. Screening for malignancy in LEMS patients who are diagnosed by RNS or positive anti-VGCC antibodies is a must.

DISORDERS OF THE SKELETAL MUSCLES

In general, myopathies are characterized by muscle weakness that is proximal in most cases. Deep tendon reflexes are normal or reduced later in the course of the disease. Sensation is preserved. Extraocular, facial, and bulbar muscles are involved in certain myopathies. Muscle diseases can be hereditary (as in muscular dystrophies, congenital myopathies, or channelopathies), inflammatory autoimmune (polymyositis, dermatomyositis, or inclusion body myositis), metabolic (glycogen or lipid storage disease), mitochondrial, toxic (statin induced), or endocrine (thyroid disease).

Muscular Dystrophies

Muscular dystrophies are genetically determined, progressive, degenerative disorders of the muscles. They are classified based on the underlying genetic and molecular deficit.

Myotonic Dystrophy

Myotonic dystrophy type 1 is the most common muscular dystrophy in adults. The prevalence is 3 to 5 per 100,000 population. It is an autosomal dominant disease that is caused by CTG triple nucleotide repeat expansions on chromosome 19q13.2. The severity of phenotype correlates with the number of repeats. The size of repeats typically increases from one generation to the next, leading to younger age of onset and more severe manifestations with every generation to come (anticipation phenomenon). Cause of death is often respiratory failure or cardiomyopathy due to conduction defect.

Clinically, patients present with facial and upper limb distal weakness mainly in the hands. Myotonic phenomenon, which is a slow and difficult relaxation of the muscle after contraction that gets better with repetition of movement, is commonly seen in hand grips and eyelid. Percussion myotonia can be seen after tapping on the abductor pollicis brevis or the tongue. Systemic manifestations include cataract, which is present in 100% of patients; cardiac conduction defect; frontal balding; temporal wasting (Figure 31–7); daytime sleepiness;

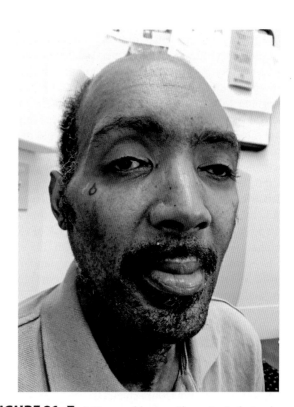

FIGURE 31–7 A 48-year-old man with myotonic dystrophy, cataracts, frontal baldness, and wasting of the temporalis, facial, and sternocleidomastoid muscles. (Reproduced with permission from Simon RP, Aminoff MJ, Greemberg DA: *Clinical Neurology*, 10th ed. New York, NY: McGraw Hill; 2018.)

hypoventilation; diabetes; hypogonadism; and gastrointestinal pseudo-obstruction due to the relatively milder smooth muscle involvement. EMG shows waxing and waning motor unit potentials, which gives the chrematistic dive bomber sound. Creatine kinase is usually mildly elevated. Genetic testing typically confirms the diagnosis. Patients should be screened annually for cataract and cardiac conduction defect. If the latter is found, cardiac pacing is lifesaving. The myotonia itself is painful and can respond to phenytoin or mexiletine. Prenatal diagnosis through amniocentesis or chorionic villous sampling is available. Myotonic dystrophy type 1 has a congenital (congenital myotonic dystrophy) form in which myotonia is not present earlier in the course.

Myotonic dystrophy type 2 is an autosomal dominant disorder that results from CCTG repeat expansions in the *CNBP* gene on chromosome 3q21. Weakness is mainly seen in the proximal limb muscles with more severe muscle pain than in type 1. Type 2 myotonic dystrophy does not have a congenital form.

Dystrophinopathies (Duchenne & Becker Muscular Dystrophies)

Dystrophinopathies are the second most common muscular dystrophies in adults. They will be discussed in Chapter 35 with the pediatric neurology topics.

Facioscapulohumeral Muscular Dystrophy

Facioscapulohumeral muscular dystrophy (FSHD) is the third most common muscular dystrophy in adults. Prevalence of FSHD is estimated to be 7 per 100,000 population. The disease follows an autosomal dominant inheritance pattern and results from reduction of the D4Z4 repeats on chromosome 4q35. As its name implies, asymmetric weakness affects facial, periscapular, biceps, and triceps muscles. Pectoral muscles are distinctly weak, yet the deltoid muscles tend to be spared. Weakness spreads caudally, with onset in the face, then the scapular region, followed by the proximal arms, and then the legs. Twenty percent of patients become wheelchair bound. Hearing loss and retinal vascular abnormalities are common extramuscular features for which patients need to be screened. Because of the lack of significant bulbar, respiratory, or cardiac involvement, life expectancy is normal. Genetic testing is the gold standard for diagnosis. Treatment is supportive, with long-term physical therapy and genetic counseling.

Channelopathies

Muscle channelopathies are a rare group of disorders caused by mutations in virtually all ion channels, including chloride, sodium, calcium, and potassium channels.

Myotonia Congenita

There are both autosomal dominant and recessive forms of the disease. They result from a mutation in the muscle chloride channel gene (*CLCN1*). Clinical and electrical myotonia is the main clinical feature with no noticeable muscle weakness. Often, patients have a generalized muscle hypertrophy. Treatment is still symptomatic using phenytoin or mexiletine.

Paramyotonia Congenita

This is another autosomal dominant disorder that results from a mutation in the voltage-gated sodium channel gene (*SCN4A*). The muscle weakness is mainly in the proximal limb muscles and is associated with stiffness. Unlike the other myotonias where there is the warm-up phenomenon, the myotonia in this disorder gets worse with continued exercise. It is also worse with exposure to cold temperature. Symptomatic treatment is the same as in myotonia congenita.

Hypokalemic Periodic Paralysis

The estimated prevalence of hypokalemic periodic paralysis is 1 per 100,000 population. Two-thirds of cases occur due to mutations in the calcium channel gene *CACNA1S* on chromosome 1q32 or the sodium channel gene *SCN4A* on chromosome 17q23. Onset is usually in the second decade of life. Patients experience attacks of variable severity, from mild weakness to outright paralysis that can last for hours or a few days. Potassium levels can drop to <3.0 mmol/L during attacks. Carbohydrate-rich food, stress, and alcohol are potential triggers of the attack. Treatment of acute episodes can be achieved by giving oral or IV potassium slowly. Patients are instructed to maintain a low-carbohydrate diet. Frequency and severity of attacks can be reduced by using carbonic anhydrase inhibitors such as acetazolamide.

Hyperkalemic Periodic Paralysis

Prevalence of hyperkalemic periodic paralysis is <1 per 100,000 population. It is caused by a mutation in the sodium channel gene *SCN4A* on chromosome 17q23. Onset is usually in the first decade of life. Episodes of weakness are shorter (minutes to hours) and more frequent than in hypokalemic periodic paralysis. Potassium levels can be >5.0 mmol/L during attacks. However, the level may not be increased during the attack at all. Fasting and ingestion of potassium-rich foods are potential triggers of the attack. Treatment of acute episodes can be achieved by giving oral carbohydrates or glucose. Patients are instructed to avoid fasting, strenuous activity, and cold. Frequency and severity of attacks can be reduced by using thiazide diuretics or acetazolamide.

SELF-ASSESSMENT QUESTIONS

1. A 65-year-old man comes to the neurology clinic for double vision that has been going on for the past 6 months. The double vision is worse at night. He also has bilateral droopy eyelids.

There is no limb weakness. He has smoked a pack of cigarettes a day for the past 40 years. On neurologic exam, he has bilateral ptosis and inability to look upward. His pupils are equal and reactive. Muscle power is normal. Deep tendon reflexes are preserved. Sensory exam is normal. Which of the following is the most likely underlying mechanism of his disease?

A. Antibody-mediated attack on the postsynaptic side of the neuromuscular junction
B. Antibody-mediated attack on the presynaptic side of the neuromuscular junction
C. Toxin-mediated attack on vesicles in the presynaptic terminal
D. Cell-mediated immune response against myelinated nerve fibers
E. Cell-mediated immune response against muscle membrane proteins

2. A 25-year-old man presents to the emergency department with a 4-day history of tingling in both legs and feet. He also has low back pain that radiates to the anterior surface of the abdomen. Three weeks earlier, he had symptoms of upper respiratory tract infection and was treated with azithromycin. He does not have any symptoms in the upper limbs. On neurologic exam, he has normal mental status. His speech and cranial nerve examinations are normal. He has mild weakness in both ankle dorsiflexors. His deep tendon reflexes are absent in the ankles and diminished in the knees on both sides. Upper limb deep tendon reflexes are preserved. What is the most likely underlying mechanism of his disease?

A. Immune attack against peripheral myelin
B. Toxin penetration through the blood–nerve barrier
C. Immune complex disposition in the wall of the epineurial blood vessels
D. Mutation in 1 of the genes coding for structural proteins of myelin

3. A 48-year-old woman is being evaluated in the neurology clinic for recent-onset right foot drop. She has a long history of dull aching low back pain. She was told that she has borderline diabetes and was advised to lose weight. She has lost 20 pounds over the past 4 months prior to presentation. She has some tingling sensation on the dorsum of the foot on the right side. On neurologic exam, she has moderate weakness in the right ankle dorsiflexors and evertors. Ankle inversion is normal. There is loss of pinprick sensation over the dorsum of the foot. Deep tendon reflexes are intact all over. Injury of which of the following structures could cause her clinical picture?

A. Right L5 nerve root
B. Lumbosacral plexus on the right side
C. Right sciatic nerve
D. Right common peroneal nerve
E. Right tibial nerve

Neurologic Infections

Shruti P. Agnihotri

- Recognize various types of neurologic infections based on localization.
- Identify the common organisms and the clinical scenarios for these infections.
- Discuss the pathology of these infections.

PREVALENCE & BURDEN

Neurologic infections remain an important cause of mortality and morbidity worldwide. Over 1.2 million cases of bacterial meningitis are estimated to occur worldwide each year. The case fatality rate for meningitis can be as high as 70% without treatment. The prevalence of central nervous system (CNS) infections varies based on geographic locations, with higher prevalence in developing areas and areas with a high incidence of human immunodeficiency virus (HIV) infection.

Neurologic infections can be caused by various pathogens, including bacteria, fungi, viruses, parasites, and prions. Common organisms and the clinical syndromes associated with each of them are discussed in this chapter. Although detailed discussion is beyond the scope of this chapter, one should be aware of emerging viruses that affect the nervous system, such as Zika virus, Nipah virus, dengue virus, and chikungunya virus.

LOCALIZATION

Pathogens can affect various parts of the nervous system, but most often, they have a certain predilection (eg, varicella-zoster virus resides in the sensory ganglia). Diffuse infection of the meninges results in meningitis, whereas infection of the brain parenchyma results in encephalitis. Encephalitides occur either due to contiguous spread from nearby structures or due to hematogenous spread. Within the brain parenchyma, certain organisms have a predilection for white matter (eg, JC virus infecting oligodendrocytes). Abscesses can occur in epidural and subdural spaces as well as in the brain parenchyma.

DISORDERS

Meningitis

Meningitis refers to an inflammatory reaction in the subarachnoid space. The clinical syndrome is that of headache, fever, and neck stiffness. Cerebrospinal fluid (CSF) shows evidence of an inflammatory reaction, as noted by elevated white blood cell counts and protein. Acute meningitis usually presents within hours to days, whereas by definition, chronic meningitis is longer than 4 weeks in duration.

Acute Meningitis

Acute meningitis is most often infectious, caused by bacteria or a virus, with noninfectious etiologies in the differential diagnosis. As noted previously, the morbidity and mortality of bacterial meningitis remain high despite widespread availability of antibiotics. Early diagnosis and treatment are imperative to reduce morbidity and mortality.

Acute bacterial meningitis is seen in all age groups. With the extensive use of the *Haemophilus influenzae* type b (Hib) vaccine, the incidence of acute bacterial meningitis in the pediatric age group has been reduced. It is now more commonly seen in young and older adults. The most common community-acquired organisms are *Streptococcus pneumoniae* (pneumococcus), *Neisseria meningitidis* (meningococcus), *Listeria monocytogenes*, group B streptococci, and *H influenzae*.

1. *S pneumoniae* is the most common bacterium, responsible for meningitis in more than half of all cases in all ages except infants younger than 2 months. Immunoglobulin deficiency, sickle cell disease, alcoholism, diabetes, and CSF leaks are risk factors for this organism.

VOCABULARY

Encephalitis: Inflammation in the brain parenchyma.

Immune reconstitution inflammatory syndrome (IRIS): Syndrome of clinical (and often radiologic) worsening after start of treatment due to a strong immune response that produces significant inflammation.

Meningitis: Inflammation of the meninges, particularly in the subarachnoid space.

Myelitis: Inflammation of the spinal cord.

Opportunistic infection: Infections occurring secondary to impairment of the immune defenses. Some examples of impaired body defenses include human immunodeficiency virus, chemotherapy and other immunosuppressive medications, organ transplantation, severe burns, leukemia, lymphoma or other malignancy, diabetes, and prolonged corticosteroid therapy.

Polymerase chain reaction (PCR): Commonly used technique for detection of organisms by amplifying their DNA.

Rhombencephalitis: Inflammation of the brainstem.

Ventriculitis: Inflammation of the lining of the ventricles.

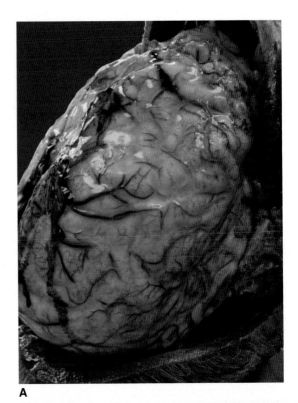

A

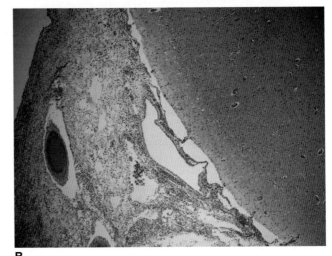

B

FIGURE 32–1 Acute purulent bacterial meningitis. **A.** The yellow-green discoloration centered around the vessels at the convexity of the right cerebral hemisphere represents an acute bacterial meningitis caused, in this case, by *Streptococcus pneumoniae*. **B.** This low-power photomicrograph depicts the cortical surface and meninges. The meninges are expanded by a cellular infiltrate, which is composed predominantly of neutrophils. Hematoxylin and eosin, 40×. (Reproduced with permission from Kemp WL, Burns DK, Brow TG: *Pathology: The Big Picture*. New York, NY: McGraw Hill; 2008.)

2. *N meningitidis* is common in adolescents and young adults. Along with *S pneumoniae*, these bacteria are responsible for >90% of cases in that age group.

3. Hib was once the most common cause of meningitis in the pediatric age group. However, with the widespread use of the Hib vaccine, the incidence has been dramatically reduced. It is now seen in nonvaccinated children and in adults.

4. *L monocytogenes* causes meningitis and meningoencephalitis in the immunocompromised. This is discussed in detail later in this chapter.

5. Group B *Streptococcus* is a cause of meningitis in the newborn. It is a common flora in the female vaginal tract and can be transmitted to the newborn during delivery.

6. Gram-negative rods (eg, *Escherichia coli*, *Klebsiella*, *Pseudomonas*) and *Staphylococcus* are causative agents in nosocomial cases. The incidence of these has been increasing. Other risk factors include diabetes, alcoholism, and cirrhosis.

The bacteria invade the subarachnoid space, causing an inflammatory response. Neutrophilic infiltrate and protein exudates cover the base of the brain and the nerve sheaths of exiting cranial nerves. Subsequently, there is infiltration of lymphocytes and histiocytes, and fibrin is deposited, resulting in a thick yellowish membrane covering the brain convexity (Figure 32–1).

Viral meningitis is more common than any other meningitis. The causative viruses are listed in Table 32–1. Some of the viruses may cause encephalitis, myelitis, or encephalomyelitis

in addition to meningitis. The most common etiologic agent for meningitis is enterovirus. Arboviruses, which require an insect vector for transmission, include West Nile virus, Japanese encephalitis, and St. Louis encephalitis. These viruses are discussed later in the chapter under viral encephalitides.

TABLE 32–1 Viruses causing acute meningitis and encephalitis in North America.

Acute Meningitis	
Common	**Less Common**
Enteroviruses (coxsackieviruses, echoviruses, and human enteroviruses 68–71)	Herpes simplex virus 1
	Human herpesvirus 6
	Cytomegalovirus
Varicella-zoster virus	Lymphocytic choriomeningitis virus
Herpes simplex virus 2	Mumps
Epstein-Barr virus	
Arthropod-borne viruses	
HIV	

Acute Encephalitis	
Common	**Less Common**
Herpesviruses	Rabies
Cytomegalovirus[a]	Eastern equine encephalitis virus
Herpes simplex virus 1[b]	Powassan virus
Herpes simplex virus 2	Cytomegalovirus[a]
Human herpesvirus 6	
Varicella-zoster virus	
Epstein-Barr virus	
Arthropod-borne viruses	Colorado tick fever virus
	Mumps
La Crosse virus	**West Nile virus**[c]
	St. Louis encephalitis virus
	Enteroviruses

[a]Immunocompromised host.

[b]The most common cause of sporadic encephalitis.

[c]The most common cause of epidemic encephalitis.

Reproduced with permission from Kasper D, Fauci A, Hauser S, et al: *Harrison's Principles of Internal Medicine*, 19th ed. New York, NY: McGraw Hill; 2015.

Herpes simplex virus (HSV) type 2 is commonly responsible for genital herpes. Some patients can develop recurrent lymphocytic meningitis due to HSV-2, known as Mollaret meningitis. Varicella-zoster virus (VZV), human herpesvirus type 6, HIV, and Epstein-Barr virus are also associated with meningitis.

Eosinophilic meningoencephalitis is seen with parasitic infections such as *Angiostrongylus cantonensis*, *Gnathostoma*, *Paragonimus*, and *Toxocara canis* and *Toxocara cati* infections. These cause cranial neuropathies and polyradiculitis. CSF shows presence of eosinophils.

Aseptic meningitis refers to meningitis seen in autoimmune disorders, following medication use (eg, intravenous immunoglobulin), or as part of neoplastic disorders.

Clinical features common in meningitis include fever, neck stiffness, headache, and altered sensorium. Altered level of consciousness is present in two-thirds of patients with bacterial meningitis but is almost never seen in viral meningitis. Seizures can occur in bacterial meningitis and portend poor prognosis. Examination shows nuchal rigidity, Kernig sign, and Brudzinski sign (**Figure 32–2**). However,

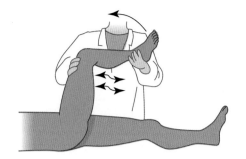

A Kernig sign

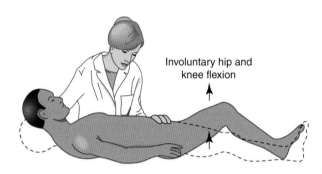

B Brudzinski sign

FIGURE 32–2 The Kernig and Brudzinski signs.

absence of these does not rule out meningitis. In viral meningitis, headache is more severe with nausea and vomiting. Lumbar puncture will often relieve the headache temporarily. Presence of diarrhea suggests viral etiologies such as enteroviruses or arboviruses. Rash may be seen with *Enterovirus*. Hemorrhagic purpura is very suggestive of meningococcemia.

Early diagnosis is very important to reduce mortality in bacterial meningitis. Imaging is helpful, but the decision on when to do it depends on the clinical scenario. Brain magnetic resonance imaging (MRI) may show signs of encephalitis, abscess, or hydrocephalus. Timely CSF evaluation is important so that cultures can be sent before prolonged antibiotic therapy and organisms are identified. Elevated opening pressure (>20 cm H$_2$O) is seen in bacterial meningitis. In addition, bacterial meningitis is characterized by polymorphonuclear pleocytosis, elevated protein concentrations, and CSF hypoglycorrhachia (low glucose). In viral meningitis, however, there is usually a mononuclear pleocytosis, and CSF abnormalities of protein and glucose concentrations are mild. Aggressive cases of viral meningitis may show an initial polymorphonuclear pleocytosis that then transforms into a lymphocytic-predominant pleocytosis over days to weeks. Gram stain is positive in 60% to 90% of cases of bacterial meningitis. The yield of Gram stain is reduced with early use of antibiotics. CSF cultures are helpful in identification of the organisms in approximately 70% of cases of bacterial meningitis. For viral meningitis, viral polymerase chain reaction (PCR) testing of CSF is helpful. Antibodies against the viruses can also be measured in the CSF. HIV testing should be routinely performed in all patients presenting with meningitis.

The choice of appropriate early treatment depends on age, immune status, and predisposing and associated conditions. The antibiotics of choice based on the organism are listed in Table 32–2. Most often, a combination of multiple drugs is used as initial therapy. Once culture results are available, only appropriate antibiotics should be continued. Corticosteroids given in addition to antibiotics have been shown to reduce morbidity and mortality in children as well as improve the functional outcome in adults. Acyclovir is used in treatment of viral meningitis caused by HSV or VZV. Antiretroviral therapy should be started in HIV patients. For meningococcal meningitis, prophylactic antibiotic treatment is given to all contacts of the patient.

Subacute & Chronic Meningitis

In subacute and chronic meningitis, the signs and symptoms evolve over a period of a few weeks and may persist for much longer. Usually, these are caused by atypical bacteria, spirochetes, or fungal agents. Autoimmune diseases such as sarcoidosis, Wegener granulomatosis, and neoplastic

TABLE 32–2 Antimicrobial therapy of central nervous system bacterial infections based on pathogen.

Organism	Antibiotic
Neisseria meningitides	
Penicillin-sensitive	Penicillin G or ampicillin
Penicillin-resistant	Ceftriaxone or cefotaxime
Streptococcus pneumoniae	
Penicillin-sensitive	Penicillin G
Penicillin-intermediate	Ceftriaxone or cefotaxime or cefepime
Penicillin-resistant	Ceftriaxone (or cefotaxime or cefepime) + vancomycin
Gram-negative bacilli (except Pseudomonas spp.)	Ceftriaxone or cefotaxime
Pseudomonas aeruginosa	Ceftazidime or cefepime or meropenem
Staphylococci spp.	
Methicillin-sensitive	Nafcillin
Methicillin-resistant	Vancomycin
Listeria monocytogenes	Ampicillin + gentamicin
Haemophilus influenzae	Ceftriaxone or cefotaxime or cefepime
Streptococcus agalactiae	Penicillin G or ampicillin
Bacteroides fragilis	Metronidazole
Fusobacterium spp.	Metronidazole

Reproduced with permission from Kasper D, Fauci A, Hauser S, et al: *Harrison's Principles of Internal Medicine*, 19th ed. New York, NY: McGraw Hill; 2015.

disorders such as lymphoma can cause chronic meningitis. These patients may not have the classic signs and symptoms of meningitis. Fever is rare. Patients will have headache, altered sensorium, and possibly seizures. Cranial nerve abnormalities can also be seen. Although pleocytosis and increased protein levels are usually found in the CSF, cultures are often negative because the organisms are usually more difficult to detect and culture. Tuberculous meningitis and various fungal meningoencephalitides are discussed later in this chapter.

Bacterial Infections of the Brain & Spinal Cord

Bacteria invade the brain or spinal cord either by hematogenous spread (emboli of bacteria or infected thrombi) or by extension from nearby structures adjacent to the brain (eg, ears and paranasal sinus infections, osteomyelitis of nearby bones). Most cases of bacteremia do not result in CNS infection. However, CNS infections can occur secondarily to pneumonia or endocarditis. Increasingly, infection in the brain is iatrogenic, occurring after cerebral or spinal surgery or in the setting of a ventriculoperitoneal shunt. Intracranially, these organisms can cause epidural abscess, subdural empyema, meningitis, septic thrombophlebitis, brain abscess, and encephalitis. Meningitis has been discussed earlier; the other conditions will be discussed later.

Abscesses: Epidural Abscess, Subdural Empyema, Brain Abscess, & Septic Thrombophlebitis

Abscess means collection of pus. Within the cranium, this can occur in different locations.

1. Epidural abscess is a collection of pus on the outer surface of the dura, separating it from the bone. This occurs secondary to infections in the ear and paranasal sinuses or as a complication from a surgical procedure. There is associated osteomyelitis of the underlying bone. Spinal epidural abscesses can occur secondary to bacteremia as well. Symptoms include local pain, fever, tenderness, and nasal or aural discharge. Rarely, seizure may occur. Spinal epidural abscess presents with back pain, radicular pain and paresis, loss of sensation, and bladder and bowel dysfunction. *Staphylococcus aureus* is most often the causative organism. CSF may show a mild inflammatory reaction. Antibiotics should be directed against the organism identified or suspected. The underlying bone may need to be removed as well. Spinal epidural abscesses almost always need surgery. Delay in treatment of spinal epidural abscesses results in permanent injury due to ischemic changes in the cord.

2. Subdural empyema is a collection of pus between the inner surface of the dura and outer surface of the arachnoid matter. This is commonly seen in children. Paranasal sinus infection is most often the cause. It is increasing in incidence secondary to increasing surgical manipulations. Organisms enter the subdural space through bone and dura or by spread from septic venous sinus thrombosis. Fever, headache, neck stiffness, and focal neurologic signs are seen. Computed

tomography (CT) scan and MRI show the pus collection along with disease in the paranasal sinuses. CSF analysis shows elevated pressure, polymorphonuclear pleocytosis in the range of 50 to 1000/μL, increased protein content, and normal glucose values. CSF culture is usually sterile. Most of these patients require burr holes in the skull to drain the pus along with broad-spectrum antibiotic coverage.

3. Septic thrombophlebitis refers to infection of the dural venous sinuses. This results from an infection of the middle ear and mastoid cells, the paranasal sinuses, or skin around the upper lip, nose, and eyes. It can also occur as a complication of meningitis, epidural abscess, subdural empyema, and brain abscess. Clinical manifestations include fever, headache, signs and symptoms of raised intracranial pressure, seizures, and focal neurologic deficits. CSF will show raised intracranial pressure, but the formula may be normal, unless there is associated meningitis or subdural empyema. Clot may be visualized on CT scan or MRI. Treatment includes large doses of antibiotics. Heparin has been used as well, unless there is associated large intracranial hemorrhage. Surgical debridement of the primary source may also be needed.

4. Brain abscess refers to collection of pus in the parenchyma of the brain. This mostly occurs via hematogenous spread from a pulmonary or cardiac source and is less likely to occur from a contiguous source. In cases of bacterial endocarditis, cerebral seeding can also occur via septic emboli. Common causative organisms are staphylococci and streptococci. These may sometimes be seen along with some anaerobic bacteria such as *Bacteroides*, *Fusobacterium*, and *Prevotella*. Fungal abscesses are discussed later in this chapter. The abscess formation starts with cerebritis (focal suppurative encephalitis), which is followed by organization wherein the center becomes necrotic and fibroblasts and granulation tissue are seen in the periphery. Brain abscesses mimic brain tumors clinically and radiologically. Headache, seizures, and focal neurologic signs are common presentation.

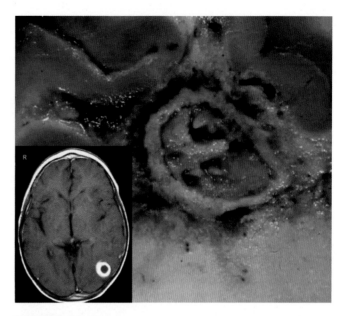

FIGURE 32–3 Bacterial brain abscess. A pus-filled abscess cavity is surrounded by a thick, vascularized, fibrous capsule at the junction of cortex and white matter. The thick fibrovascular capsule brightly enhances in the brain magnetic resonance imaging scan (*inset*). (Reproduced with permission from Reisner H. *Pathology a Modern Case Study*, 2nd ed. New York, NY: McGraw Hill; 2020.)

Fever and leukocytosis may not be present, except when there is an active systemic source of infection. MRI shows increased T2 signal within the abscess cavity as well as surrounding edema. The capsule rim is hypointense on T1 but enhances with gadolinium (Figure 32–3). Abscesses show restricted diffusion. Blood cultures and lung scan are helpful to identify the source. Patients often undergo biopsy or surgical excision for diagnosis. Treatment includes broad-spectrum antibiotics. Steroids and mannitol may be needed if there is mass effect. Stereotactic needle aspiration is preferred over excision for deep abscesses.

CASE 32–1

An 18-year-old male student presents to the emergency department with complaints of fever and a new headache for the past 3 days. The headache is severe, frontal in location, and associated with photophobia and neck stiffness. His past medical history is significant only for asthma, for which he had completed a 5-day course of prednisone a week prior to this presentation. Upon examination, he is noted to have a temperature of 101°F. The remainder of the vital signs and systemic examination are normal. Neurologic examination is normal except for neck rigidity with positive Kernig sign and Babinski sign on the right. Computed tomography scan without contrast shows a hypodensity in the left periventricular area, abutting the left lateral ventricle. Magnetic resonance imaging shows a round T2 hyperintense lesion in the left

parietal lobe, abutting the left lateral ventricle with surrounding vasogenic edema. There is restricted diffusion in the lesion and ring enhancement upon contrast administration. The patient receives antibiotic coverage with vancomycin and ceftriaxone for suspected brain abscess. Cerebrospinal fluid (CSF) analysis shows a white blood cell count of 13,000/μL with 88% neutrophils and 12% lymphocytes, protein of 293 mg/dL, and glucose of 4 mg/dL with serum glucose of 82 mg/dL. Gram stain of the CSF shows gram-positive cocci in pairs. CSF culture is negative. Blood cultures, chest x-ray, and transesophageal echocardiogram are negative. The patient improves significantly by day 3 of hospitalization and is continued on vancomycin and ceftriaxone for 14 days for early stages of brain abscess likely due to pneumococcus.

Atypical Bacterial Organisms

Tuberculosis

Mycobacterium tuberculosis is an acid-fast organism that causes systemic infection. CNS involvement occurs in approximately 1% to 5% of patients with tuberculosis. The incidence of tuberculosis in the United States has decreased significantly over time, but it remains a huge burden globally, especially in developing countries. Young children and immunosuppressed individuals are at highest risk. Acquired immunodeficiency syndrome (AIDS) led to a dramatic increase in the incidence of tuberculosis. CNS involvement occurs via hematogenous spread.

1. **Tuberculous meningitis:** There is bacterial seeding of the meninges and subpial regions of the brain with the formation of tubercles (Rich foci). One or more of the tubercles may rupture and release bacteria into the subarachnoid space. A dense, gelatinous exudate, sometimes in the form of multiple small abscesses, forms along the base of the brain. When this covers the choroid plexus and basal subarachnoid cisterns, CSF flow is obstructed and hydrocephalus develops. Vasculitis may occur, causing strokes commonly in the basal ganglia and upper brainstem. Clinical presentation is subacute compared to bacterial meningitis. Early symptoms include low-grade fever, malaise, headache, lethargy, confusion, and stiff neck. Cranial nerve palsies and papilledema can be present by the time the patient comes to medical attention.

2. **CNS tuberculomas:** These are granulomatous tuberculous foci that may occur concurrently or separately from tuberculous meningitis. These form anywhere in the brain, along the meninges, or in the spinal cord. They cause symptoms of space-occupying lesions and can cause hydrocephalus depending on the location.

3. **Spinal tuberculosis:** The spinal cord can be involved due to the meningeal exudate invading the parenchyma of the spinal cord or due to compression from osteomyelitis of the vertebrae (Pott disease) or an epidural abscess. Patients often present with signs and symptoms of posterior and lateral cord involvement along with nerve root involvement.

MRI of the brain can show basal leptomeningeal enhancement, which is often thick and irregular; hydrocephalus; and strokes in the basal ganglia and midbrain (**Figure 32–4**). CNS tuberculomas may present as multiple ring-enhancing lesions on the MRI. CSF in tuberculous meningitis shows lymphocytic pleocytosis with elevated protein (between 100 and 200 mg/dL) and low glucose. The glucose level may not be reduced in CNS tuberculomas. CSF culture of *M tuberculosis* is the gold standard for diagnosis of CNS tuberculosis. However, the cultures take 2 to 8 weeks to grow. Large-volume CSF tap, increasing time for examination of CSF smears, and repeating lumbar puncture can improve the yield. CSF PCR for *M tuberculosis* has low sensitivity. Patients infected with HIV may have atypical CSF and neuroimaging findings.

Treatment regimen for CNS tuberculosis is the same as for pulmonary tuberculosis but requires a longer duration of

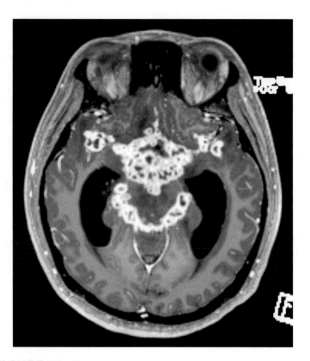

FIGURE 32–4 Magnetic resonance imaging in tuberculous meningitis showing gadolinium enhancement of the basal meninges, reflecting microabscesses and intense inflammation, accompanied by hydrocephalus and cranial nerve palsies. (Reproduced with permission from Ropper AH, Samuels MA, Klein JP: *Adams and Victor's Principles of Neurology,* 11th ed. New York, NY: McGraw Hill; 2019.)

9 to 12 months. A 4-drug combination of isoniazid, rifampin, ethambutol, and pyrazinamide is used for the first 2 months, followed by rifampin and isoniazid. Corticosteroids used in the initial phase of treatment reduce mortality. Drug resistance is associated with higher mortality, and second-line agents should be used in these cases. Overall mortality is approximately 10% with CNS tuberculosis.

Leprosy

Also known as Hansen disease, leprosy is caused by *Mycobacterium leprae*, which is extremely slow growing. It is a very common cause of neuropathy in developing countries. In North America, it is mostly seen in immigrants and is uncommon. It has a long incubation period. It affects skin, superficial cutaneous nerves, and later peripheral nerves, eyes, and testes. The clinical spectrum ranges from tuberculoid leprosy (patients have good immune response, few lesions, and few bacteria in the lesions) to lepromatous leprosy (patients have poor immune response and multiple skin lesions with demonstrable bacteria). There is loss of sensation to pinprick and temperature in the areas of the skin lesions or beyond. This initially involves the cooler surfaces of the body, such as the ears and dorsal surfaces of the hands, feet, forearms, and anterolateral legs, and then later involves the nose, malar areas, lateral trunk, and buttocks. Focal neuropathies such as ulnar neuropathy above the elbow, peroneal neuropathy at the fibular head, or facial neuropathy can occur. Finding acid-fast bacteria on the skin smear or biopsy is diagnostic. Treatment includes rifampin with dapsone for tuberculoid leprosy, and clofazimine is added to that regimen for lepromatous leprosy.

Listeriosis

L monocytogenes causes a meningoencephalitis in immunocompromised individuals, newborns, and pregnant women. Specifically, it causes rhombencephalitis. This manifests as fever, headache, nausea, and vomiting, followed by cranial nerve palsies, cerebellar dysfunction, and hemiparesis. MRI may show abnormal T2 signal in the brainstem after few days of illness. CSF cultures may reveal the organism in about half of the cases. Treatment includes ampicillin with gentamicin. Immunocompromised patients can have fatal outcomes. Having a high degree of suspicion in immunocompromised patients can help to institute early treatment, which reduces mortality.

Mycoplasma Infection

Mycoplasma pneumoniae is a common cause of pneumonia in adults, often referred to as "walking pneumonia." It is associated with a wide variety of neurologic complications, occurring in up to 5% of cases. These include Guillain-Barré syndrome, cranial neuritis, acute myositis, aseptic meningitis, transverse myelitis, global encephalitis, seizures, cerebellitis, acute disseminated encephalomyelitis, and acute hemorrhagic leukoencephalitis (Hurst disease). The exact underlying mechanism is not clearly understood, but some of these complications are likely postinfectious, occurring secondary to molecular mimicry. In other instances, mycoplasmal DNA has been isolated from CSF. In acute hemorrhagic leukoencephalitis, MRI will show T2 signal hyperintensities within the white matter along with some hemorrhage on susceptibility-weighted imaging. CSF will show mild lymphocytic pleocytosis along with elevated protein. Rising titers of serum immunoglobulin (Ig) M and IgG antibodies or demonstration of cold agglutinins can help with the diagnosis. Antibiotic treatment can help eliminate respiratory infection but is not helpful for the neurologic complications. Steroids, plasma exchange, and sometimes intravenous immunoglobulin are used. Most patients recover well, although the recovery may be prolonged.

Cat Scratch Fever

Cat scratch fever refers to encephalitis with very high fever after a scratch or bite from a cat caused by *Bartonella henselae*, a gram-negative bacillus. Patients present with lymphadenopathy in the drainage area of the scratch, confusion, and high-grade fever, followed by seizures and status epilepticus. In severely immunocompromised patients, this can also cause vasculitis. Treatment includes azithromycin or doxycycline. Most patients recover well.

Diseases Caused by Bacterial Exotoxins

There are 3 types of exotoxins that are very potent and have strong effects on the nervous system. They cause diphtheria,

tetanus, and botulism. These are discussed in the following sections.

Diphtheria

Diphtheria is an acute, contagious disease caused by the gram-positive bacillus *Corynebacterium diphtheriae*. The most common clinical presentation is the characteristic pseudomembranous pharyngitis. The bacteria produce an exotoxin called diphtheria toxin, which is responsible for cardiac and neurologic complications in approximately 20% of cases. Palatal paralysis occurs around weeks 3 to 5 after onset of initial symptoms. This can be accompanied by other cranial neuropathies. Late complications (weeks 5 to 8) include an acute demyelinating sensorimotor polyneuropathy causing an ascending paralysis similar to Guillain-Barré syndrome. In severe cases, paralysis of the diaphragm and respiratory failure can occur as can autonomic instability.

Diagnosis is based on isolation of the bacteria from nasopharyngeal swabs of patients or immediate contacts of patients. CSF findings are similar to those seen in Guillain-Barré syndrome, with mild lymphocytic pleocytosis but a disproportionate increase in protein content. Treatment for neurologic complications is supportive care. Use of antitoxin within 48 hours of the earliest symptoms of the primary diphtheritic infection lessens the incidence and severity of the peripheral nerve complications. Immunization with diphtheria toxoid to prevent diphtheria is the only effective measure. Booster doses are needed every 10 years after initial immunization.

Botulism

Clostridium botulinum is a spore-forming, anaerobic, gram-positive bacillus that produces botulinum toxin. It is the most potent toxin known to mankind and is responsible for causing botulism. In infantile botulism, ingested bacterial spores germinate in the gastrointestinal tract where they produce toxin that is systemically absorbed. In the United States, infant botulism is most often associated with consumption of honey, which should be avoided before the age of 12 months. In adults, the most common cause is improper canning of foods, which allows growth of the anerobic organism. Rarely, an infected wound is the source. The toxin acts at the neuromuscular synapse, interfering with the release of acetylcholine from the peripheral motor nerves. Initial symptoms include blurred vision and diplopia. Prominent bulbar symptoms, along with external ophthalmoplegia, dysarthria, dysphonia, and dysphagia, lead one to consider myasthenia gravis as the diagnosis. However, patients with botulism also have loss of accommodation and unreactive pupils. Limb paralysis can progress to respiratory muscle weakness, causing respiratory insufficiency. Deep tendon reflexes are diminished to absent. Patients may also have autonomic symptoms such as dry mouth, fixed dilated pupils, constipation, paralytic ileus, and urinary retention.

CSF examination is normal in botulism. Nerve conduction studies will show low-amplitude compound muscle action potentials (CMAPs). Repetitive nerve stimulation at 30 to 50 Hz for 10 seconds shows an increment in CMAPs (unlike in myasthenia gravis). Isolating the bacteria from serum, stool, food samples, or wound material is diagnostic. Antitoxin should be administered as soon as the diagnosis is made. Patients often require intensive management, especially for respiratory function. Enemas and emetics to remove unabsorbed toxin from the gut should be considered. Drugs causing neuromuscular blockade should be avoided.

Tetanus

Tetanus is a vaccine-preventable disease caused by the exotoxin of the anaerobic spore-forming bacillus *Clostridium tetani*. It is extremely rare in the United States due to effective immunization. However, in developing countries, it is still a common occurrence in newborns (tetanus neonatorum) of unimmunized mothers, where the spores enter via an umbilical cord cut with unclean blades. The spores remain dormant in the soil for many years. Once the spores enter the body through a penetrating wound, they convert to a vegetative state and produce the exotoxin tetanospasmin. The toxin causes blockade of the release of the neurotransmitter γ-aminobutyric acid (GABA). This causes both agonist and antagonist muscle contractions, leading to the characteristic muscle spasms of tetanus. These contractions can initially be limited to the area near the wound site. This is followed by rigidity of axial muscles of neck, back (opisthotonos), and abdomen. An early manifestation of generalized tetanus is rigidity of the masseter muscles (trismus, also known as lockjaw). *Risus sardonicus* refers to distinct straightening of the upper lip causing a grimacing posture due to contraction of facial muscles. The muscle spasms can be severe enough to cause fractures. Minimal external stimulus can provoke tonic contractions that are extremely painful. Spasms of the pharyngeal, laryngeal, or respiratory muscles result in dysphagia, dysarthria, and asphyxia. Autonomic instability with blood pressure and heart rate fluctuations, profuse sweating, and increased salivation can also be seen. Fever and pneumonia are common complications.

Treatment is aimed at eliminating the bacteria as well as neutralizing the toxin. A single dose of antitoxin is given intravenously as well as locally around the wound after surgical debridement of the wound. Metronidazole or penicillin is used as well to help eliminate any vegetative bacteria. An important aspect is supportive care with benzodiazepines, neuromuscular-blocking agents, ventilatory support, and care for autonomic instability. Overall mortality rate is approximately 50%. Neonatal tetanus carries a very high mortality. The key is prevention with tetanus toxoid. Booster doses are needed every 10 years.

Spirochetal & Rickettsial Infections

Spirochetes are long, slender bacteria that cause Lyme disease, syphilis, leptospirosis, and relapsing fever in humans. The first 3 conditions have neurologic complications and are discussed in the following sections.

Lyme Disease

Lyme disease is caused by *Borrelia burgdorferi* in North America and Europe. whereas *Borrelia afzelii* and *Borrelia garinii* are responsible for Lyme disease in Europe and Asia. In North America, Lyme is transmitted by the deer tick *Ixodes scapularis*. In the United States, it is endemic in the Northeast and Upper Midwest regions, with most cases occurring in late spring and early summer. The initial manifestation is a characteristic skin lesion at the site of a tick bite called erythema migrans. Neurologic involvement occurs in up to 15% of untreated patients, weeks after initial infection. This manifests as facial nerve palsy, lymphocytic meningitis, and radiculoneuritis. CSF analysis shows lymphocytic pleocytosis, moderate increase of protein level, and a normal glucose level. Enzyme immunoassay is performed first, followed by Western blot testing for IgM and IgG antibodies. Intrathecal antibody production is considered present if the antibody titer in the CSF exceeds the titer in serum. Treatment for facial palsy is doxycycline 100 mg twice a day for 14 days. However, for meningitis or radiculoneuritis, ceftriaxone 2 g/d for 14 days is thought to be more effective.

Neurosyphilis

Neurosyphilis is a complication of syphilis occurring at any point during the course of the disease. Overall incidence has reduced dramatically since the use of penicillin. However, recently, there has been an increase in early syphilis cases, especially in HIV-positive patients. *Treponema pallidum*, the causative organism, is transmitted sexually and invades the brain early in the course of the disease. In the early stages of neurosyphilis, meninges and blood vessels are affected. In the late stages, spinal cord and brain parenchyma are affected, although the underlying mechanism for these symptoms is also chronic meningitis.

1. Asymptomatic syphilitic meningitis occurs in the early stages, with patients having no neurologic symptoms but having serologic or clinical evidence of syphilis, or both, and CSF pleocytosis, elevated protein, or reactive CSF Venereal Disease Research Laboratory (VDRL) test. Treatment at this stage prevents progression to symptomatic stages.

2. Symptomatic syphilitic meningitis also occurs in the early stage, within a year of infection. Besides signs and symptoms of meningitis, other findings include papilledema, confusion, and cranial nerve palsies, particularly involving cranial nerves II, VII, and VIII. The meningitis can be localized, producing mass-like lesions that are called syphilitic gummas.

3. Meningovascular neurosyphilis develops within months to years of initial infection. It can cause arteritis and stroke affecting vessels of the brain and, less commonly, the spinal cord. Middle cerebral artery territory strokes are most common.

4. Tabes dorsalis, also known as locomotor ataxia, occurs many years after the initial infection. It is seen less frequently

since the use of antibiotics. Clinical features include abnormal papillary response (Argyll Robertson pupils), optic atrophy, sensory changes, lancinating pain, and bowel and bladder dysfunction. Early sensory changes include paresthesia or hyperesthesia in radicular distributions. Later, pain, vibration, and tactile sensations and reflexes are lost. Gait ataxia is the most predominant symptom. This occurs due to degeneration of the posterior columns.

5. Syphilitic dementia, also known as general paresis or dementia paralytica, occurs 5 to 25 years after the initial infection. It is seen rarely these days due to use of antibiotics. Early in the course, patients have mild memory issues and personality changes. However, as the disease progresses, they develop various psychiatric syndromes and severe memory problems progressing to frank dementia. Pathologic correlates include meningeal thickening, brain atrophy, ventricular enlargement, and granular ependymitis.

Testing for syphilis includes nontreponemal tests, such as rapid plasma reagin and the VDRL test, and treponemal tests, such as the fluorescent treponemal antibody absorption test and the *T pallidum* particle agglutination assay. Serum reactivity to the nontreponemal tests suggests exposure to syphilis. However, these can be false positive and can also be false negative in the late stages of neurosyphilis. CSF reactivity to the nontreponemal tests is virtually diagnostic of neurosyphilis. The treponemal tests are positive in almost all patients with neurosyphilis. Because asymptomatic neurosyphilis can be recognized only by the changes in the CSF, all patients with cutaneous syphilis are recommended to have a CSF analysis.

All forms of neurosyphilis are treated with penicillin G, given intravenously in a dosage of 18 to 24 million units daily for 10 to 14 days. Ceftriaxone is an alternative. However, penicillin is preferred even in patients with allergy; they should ideally undergo desensitization.

Leptospirosis

This extremely rare disease is caused by *Leptospira interrogans* and is a zoonotic infection seen in humans with occupational exposure to infected animals. In recent years, it has been seen with adventure sports resulting in exposure to mud and soil. It causes a biphasic illness with both meningitis and hepatitis. It has a benign course in most cases; approximately 10% of patients have a dramatic presentation with hepatic and renal involvement.

Rocky Mountain Spotted Fever

Rocky Mountain spotted fever (RMSF) is caused by *Rickettsia*, which are obligate intracellular bacteria requiring insect vectors for transmission. RMSF is transmitted by a painless tick bite and is commonly seen in the states of Tennessee, North Carolina, Virginia, and Maryland. It causes meningitis along with a rash. The rash typically begins on the wrists and ankles and then spreads centrally to the face, chest, and abdomen. In the early stages of the disease, serologic tests have low sensitivity. Biopsy of the skin lesions can be helpful. Doxycycline is the treatment of choice. Neurologic complications are rare, and the case fatality rate is close to 10%.

Fungal Infections

Fungal infections in the CNS are usually secondary to systemic fungal infections and are much rarer than bacterial infections. Most of the fungal infections involving the nervous system are opportunistic infections such as candidiasis, aspergillosis, mucormycosis, and actinomycosis. Cryptococcal infection can occur in immunocompetent patients as well. Fungal meningitis is insidious in onset and mimics tuberculous meningitis in terms of the clinical, radiologic, and CSF findings. In immunocompromised states, CSF pleocytosis may be minimal or absent.

Cryptococcosis

Cryptococcosis is one of the most common fungal infections in the brain, causing a granulomatous meningitis as well as nodules in the brain known as cryptococcomas. The causative organism is a ubiquitous fungus named *Cryptococcus neoformans*. Cryptococcal meningitis often presents subacutely with signs and symptoms of raised intracranial pressure and confusional state. Fever, meningismus, and cranial nerve palsies are infrequent, which makes it harder to diagnose this condition. Deep territory strokes due to meningovascular involvement often present with hemiparesis. In a few cases, this may be an indolent infection, with a course spread over few months. Imaging may show leptomeningeal enhancement, which can be nodular, and hydrocephalus may be present. CSF analysis will show a polynuclear pleocytosis turning into a lymphocytic pleocytosis as the disease progresses. However, the pleocytosis may be minimal in immunocompromised states. Detection of cryptococcal antigen in the CSF by latex agglutination is the test of choice because it has high sensitivity, is easily available, and provides rapid results. India ink preparations have a sensitivity of approximately 75% (Figure 32–5). Fungi may be seen on biopsy samples (Figure 32–6). It is imperative to start treatment early to prevent mortality. The combination of amphotericin B and flucytosine is used in immunocompetent patients for at least 6 weeks. In AIDS patients, fluconazole is added after 2 weeks for a prolonged course. Serial lumbar punctures are needed sometimes to reduce the intracranial pressure.

Candidiasis

Candida albicans is a ubiquitous fungus and a common cause of fungal infection in the body. CNS involvement is rare, occurring mostly in immunocompromised patients as part of disseminated candidiasis. It can produce meningitis, meningoencephalitis, or abscesses. CSF analysis shows a polynuclear or lymphocytic pleocytosis, elevated protein, and some reduction in glucose. CSF Gram stain will show the yeast in a minority of the cases, and cultures may also be negative. The yield is increased by performing a large-volume tap and using the sediment for culture. CSF 1,3-β-D-glucan detects fungal

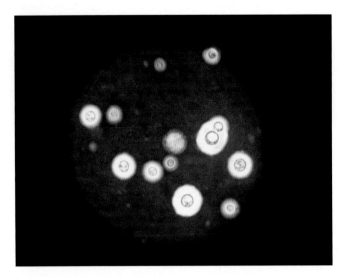

FIGURE 32–5 India ink preparation. *Cryptococcus neoformans* seen as encapsulated yeast on India ink preparation of the cerebrospinal fluid from an HIV patient with cryptococcal meningitis. (Reproduced with permission from Knoop KJ, Stack LB, Storrow AB, et al: *The Atlas of Emergency Medicine*, 4th ed. New York, NY: McGraw Hill; 2016. Photo contributor: Seth W. Wright, MD.)

cell wall component and is useful for diagnosis, although it is a nonspecific test. Treatment is with amphotericin B and flucytosine. The prognosis is generally poor despite treatment.

Aspergillosis

Aspergillus is a common mold that is present throughout the world. In immunosuppressed patients, it can invade the blood vessels (infectious vasculitis). It can have a contiguous spread

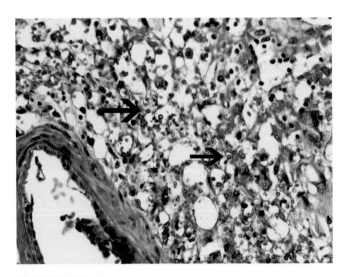

FIGURE 32–6 Cryptococcal meningitis. This high-power photomicrograph of the meninges, stained with mucicarmine, highlights encapsulated and budding yeast forms. In cryptococcal meningitis, an opportunistic disorder most commonly associated with HIV infection, there is minimal inflammatory reaction. The capsule of *Cryptococcus neoformans* stains with mucicarmine (*arrows*). Mucicarmine, 400×. (Reproduced with permission from Kemp WL, Burns DK, Brow TG: *Pathology: The Big Picture*. New York, NY: McGraw Hill; 2008.)

from the nasal sinuses with subsequent skull base involvement or a hematogenous dissemination. This can lead to cavernous sinus thrombosis and cranial nerve palsies, which can be indolent. In the brain, it causes ischemic or hemorrhagic strokes, abscesses, or mass-like lesions and rarely a meningoencephalitis. MRI can show ring-enhancing lesions, which represent abscesses. Strokes can also be seen. Hemorrhage within the lesions is suggestive of angioinvasive organisms. Associated sinonasal disease on imaging can provide clues to the diagnosis. Definitive diagnosis is made on histopathology and tissue culture. Serum galactomannan and 1,3-β-D-glucan help in diagnosis. Voriconazole is the drug of choice; other agents include amphotericin B, itraconazole, and posaconazole. Adjunctive surgery may help reduce the mortality.

Mucormycosis

Mucormycosis caused by *Mucorales* is an angioinvasive disease that is similar to aspergillosis but is very aggressive and responds poorly to voriconazole. In addition to the previously described risk factors associated with immunosuppression, diabetic ketoacidosis and corticosteroid-associated hyperglycemia, intravenous drug use, and iron overload states are unique risk factors for mucormycosis. It often presents with involvement of the retinal arteries, leading to sudden blindness. Once the brain is involved, few patients survive. Treatment with amphotericin B and posaconazole and rapid correction of underlying risk factors have resulted in survival in some cases.

Coccidioidomycosis, Histoplasmosis, & Blastomycosis

These are dimorphic fungi, entering the lungs through inhalation. Each fungus is endemic to certain regions in North America: *Blastomyces dermatitidis* in the US midwestern states and Canadian provinces that border the Great Lakes, as well as southeastern and south central states; *Histoplasma capsulatum* around the Ohio and Mississippi River basins; and *Coccidioides immitis* in the arid southwestern United States. CNS involvement occurs as a complication of disseminated disease in 5% to 10% of cases, producing chronic meningitis or sometimes focal mass-like lesions in the brain. These fungi mimic CNS tuberculosis in regard to clinicopathologic and imaging aspects as well as on CSF analysis. Diagnosis can be difficult in these cases. Urine, serum, and CSF *Histoplasma* galactomannan antigen (quantitative enzyme immunoassay) may be positive in some cases. CSF culture requires multiple high-volume taps to increase the yield. Histopathology and culture of biopsy tissue may be positive. Amphotericin B followed by itraconazole is the treatment of choice. Lifelong suppressive therapy may be needed in some patients.

Protozoal & Parasitic Infections
Toxoplasmosis

The disease caused by *Toxoplasma gondii* is seen in 2 circumstances: congenital and late acquired. The late acquired infection usually occurs in the setting of immunosuppression and is discussed later in this chapter. Congenital infection occurs when the mother develops initial infection during pregnancy. Manifestations include microcephaly, hydrocephalus, cerebral calcifications, and chorioretinitis. The consequences are fatal in most infants; others survive with significant mental and motor disabilities.

Amebic Encephalitis

This is a very rare but fatal disease, caused by free-living amoebae such as *Naegleria*, *Acanthamoeba*, or *Balamuthia*. These are acquired by swimming in warm fresh water. The clinical manifestations and the CSF findings resemble those of acute bacterial meningitis. Wet CSF preparation can show the mobile trophozoites, but a high degree of suspicion is often needed to look for them. Pathology shows necrotizing meningoencephalitis with microabscesses. The organisms are often mistaken for macrophages or cellular debris. The disease has a very fulminant course, and even early treatment is rarely effective.

Neurocysticercosis

Cysticercosis is not endemic in the United States but is seen more frequently now due to immigration from the endemic countries of Central and South America and Asia. It is caused by larval stages of *Taenia solium* and may be acquired by consumption of undercooked pork or other carnivore meat. CNS manifestations occur due to cyst formation, the resulting inflammatory response, and calcification in the subarachnoid space along the brain or the spinal cord. There are usually multiple lesions. If they are located in the intraventricular space, they may obstruct CSF flow, causing hydrocephalus. There is a more fulminant form of the disease, known as the racemose type, in which there is a strong inflammatory response to the cysts in the subarachnoid space causing severe arachnoiditis, vasculitis resulting in hydrocephalus, cranial nerve palsies, and strokes. The inactive form is a result of calcifications and

is a common cause of seizures in endemic countries. CT scan and MRI show multiple calcified lesions in the inactive stage. Scolex may be visualized prior to calcification. During the active stage, contrast enhancement is noted (Figure 32–7). Treatment with albendazole or praziquantel is effective. Corticosteroids are added to the initial phase of treatment when there is significant inflammatory response.

Schistosomiasis

Schistosomiasis is caused by *Schistosoma japonicum* or rarely by *Schistosoma haematobium* or *Schistosoma mansoni*. The disease is rare in North America (seen mostly in travelers) but is common in sub-Saharan countries and other tropical countries. Brain lesions occur due to egg deposition in blood vessels, resulting in ischemia and necrosis in the parenchyma along with an inflammatory response by eosinophils and giant cells. Neurologic symptoms such as headache, seizures, and focal signs usually develop months after exposure. *S mansoni* in particular localizes in the spinal cord and conus medullaris, affecting bladder control and causing radicular symptoms in legs. Eosinophil count is increased in blood as well as CSF. Imaging will show the lesion along with surrounding edema and contrast enhancement. Treatment is with praziquantel and corticosteroids.

Malaria

Although very rare in the United States, malaria is very prevalent in tropical countries and can be fatal. Cerebral malaria is caused by *Plasmodium falciparum*. Children are more susceptible and present with fever, headache, and confusion that rapidly progress to seizures and coma. There is significant cerebral edema due to blockage of the capillaries and venules by the infected red blood cells. Treatment instituted based on knowledge of resistance patterns in the endemic area using antimalarial agents such as mefloquine, artemether, atovaquone, and others.

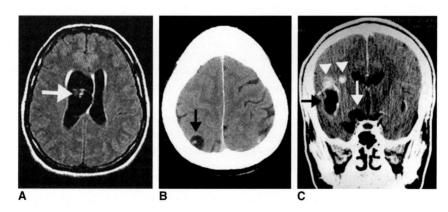

FIGURE 32–7 Neurocysticercosis is caused by *Taenia solium*. Neurologic infection can be classified based on the location and viability of the parasites. When the parasites are in the ventricles, they often cause obstructive hydrocephalus. *Left:* Magnetic resonance imaging showing a cysticercus in the lateral ventricle, with resultant hydrocephalus. The *arrow* points to the scolex within the cystic parasite. *Center:* Computed tomography showing a parenchymal cysticercus, with enhancement of the cyst wall and an internal scolex (*arrow*). *Right:* Multiple cysticerci, including calcified lesions from prior infection (*arrowheads*), viable cysticerci in the basilar cisterns (*white arrow*), and a large degenerating cysticercus in the Sylvian fissure (*black arrow*). (Parts A and B, reproduced with permission from Jameson J, Fauci AS, Kasper DL, et al: *Harrison's Principles of Internal Medicine*, 20th ed. New York, NY: McGraw Hill; 2018; part C, reproduced with permission from Bandres JC, White AC Jr, Samo T, et al: Extraparenchymal neurocysticercosis: report of five cases and review of management, *Clin Infect Dis*. 1992 Nov;15(5):799-811.)

Viral Infections

Viral infections are the most common infections in the nervous system. Various different agents and their syndromes are described in the following sections.

Poliomyelitis

Poliomyelitis is an infection of the anterior horn cells resulting in acute flaccid paralysis. Historically, this was most commonly caused by poliovirus. However, with eradication of this virus from most of the world, other viruses have been identified as potential etiologic agents leading to the same syndrome. These include coxsackievirus A and B, West Nile virus, and Japanese encephalitis. In recent times, there has been an increase in incidence, and enteroviruses are implicated. Involvement of the diaphragmatic muscles or brainstem is concerning. Management includes supportive care.

Viral Encephalitides

Viral encephalitis can occur with or without meningitis. Most viruses that cause meningitis can cause encephalitis as well. However, there are other viruses, especially arboviruses, that cause encephalitis without meningeal signs. Clinical features include confusion, seizures, coma, abnormal movements, cranial nerve palsies, and abnormal reflexes. MRI can be normal or show T2 signal abnormalities in the areas affected, with or without enhancement. CSF demonstrates pleocytosis and elevated protein. CSF PCR helps in the identification of the culprit virus.

Arboviral encephalitis refers to encephalitides caused by viruses transmitted via mosquitoes. West Nile, St. Louis, California, and La Crosse viruses are seen in the United States. West Nile virus also causes an acute flaccid paralysis in addition to the encephalitis. In the brain, it has a predilection for the deep nuclei. Eastern equine encephalitis, although rare, can be very devastating with high morbidity and mortality rates. La Crosse encephalitis is more common in children and has a benign course. Japanese encephalitis is the most common arboviral encephalitis outside of North America, especially in Asia.

Postinfectious encephalomyelitis can be seen after a viral infection that incites an autoimmune reaction. The virus is not present in the neural tissue. This is difficult to distinguish from an infectious encephalitis. Acute disseminated encephalomyelitis is a postinfectious complication seen most commonly in young patients and is characterized by demyelination.

Herpes simplex encephalitis is the most common of the viral encephalitides. This is almost always caused sporadically by the HSV-1 virus. The virus has a strong predilection for the temporal lobes and insula. The disease evolves over a few days, manifesting with fever, headache, confusion, seizures, and coma. Temporal lobe features such as hallucinations, aphasia, and delirium are also noted. Pathology includes hemorrhagic necrosis of the brain tissue. CSF findings are notable for presence of red blood cells, xanthochromia, and lymphocytic pleocytosis. MRI shows T2 signal abnormalities in the temporal lobe and may show evidence of hemorrhage as well. It is imperative to treat patients early on with intravenous acyclovir, even before the CSF HSV PCR results are returned, because the condition can be fatal.

Varicella-Zoster Syndromes

Varicella-zoster infection occurs due to reactivation of the VZV and is 1 of the most common viral infections, with a higher incidence in the elderly. The virus is thought to be latent in the sensory ganglia following primary infection. Reactivation can cause various syndromes, as discussed in the following text.

Shingles refers to the cutaneous manifestation of a vesicular rash in a dermatomal distribution, along with pain and itching. Zoster ophthalmicus occurs as a result of involvement of the ophthalmic division of the trigeminal nerve, resulting in pain and rash over the forehead and face. This is particularly concerning due to possibility of blindness from corneal involvement. Ramsay Hunt syndrome is involvement of the facial nerve, resulting in facial palsy and herpetic eruption in the external auditory canal. Postherpetic neuralgia is a severe neuralgic pain that can follow shingles, with an incidence of >40% in patients over age 60 years. Other complications include VZV poliomyelitis, VZV radiculomyelitis, VZV leptomeningitis, and VZV vasculopathy. Of these, VZV vasculopathy is the most serious complication. Inflammation of the blood vessels in the brain causes stroke-like manifestations as well as encephalopathy, leading to coma and potentially death if not treated early.

CSF analysis shows lymphocytic pleocytosis and elevated protein, but in some cases, it can be normal. CSF VZV PCR and VZV antibody testing are helpful in diagnosis. Acyclovir is the antiviral of choice for all VZV syndrome. Use of acyclovir during the acute phase of shingles reduces the duration of postherpetic neuralgia. Serious complications such as myelitis and vasculopathy need intravenous and higher doses of acyclovir along with intravenous steroids.

Subacute Sclerosing Panencephalitis

Subacute sclerosing panencephalitis is an encephalitis due to slow persistent infection with the measles virus. This is rare in developed countries but can be seen in developing countries where primary measles infection is common. This is seen commonly in older children, sometimes in young adults who have a history of measles infection. Presentation includes cognitive and personality changes, followed by seizures, myoclonus, and hyperreflexia. This progresses to unresponsiveness, autonomic dysfunction, and death within 1 to 3 years of onset. This condition is always fatal, and measles vaccine is the only preventive measure.

Rabies

Rabies is a fatal encephalitis caused by rabies virus, a rhabdovirus. It is rare in the United States and is transmitted by wild animals such as bats, raccoons, skunks, and foxes. It is more common in certain developing countries, where it is transmitted by bites of stray dogs. The incubation period can be a few weeks to months. There is an encephalitic form (primarily a rhombencephalitis) and a paralytic form. In encephalitic form, symptoms include fever, headache, agitation, throat spasms when attempting to

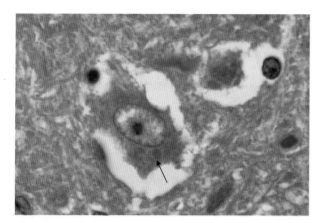

FIGURE 32–8 Rabies virus—Negri body. *Arrow* points to a Negri body, an inclusion body in the cytoplasm of an infected neuron. (Reproduced with permission from Public Health Image Library, Centers for Disease Control and Prevention.)

swallow water (hydrophobia), and diplopia followed by seizures and coma. The paralytic form is characterized by sensory or motor symptoms in the bitten limb, progressing to flaccid paralysis. The disease is almost always fatal after onset of symptoms. Antemortem diagnosis is made by antigen detection tests in the CSF or by biopsy of skin or brain. Postmortem examination shows mononuclear infiltration, perivascular cuffing, and characteristic Negri bodies, which are intracytoplasmic inclusions of viral nucleocapsid proteins (Figure 32–8). Treatment includes proper cleaning of the wound and postexposure vaccination.

HIV & the Nervous System

HIV is a retrovirus that causes reduction in the CD4 T-cell count. When the infection is advanced and the counts are severely suppressed, it causes profound immunosuppression. This in turn leads to opportunistic infections and peculiar neoplasms. HIV itself enters the nervous system early in the infection phase and can cause various neurologic manifestations. These are outlined in Table 32–3, and some are discussed in detail in the following sections.

HIV in the Nervous System

Acute infection with HIV can cause various neurologic syndromes. It is important to recognize these and test for HIV, because these illnesses are nonspecific and patients will often recover fully only to develop HIV-associated complications later on. These manifestations include meningitis, meningoencephalitis, myelopathy, and an acute demyelinating polyneuropathy similar to Guillain-Barré syndrome.

HIV-associated neurocognitive disorders are a group of disorders encompassing the spectrum from mild cognitive impairment to AIDS dementia complex. The incidence of AIDS dementia complex has been reduced dramatically with the use of combined antiretroviral regimens. However, mild cognitive impairments are very common even in patients who are virologically suppressed. In patients with high HIV viral load, manifestations include forgetfulness, apathy, and gait

TABLE 32–3 Neurologic complications of HIV-AIDS.

Brain
Encephalitis
HIV encephalitis
Cytomegalovirus encephalitis
Varicella zoster virus encephalitis
Herpes simplex virus encephalitis
Focal lesion
Cerebral toxoplasmosis
Brain lymphoma
Progressive multifocal leukoencephalopathy
Cryptococcoma
Bacterial brain abscess
Tuberculoma
Cerebrovascular disorders—nonbacterial endocarditis, cerebral hemorrhages associated with thrombocytopenia, and vasculitis
HIV dementia
Spinal cord
Vacuolar myelopathy
Herpes simplex or zoster myelitis
Meningitis
Acute and chronic lymphocytic meningitis
Cryptococcal and other fungal types
Tuberculous
Syphilitic
Herpes zoster
Peripheral nerve and root
Distal sensory polyneuropathy
Herpes zoster
Cytomegalovirus lumbar polyradiculopathy
Acute and chronic inflammatory polyneuritis
Mononeuritis multiplex
Sensorimotor demyelinating polyneuropathy
Diffuse infiltrative lymphocytic syndrome (DILS)
Leprosy
Muscle
Polymyositis and other myopathies (including drug induced)

Reproduced with permission from Ropper AH, Samuels MA, Klein JP: *Adams and Victor's Principles of Neurology*, 11th ed. New York, NY: McGraw Hill; 2019.

ataxia and can progress to mutism and paraplegia in the late stages. CSF studies can be normal or show elevated protein and low-grade lymphocytic pleocytosis. HIV can be detected in CSF when patients are not virologically suppressed. MRI shows symmetric T2 hyperintensity in the periventricular white matter, which is typically nonenhancing (Figure 32–9). Patients with HIV also have significant brain atrophy. Pathology shows diffuse atrophy and pallor in the white matter. Microscopically, there are perivascular lymphocytic infiltrates, microglial nodules, foamy macrophages, and multinucleated giant cells. Treatment includes antiretroviral agents with good CNS penetration.

HIV myelopathy can occur in isolation or in combination with AIDS dementia complex in the late stages of the disease.

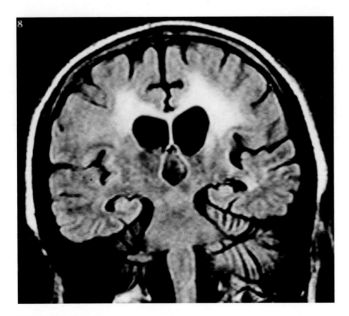

FIGURE 32–9 Magnetic resonance imaging of HIV leukoencephalopathy. There are large areas of white matter change that underlie 1 form of AIDS dementia; cortical atrophy and ventricular enlargement are evident. (Reproduced with permission from Ropper AH, Samuels MA, Klein JP: *Adams and Victor's Principles of Neurology*, 11th ed. New York, NY: McGraw Hill; 2019.)

It bears a striking clinical and pathologic resemblance to the subacute combined degeneration seen in vitamin B_{12} deficiency.

Peripheral neuropathy is common in HIV patients, including patients who are virologically suppressed in the blood. The virus has been isolated from the peripheral nerves. The most common type is the distal symmetric axonal sensory polyneuropathy, which predominantly involves the small fibers. Patients typically present with painful dysesthesias. Treatment remains symptomatic, in addition to antiretrovirals. Some older retroviral agents such as lamivudine and didanosine were associated with peripheral neuropathy, but these are rarely used now.

HIV myopathy can occur at any stage of HIV illness. A polymyositis-like presentation is noted that improves with corticosteroid therapy. Zidovudine, an older retroviral agent, has been associated with mitochondrial myopathy.

Opportunistic Infections & Neoplasms in HIV Affecting the Nervous System

CNS Toxoplasmosis Toxoplasmosis is one of the most common infectious complications of HIV and is caused by the parasite *T gondii*. Cats are a natural host for the parasite, and handling cat feces is a risk factor, but other sources may also be present. Initial infection is often asymptomatic. Most cases in adults are due to reactivation. The disease may present as a fulminating encephalitis or as focal abscesses. Patients often present with seizures, confusion, and coma. CT scan and MRI show multiple ring-enhancing lesions with surrounding edema and mass effect. The abscesses have a predilection for the basal ganglia. A rising antibody titer can aid in the diagnosis but may not always be present in immunocompromised patients. CSF shows elevated protein and lymphocytic pleocytosis. When patients with HIV

develop multiple nodular or ring-enhancing brain lesions, they are treated presumptively for toxoplasmosis. If there is no clinical response within 10 to 14 days, further evaluation for CNS lymphoma (including biopsy) should be undertaken. Treatment includes oral sulfadiazine and pyrimethamine.

Cryptococcal Disease Cryptococcal meningitis is a common fungal infection in HIV patients. Rarely, cryptococcomas also occur. In HIV patients, the signs and symptoms of meningitis may not be obvious and the disease may have an indolent course. There is a high risk of immune reconstitution inflammatory syndrome (IRIS), and hence, initiation of antiretroviral therapy is delayed in these patients.

Varicella-Zoster Infection Shingles is common in HIV patients, with a greater risk of recurrence compared to non-HIV patients. Multidermatomal involvement and disseminated VZV are seen with low CD4 T-cell counts (**Figure 32–10**). Severe complications of VZV, such as VZV vasculopathy and VZV myelopathy, occur more frequently in patients with AIDS.

Cytomegalovirus Encephalitis Cytomegalovirus (CMV) encephalitis is a common nonfocal neurologic infections in patients with AIDS. The virus reactivates typically in late stages of AIDS illness. CMV retinitis often accompanies the encephalitis. CMV can also cause a painful polyradiculitis. The virus has a predilection for the ventricle linings, causing a ventriculitis. MRI shows T2 hyperintensities and gadolinium enhancement along the ventricles. CSF shows elevated red blood cells, xanthochromia, and lymphocytic pleocytosis and elevated proteins. CSF CMV PCR is helpful for diagnosis because the viral cultures can be negative and take a long time to grow. Treatment includes ganciclovir and foscarnet. However, there is high morbidity and mortality in immunocompromised patients.

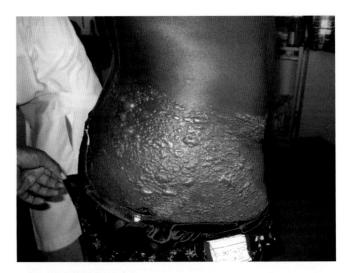

FIGURE 32–10 Varicella-zoster virus—multiple dermatomes. Severe painful shingles (vesicles and bullae) spanning multiple cutaneous dermatomes in this HIV patient. (Reproduced with permission from Knoop KJ, Stack LB, Storrow AB, et al: *The Atlas of Emergency Medicine*, 4th ed. New York, NY: McGraw Hill; 2016. Photo contributor: John O'Mara, MD.)

Progressive Multifocal Leukoencephalopathy Progressive multifocal leukoencephalopathy (PML) is an opportunistic infection caused by JC virus (JCV). Primary infection with JCV is asymptomatic. When the surveillance by the T cells in the brain is altered, as in HIV or with use of certain medications such as natalizumab (disease-modifying agent for multiple sclerosis) or in certain leukemias and lymphomas, JCV reactivates in the brain, leading to PML. It primarily infects the oligodendrocytes, resulting in demyelination. Clinical features include cerebellar ataxia, aphasia, tremors, hemiparesis, visual field deficits, and cognitive and personality changes. MRI shows T2 hyperintensity in the white matter, which can be multifocal (Figure 32–11). The lesions generally do not enhance. Basic CSF studies are normal. CSF JCV PCR helps in the diagnosis. Brain biopsy or autopsy will show the characteristic features of demyelination, bizarre reactive astrocytes, and enlarged oligodendrocytes with inclusion bodies (Figure 32–12). There is no specific treatment for PML. Reversal of immunosuppression when possible, such as treatment of HIV with antiretroviral agents or withdrawal of immunosuppressing agent, is the key. When the immune system reconstitutes rather rapidly (eg, increasing CD4 counts with use of antiretroviral agents in HIV or after withdrawal of natalizumab), PML-IRIS develops. There is clinical and radiologic worsening that can be fatal.

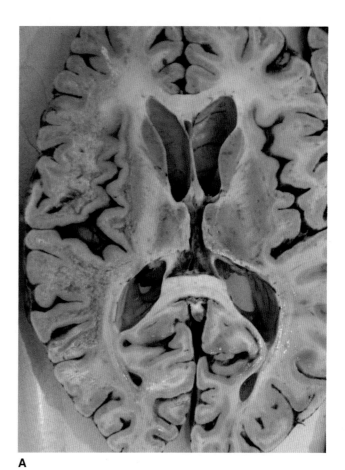

A

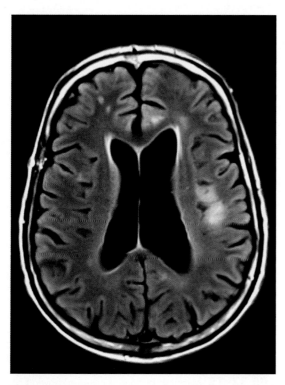

FIGURE 32–11 Progressive multifocal leukoencephalopathy (PML). T2-weighted fluid-attenuated inversion recovery magnetic resonance imaging demonstrates multiple subcortical white matter lesions in both hemispheres (*top panel*) and in the left pons (*bottom panel*) in a 31-year-old male with AIDS. The lesions did not enhance. (Reproduced with permission from Ropper AH, Samuels MA, Klein JP: *Adams and Victor's Principles of Neurology*, 11th ed. New York, NY: McGraw Hill; 2019.)

B

FIGURE 32–12 Progressive multifocal leukoencephalopathy. **A.** Gross pathology. Large areas of demyelination are seen in the subcortical white matter area. **B.** Histologic section shows infected enlarged oligodendrocytes within an area of demyelination. (Part B, reproduced with permission from Kleinschmidt-DeMasters BK, Rodriguez FJ, Tihan T: *Diagnostic Pathology: Neuropathology*, 2nd ed. Philadelphia, PA: Elsevier; 2016.)

Tuberculosis Tuberculosis is the most common complication of HIV in developing countries. CNS manifestations include tuberculous meningitis and tuberculomas. Some authors argue that the disease presents a more fulminant course in HIV patients. Multidrug-resistant tuberculosis is also noted in HIV patients.

Syphilis Neurosyphilis manifesting as meningitis and vasculopathy has a higher incidence in patients with HIV. An aggressive course of the disease with a higher incidence of strokes and dementia is described in AIDS patients. Longer courses of antibiotics are needed in these patients because there is a higher incidence of relapse and resistance to treatment. Serial measurements of antibody titers help guide the course of treatment.

Primary CNS Lymphoma Primary CNS lymphoma has a particularly high incidence in patients with AIDS or who are otherwise immunosuppressed. It can be solitary or multifocal and can occur in the cerebral hemispheres or the cerebellum and brainstem. These lymphomas arise from B lymphocytes or lymphoblasts. The Epstein-Barr virus genome has been detected in these tumors and is thought to be pathogenic. MRI features are indistinguishable from toxoplasmosis. Corticosteroids help initially, but relapse occurs soon after. Definitive treatment includes chemotherapy.

Prion Diseases

A prion is an abnormally folded protein that is infectious and pathologic due to its ability to propagate. It differs from a virus due to lack of nucleic acids. Prion diseases can be sporadic or sometimes inherited. Together known as transmissible spongiform encephalopathies (TSEs), this group includes Creutzfeldt-Jakob disease (CJD), Gerstmann-Sträussler-Scheinker syndrome, kuru, and fatal familial insomnia. CJD is the most common and important prior disease in humans. In addition to their infectious forms, prion diseases can occur sporadically (due to spontaneous misfolding of prion protein, PrP) or in familial forms (due to mutations in *PRNP*, the PrP gene).

Creutzfeldt-Jakob Disease

CJD is characterized by rapidly progressive dementia associated with myoclonic jerks. It is most often sporadic. Iatrogenic cases have been linked to use of human growth hormone from cadaveric sources and corneal and dural graft transplants from infected patients. Variant CJD occurs in younger individuals and is thought to be related to ingestion of cow meat infected with bovine spongiform encephalopathy (or mad cow disease), a form of TSE in cows. Clinical features include cognitive changes, confusion, hallucinations, visual disturbance, and ataxia. Over weeks to months, it progresses to dementia followed by worsening myoclonic jerks. Coma ensues and eventually leads to death. MRI of the brain shows hyperintensity on T2 images in the lenticular nuclei as well as on diffusion-weighted images in contiguous bands in the cortex and basal ganglia (**Figure 32–13**). Electroencephalography shows a characteristic pattern of periodic sharp wave complexes on a low-voltage, slow background. Routine CSF studies are normal. CSF 14-3-3

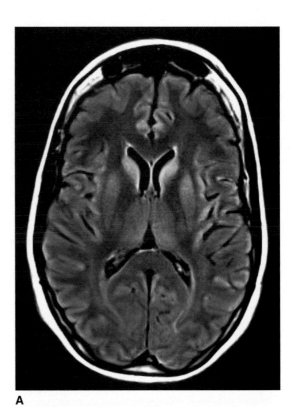

A

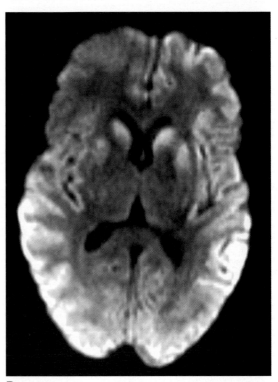

B

FIGURE 32–13 Magnetic resonance imaging showing T2 signal changes in the striatum in a patient with sporadic Creutzfeldt-Jakob disease (**A**) of 1 month in duration. Diffusion-weighted imaging sequence showing restriction of diffusion in contiguous bands of cortex and in the striatum (**B**) in the same patient. (Reproduced with permission from Ropper AH, Samuels MA, Klein JP: *Adams and Victor's Principles of Neurology*, 11th ed. New York, NY: McGraw Hill; 2019.)

protein may be elevated, but this test identifies fragments of normal brain protein, not the prion, and is not specific for CJD. CSF enolase and CSF tau are also elevated, suggesting neuronal injury. CSF real-time quaking-induced conversion test detects prion seeding and should be performed when CJD is suspected. The disease is fatal, and autopsy shows diffuse changes in the cortex with microscopic vacuoles in the cytoplasmic processes of glia cells and dendrites of nerve cells leading to a sponge-like appearance of the brain.

SELF-ASSESSMENT QUESTIONS

1. Tabes dorsalis is a late complication of which systemic infection?
   A. Syphilis
   B. Lyme disease
   C. Human immunodeficiency virus
   D. Varicella zoster virus

2. Which of the following arboviruses can cause meningoencephalitis?
   A. West Nile virus
   B. JC virus
   C. St. Louis encephalitis virus
   D. A and B
   E. A and C

3. What is the characteristic imaging finding in neurocysticercosis?
   A. Strokes in basal ganglia
   B. Multiple small calcified lesions
   C. Solitary mass-like lesions
   D. None of the above

4. What is the mode of transmission for Lyme disease?
   A. Mosquito bite
   B. Airborne transmission
   C. Tick bite
   D. Ingestion of infected meat

Neurotrauma

Angela Hays Shapshak

- Explain the distinction between primary and secondary brain injury.
- Define *intracranial pressure (ICP)* and *cerebral perfusion pressure (CPP)*, and understand the relationship between the 2 pressures.
- Discuss the Monro-Kellie doctrine and its implications for management of intracranial hypertension.
- Understand the diagnosis of *concussion*, or *postconcussive syndrome*, and discuss return-to-play criteria for injured athletes.
- Understand the clinical features of acute spinal cord injury (SCI), including *spinal shock* and *neurogenic shock*.

PREVALENCE & BURDEN

Traumatic brain injury (TBI) is a global health problem and one that has generated increasing public attention over the past several years. Overall, the most common cause of TBI in civilian populations is motor vehicle collision; falls constitute the second largest category, followed by self-inflicted injuries and assault. In the United States, approximately 1.4 million individuals sustain TBIs each year. Of those, approximately 235,000 require hospitalization, and 50,000 result in death. TBI can result in significant long-term motor, cognitive, and behavioral impairment; >3 million TBI survivors in the United States are living with chronic disabilities as a result of their injuries. Because traumatic injuries often affect patients who are young and otherwise healthy, it is a costly disease: The estimated annual costs of TBI, including lost productivity, exceed $76 billion.

Similarly, traumatic injury to the spinal cord can have devastating, life-long effects. Trauma is the leading cause of acute myelopathy in the United States, resulting in about 54 cases per 1 million people annually. The prevalence of spinal cord injury (SCI) in the United States is estimated at approximately 250,000 individuals. As with TBI, SCI often affects young adults: The average age of victims, according to the National Spinal Cord Injury Database, is 40.2 years. However, the rate of SCIs in the elderly has been increasing, largely related to falls. Unsurprisingly, the sequelae of SCI depend on the location and extent of the injury, with complete cervical cord lesions resulting in the most severe deficits. Unfortunately, this is not an uncommon

scenario. Nationally, 30.1% of SCI patients at discharge demonstrate incomplete quadriplegia; 25.6% have complete paraplegia; 20.4% have complete quadriplegia; and 18.5% have incomplete paraplegia. Less than 1% of SCI patients recover full neurologic function at the time of hospital discharge.

TRAUMATIC BRAIN INJURY

Classification

Traumatic brain injury is a broad term used to describe the diverse pathologic changes that may occur when the cranium is subjected to external forces. The specific injuries sustained by an individual can vary widely depending on the mechanism of the insult; for example, the magnitude, duration, and orientation of the force applied to the cranium have a significant impact on the nature of the resulting lesion(s). Due to the heterogeneous nature of TBI, a variety of classification schemes have arisen. TBI can be classified according to mechanism of injury, morphology of the injury, or clinical severity. With respect to mechanism of injury, TBI can be divided into penetrating versus blunt trauma or open versus closed lesions. In an open wound, components of the intracranial compartment are open to the environment, leading to a higher incidence of infection. Penetrating trauma produces exclusively open injuries, such as those resulting from knife or gunshot wounds; blunt trauma, on the other hand, can result in open or closed wounds.

VOCABULARY

Cerebral contusion: A focal brain injury characterized by extravasation of blood into the brain tissue from small perforating vessels.

Concussion: Alteration of consciousness following blunt-force trauma to the cranium.

Hematomyelia: Hemorrhage into the spinal cord parenchyma.

Herniation: The abnormal protrusion of brain tissue from 1 intracranial compartment into an adjacent anatomic space, a potentially lethal complication of cerebral edema or space-occupying intracranial lesions.

Hydrocephalus: An abnormal increase in the amount of cerebrospinal fluid, accompanied by enlargement of the ventricles (ventriculomegaly).

Intracranial pressure: The pressure within the skull.

Subluxation: A partial dislocation; within the spine, this term generally refers to displacement of one vertebral body relative to the adjacent vertebra.

Syringomyelia: The clinical syndrome resulting from formation of a fluid-filled cavitation, or syrinx, within the spine.

Ventriculostomy: The surgical placement of an opening into the cerebral ventricles for drainage of spinal fluid.

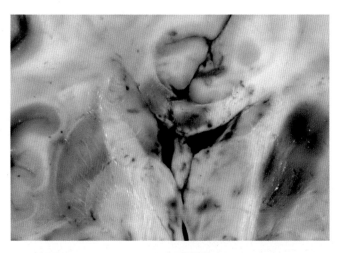

FIGURE 33–1 Gross image demonstrating deep cerebral microhemorrhages typical for patients with diffuse axonal injury. (Reproduced with permission from Reisner H. *Pathology a Modern Case Study*, 2nd ed. New York, NY: McGraw Hill; 2020.)

diffuse axonal injury (Figure 33–1). With increasing magnitude of inertial forces, progressively deeper brain structures show signs of injury. In clinical practice, most severe brain injuries are caused by the impact of the head against a solid object at high velocity, which can often result in a combination of focal and diffuse pathology.

Injuries to intracranial vascular structures can carry considerable morbidity and mortality and must be recognized promptly. *Subdural hematomas* (Figure 33–2), which result

With respect to lesion morphology, TBI can be classified as intracranial or extracranial. Extracranial brain injuries generally include factures of the skull base or cranial vault. Fractures of the cranial vault may further be classified as open or closed and depressed or nondepressed; depressed skull fractures are more likely to be associated with injuries of underlying brain parenchyma or vascular structures. Intracranial injuries may include lesions of the brain parenchyma as well as injuries to intracranial blood vessels. Injuries of the brain parenchyma may be focal or diffuse. Focal injuries often result from linear acceleration or deceleration of the skull and its contents. For example, a direct localized blow to the cranium may result in a depressed skull fracture with a focal contusion or hematoma in the underlying brain tissue. *Contusions* are "bruises" of the brain tissue, characterized by extravasation of blood from small perforating vessels, whereas hematomas are larger hemorrhages within the brain parenchyma. When this sort of injury occurs at the site of impact, it is often referred to as a *coup injury*. *Contrecoup injuries* occur opposite the site of initial impact and are thought to result from rapid deceleration, which produces differential movement of the brain within the skull. As a result, this causes neuronal structures to collide against the interior of the skull, resulting in focal injuries remote from the site of impact. In contrast, rotational or angular acceleration often results in diffuse brain injuries. This causes shearing of different brain layers in relation to each other, resulting in disruption of axons known as

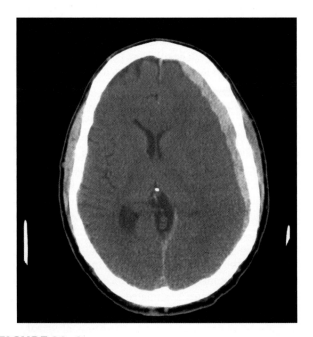

FIGURE 33–2 Head computed tomography demonstrating a left frontotemporoparietal acute subdural hematoma with mass effect and mild midline shift. Subdural hematomas do not respect suture lines and are typically crescent shaped. (Reproduced with permission from Hall JB, Schmidt GA, Kress JP: *Principles of Critical Care*, 4th ed. New York, NY: McGraw Hill; 2015.)

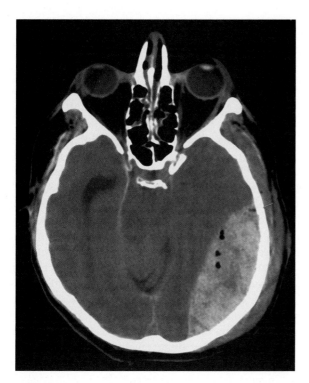

FIGURE 33–3 Epidural hematoma. A lens-shaped epidural hematoma is seen on the left. The quadrigeminal cistern should be seen on this slice and is completely effaced, suggesting herniation. (Reproduced with permission from Knoop KJ, Stack LB, Storrow AB, et al: The *Atlas of Emergency Medicine*, 4th ed. New York, NY: McGraw Hill; 2016. Photo contributor: Lawrence B. Stack, MD.)

TABLE 33–1 Glasgow Coma Scale.

Eye opening	Spontaneous	4
	To verbal command	3
	To pain	2
	None	1
Verbal responsiveness	Oriented	5
	Confused	4
	Inappropriate words	3
	Incomprehensible sounds	2
	None	1
Motor response	Obeys	6
	Localizes	5
	Withdraws (pain)	4
	Flexion (pain)	3
	Extension (pain)	2
	None	1

Adapted with permission from Teasdale G, Jennett B: Assessment of coma and impaired consciousness. A practical scale, *Lancet*. 1974 Jul 13;2(7872):81-84.

from blood collecting in the subdural space, are the most common focal traumatic intracranial lesion. They may arise from bleeding related to torn bridging veins between the cerebral cortex and the venous sinuses or from lacerations of cortical blood vessels. On neuroimaging, subdural hematomas appear as a convex lesion overlying the surface of the brain. They may be associated with underlying cerebral contusions or lacerations. *Epidural hematomas* (Figure 33–3) result from accumulation of blood between the skull and the dura, usually secondary to laceration of the middle meningeal artery. This type of hemorrhage results in a lens-shaped or convex lesion on brain imaging sometimes associated with an overlying skull fracture. *Subarachnoid hemorrhages* are also commonly seen in TBI, either in isolation or in conjunction with cerebral contusions or hematomas. Unlike aneurysmal subarachnoid hemorrhages, which are discussed in Chapter 24, traumatic subarachnoid hemorrhages tend to localize to the cerebral convexities.

In practice, the most common way to classify TBI is based on clinical severity. There are several classification schemes in use, but the most widely used system is the Glasgow Coma Scale (Table 33–1). The Glasgow Coma Scale (GCS) is the sum of 3 scores that are obtained by examining the patient's response to verbal or tactile stimulation. The assessment should be performed after the patient has been adequately resuscitated because hypotension or hypoxia can confound the neurologic evaluation. The examiner evaluates the patient's eye opening, verbal response, and motor response, as described in Table 33–1. The maximum (best) score is 15; the minimum possible score is 3. In the event that the patient is intubated at the time of evaluation, he or she is given a 1 for the verbal item and the score is appended with the modifier "T" to denote intubation. Generally speaking, a GCS score ≤8 is considered consistent with coma. The initial, postresuscitation GCS score has been shown to correlate with neurologic outcome; in particular, the motor response is an important prognostic indicator. Using the GCS, brain injury can be classified as mild (GCS score of 13 to 15), moderate (GCS score of 9 to 12), or severe (GCS score of 3 to 8).

Pathophysiology

To discuss the pathophysiology and clinical management of patients with TBI, it is necessary to distinguish between *primary* and *secondary* brain injury. A *primary* injury is pathologic damage that occurs at the time of impact; this may include cerebral contusions, lacerations, and/or diffuse axonal injury that results from the initial insult. *Secondary* brain injury refers to the downstream processes that occur in the CNS in response to the primary injury. Mechanisms of secondary brain injury include oxidative stress; loss of autoregulation in the cerebral vasculature; induction of apoptosis, leading to neuronal cell loss; and release of cytotoxic amino acids. A complete discussion of the various pathways contributing to secondary brain injury is beyond the scope of this chapter, but it is important to understand 2 critical topics: *cerebral edema* and *intracranial pressure* (ICP).

The end result of many of the pathways involved in secondary brain injury is an increase in brain water content, resulting in cerebral edema. There are 2 main mechanisms underlying the development of cerebral edema in the injured brain. *Cytotoxic edema* is cell swelling related to intracellular processes such as oxidative injury and ischemia. *Vasogenic edema* is predominantly extracellular and is related to endothelial damage within the blood vessel walls. Cerebral edema can contribute to secondary brain injury by causing increases in ICP. Because the brain is located within the rigid confines of the skull, the volume of the intracranial contents must remain constant. This concept is known as the Monro-Kellie doctrine, and can be expressed mathematically as:

$$V_{intracranial} = V_{brain} + V_{CSF} + V_{blood} + V_{mass\ lesion}$$

Under normal circumstances, the intracranial contents include brain tissue, cerebrospinal fluid (CSF), and blood (arterial and venous). In the event that a mass lesion is added to the intracranial compartment, the volume of brain, blood, or spinal fluid must decrease; if this does not occur, the ICP will increase. In a trauma patient, an epidural hematoma, subdural hematoma, intraparenchymal hematoma, or cerebral contusion can act as an intracranial mass lesion; a focal area of cerebral edema can function similarly. In this setting, CSF and eventually venous blood are displaced from the intracranial compartment to compensate, while maintaining relatively normal ICPs. However, if the mass lesion continues to grow, these compensatory mechanisms will be overwhelmed, and the ICP will begin to rise exponentially (Figure 33–4).

Elevated ICP can exacerbate secondary brain injury by worsening cerebral ischemia. The cerebral vasculature is governed by powerful autoregulatory mechanisms that ensure that the cerebral blood flow, or CBF, remains relatively constant during a broad range of physiologic circumstances. The *cerebral perfusion pressure* (CPP) is the pressure gradient driving blood flow to the brain tissue. It is determined by the difference between the *mean arterial pressure* (MAP) and the ICP:

$$CPP = MAP^* - ICP$$
$$^*MAP = [systolic\ blood\ pressure$$
$$+ (2 \times diastolic\ blood\ pressure)] \div 3$$

Under normal circumstances, cerebral autoregulatory mechanisms ensure that cerebral blood flow is preserved as long as the CPP is between 50 and 150 mm Hg. Outside of that range, the relationship between cerebral blood flow and CPP becomes linear (Figure 33–5). As a consequence, patients with significant intracranial hypertension (high ICPs) or systemic hypotension (inadequate MAPs) are at risk of global cerebral ischemia. This concept has profound implications for the clinical management of patients with severe brain injuries. The main goal of prehospital and emergency department resuscitation efforts is to maintain adequate systemic blood pressures, in an effort to avoid compromised cerebral perfusion. In the setting of a confirmed TBI, efforts to minimize secondary brain injury often revolve around management of ICP and optimization of CPP; these strategies will be discussed in more detail later in this chapter.

Mass lesions can also contribute to neurologic injury by causing compression of adjacent structures. The intracranial compartment is divided into several smaller compartments by the rigid fibrous structures, the falx cerebri and the tentorium cerebelli. The accumulation of a hematoma or significant cerebral edema in 1 of these intracranial compartments can cause the formation of a pressure gradient, which can cause *herniation* of cerebral or cerebellar structures into adjacent compartments (Figure 33–6). These tissue shifts can compress arteries against falx, resulting in cerebral infarctions. More critically, the herniated tissue can compress vital structures in the brainstem, which can result in cardiovascular and

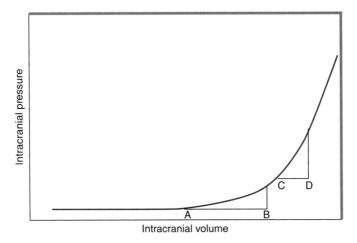

FIGURE 33–4 Intracranial compliance curve. The Monro-Kellie doctrine states that the skull is rigid and brain, cerebrospinal fluid (CSF), and blood are incompressible structures; therefore, an increase in any intracranial component must be accompanied by displacement of brain, CSF, or blood, or an increase in intracranial pressure (ICP). Once the ICP increases and compliance is reduced, smaller changes in volume can cause relatively larger changes in ICP (A-B vs C-D). Likewise, only small amounts of CSF drainage can lead to large decreases in ICP. (Reproduced with permission from Hall JB, Schmidt GA, Kress JP: *Principles of Critical Care*, 4th ed. New York, NY: McGraw Hill; 2015.)

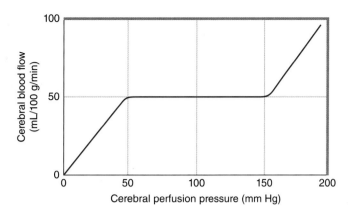

FIGURE 33–5 Cerebral autoregulation. Cerebral blood flow is tightly linked to the cerebral metabolic rate in normal brain tissue over a wide range of mean arterial pressure and cerebral perfusion pressure. (Reproduced with permission from Hall JB, Schmidt GA, Kress JP: *Principles of Critical Care*, 4th ed. New York, NY: McGraw Hill; 2015.)

respiratory compromise and eventually death. There are several recognized *herniation syndromes*, which will be discussed in the next section.

Clinical Presentation

The clinical presentation of the patient with TBI is as variable as the pathologic manifestations discussed earlier. As with all neurologic disorders, the presenting symptoms are determined by the location of the injury. Certain cerebral structures, most notably the anterior temporal lobes, the inferior frontal lobes, and the olfactory nerves, are particularly vulnerable to damage due to collision with the skull base. Consequently, patients with mild to moderate closed head injury often present with confusion and/or amnesia for the event. Anosmia is also common. The term *concussion* is often used to refer to

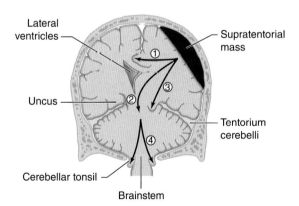

FIGURE 33–6 Anatomic basis of herniation syndromes. An expanding supratentorial mass lesion may cause brain tissue to be displaced into an adjacent intracranial compartment, resulting in (1) cingulate herniation under the falx, (2) downward transtentorial (central) herniation, (3) uncal herniation over the edge of the tentorium, or (4) cerebellar tonsillar herniation into the foramen magnum. Coma and ultimately death result when (2), (3), or (4) produces brainstem compression. (Reproduced with permission from Simon RP, Aminoff MJ, Greemberg DA: *Clinical Neurology*, 10th ed. New York, NY: McGraw Hill; 2018.)

temporary alteration of consciousness related to a closed head injury in the presence of a normal head computed tomography (CT) scan. Patients with concussion may experience loss of consciousness or confusion, headache, and memory loss. The duration of posttraumatic amnesia is generally related to the severity of the injury. Most patients will eventually recover completely; however, in severe cases, patients may go on to develop *postconcussive syndrome*. Postconcussive syndrome is characterized by headaches, depression, fatigue, and emotional lability; treatment is predominantly supportive. In recent years, investigators have called attention to the problem of concussion in athletes, where head injuries are common and often underrecognized. This is problematic because the injured brain remains highly sensitive to subsequent injury in the days to weeks following a concussion. If an athlete sustains a second closed head injury too soon following a concussion, *second impact syndrome* can develop. Although rare, this is characterized by severe and sometimes catastrophic cerebral edema, which has resulted in death in some young athletes. As a result, the Centers for Disease Control and Prevention recommends at least 24 hours of physical and cognitive rest following any closed head injury. Patients may begin to resume usual activities in a stepwise fashion once they are completely symptom free.

Patients with mild closed head injury who did not lose consciousness and have returned to baseline (ie, GCS score of 15) may not require inpatient observation; however, they should be supervised by a responsible caregiver for at least 24 hours after the injury. This is because patients with expanding mass lesions, classically epidural hematomas, sometimes present with a *lucid interval*. The patient initially appears to recover from the injury within minutes to hours, but later begins to develop an altered level of consciousness as the mass lesion expands. This should prompt return to the emergency department for urgent neuroimaging, as it may signal a neurosurgical emergency.

Generally, patients with altered cognition, penetrating brain injury, focal findings on neurologic examination, or clinical suspicion for increased ICP require neuroimaging, typically with CT, to evaluate for focal brain pathology. Clinical signs of increased ICP may include nausea and vomiting, depressed level of consciousness, and/or cranial nerve abnormalities. Patients with diffuse cerebral edema are prone to developing lateral rectus palsies, due to stretching of the abducens nerve along the base of the skull. Pupillary dilation can be a sign of *uncal herniation*, caused when a supratentorial mass lesion causes the uncus of the temporal lobe to herniate transtentorially. This compresses the oculomotor nerve against the tentorium, resulting in loss of parasympathetic input to the ipsilateral pupil. The pupil becomes dilated as a result of unopposed sympathetic innervation. With progressive uncal herniation, the motor fibers of cranial nerve III become involved, leading to inferolateral eye deviation. The posterior cerebral artery, which runs adjacent to cranial nerve III, may also be compressed. Eventually, compression of the ipsilateral cerebral peduncle can produce contralateral hemiparesis. *Subfalcine herniation* occurs when a mass lesion in 1 cerebral hemisphere produces herniation of the cingulate gyrus beneath the falx. In the process, the anterior communicating artery can be compressed against the edge of the falx, which can result in infarction. *Central herniation* occurs when a large supratentorial mass forces the thalamus and midbrain downward, through the tentorial notch. This results in compression of the brainstem, producing a depressed level of consciousness. Pupils will generally be midrange or small, due to loss of sympathetic innervation from the midbrain. Cheyne-Stokes respirations, characterized by periods of rapid, deep breaths punctuated by brief apneic spells, may be seen. In *tonsillar herniation*, the cerebellar tonsils herniate through the foramen magnum, resulting in compression of the cervicomedullary junction. This can produce coma, hypertension, Cheyne-Stokes respirations, central hypoventilation, and cardiac effects. Uncal herniation, central herniation, and tonsillar herniation can all lead to brain death due to brainstem compression if not recognized and treated promptly.

Clinical Management

In patients with severe TBI, especially if there is clinical concern for elevated ICP, acute management is focused on minimizing the potential for secondary brain injury. In the initial stages, these efforts center on stabilizing the patient's vital signs in order to prevent cerebral hypoxia and/or cerebral ischemia. The brain is highly metabolically active; despite constituting <2% of total body weight, it is accounts for 20% of total body oxygen consumption. Therefore, it is extremely susceptible to injury from lack of oxygen. A hypoxic insult can result from reduced cerebral blood flow or from impaired oxygen-carrying capacity in the setting of preserved cerebral blood flow. Cerebral blood flow is reduced in the setting of systemic hypotension or when CPP is compromised as a result of intracranial hypertension, as discussed earlier. Similarly, systemic hypoxemia can result in cerebral hypoxia and has been correlated with adverse outcomes in TBI survivors. Severe anemia is also

a contributing factor due to reduced oxygen-carrying capacity. Because many patients with TBI have other associated injuries to the thorax, abdomen, or limbs, they are at risk of hypoxemia and hemorrhagic shock. Prehospital guidelines from the Brain Trauma Foundation emphasize the need to monitor blood

---

CASE 33–1

A 35-year-old woman was involved in a motor vehicle collision in which she was a passenger on a motorcycle that was struck by an oncoming car. She was not wearing a helmet. She was thrown a considerable distance from the motorcycle and sustained a severe closed head injury, with an initial Glasgow Coma Scale score of 6 upon evaluation by emergency personnel. She was intubated in the field due to impaired airway protection, immobilized using a cervical collar and a spine board, and transported to the nearest Level I trauma center. In the emergency department, she was resuscitated and stabilized. Computed tomography (CT) scans revealed no evidence of spinal injury; however, the CT of the head was suggestive of diffuse axonal injury. Due to her poor exam and the abnormal imaging findings, an external ventricular drain was placed for monitoring of intracranial pressure (ICP). She was admitted to the neurosciences intensive care unit for further management. There, she remained comatose and critically ill due to respiratory failure and worsening cerebral edema. Within 48 hours of admission, she began to develop elevated ICPs. Initially, these could be managed with optimization of sedation and analgesia, along with positioning to maintain venous outflow from the cranial vault; however, by hospital day 3, she was requiring frequent doses of mannitol as well as an infusion of hypertonic saline to maintain an ICP <25 mm Hg. Some additional improvement was seen with drainage of cerebrospinal fluid, but eventually, the decision was made to induce pharmacologic coma with an infusion of pentobarbital. Continuous electroencephalography was used to monitor her response to therapy and optimize the dose of the drug. Vasopressors were initiated in an effort to ensure that adequate cerebral perfusion pressure was maintained. Within several days, the barbiturates were able to be weaned, and ICPs remained well controlled. She required a tracheostomy and percutaneous gastrostomy tube due to prolonged dependence on mechanical ventilation, but with time, her exam began to improve. By hospital day 16, she had begun to show evidence of intermittently following commands, and by hospital day 21, she was successfully weaned from the ventilator. She was subsequently discharged to a subacute rehabilitation center. Six months after the injury, she was ambulatory and had regained language function. Family members reported frequent headaches, depression, and impulsivity but noted that she was independent for activities of daily living and was investigating the possibility of returning to work as a waitress part time.

pressure and oxygen saturation frequently and to provide supportive care as required to maintain oxygen saturation >90% and systolic blood pressure >90 mm Hg.

ICP monitoring should be considered in patients in whom there is a high clinical suspicion for intracranial hypertension. This includes patients who remain comatose following adequate resuscitation and have abnormalities visible on CT scan. A variety of ICP monitors are available, as shown in Figure 33–7. An intraventricular catheter, also known as a *ventriculostomy* or *external ventricular drain*, has the advantage of allowing drainage of CSF in addition to monitoring of ICP. CSF drainage can be useful for treating raised ICP, as well as managing *hydrocephalus*. Hydrocephalus is an abnormal accumulation of spinal fluid, which can result from impaired CSF circulation or reabsorption. It can produce ventriculomegaly and contribute to intracranial hypertension, although it can occur in the absence of elevated ICP. In trauma patients, hydrocephalus can be associated with hemorrhage into the ventricles or subarachnoid space, which can disrupt CSF absorption. It can also arise due to brainstem compression, resulting in occlusion of the cerebral aqueduct or the fourth ventricle.

Managing intracranial hypertension requires reducing the volume of the contents in the intracranial space. If there is a pathologic mass lesion, such as an epidural or subdural hematoma, this can be accomplished by surgical evacuation. In the absence of a pathologic mass lesion, management strategies focus on reducing the volume of blood, brain, or CSF, as inferred from the Monro-Kellie doctrine. CSF can be drained using a ventriculostomy, if available. Reducing the volume of

venous blood in the intracranial compartment can be accomplished by taking steps to promote venous outflow, such as elevating the head of the bed, removing or loosening devices that may compress the jugular veins, and optimizing analgesia and sedation in order to prevent elevations of intrathoracic or intra-abdominal pressure.

Reducing the volume occupied by the brain itself is accomplished by taking steps to minimize cerebral edema by using a strategy known as *osmotherapy*. Osmotherapy relies on the presence of the blood–brain barrier, which acts as a semipermeable membrane. By increasing the osmolarity of the plasma, the clinician can create an osmotic gradient across the blood–brain barrier, which will act to draw water out of the brain tissue. This can be accomplished using an intravenous infusion of a substance to which the blood–brain barrier is impermeable; the 2 most commonly used substances are mannitol and hypertonic sodium chloride. Mannitol is a metabolically inert sugar that acts as an osmotic diuretic and is excreted by the kidneys. It is usually given as an intravenous bolus, either in response to clinical signs or symptoms of herniation or to treat elevated ICP. Hypertonic saline can be used as a continuous infusion or as a bolus in the setting of acute intracranial hypertension. Concentrations of >3% sodium chloride must be given through a central line.

In the event that other measures have failed, clinicians may attempt to lower the volume of the arterial blood in the intracranial compartment. This is done by making use of metabolic autoregulation of the cerebral vasculature. As discussed in Chapter 24, the cerebral vasculature is sensitive to

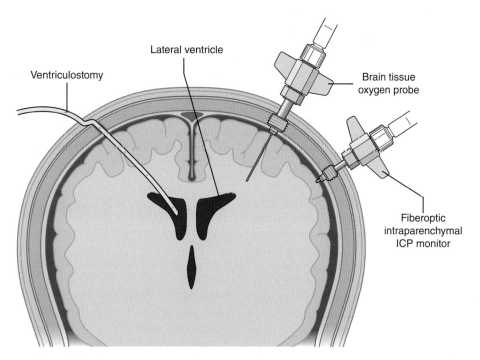

FIGURE 33–7 Intracranial pressure (ICP) and brain tissue oxygen monitoring. A ventriculostomy allows for drainage of cerebrospinal fluid to treat elevated ICP. Fiberoptic ICP and brain tissue oxygen monitors are usually secured using a screwlike skull bolt. (Reproduced with permission from Jameson J, Fauci AS, Kasper DL, et al: *Harrison's Principles of Internal Medicine*, 20th ed. New York, NY: McGraw Hill; 2018.)

a variety of metabolic factors including pH, potassium, carbon dioxide, and nitric oxide. The cerebral arterioles dilate in response to CSF acidosis, indicating oxygen-starved brain tissue, and in the setting of increased metabolic demand. Physicians can therefore induce cerebral vasoconstriction by suppressing brain metabolism or by inducing CSF alkalosis. Suppressing brain metabolism generally requires induction of a *pharmacologic coma*: The physician uses a continuous infusion of a powerful sedative, generally a barbiturate, to suppress cerebral activity. Pentobarbital is the most commonly used agent in the United States. Barbiturates can be very effective in managing intracranial hypertension, and in experimental settings, there are indications that they reduce cerebral edema formation and minimize free radical–mediated lipid peroxidation. However, they have a number of systemic side effects, including systemic hypotension, bone marrow suppression, and disruption of gastrointestinal motility. As a consequence, this strategy must be used cautiously. Continuous electroencephalography is necessary to appropriately guide therapy in order to ensure that adequate suppression of cerebral metabolism is achieved using the minimum effective dose of barbiturates to minimize adverse effects.

Systemic hyperventilation is another method by which cerebral arterial blood volume can be reduced. Hyperventilation produces a systemic respiratory alkalosis, which in turn reduces the pH of the CSF. CSF alkalosis results in cerebral vasoconstriction, thereby lowering cerebral blood volume and temporarily lowering ICP. However, reducing cerebral blood flow for an extended period of time without suppressing cerebral metabolism can precipitate cerebral ischemia. Furthermore, the benefits of hyperventilation are short lived: The choroid plexus acts to correct the pH of the CSF fairly rapidly, which reverses the vasoconstriction. As a consequence, prophylactic or prolonged hyperventilation is not recommended, although it can be used as a short-term temporizing measure while more definitive interventions are being initiated.

Finally, clinicians must be aware of other complications of TBI that can exacerbate secondary brain injuries. Seizures, in particular, are common; as many as 16% of patients with TBI may experience early seizures, defined as those occurring within the first week. Seizures are important to recognize because they can contribute to neuronal injury, exacerbate intracranial hypertension, and contribute to systemic complications. Current guidelines recommend prophylactic antiepileptic treatment for 7 days in patients who are admitted with severe TBI; long-term therapy is not required unless seizures occur outside of the acute phase. In addition, TBI patients are susceptible to systemic complications of immobility, including thromboembolic events and infection. Fever is 1 factor that can exacerbate secondary brain injury; hyperpyrexia has been shown to correlate with poor outcomes in TBI survivors. TBI patients who require hospital admission are best managed in experienced centers where advanced monitoring techniques can be used to optimize brain recovery.

Long-Term Sequelae

Much of the literature on management of TBI focuses on the acute phase; however, in recent years, there has been an increased recognition of long-term sequelae seen in TBI survivors. Posttraumatic epilepsy (PTE) is 1 well-recognized complication. Unlike seizures in the acute phase of illness, PTE may present months or years after the initial brain injury. Estimates of incidence vary considerably depending on the population being studied, but subsequent development of PTE is more likely in patients with penetrating injuries and in survivors of severe closed head injuries. Although many of these patients will experience good seizure control with antiepileptic therapy, a significant minority may develop treatment-resistant epilepsy, which can have a significant adverse impact on quality of life.

Cognitive and behavioral disorders are also commonly reported in TBI survivors. Again, patients with a history of penetrating trauma and those who survive a severe closed head injury are at highest risk; however, moderate TBI poses some risk as well. Language difficulties, memory impairment, and mood disturbances are among the most common complaints. Although there is little evidence that a single episode of mild TBI can produce durable cognitive deficits, there is evidence that mild and moderate brain injuries are associated with an increased risk of dementia. The incidence of dementia of Alzheimer type is increased in patients with a history of head trauma, with survivors of moderate TBI carrying more than twice the risk of the general population. The impact of recurrent head injuries can be even more profound. Chronic recurrent head injuries result in a unique degenerative neurologic condition, first recognized in boxers; it was initially termed *dementia pugilistica*, but the term *chronic traumatic encephalopathy* (CTE) is now preferred. CTE is characterized by memory deficits, impaired executive function, and poor attention; impulsivity, paranoia, and anxiety may also be reported. Pathologic examination reveals phosphorylated tau inclusions within neurons and astrocytes around small vessels within the depths of the cortical sulci. This pattern is increasingly recognized among combat veterans and athletes involved in contact sports and is gaining recognition as a public health concern.

TRAUMATIC SPINE INJURY

Classification

Like TBI, SCI can be classified according to anatomic features, mechanism of injury, and clinical severity (Figure 33–8). Isolated injuries to the spinal cord itself are uncommon; typically, there is associated damage to the vertebral column and ligamentous structures as well. Bony injuries may include fractures and/or dislocations. Blunt-force injury to the spinal column that is sufficient to disrupt bone and ligament can result in *subluxation* (Figure 33–9), or displacement of the vertebral body relative to the adjacent levels. This in turn may produce narrowing of the spinal canal, which can compress the spinal cord itself. Compression of the cord can also result from retropulsion of bone fragments into the canal following a fracture; this is commonly seen in *burst fractures* (Figure 33–10), which may occur following a direct axial load on the vertebral column. Most closed spinal injuries involve some combination of vertical compression associated with flexion or hyperextension, which often occurs in motor vehicle collisions, falls, and diving accidents. Flexion injuries cause an axial load on the vertebral bodies and distract the posterior cord and interspinous ligaments. This can cause displacement of the facet joints, producing so-called "jumped" facets. Hyperextension has the opposite effect, compressing elements of the posterior vertebral column and causing distraction anteriorly. Hyperextension in particular can result in cord injury without damage to the bony structures; this results when the ligamentum flavum and other ligamentous elements

are disrupted, allowing transient vertebral dislocation. Compression or shearing of the spinal column results in hemorrhage within the cord parenchyma, known as *hematomyelia*. Cord edema, with or without hematomyelia, is also common. Penetrating injuries, such as those resulting from a bullet or knife wound, may result in spinal cord lacerations or complete transection of the cord. Specific clinical syndromes will be discussed in subsequent sections.

1122In terms of clinical severity, injuries to the spinal cord can be classified as complete injuries, in which no spinal cord function is detectable below the level of the lesion, and incomplete injuries, in which there is some degree of preserved function below the lesion. The American Spinal Injury Association (ASIA) has established standards for classification of spinal injuries according to a 5-point scale (see Figure 33–8). The ASIA A classification represents complete spinal cord injuries. ASIA B includes patients in whom sensory function is

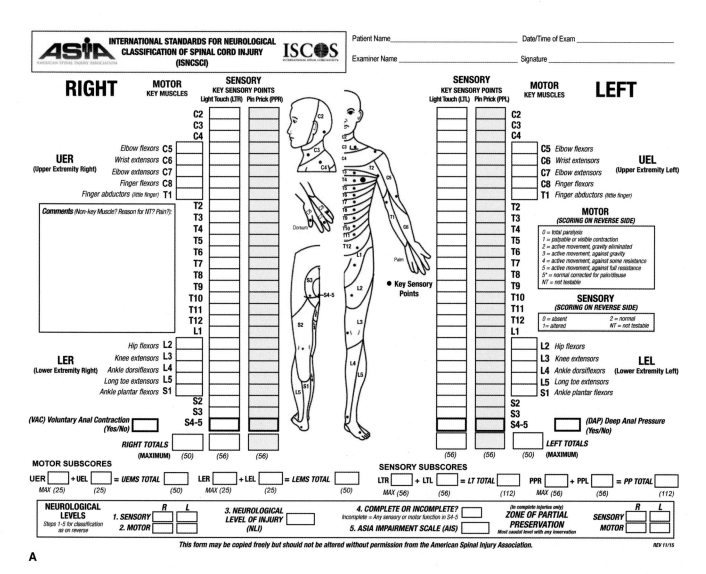

FIGURE 33–8 International Standards for Neurological Classification of Spinal Cord Injury (ISNCSCI) Worksheet. (Reproduced with permission from Kirshblum SC, Burns SP, Biering-Sorensen F, et al: International standards for neurological classification of spinal cord injury (revised 2011), *J Spinal Cord Med*. 2011 Nov;34(6):535-546.)

Muscle Function Grading

0 = total paralysis

1 = palpable or visible contraction

2 = active movement, full range of motion (ROM) with gravity eliminated

3 = active movement, full ROM against gravity

4 = active movement, full ROM against gravity and moderate resistance in a muscle specific position

5 = (normal) active movement, full ROM against gravity and full resistance in a functional muscle position expected from an otherwise unimpaired person

5* = (normal) active movement, full ROM against gravity and sufficient resistance to be considered normal if identified inhibiting factors (i.e. pain, disuse) were not present

NT = not testable (i.e. due to immobilization, severe pain such that the patient cannot be graded, amputation of limb, or contracture of > 50% of the normal ROM)

Sensory Grading

0 = Absent

1 = Altered, either decreased/impaired sensation or hypersensitivity

2 = Normal

NT = Not testable

When to Test Non-Key Muscles:

In a patient with an apparent AIS B classification, non-key muscle functions more than 3 levels below the motor level on each side should be tested to most accurately classify the injury (differentiate between AIS B and C).

Movement	Root level
Shoulder: Flexion, extension, abduction, adduction, internal and external rotation **Elbow:** Supination	C5
Elbow: Pronation **Wrist:** Flexion	C6
Finger: Flexion at proximal joint, extension. **Thumb:** Flexion, extension and abduction in plane of thumb	C7
Finger: Flexion at MCP joint **Thumb:** Opposition, adduction and abduction perpendicular to palm	C8
Finger: Abduction of the index finger	T1
Hip: Adduction	L2
Hip: External rotation	L3
Hip: Extension, abduction, internal rotation **Knee:** Flexion **Ankle:** Inversion and eversion **Toe:** MP and IP extension	L4
Hallux and Toe: DIP and PIP flexion and abduction	L5
Hallux: Adduction	S1

ASIA Impairment Scale (AIS)

A = Complete. No sensory or motor function is preserved in the sacral segments S4-5.

B = Sensory Incomplete. Sensory but not motor function is preserved below the neurological level and includes the sacral segments S4-5 (light touch or pin prick at S4-5 or deep anal pressure) AND no motor function is preserved more than three levels below the motor level on either side of the body.

C = Motor Incomplete. Motor function is preserved at the most caudal sacral segments for voluntary anal contraction (VAC) OR the patient meets the criteria for sensory incomplete status (sensory function preserved at the most caudal sacral segments (S4-S5) by LT, PP or DAP), and has some sparing of motor function more than three levels below the ipsilateral motor level on either side of the body.
(This includes key or non-key muscle functions to determine motor incomplete status.) For AIS C – less than half of key muscle functions below the single NLI have a muscle grade ≥ 3.

D = Motor Incomplete. Motor incomplete status as defined above, with at least half (half or more) of key muscle functions below the single NLI having a muscle grade ≥ 3.

E = Normal. If sensation and motor function as tested with the ISNCSCI are graded as normal in all segments, and the patient had prior deficits, then the AIS grade is E. Someone without an initial SCI does not receive an AIS grade.

Using ND: To document the sensory, motor and NLI levels, the ASIA Impairment Scale grade, and/or the zone of partial preservation (ZPP) when they are unable to be determined based on the examination results.

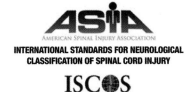
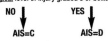

INTERNATIONAL STANDARDS FOR NEUROLOGICAL CLASSIFICATION OF SPINAL CORD INJURY

Steps in Classification

The following order is recommended for determining the classification of individuals with SCI.

1. Determine sensory levels for right and left sides.
The sensory level is the most caudal, intact dermatome for both pin prick and light touch sensation.

2. Determine motor levels for right and left sides.
Defined by the lowest key muscle function that has a grade of at least 3 (on supine testing), providing the key muscle functions represented by segments above that level are judged to be intact (graded as a 5).
Note: in regions where there is no myotome to test, the motor level is presumed to be the same as the sensory level, if testable motor function above that level is also normal.

3. Determine the neurological level of injury (NLI)
This refers to the most caudal segment of the cord with intact sensation and antigravity (3 or more) muscle function strength, provided that there is normal (intact) sensory and motor function rostrally respectively.
The NLI is the most cephalad of the sensory and motor levels determined in steps 1 and 2.

4. Determine whether the injury is Complete or Incomplete.
(i.e. absence or presence of sacral sparing)
*If voluntary anal contraction = **No** AND all S4-5 sensory scores = **0** AND deep anal pressure = **No**, then injury is **Complete**.*
*Otherwise, injury is **Incomplete**.*

5. Determine ASIA Impairment Scale (AIS) Grade:

Is injury **Complete**?   If YES, AIS=A and can record ZPP (lowest dermatome or myotome on each side with some preservation)

NO ↓

Is injury Motor **Complete**?   If YES, AIS=B

NO ↓   (No=voluntary anal contraction OR motor function more than three levels below the motor level on a given side, if the patient has sensory incomplete classification)

Are <u>at least</u> half (half or more) of the key muscles below the <u>neurological</u> level of injury graded 3 or better?

NO ↓   **YES** ↓
AIS=C   AIS=D

If sensation and motor function is normal in all segments, AIS=E

Note: AIS E is used in follow-up testing when an individual with a documented SCI has recovered normal function. If at initial testing no deficits are found, the individual is neurologically intact; the ASIA Impairment Scale does not apply.

B

FIGURE 33–8 *(Continued)*

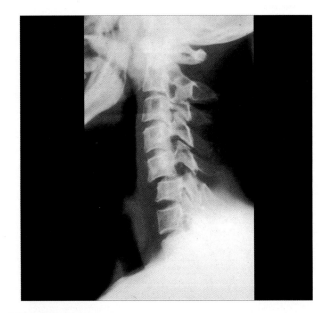

FIGURE 33–9 Subluxation.

preserved in the sacral regions. Groups C and D have differing degrees of preserved motor function, and patients classified as ASIA E have normal neurologic exams. This classification scheme has prognostic implications; not surprisingly, ASIA C, D, and E injuries have the best prognosis for neurologic recovery. In the setting of an acute injury, patients often present in *spinal shock*, where all motor, sensory, and autonomic function is lost below the level of the lesion. The duration of spinal shock is somewhat variable, but the motor and sensory findings may begin to resolve within the first several hours, although the autonomic symptoms can persist for somewhat longer. Consequently, the ASIA Impairment Scale is typically assessed >24 hours after the injury, after the patient has been stabilized.

Clinical Syndromes

The clinical findings associated with an acute spine injury are determined by the level of the lesion. Motor nerve root damage can occur due to neuroforamenal stenosis resulting

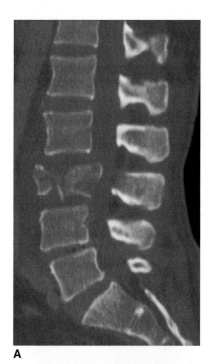

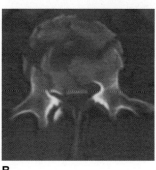

FIGURE 33–10 Burst fracture. (Reproduced with permission from Hall JB, Schmidt GA, Kress JP: *Principles of Critical Care*, 4th ed. New York, NY: McGraw Hill; 2015.)

from fractures or disk fragments; injury to the nerve root itself or to the anterior horn of the spinal cord will produce lower motor neuron findings in the affected muscle groups. Damage to the corticospinal tracts produces upper motor findings distal to the lesion. Injuries to the upper portion of the cervical cord result in quadriplegia; lesions at C3 and above also result in respiratory dysfunction secondary to diaphragmatic paralysis, as the phrenic nerve receives innervation from the third, fourth, and fifth cervical segment. Patients with lesions from C3 through T4 may have lesser degrees of respiratory compromise due to loss of innervation of the intercostal muscles, which reduces vital capacity and impairs the ability cough. Lower cervical lesions result in hand and leg weakness, with preserved function in the proximal upper extremities. Traumatic lesions to the thoracic spine are somewhat less common than injuries in the cervical and lumbar segments, because the spinal column in the thorax is stabilized by the rib cage. However, when they do occur, complete injuries result

in paraplegia with a sensory level apparent in a dermatomal distribution along the trunk. *Conus medullaris syndrome* can result from injuries at the level of the thoracolumbar junction. In adults, the spinal cord usually terminates at about the level of the L1 vertebral body. Therefore, injuries at T11–L1 present with a combination of lower motor neuron findings, due to involvement of nerve roots that exit the canal more distally, as well as upper motor neuron findings affecting the sacral segments. A complete lesion of the conus will present acutely with flaccid paralysis of the legs and loss of tone in the anal sphincter, accompanied by bladder and bowel incontinence. With time, a combination of muscle atrophy and spasticity develops; extensor plantar responses are often present, and the patient will develop a neurogenic bladder. If incomplete, a patient with a conus lesion may have preserved sensation in the perineum, which is known as sacral sparing. Lesions below the level of L1 involve the nerve roots in the cauda equina. Like conus lesions, patients with acute complete cauda equine injuries present acutely with loss of bowel and bladder function and flaccid paraplegia. However, occasionally central disk herniation at the level of L4–L5 or L5–S1 may compress the sacral nerve roots, which are located centrally, while sparing the more lateral lumbar fibers. This can result in profound bladder and bowel dysfunction with relative preservation of motor strength in the legs. Therefore, it is critical to perform a thorough neurologic examination, including an assessment of rectal tone and perineal sensation, in every patient who is suspected of having an SCI.

There are several patterns of incomplete cord injuries that are important to recognize clinically (Figure 33–11). The *Brown-Sequard syndrome* results from a spinal cord hemisection, typically as a result of a penetrating injury. Disruption of the corticospinal tract produces ipsilateral loss of motor function distal to the lesion, whereas interruption of the dorsal columns results in ipsilateral loss of light touch, proprioception, and vibration. However, because fibers of the spinothalamic tract decussate at the level of entry into the cord, patients with Brown-Sequard syndrome will demonstrate contralateral loss of pain and temperature sensation. *Anterior cord syndrome* can result from an acute disk herniation or from retropulsion of bone fragments into the canal, often due to flexion and compression of the spinal column. This results in loss of motor function, due to involvement of the corticospinal tracts, and absence of pain and temperature sensation, due to bilateral disruption of the spinothalamic tracts. Light touch, vibration, and proprioception are preserved, due to sparing of the dorsal columns. Infarction in the territory of the anterior spinal artery infarction, as discussed in Chapter 24, is another cause of this syndrome. *Posterior cord syndrome* is rare, although it has been described in the setting of hyperflexion injuries. It is characterized by loss of light touch, vibration, and proprioception due to damage to the posterior columns; motor function is typically spared. Hyperextension injuries of the cervical spine can result in *central cord syndrome,* characterized by a pattern of weakness in which the arms are disproportionately affected, with

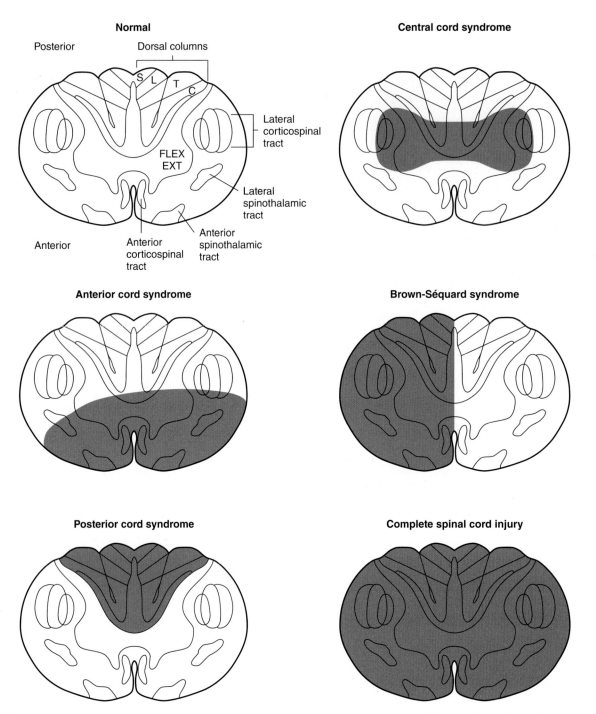

FIGURE 33–11 Diagrams illustrating cross-sectional views of the normal and injured spinal cord. The diagram of the normal spinal column shows the segmental arrangement (C, cervical; L, lumbar; S, sacral; T, thoracic) and the area of flexors and extensors (FLEX and EXT). Central cord syndrome, anterior cord syndrome, Brown-Sequard syndrome, and posterior cord syndrome are incomplete injuries, with affected areas shaded. In complete spinal cord injury, all areas are affected. (Reproduced with permission from Skinner HB, McMahon PJ: *Current Diagnosis & Treatment in Orthopedics*, 5th ed. New York, NY: McGraw Hill; 2014.)

relative sparing of the legs. Pain and temperature sensation may be impaired, and patients may complain of dysesthesia or allodynia, particular in the upper extremities. Vibration, light touch, and position sense are typically preserved, as are bowel and bladder function. This syndrome is most commonly seen in elderly patients, especially those with preexisting cervical

canal stenosis. There has been considerable debate about the precise pathophysiology, although it is often attributed to edema or hematomyelia affecting the central region of the cord. The pattern of weakness and sensory loss is often attributed to somatotopic organization of fibers within the corticospinal and spinothalamic tracts, with cervical fibers located medially. Involvement of the spinal cord gray matter has also been implicated. A similar clinical presentation, in this case known as *cruciate paralysis,* can be seen with injuries to the craniocervical junction. It is thought to result from compression of the corticospinal tract just caudal to the pyramidal decussation, which may occur with displacement of the odontoid process. The clinical features are thought to result from somatotopic organization of upper extremity and lower extremity fibers through the medulla and the corticospinal tracts in the upper cord. Specifically, upper extremity fibers are thought to decussate superior to the lower extremity fibers and occupy a medial position in the corticospinal tract starting at the level of C1. Lower extremity fibers cross inferiorly, around the C1–C2 junction, and continue to run lateral to the upper extremity fibers in the cervical spine. Acutely, cruciate paralysis and central cord syndrome present with similar clinical features; however, injuries to the craniocervical junction may result in lower cranial nerve dysfunction. Sensory abnormalities over the face may also be present, due to involvement of the spinal tract of the trigeminal nerve. More severe injuries of the craniocervical junction can be life threatening, resulting in quadriplegia, respiratory arrest, and hemodynamic instability.

Although injuries to the descending tracts in spinal cord constitute upper motor neuron lesions, the classic upper motor neuron findings (spasticity, increased muscle tone, and hyperreflexia) do not develop until weeks or months after the initial injury. In the acute period, mild to moderate spine injury presents with decreased motor strength and/or sensory abnormalities distal to the level of the lesion. Severe injuries, however, can present with *spinal shock.* In this scenario, all motor and sensory function below the level of the injury is lost, and spinal reflexes are completely absent. The patient will demonstrate flaccid paraplegia or quadriplegia, depending on the level of the injury. Disruption of autonomic function is frequently present; this may present as loss of sweating and piloerection, impaired vasomotor tone, and loss of peristalsis. Atony of the detrusor muscle results in overflow incontinence, in which the bladder distends until the intravesicular pressure is high enough to overcome the resting tone of the urethral sphincter. Profound hypotension may result due to loss of vasomotor tone; bradycardia is often present due to unopposed vagal nerve activity. It is important to differentiate hypotension secondary to neurologic injury, sometimes called *neurogenic shock,* from other causes of hypotension, such as cardiogenic shock, hemorrhagic or hypovolemic shock, and septic shock. The presence of bradycardia with warm flushed skin is suggestive of a neurologic etiology. Spinal shock is much more common and severe in cervical spine injuries, although it can occur in lesions to the thoracic spine; it is rarely seen with injuries confined to lumbar segments. It is important to recognize clinically because severe spinal shock can cause a serious, although incomplete, injury to be mistakenly characterized as a complete lesion. In addition, it has implications for patient management. Like the injured brain, the injured spinal cord is highly susceptible to secondary injury due to hypotension;

consequently, appropriate hemodynamic support is critical in hypotensive patients in order to prevent worsening cord injury.

Clinical Management

As with any medical emergency, the first priority is stabilization of the airway, followed closely by appropriate hemodynamic support. Patients with injuries to the upper cervical spine often require intubation due to respiratory compromise. Effort should be made to accomplish this with the spine in neutral position to avoid further spinal injury resulting from neck extension during intubation. In the setting of hypotension, aggressive fluid resuscitation is needed to achieve hemodynamic stability. It is important to try to distinguish between neurogenic shock and other causes of hypotension, in part because neurogenic shock may not respond to fluid resuscitation alone; vasopressors may be required. As soon as feasible, the spinal column should be immobilized to minimize the possibility of further impingement of the spinal canal. A cervical collar may be used to stabilize the cervical spine. If the patient is being transported from the field, he or she should be placed on a spine board, to which the head is secured. Subsequent evaluations and procedures should use spine precautions, in which the cervical and lumbar spine are maintained in a neutral position, until the possibility of a clinically significant spine injury has been excluded. The process of rolling or turning an injured patient while maintaining spine precautions is often called "logrolling."

In an alert patient, it is helpful to obtain information about the mechanism of injury, as well as any subjective symptoms, such as neck or back pain, numbness, or weakness, that the patient may be experiencing. The back and neck should be examined for visible deformity and palpated to assess for point tenderness, a palpable "step-off" between vertebrae, or gaps between spinous processes. Motor power should be evaluated in each muscle group, and graded on a scale from 0 to 5, as follows:

0: Total paralysis, no contraction is palpable

1: Active muscle contraction can be visualized or palpated

2: Active muscle activation, sufficient to move the joint through the full range of motion when gravity is eliminated

3: Active muscle activation, sufficient to move the joint through the full range of motion against gravity

4: Active muscle activation sufficient to move against some resistance

5: Normal muscle activation with full strength.

A thorough sensory examination, including vibration, light touch, pinprick, and joint position sense, should be performed if possible. Deep tendon reflexes should also be assessed. Finally, it is critical to evaluate the motor and sensory function of the sacral nerve roots in every patient with suspected spine injury. This evaluation should include perineal sensation and rectal tone. It is also useful to document lower sacral reflexes, such as the anal wink and the bulbocavernosus reflex. Unfortunately, many patients with traumatic injuries to the spine also have other concurrent injuries, including TBI, which may confound the exam. In that case, the neurologic assessment might be limited to evaluating motor response to central and peripheral pain; however, rectal tone and spinal reflexes must still be assessed.

Once the patient has been physiologically stabilized, spinal imaging is often obtained. CT scans are useful for evaluating bony injuries, such as fractures and dislocations. CT is useful for evaluating vertebral alignment, encroachment of bony fragments on the spinal canal, and distraction between vertebral bodies. CT angiography may be ordered in patients who are found to have bony injuries of the cervical spine and/or the base of the skull, because these lesions are occasionally accompanied by injuries to the vertebral arteries or the carotid arteries because they course through the neck. Although a CT of the neck may provide some clues as to the presence of a ligamentous injury, it does not permit visualization of ligaments or intervertebral disks; it is also inadequate for evaluating nerve roots or the spinal cord parenchyma. Magnetic resonance imaging (MRI) may be useful in situations in which the exam suggests spinal cord compromise but initial CT imaging proves unrevealing. Using MRI, it is possible to directly visualize spinal cord transection, edema, hematomyelia, and other intramedullary lesions. It can also provide information regarding injury to ligamentous structures, such as the transverse dental ligament, anterior and posterior longitudinal ligaments, and interspinous ligaments. MRI also enables detection of cord compression due to extramedullary lesions such as epidural hematomas and herniated disk fragments. In patients who have contraindications to MRI, a CT myelogram may provide information about compression of the thecal sac. This is performed by injecting contrast material into the epidural space prior to imaging. It allows visualization of the spinal column and nerve roots and aids in identifying compressive lesions, but it does not provide information about the cord parenchyma or ligamentous structures. As a consequence, MRI is preferred when feasible.

It is important to note that neuroimaging is not a substitute for a thorough evaluation by a qualified clinician. Because patients with SCI so often suffer from other associated injuries, these patients are best managed by multidisciplinary teams at experienced centers. Early evaluation by a neurosurgeon or orthopedic spine surgeon is necessary to determine whether surgical intervention and/or external stabilization is required. A comprehensive discussion of operative management of SCIs is beyond the scope of this chapter, but generally speaking, the goals of operative intervention include decompression of the spine and nerve roots, as well as stabilization of unstable injuries to the vertebral column. There is considerable debate about the optimal timing of spine surgery, but some evidence exists that early decompression may be warranted, especially for patients with incomplete cord lesions. Unstable injuries may be managed

conservatively, with external fixation, or surgically, with internal fixation. Decisions regarding the timing and necessity of surgical treatment are best made on a patient-specific basis. For SCI patients who initially present to centers without access to spine surgeons, urgent transfer to an appropriate trauma center should be considered.

The medical management of SCI patients, as with TBI patients, is predominantly directed at preventing secondary injury and managing or preventing medical complications. The injured spine is highly susceptible to ischemia, so adequate hemodynamic support is critical. Maintaining systolic blood pressure >90 mm Hg is required at a minimum; in cases

CASE 33-2

A 19-year-old man was discovered by his friends after diving off a pier into shallow water. Emergency personnel arrived at the scene quickly and found him to be hypoxemic and hypotensive, with labored respirations. Due to the mechanism of injury, concern for a cervical spine lesion was high. They were able to secure an airway while maintaining the cervical spine in neutral position. Intravenous access was obtained, and fluid resuscitation was initiated in an effort to correct his hypotension; supplemental oxygen and positive-pressure ventilation were employed to ensure adequate oxygenation. Upon arrival in the emergency department, he was alert and able to make eye contact with examiners and follow some commands. He was able to shrug his shoulders and adduct the arms easily. He could weakly flex the elbows with gravity eliminated; however, no movement was noted in the forearms or hands, and the legs were also flaccid. The biceps tendon reflex was present, although it appeared weak; other deep tendon reflexes were found to be absent. He was able to indicate with eye blinks that he appreciated pinprick sensation over the neck, shoulders, and the lateral portion of his arms; however, sensation was considerably diminished below the level of the clavicle. Rectal tone was absent, and the patient did not have preserved sacral sensation. Computed tomography imaging of the cervical spine demonstrated a C4 burst fracture with retropulsion of bony fragments into the spinal canal. Neurosurgery was promptly consulted and opted for early surgical decompression and stabilization. Intraoperatively, vasopressors were used to maintain adequate spinal cord perfusion. Postoperatively, the patient remained quadriplegic and showed evidence of spinal shock; however, over the next several days, he began to demonstrate return of sensation over his anterior chest wall and improved strength in his biceps muscles bilaterally. He was successfully weaned from mechanical ventilation and transferred to an acute rehabilitation center.

of neurogenic shock, vasopressors may be required. There is some evidence that patients with SCI may have improved outcomes with mild induced hypertension (ie, a MAP of ~85 to 90 mm Hg) in the first week after injury. Although this is not universally accepted, it is practiced in some centers provided that the patient does not have any contraindications. Two trials in the 1990s purported to demonstrate a benefit of high-dose methylprednisolone treatment for acute SCI; however, the clinical benefit was modest, and the results of these trials have been extensively criticized due to methodologic issues. It is clear that high-dose steroids increased the rate of medical complications in trial participants, and consequently, the use of steroids in acute SCI is no longer recommended.

Patients with acute cervical injuries will generally require management in a critical care unit due to the potential for hemodynamic instability and respiratory compromise. Like TBI patients, SCI patients are at risk of complications of immobility, such as nosocomial infections, pressure ulcers, and thromboembolic complications. They also have a high incidence of gastrointestinal and urinary dysfunction. Foley catheters are typically required in the acute phase to decompress the bladder and enable accurate assessment of volume status. A nasogastric tube may be necessary to decompress the stomach, and a bowel regimen should be instituted early to prevent constipation. The gastroparesis generally resolves within a few days, enabling initiation of enteral nutrition either by mouth or via feeding tube. Pneumatic compression devices are required at all times, unless contraindicated, to mitigate the risk of deep venous thrombosis and pulmonary emboli. In most patients, pharmacologic prophylaxis can be initiated within 72 hours. Diligent nursing care is required to prevent skin breakdown and minimize the risk of hospital-acquired infection. When the patient is clinically stable, transitioning to use of intermittent straight catheterization for management of urinary retention is favored to prevent the development of urinary tract infections. Early mobilization, to the extent that the patient is able, is important for pulmonary toilet, prevention of muscle wasting, and minimization of other complications associated with immobility.

Long-Term Sequelae

Over time, the flaccid paralysis common in the setting of acute spinal injury evolves into a spastic paralysis more consistent with upper motor neuron pathology. Patients develop increased muscle tone and deep tendon reflexes, as well as pathologic reflexes such as the Babinski sign. The bladder, which is initially atonic, also becomes spastic, resulting in intermittent reflexive bladder emptying. Occasionally, detrusor dysynergy can develop, in which the detrusor muscle reflexively contracts against a closed urethral sphincter, resulting in urinary retention. Close attention to voiding is necessary in order to detect urinary retention, which may predispose to infection, and can result in hydronephrosis and renal injury if left untreated. Bowel complications, including constipation

and incontinence, are also common. Often these can be addressed with a combination of stool softeners and prokinetic agents. Pain is a common complication of chronic SCI, resulting both from muscle spasms and sensory abnormalities. Muscle spasms are often treated with muscle relaxants, such as baclofen, which can be administered orally or through an implanted pump designed to permit intrathecal administration. In some instances, injection of botulinum toxin can be beneficial. Patients may also develop neuropathic pain, often described as a burning sensation, which can be very distressing. A variety of pharmacologic interventions have been used to treat neuropathic pain, including several antiepileptic agents and tricyclic antidepressants.

One of the most clinically important consequences of chronic SCI is *autonomic dysreflexia*. This term describes an episodic sympathetic response to sensory stimuli applied below the level of the lesion; it can be seen in patients with lesions at T6 or above. It occurs when a stimulus below the level of the lesion, often a due to a distended bladder or rectum, provokes a pathologic sympathetic response via spinal reflexes. The impulse travels via paraspinal sympathetic ganglia, causing vasoconstriction below the level of the lesion. The resulting hypertension results in vagal stimulation by way of the carotid bodies, which produces bradycardia and pupillary constriction. Flushing and sweating may be visible above the level of the lesion, due to unopposed parasympathetic function; however, below the lesion, piloerection and anhidrosis will be noted. The splanchnic vascular bed, which receives its innervation from the T5–T9 spinal levels, represents a high-volume vascular reservoir. Consequently, unopposed sympathetic input to the abdominal viscera can provoke a hypertensive crisis, which may be life threatening if not treated promptly. Patients may develop hypertensive encephalopathy, intracranial or retinal hemorrhages, pulmonary edema, and cardiac or renal complications. The hypertensive crisis typically resolves when the precipitating stimulus is removed. Antihypertensive medications may be required, but short-acting agents should be chosen to prevent hypotension from developing once the underlying cause of the episode has been addressed.

The development of a syrinx is another potential long-term complication of traumatic SCI that deserves mention. A *syrinx* is a fluid-filled cavitation within the cord parenchyma that can develop months or years after the initial injury. It typically originates at the level of the injury and can extend either rostrally or caudally. It can present with signs and symptoms of progressive myelopathy. Often the initial symptoms involve sensory changes, including neuropathic pain, due to the involvement of the spinothalamic tracts; a decline in motor function can occur as the syrinx enlarges. This complication is fairly rare, occurring in approximately 3% of SCI survivors. However, it is important to recognize it promptly because *syringomyelia* can be treated with shunting, which can halt the progression and perhaps relieve some of the symptoms.

Unfortunately, the prognosis for neurologic recovery following a complete spinal cord lesion remains poor. However, many patients with incomplete lesions have the potential to make significant strides with aggressive physical and occupational therapy. Even patients with complete SCIs may demonstrate some degree of functional improvement despite the lack of any measurable recovery of neurologic function. Advances in rehabilitation techniques, technology, and assistive devices have contributed to continued improvements in quality of life for survivors. Consequently, it is possible for even patients with lower cervical spine injuries to regain considerable independence.

SELF-ASSESSMENT QUESTIONS

1. A 19-year-old bicycle messenger is brought to the emergency department (ED) by bystanders after inadvertently running his bike into a sign. Unfortunately, he was not wearing a helmet. Upon arrival in the ED, the patient is somnolent and mumbling. He opens his eyes when his name is called and says occasional words, but he does not answer orientation questions appropriately. He does not follow commands, although he reaches up to grab the examiner's hand when noxious stimulation is applied. What would this patient's Glasgow Coma Scale (GCS) score be?

   A. 2
   B. 11
   C. 15
   D. 9

2. A 36-year-old woman is involved in a motor vehicle collision. She is intubated upon arrival in the emergency department due to her depressed neurologic status. Upon arrival in the intensive care unit, an external ventricular drain is placed; her intracranial pressure is found to be 19 mm Hg. Her mean arterial pressure is 58 mm Hg. What is her cerebral perfusion pressure (CPP)?

   A. 39 mm Hg
   B. 72 mm Hg
   C. 58 mm Hg
   D. Equivalent to her central venous pressure

3. For the patient in Question 2, what is the most appropriate next step in management?

   A. Hyperventilate to induce cerebral vasodilation
   B. Remove cerebrospinal fluid to achieve a CPP of 50 to 70 mm Hg
   C. Support her blood pressure, with fluids and/or vasopressors, to maintain CPP of 50 to 70 mm Hg
   D. Start steroids to treat cerebral edema

4. A 70-year-old man with a history of cervical radiculopathy trips over his cat, which causes him to fall forward and hit his forehead on the seat of a nearby chair. He arrives in the emergency department complaining of bilateral hand numbness and burning. The emergency physician finds that he has minimal 2/5 grip strength in his hands bilaterally, 3/5 wrist extension bilaterally, and weak interossei bilaterally. Motor strength in the legs is normal. Which clinical syndrome is most consistent with this presentation?

   A. Central cord syndrome
   B. Brown-Sequard syndrome
   C. Cauda equina syndrome
   D. Pseudotumor cerebri

Sleep Disorders

Joseph T. Daley

O B J E C T I V E S

After studying this chapter, the student should be able to:

- State the physiologic characteristics of sleep stages and what constitutes normal sleep.
- Describe the neural mechanisms underlying sleep–wake regulation in the brain.
- Display an understanding of the diagnosis and classification of common sleep disorders.
- Describe the effects on sleep and the mechanisms of action of commonly prescribed medications for sleep and sleep disorders, as well as commonly used nonprescription agents.

Sleep can be defined as a physiologic state characterized by behavioral quiescence and reduced awareness of sensory inputs that can be reversed by a stimulus of sufficient magnitude. For centuries, sleep was thought of as a passive state, the absence of wakefulness, when your mind and body turned off until it was time to start another day. Modern medicine, however, has given us great insight into the fact that sleep is a very active process, with distinct stages regulated by the complex interaction of a myriad of neurologic, metabolic, and behavioral factors. Like food and water, sleep is an essential physiologic process that is regulated by a homeostatic drive—if you get too little of it for a period of time, you want more of it in the future. This chapter discusses the complexity of the state of sleep, building on the introduction in Chapter 23, and introduces various pathologic and nonpathologic conditions associated with sleep.

The breakthroughs in neurophysiology necessary to examine sleep occurred relatively recently. In 1934, Hans Berger first described the potentials that can be observed by comparing 2 points on the scalp above the brain, waves we commonly refer to as the electroencephalogram (EEG). In 1936, Frederic Bremer noticed that transection of the brain at the level of the rostral midbrain in experimental animals produced a slow, rhythmic pattern on the EEG, whereas transection lower in the caudal membrane allowed the brain to maintain the EEG typically seen in wake. Building on this work, in 1946, Giuseppe Moruzzi and Horace Magoun first described an area in the midbrain-pontine junction they called the reticular activating system,

which is necessary for keeping an animal awake. The first published description of a substate during sleep associated with the highest amount of dream recall, termed *rapid eye movement* (REM) sleep due to the characteristic saccadic movements seen, was by William Dement and Nathaniel Kleitman in 1956. Since that time, there have been a great many discoveries identifying what brain areas are responsible for the control of these processes.

PREVALENCE & BURDEN

The sleep disorders discussed in this chapter range from very common to very rare. Obstructive sleep apnea (OSA) is believed to affect approximately 25% of adults between the ages of 30 and 70 years. Because of the role that obesity plays in the pathophysiology of this disorder, the incidence of OSA has been steadily increasing over the past several decades. Restless legs syndrome (RLS) has an estimated prevalence of 15% in North America, although the studies reporting on this vary widely depending on the diagnostic criteria used. Enuresis affects a similar fraction of children, approximately 15%. At the other end of the spectrum, narcolepsy is far less common, with an estimated prevalence of 0.05%.

None of the sleep disorders discussed in this chapter are progressively fatal conditions, like those discussed in the chapter on neurodegeneration. However, several studies have described a U-shaped curve when investigating the relationship between sleep duration and mortality; those with too little or too much sleep are at an increased risk of death from all causes. Multiple retrospective studies have demonstrated that moderate or severe OSA is a risk factor for all cardiovascular mortality, as well as the specific conditions of myocardial infarction and stroke. Those same studies show that this risk attributable to OSA can be ameliorated by treatment, so this is an important modifiable risk factor that should be evaluated and addressed. Furthermore, depending on the situation in which patients find themselves, hypersomnolence resulting from any of the myriad of causes detailed later in this chapter can clearly have fatal consequences. This applies to physicians, both in training and beyond, as well as their patients.

LOCALIZATION: NEURAL REGULATION OF SLEEP–WAKE STATES

Before one can understand the pathologic aspects of sleep medicine, there must be an explanation of the basic neuroanatomy of sleep–wake states as well as the systems that control the timing of these behaviors.

Wake-Promoting Nuclei & Their Neurotransmitters

The first category of wake-promoting cells consists of a group of nuclei containing monoaminergic neurotransmitters. Cells of the dorsal raphe contain serotonin, cells of the locus coeruleus contain norepinephrine, cells of the ventrolateral periaqueductal gray contain dopamine, and cells of the tuberomammillary nucleus contain histamine. The neurons in these areas all share the same pattern of firing across the states: highly active when we are awake, dramatically reduced as we fall asleep, and then virtually silent during REM sleep. Many medications used to promote wakefulness increase these substances (eg, stimulants that increase the amount of dopamine and norepinephrine in the synapse). Conversely, substances that block the signaling of these substances produce drowsiness (eg, antihistamines such as diphenhydramine, the active ingredient in most over-the-counter sleep aides).

The other chief wake-promoting neurotransmitter is acetylcholine. This substance can be found in the pedunculopontine tegmental nucleus in the midbrain-pontine junction and the nucleus basalis of Meynert in the forebrain. These neurons are highly active in wakefulness, and their rates are dramatically reduced in non-REM sleep. However, unlike the monoaminergic nuclei, the cholinergic cells have increased firing rates during REM sleep. These cholinergic, "REM-on" neurons are believed to regulate the active-appearing EEG characteristic of REM and also activate the pathways responsible for the atonia seen in REM sleep.

Sleep-Promoting Area of the Brain

In contrast to the widespread redundancy of wakefulness and attention, there is only 1 area in the brain that contains neurons that are active solely during sleep: the ventrolateral preoptic (VLPO) nucleus of the hypothalamus. These neurons contain γ-aminobutyric acid (GABA), which is the main inhibitory transmitter of the brain, and they project to the wake-promoting areas, turning them off during sleep. It is hypothesized that the wake-active and sleep-active neurons oppose each other directly to provide a stable switching mechanism between behavioral states.

In addition to the neuroanatomically specific GABA in the VLPO, the other neuromodulator that promotes sleep in the brain is adenosine. It is believed that through metabolism in the brain, as adenosine triphosphate is metabolized to adenosine diphosphate, circulating levels of adenosine in the cerebrospinal fluid increase. Adenosine is released through extrasynaptic mechanisms and has wide reaching effects, particularly by down-modulating the activity of wake-promoting neurons in the cholinergic basal forebrain. This is believed to underlie the sleepiness we feel as we remain awake throughout the day and is even more pronounced during sleep deprivation.

TECHNIQUES IN SLEEP MEDICINE

Because sleep is such a multifactorial process, the first place to start in the accurate diagnosis of sleep disorders is a careful history. A sleep-focused history should include all of the following questions: What time does the patient get into bed? How long does it take the patient to fall asleep? Once the patient is asleep, how many times does the patient wake up? How long does it then take the patient to get back to sleep? What time does the patient finally get up to start the day? In addition, it is important to know whether the patient takes naps, and if so, for how long, how frequently, and at what time. In addition to napping, unintended sleep episodes, particularly those that occur while driving or in other dangerous situations, should be queried. Other factors that can affect sleep should also be identified, such as the sleep environment. Does the patient share the bed with a spouse, pet, or child(ren)? The activities that precede bedtime or that are performed during nighttime arousals can also be an opportunity for intervention to improve sleep onset and continuity. For example, studying neurology review materials immediately before bedtime can contribute to insomnia. One should review the contribution of the alerting or sedating effects of the patient's medications to the patient's complaints. In addition, the use of over-the-counter sleep aids, alcohol, caffeine, and illicit drugs should be ascertained, because all of these substances can impact the patient's sleep and daytime alertness. As discussed thoroughly in Chapter 23, the timing of sleep and the timing of the patient's work shift may also contribute to the patient's level of alertness and any sleep-related complaints.

The current standard for sleep–wake diagnostic testing is polysomnography, during which various physiologic signals are recorded and then used to identify what state the patient is experiencing, using 30-second epochs. There are 3 key variables on which the criteria for sleep staging are based: EEG (brain waves), the electrooculogram (EOG; eye movements), and the electromyogram (EMG; muscle activity). Using specific characteristics of these signals allows us to categorize behavior into 1 of the following 5 states: wake, N1, N2, N3, and REM sleep (Figure 34–1). Together, N1, N2, and N3 are collectively known as non-REM sleep.

1. **Wake** (Figure 34–1A): Wakefulness is characterized by low-amplitude, fast-frequency EEG. Muscle tone is high, eye movements are large and brisk, and blinking is also observed. Another feature on EEG that helps to identify wakefulness is the alpha rhythm, which is a synchronous 9- to 10-Hz brainwave pattern that appears most predominantly over the occipital cortex when the patient is sitting quietly with his or her eyes closed.

2. **N1** (Figure 34–1B): Stage N1 marks the transition from wake to sleep. It is characterized by a slower EEG with higher amplitude than when awake, the absence of the alpha rhythm, a slight decrement in muscle tone, and slow, rolling eye movements. Typically, approximately 5% to 10% of sleep is spent in this stage.

3. **N2** (Figure 34–1C): Stage N2 is the stage of sleep during which most of the night is spent. The muscle tone is more clearly reduced from waking, and eye movements are absent. There are 2 prominent findings on the EEG that help identify N2: K complexes and spindles. K complexes are large, bi- or triphasic potentials with an initial negative deflection, followed by a positive deflection, lasting about 0.5 seconds. Spindles are brief 1- to 2-second bursts of higher frequency activity (11 to 16 Hz). They are named for their shape, like the spindle on a loom, and originate in the reticular nucleus of the thalamus. About 45% to 55% of an adult's sleep is spent in N2.

4. **N3** (Figures 34–1D **and** 34–1E): Stage N3 comprises what is traditionally referred to as *slow-wave sleep*. There may be a further decrease in EMG tone seen in this stage, and eye movements are also absent. The EEG consists of large-amplitude slow waves (also called delta waves), which occur at 1 to 3 Hz. This stage is also referred to as *deep sleep*, because the threshold to arouse someone is often the highest from N3 sleep when compared to any other stage. Approximately 15% to 20% of the night is spent in this stage in adults.

5. **REM** (Figure 34–1F): REM sleep is the stage during which we do most of our dreaming. Aside from a few twitches, the EMG is normally silent during REM sleep (termed *atonia*). The EOG demonstrates multiple fast saccadic movements, which give this state its name. The EEG of REM sleep is most like wakefulness or stage 1, with faster rhythms of lower amplitude than either N2 or N3 sleep, indicating a higher amount of desynchronized neural activity. This stage composes 20% to 25% of adult sleep.

Once a night in the lab has been scored according to the above criteria, we can use these data to compose a hypnogram that shows what stage the patient is in on the y-axis by time of night on the x-axis (Figure 34–2). It is normal to cycle from wake, through the stages of non-REM sleep, and then to REM sleep several times throughout the night, in 90- to 120-minute intervals. Periods of N3 are typically longer in the beginning of the night, whereas REM sleep is more prevalent at the end of the night. This provides a view of the entire night's worth of sleep. As one can see from Figure 34–2, sleep architecture changes across the lifespan. It is normal for the elderly patient to have less stage N3 sleep, less REM sleep, and more sleep disruptions.

The nocturnal polysomnogram remains the standard diagnostic testing modality in sleep medicine. In addition to the 3 variables discussed earlier for sleep staging (EEG, EOG, and EMG), an in-lab test includes monitoring of the patient's oxyhemoglobin saturation, respiratory effort, and airflow to assess for sleep apnea. The combined number of apneas (pauses in breathing ≥10 seconds) and hypopneas (periods of shallower than normal breathing) per hour is the apnea-hypopnea index (AHI), and is normally <5. The EMG of the submentalis muscle in the chin is used for sleep staging, and the EMG of each anterior tibialis muscle is monitored to look

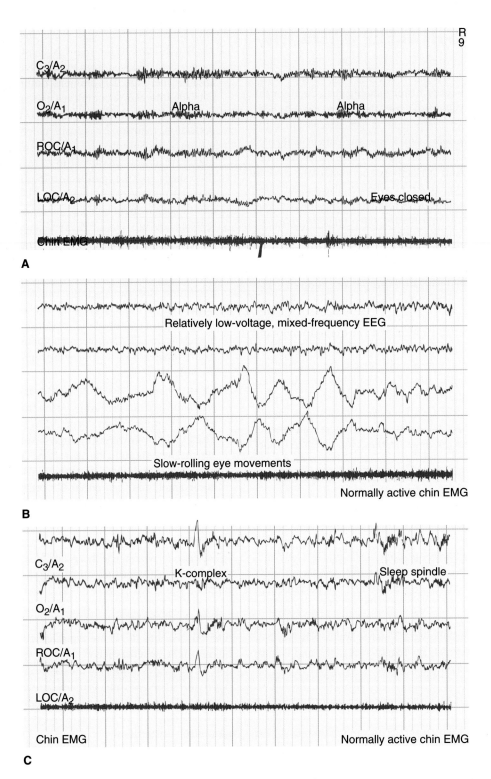

FIGURE 34–1 Representative polysomnographic recordings from adults in the awake state and various stages of sleep. **A.** Awake state (with eyes closed). Alpha rhythms are prominent in electroencephalogram (EEG). Normally active chin EMG. **B.** Stage 1 (N1) sleep. Characterized by slower frequency EEG and slow rolling eye movements. **C.** Stage 2 (N2) sleep, characterized by appearance of high-amplitude K-complex waves and bursts of 11- to 16-Hz waves (sleep spindles) on a background of low frequency. **D.** Stage 3 (N3) sleep. Appearance of high-voltage slow (delta) waves. **E.** Deepest stage of N3 sleep, with predominant delta-wave activity occupying 50% of a 30-second tracing. **F.** Rapid eye movement (REM) sleep, characterized by episodes of REM and occasional muscle twitches in an otherwise flat chin electromyogram (EMG). Technical note: Four sites from the same montage are illustrated in each recording: C₃/A₂, left central to right mastoid; O₂/A₁, right occipital to left mastoid; ROC/A₁, right outer canthus to left mastoid; LOC/A₂, left outer canthus to right mastoid. A chin EMG tracing is added to each recording.

(Adapted with permission from Butkov N. *Atlas of Clinical Polysomnography*, Volume 1. Medford, OR: Synapse Media; 1996.)

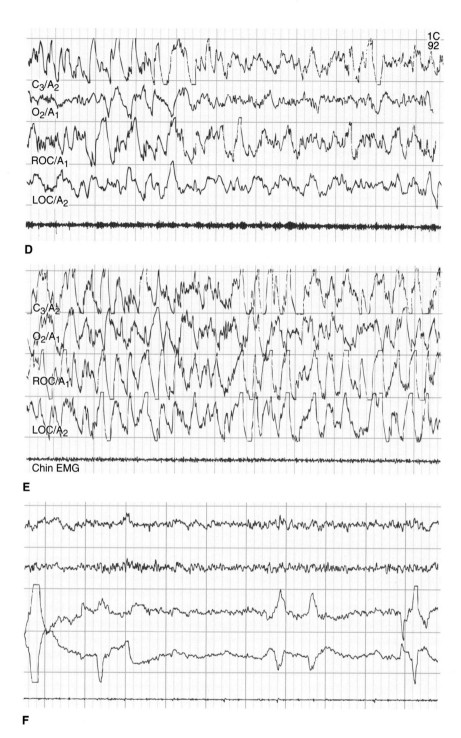

FIGURE 34–1 (*Continued*)

for leg movements, which will be covered later in this chapter. Often, video is kept of the patient at night so that any unusual behaviors can be analyzed and compared with the rest of the sleep recording to help determine the underlying etiology of these episodes.

In addition to the use of the nocturnal polysomnogram to evaluate sleep disorders at night, 2 tests are performed to assess daytime sleepiness/alertness. The most common evaluation performed is the multiple sleep latency test (MSLT). In this procedure, after the patient spends a night in the sleep lab to evaluate for the presence of sleep disorders, the patient is given several nap opportunities spaced apart by 2 hours. Each nap opportunity lasts 20 minutes, and if sleep onset is not observed, the lights are turned back on and the patient is kept awake until the next nap. If sleep is observed, then the patient is given 15 minutes to nap, during which time the

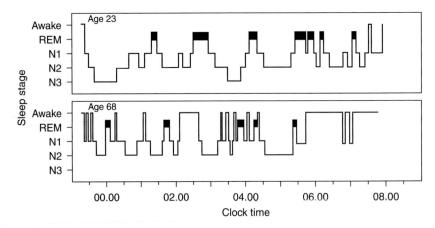

FIGURE 34–2 Sleep–wake architecture. Alternating stages of wakefulness, the 3 stages of non–rapid eye movement (REM) sleep (N1 to N3), and REM sleep (*solid bars*) occur over the course of the night for representative young and older adult men. Note the periodic cycles from wake to non-REM to REM sleep repeated throughout the night. Common changes seen in the aging population include reduction of REM and stage N3 sleep, frequent spontaneous awakenings, early sleep onset, and early-morning awakening. (Reproduced with permission from the Division of Sleep and Circadian Disorders, Brigham and Women's Hospital.)

presence of daytime REM sleep can be observed. The average latency to sleep across the nap opportunities is calculated, as is the number of REM onsets observed in the naps. Average sleep latency of >10 minutes is considered normal, whereas a latency of <8 minutes is considered consistent with hypersomnolence. The presence of 2 or more REM onsets during the daytime naps is also considered pathologic and is consistent with the diagnosis of narcolepsy, which will be discussed in detail later in this chapter.

The second test is a test to assess the patient's ability to stay awake, known as the maintenance of wakefulness test. In this test, the lights are turned out for 40 minutes at 2-hour intervals. However, in this case, the patient is instructed to stay awake. Normal sleep latency on this test is >20 minutes. This test is most often used in patients with underlying sleep disorders to ensure that their treatment is effectively treating daytime somnolence when their occupation demands sustained alertness (eg, airline pilots who are being treated for OSA).

SLEEP DISORDERS

Sleep-Disordered Breathing

The most common disorder treated by sleep physicians is sleep apnea. Sleep apnea can be divided into 2 separate entities with very different physiologic mechanisms: OSA and central sleep apnea (CSA).

OSA

As the name implies, OSA is caused by airway obstruction, typically by narrowing or collapse of the posterior oropharynx. An example of an obstructive event is illustrated in Figure 34–3. The patient is trying to breathe but not getting enough air. There are several factors that explain why this only happens during sleep: (1) When you lie down, gravity works

to narrow the airway, particularly when supine; and (2) as mentioned earlier, muscle tone drops when we fall asleep, and this applies to the muscles that serve to keep the throat open as well. These factors also contribute to snoring; however, it is estimated that about 20% of all snorers have OSA. As one might predict based on this mechanism, OSA is often more severe when patients are in REM sleep and their muscle tone is at the lowest. These breathing events often have consequences, including a drop in oxyhemoglobin saturation that typically returns to baseline as the patient responds with hyperventilation and brief arousals on EEG.

CSA

Unlike OSA, where the abnormality in breathing arises from obstruction, CSA is characterized by breathing pauses caused by a reduction in the brainstem-mediated drive to breathe. Thus, the difference between OSA and CSA lies in the presence or absence of respiratory effort; in OSA, the patient is trying to inhale, but there is obstruction, whereas in CSA, there is no signal coming from the brain to inspire (Figure 34–4). The symptoms and consequences of CSA, however, can be exactly the same: increased sleep disruption and daytime sleepiness. The most common causes of CSA are brainstem stroke or brainstem tumors, which can affect the respiratory centers, as well as congestive heart failure.

Treatment of OSA

First-line therapy for OSA is continuous positive airway pressure (CPAP). CPAP works by blowing air at a sufficient pressure to keep the back of the throat open when the patient is asleep, aiming to eliminate the obstructive events and remove the frequent oxyhemoglobin desaturations and arousals. Effective treatment involves wearing a mask on the face nightly with all sleep. There are alternatives to CPAP, but they are less effective. These include oral appliances that fit in the upper and lower teeth and are worn at night. These work

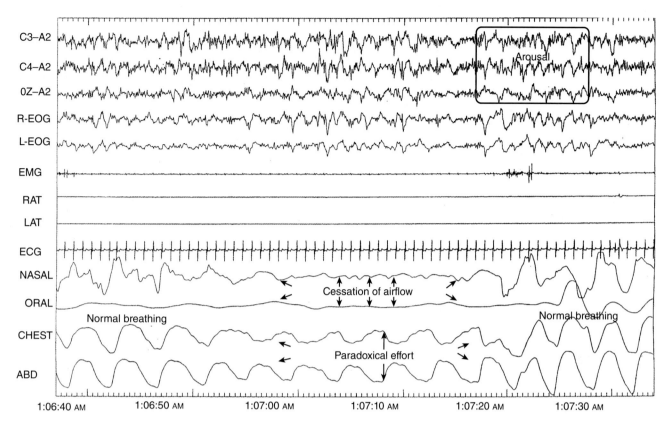

FIGURE 34-3 Obstructive apnea. During the apneic episodes, there is abnormal airflow (both oral and nasal) with paradoxical motion of the rib cage and abdomen. At the end of the apneic episode, there is a burst of electromyogram (EMG) activity at the arousal. Following the arousal, respiration resumes with synchronous movements of the rib cage and abdomen. The polysomnography traces from the top down are as follows: 3 electroencephalogram (EEG) channels (C3–A2, C4–A2, OZ–A2); 2 electrooculogram (EOG) channels (R and L); submental EMG; right and left anterior tibialis EMG (RAT, LAT), electrocardiogram (ECG); nasal and oral airflow; and chest and abdominal (ABD) motion. (Reproduced with permission from Grippi MA, Elias JA, Fishman JA, et al: *Fishman's Pulmonary Diseases and Disorders*, 5th ed. New York, NY: McGraw Hill; 2015.)

by positioning the jaw forward, widening the airway and stiffening the walls to reduce collapse. Another alternative is oral surgery to achieve the same goal of widening the airway, but in a more permanent manner by removing tissue or changing the surrounding structures (eg, removing a portion of the soft palate [uvulopalatopharyngoplasty] and base of the tongue, or maxillomandibular procedures to widen the oral cavity). These alternatives work about half of the time and are more effective in patients with mild or moderate OSA. The newest method of treating OSA is the hypoglossal nerve stimulator, which is essentially a pacemaker for the tongue. This implanted device is turned on at night and uses stimulation of the distal branch of cranial nerve XII to move the tongue forward during inspiration, alleviating potential obstructive events. This is clearly more invasive and expensive than CPAP but can be a good treatment option for the appropriate patient when all else fails.

Hypersomnolence

The initial evaluation of a patient with excessive daytime sleepiness must also include a careful history. By far, the most common cause of excessive daytime sleepiness in our society is sleep deprivation. We all know that if we stay up all night, our subjective level of alertness will be impaired, as well as our performance in tasks that require attention, reaction time, or memory. A less widely recognized fact is that chronic partial sleep deprivation can cause a cumulative effect over time that is just as detrimental. For example, approximately 2 weeks of restriction to 6 hours in bed every night without the opportunity for recovery caused the equivalent impairment as 1 full night spent awake. Further reduction of time in bed to 4 hours nightly produced similar deficits in about a week. The deficits in performance following sleep deprivation have been demonstrated to be equivalent to being legally inebriated. Thus, this can be an important factor in both a patient's health and in public safety.

Some medical conditions can produce hypersomnolence and fatigue, such as hypothyroidism. In addition, misalignment of the circadian rhythm (discussed in detail in Chapter 23) with a patient's behavioral schedule can also produce daytime sleepiness. For example, a teenager whose brain would prefer to be asleep from 1 am until 9 am will certainly experience somnolence if the teenager's first class in the morning starts at 8 am. Mood disorders, such as depression, can present with complaints such as lack of energy and anhedonia,

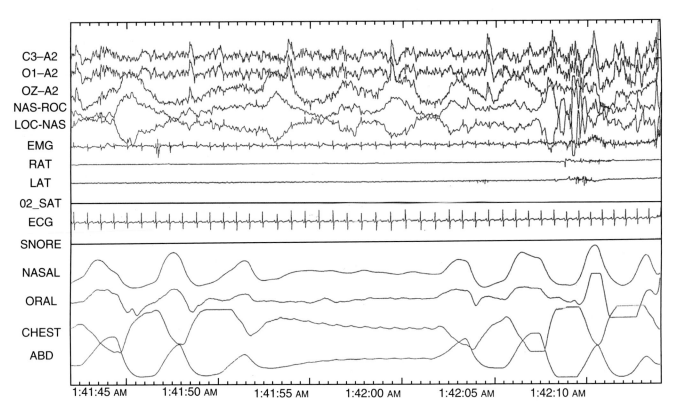

FIGURE 34–4 Central apnea. During the apneic episodes, there is lack of airflow without rib cage or abdominal motion. At the end of each apneic episode there is a burst of electroencephalogram (EEG) activity consistent with an arousal. The polysomnography traces from the top down are as follows: 3 EEG channels (C3–A2, O1–A2, OZ–A2); 2 EOG channels (NAS-ROC and LOC-NAS); submental electromyogram (EMG); right and left anterior tibialis EMG (RAT and LAT); oxyhemoglobin saturation (O2_SAT); electrocardiogram (ECG); snoring channel (SNORE); nasal airflow (NASAL); oral thermistor (ORAL); and chest and abdominal motion (CHEST and ABD). (Reproduced with permission from Grippi MA, Elias JA, Fishman JA, et al: *Fishman's Pulmonary Diseases and Disorders*, 5th ed. New York, NY:McGraw Hill; 2015.)

which often may be mistaken for sleepiness. Finally, sleep disorders that affect sleep at night, as in the sleep-disordered breathing conditions discussed earlier, can clearly produce daytime sleepiness.

Hypersomnias

Once a careful history and medical examination have ruled out common causes of sleepiness, sleep laboratory evaluation, as discussed earlier, is indicated. In the absence of nocturnal sleep disorders (or when other nocturnal sleep disorders are well controlled), excessive daytime sleepiness as measured by the MSLT falls into 2 main disorders: narcolepsy and idiopathic hypersomnia. The differentiation between these disorders is made based on the presence or absence of REM during daytime naps on the MSLT.

Narcolepsy

Narcolepsy is characterized by a clinical tetrad of symptoms: (1) excessive daytime sleepiness, (2) hypnagogic or hypnopompic hallucinations, (3) sleep paralysis, and (4) cataplexy. Hypnagogic and hypnopompic hallucinations are often visual disturbances that happen at sleep onset or sleep offset,

respectively. Sleep paralysis is the experience of waking from sleep and being unable to move one's limbs or to otherwise communicate, typically lasting <1 minute. Finally, cataplexy is the sudden onset of loss of muscle tone, typically triggered by humor or other emotion. It is important to note that narcolepsy can be found either with or without cataplexy. However, of these 4 cardinal symptoms, cataplexy is the only symptom that is specific to narcolepsy. The other 3 can all be found in a myriad of other disorders that cause disruptions at night, in sleep deprivation, or even in rare isolated episodes in a normal patient.

A neuroanatomic basis for narcolepsy with cataplexy has been identified. Investigations of animal models identified a neuropeptide called orexin found in the lateral hypothalamus that is responsible for the excessive sleepiness and cataplexy found in this disorder. Further investigations in human patients found that orexin is undetectable in the cerebrospinal fluid of patients with narcolepsy with cataplexy. However, only 1 patient has been identified with a direct genetic mutation in this protein or its receptors. Several lines of evidence point to a possible autoimmune cause for this rare disorder. Conversely, idiopathic hypersomnia does not have as clear a neuroanatomical basis.

Treatment of Hypersomnia

Idiopathic hypersomnia and narcolepsy share the same treatments with a few exceptions. Commonly used medications to treat excessive daytime sleepiness include modafinil and armodafinil, which work by preventing dopamine reuptake in the synapse, increasing the levels of this wake-promoting neurotransmitter. Amphetamine, dextroamphetamine, and methylphenidate all work by blocking the reuptake of dopamine, serotonin, and norepinephrine.

One medication used uniquely in narcolepsy with cataplexy is sodium oxybate. This is an agonist of the GABAergic system that enhances inhibition in the brain. Sodium oxybate is taken at night; it enhances sleep and reduces excessive sleepiness in narcoleptic patients. In addition, although it has a very short half-life, sodium oxybate can have dramatic effects on a patient's cataplexy during the daytime as well. Other medications that can reduce cataplexy include selective norepinephrine reuptake inhibitors and selective serotonin reuptake inhibitors (eg, venlafaxine or fluoxetine).

Restless Legs Syndrome & Periodic Limb Movements

Another subset of sleep disorders involves the sensory and motor systems of the limbs. Restless legs syndrome (RLS; also known as Willis-Ekbom disease) is a sensory phenomenon that has several characteristic features to distinguish it from other sensory disorders. In this condition, sensations (patients may describe pain, numbness, tingling, or even just the need to move) are present at rest or during periods of inactivity, are worse at night, and are relieved by movement. RLS can be a primary disorder, or it can be found secondarily to other medical conditions. The most common causes of secondary RLS are neuropathy, iron deficiency, end-stage renal disease or pregnancy.

In contrast, periodic limb movements of sleep (PLMS) are stereotypical leg movements characterized by flexion at the hip and knee and dorsiflexion of the ankle occurring during sleep. In some cases, these limb movements go unnoticed by the patient, and in others, they can cause significant arousals, disrupted sleep, and daytime sleepiness. RLS and PLMS often overlap, with 80% of patients with RLS demonstrating PLMS, but just 20% of patients with PLMS experiencing the symptoms of RLS.

Treatments for these 2 conditions overlap as well. One category of medications used is D_2 dopamine receptor agonists, including pramipexole and ropinirole. In contrast to their use in Parkinson disease, these medications are typically given at lower doses for RLS/PLMS and only once a day at bedtime, targeted to the time of symptom occurrence. Another dopaminergic option is rotigotine, available in a once-daily transdermal patch. The second category of medications that have proven useful in these disorders are the $\alpha_2\delta$ calcium channel ligands gabapentin enacarbil and pregabalin. When these agents have failed, other effective treatments

that have been described include benzodiazepines, opioid agents, clonidine, and carbidopa/levodopa. However, these choices are supported by less experimental evidence and have a greater risk of side effects than either class of first-line agents.

Parasomnias

Parasomnias are a broad category of disorders that encompass abnormal behaviors during sleep. They can be benign, or they can be signs of an underlying disorder. There are parasomnias that are more common in children or more common in adults. Another categorization of parasomnias is derived from what stage of sleep they commonly arise from—non-REM or REM sleep. These disorders are described in the following paragraphs.

Hypnic jerks, or hypnagogic myoclonus, are brief sudden movements that occur at sleep onset. They are typically associated with the sensation of kicking or falling. These are benign and common but should be differentiated from myoclonic seizures, which can occur throughout the night.

Sleep walking is a non-REM parasomnia that is far more common in children than adults. It is also a benign condition, although it can lead to sleep-related injury, for instance falling down the stairs. Typically, these episodes are rare and go away as the child ages. Sleep walking in adults can be associated with other sleep disorders that produce frequent nocturnal arousals (eg, OSA), and thus may trigger further evaluation. In addition, medications such as zolpidem can trigger such episodes. Treatment includes adjusting medications that could be the cause, securing the bedroom environment for potential hazards, using bed alarms that go off to alert others that the patient is out of bed, and preventing access to stairs with a door lock or gate. In rare cases, pharmacologic treatment may be indicated, the most common of which is a benzodiazepine such as clonazepam.

Night terrors are a non-REM parasomnia that typically occur in the pediatric population. These episodes typically arise from stage N3 sleep and are associated with the child arising from sleep, crying, and appearing upset and inconsolable. The child does not interact normally with the environment or the caregiver who enters, and this can last for several minutes, ending with the child returning to sleep. The patient does not remember these episodes. Typically, these resolve late in childhood. Other than reassurance and avoiding sleep deprivation, which can make these episodes more common, no treatment is typically indicated.

Confusional arousals are very similar to night terrors, in that they are another non-REM parasomnia that arise from stage N3 sleep. These are more common in children than adults and are characterized by periods of diminished responsiveness, disorientation, and inability to be redirected. To an outside observer, the patient appears to be awake but is not acting normally. The episodes typically last minutes but can be much longer, and as with night terrors, the patient is amnestic for these events. These episodes can be exacerbated by many factors: sleep deprivation, shift work, alcohol, and stress. When found in adults, a sleep study is indicated to evaluate for another sleep disorder, such as sleep apnea or PLMS, that could potentially be provoking these episodes.

Nightmares are a REM-associated parasomnia that occur more commonly in children than adults. Typically, reassurance is all that is needed to treat nightmares for most sufferers, young and old. However, in patients with posttraumatic stress disorder, nightmares may occur so frequently that they contribute to the patient's insomnia, insufficient sleep, and daytime fatigue. When nightmares are contributing to such morbidity, there are treatment options. One is imagery rehearsal therapy, where the patient is asked to write out the nightmare and then rescript the ending to a happier, less distressing one. The patient then "rehearses" the rescripted dream each night before bedtime. Another option is pharmacotherapy with the α_1-adrenergic antagonist prazosin. Studies have demonstrated that, taken nightly, this medication reduces nightmare frequency dramatically and reduces the distress that any remaining nightmares have.

REM sleep behavior disorder (RBD), as the name implies, is a REM sleep–associated parasomnia in which patients act out their dreams. It is more common in men than women, and peak incidence is in the elderly. As mentioned earlier, a key feature of REM sleep is atonia, or the paralysis of the muscles of the arms and legs. In this condition, that aspect of REM sleep is impaired, and thus, the patient moves and acts out while he or she is asleep. Frequently, the patient's actions include violent behavior, such as kicking and punching, along with shouting, lasting up to several minutes. Upon awakening, the patient is not aware of what happened in the room but may be able to recall a dream in which he or she was fighting off an attacker. The risk of this condition includes sleep-related injury to the patient or the patient's bed partner. A sleep study is indicated for patients with this presentation, because there is a phenomenon termed *pseudo-RBD*, where episodes of dream enactment are triggered by other disruptions in REM sleep, such as those seen in sleep-disordered breathing.

Studies have shown that RBD is associated with several neurodegenerative conditions discussed in Chapter 29. In the case of Parkinson disease and dementia with Lewy bodies, RBD is likely to precede the motor manifestations and diagnosis of these conditions by years. With multiple systems atrophy, another condition characterized by the abnormal inclusions of α-synuclein, RBD typically develops at the same time as the motor symptoms. Studies have indicated that the atonia-producing centers in the brainstem may be involved in these conditions, giving rise to this problem in these patients.

Treatment of this disorder is typically with clonazepam 0.5 to 1.5 mg nightly at bedtime. If that fails or in a patient with a higher concern of increased falls or the cognitive side effects of clonazepam, melatonin at bedtime has also been described as effective in several case reports and series.

Nocturnal enuresis is a common sleep disorder in children. The child must be at least 6 years old for this diagnosis to apply. This can be divided into primary enuresis (a child who has never been dry for >6 months) or secondary enuresis (when bed wetting occurs after the child has been dry for ≥6 months). Primary enuresis is far more common (85% of cases) and is less likely to be associated with pathologic conditions. Most primary enuresis resolves on its own as the child ages (at a rate of about 15% per year). First-line treatment is behavioral adaptation, avoiding drinking at bedtime, and avoiding substances that can increase urine output (most commonly caffeine). Other treatments include moisture alarms on the bed and, at times, the use of desmopressin, a synthetic antidiuretic hormone analog, which can be administered orally or as a nasal spray.

SLEEP PHARMACOLOGY

In addition to the many agents discussed earlier in the context of sleep disorders, it is important for healthcare providers be familiar with the effects of over-the-counter agents on sleep and wake, as well as the medications commonly used as sleep aids.

Nonprescription Substances That Affect Sleep–Wake Regulation

Caffeine

Caffeine is the most widely self-administered agent to enhance daytime alertness. It has been shown in many studies to suppress sleep in both humans and animal models. Pharmacologically, caffeine is an antagonist at the adenosine receptor. Thus, it serves to block the sleep-promoting properties of this neurotransmitter. Although caffeine is a nonselective adenosine antagonist, it has been shown that it is the A_{2A} adenosine receptors that mediate the wake-promoting effects of this substance. The half-life of caffeine is between 5 and 6 hours, so caffeine ingested in the early afternoon can still be exerting its effects on a patient's sleep at bedtime. In addition to the most common beverages that come to mind (eg, coffee, tea, caffeinated soft drinks), chocolate also contains a significant amount of caffeine that can contribute to difficulty getting to sleep. Aside from the wake-promoting effects of caffeine, it can also disrupt sleep by contributing to the symptoms of patients with RLS.

Ethanol

Ethanol exerts its chemical effects as an agonist of GABA receptors, enhancing inhibitory transmission. This can decrease sleep latency but also has potent effects later in the night, making its use as a sleep aid counterproductive. Ethanol increases nocturnal arousals and suppresses REM sleep. In addition, alcohol makes snoring worse and makes OSA more severe as well. Ethanol is another substance that exacerbates RLS. Using alcohol to get to sleep has been identified as an important risk factor for the development of alcohol dependence and thus should be avoided.

Diphenhydramine

The active ingredient in most over-the-counter sleep aids is diphenhydramine. The mechanism of action is through the blockade of histamine receptors at the H_1 receptor. It can be very effective at reducing sleep onset latency but has many caveats. First, it has been shown to exacerbate snoring, sleep apnea, and RLS, just like ethanol. Second, diphenhydramine has strong anticholinergic side effects (ie, urinary retention, constipation, and detrimental effects on cognition). For this reason, over-the-counter sleep aids should largely be avoided by the elderly.

Commonly Used Prescription Sleep Aids

Nonbenzodiazepine GABA Agonists

This category of medications includes zolpidem, zopiclone, and zaleplon. They all work to reduce sleep onset latency. As the category name implies, these agents work at GABA receptors but not at the same molecular site as benzodiazepines. This is thought to underlie their improved side effect profile and the reduced risk of habit formation that comes with these medications. All of these agents may increase somnolence in the morning after taking them, especially if they are taken later in the night, and this may increase the risk of accidents from drowsy driving the morning after administration. Zolpidem is associated with the side effect of parasomnias, such as sleep walking or sleep eating. It is important to note that US Food and Drug Administration (FDA) approval for these agents is limited to short-term usage (2 to 4 weeks); however, they are often prescribed to patients for months or years. There is always a risk of developing tolerance over time, causing an agent to lose its effectiveness.

Benzodiazepines

This class of medications remains widely prescribed as sleep aids. The most commonly used examples are triazolam and temazepam. These medications have a worse side effect profile than the nonbenzodiazepine GABA agonists, with an increased risk of falls and cognitive side effects, particularly in the elderly. They also have a greater potential for dependence and abuse. In addition, benzodiazepines suppress respiratory drive, and thus can exacerbate snoring and sleep apnea. However, due to their anxiolytic properties, they are still commonly used as sleep aids when the goal is to treat both problems with a single agent. Often, one will encounter benzodiazepines with a longer half-life prescribed as sleep

aids in off-label use. This enhances the risk of side effects and prolonged drowsiness into the morning and should be avoided.

Antidepressants

Because of the frequent comorbid conditions of mood disorders and insomnia, sedating antidepressants are commonly used at bedtime to attempt to ease the patient's sleep difficulties while also treating the mood disorder. One class of medications in this category are the tricyclic compounds, including amitriptyline and nortriptyline. The limitation of these agents is their potent anticholinergic effects. Another tricyclic used in sleep is low-dose doxepin, which is believed to exert its primary effect at these doses as a histamine H_1 receptor blocker. Trazodone, whose mechanisms are more poorly defined, is another antidepressant often used off label as a sleep aid. One advantage of this agent is that it does not have anticholinergic side effects. Thus, it is often applied short term in the inpatient setting, where delirium caused by the abrupt initiation of effective doses of other agents is a potential consequence.

Orexin Antagonists

Suvorexant, the only medication currently in this category, works as an antagonist at both receptors for orexin, the OX_1 and OX_2 receptors. Much like many of the previously mentioned agents, this agent can be associated with continued hypersomnolence in the morning in a dose-dependent manner. Suvorexant has also been approved for short-term use in insomnia.

Melatonin Receptor Agonists

Ramelteon is the only agent available in this category and exerts its effects as an agonist at the melatonin MT_1 and MT_2 receptors. It is 1 of the few sleep aids with FDA approval for use for a longer term than 2 to 4 weeks. In addition, it has a better side effect profile and can be used in patients in whom the increased risks of cognitive side effects and of falls associated with most other agents are unacceptable.

CONCLUSION

In summary, sleep is a physiologic process that is vital to daytime behavior and performance, and that exhibits a homeostatic drive to replace a deficiency in the past with an increase in the future. It is an important aspect of the patient's health that is often overlooked when we focus on the patient's daytime symptomology, yet it has important implications for both normal functioning and in pathologic states. An understanding of common sleep disorders and their treatment provides an important tool to help physicians ameliorate the cause of the patient's morbidity and potentially identify the warning signs of other conditions.

CASE 34-1

A 66-year-old man with type 2 diabetes mellitus, hypertension, known obstructive sleep apnea, reflux, arthritis, vitamin B_{12} deficiency, and depression, who is on continuous positive airway pressure (CPAP), presents with complaints of difficulty falling asleep that has persisted for years.

His troubles began over 10 years ago, when he retired from work. He lost his typical sleep–wake routine and exhausting work schedule and began staying up later and sleeping during the day. He leads a sedentary lifestyle. He gets into bed around midnight or later and can lie there for hours. He has a very active mind, and this often prevents him from falling asleep. In addition, he reports that while awake, when he lies still, his legs jerk. Rarely, this can involve his arms as well. He endorses the "need to move," and if he stands and walks, this jerking goes away and the need to move temporarily subsides. This sensation is present whenever he is inactive but is much worse at night as he is trying to fall asleep and is present on a nightly basis.

He uses his CPAP every night. Once he does get to sleep, he wakes up several times a night for unknown reasons. He awakens after 3 to 4 hours of sleep and feels unrefreshed. He states that he feels tired all day and falls asleep when he is sitting still, for instance when watching TV or reading, even when these activities involve his favorite subjects. He denies drowsy driving.

His initial sleep study was 4 years prior to his evaluation. It demonstrated moderate sleep apnea, with an apnea-hypopnea index of 24 events per hour. CPAP of 9 cm H_2O was shown to be effective. Given his continued complaints of poor-quality sleep and daytime sleepiness, an attempt was made to get a repeat sleep study, but he only slept for 15 minutes.

He reports that his previous physician prescribed trials of ropinirole and pramipexole in the past for his legs, both of which caused both nausea and visual hallucinations at effective doses. He has also tried several sleep aids in the past, including zolpidem and zaleplon, without getting any relief.

His current medications are Actos (pioglitazone), metformin, Cozaar (losartan), furosemide, aspirin, Synthroid (levothyroxine), Allegra (fexofenadine), Prevacid (lansoprazole), a multivitamin, and iron 325 mg daily.

Examination is notable for a body mass index of 35 kg/m², difficulty visualizing the soft palate, and marked macroglossia. Neurologic exam shows decreased vibration at the ankles bilaterally. Otherwise, the exam is within normal limits.

Discussion

This patient seems to have 3 common sleep disorders. The first is obstructive sleep apnea (OSA). In addition, he describes insomnia, which is difficulty falling or staying asleep. It is very common for patients to describe difficulty turning off their thoughts at night. Finally, restless legs syndrome (RLS; or Willis-Ekbom disease) also appears to be playing a role in his inability to fall asleep.

Thus, the plan for this patient should be designed to address these 3 conditions. From the perspective of his OSA, he states he is using his CPAP nightly. A repeat polysomnogram should be arranged to verify the effectiveness of his current CPAP, because if his OSA is insufficiently treated, this could be contributing to his disrupted sleep and daytime sleepiness. Second, follow-up with a psychologist should be arranged for cognitive-behavioral therapy for insomnia. It is not uncommon for insomnia medications to fail, and behavioral therapy has been shown to be as equally effective as medications. Third, since the patient failed dopamine agonist therapy for RLS in the past, he should be prescribed gabapentin enacarbil nightly for his restless legs.

Outcome

After the treatment plan was instituted, the patient returned to clinic about 2 months later. He told his physician that he had cancelled both the appointment for the sleep study and the consultation with the psychologist. Once an effective dose of the gabapentin enacarbil was achieved, he noted an immediate change in his sleep quantity and quality and a decrease in his daytime sleepiness. With his leg symptoms controlled, he was falling asleep easier, regularly at around 11 pm; getting 6 to 7 hours of sleep; and feeling far less sleepy during the day.

SELF-ASSESSMENT QUESTIONS

1. A 22-year-old patient presents to your clinic with several complaints. He states that he is sleepy all of the time, and his course work in college is suffering because of his inability to stay awake during class or exams. He has episodes when he wakes up during sleep and sees thing in the room that are not there. He also has periods when he wakes from sleep and cannot move his arms or legs. He noticed an episode last week where he could not stand up or keep his eyes open for several minutes after his roommate told him a joke. His disorder is associated with a reduction of neurons containing which neurotransmitter?

   A. Norepinephrine
   B. Orexin
   C. Vasopressin
   D. Enkephalin
   E. Serotonin

2. For the past 3 months, a 72-year-old man has had episodes during sleep in which he exhibits violent behaviors, including kicking his bed partner and shouting out. He appears to be asleep

or confused during these episodes. He is unable to recall what happened in the room, but he reports having dreams of fighting off an attacker on the nights that these episodes take place. Which of the following disorders is most likely to develop years later in this patient?

A. Amyotrophic lateral sclerosis
B. Schizophrenia
C. Obstructive sleep apnea (OSA)
D. Parkinson disease
E. Cataplexy

3. A 53-year-old woman reports over 5 year of abnormal sensations in her legs occurring mostly in the evening when she is trying to fall asleep. She describes the sensations as "crawling and tingling" in her calves. If she stands up and walks around, she gets immediate relief, but the symptoms recur when she lies down. The symptoms are becoming progressively more severe and are quite disruptive to her sleep. Her neurologic examination is normal. Which of the following additional clinical features or findings would most likely be present in this patient?

A. Hepatic dysfunction
B. Iron deficiency
C. Loud snoring
D. Polycythemia
E. Somnambulism

4. Which of the following is an electroencephalogram (EEG) characteristic that helps define stage N2 sleep?

A. Posterior occipital sharp transients
B. Delta activity
C. K complexes
D. Alpha rhythm
E. Sawtooth waves

Pediatric Neurology

Lydia Marcus

- Identify various neural tube defects and their associated congenital malformations.
- Understand the genetic defects and clinical presentations of neurogenetic syndromes.
- Identify the underlying pathophysiology, clinical presentation, and treatment for a variety of metabolic disorders.
- Appreciate the difference between dysmyelinating and demyelinating disorders.
- Understand the clinical manifestations of common pediatric epilepsy syndromes.

PREVALENCE & BURDEN

Pediatric neurology encompasses a vast array of disorders spanning all subspecialties of neurology, yet the pathophysiology, diagnosis, and treatment of neurologic disorders in children are often unique and require special attention. Although as a whole, pediatric neurologic disorders are less prevalent and burdensome than neurologic disorders in the adult population, they are nonetheless an important cause of chronic morbidity in children.

The most common chronic pediatric neurologic disorder is pediatric epilepsy, occurring in 0.5% to 1% of the pediatric population and accounting for approximately 15% of all epilepsy patients. The cost of pediatric epilepsy in the United States is approximately $20,000 per child in the first year after diagnosis. Cerebral palsy (CP) is the most common developmental disability in children, with a prevalence of 2 to 3 per 1000 children and occurring at an incidence between 8,000 and 10,000 children per year. The lifetime economic cost of CP in the United States has been estimated to be almost $1 million per child.

Although individually they are extremely rare, the wide array of metabolic disorders or inborn errors of metabolism have a collective incidence of 1 in 800 to 2500 births per year. Despite a low prevalence at approximately 0.3%, they account for 3.5% of neonatal deaths, indicating a disproportionately high mortality rate due to these disorders. Congenital anomalies have an even higher mortality rate, accounting for 17% to 42% of neonatal deaths worldwide, or 300,000 infants every year. Early detection and treatment of pediatric neurologic disorders are essential to reduce both the mortality and morbidity of these disorders.

CONGENITAL MALFORMATIONS

The neural tube, which is the precursor of the central nervous system in the embryo, forms during the process of neurulation in the third and fourth weeks of development. A **neural tube defect** occurs when there is incomplete closure of the neural tube during this process. There are many forms of neural tube defects, which are differentiated based on the location and severity of the defect and protrusion of underlying tissues. The mildest forms of hindbrain anomalies are spina bifida occulta and spina bifida cystica, in which there is a protrusion of tissue through the defect. In **spina bifida occulta,** there is simply a failure of the vertebral arches to fuse. This defect can occur anywhere along the spine but usually occurs in the lumbar region. There can often be an overlying tuft of hair, dermal sinus, dimple, or skin tag, but otherwise, it is asymptomatic. This defect is relatively common, affecting up to 24% of the population. If there is an associated underlying spinal cord malformation, the defect is considered an occult spinal dysraphism. In a **meningocele**, there is herniation of

VOCABULARY

Cerebral palsy/static encephalopathy: A permanent and nonprogressive disability resulting from brain damage before, during, or shortly after birth, often involving motor or speech impairment.

Congenital: Existing at or dating from birth; acquired during intrauterine development rather than inherited.

Congenital myopathy: A muscle disorder present at birth, involving a defect in a muscle protein.

Cryptogenic: Of obscure or unknown origin.

Genotype: The genetic code responsible for a particular trait.

Holoprosencephaly: A disorder caused by the failure of the embryonic forebrain to sufficiently divide into 2 cerebral hemispheres, leading to defects in both brain and facial structures.

Hydrocephalus: A condition of abnormal accumulation of cerebrospinal fluid in the ventricles of the brain, which can lead to macrocephaly and potentially brain damage.

Hypertonia: The presence of increased muscle tone, or excessive resistance to stretch in a muscle.

Hypotonia: The presence of low muscle tone, or low resistance to stretch in a muscle.

Leukodystrophy: A group of disorders characterized by degeneration of myelin in the brain, spinal cord, and peripheral nerves; also known as dysmyelinating disorders.

Lissencephaly: A neuronal migration disorder involving a smooth cerebral cortex with few or no convolutions.

Meningocele: A protrusion of the meninges through a defect in the skull or the spinal column, forming a cyst filled with cerebrospinal fluid.

Muscular dystrophy: A hereditary condition involving progressive muscular wasting, characterized by degeneration of muscle fibers and usually involving a deficiency of a muscle protein.

Pachygyria: A congenital brain malformation involving unusually thick, broad, and few gyri; considered to be a form of incomplete lissencephaly.

Phenotype: The physical expression or characteristics of a particular trait.

Semiology: The study of signs; in epilepsy, it refers to clinical signs and other aspects of the clinical presentation of a seizure.

Spasticity: A velocity-dependent increase in muscle tone in response to passive movement.

Spina bifida: A congenital cleft or incomplete closure of the neural tube during embryonic development, resulting in a protrusion of the meninges and/or the spinal cord.

Syringomyelia: A chronic progressive disease due to longitudinal cyst formation in the spinal cord, leading primarily to weakness and numbness of the upper extremities.

---

the underlying meninges (but not the spinal cord) through the defect. In the most severe form of hindbrain anomaly, **myelomeningocele**, both the meninges and spinal cord protrude through the defect into an external sac. This defect is almost always symptomatic, with paralysis and sensory loss below the level of the defect.

Forebrain anomalies are more variable than hindbrain anomalies and include anencephaly, holoprosencephaly, septooptic dysplasia, and agenesis of the corpus callosum. The most severe forebrain anomaly is **anencephaly**, which arises from a complete failure of the anterior neural tube to close in the third and fourth weeks of development. In this anomaly, there is a defect in the scalp, skull, and meninges with absence of both cerebral hemispheres. This defect is often noted on second-trimester ultrasound and can be confirmed prior to delivery with elevated α-fetoprotein levels in the amniotic fluid. Infants with anencephaly are either stillborn or die shortly after birth.

In **holoprosencephaly**, there is a failure of the prosencephalon (embryonic forebrain) to separate into cerebral hemispheres. This defect can have varying severity depending on the degree of the separation failure. Alobar holoprosencephaly is the most severe form, in which there is only a single cerebral structure. In semilobar holoprosencephaly, there is posterior cleavage, but the lobes are severely underdeveloped. In lobar holoprosencephaly, the least severe form, the frontal lobes are often well developed but other cerebral defects such as agenesis of the corpus callosum, cleft lip or palate, or facial anomalies (cyclopsia, single central incisor) are present.

Septo-optic dysplasia, another midline defect, involves hypoplasia of the optic nerves, hypothalamus, and pituitary glands. It is often associated with other midline anomalies such as agenesis of the corpus callosum or septum pellucidum, as well as blindness, seizures, and intellectual disability. **Agenesis of the corpus callosum** arises from disruption of porencephalic segmentation between 10 and 12 weeks of gestation. There can be varying degrees of agenesis, from complete to partial, in which there is only thinning or segmental loss of the corpus callosum. This defect is often associated with Chiari II malformations, as well as multiple genetic and metabolic syndromes.

Congenital microcephaly is defined as an occipitofrontal circumference (OFC) <2 to 3 standard deviations below the mean for gestational/chronologic age and sex. This disorder can arise from multiple etiologies, including fetal alcohol syndrome, TORCH infections (toxoplasmosis, other [syphilis, varicella-zoster, parvovirus B19], rubella, cytomegalovirus, and herpes), maternal radiation or toxin exposure, familial microcephaly, trisomy and deletion syndromes, neural tube defects, or metabolic disorders. It is usually associated with cognitive impairment, but up to 7.5% of children with microcephaly have normal intelligence.

Macrocephaly, generally defined as an OFC >2 standard deviations above the mean, also has many different etiologies. The most common cause is benign familial macrocephaly, often suggested by above average parental head circumference. Macrocephaly can also be associated with neurocutaneous disorders, leukodystrophies, infections (meningitis, abscess, and subdural effusion), hydrocephalus, fragile X, metabolic diseases (maple syrup disease, lysosomal storage diseases, mucopolysaccharidoses, Tay-Sachs disease), and toxins (vitamin A, lead, tetracyclines).

In **lissencephaly**, a disorder of neuronal migration, the surface of the cerebral cortex is smooth with no gyri and sulci. Additionally, the cerebral cortex is thicker than normal, but with only 4 primitive neuronal layers rather than the typical 6 layers. When a few primary gyri and sulci are present, the disorder is known as **pachygyria**. Lissencephaly is associated with microcephaly, polyhydramnios, facial anomalies, severe intellectual disability, and seizures.

Posterior fossa malformations include Chiari type I and type II malformations and Dandy-Walker syndrome. In the Chiari

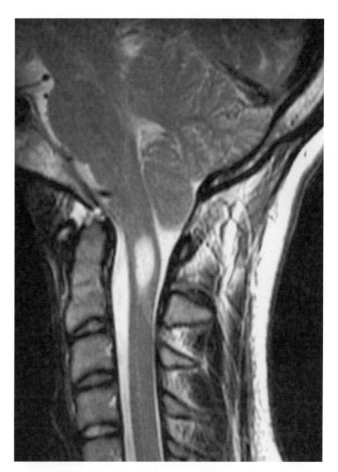

FIGURE 35–1 Chiari-type malformation and developmental syringomyelia. T2-weighted magnetic resonance imaging of the low-lying cerebellar tonsils below the foramen magnum and behind the upper cervical cord and the syrinx cavity in the upper cord. (Reproduced with permission from Ropper AH, Samuels MA, Klein JP: *Adams and Victor's Principles of Neurology*, 11th ed. New York, NY: McGraw Hill; 2019.)

CASE 35–1

An 11-year-old boy is referred to a pediatric neurologist for bilateral arm numbness and weakness. He has complained of numbness and pain in both arms for a few months, primarily in his shoulders. Over the past few weeks, he has had trouble raising his arms above his head, and his parents have noticed he frequently drops objects. He often complains of posterior headaches and neck pain. His parents report that he sometimes chokes on his food and snores when he sleeps. He was adopted from China at the age of 2 years, and there are no medical records prior to adoption, but his parents were told he had a "back surgery" soon after birth. He was daytime potty trained at age 3 years but continued to wet the bed regularly until the age of 6. His physical exam is significant for decreased sensation in bilateral arms to temperature, anodynia in his shoulders, and 4/5 strength in all muscle groups in both arms. He has mild dysmetria with finger to nose testing bilaterally and nystagmus on horizontal far gaze. His neurologist orders a magnetic resonance imaging scan, which reveals the image shown in **Figure 35–1**.

The patient is diagnosed with a Chiari II malformation with an associated syrinx. The "back surgery" in infancy was most likely to correct a myelomeningocele, the neural tube defect associated with this malformation. His symptoms of arm pain, numbness, and weakness are due to the syrinx, as expansion of the central canal of the spinal cord causes a cape-like distribution of numbness, pain, and eventually weakness. Herniation of the cerebellar tonsils can cause nystagmus, ataxia, and dysmetria. Compression and elongation of the medulla can cause dysphagia, dysarthria, and obstructive sleep apnea. If severe enough, treatment involves occipital decompressive surgery to relieve compression of the brainstem.

malformations, there is a skull defect causing displacement (at least 5 mm) of the cerebellar tonsils into the foramen magnum. This displacement can lead to blockage of the flow of cerebrospinal fluid (CSF), which in turn can lead to a **syrinx** or **syringomyelia**, a fluid-filled cyst within the spinal cord. **Chiari type II** malformation is the more common form, with associated myelomeningocele in addition to the displacement of the cerebellum and medulla into the cervical canal. The upper medulla and lower pons are often elongated and thinned. The malformation is typically associated with hydrocephalus and aqueductal stenosis, as well as cortical dysgenesis or bony anomalies in a large majority of patients. **Chiari type I** is a milder malformation, with only an elongated but not displaced medulla and no associated myelomeningocele. This malformation is often asymptomatic, although patients can complain of headache, neck pain, ataxia, dysphagia, and nystagmus (Figure 35–1).

Dandy-Walker syndrome is characterized by cerebellar vermis hypoplasia with cystic dilatation of the fourth ventricle. An elevated tentorium, hydrocephalus, and agenesis of the corpus callosum are also commonly seen in this syndrome.

Symptoms include lethargy, vomiting, cranial neuropathies, ataxia, and incoordination (Figure 35–2).

Congenital hydrocephalus is caused by excessive accumulation of CSF in the ventricular system, which causes increased intracranial pressure and eventually ventricular

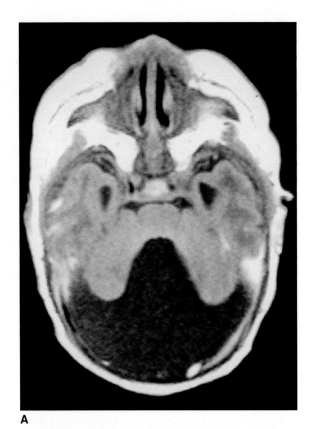

A

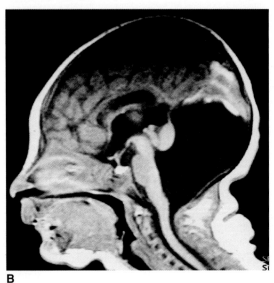

B

FIGURE 35–2 Dandy-Walker syndrome. Magnetic resonance imaging showing agenesis of the midline cerebellum and large midline cyst, representing the greatly dilated fourth ventricle, which occupies almost the entire posterior fossa. **A.** Axial view. **B.** Sagittal view. (Reproduced with permission from Ropper AH, Samuels MA, Klein JP: *Adams and Victor's Principles of Neurology*, 11th ed. New York, NY: McGraw Hill; 2019.)

dilatation. The disorder can be divided into the **communicating** form (impaired absorption of CSF by arachnoid granulations) and the **noncommunicating** form (structural blockage of CSF circulation, usually due to aqueductal stenosis). Hydrocephalus has many varied etiologies, including malformations (especially Chiari type II), familial aqueductal stenosis, infection, neoplasm, hemorrhage, or vascular malformation. It can be asymptomatic if mild, with the more severe forms presenting with macrocephaly, irritability, poor feeding, spasticity, headache, seizures, ataxia, and visual disturbances.

Static encephalopathy and **cerebral palsy** are both terms used to describe brain damage sustained pre-, peri-, or postnatally, causing a nonprogressive neuromotor impairment. For an impairment to qualify as CP, it must be diagnosed by age 2, and the child must have stable nonprogressive symptoms; some mild forms may show improvement at later ages. In more severe forms of CP, multiple comorbidities can be seen, including intellectual disability, epilepsy, speech/language deficits, vision/hearing deficits, behavioral problems, and autism spectrum disorder. Etiologies of CP include prematurity, hypoxic-ischemic encephalopathy (HIE), infections, genetic disorders, and malformations. CP can be classified into 3 major groups defined by motor impairment: spastic, athetoid/dyskinetic, and hypotonic/ataxic. Spastic CP can be further divided based on which limbs are affected. In **spastic diplegia/paraplegia**, there is weakness in all extremities but more so in the legs than in the arms. This is the most common form of CP and usually not associated with speech or cognitive impairment. In **spastic hemiplegia**, there is weakness primarily on one side of the body. This type is often due to perinatal stroke or hemorrhage and is frequently associated with focal seizures, and children will typically walk. The most severe form of spastic CP is **spastic quadriplegia**, which involves weakness in all 4 extremities and is usually associated with severe developmental delay, speech impairment, and seizures. **Athetoid/dyskinetic CP** is caused by basal ganglia lesions from kernicterus or HIE and causes dystonia, athetosis, and chorea, which are often very difficult to manage. Because kernicterus is becoming less common in neonates with better early management of hyperbilirubinemia, this is becoming a rarer form of CP. The least common form of CP is **ataxic/hypotonic CP**, which is associated with a cerebellar malformation. Clinical features include ataxia, hypotonia with hyperactive reflexes, cognitive impairment, tremor, dysarthria, abnormal eye movements, and episodic apnea.

NEUROGENETIC SYNDROMES

Many genetic syndromes have neurologic sequelae, ranging from mild intellectual disability or developmental delay to epilepsy, brain malformations, and ataxia. This section aims to review the most common and well-recognized neurogenetic syndromes presenting in pediatric patients, specifically with regard to their neurologic deficits.

Trisomies are all genetically characterized by an extra copy of a particular chromosome. Although trisomy can occur with any chromosome, in most cases, the result is lethal and the pregnancy does not result in a live birth. The 3 most common autosomal (nonsex) trisomies that result in live births are trisomy 21 (also known as Down syndrome), trisomy 18 (Edward syndrome), and trisomy 13 (Patau syndrome).

Both **Edward syndrome** and **Patau syndrome** are relatively rare, and although infants are often viable at birth, their life expectancy is generally a few months to a year. They are both clinically characterized by severe mental retardation, rocker bottom feet, and microcephaly, with Edward syndrome infants exhibiting a long, narrow head and clenched fists and Patau syndrome infants often exhibiting holoprosencephaly, cleft lip or palate, polydactyly, and congenital cardiac defects.

Down syndrome is the most common chromosomal abnormality, as well as the most common cause of congenital intellectual disability. The risk of Down syndrome increases significantly with advanced maternal age (over age 35 years); however, the majority of infants with Down syndrome are born to mothers under the age of 35 years. Down syndrome is typically due to trisomy 21, although it can also be the result of nonreciprocal translocation or mosaicism. Prenatal screening of maternal serum can be done with the "quad screen"; low α-fetoprotein and estriol levels together with elevated β-human chorionic gonadotropin and inhibin A levels suggest Down syndrome. Prenatal ultrasound will often demonstrate increased nuchal translucency. Definitive testing is done by cytogenetic analysis of amniotic fluid or infant blood after birth.

Clinically, Down syndrome is characterized by prominent epicanthal folds, a single palmar crease (previously known as a simian crease), flat facies, an open mouth with a protruding fissured tongue, low hairline, redundant neck tissue, short stature, obesity, hypotonia, and intellectual disability. These patients are at higher risk for many multisystem disorders including thyroid disease, diabetes, acute lymphoblastic leukemia, acute myeloid leukemia, Alzheimer disease (above age 35 years), congenital heart disease (particularly atrial and ventricular septal defects), duodenal atresia, Hirschsprung disease, epilepsy, cataracts, glaucoma, hearing loss, autism, and atlantoaxial subluxation. Life expectancy previously was around 20, but with improved screening tools and medical management, it has been increased to up to 50 to 60 years (Figure 35–3).

Trinucleotide repeat disorders are the result of an expansion of a trinucleotide in a certain gene that exceeds the normal threshold for a repeat in that gene. Trinucleotide disorders common in adult populations are Huntington disease and the spinocerebellar ataxias, discussed in Chapter 28, "Movement Disorders." Two trinucleotide repeat disorders commonly diagnosed in children are fragile X syndrome and Friedreich ataxia.

Fragile X syndrome is associated with a repeat of the trinucleotide CGG in the *FMR1* (fragile X mental retardation 1) gene on the X chromosome. It is much more commonly seen in males than females. The length of the repeat is associated with the severity of disease, with short repeats being subclinical and longer repeats causing chromosomal breakage (appearing to be "fragile" on cytogenetic testing) and associated with more severe intellectual disability. Fragile X syndrome is the second most common genetic cause of intellectual disability after Down syndrome. The most common characteristics besides intellectual disability include a long face with a prominent jaw and large ears, large testes (macro-orchidism), hypotonia, autism (up to 30% to 70%), joint laxity, and epilepsy.

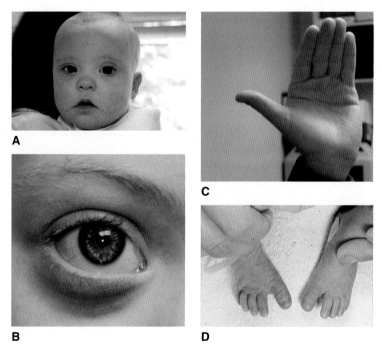

FIGURE 35–3 Down syndrome. **A.** Typical facial features. **B.** Eye showing Brushfield spots (small light colored spots within the iris due to focal dysplasia of the connective tissue). **C.** Single transverse palmar (simian) crease. **D.** Wide gap between first and second toes. (Reproduced with permission from Schaefer GB, Thompson JN: *Medical Genetics: An Integrated Approach.* New York, NY: McGraw Hill; 2014.)

In **Friedreich ataxia**, the trinucleotide GAA is repeated in the *FXN* gene, which codes for the mitochondrial protein frataxin. Frataxin is expressed in all organ systems; therefore, this disorder causes multisystem dysfunction including heart disease, diabetes, and skeletal, visual, and auditory abnormalities. Cognitive function is preserved, however. In the nervous system, the mutated protein causes progressive degeneration of sensory neurons in the spinal cord and cerebellum, leading to severe ataxia, with patients usually being wheelchair bound within 15 years of diagnosis.

Genomic imprinting refers to an epigenetic phenomenon in which a gene is "tagged" by methylation by its parent of origin and either expressed or silenced based on that tag. The most famous neurogenetic disorders exhibiting imprinting are Prader-Willi syndrome and Angelman syndrome. These syndromes can be thought of as reciprocals, because they are both associated with a deletion of a portion of chromosome 15 (15q11-13) and inactivation of that portion on the alternate chromosome. In **Prader-Willi syndrome**, there is deletion of the paternal portion of chromosome 15 with epigenetic inactivation (or imprinting) of the maternal chromosome (although the syndrome can also manifest from uniparental disomy in which both chromosomes are inherited from the mother). In **Angelman syndrome**, the reverse occurs: There is a maternal deletion of the portion of chromosome 15 with inactivation of the paternal chromosome (or uniparental paternal disomy). Strangely, many of the clinical features of the 2 syndromes are markedly different, even though both syndromes have no working 15q11-13 regions. Children with Prader-Willi syndrome exhibit hyperphagia, obesity, hypersomnolence, hypotonia, hypogonadism, small feet and hands, intellectual disability, and seizures. Although children with Angelman syndrome also exhibit intellectual disability and seizures, they are more specifically characterized by hyperexcitability, inappropriate laughter, gait ataxia, jerky movements (thus the historic name "happy puppet"), hand flapping, a fascination with water, and sleep difficulties.

Rett syndrome is a neuropsychiatric disorder caused by a sporadic mutation in the *MECP2* gene on the X chromosome. It is almost exclusively seen in females, as most males with the disorder die in utero or shortly after birth. The syndrome follows a progressive course of initially normal development, followed by decelerated brain growth between 2 and 5 months of age. Children then begin to show developmental stagnation followed by regression of intellectual, social, speech, and motor abilities with significant irritability between 12 and 18 months. Children will also exhibit stereotyped hand movements, seizures, constipation, scoliosis, and respiratory abnormalities. Most children have no verbal skills and are not able to walk.

METABOLIC DISORDERS/INBORN ERRORS OF METABOLISM

Inborn errors of metabolism constitute a wide-ranging group of inherited disorders involving abnormalities in the chemical reactions of metabolic pathways. Many metabolic disorders have some neurologic sequelae, and this section attempts to review the major disorders that present in infancy or childhood with neurologic symptoms. The most common presenting symptoms of metabolic disorders in infants are relatively nonspecific and include lethargy, poor feeding, vomiting, hypotonia, jaundice, and seizures.

Lysosomal Storage Diseases

The lysosome is an organelle that uses enzymes to break down biomolecules entering the cell. In **lysosomal storage diseases**, one of the enzymes involved in this degradation process is defective, leading to accumulation of the biomolecules in the cell and eventually cell death. Patients of Ashkenazi Jewish descent are at increased risk for many of these diseases, including Tay-Sachs, Niemann-Pick, and Gaucher. Krabbe disease and metachromatic leukodystrophy, both lysosomal storage diseases causing leukodystrophy, will be covered later in the dysmyelinating disorders section of this chapter.

Tay-Sachs disease is caused by a deficiency of the enzyme hexosaminidase A, which leads to the accumulation of GM_2 ganglioside. In addition to developmental delay, progressive neurodegeneration, and epilepsy, the disease is characterized by a macular cherry red spot, blindness, and an excessive startle in infants. Lysosomes will have the appearance of onion skin, and foamy leukocytes will be noted on peripheral smear. The life expectancy is usually 2 to 5 years for the infantile form. The juvenile form, characterized by juvenile- or adult-onset ataxia, dementia, epilepsy, and proximal muscle weakness, has a variable life expectancy.

Niemann-Pick disease is due to a deficiency of sphingomyelinase, which leads to accumulation of sphingomyelin. This buildup is prominent in macrophages, causing the appearance of "foam cells." Clinical symptoms include failure to thrive, hypotonia, blindness, developmental regression, hepatosplenomegaly, and, as in Tay-Sachs disease, blindness and a macular cherry red spot (Figure 35–4). Life expectancy is <1 year for the infantile form and around 15 years for the juvenile form.

Gaucher disease is the most common of the lysosomal storage diseases and is caused by β-glucosidase (glucocerebrosidase) deficiency, leading to the accumulation of glucocerebroside. There are 4 forms—infantile, juvenile, adult, and adult nonneuronopathic—which decrease in severity as the age of onset increases. Gaucher cells, which are macrophages with the appearance of crumpled tissue paper, can be noted on peripheral smear.

Fabry disease, the only X-linked recessive lysosomal storage disease, is due to α-galactosidase A deficiency, which causes accumulation of glycosphingolipids in the central and peripheral nervous systems, as well as in the skin, kidneys, and blood vessels, leading to multisystem organ dysfunction. Symptoms include severe acroparesthesias, abdominal pain, anhidrosis with heat intolerance and fever, hearing loss, truncal angiokeratomas, and cardiac and renal disease. Patients often can live to middle age.

In **Farber disease**, ceramidase deficiency leads to accumulation of ceramide in cells. It is clinically characterized by joint pain and swelling, subcutaneous nodules, hepatosplenomegaly, dysphagia, cardiomyopathy, limb or tongue edema,

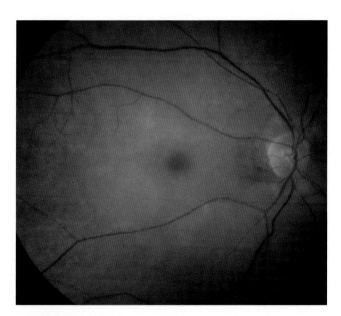

FIGURE 35–4 Cherry red spot at the macula and cloudy swelling of the macula in a patient with central retinal artery occlusion due to embolus originating from a carotid artery atheromatous plaque. (Reproduced with permission from Kasper D, Fauci A, Hauser S, et al: *Harrison's Principles of Internal Medicine*, 19th ed. New York, NY: McGraw Hill; 2015.)

variable mental retardation, macular cherry red spot, and pulmonary granulomas. Life expectancy is <2 years, with death usually due to lung disease.

Mucopolysaccharidoses

Mucopolysaccharidoses are a subset of lysosomal storage diseases characterized by a deficiency of lysosomal enzymes involved in the degradation of glycosaminoglycans. The 2 most well-known diseases with neurologic features in this category are **Hurler syndrome** and **Hunter syndrome**. Both syndromes involve accumulation of heparan sulfate and dermatan sulfate. In Hurler syndrome, this is due to a deficiency of α-L-iduronidase, whereas in Hunter syndrome, it is due to a deficiency of iduronate sulfatase. The syndromes can be distinguished based on their clinical symptoms. In Hurler syndrome, patients exhibit intellectual disability, gargoylism (coarse facies), dwarfism, hydrocephalus, corneal clouding, deafness, vertebral/hand deformities, hepatosplenomegaly, and developmental regression around age 2 years, with death usually in the first decade. Hunter syndrome is clinically similar to Hurler syndrome, although symptoms are generally milder (particularly intellectual disability), and there is no corneal clouding. Patients with Hunter syndrome can also exhibit more behavioral problems including attention-deficit/hyperactivity disorder, obsessive-compulsive disorder, aggression, and autism (Figure 35–5).

Peroxisomal Disorders

The peroxisome is an organelle with a variety of functions including breakdown of fatty acids and amino acids, reduction of reactive oxygen species, and synthesis of lipids. **Refsum disease**

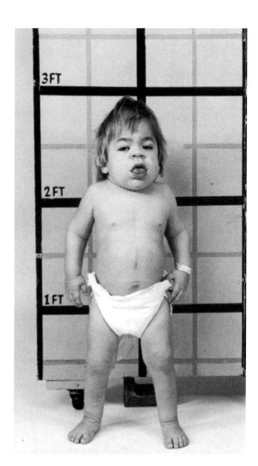

FIGURE 35–5 Mucopolysaccharidosis type IH (Hurler syndrome) in a 4-year-old boy. The diagnosis was made at the age of 15 months, at which time he had developmental delay, hepatomegaly, and skeletal involvement. At the time of the picture, the patient had short stature, an enlarged tongue, persistent nasal discharge, stiff joints, and hydrocephalus. Verbal language skills consisted of 4 or 5 words. The patient had a severe hearing loss and wore hearing aids. (Reproduced with permission from Valle D, Antonarakis S, Ballabio A, et al: *The Online Metabolic and Molecular Bases of Inherited Disease.* New York, NY: McGraw Hill; 2019.)

is caused by a defect in the phytanoyl-coenzyme A hydroxylase enzyme, which leads to accumulation of phytanic acid. Because phytanic acid is not synthesized by the body, this disease can be managed solely by avoiding phytanic acid in the diet. The disease is clinically characterized by retinitis pigmentosa with night blindness, hypotonia, hearing loss, ataxia, peripheral neuropathy, psychiatric symptoms, ichthyosis, and bone deformities. Symptoms typically worsen with fasting. Zellweger disease, a peroxisomal disorder and a leukodystrophy, will be covered later in the dysmyelinating disorders section.

Organic Acidemias

Organic acidemias refer to metabolic disorders in which the metabolism of amino acids is dysfunctional. **Homocystinuria** can be caused by a variety of enzyme deficiencies, all of which lead to excess homocysteine, which in turn makes cystine essential. The clinical onset is often variable, and symptoms include intellectual disability, psychiatric disorders, epilepsy, osteoporosis, tall stature (often Marfan-like), lens subluxation, glaucoma, kyphosis, atherosclerosis (leading to early myocardial infarction and stroke), and hypercoagulability (leading to deep venous thrombosis or venous sinus thrombosis). The disease is treated with vitamin B₆ and vitamin C, as well as a protein-restricted diet.

In **Maple syrup urine disease (MSUD)**, a deficiency of α-ketoacid dehydrogenase inhibits the breakdown of the branched-chain amino acids leucine, isoleucine, and valine. Children with this disease will present between 6 and 24 months with attacks of ataxia, irritability, and lethargy, with severe metabolic acidosis triggered by stress. During the attacks, the patient's urine will smell of maple syrup. If untreated, MSUD can lead to spasticity, opisthotonos, seizures, and neurodegeneration. Treatment consists of protein restriction, particularly of the branched-chain amino acids.

Phenylketonuria is a disease in which the conversion of phenylalanine to tyrosine is inhibited due to a deficiency of either phenylalanine hydroxylase or tetrahydrobiopterin cofactor. The resultant buildup of phenylalanine eventually leads to phenylketonuria. Symptoms include intellectual disability, failure to thrive, epilepsy, behavior problems, eczema, pale skin and hair with blue eyes, and a musty body odor. Magnetic resonance imaging (MRI) will often show progressive basal ganglia calcification. Testing for this disease is part of the newborn screen, and treatment includes avoiding phenylalanine and increasing tyrosine in the diet.

Purine Salvage Deficiencies

The purine salvage pathway produces the nucleotides purine and pyrimidine from the breakdown process of other nucleotides. The most well-known purine salvage deficiency is Lesch-Nyhan syndrome, an X-linked recessive disorder in which there is defective purine salvage leading to excessive uric acid production. These children exhibit symptoms including hypotonia, intellectual disability, gout, nephrolithiasis, hyperuricemia, choreoathetosis, and spasticity. They also exhibit significant aggressive and self-mutilation behaviors including finger and lip biting. Treatment is limited to symptomatic treatment such as allopurinol for gout, benzodiazepines for aggression, and physical restraints and removal of dentition for self-mutilating behaviors. Life expectancy is generally limited to 10 to 20 years.

NEUROCUTANEOUS SYNDROMES

Neurocutaneous syndromes, also known as phakomatoses (from *phakos*, Greek for lentil or lens), include a variety of central nervous system syndromes with cutaneous and often ophthalmologic findings. Because both the nervous system and cutaneous system develop from the embryonic neural crest cells, these syndromes are all due to abnormal neural crest cell migration, formation, or differentiation. Many neurocutaneous disorders are associated with neoplasms and will thus be covered in Chapter 25, "Neurooncology." These include neurofibromatosis type I and type II, Sturge-Weber syndrome, von Hippel-Lindau, and tuberous sclerosis. Ataxia telangiectasia will be covered here.

Ataxia telangiectasia is a multisystem disorder involving progressive ataxia, choreoathetosis, anterior horn cell loss, and oculocutaneous telangiectatic lesions of skin. Patients can also exhibit immunodeficiency secondary to thymic hypoplasia and are at increased risk of neoplasms. The disease presents in the first few years of life with truncal ataxia followed by extremity ataxia. Patients are often hypotonic with decreased reflexes and exhibit drooling and significant dysarthria.

NEUROMUSCULAR DISORDERS

It is perhaps easiest to divide the neuromuscular disorders based on which segment of the lower motor neuron and muscle is affected (Figure 35–6). From proximal to distal, these categories include motor neuron disorders, peripheral

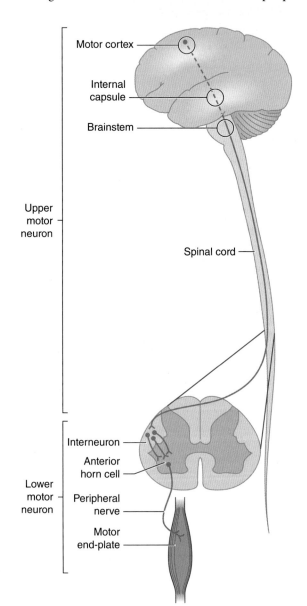

FIGURE 35–6 Anatomic basis of the upper motor neuron and lower motor neuron concepts. (Reproduced with permission from Simon RP, Aminoff MJ, Greemberg DA: *Clinical Neurology*, 10th ed. New York, NY: McGraw Hill; 2018.)

neuropathies, neuromuscular junction disorders, and muscle disorders. The most important motor neuron disorders in pediatrics are the **spinal muscular atrophies**, a group of disorders characterized by progressive degeneration of anterior horn cells of the spinal cord and brainstem motor nuclei. The most common inherited peripheral neuropathy is **Charcot-Marie-Tooth disease.** These disorders are covered in Chapter 31, "Neuromuscular Disorders."

Neuromuscular junction disorders are caused by dysfunction of neurotransmitter release, binding, or reuptake at the neuromuscular junction. In the pediatric population, the most common neuromuscular junction disorders are transient neonatal myasthenia gravis, congenital myasthenia gravis, juvenile myasthenia gravis, and botulism. In **transient neonatal myasthenia gravis,** an infant born to a mother with myasthenia gravis will have symptoms of the disease soon after birth due to transplacental transfer of acetylcholine receptor (AChR) antibodies. This can be seen in 10% to 20% of infants born to myasthenic mothers (whether symptomatic or in remission), and symptoms are seen within 48 hours of delivery. Infants will initially be normal, then begin to show signs of poor feeding, weak cry, generalized weakness, and respiratory insufficiency. The symptoms can last from days to weeks and sometimes require supportive care such as ventilation. Treatment with acetylcholinesterase inhibitors improves symptoms in the short term; however, as the mother's AChR antibodies are washed out of the infant's system, the symptoms will completely resolve.

Congenital myasthenia gravis actually refers to a diverse group of disorders with similar clinical presentations. Infants can be either asymptomatic or symptomatic in the neonatal period, with symptoms including extremity weakness, bulbar weakness, respiratory insufficiency, and delayed motor development. Typical myasthenic symptoms of ophthalmoplegia, fatigability, and ptosis are also common. Because this disease is not due to AChR antibody production, AChR antibodies will be negative. Instead, congenital myasthenia gravis is due to a variety of gene mutations of presynaptic, synaptic, and postsynaptic proteins. Interestingly, depending on which protein is affected, pyridostigmine can either improve or worsen symptoms.

Juvenile myasthenia gravis is more closely related to the adult-onset form, because it is due to antibodies directed against the postsynaptic AChR or the muscle-specific kinase (MuSK) receptor. MuSK receptor antibodies lead to a more severe disease with more oculobulbar symptoms and are generally less responsiveness to pyridostigmine. Juvenile myasthenia gravis is seen more commonly in Asian populations; usually occurs in children between 5 and 10 years old; and can be associated with rheumatoid arthritis, dermatomyositis, or thyroid disease. Onset of symptoms can be rapid or insidious and often occur after a viral infection. The most common presentations are ocular symptoms such as ophthalmoplegia or strabismus. Patients also exhibit generalized weakness, fatigability, hypophonia, and dysphagia. Weakness typically fluctuates during the day, with worsening toward the end of the day,

and improves with rest. A *myasthenic crisis* refers to a rapid worsening of symptoms with respiratory failure requiring ventilator support. A crisis can be triggered by heat, illness, medication changes, and multiple medications (β-blockers, calcium channel blockers, and fluoroquinolones, among others). Treatment of juvenile myasthenia gravis, as in the adult-onset form, can be divided into symptomatic treatment (pyridostigmine) and immunotherapy (prednisone, mycophenolate, azathioprine, intravenous immunoglobulin, thymectomy, and plasma exchange).

Botulism is a disease caused by the ingestion of the spores of *Clostridium botulinum* from the soil or the preformed bacterial toxin from canned goods or honey. This bacterium is commonly found in soil, primarily in Utah, California, and Pennsylvania. Over 70% of cases of botulism occur in infants between the ages of 2 and 4 months. About a third of the infantile cases are due to honey ingestion, prompting the recommendation to avoid feeding honey to infants before the age of 1 year. Botulinum toxin binds to the presynaptic terminal and inhibits release of acetylcholine, causing weakness of both striated and smooth muscles. Symptoms develop between 6 and 48 hours after ingestion and begin with cranial nerve involvement (afferent pupillary defect, ptosis, ophthalmoplegia, poor feeding, weak cry). This in turn leads to hypotonia, constipation, and urinary retention (due to smooth muscle involvement), and eventually progresses to generalized descending paralysis and respiratory failure. Diagnosis is typically made by stool culture and stool analysis for toxin. Infants are treated with botulinum immunoglobulin, whereas older children and adults are treated with botulinum antitoxin. Gentle stomach lavage and enemas can also be used to decrease absorption. The prognosis is relative to the amount of toxin that is absorbed or ingested. Patients can have a complete recovery; however, if large amounts are ingested, then patients can die within a few days due to cardiovascular or respiratory failure. Other forms of botulism are discussed in Chapter 32, "Neurologic Infections."

There are a wide variety of pediatric muscle disorders, as most are genetic disorders with childhood presentations. The muscular dystrophies (MDs) are the most well known, but these disorders also include congenital myopathies, myotonia congenita, and myotonic dystrophy. The latter 2 are covered in Chapter 31, "Neuromuscular Disorders."

The 2 most common MDs are Duchenne MD and Becker MD. **Duchenne MD** is an X-linked disorder seen almost exclusively in males. It is due to a deletion of the dystrophin gene (*DMD*) located on chromosome Xp21, which encodes the protein dystrophin. Dystrophin connects the cytoskeleton of muscle fibers to the basal lamina, the absence of which causes an excess of calcium influx into the cell and subsequent damage to the mitochondria. Symptoms are usually evident between the ages of 2 and 5 years and initially consist of delayed ambulation and difficulty with climbing or rising from the floor or seated positions, resulting in the Gowers sign (Figure 35–7).

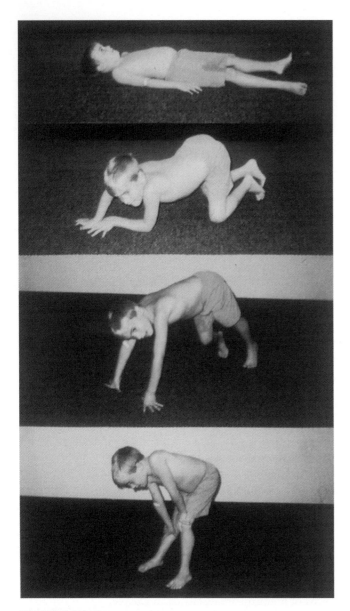

FIGURE 35-7 Gowers sign showing a patient using his arms to climb up the legs in attempting to get up from the floor. (Reproduced with permission from Jameson J, Fauci AS, Kasper DL, et al: *Harrison's Principles of Internal Medicine*, 20th ed. New York, NY: McGraw Hill; 2018.)

Children exhibit proximal muscle weakness, a waddling gait, lumbar lordosis, decreased patellar reflexes, pseudohypertrophy of calves and deltoids, and contractures of hamstrings and Achilles tendon, leading to toe walking. Some degree of intellectual disability is usually seen in children with Duchenne MD. As the disease progresses, children can develop cardiomyopathy, gastrointestinal hypomotility, respiratory insufficiency, and scoliosis. Creatine kinase (CK) serum levels will be 10 to 30 times above normal as a result of muscle breakdown. Diagnosis was previously made with muscle biopsy but is now typically made with genetic testing. Corticosteroids were the only known therapy to stabilize or improve strength. Recently, eteplirsen, an antisense oligonucleotide that mediates skipping

of *DMD* exon 51, has been approved for the ~13% of DMD patients with a mutation amenable to this approach. Patients are recommended to avoid high-resistance exercise (which can accelerate muscle damage); anticholinergic medications or general anesthesia should also be avoided because these patients are at risk of malignant hyperthermia. If untreated, patients are usually wheelchair bound by age 12 or 13. Treatment with steroids can prolong ambulation by up to 5 years; however, patients usually die in the second or third decade due to cardiac or respiratory disease.

Becker MD is similar to Duchenne MD in that it is an X-linked disorder due to a mutation of the dystrophin gene at Xp21.2. Clinical symptoms are similar to Duchenne MD as well, including proximal weakness, pseudohypertrophy, and elevated CK levels. However, in Becker MD, symptoms are often not present until children are in their second decade, and they will often continue to walk independently until their third decade. These patients generally have more severe cardiac disease than patients with Duchenne MD, and they are generally of normal intellect. Treatment for Becker MD is the same as for Duchenne MD, but overall, the prognosis is better with survival into adulthood.

Congenital myopathies include disorders due to a defective protein, rather than a deficiency of a protein as in MDs. These disorders are often noticeable in the neonatal period and have variable progression of symptoms. **Nemaline myopathy** derives its name from the Greek *nema*, or thread, due to the red staining "rods" (type I muscle fibers) seen in abnormal muscle fiber aggregation on muscle biopsy. There are 6 clinical forms of nemaline myopathy, ranging from the most severe infantile form that presents with a severely hypotonic infant to the milder adult-onset form with a "dropped head" sign. The primary symptom is muscle weakness, which can be of variable intensity. Patients can also exhibit skeletal abnormalities, arthrogryposis, cardiomyopathy, and ophthalmoplegia.

Central core disease was the first described congenital myopathy. The name refers to muscle biopsy findings, in which the center of the muscle cell is devoid of mitochondria and enzymes, leaving an empty-appearing "core." It is clinically characterized by proximal extremity and facial weakness, muscle cramps, hypotonia, decreased reflexes, delayed motor development, and skeletal abnormalities such as scoliosis and hip dislocation; however, up to a third of patients can have no clinical symptoms. These patients are also at increased risk for malignant hyperthermia.

DYSMYELINATING/ DEMYELINATING DISORDERS

White matter refers to the myelinated tracks of neurons in the brain and is responsible for relaying information between different parts of the brain and spinal cord. Disruption of myelin, whether intrinsic or acquired, can cause a variety of symptoms and presentations depending on the degree and location of the damage. In children, white matter disease can be divided between the leukodystrophies, a group of disorders in which the maturation and development of myelin is disrupted, and acquired demyelinating diseases. Almost all of the more common demyelinating diseases seen in adults, such as multiple sclerosis, optic neuritis, neuromyelitis optica, and transverse myelitis, are also seen in children; however, these diseases are covered thoroughly in Chapter 30, "Neuroimmunology and Neuroinflammatory Disorders."

Adrenoleukodystrophy is an X-linked hereditary leukodystrophy in which an enzyme responsible for breakdown of very-long-chain fatty acids is defective, causing buildup of those fatty acids in the brain, which subsequently leads to myelin damage. This defective enzyme is also active in the adrenal cortex and Leydig cells of the testes, leading to damage in those organs as well. MRI findings include primarily posterior and periventricular involvement with contrast enhancement of the lesions. Children will develop motor regression, behavioral problems (aggression, withdrawal, memory deficits, and eventually dementia), chronic progressive spastic paraparesis, vision loss with optic nerve atrophy, deafness, dysphagia, gait disturbance, seizures (often late in the course), and, as the name implies, signs of adrenal failure (fatigue, vomiting, hyperpigmentation, and salt craving). Multiple subtypes are described, including childhood, adolescent, adrenomyeloneuropathy, adrenal insufficiency alone, and even an asymptomatic form. Treatment is usually with "Lorenzo's oil," a combination of fatty acids that competitively inhibit the enzyme responsible for the production of very-long-chain fatty acids. The disease course is nonetheless progressive and relentless, with death often within 1 to 10 years of onset.

Metachromatic leukodystrophy, an autosomal recessive disorder, is caused by a deficiency of the arylsulfatase A enzyme, leading to cerebroside sulfate accumulation, which in turn impairs myelin production. It is also considered a lysosomal storage disease, because the breakdown of cerebroside sulfate occurs in the lysosome. On MRI, diffuse white matter abnormalities are seen with sparing of U-fibers (short association fibers connecting adjacent gyri). This disease causes both central and peripheral nervous system demyelination. As in adrenoleukodystrophy, the buildup of the fatty acid occurs in other organ systems and leads to damage of the kidneys, pancreas, adrenal glands, and liver. Clinically, children with metachromatic leukodystrophy exhibit behavioral disturbances, ataxia, hyperreflexia, and dementia.

Krabbe disease is another leukodystrophy caused by an inborn error metabolism, in this case a sphingolipidosis with accumulation of galactocerebroside due to a mutation of the galactocerebrosidase enzyme. MRI findings include posterior-predominant periventricular white matter lesions with no contrast enhancement. Clinical features include developmental regression, spasticity, opisthotonos (extreme spasticity and hyperextension), seizures, and optic atrophy with death usually by the age of 2 years.

Alexander disease is associated with mutations on the *GFAP* (glial fibrillary acidic protein) gene on chromosome 17q21 and is most often a sporadic mutation. Histologically, Rosenthal fibers (eosinophilic inclusions) can be seen in astrocyte footplates, as well as subpial, subependymal, and perivascular distributions. Demyelination is also noted in these same areas, with a primarily anterior predominance. Three variants exist, the most common of which is the rapidly progressive infantile form. This form presents in the first 2 years of life with psychomotor retardation, megalencephaly, seizures, and spasticity, and has a life expectancy of <5 years. The juvenile form presents between age 4 years and the early teens and has a slower course. These patients usually do not have seizures but have prominent bulbar or pseudobulbar symptoms such as dysphagia, nystagmus, hypophonia, ptosis, and facial diplegia, as well as ataxia, spasticity, and weakness. The adult-onset form is rare and generally presents with bulbar symptoms, ataxia, spasticity, with variable intellectual disability.

The 2 acquired demyelinating diseases covered in this chapter are acute disseminated encephalomyelitis (ADEM) and subacute sclerosing panencephalitis (SSPE). Other forms are discussed in Chapter 30.

ADEM is characterized by acute, widespread autoimmune demyelination of the central nervous system. Seventy-five percent of cases of ADEM are postinfectious, with the other 25% developing within 3 months of vaccines (measles, mumps, rubella, rabies, influenza, and smallpox). Clinical criteria for ADEM include the following: acute/subacute onset; the first clinical attack of demyelination/inflammation of the central nervous system; polyfocality; polysymptomatic (cranial neuropathies, meningismus, nausea/vomiting, optic neuritis, hemiparesis, pyramidal signs, ataxia, seizures, transverse myelitis); and encephalopathy (acute behavior change or altered consciousness). MRI of the brain will show large, multifocal, hyperintense, bilateral asymmetric lesions, rarely with contrast enhancement. The lesions can occur almost anywhere (supratentorial, infratentorial, or involving the basal ganglia or thalamus). The mortality rate for ADEM is quite high at 10% to 30% and can be even higher if the disease was preceded by measles infection.

SSPE, also known as Dawson disease or subacute inclusion body encephalitis, is a progressive neurodegenerative disease caused by a defective measles virus. Luckily, the incidence of this disease has significantly decreased with widespread use of the measles vaccine. Children under age 12 years are primarily affected, and symptoms include poor memory and behavior changes leading to progressive dementia, incoordination, ataxia, myoclonus, and seizures. The terminal stage is characterized by rigid quadriplegia. The course can be rapidly progressive or, more commonly, prolonged over many years. Treatment includes antiviral and immunomodulating medications, and if treated early in the course, children can recover or halt progression of the disease. If not caught early, patients often die within 3 years.

PEDIATRIC EPILEPSY

Much of epilepsy seen in children can also be seen in adult epilepsy, such as simple or complex partial epilepsy or primary generalized epilepsies, and is covered in great detail in Chapter 27, "Epilepsy." However, there are certain epilepsy phenotypes and syndromes that are specific to pediatric epilepsy and will be covered here.

A **febrile seizure** refers specifically to a seizure provoked by fever in the pediatric population between the age of 6 months and 6 years. Febrile seizures are subdivided between *simple febrile* and *complex febrile* seizures. Simple febrile seizures, which account for 80% to 90% of all febrile seizures, refer to febrile seizures that are <15 minutes in duration, have a generalized semiology, and occur only once in a 24-hour period. Conversely, complex febrile seizures refer to febrile seizures lasting >15 minutes, occur more than once in a 24-hour period, and have focality (focal semiology, secondary generalization, or an associated Todd paralysis). Febrile seizures are often provoked by upper respiratory infections, acute otitis media, gastroenteritis, or roseola infection. Up to one-third of children will have recurrent febrile seizures, with an increased risk in those with a family history of febrile seizure, a first episode prior to age 18 months, or a low peak temperature with the seizure. In children who have had 1 febrile seizure, there is no increased risk of developing epilepsy compared to the general population. If a child has recurrent febrile seizures, however, their risk of epilepsy doubles to 2% to 3%. If a child has a family history of epilepsy, a complex febrile seizure, or any neurologic abnormality prior to the seizure, their risk of developing epilepsy is increased to 10% to 13%. Febrile seizures are rarely treated with maintenance antiepileptic medications, although rescue medications such as rectal diazepam can be prescribed for seizures lasting >5 minutes. Round-the-clock antipyretics have not been proven to be effective, and reassurance and education of parents are paramount.

Infantile spasms are a distinctive seizure type seen in West syndrome, which is defined as the triad of infantile spasms, psychomotor regression, and a hypsarrhythmia pattern on electroencephalography (EEG). Patients typically develop spasms between 4 and 8 months of age, with episodes of brief tonic or clonic spasms of truncal and/or upper extremity flexion or extension. The spasms can cluster, be followed by fussiness, or occur on awakening from sleep. *Hypsarrhythmia* on EEG is characterized by interictal high voltage, disorganized activity, and an ictal electrodecremental response (generalized attenuation of voltage across all EEG leads during a seizure). West syndrome is often symptomatic and caused by a pre-, peri-, or postnatal insult; a genetic condition; a metabolic syndrome; tuberous sclerosis; or a cerebral malformation. Initial treatment with a course of adrenocorticotropic hormone (ACTH) or prednisone is standard of care, followed by long-term treatment with an antiepileptic medication such as topiramate. Prognosis is overall poor, although somewhat better if spasms are cryptogenic rather than symptomatic, with good developmental outcomes in approximately 5% of patients.

Lennox-Gastaut syndrome (LGS) is a pediatric epilepsy syndrome characterized by the triad of multiple seizure types (eg, tonic, atypical absence, myoclonic, atonic), cognitive impairment, and a typical EEG pattern of slow spike wave activity. The seizures are generally refractory to medication and often require nonpharmacologic treatments such as corpus callosotomy, vagal nerve stimulation, or ketogenic diet. Patients typically develop LGS between 2 and 8 years of age, and up to one-fifth of cases are preceded by West syndrome. Patients often have comorbid psychiatric illness including psychosis.

Landau-Kleffner syndrome (LKS), also known as acquired epileptic aphasia, refers to a rare childhood disorder involving acquired receptive aphasia and EEG abnormalities with electrographic status epilepticus of sleep (ESES). Children can develop clinical seizures (usually focal) but do not always have seizures. These children usually have normal language development until around 3 to 5 years of age. The first sign of aphasia is usually *auditory verbal agnosia* with inability to understand speech. This is often misinterpreted as hearing loss or autism, and delayed diagnosis can lead to long-term language deficits. Personality changes and hyperactivity can be seen in up to half of children with LKS, but intellectual disability is not associated with the syndrome. Treatment is with antiepileptic medications, and steroids and ACTH have also been shown to be beneficial. ESES often improves by puberty, but most children will have significant residual language deficits.

The most common epilepsy syndrome of childhood is **benign Rolandic epilepsy**, also known as **benign childhood epilepsy with centrotemporal spikes,** which accounts for 10% to 15% of all childhood epilepsies. As the name implies, this is a benign syndrome that typically resolves by puberty with no residual neurodevelopmental deficits. Children usually develop seizures between 7 and 9 years of age. Seizures are almost always nocturnal and involve unilateral facial and upper extremity jerking or sensory changes, hypersalivation, or oropharyngeal symptoms. Patients typically retain awareness during the seizures, although they can secondarily generalize during sleep. On EEG, interictal unilateral or bilateral centrotemporal spikes can be seen with prominent sleep activation and an otherwise normal background. Because these seizures are usually rare, are limited to sleep, and do not cause long-term deficits, most children are not treated with antiepileptic medications. If the seizures are frequent or prolonged, secondarily generalize, or occur while awake, then they can be medically treated.

Panayiotopoulos syndrome is another fairly common benign nocturnal epilepsy syndrome of childhood. Seizures can be convulsive but most often have autonomic features including vomiting, pallor, flushing, hypersalivation, incontinence, and headache. Seizures in Panayiotopoulos syndrome are long, often lasting >30 minutes. EEG will show occipital-predominant spike-and-wave activity. Half of children with this syndrome will have <5 seizures, and will achieve remission typically within 2 years.

Childhood absence epilepsy (CAE) is an idiopathic generalized epilepsy with absence seizures occurring in children between the ages of 4 and 10 years. Absence seizures generally last between 5 and 15 seconds and involve abrupt behavioral arrest, staring, and sometimes automatisms followed by immediate return to baseline. These seizures can occur up to hundreds of times a day. Hyperventilation will typically provoke seizures, and EEG will show a typical generalized 3-Hz spike-and-wave pattern with an otherwise normal background. Children with CAE are usually developmentally normal, although can have learning disabilities due to frequent seizures. CAE is treated with ethosuximide, valproic acid, and lamotrigine. About 40% of children will not respond to the first antiepileptic medication; however, up to two-thirds of children will grow out of their seizures by adolescence.

Although most children with CAE will outgrow their seizures, up to 15% will go on to develop **juvenile myoclonic epilepsy (JME)**. JME occurs in adolescents and is characterized by multiple seizure types including absence seizures, myoclonic seizures, and tonic-clonic seizures. Myoclonic seizures are most noticeable on awakening, and seizures are provoked by sleep deprivation, stress, alcohol, and photosensitivity. As in CAE, children with JME are usually neurodevelopmentally normal. Unlike CAE, however, patients rarely outgrow their seizures and will require lifelong antiepileptic treatment.

SELF-ASSESSMENT QUESTIONS

1. A 4-year-old boy presents to his pediatrician after his parents notice he has trouble rising from a seated position. They have also noticed he tends to walk on his toes, falls easily if jostled, and tires quickly when he walks. On further questioning, they report that he crawled late and did not walk until 18 months of age. His verbal and social skills are normal, and he was toilet trained by age 2.5 years. On exam, he has decreased patellar reflexes, 4/5 strength in his proximal leg muscles, and an exaggerated lumbar lordosis. What is the best first test to order?

   A. Magnetic resonance imaging (MRI) of brain with and without contrast
   B. MRI of lumbar spine
   C. Nerve conduction studies of his lower extremities
   D. Creatine kinase (CK) level

2. A 2-year-old girl is brought to the emergency department (ED) by her parents after she had an episode at home of arm and leg stiffening followed by eye rolling and whole-body rhythmic jerking lasting 3 minutes. They report she had a similar episode a few months ago lasting about 30 seconds associated with an upper respiratory infection and fever. In the ED, she is febrile to 102°F but otherwise awake, alert, and without any focal neurologic deficits. She has no significant medical history and normal development. Her parents report that recently she has had a runny nose and cough and has been pulling on her ears. Lab work in the ED, including electrolytes, complete blood count, and urinalysis, is unremarkable. What is the next best step?

   A. Stat head computed tomography (CT)
   B. Lumbar puncture
   C. Reassurance
   D. Start antiepileptic medication

3. A child presents to her pediatrician for her 12-month check-up. Her parents report that although she had normal development until around 6 months of age, she is not yet walking, has no words, and in fact has stopped babbling. She no longer makes eye contact regularly and has frequent prolonged screaming fits and inconsolable crying. On review of her growth chart, her weight and height have continued to be average, but her head circumference has fallen to the fifth percentile. On exam, she is hypotonic throughout and makes frequent repetitive hand wringing movements. What is the genetic mutation associated with this disorder?

   A. *FMR1* gene mutation
   B. *MECP2* gene mutation
   C. Chromosome 15 uniparental disomy
   D. *FXN* gene mutation

SECTION VI

Ear & Eye Disorders

Neurotology & Ear Disorders

Yoon-Hee Cha

- Recognize the common signs and symptoms of external and middle ear disease, particularly those that may lead to prolonged morbidity if misdiagnosed.
- Understand the patterns in symptoms associated with cochlear and vestibular dysfunction.
- Appreciate risk factors for avoidable causes of ear injury, such as barotrauma, head injury, noise exposure, and ototoxic medications.

PREVALENCE & BURDEN

Disorders of the ear and their central connections are common contributors to morbidity throughout the human life span, beginning with congenital deafness and progressing with age to childhood ear infections, viral reactivation syndromes, and noise- and age-related hearing loss. Childhood middle ear infections (otitis media) alone affect 5 out of every 6 children before the age of 6 years. Noise-related hearing loss affects >15% of adult men and almost 10% of adult women, and severe hearing loss affects >35% of the elderly. Dizziness of all causes affects about 30% of adults in any age group, and inner ear–specific causes such as benign paroxysmal vertigo affect >25% of individuals over the age of 75 years. These disorders will inflict a higher and higher burden on public health because of the aging of the population. Rapid recognition of symptoms that implicate structural ear injury as well as preventable contributors of neurotologic disease are key to preventing long-term morbidity.

LOCALIZATION

Disorders of the external and middle ear are characterized by physical manifestations and typically unilateral symptoms that make localization unambiguous. Auditory symptoms, when unilateral, are fairly easily localized to the affected side. The strong bilateral representation of central cochlear projections makes unilateral auditory symptoms unusual for central lesions.

Vertigo, dizziness, and spatial misperception can be due to either peripheral (inner ear) or central causes, and making this distinction can be challenging. The vestibular system maintains a fair degree of lateralization all the way to the cerebral cortex but the projections within the cerebral cortex are diffuse. This relates to the variety of central lesions that can create motion perception disorders. When paired with unilateral auditory symptoms in the absence of any central findings, the localization of vertigo is typically the inner ear. In the absence of auditory symptoms, a careful evaluation of other central features needs to be performed in order to distinguish peripheral versus central causes of motion misperception.

DISORDERS OF THE EAR

Infectious & Inflammatory Disorders of the Ear

Chondritis

Chondritis, specifically *auricular chondritis*, as it pertains to this section, refers to inflammation of the cartilage of the external ear (Figure 36–1A). It is usually the sequela of perichondritis. The perichondrium is the layer of tissue over the cartilage that provides it nutrients. Causes of chondritis largely fall into traumatic, infectious, and autoimmune categories. Chondritis can be caused by trauma to the ear such as ear piercing through the cartilage of the helix rather than the earlobe. Piercing through the earlobe does not involve cartilage and is not a risk for chondritis. Chronic pressure on

VOCABULARY

Cochlea: The sensory organ of hearing. It is a spiral structure that makes 2.5 turns around a central axis, with each portion tuned to a specific frequency. The rings consist of 3 fluid-filled chambers that serve to translate mechanical vibrations from the oval window into electrical signals through movement of hair cells embedded in the organ of Corti.

Dizziness: A sense of disturbed or impaired spatial orientation not involving a false sense of motion.

External ear: Otherwise known as the pinna or auricle, it is the cartilaginous portion of the auditory system that is outside of the head.

Inner ear: The innermost part of the ear; it is surrounded by the otic capsule and houses the cochlea, the 3 semicircular canals, and otolith organs (utricle and saccule).

Middle ear: The central portion of the human auditory system that resides between the tympanic membrane and the oval window. It houses the ossicular chain (malleus, incus,

and stapes) and is connected to the nasopharynx through the eustachian tube.

Otolith organs: Composed of the utricle and saccule, the gravity-sensing organs of the inner ear. The utricle is more sensitive to horizontal accelerations, and the saccule is more sensitive to vertical accelerations.

Semicircular canals: Three interconnected tubular structures that contain endolymphatic fluid and translate angular acceleration movements of the head to the vestibular nerve. The horizontal, posterior, and superior (ie, anterior canal) canals sit orthogonally to each other, allowing head motion information to be encoded in 3 planes.

Vertigo: A false sense of motion, involving either an internal perception of self-motion or an external perception of environmental motion.

Vestibulocochlear nerve: The eighth cranial nerve, it is comprised of the cochlear and vestibular branches.

---

the external ear from frequent cell phone use, wearing tight headbands around the ear, and sleeping on the involved ear are risk factors for a related disorder *chondrodermatitis nodularis helicis*, the formation of small nodules on the helix. Infections can occur as an extension of otitis externa or as superimposed infections from broken skin due to atopic, contact, or photoallergic dermatitis; radiation exposure; or psoriasis. The key autoimmune disorder that is associated with auricular chondritis is relapsing polychondritis. Polychondritis also affects

the cartilage of the nose, eustachian tube, laryngotracheal tree, heart valves, and joints. Treatment is aimed at reducing pain and avoidance of inciting factors.

Mastoiditis

Mastoiditis is inflammation of the mastoid air cells, the aerated portion of the temporal bone that lies just posterior to the pinna. Mastoiditis most frequently accompanies an episode of acute otitis media (AOM) and is thus etiologically

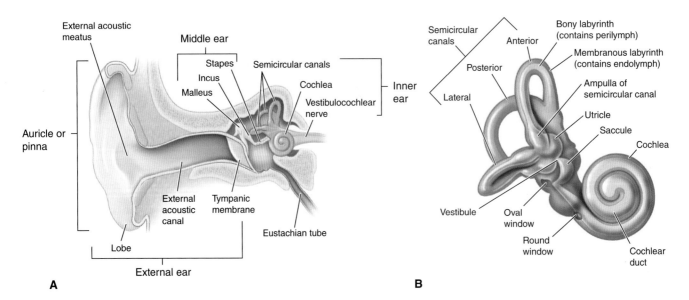

A

B

FIGURE 36–1   Coronal section through the temporal bone showing structures through (**A**) the external canal, middle ear, and inner ear and (**B**) high resolution of the inner ear. (Reproduced with permission from Jameson J, Fauci AS, Kasper DL, et al: *Harrison's Principles of Internal Medicine*, 20th ed. New York, NY: McGraw Hill; 2018.)

related. The most common symptoms are pain behind the pinna in addition to the symptoms of AOM. Uncomplicated cases may be managed with oral antibiotics directed toward typical AOM pathogens (see next section on otitis media). If left untreated, mastoiditis can lead to swelling, deformation, and abscess formation, causing an anterior deflection of the pinna. Infections can spread to the occipital bone, sigmoid sinus, cerebellum, parotid glands, and neck and can thus be complicated by more extensive osteitis and neurologic symptoms such as headache, vertigo, ataxia, diplopia, and facial palsy. Mastoidectomy, or removal of the infected air cells, is rarely performed in situations of early diagnosis and treatment with antimicrobials. However, in cases of local invasion or severe pain, the infected area may need surgical debridement and tympanostomy to drain fluid in the middle ear both for diagnostic (to culture organism) and therapeutic purposes (to allow drainage and provide access to antimicrobial drops).

Otitis Media

Otitis media refers to inflammation of the middle ear that can be caused by different etiologies, the most common of which is bacterial infections (see Figure 36–1A). AOM typically occurs in children younger than 7 years of age and is associated with fever and ear pain (otalgia) along with other signs of infection such as irritability and anorexia. The normally gray translucent tympanic membrane becomes erythematous and bulging in AOM. A conductive hearing loss due to fluid in the middle ear space is common. The most common bacterial organisms causing AOM are *Streptococcus pneumoniae*, *Haemophilus influenzae*, and *Moraxella catarrhalis*. Otitis media with effusion refers to fluid in the middle ear space that does not imply an actual infection but can follow an episode of AOM. It was previously termed *serous* or *secretory otitis media*. Chronic suppurative otitis media refers to middle ear inflammation that persists for >6 weeks and is associated with otorrhea (drainage). Anatomic abnormalities and upper respiratory infections that impair eustachian tube functioning and host immune deficiencies are risk factors for developing and maintaining middle ear inflammation and infection. Invasion of the infection into deeper tissue is a process referred to as **malignant otitis media** or **necrotizing otitis media** and is a life-threatening condition that should be considered in patients with severe deep pain, with structural abnormalities of the temporal bone (eg, prior surgery or radiation to the skull base), or who are immunocompromised (eg, patients with human immunodeficiency virus [HIV] or diabetes or on chronic steroids).

Otitis Externa

Otitis externa (OE) refers to inflammation of the external auditory canal that can be caused by different etiologies including bacterial or fungal infections or skin disorders causing eczema (eg, psoriasis) or dermatitis (eg, allergic or contact). Although it is colloquially referred to as *swimmer's ear*,

any condition that causes high humidity and maceration of the external canal, such as frequent water exposure and trapped fluid behind cerumen or foreign objects (eg, hearing aids), can cause OE. The most common bacterial pathogens are *Pseudomonas aeruginosa* and *Staphylococcus aureus*, whereas the most frequent fungal pathogen is *Aspergillus*. The external canal and the surrounding pinna and tragus can be painful to touch in OE, and OE can be associated with redness, fever, and discharge as well as more serious complications such as mastoiditis, cellulitis, and osteomyelitis. Recurrent OE can lead to external canal stenosis. Although most cases of OE can be managed with topical antibiotics, severe cases require imaging to rule out local invasion as well as debridement and systemic antibiotics.

Labyrinthitis

Labyrinthitis is an inflammation or infection of the inner ear structures, which include the semicircular canals, the otolith organs (utricle and saccule), and the cochlea (see **Figures** 36–1A and 36–1B). It may also be known as *otitis interna* in older textbooks. The prominent symptoms of labyrinthitis are severe rotational vertigo and hearing loss, often leaving permanent vestibular and hearing impairment. Direct infection of the inner ear by bacteria can occur as a consequence of meningitis, otitis media, or mastoiditis via spread through existing channels such as the internal auditory canal or cochlear aqueduct, or by dehiscence of the temporal bone due to overwhelming inflammation. Viral infection can occur either by direct spread through these pathways or by reactivation of a latent infection (eg, herpes simplex virus, varicella) lying dormant in the spiral and vestibular ganglion. Congenital or perinatal infections such as rubella, mumps, or measles can also damage the contents of the labyrinth. In general, the same pathogens that cause upper respiratory infections, meningitis, and otitis media are culprits in labyrinthitis, which, except in the case of viral reactivation, occurs as a process secondary to another infection. Serous labyrinthitis occurs as inflammatory mediators cross into the labyrinth through the round window without direct infection.

The main differential diagnosis to consider in cases of labyrinthitis is ischemic injury to the inner ear from occlusion of the anterior inferior cerebellar artery (a branch of the basilar artery), which serves the labyrinthine artery, because both can cause concurrent vertigo and hearing loss. In ischemia, however, the symptoms come on acutely and are maximal at onset, whereas labyrinthitis symptoms build subacutely. A Ménière attack can mimic labyrinthitis at its onset, but episodes are usually self-limited, resolve in less than a day (typically lasting about 5 to 6 hours), and are not associated with deafness. However, Ménière disease can develop as a consequence of a prior episode of labyrinthitis. Labyrinthitis and vestibular neuritis are distinct, as the latter refers to inflammation of the vestibular nerve rather than the contents of the inner ear and thus leads to vertigo and vestibulopathy without hearing loss.

Neoplasms

Vestibular Schwannomas

Vestibular schwannomas are peripheral nerve sheath tumors that arise from the covering of the vestibular nerve and compose approximately 8% of all intracranial tumors. They have been incorrectly called acoustic neuromas historically, which is a misnomer because the tumors neither arise from an acoustic (ie, hearing) nerve nor grow from the nerve itself. They are slow-growing tumors that generally present with unilateral hearing loss due to progressive compression of the paired cochlear nerve. Approximately 95% of cases of vestibular schwannomas present with progressive asymmetric hearing loss, 75% with tinnitus, and approximately 57% with various kinds of dizziness and gait instability. Actual rotational vertigo occurs in approximately 15% of patients. Overall, these are rare tumors, with an incidence of approximately 1 to 2 per 100,000 persons. Therefore, even in patients who present with asymmetric hearing loss to otolaryngology clinics, vestibular schwannomas account for <3% of cases. They usually start growing within the internal auditory canal (termed *intracanalicular*) and then grow more medially toward the brainstem (termed *extracanalicular*). When large, vestibular schwannomas can grow into the cerebellopontine angle and be associated with other neurologic abnormalities such as compression of other cranial nerves, most commonly the trigeminal or facial nerves, or compression of the cerebellum causing cerebellar ataxia. If left unchecked, large tumors can obstruct the normal efflux of cerebrospinal fluid, leading to hydrocephalus.

The tumors are slow growing and benign and are often managed with observation. Timing of intervention either with surgery or radiation is done through consultation with an otolaryngologist and close monitoring of hearing function. Occasionally, during growth in the intracanalicular phase, the tumors can compress their own vascular supply, leading to infarction of the vestibulocochlear nerve and sudden deafness and vertigo. Vestibular schwannomas are typically found sporadically, presenting generally between the ages of 30 and 60 years with an equal prevalence in males and females. However, it is believed that the same loss of function of a tumor suppressor gene on chromosome 22 (*NF2*) that occurs in neurofibromatosis type 2, an autosomal dominantly inherited genetic disorder causing bilateral vestibular schwannomas, may also be relevant to sporadic cases of vestibular schwannomas.

Neurofibromatosis Type 2

Neurofibromatosis type 2 (NF2) is an autosomal dominantly inherited disorder due to mutations, duplications, deletions, or ring formation of the *NF2* gene located on chromosome 22. *NF2* encodes for the tumor suppressor protein merlin, which, when dysfunctional, leads to the development of a variety of central nervous system tumors. Diagnostic criteria for NF2 are met when the patient either has bilateral vestibular schwannomas present before the age of 30 years or presents with a combination of a positive family history, a unilateral vestibular schwannoma, or another intracranial tumor such as a meningioma, ependymoma, glioma, neurofibroma, or astrocytoma. Posterior subcapsular lens opacities of the eye and mononeuropathies are also frequent in NF2. Fifty-percent of cases of NF2 occur sporadically through de novo mutations, and 50% are associated with a positive family history. Treatment is symptomatic for each associated tumor. Vigilance for spinal cord involvement should be high in patients presenting with back pain, dermatomal cutaneous symptoms, and bowel or bladder dysfunction. Unlike neurofibromatosis type 1, which has strong cutaneous manifestations such as neurofibromas and café-au-lait spots, NF2 manifests a relative paucity of cutaneous abnormalities.

Cholesteatomas

Cholesteatomas are benign but locally destructive growths of squamous epithelial cells that collect either in the middle ear or mastoid air cells. Although cholesteatomas can be congenital, most are acquired. Progressive retraction of the tympanic membrane from negative pressure in the middle ear, frequently from eustachian tube dysfunction or otitis media, can render a tear in the tympanic membrane, allowing skin cells to enter into the middle ear. Continued sloughing of these skin cells increases the size of the cholesteatoma, which can cause mechanical pressure on the ossicular chain, leading to conductive hearing loss. The most common presenting sign of a cholesteatoma is a painless discharge through a perforated tympanic membrane. Cholesteatomas can become infected, but because they do not have a blood supply, infections are not responsive to antibiotics. Almost all cholesteatomas are treated with surgical removal. Unchecked cholesteatomas can become locally invasive and grow into the temporal bone, leading to complications such as meningitis and sigmoid sinus thrombosis. They are otherwise easy to diagnose by an otolaryngologist through a combination of direct inspection of the external ear canal, audiometry, and sometimes computed tomography of the temporal bones.

Hearing Loss & Deafness

Significant hearing loss affects about one-third of adults over the age of 65 years globally and increases in prevalence with age. Hearing loss can be conductive, sensorineural, or mixed. Conductive hearing loss occurs when there is impaired transmission of sound pressure energy in the pathway between the external canal, the middle ear ossicles, and the oval window at the base of the stapes (see Figure 36–1A). Common causes of conductive hearing loss include foreign bodies in the external canal, impacted cerumen, perforated tympanic membrane, AOM, otitis media with effusion, ossicular disruption due to head trauma, cholesteatomas, otosclerosis, and congenital malformations of the temporal bone or middle ear.

Sensorineural hearing loss involves dysfunction of the inner ear apparatus that performs the mechanoelectrical transduction of auditory information to the brain. Damage to the hair cells in the cochlea or injury of the cochlear nerve leads to sensorineural hearing loss. A characteristic of sensorineural

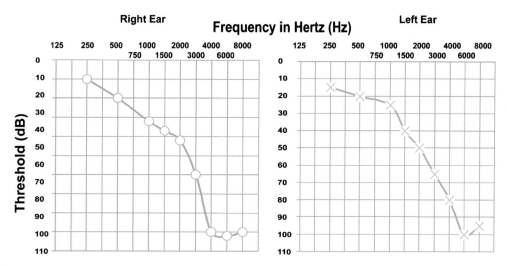

FIGURE 36–2 Audiogram of the right and left ears showing a "down-sloping" pattern of hearing loss in each. Pure-tone frequencies are represented from left to right. Increasing intensities are represented from top to bottom. This audiogram shows that higher intensities at the higher frequencies are needed for this patient to detect the sound, typical of age-related hearing loss. Hearing detection at 20 dB or lower is considered normal. (Reproduced with permission from Halter JB, Ouslander JG, Studenski S, et al: *Hazzard's Geriatric Medicine and Gerontology.* 7th ed. New York, NY: McGraw Hill; 2017.)

hearing loss is poor speech discrimination even at an audible speech detection threshold. Common causes of sensorineural hearing loss include age-related hair cell degeneration, noise exposure, genetics, autoimmune disorders, tumors compressing the cochlear nerve (typically a vestibular schwannoma), Ménière disease, and exposure to ototoxic medications.

Hearing levels are measured on a logarithmic scale at different frequencies (Figure 36–2). A typical clinical audiogram tests hearing thresholds from 250 to 8000 Hz. Hearing thresholds are measured in decibels (dB), a ratio of the sound intensity of a presented sound relative to a set of internal sounds calibrated in the testing device. Each 10 dB of hearing represents an amplification of 10 times, meaning that 30 dB represents 10 times the sound energy at 20 dB and 100 times the sound energy at 10 dB. A measure of 3 dB represents an approximately 2-fold difference in sound energy. The sound pressure level at which a patient can hear a tone is referred to as the hearing threshold; thresholds at each frequency are tested individually, generally in 5- to 10-dB increments.

Permanent damage to cochlear hair cells can be incurred with extremely brief amounts of loud noise exposure. The duration of exposure and the sound pressure level needed to induce permanent damage are inversely related. A 90-dB sound (eg, as loud as a motorcycle) requires 8 hours of exposure, whereas a 110-dB sound (eg, a rock concert) requires just 30 minutes to induce permanent hair cell damage. Hearing thresholds can be tested to 120 dB, but for practical purposes, a hearing level that requires a sound intensity of >70 dB for perception qualifies as severe hearing loss.

Age-related sensorineural hearing loss preferentially affects the higher frequencies (see Figure 36–2). Because audiograms are written with increasing frequencies from left to right and sound thresholds increasing from top to bottom, a "down-sloping" pattern is described for age-related hearing

loss. In contrast, noise-related hearing loss typically creates a "notched" pattern in the 4000 to 6000 Hz range and a recovery at 8000 Hz. The hearing loss of Ménière disease preferentially affects the lower frequencies (although it can be of any pattern), which gives rise to an "up-sloping" pattern. Hearing loss that is most prominent in the midfrequencies is typical of congenital hearing loss and is reported as a "cookie bite" pattern. Hearing detection at 20 dB or lower is considered within normal limits. Regular human conversation occurs at about 20 to 40 dB, so hearing loss beyond this level will interfere with normal speech. Very loud talking or shouting is in the range of 60 to 70 dB. When hearing thresholds are beyond this level, the hearing is considered nonserviceable.

Hearing loss may be congenital, occurring in about 0.1% to 0.3% of births. Congenital hearing loss may be associated with infections, syndromic genetic causes, and nonsyndromic causes. In utero infections, particularly with cytomegalovirus, rubella (German measles), and lymphocytic choriomeningitis virus, are the most common acquired congenital causes. HIV and herpes simplex virus types 1 and 2 are associated with both congenital and acquired hearing loss, whereas varicella (chickenpox), mumps, measles (rubeola), and West Nile virus are associated with acquired postnatal hearing loss. Genetic factors account for about 50% of the risk of hearing loss and may play a role in the vulnerability to hearing loss in the elderly. Autosomal recessive, autosomal dominant, X-linked, and mitochondrial modes of inheritance have all been reported, and there are presently >100 genes that have been implicated in genetic contributions to hearing loss. Most genetic causes of hearing loss (about 80%) are nonsyndromic (ie, not associated with other clinical features). About half of the mutations that are associated with hearing loss are in the gap junction protein connexin-26 (also known as GJB2). Mutations in actin, collagen, and other connexin proteins make up the majority of

CASE 36–1

A 50-year-old man has noticed progressive difficulty following conversations. This is particularly difficult in noisy environments such as restaurants. Because he frequently misses key elements of conversations, he often asks questions repeatedly and finds this to be embarrassing. He has become less involved in social functions. He had worked as a roofer all his life using a nail gun several hundred times a day, but he never used ear protection. His mother had also suffered from hearing loss starting from the age of 50 years. He has tried hearing aids but is variably compliant in using them.

Discussion

Sensorineural hearing loss affects about 35% of people over the age of 65 years. Latent genetic factors may be an important contributor to the vulnerability of hearing loss from acquired factors such as noise exposure and age. Patients with hearing loss may find hearing amplification systems helpful. However, they do not separate background from foreground sounds nor are they able to perform selective frequency amplification on a situation-to-situation basis, as the normal feedback system of the human inner ear is able to achieve. This contributes to poor adherence. Untreated hearing loss can lead to embarrassment and social isolation and is thus important to recognize and prevent when possible.

other genetic loci. Mutations that follow an autosomal dominant inheritance pattern are termed *DFNA*; mutations that follow an autosomal recessive pattern are termed *DFNB*; and mutations that follow an X-linked pattern are termed *DFN*.

Deafness is a common feature of syndromic genetic disorders, particularly those associated with dysmorphic facial features, retinal disorders, renal dysfunction, and neuropathy. Among these are Pendred syndrome, in which sensorineural hearing loss is associated with thyroid dysfunction; Alport syndrome, which is associated with renal dysfunction; and Usher syndrome, which is associated with retinitis pigmentosa and variable degrees of concurrent vestibular dysfunction. Hearing loss is typical of mitochondrial disorders such as myoclonic epilepsy with ragged red fibers (MERRF), mitochondrial encephalomyopathy lactic acidosis and stroke-like episodes (MELAS), and Kearns-Sayre syndrome. Structural abnormalities of the inner ear can occur in isolation such as in Mondini dysplasia, in which development is arrested before the usual 2.5 turns of the cochlea are completed. Enlarged vestibular aqueducts (the channel between the inner ear and the endolymphatic sac) can occur in isolation or be a part of the Pendred syndrome. They can lead to both hearing loss and vestibular dysfunction.

Hearing amplification can increase sound detection by 100 to 1000 times. However, it does not improve discrimination of foreground from background noise, like attending to a particular individual's voice in a noisy environment. Although different frequencies can be amplified specifically by modern hearing aids, they cannot make the moment-by-moment frequency-specific tuning adjustments performed by the native outer hair cells, which are typically damaged by most causes of sensorineural hearing loss. If the hearing loss is conductive and the sound amplification pathway cannot be repaired, a bone-anchored hearing aid can be used to bypass the regular conduction pathway and directly conduct sound through the skull into the inner ear. A cochlear implant can bypass the normal cochlear apparatus in the case of severe sensorineural hearing loss.

Otosclerosis

Otosclerosis is a rare progressive disorder in which remodeling of the middle ear ossicles (malleus, incus, and stapes) and otic capsule (the bone surrounding the cochlea and semicircular canals) results in a mixture of both conductive and sensorineural hearing loss. The remodeling process begins in adolescence and the early 20s through an early phase called *otospongiosis*, in which the bone is actively remodeling and may be soft. During this time, sensorineural hearing loss may start. Attempts to harden the bone during this vulnerable time with treatment with fluoride have had mixed results. As the disease progresses, the ossicles fuse and become unable to effectively transmit the mechanical vibrations of the eardrum to the oval window. One of the most common places in which problematic fusion occurs is at the baseplate of the stapes at its interface with the oval window. Stapedectomy, a surgical technique that replaces the native stapes with a prosthetic, is used as a temporizing measure to improve the conductive hearing loss component. The disorder progresses into a mixed stage and generally plateaus in the late 30s. Imbalance may be a feature of otosclerosis as the vestibular apparatus also becomes affected. Hearing aids for amplification may be helpful (eg, with a bone-anchored hearing aid), particularly in overcoming the conductive hearing loss component. Regular amplification for the sensorineural hearing loss component is generally less effective, especially because sensorineural hearing loss is associated with poor speech discrimination. Hormones, particularly estrogen, play an important role in the pathogenesis of otosclerosis because the disease tends to worsen in pregnancy and is twice as common in women as in men. There is evidence that otosclerosis is inherited in an autosomal dominant manner with reduced penetrance. This diagnosis should be suspected in individuals with a family history of hearing loss. There is evidence for vascular and infectious etiologies that contribute, particularly the measles virus. Clinically, the prevalence of clinical otosclerosis is much less than 1%, and it appears to be declining in incidence, a phenomenon that has been ascribed to the spread of the measles, mumps, rubella (MMR) vaccine. However, temporal bone studies show that up to 10% of individuals have some evidence of otosclerosis.

Tinnitus

Tinnitus is the abnormal perception of sound in the absence of an external auditory stimulus. The vast majority of cases of tinnitus are experienced as a subjective perception, with only rare cases also audible by the examiner. These rare cases of objective tinnitus are typically caused by muscular contractions or by the transmission of the sounds in blood vessels. Subjective tinnitus is usually described as a whistling, hissing, chirping, or buzzing perception when experienced in association with sensorineural hearing loss. Tinnitus that is described as roaring or rumbling should raise concerns for endolymphatic hydrops or abnormal intracranial pressure. Because the endolymphatic canal is a potential space that connects the intracranial space to the inner ear, pressure changes in the intracranial cavity (high or low) can affect inner ear pressure and cause tinnitus. Tinnitus affects about 30% of adults either chronically or intermittently, typically being most prominent in very quiet environments. However, about 3% to 5% of adults are chronically affected by tinnitus, and 1% are affected to the point of significant impairment of daily functioning. When severe, tinnitus can contribute to cognitive dysfunction, depression, feelings of helplessness, and difficulty with sleeping. About 90% of cases of tinnitus are associated with sensorineural hearing loss, and thus, it is more common in older patients. Noise exposure, even short periods of very loud sounds (eg, rock concerts, jackhammers, gun firing), can induce hair cell damage and cause prolonged tinnitus. The present dominant theory of tinnitus involves the remapping of the tonotopic map of the auditory cortex. However, since tinnitus can occur in the absence of hearing loss, there are likely different mechanisms. If tinnitus is unilateral, a search should be made for structural damage to the cochlear apparatus, including the eighth nerve, and for vascular malformations at the skull base. Dozens of medications can potentially cause tinnitus, but the most common are salicylates (eg, aspirin), loop diuretics (eg, furosemide), and quinine. Some patients are less able to mask out normal physiologic sounds such as the venous hum from the jugular vein, and high-flow states such as anemia, high-output heart failure, thyrotoxicosis, and pregnancy can be associated with pulsatile tinnitus.

Treatment for tinnitus remains fairly limited. Presenting the patient with a range of sound frequencies and matching the one that masks the internal perception can map the tinnitus frequency. Theoretically, the bandwidth of the subjectively experienced tinnitus should be masked by presentation of the same frequency. This is the principle by which frequency-specific masking devices are used therapeutically. Broadband white noise generators may be just as effective, however. Hearing aids may help to increase ambient sounds to avoid the central remapping process and drown out the internal perception. A form of cognitive-behavioral therapy called tinnitus retraining therapy attempts to enhance habituation to the tinnitus so that the tinnitus is no longer perceived to be threatening and can be ignored.

Disorders of Balance & Spatial Orientation

Vertigo

Vertigo, as defined in the International Classification of Vestibular Disorders, is any false sense of motion and is further divided into internal vertigo, in which the perception is of self-motion, and external vertigo, in which the perception is of movement of the surround. It can be spinning or nonspinning. In the case of nonspinning vertigo, the perceived motion can be swaying, bobbing, tilting, or sliding. Both internal and external vertigo are further defined as spontaneous, triggered, positional, head motion induced, visually induced, sound induced, Valsalva induced, and orthostatic. The term *vertigo* is distinct from the term *dizziness*, which is defined as a sense of disturbed or impaired spatial orientation not involving a false sense of motion. It includes all the same subcategories as vertigo. Both vertigo and dizziness should be considered distinct from unsteadiness and primary visual symptoms such as oscillopsia or visual tilt.

Benign Paroxysmal Positional Vertigo

Benign paroxysmal positional vertigo (BPPV) is an episodic disorder in which brief spells of vertigo are triggered by head movement. BPPV is a common disorder that increases in prevalence with age. About 25% of individuals over the age of 75 years will experience at least one episode of BPPV. Risk factors for the development of BPPV include older age, head trauma, osteoporosis, prior injury to the inner ear, and a history of migraine headaches. Calcium carbonate crystals that are normally embedded in the macula of the utricle become dislodged and fall into the semicircular canals (Figure 36–3). Because of the dependent orientation of the posterior canal, the particles fall into this canal about 85% to 90% of the time. The horizontal canal is affected in 10% to 13% of cases, and the anterior canal is affected in about 1% of cases. Because of the higher density of the particles in relation to the endolymphatic fluid, they settle into the most dependent part of the canal whenever the head is moved. When the individual moves his or her head horizontally, the most dependent portion does not change. Therefore, it is unusual for horizontal head movements to trigger BPPV spells. When the head is moved vertically, however, the most dependent part of the

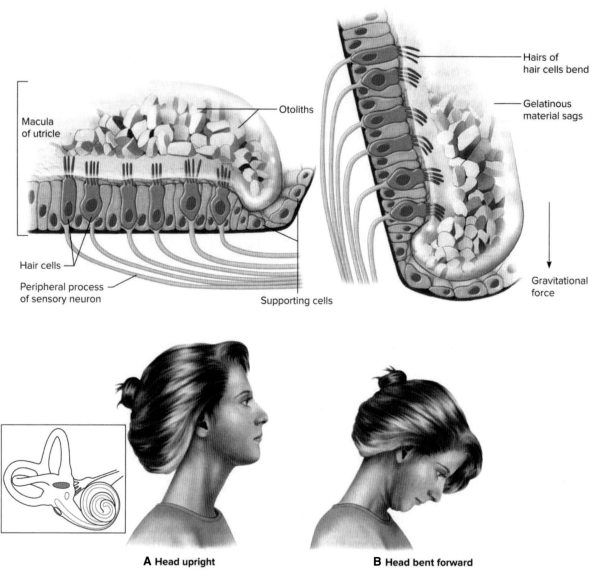

A Head upright   **B Head bent forward**

FIGURE 36–3 Close-up of the macula of the utricle. The heavy otoliths on the macula create a shear force as they are pulled down by gravity when the head is tilted, causing deflection of the hair cells and relaying of gravity-related head position information. In benign paroxysmal positional vertigo, the otoliths of the utricle become dislodged and fall into the semicircular canal, typically in the posterior canal. (Reproduced with permission from Shier D, Butler J, Lewis R. *Hole's Human Anatomy & Physiology*, 15th ed. New York, NY: McGraw Hill; 2019.)

canal shifts, and the particles slide to the new more dependent position. In this process, the endolymphatic fluid is moved, which causes deflection of the cupula, stimulation of the hair cells, and activation of the vestibular nerve. The result is vertigo and nystagmus that beats in the direction dictated by the involved canal. For the posterior and anterior canal, it is a torsional vertical nystagmus (upbeat for posterior, downbeat for anterior). For the horizontal canal, it is a horizontal nystagmus. The typical movements that trigger BPPV are extending the head back, lying down (eg, in bed), and arising from a recumbent position. The posterior semicircular canal lies 45 degrees off the sagittal plane. Thus, rolling over to the side of the affected ear also triggers vertigo with posterior canal involvement.

In many cases, BPPV will resolve on its own through reabsorption of the calcium carbonate particles back into the endolymphatic fluid. The average duration of symptoms of posterior canal involvement is 39 days, and the average duration of horizontal involvement is 16 days. Posterior canal BPPV is diagnosed through bedside positional testing, eponymously known as the Dix-Hallpike maneuver. In this maneuver, the patient is seated on a table facing the examiner with the patient's head turned 45 degrees toward the examiner. The examiner then lowers the patient's head down to a head-extended position. The side to which the patient is turning is the side being tested. In the case of a right-sided BPPV of the posterior canal, nystagmus that beats counterclockwise with an upbeat component will be triggered. When the left side is involved, the nystagmus is clockwise with an upbeat component. There is usually a slight delay in the onset of the nystagmus, which typically lasts <20 seconds. In horizontal canal BPPV, the patient is laid supine. The head is turned to the right for about 1 minute and then to the left for about 1 minute. The nystagmus that is elicited is a geotropic beating nystagmus. In the right ear down position, the nystagmus beats toward the right ear. In the left ear down position, the nystagmus beats toward the left ear. In a related disorder called *cupulolithiasis*, the calcium carbonate crystals become stuck on cupula of the horizontal canal. In this case, the triggered nystagmus is apogeotropic, meaning that it beats to the left when the patient is lying with the right ear down and it beats to the right when the patient is lying with the left ear down.

BPPV can be easily treated with a variety of canalith liberatory maneuvers that attempt to roll the particles out of the semicircular canals back into the utricle. In the case of posterior canal involvement, after the initial Dix-Hallpike test is done, the patient is rolled over to the opposite side until another burst of vertigo is elicited. Then the patient is sat up. In the case of horizontal BPPV, the patient is rolled in a "barbeque-roll" maneuver toward the unaffected ear. BPPV can recur, with a general recurrence rate of about 50% within 5 years, although about 80% of these recurrences happen within the first year.

Vestibular Neuritis

Vestibular neuritis has an incidence of about 3.5 in 100,000 people and occurs through reactivation of herpes simplex virus in the vestibular ganglion, leading to an inflamed and consequently demyelinated nerve. Clinically, affected individuals present with the subacute onset of isolated spinning vertigo. If there are concurrent auditory symptoms, then labyrinthitis and Ménière disease should also be considered. If the onset of vertigo is hyperacute, a cerebellar infarction should be considered in the differential diagnosis. In the acute phase, relative dysfunction of the affected vestibular nerve leads to a spontaneous nystagmus that beats away from the affected ear. Central compensation begins rather rapidly, so after a few days, this spontaneous nystagmus may only be seen when visual fixation is removed (eg, if the patient is placed in the dark or when the patient is wearing Frenzel lenses). The initial symptoms of vertigo are typically prostrating, but recovery occurs within several days, and most patients are ambulatory within a week. Recurrences are very uncommon, typically at a rate of about 1% to 2% within 10 years. Therefore, "recurrent" vestibular neuritis should only be diagnosed when there is laboratory evidence of a new vestibular paresis. Although the majority of patients recover without residual symptoms, about 30% of patients with vestibular neuritis can be left with persistent head motion–triggered dizziness and may have a difficult time participating in activities that involve a lot of fast head movements. Vestibular neuritis is pathophysiologically similar to Bell palsy, and there is similar evidence that treatment with steroids within the first 3 days is helpful in maintaining long-term vestibular function, although whether this translates to improved functional status of the patient is still ambiguous.

Ménière Disease

Ménière disease is the eponymous term for idiopathic endolymphatic hydrops, a syndrome of episodic inner ear dysfunction leading to attacks of severe vertigo, tinnitus, aural

CASE 36–2

A 50-year-old man presents with the gradual onset of severe room-spinning vertigo. He notes that the symptom started around 1 pm, and by the evening, he was so vertiginous that he could not stand. Nausea and vomiting ensued. He denies hearing loss, tinnitus, and ear fullness. He could only slow down the spinning by staring at a point on the wall. He notes being ill with an upper respiratory illness about 2 weeks prior to the onset of the vertigo. His exam is significant for a spontaneous right-beating nystagmus that increases on gaze to the right and decreases on gaze to the left. On head impulse testing, he has a catch-up saccade on head thrust to the left. Other cranial nerve, motor, sensory, and coordination tests are normal. He can stand with his eyes open, but when his eyes are closed, he falls to the left.

Discussion

This is a classic example of vestibular neuritis, in this case of the left vestibular nerve. The onset is subacute, progressing over hours, and culminates in severe prostrating vertigo. There are no auditory symptoms such as tinnitus, hearing loss, or aural pressure. If there were features of these, then either Ménière disease or labyrinthitis should be considered. Each vestibular system deviates the eyes conjugately away from itself, and thus, a corrective saccade to a neutral position will be toward the healthy ear. Therefore, a spontaneous right-beating nystagmus indicates that the healthy ear is the right ear. Visual fixation will suppress a peripheral nystagmus, and patients will often learn to focus on a stationary object, such as a point on the wall, in order to suppress the nystagmus and the vertigo. Normally, the vestibulo-ocular system is so efficient that if an individual is asked to look straight ahead while the head is being quickly accelerated to 1 side, the eyes will make an instantaneous adjustment in the opposite direction in order to keep fixation straight. If the vestibular nerve is inflamed and demyelinated, conduction of high acceleration information through the vestibular nerve to the brainstem and to the extraocular muscles will be slowed. Thus, on head thrust toward the impaired side, the eyes will move with the head and then make an adjustment back to midline. This adjustment is termed a *catch-up saccade* and is the classic sign of an acute peripheral vestibular injury.

fullness, and hearing loss. The attacks typically last from 20 minutes to up to 5 to 6 hours and are thought to be due to congestion of the endolymphatic space. Endolymphatic hydrops can result from a variety of insults to the inner ear including ischemic, inflammatory, and infectious causes that lead to disrupted fluid balance. The term *Ménière disease* is reserved for cases of endolymphatic hydrops without a known proximate cause, whereas hydrops that develops after a known injury is frequently referred to as *delayed endolymphatic hydrops*. The fluid channels within the cochlea are separated into 3 compartments—the scala vestibuli, scala media, and scala tympani. The scala vestibuli and tympani contain perilymph, a fluid that resembles extracellular fluid in other parts of the body, being high in sodium (140 mM) and low in potassium (5 mM). In contrast, the endolymphatic fluid within the scala media is very high in potassium (150 mM) and low in sodium (1 mM). The auditory sensory apparatus, the organ of Corti, resides in the scala media and consists of the basilar membrane, the inner and outer hair cells, the overlying tectorial membrane, and the innervating neural structures. Dysregulation of the finely tuned fluid dynamics within this 3-compartment system leads to congestion within the endolymphatic space and disruption of normal auditory processing. Postmortem series show, however, that histologic evidence of hydrops can exist in the temporal bones of people who had no clinical evidence of hydrops attacks in their lifetimes.

Early in the course of endolymphatic hydrops attacks, the tinnitus is often described as a low-frequency "roaring" sound. In addition, in the early stage of hearing loss, the audiogram shows an up-sloping pattern indicating decreased hearing in the lower frequencies. As attacks accumulate, the tinnitus and hearing loss assume a mixed pattern. The consumption of high-salt foods, stress, and sleep deprivation are known triggers of attacks of endolymphatic hydrops. Therefore, medical management consists of limiting dietary salt, using a diuretic, and controlling stress reactions. Most cases of endolymphatic hydrops do remit naturally as the inner ear becomes progressively more damaged with each episode and is subsequently less able to generate attacks. Temporizing measures include intratympanic dexamethasone injections. Surgical interventions for intractable cases of vertigo include ablation of the labyrinth with gentamicin and vestibular nerve section, which are considered hearing-preserving measures, although each does carry a risk of hearing loss. Labyrinthectomy is considered an option if there is nonserviceable hearing.

Motion Sickness

Motion sickness is the feeling of unwellness that occurs during and often for some time after exposure to passive motion. Symptoms may include nausea, stomach awareness, sweating, headache, or drowsiness. It can occur with water, air, or land travel. Although exposure to rapid motion, such as on roller coaster rides, can be a potent motion sick inducer, motion sickness is most acutely induced with very-low-frequency oscillating motion with a peak at around 0.2 Hz. This may explain why wavelike motion is the most common trigger for motion sickness. Motion sickness is more common in women, with susceptibility decreasing with age, and children between the ages of 5 and 12 years. Individuals with bilateral vestibular loss are resistant to motion sickness induced by body motion. However, they can still be quite sensitive to visual motion–induced feelings of nausea. Motion sickness triggered by exposure to visual motion is most typically experienced by looking at large-screen televisions and movie screens and, more frequently in the modern day, through virtual reality and full visual field immersive simulation experiences. Several theories have been presented through the years to explain why the motion sickness reaction exists. One intuitive theory proposes that a feeling of unwellness is the natural consequence of a conflict between visual and vestibular motion information, such as when one is reading in a car. The vestibular system indicates that the car is moving, while the visual system indicates that the person is not.

The vestibular system adapts to constant velocity very quickly, so this explanation is not wholly adequate. Being able to predict the motion can reduce motion sickness, so cognitive control mechanisms are important (eg, drivers are less motion sick than passengers). Habituation to the motion over time reduces the incidence of motion sickness, a phenomenon seen in novice versus experienced sailors. Vestibular suppressants are typically used to prevent motion sickness in the short term. Most have either anticholinergic or antihistaminergic effects. Common motion sickness treatments include scopolamine patches and pills, meclizine, dimenhydrinate, and promethazine.

Traumatic & Mechanical Disorders

Barotrauma

Barotrauma refers to injury to external, middle, or inner ear structures due to exposure to rapid pressure differentials for which there is inadequate time to accommodate or there are physical obstructions to pressure relief. Pressure-related injury can occur from external forces, such as exposure to explosions, direct trauma to the head, rapid descent in altitude, or diving into water. Injury can also come internally during forceful sneezes or the Valsalva maneuver. Mild barotrauma is associated with pain, feelings of ear fullness, and conductive hearing loss. The most common etiology is the inability to equalize middle ear pressure with atmospheric pressure when descending in altitude. The typical scenario is in the setting of eustachian tube dysfunction and otitis media.

More severe barotrauma can cause tears in the tympanic membrane, dislodged ossicles in the middle ear, or dehiscence of the bony integrity of the otic capsule creating connections with the middle ear, as in the case of perilymphatic fistulas, or with the intracranial space, as in the case of superior (ie, anterior) canal dehiscence. Conductive hearing loss occurs when injury is limited to the external and middle ears, whereas sensorineural hearing loss is typical of perilymphatic fistulas in which the inner ear and middle ear are connected by a "third" window (which is distinct from the oval window and the round window). Superior canal dehiscence leads to sound- and pressure-related spells of vertigo (ie, the patient develops vertigo when exposed to sudden loud noises or when performing maneuvers that raise intracranial pressure such as coughing, sneezing, or bearing down). The vertigo occurs because pressure from the intracranial space is transmitted into the superior canal through that third window.

Perforation of Tympanic Membrane

The tympanic membrane (eardrum) separates the external auditory canal from the middle ear (see Figure 36–1). The outer surface layer is made up of squamous cells similar to what makes up skin. The *pars tensa* portion has a fibrous middle layer and an inner mucosal layer. The *pars flaccida* portion only has the inner and outer layers and is thus flaccid. The tympanic membrane transmits sound vibrations entering the external canal to the middle ear ossicles and ultimately to the cochlea through the oval window. The tympanic membrane can be ruptured either from external trauma or from increased pressure in the middle ear, resulting in conductive hearing loss. The *pars tensa* is more commonly ruptured than the *pars flaccida*. Common causes of trauma include direct injury from objects inserted into the external canal, such as bobby pins or cotton swabs, and barotrauma from the ear being struck or exposed to sudden high pressure such as from explosions, rapid descent on diving, and head injury. Otitis media can cause the tympanic membrane to rupture, causing otorrhea, otalgia, and loss of hearing. Situations in which middle ear pressure cannot equilibrate with atmospheric pressure because of eustachian tube dysfunction raise the risk of a perforation. Small tympanic membrane perforations may heal naturally within several weeks, but larger holes may need to be patched by an otolaryngologist, a process called *tympanoplasty*. During the healing period, water and potentially infectious agents must be prevented from entering the middle ear and damaging the ossicles. Incisions in the tympanic membrane (ie, tympanostomy or myringotomy) and placement of pressure-equalization tubes may be performed by otolaryngologists in order to prevent recurrent otitis media.

Foreign Body in Ear

A variety of small foreign objects may enter the external ear canal either intentionally or unintentionally. The risk starts once babies can develop a pincer grasp to hold things such as raisins, pencil erasers, and small toys, and they inadvertently place them in the ear. The risk of foreign bodies is highest in the 4- to 8-year age group, generally because of insertion of jewelry, rocks, nuts and other organic material, and pieces of small toys. In adults, the dislodged tips of cotton swabs, insects, and loosened batteries of hearing aids are more common. Intentional placement of vegetable material such as herbs and leaves and the practice of ear candling for purported therapeutic purposes are other considerations. The existence of foreign bodies in the ear may not be noticed by the patient, particularly by children. However, common symptoms include itching, feeling of fullness, conductive hearing loss, pain, and the production of foul odors. Care must be taken in removal of foreign objects not to abrade the skin of the external canal. Organic material may increase in size when the ear is irrigated, making removal more difficult. Consideration for whether the tympanic membrane is compromised must be made when attempting to irrigate out the foreign body and particularly when the object itself may be stuck onto the tympanic membrane such as with pieces of glue, gum, or the hook of a sharp object. Potentially corrosive objects such as dislodged batteries should be removed with direct visualization from a healthcare professional with experience in this procedure.

Impacted Cerumen

Cerumen (earwax) is a natural product of the external ear and is made up of sloughed skin cells, hair, and secretions of the sebaceous and apocrine sweat glands of the ear. The quantity, color, and content of cerumen vary greatly between individuals and across races. Cerumen is naturally acidic and plays an important role in protecting against exogenous pathogens that can cause OE. The natural growth of skin cells and jaw movement push cerumen to the opening of the external ear canal until it falls out. Exuberant clearance of cerumen can increase the risk of subsequent OE by removing an important protective barrier against the invasion of common pathogens that colonize the skin such as *Pseudomonas* and *Staphylococcus*.

Although the external ears generally do not have to be cleared of cerumen, certain conditions increase the probability of cerumen impaction. Cerumen impaction can lead to conductive hearing loss, tinnitus, discomfort, foul odors, and even chronic cough and increased vagal tone due to the innervation of the external canal by the vagus nerve. Risk factors for cerumen impaction include frequent probing of the external canal with foreign objects that push the cerumen in more deeply, the use of hearing aids, and anatomic irregularities that prevent normal clearance. Residents of nursing homes, hospitalized patients, developmentally delayed individuals, and children are at particularly high risk. Impacted cerumen can be manually extracted with cerumen scoops or forceps by a healthcare provider under direct visualization. Because cerumen can become quite hard, cerumenolytics such as docusate, hydrogen peroxide, acetic acid, saline, and even water can be used ahead of manual removal or irrigation. The practice of ear candling may worsen cerumen impaction and may also lead to skin burns. There is no evidence that it helps with cerumen clearance. Care must be taken not to disturb the tympanic membrane, which if disturbed can cause pain and risk perforation.

Lacerations & Avulsions

Given its exposed position on the head, the auricle (external ear) can be easily traumatized by bites, burns, or crush and shear forces that are associated with head injury. The skin of the auricle is highly vascular and generally heals well when repaired. The underlying cartilage, however, is avascular and is dependent on the overlying skin for its blood supply. Chondritis may occur as a consequence of trauma to the auricle that results in breaking of the overlying skin. During repair of the auricle, care must be taken to avoid cutting through the cartilage and creating pockets of devitalized tissue that may become foci for infections.

Eustachian Tube Disorders

The eustachian tube connects the middle ear and the nasopharynx and functions to equalize the pressure in the middle ear to atmospheric pressure, protect the middle ear from pathogens from the nasopharynx, and aid in clearing the middle ear of fluid and debris. The middle ear tends to develop progressive negative pressure from mucosal gas exchange and requires periodic equilibration with the nasopharynx to maintain normal pressure. The bony upper third of the eustachian tube is part of the temporal bone, whereas the lower two-thirds is cartilaginous and is kept open by the contraction of the levator veli palatini and the tensor veli palatini. It otherwise remains closed at rest. Symptoms of eustachian tube dysfunction include a feeling of pressure or fullness of the ear, often associated with "popping" or "crackling" sounds, and pain. Symptoms can occur at normal atmospheric pressure or be induced by changes in ambient pressure such as on airplane descent or deep-water diving. Patients may complain of feeling like the ear is under water and that they can hear their own voice inside their heads (autophony). Autophony is particularly common with patulous eustachian tubes (ie, when the tube stays patent at baseline, causing sound and pressure in the nasopharynx to be transmitted directly into the middle ear). Patulous tubes are associated with frequent sniffing and Valsalva maneuvers in an attempt to clear the middle ear. Risk for eustachian tube dysfunction is increased by recurrent otitis media, upper respiratory infections, allergic rhinitis, gastroesophageal reflux, and nasopharyngeal surgery. Significant weight loss and dehydration may be additional risk factors.

Adverse Effects of Drugs on the Ear

Although there are >100 medications that are associated with damage to the inner ear, there are 4 major classes of ototoxic medications: aminoglycoside antibiotics, loop diuretics, anticancer agents, and salicylates. Among these, aminoglycosides are the most commonly associated with medication-induced ototoxicity. These medications may also cause nephrotoxicity. Some agents are preferentially cochleotoxic, causing hearing loss and tinnitus, whereas others are more vestibulotoxic, causing dizziness and imbalance. The main mechanism of injury appears to be free radical damage either directly to the cochlear and vestibular hair cells or to the stria vascularis, the epithelial layer that produces endolymphatic fluid. When cochleotoxic medications produce tinnitus, it is typically reversible with rapid cessation of the medication. However, concurrent hearing loss is usually permanent, so care must be taken to recognize any early symptoms of ototoxicity in order to avoid irreversible

injury. Hearing loss typically starts in the very high frequencies (>4000 Hz) and may be missed if attention is only paid to voice recognition. Vestibulotoxicity tends to be permanent, with damage that increases with longer exposure. Therefore, vigilance should be high for early signs of vestibulotoxicity, especially in patients who are not mobile and therefore not able to manifest gait imbalance. Symptoms of vestibulotoxicity include blurred vision with head movement, oscillopsia, and gait imbalance. Because the damage is bilateral, patients will typically not complain of vertigo. Risk factors for ototoxicity include longer exposure to the offending agent, exposure to high doses, concurrent treatment with 2 or more ototoxic medications, renal dysfunction, older age, and preexisting inner ear disease. Even after an offending agent is stopped, damage to the inner ear can continue for months, so long-term monitoring is recommended when signs of ototoxicity are discovered.

The most commonly used aminoglycoside antibiotic is gentamicin, which preferentially causes vestibulotoxicity; cochleotoxicity occurs in about 10% of cases. Therefore, monitoring for ototoxicity in patients on gentamicin should involve screening for bilateral vestibular failure (eg, a slowed vestibulo-ocular reflex [VOR]). A quick and sensitive bedside test for vestibular dysfunction is to test vision with a hand-held eye chart and compare visual acuity when the head is still versus when the patient's head is shaken horizontally at 2 Hz. Losing >2 lines of visual acuity with head shaking signifies a slowed VOR and should prompt a modification of therapy. Streptomycin is even more vestibulotoxic than gentamicin and thus rarely used clinically, except in some cases of tuberculosis. Amikacin, neomycin, kanamycin, and tobramycin are preferentially cochleotoxic and are rarely used systemically, although amikacin is occasionally used to treat particularly severe gram-negative infections.

Acetylsalicylic acid (ie, aspirin) is usually not problematic at doses used for common clinical indications such as for its analgesic, antipyretic, or antiplatelet aggregation properties, but at higher doses, such as those used to treat rheumatologic disorders, it can lead to bothersome tinnitus and even hearing loss. These symptoms typically have a rapid onset and resolve with cessation of the offending agent if it is stopped before hearing loss ensues. Similarly, loop diuretics such as furosemide, bumetanide, and ethacrynic acid can cause tinnitus and hearing loss, which are usually reversible if stopped early. However, the hearing loss may be permanent in the setting of concurrent renal failure, prior hearing loss, or concurrent treatment with other ototoxic medications.

The platinum-based anticancer medications cisplatin and, to a lesser degree, carboplatin are the 2 antineoplastic agents that are most frequently associated with ototoxicity. The rate of ototoxicity for cisplatin is >60%, a rate so high that baseline and periodic audiograms are recommended for treatment with this agent. Damage to the stria vascularis and hair cells occurs through free radical production and apoptosis, a process that can trigger further injury even after the agents are out of the systemic circulation. Therefore, audiograms are required even months after cessation of treatment.

CASE 36–3

A 40-year-old woman was admitted for gram-negative sepsis following infection of a dialysis catheter. She had been receiving hemodialysis for renal failure for several years. After she was stabilized, she was sent home to receive intravenous gentamicin through a peripherally inserted central catheter line. Hearing was checked daily, and she reported no change. About 4 weeks into treatment, she noted that the room looked like it was bouncing when she walked. She had a hard time reading her newspaper, thinking that the words were blurred when she moved her head. She had a particularly difficult time walking in the evening as the sun went down.

Discussion

This patient has gentamicin-related bilateral vestibulopathy. Renal failure, intravenous treatment, long duration of treatment, high peak doses, concurrent use of other ototoxic medications, and older age are risk factors. There is general knowledge that aminoglycosides are ototoxic, and medical staff often dutifully check hearing. However, hearing loss is the minor concern in gentamicin ototoxicity; the major concern is vestibular injury. The patient's clinical symptoms are consistent with bilateral vestibular dysfunction, namely in the development of oscillopsia (bouncing vision with head movement) and head-triggered visual blurring, signifying a slowed vestibulo-ocular reflex (VOR). Her gait is impaired in low light because she has become more dependent on vision to maintain balance.

SELF-ASSESSMENT QUESTIONS

1. A 75-year-old man was turning over in bed one night to turn off his reading light. He experienced a brief spell of rotational vertigo lasting about 20 seconds. He decided to go to sleep. In the morning, as he was arising from bed, he had a recurrence of the vertigo, again lasting about 20 seconds. After the vertigo subsided, he got out of bed. His gait was not impaired, and he was able to perform his usual morning activities. However, when he reached for his cereal box in the cupboard above him, he had a recurrence and nearly fell over. There were no auditory, motor, sensory, or coordination problems otherwise. What is the most likely diagnosis?

   A. Benign paroxysmal positional vertigo (BPPV)
   B. A brainstem stroke
   C. Vestibular neuritis
   D. Ménière disease

2. A 20-year-old woman presents with a constant feeling like her ears are plugged and frequently hears a popping or crackling sound in her ears. She notices that when she takes a deep breath she can hear the sound of her breathing, and she finds this very distracting. She is constantly sniffling. She notes having had frequent ear infections as a child. What is the most likely diagnosis?

   A. Otitis media
   B. Eustachian tube dysfunction
   C. Chondritis
   D. Mastoiditis

3. An 18-year-old man presents with bilateral ear pain. He is a swimmer on his high school swim team and is in the water every day. In the winter, he puts a ski cap on over his head after his morning swim. He has noticed that an unpleasant smell is coming from his ears. On exam, the external canals are red and narrowed. He winces when the pinna is touched. He has as a mild fever of 100°F. What is the most likely diagnosis?

   A. Otitis media
   B. Labyrinthitis
   C. Perforated tympanic membrane
   D. Otitis externa (OE)

Ocular Disorders

Brian Samuels

- Understand the basic optics of the eye, including the optics of common refractive errors.
- Understand basic eyelid, orbit, and ocular anatomy, as well as some of the common ocular disorders associated with each tissue.
- Understand the role of the primary care physician in the treatment and diagnosis of some of the more common ocular pathologies, as well as have a basic understanding of when an ophthalmology consult is recommended.

PREVALENCE & BURDEN

There are >35 million individuals throughout the world who are legally blind and an additional 240 million individuals who are classified as having low vision. In the United States alone, the prevalence of blindness and low vision in middle-aged adults and the elderly is approximately 1 and 3 million people, respectively. Although we often focus on the physical burden the visually impaired experience when trying to function in a world that relies heavily on visual cues, we often fail to consider the full emotional impact of vision loss. When asked, many individuals state that their top health-related fear is loss of vision, above loss of a limb, being diagnosed with cancer, or even death. As one might expect, individuals who experience significant vision loss are at a much greater risk of developing depression. Further, although it is understood that loss of vision will have tremendous impact on the life of a visually impaired individual, it is also important to appreciate the impact on the family members and friends who help with their routine care. In many countries, it is the cultural norm for a family member to assume a full-time caretaking role to assist a visually impaired relative. Depending on the age of the individual with vision loss and the chosen caretaker, 1 or possibly 2 people may be removed from the workforce. Thus, not only are there personal health implications, there are also broad economic impacts of vision loss as well.

OPTICS & REFRACTIVE ERRORS

The eye is a specialized neurosensory organ whose primary purpose is to gather and process light stimuli emerging from the visual field and convert it into an electric signal that can be modified and propagated along the visual pathway to neurons in the brain for higher order processing. The first critical step is to focus the incoming light onto the retinal photoreceptors. The eye has a refractive power of approximately +60 diopters; with two-thirds of the refractive power being generated by the cornea and one-third of the refractive power being generated by the natural lens. If the axial length is matched correctly to the refractive power of the eye, parallel beams of light from a distant object (greater than approximately 20 feet away) will be perfectly focused on the retinal plane, and a clear image should be perceived by the individual. When the refractive power and axial length are matched, the person is said to be emmetropic. A mismatch between the refractive power of the eye and the axial length results in refractive errors (Figure 37–1) and the perception of a blurred image. Myopia, or nearsightedness, is a case where the refractive power of the eye in relation to the axial length is too long and the light is focused in front of the retinal plane. Lenses or contacts that cause divergence of light (ie, negative power) are used to correct this problem. Hyperopia, or farsightedness, is the opposite. The refractive power of the eye in relation to the axial length is too low, and the light is focused behind the retinal plane. Lenses or contacts that cause

VOCABULARY

Amblyopia: Permanent visual impairment in an anatomically normal eye that is caused by an abnormal development of the visual pathway and vision processing centers during childhood.

Axial length: The distance from the front of the corneal surface to the retinal plane.

Blindness: The best corrected visual acuity of an individual's better seeing eye is 20/200 or worse.

Low vision: The best corrected visual acuity of an individual's better seeing eye is 20/40 or worse.

Strabismus: A misalignment of the eyes that causes an inability to fixate both eyes on a single focal point or object at the same time.

Visual acuity: The ability of an individual to distinguish between 2 points or identify a specific shape at a certain distance relative to a standard "normal" individual. Someone with 20/40 vision would need to stand at 20 feet in order to distinguish an object that someone with normal vision could distinguish at 40 feet.

Visual field: The complete area that a single eye can see when the eye is held in a fixed position. The visual field of an eye comprises the full central and peripheral vision.

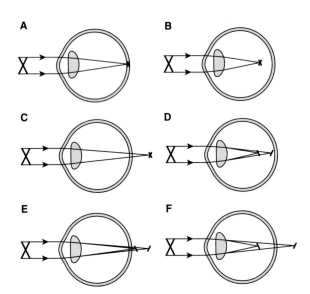

FIGURE 37–1 Different refractive states of the eye. **A.** Emmetropia. Image plane from parallel rays of light are focused on retina. **B.** Myopia. Image plane focuses anterior to retina. **C.** Hyperopia. Image plane focuses posterior to retina. **D.** Astigmatism, myopic type. Images in horizontal and vertical planes focus anterior to retina. **E.** Astigmatism, hyperopic type. Images in horizontal and vertical planes focus posterior to retina. **F.** Astigmatism, mixed type. Images in horizontal and vertical planes focus on either side of retina. (Reproduced with permission from Hay WW Jr, Levin MJ, Deterding RR, et al: *Current Diagnosis & Treatment: Pediatrics*, 23rd ed. New York, NY: McGraw Hill; 2016.)

light to converge (ie, positive power) are used to treat hyperopia. If the cornea or lens imparts dissimilar refractive powers along different axes, this is termed *astigmatism*. There will be 2 focal lines generated, typically 90 degrees from each other, at different distances along the visual axis. The location of those focal lines either in front of, behind, or straddling the retinal plane determines the type of astigmatism. Astigmatism is corrected using lenses or contacts that provide different powers in different axes. Although refractive errors can be temporarily corrected using glasses or contact lenses, patients often consider elective refractive surgery, such as laser-assisted in situ keratomileusis (LASIK) for more permanent correction of refractive errors.

In most instances, refractive errors are corrected so that objects at a distance are in focus. In order to focus on near objects, we need to increase the refractive power of the eye, a process called *accommodation*. To focus on a near object, the ciliary muscle contracts and reduces the tension on the zonules that hold the lens in place. When zonular tension is reduced, the lens assumes a more convex shape, thus increasing its refractive power. As we age, the lens naturally becomes less compliant and loses the ability to change shape. This loss of accommodative power and inability to focus on near objects as we age is termed *presbyopia*. Typically, it is not clinically significant until the mid-40s, at which time reading glasses or bifocal lenses are prescribed.

ORBIT & EYELID

Orbit

The bony orbit is made of 7 bones—the frontal, zygomatic, maxillary, sphenoid, ethmoid, palatine, and lacrimal bones. These create a pear-shaped cavity that contains the globe, a portion of the optic nerve, the extraocular muscles, blood vessels, nerves, and adipose tissue. With a 35- to 40-mm opening, the eye is relatively well protected, but there is still a risk for significant injury from small objects or blunt force trauma to the globe and orbit.

Orbital Fractures

Orbital rim and wall fractures can occur with direct blows to the periorbital region. Although rim fractures often occur as a result of the direct impact, fractures to the orbital walls are often secondary to increased orbital pressure as a result of globe retropulsion and compression of the orbital tissues. The elevated tissue pressure is significant enough to fracture or "blow out" the orbital wall, with the medial orbit and floor being at greatest risk. In many cases, the wall fracture immediately self-reduces and heals with conservative management. It is recommended that patients avoid blowing their nose or performing Valsalva maneuvers to prevent air within the sinuses being forced into the orbit. In addition, oral antibiotics should be considered for medial and floor fractures to prevent sinus contents from seeding the orbital tissue and causing an infection. Because the wall fractures quickly self-reduce,

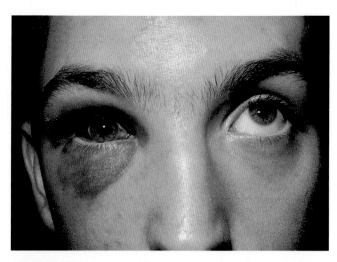

FIGURE 37–2 The right inferior rectus muscle is entrapped within this patient's orbital floor fracture, limiting upward gaze. (Reproduced with permission from Knoop KJ, Stack LB, Storrow AB, et al: *The Atlas of Emergency Medicine*, 4th ed. New York, NY: McGraw Hill; 2016. Photo contributor: Lawrence B. Stack, MD.)

the greatest concern is herniation and incarceration of orbital tissue into the fracture site. Herniated tissue is often seen on orbital computed tomography (CT), but ocular examination will also reveal restriction of eye movements (Figure 37–2). If the rectus muscle is incarcerated, the oculocardiac reflex may be stimulated, resulting in nausea, vomiting, and bradycardia. This would prompt an evaluation for surgical removal of incarcerated tissue and repair of the fracture. Otherwise, many fractures are self-limited and heal without complication.

Injuries to the Orbital Globe

If the orbital bones do not manage to protect the eye, the globe itself can be injured as a result of a direct impact as well. Smaller objects may cause lacerations of the conjunctiva, cornea (Figure 37–3), and sclera. In addition, direct impacts can also cause pressure to build rapidly inside the eye and result in a posterior rupture of sclera. The sclera is most vulnerable directly behind the extraocular muscle insertions where it is the thinnest; however, ruptures can occur at any location. Any trauma resulting in a full-thickness laceration or rupture of the eye is termed an *open globe injury* and requires emergent surgical intervention.

Even without a rupture of the scleral coat or cornea, blunt trauma can cause significant injuries to internal ocular structures and bleeding inside the eye. A **hyphema** can form when blood accumulates in the anterior chamber of the eye (Figure 37–4). This blood can clog the natural drainage system of the eye and result in secondary glaucoma. It is imperative to determine the sickle cell status in any patient with a hyphema because sickled red blood cells have a much higher probability of clogging the outflow pathway and causing problems. Further, carbonic anhydrase inhibitors should be avoided in sickle cell patients with hyphemas due to their potential for exacerbating the sickling of red blood cells.

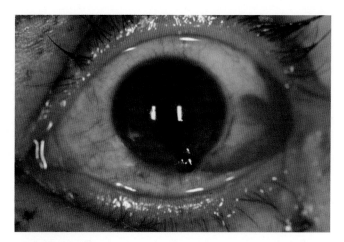

FIGURE 37–3 Trauma to the eye resulting in an open globe injury with extrusion of some of the iris through the corneal wound. Note the abnormal, teardrop pupil. There is conjunctival injection (superior, medial [left side], and inferior) and subconjunctival hemorrhage (temporal, right side) causing this red eye. (Reproduced with permission from Usatine RP, Smith MA, Mayeaux EJ, Chumley HS: *The Color Atlas and Synopsis of Family Medicine*, 3rd ed. New York, NY: McGraw Hill; 2019. Photo contributor: Paul D. Comeau.)

Infections of the Orbit

Orbital and ocular infections are not uncommon and require a thorough ocular examination and often radiologic imaging to provide an accurate diagnosis. Orbital infections are divided into 2 categories—preseptal and postseptal—based on their relationship to the orbital septum. The septum is a fibrous sheet that separates the orbit and eyelid and serves as a relative barrier to the spread of infection. Preseptal cellulitis often results from minor lid trauma or an abrasion. Due to the mechanism of injury, the most likely organism causing preseptal cellulitis is *Staphylococcus aureus*. Patients are often

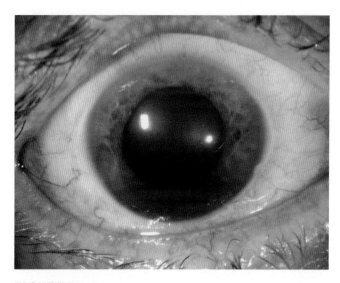

FIGURE 37–4 This hyphema, consisting of red blood cells, has completely layered out in the anterior chamber. (Reproduced with permission from Knoop KJ, Stack LB, Storrow AB, et al: *The Atlas of Emergency Medicine*, 4th ed. New York, NY: McGraw Hill; 2016. Photo contributor: Brice Critser, CRA, The University of Iowa and EyeRounds.org.)

febrile and present with eyelid erythema and edema as well as discomfort. Preseptal cellulitis can often be managed with oral antibiotics; however, intravenous (IV) antibiotics may be necessary in patients who do not respond to oral medications. Orbital cellulitis involves an infection posterior to the orbital septum. Often, orbital cellulitis results from direct extension of a sinus infection through the bony wall into the orbital cavity. Presence of a subperiosteal abscess along the orbital wall must be ruled out with imaging. The most common organisms are *S aureus*, *Streptococcus pneumoniae*, and occasionally fungi. Patients are often febrile and present with decreased vision, proptosis, restricted eye movements, pain with eye movement, lid edema, erythema, and possibly a relative afferent pupillary defect.

Treatment for orbital cellulitis requires IV antibiotics. Depending on the age of the patient and suspected pathogen, drainage of the periosteal abscess may be required. Finally, endophthalmitis, an infection inside the globe, constitutes a significant threat to vision. Although there are multiple potential etiologies, immediate postoperative (*Staphylococcus epidermidis*, *S aureus*, *Streptococcus* species, and *Pseudomonas*), traumatic (*Bacillus*, *S epidermidis*, *Streptococcus* species, *S aureus*), and endogenous seeding (*Candida*) are the most common. Late postoperative endophthalmitis, >6 weeks after surgery, is often caused by *Propionibacterium acnes*. Prevention is key to avoiding postoperative endophthalmitis. Use of 5% betadine solution as part of the surgical site preparation has been proven to significantly decrease postoperative endophthalmitis rates. Patients often present with pain and decreased vision. Ocular examination reveals intraocular inflammation and potentially a hypopyon, layering of white blood cells in the anterior chamber (Figure 37–5). A vitreous

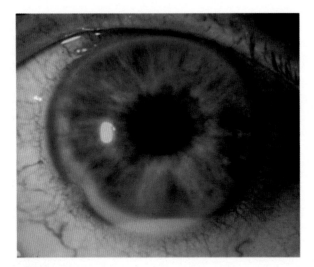

FIGURE 37–5 Hypopyon in a patient with Behçet disease, consisting of white blood cells layered out in the inferior portion of the anterior chamber. (Reproduced with permission from Riordan-Eva, P, Augsburger JJ: *Vaughan & Asbury's General Ophthalmology*, 19th ed. New York, NY: McGraw Hill; 2018.)

or aqueous humor sample should be taken for cultures and sensitivities, and intravitreal antibiotics should be given. In addition, topical and systemic antibiotics should be added depending on the presentation. If vision is reduced to light perception or worse, removal of the vitreous via vitrectomy in addition to aggressive antibiotic treatment has been shown to be beneficial.

Orbital Pseudotumor

Idiopathic orbital inflammation, or orbital pseudotumor, is inflammation of the orbital tissues of unknown etiology. Diagnosis is often challenging. Patients often present with afebrile lid edema and erythema, restricted eye movement, proptosis, orbital pain, diplopia, and changes in vision. CT scans of the orbit show enlargement of the extraocular muscles (orbital myositis) and their respective tendons, enhancement of the sclera, and often enlargement of the lacrimal gland. The differential diagnosis must include preseptal and orbital cellulitis as well as thyroid eye disease (Graves ophthalmopathy). Graves patients will present with relatively painless proptosis, diplopia, strabismus, restricted eye movement, and CT evidence of orbital myositis that spares the tendons. Antibiotics are ineffective in orbital pseudotumor; however, systemic steroids often cause a rapid improvement in symptoms. In patients nonresponsive to steroid treatment, systemic chemotherapy may be required.

Eyelids

The eyelids serve multiple purposes. In addition to protecting the globe, the eyelids also assist in spreading the natural tears over the surface of the cornea. Blinking creates a natural pumping action that propels tears medially along the lid margin to the punctum. Tears enter the canalicular system and are transported through the nasolacrimal sac and duct before entering the nose at the inferior turbinate. A functional tear drainage system is integral to maintaining good vision and comfort.

Similar to the globe, the eyelids are at risk for injury by both blunt and sharp objects. Laceration of the eyelid typically requires a layered closure with sutures, with special attention being paid to the horizontal realignment of the eyelid structures. The key is to recognize when the lid margin and/or the tear drainage system (ie, the canaliculus) have been violated. The upper and lower punctum should be cannulated to ensure they are patent and intact. Any canalicular involvement (Figure 37–6) requires intubation and temporary stenting of the tear drainage system during closure to prevent scaring, permanent closure, and development of excessive tearing known as **epiphora**.

Various pathologies involving the eyelid margins can cause significant issues. Inflammation of the eyelid margin, known as **blepharitis**, can have several causes. If the inflammation is toward the anterior surface, the most common culprits include *Staphylococcus* infections or a dandruff-type reaction known as *seborrheic blepharitis*. Inflammation of the

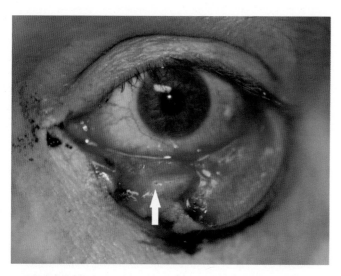

FIGURE 37–6 This complex eyelid laceration shows the displaced inferior punctum (*arrow*). This laceration clearly violates the canalicular structures. (Reproduced with permission from Knoop KJ, Stack LB, Storrow AB, et al: *The Atlas of Emergency Medicine*, 4th ed. New York, NY: McGraw Hill; 2016. Photo contributor: Harold Lee, MD.)

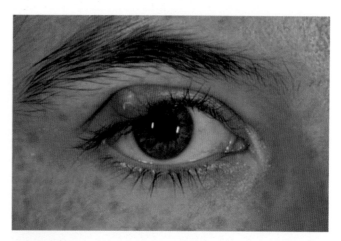

FIGURE 37–7 Chalazion of right upper lid. (Reproduced with permission from Riordan-Eva, P, Augsburger JJ: *Vaughan & Asbury's General Ophthalmology*, 19th ed. New York, NY: McGraw Hill; 2018.)

posterior margin of the eyelid is often the result of Meibomian gland inflammation. Patients often report itching, burning, and a foreign body sensation. Inspection of the lid margin shows roughening, crusting, and scaling along the lid margin, clogged or capped Meibomian glands, and a foamy tear layer. Conservative treatment with baby shampoo lid scrubs (50% dilution with water) and topical antibiotics is often curative. Oral antibiotics and addition of steroids may be necessary in some cases.

Infection or obstruction of the glands within the eyelid can cause an acute, severe inflammatory response. Involvement of the glands of Zeiss and the Meibomian glands results in an external **hordeolum** and **chalazion,** respectively. Each presents with a focal, red, painful swelling at or just behind the lid margin. Often, capped glands can be seen at the lid margin. Chalazions (Figure 37–7), which are most often inflammatory and not infectious, are treated conservatively with warm compresses and baby shampoo lid scrubs. If conservative treatment is not successful, surgical incision and curettage are performed. A similar regimen is prescribed for an external hordeolum; however, because of a higher likelihood of infectious etiology, antibiotics are also prescribed. If a chalazion or hordeolum recurs in the same location, a biopsy should be done to rule out a sebaceous carcinoma.

OCULAR COAT & ANTERIOR SEGMENT

The ocular coat consists of the cornea and sclera, the structures that maintain the outer shape of the eye. The anterior segment of the eye is composed of all of the structures anterior to the vitreous face, including the cornea, anterior chamber, drainage angle of the eye (trabecular meshwork and Schlemm's canal), iris, ciliary body, and the lens.

Ocular Coat & Conjunctiva

The conjunctiva is a continuous layer of tissue composed of nonkeratinized stratified columnar epithelium that lines the back of the eyelids (palpebral conjunctiva), the fornix, and the surface of the globe (bulbar conjunctiva) before terminating at the limbus. The conjunctival goblet cells secrete mucin into the tear film, helping the fluid distribute evenly over the surface of the eye. Typically, the conjunctiva is relatively transparent, allowing the white sclera to be seen underneath.

"Red eye" is a common chief complaint among patients and carries an extensive differential diagnosis. One of the most common causes of redness and irritation is **conjunctivitis**. Viral conjunctivitis (ie, "pink eye") is caused by the adenovirus (Figure 37–8) and produces discomfort, watery discharge, and photophobia. Often viral conjunctivitis begins unilaterally and then becomes bilateral due to auto-inoculation of the fellow eye. Treatment is supportive, with cool compresses and artificial tears. Frequent hand washing with frequent changes of sheets and towels is advised. In addition, patients should be instructed to avoid touching their eyes to prevent spread. This can be contrasted with bacterial conjunctivitis, which is associated with more purulent discharge (Figure 37–9). Rapidly progressing conjunctivitis with copious discharge and preauricular lymphadenopathy is concerning for *Neisseria gonorrhoeae* infection. More moderate discharge and slower development could be caused by *S pneumoniae, Staphylococcus* species, *Haemophilus influenzae,* or *Pseudomonas*. All suspected bacterial conjunctivitis should be treated with topical antibiotics. Cultures can be obtained if empiric treatment is not working or the infection recurs.

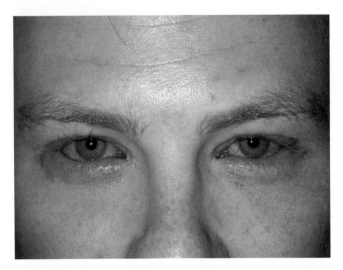

FIGURE 37–8 Bilateral viral conjunctivitis in a 41-year-old man. (Reproduced with permission from Usatine RP, Smith MA, Mayeaux EJ, Chumley HS: *The Color Atlas and Synopsis of Family Medicine*, 3rd ed. New York, NY: McGraw Hill; 2019. Photo contributor: Richard P. Usatine, MD.)

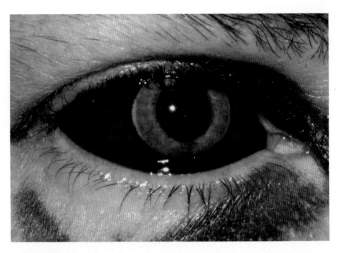

FIGURE 37–10 A 360-degree subconjunctival hemorrhage is seen in this patient after blunt trauma to the eye and orbit. Note that the hemorrhage stops abruptly at the limbus. (Reproduced with permission from Knoop KJ, Stack LB, Storrow AB, et al: *The Atlas of Emergency Medicine*, 4th ed. New York, NY: McGraw Hill; 2016. Photo contributor: Brice Critser, CRA, The University of Iowa and EyeRounds.org.)

Allergic conjunctivitis can be mistaken for viral conjunctivitis due to its similar appearance. Allergic conjunctivitis is a type I hypersensitivity reaction to various allergens. Patients present with conjunctival injection, conjunctival edema (chemosis), itching, and watery discharge. Many patients will admit to seasonal allergies and may have associated allergic rhinitis. Patients with a medical history of eczema or asthma are at risk for atopic keratoconjunctivitis, which is a combination of type I and IV hypersensitivity reactions.

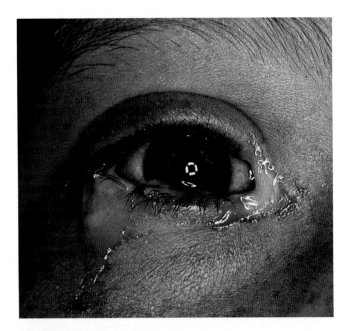

FIGURE 37–9 Mucopurulent discharge, conjunctival injection, and lid edema are noted in a pediatric patient with bacterial (*Haemophilus influenzae*) conjunctivitis. (Reproduced with permission from Knoop KJ, Stack LB, Storrow AB, et al: *The Atlas of Emergency Medicine*, 4th ed. New York, NY: McGraw Hill; 2016. Photo contributor: Frank Birinyi, MD.)

Atopic conjunctivitis can progress to cause foreshortening of the conjunctival fornix, symblepharon formation, and corneal scaring. Finally, patients can develop giant papillary conjunctivitis as a reaction to the presence of a chronic foreign body (eg, contact lenses or nondissolvable sutures postoperatively). Papillae are best seen by everting the lid and looking for a cobblestone appearance on the tarsal surface. Treatment for allergic conjunctivitis is supportive with cool compresses and artificial tears, which help dilute the allergen burden. In addition, use of topical and systemic antihistamines and topical mast cell stabilizers can be beneficial. Topical nonsteroidal anti-inflammatory drugs and steroids can be used sparingly for refractory cases.

Subconjunctival hemorrhages can be striking in their appearance (Figure 37–10) but are usually benign. The hemorrhage arises from blood vessels either within the conjunctiva or the sclera that bleed into the space between the 2 tissues. Often no etiology can be found; however, eye rubbing and Valsalva from coughing or emesis are common. Trauma can lead to subconjunctival hemorrhage as well. Depending on other ophthalmic exam findings, the presence of 360 degrees of subconjunctival hemorrhage around the cornea after ocular trauma warrants strong consideration for surgical exploration to rule out a ruptured globe.

Pinguecula and **pterygium** are relatively benign growths that are commonly seen on the conjunctiva. A pinguecula is a small whitish-yellow spot located near the corneal limbus. It appears nasally more often than temporally and represents an accumulation of protein, calcium, or fat in the conjunctiva. Pingueculae are completely benign. A pterygium is a triangular or wing-shaped growth that extends from the perilimbal conjunctiva onto the cornea (Figure 37–11). It is thought to be exacerbated by long-duration exposure to arid climates, ultraviolet light, and wind (thus its nicknames of "farmer's eye"

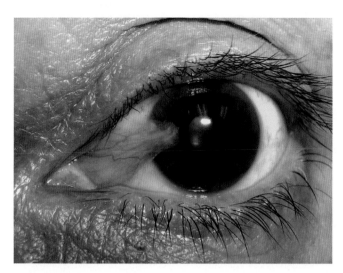

FIGURE 37–11 This fibrovascular pterygium has grown onto the cornea but has not yet obscured the visual axis. The pterygium has the shape of a bird's wing, the literal definition of "pterygium." (Reproduced with permission from Usatine RP, Smith MA, Mayeaux EJ, Chumley HS: *The Color Atlas and Synopsis of Family Medicine*, 3rd ed. New York, NY: McGraw Hill; 2019. Photo contributor: Richard P. Usatine, MD.)

and "surfer's eye"). As the growth progresses, it can induce significant astigmatism and encroach on the visual axis. If vision becomes affected, surgical excision is warranted; however, pterygia often recur.

Maintaining adequate hydration of the ocular surface is critical for good vision and comfort. Dry eyes, known as **keratoconjunctivitis sicca**, is a relatively common finding. Patients complain of a foreign body sensation, burning, or dryness, which is often worse late in the day or when doing activities that require visual concentration such as driving, watching television, reading, or working on the computer. Several clinical tests are useful in diagnosing dry eyes. Tear breakup times of <10 seconds are considered abnormal. Schirmer testing involves placement of a filter paper strip inside the temporal lower eyelid. Less than 10 mm of wetting after 5 minutes is considered abnormal. On examination at the slit lamp, a decreased tear lake can be seen. In addition, dryness can cause small punctate epithelial erosions that expose the underlying basement membrane. Fluorescein dye stains the basement membrane yellow under a cobalt blue light; thus, a yellow speckled pattern is indicative of dry eyes. Rose bengal and lissamine green can be used to stain devitalized corneal cells as well. Treatment starts with topical application of artificial tears and/or ointments for hydration. If this is insufficient, topical cyclosporine can be prescribed to increase tear production. For more severe cases, punctal occlusion may be necessary and serum autologous tears can be tried. Often patients find the use of a humidifier in the house helpful as well.

Cornea

The cornea is approximately 12 mm in diameter and has a central and peripheral thickness of approximately 540 μm

and 1 mm, respectively. The cornea is composed of 5 layers that can be remembered by the mnemonic ABCDE: anterior epithelium, Bowman membrane, corneal stroma, Descemet membrane, and endothelium. The highly organized arrangement of the stromal collagen fibrils, glycosaminoglycans, and other components is critical to maintaining corneal transparency. In addition, the cornea is densely innervated; thus, it is highly sensitive.

Corneal abrasions are relatively common and can be caused by a variety of objects, with fingernails, tree branches or foliage, and makeup applicators being common culprits. Often patients present with severe pain, tearing, conjunctival injection, and photophobia. Application of a drop of topical anesthetic often brings immediate relief of symptoms. Ocular examination should include placing a drop of fluorescein in the eye and examining under magnification. A slit lamp is preferable; however, the cobalt light of the direct ophthalmoscope and a magnifying lens can be used. Again, the abrasion will appear bright yellow as the epithelial disruption allows the fluorescein to stain the underlying basement membrane (Figure 37–12). In addition, there may be cells observed in the anterior chamber. The lids should be everted to examine for foreign bodies trapped in the fornix or on the palpebral conjunctiva behind the tarsus. Most foreign bodies can be removed with a cotton-tipped applicator. A corneal foreign body requires specialized attention, and removal should be done by an ophthalmologist at the slit lamp or in the operating room if there is concern for full-thickness penetration of the cornea. Topical antibiotics should be administered, with a fourth-generation fluoroquinolone used for any abrasions caused by vegetable matter or in contact lens wearers to prevent *Pseudomonas* infection. A bandage contact lens or patching overnight may be used in cases of extreme discomfort but only if reexamination the following day is possible. Cycloplegia can reduce photophobia caused by ciliary muscle spasm. Steroids are contraindicated because they will slow the healing of the epithelium. Finally, numbing drops such as proparacaine are never prescribed for a patient because repeated use is toxic to the epithelium and will worsen the condition.

Corneal ulcerations can have a devastating impact on visual acuity when the ulcer or residual scar is located in the visual axis (Figure 37–13). A complete discussion on the types of noninfectious corneal ulcers and their pathogenesis is beyond the scope of this chapter; however, a basic understanding of infectious keratitis is important. Patients typically present with a history of corneal trauma or contact lens wear, but severe keratoconjunctivitis sicca or eyelid abnormalities can predispose to infections as well. *Staphylococcus*, *Streptococcus*, *Pseudomonas*, and *Moraxella* species are some of the most common culprits after the epithelium has been disrupted. However, there are some bacteria, such as *N gonorrhoeae* and *Corynebacterium diphtheriae*, that can penetrate an intact epithelium and cause ulceration. Patients often have redness, photophobia, watering or discharge, and decreased visual acuity if the central axis is involved. Ocular examination should include staining with fluorescein to determine whether an epithelial defect is present

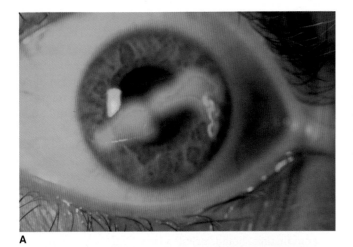

A

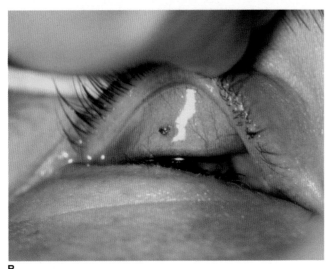

B

FIGURE 37–12 Corneal abrasion. **A.** This corneal abrasion obscures the visual axis and will benefit from close follow-up with an ophthalmologist to ensure adequate healing. **B.** Eversion of the upper eyelid reveals a retained foreign body. Without removal, this would likely continue to abrade the cornea with each blink or eye movement. (Reproduced with permission from Knoop KJ, Stack LB, Storrow AB, et al: *The Atlas of Emergency Medicine*, 4th ed. New York, NY: McGraw Hill; 2016. Photo contributor: Lawrence B. Stack, MD.)

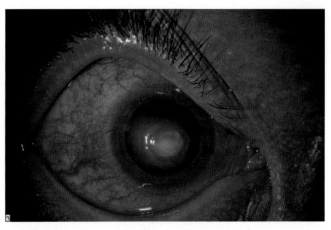

FIGURE 37–13 Diffuse conjunctival injection and cloudy cornea demonstrating keratitis with corneal ulcer formation and a leucocyte infiltrate. (Reproduced with permission from Usatine RP, Smith MA, Mayeaux EJ, Chumley HS: *The Color Atlas and Synopsis of Family Medicine*, 3rd ed. New York, NY: McGraw Hill; 2019. Photo contributor: Paul D. Comeau.)

CASE 37–1

A 21-year-old college student presents to the emergency department with decreased vision, photophobia, and a red, painful eye. Past medical history is unremarkable; however, the patient admits to sleeping in her contact lenses most nights. Visual acuity is measured as 20/400 with the patient wearing her glasses. One drop of pro-paracaine is placed in the eye. A fluorescein dye strip is used to instill fluorescein. Slit-lamp examination reveals conjunctival injection, a central corneal ulcer with a 2.0 × 2.0 mm epithelial defect, and 2.2 × 2.5 mm stromal infil-trate. There is 20% thinning of the corneal stroma. There is an anterior chamber cell with a 0.5-mm hypopyon. The iris is flat and round, and the lens is clear. There is no evi-dence of posterior segment involvement. Corneal scrap-ings are taken for Gram stain and cultures. The patient is started on fortified vancomycin and tobramycin every 5 minutes × 6 in the hospital. The patient is discharged with instructions to alternate the 2 drops every 30 minutes and is instructed to return daily for examination. On the third day, the cultures reveal *Pseudomonas* infection, and the epithelial defect and stromal infiltrate have started to heal. Steroids are started, and the antibiotic is switched to a fluoroquinolone. The patient is followed closely through her lengthy course. Eventually, the antibiotics are stopped and steroids are tapered. The ulcer is controlled, and the cornea does not perforate. Although steroids reduce the scar, its central location results in a best corrected visual acuity of 20/50. Although the bacterial keratitis has been successfully treated, the patient will likely need a corneal transplant if she hopes to improve her vision further. Unfortunately, sleeping in contact lenses can have very serious consequences.

and look for corneal opacification. The baseline size and shape of both the epithelial defect and infiltrate should be recorded, along with the degree of corneal thinning. Presence or absence of an anterior chamber reaction and hypopyon should also be noted. Corneal scrapings are obtained and sent for cultures and staining (Gram +/– Giemsa stain). Patients are typically treated empirically with fortified antibiotics if the ulcer is >1 mm. Ini-tially, vancomycin (or cefazolin) and tobramycin are alternated every 30 minutes to 1 hour and then tapered as improvement is noted. If the patient is a contact lens wearer, the contacts should be cultured and discarded. New contacts should not be worn until the infection is completely resolved. Further, contact lens wearers who sleep in their contacts should be educated on the dangers associated with that practice. Steroids can help mini-mize permanent scaring and opacification, but they should not be started until there is definitive evidence of improvement

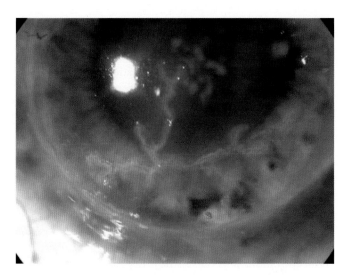

FIGURE 37–14 This close-up view of an eye with herpetic keratitis shows the branching pattern of a viral dendrite after installation of fluorescein stain and illumination with a cobalt blue light. (Reproduced with permission from Riordan-Eva P, Augsburger JJ: *Vaughan & Asbury's General Ophthalmology*, 19th ed. New York, NY: McGraw Hill; 2018.)

(typically after about 48 hours). For ulcers refractory to antibiotic therapy, one must consider a fungal or protozoan (*Acanthamoeba*) species.

Although bacterial **keratitis** can have devastating impacts on vision, herpetic keratitis is actually the leading cause of infectious corneal blindness, with herpes simplex virus (HSV) type 1 infection being more common than HSV type 2. The classic dendritic staining pattern after application of fluorescein is pathognomonic for HSV keratitis (Figure 37–14); unfortunately, this presentation is not common. Often patients present with unilateral vesicular blepharitis or follicular conjunctivitis that can be confused with other forms of conjunctivitis. Epithelial keratitis is also common with stromal infiltration, but conjunctivitis may be absent in these cases. HSV keratitis is often recurrent as a result of virus reactivation and must be monitored closely. Treatment often is based on presentation but typically involves the use of topical antivirals (ganciclovir). Use of steroids has been shown to be beneficial for stromal involvement but should be monitored closely due to the potential adverse effects (eg, glaucoma, secondary bacterial keratitis, corneal perforation). Oral acyclovir has been shown to reduce the rate of recurrence, so patients are often treated for at least 1 year prior to attempting to taper the oral medications.

Herpes zoster infection of the eye, herpes zoster ophthalmicus (HZO), is due to the reactivation of the varicella virus within the trigeminal nerve. Although reactivation in the ophthalmic branch (V_1) is the most likely to cause of ocular involvement, reactivation in the maxillary (V_2) and mandibular (V_3) branches can also lead to HZO. Presence of the Hutchinson sign (Figure 37–15), defined as vesicular lesions on the side or tip of the nose, makes ocular involvement more likely. The HZO vesicular rash respects the midline. Treatment involves use of acyclovir, if it can be started within

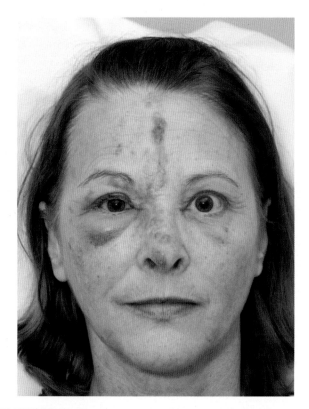

FIGURE 37–15 This classic herpes zoster ophthalmicus vesicular rash is in the ophthalmic division (V_1) of the trigeminal nerve. The presence of the lesion near the tip of the nose (Hutchinson sign) increases the risk of ocular involvement. (Reproduced with permission from Knoop KJ, Stack LB, Storrow AB, et al: *The Atlas of Emergency Medicine*, 4th ed. New York, NY: McGraw Hill; 2016. Photo contributor: Lawrence B. Stack, MD.)

48 to 72 hours of the first vesicle appearance. In addition, oral steroids can also be used and have been shown to reduce the duration of the disease. Topical antibiotics may be applied to the eye for secondary infections and cycloplegia for photophobia. In addition to ocular involvement, postherpetic neuralgia is a major concern and may require consultation with a neurologist or pain specialist. For this reason, the varicella vaccine should be given to the elderly in order to help prevent HZO.

Finally, **chemical burns** to the eye require immediate attention. If patients contact the physician by phone prior to presenting to the clinic or emergency department, they should be instructed to wash the eye out for several minutes before traveling to the physician with any clean source of water immediately available. In addition, the patient should be instructed to bring in the label or a picture of the offending agent if possible. Acids will denature and precipitate corneal proteins, which can create a protective barrier that prevents deeper penetration. Alkali chemicals, on the other hand, will only denature the proteins and saponify fat. The lack of protein precipitation allows for deeper penetration (Figure 37–16). Thus, alkali burns are often considered more worrisome. Treatment involves placing a drop of topical anesthetic into the eye, testing the pH (normal 7.4), and then using copious irrigation with lactated Ringer's or saline until the pH normalizes. A Morgan lens is helpful. If trouble normalizing

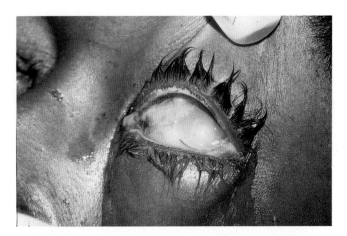

FIGURE 37–16 Diffuse opacification of the cornea occurred from a "lye" (alkali) burn to the face. (Reproduced with permission from Knoop KJ, Stack LB, Storrow AB, et al: *The Atlas of Emergency Medicine*, 4th ed. New York, NY: McGraw Hill; 2016. Photo contributor: Stephen W. Corbett, MD.)

the pH is noted, a cotton-tipped applicator or glass rod can be used to clear the fornix of any residual solid chemical that may be trapped. After the pH is normalized, the patient should be given topical antibiotics and cycloplegics. Addition of steroids, antiglaucoma medications, ascorbate and/or citrate, and collagenase inhibitors may be necessary depending on the severity of the burn. It is important to watch for cicatricial conjunctival changes and break any adhesions that begin to form during the healing process. Many patients will eventually need corneal transplants; however, success rates are highly variable depending on the severity of the chemical burn.

Lens

The lens of the eye is typically transparent and works in concert with the cornea to focus light on the retina. The lens has essentially 3 layers: a central nucleus, a surrounding cortex, and an outer lens capsule. An opacification in any layer of the lens is called a **cataract,** and it can be detected on examination by a reduction of the red reflex with direct ophthalmoscopy or direct observation at the slit lamp. Regardless of the etiology or location, the common end result of a cataract is light being scattered instead of focused on the retina. This results in the perception of a degraded image and decreased visual acuity. Cataract removal is an outpatient procedure and is the most common surgery performed in the United States. Cataract development is a natural process that is often first noted on examination around the age of 50 years. However, the rate of progression and degree of visual dysfunction is highly variable. The only method to treat cataracts is surgical removal of the natural crystalline lens while attempting to spare the lens capsule. A new artificial lens is then placed inside the capsular bag for support. Cataract surgery is only recommended when the cataract has become visually significant, which typically means best corrected visual acuity of 20/40 or worse *and* a functional complaint. Common functional complaints include the inability to drive at night due to headlight glare,

the inability to read, and the inability to see the television or computer clearly. Although cataract development is typically a natural process of aging, formation can be caused or accelerated by various diseases and medications, including ocular trauma, diabetes, uveitis, steroid use, radiation exposure, atopic dermatitis, Down syndrome, myotonic dystrophy, neurofibromatosis type 2, retinitis pigmentosa, Werner syndrome, and Wilson disease, among others. Special consideration is given to congenital cataracts, which are present at birth. It is imperative that primary care physicians check for cataracts in all children by observing the red reflex, because missing the diagnosis can result in permanent vision loss (amblyopia; see section later in this chapter on amblyopia).

The lens is typically centered along the visual axis in line with the pupil. It is held into position by zonular fibers that connect from the lens capsule near the equator to the ciliary body located behind the iris 360 degrees. Zonular disruption can result in subluxation or dislocation of the lens, known as **ectopia lentis**. The most common causes are ocular trauma (Figure 37–17), Marfan syndrome (typically superior subluxation), homocystinuria (typically inferior subluxation), aniridia, Weill-Marchesani syndrome, microspherophakia, and syphilis, among others.

Iris

The iris is a flat, round structure attached to the sclera and ciliary body near the corneoscleral junction. The iris has a central opening, the pupil, which can be dilated or constricted by activation of the dilator pupillae or sphincter muscles, respectively. The ability to regulate the size of the pupil is

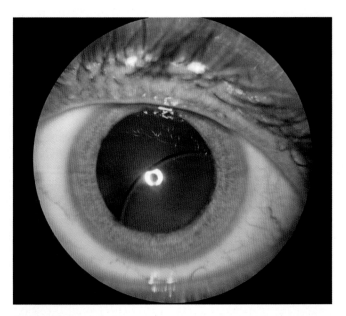

FIGURE 37–17 The crescentic edge of this dislocated crystalline lens is visible within the pupil and creates an abnormal red reflex. (Reproduced with permission from Knoop KJ, Stack LB, Storrow AB, et al: *The Atlas of Emergency Medicine*, 4th ed. New York, NY: McGraw Hill; 2016. Photo contributor: Thomas Egnatz, CRA.)

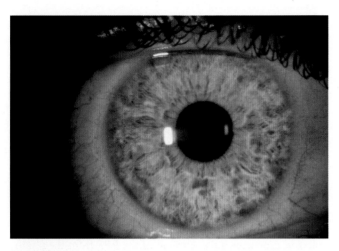

FIGURE 37–18 Lisch nodules (melanotic hamartomas of the iris) are clear yellow-to-brown, dome-shaped elevations that project from the surface of this blue iris. These hamartomas are the most common type of ocular involvement in neurofibromatosis type 1 and do not affect vision. (Reproduced with permission from Usatine RP, Smith MA, Mayeaux EJ, Chumley HS: *The Color Atlas and Synopsis of Family Medicine*, 3rd ed. New York, NY: McGraw Hill; 2019. Photo contributor: Paul D. Comeau.)

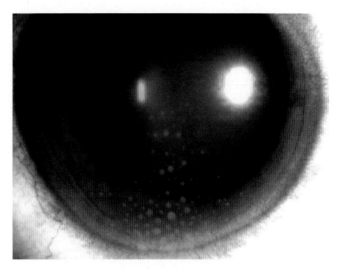

FIGURE 37–19 These granulomatous keratic precipitates are located on the inferior corneal endothelium (Arlt triangle) in a patient with uveitis. (Reproduced with permission from Riordan-Eva, P, Augsburger JJ: *Vaughan & Asbury's General Ophthalmology*, 19th ed. New York, NY: McGraw Hill; 2018.)

critical for allowing us to obtain good vision in a variety of light intensities. Eye color is determined by the amount of pigment contained in the iris, with lighter colored eyes (blue and green) having less pigment than darker (brown) eyes. The iris can obtain pathology related to systemic diseases. An excellent example of this is neurofibromatosis type 1, which is caused by a mutation in the neurofibromin 1 (*NF1*) gene located on chromosome 17. Neurofibromatosis type 1 results in multiple nervous system tumors throughout the body. In addition to skin neurofibromas, café-au-lait spots, and plexiform neurofibromas, patients will often have evidence of Lisch nodules (Figure 37–18) on the iris. These are iris hamartomas composed of dendritic melanocytes and appear as raised pigmented spots on the surface of the iris. They do not affect vision and are considered benign.

Uvea

The uvea, Latin for "grape," or uveal tract is composed of the iris, ciliary body, and choroid. These 3 structures compose a heavily pigmented, central layer in the eye and are occasionally susceptible to inflammation called **uveitis**. When the inflammation is isolated to the structures in front of the lens (ie, the iris and ciliary body), we often call this *anterior uveitis* or *iridocyclitis*. Patients often present with a complaint of decreased vision, pain, redness, and photophobia. Examination at the slit lamp is critical for diagnosis. The redness is often caused by ciliary flush, or dilation of the vessels close to the corneoscleral junction. The conjunctiva and outer layer of the sclera (episclera) may also be involved. The key aspect of the examination is observation of white blood cells floating in the anterior chamber or precipitation of those cells on the iris (iris nodules) or the cornea (keratic precipitates). Because of the natural convection current and aqueous movement in

the eye, keratic precipitates are most often found in the inferior quadrant, known as the Arlt triangle (Figure 37–19). The majority of uveitis cases are idiopathic. Because a laboratory workup is only successful in approximately half of the cases, the first occurrence is often treated empirically, and only those individuals with recurrences have laboratory work completed. The full list of known causes of anterior uveitis is extensive, but some of the most common causes include human leukocyte antigen B27–associated uveitis (ankylosing spondylitis, Reiter syndrome/reactive arthritis, psoriatic arthritis, and inflammatory bowel disease), sarcoid, syphilis, tuberculosis, Behçet disease, juvenile rheumatoid arthritis, Fuchs heterochromic iridocyclitis, Lyme disease, herpetic infections, trauma, and others. Posterior uveitis is associated with inflammation of structures posterior to the lens, including vitreous cell or fibrin, inflammation of the retinal layer (vasculitis, exudation, retinitis, and retinal pigmented epithelial changes), and/or choroidal involvement (choroiditis or choroidal detachment). Again, the differential diagnosis for posterior uveitis is extensive, but some of the more common causes are toxoplasmosis, retinal vasculitis, sarcoid, tuberculosis, syphilis, Behçet disease, Vogt-Koyanagi-Harada disease, presumed ocular histoplasmosis, Eales disease, Lyme disease, amyloidosis, various forms of choroiditis (eg, birdshot, multifocal choroiditis, toxocariasis), various forms of retinitis (eg, cytomegalovirus, cysticercosis, onchocerciasis, acute retinal necrosis, candidiasis, *Bartonella henselae* [cat scratch disease]), and multiple sclerosis.

Treatment for known causes of uveitis, such as infectious agents, is guided by the pathogen. In addition, the goal of all uveitis treatment is to reduce the inflammation. This is typically accomplished through the liberal use of steroids in the form of topical drops, periocular injections, intraocular injections, oral steroids, or implantation of a steroid-eluting pellet into the vitreous cavity. There is always a concern for secondary, steroid-induced glaucoma, so the intraocular pressure should be checked regularly. If steroids alone do not control the inflammation, systemic immune suppressants may be needed. In addition, in the setting of an acute episode, cycloplegics are often prescribed to reduce pain and avoid the development of a small fixed pupil as a result of adhesions between the pupillary margin and the lens capsule, known as *posterior synechiae*.

POSTERIOR SEGMENT

The posterior segment is made up of the structures located behind the lens of the eye. These include the vitreous, retina, choroid, and optic nerve.

Vitreous

The vitreous is a transparent gel. It is made up of 98% to 99% water, whereas the remaining 1% to 2% is an extracellular matrix consisting of fibrillar proteins (primarily collagen) and glycosaminoglycans (primarily hyaluronan), among other substances. The vitreous is most strongly attached to the retina at the optic nerve, blood vessels, and the ora serrata, which is the anterior termination of the retina. Although the vitreous typically remains clear, opacification of the vitreous can cause patients to notice a change in their vision. As a natural part of aging, the vitreous will go through a process of liquefaction and condensation. Usually around the age of 60 years, the vitreous will begin to pull away from its retinal and posterior pole attachments. Traction on the retina during this process can result in a perception of "flashes of light" known as photopsias. If small condensations of vitreous remain suspended just above the sensory retina after vitreal detachment, they can cast small shadows onto the retina that are perceived as "floaters." Although a posterior vitreal detachment or vitreous degeneration is typically benign, the process of separating the vitreoretinal interface can cause breaks in the retinal vessels or a hole to be torn in the retina. Vitreous hemorrhage, regardless of the cause (eg, vitreous degeneration, hypertension, diabetes), can obscure the vision. Often the blood will layer out inferiorly until it is reabsorbed as long as the patient keeps his or her head upright and stable.

Retina

The neurosensory retina typically lines the inner wall of the eye between the vitreous and the choroid. The retinal layers from the innermost to outermost include the following: (1) retinal nerve fiber layer composed of ganglion cell axons; (2) ganglion cell layer composed of ganglion cell nuclei; (3) inner plexiform layer composed of bipolar and amacrine cell axons plus ganglion cell dendrites; (4) inner nuclear layer composed of horizontal, bipolar, and amacrine cell nuclei; (5) outer plexiform layer composed of photoreceptor axons plus horizontal and bipolar cell dendrites; (6) outer nuclear layer composed of photoreceptor cell bodies; (7) photoreceptor layer composed of

inner and outer segments of the photoreceptors; and (8) retinal pigmented epithelium (RPE). Thus, light must travel through nearly all of the retinal layers prior to activating photoreceptor opsin pigments that initiate the process of turning light into an electrical signal, a process known as *phototransduction*.

There are several pathologies of the retina that can have a dramatic effect on vision. Occasionally, the retina will become detached. The most common cause of **retinal detachment** is the development of a hole or tear in the retina. Holes and tears can be caused by a variety of conditions, including vitreous degeneration and traction on the retina, as mentioned previously; trauma; lattice degeneration (thin peripheral retina); high myopia; and previous ocular surgery. Once a hole or tear develops, aqueous fluid or liquefied vitreous can enter the hole and propagate a detachment of the RPE from the photoreceptor layer (Figure 37–20). The detached retina will result in loss of vision from the corresponding visual field that is typically focused on that portion of the retina. If the retina remains intact over the macula and fovea, visual acuity is usually spared. If the fovea is involved, visual acuity will be significantly decreased. Therefore, patients experiencing flashes of light, new floaters, or the feeling like a curtain is coming over their vision should be instructed to see an eye care specialist for evaluation immediately. Evaluation requires a dilated examination with indirect ophthalmoscopy including scleral depression to examine the peripheral retina, where breaks mainly occur. If a clear view cannot be obtained by direct examination, an ultrasound of the eye can be completed. A detached retina will show up as a hyperechoic membrane within the vitreous space. Treatment of retinal detachment often includes a core vitrectomy, removal of subretinal fluid, laser cerclage around the hole, and introduction of gas into the eye to press the retina

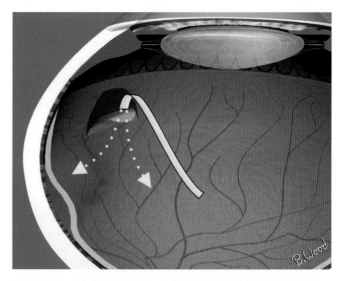

FIGURE 37–20 An illustration of liquid vitreous passing through a horseshoe retinal tear causing a retinal detachment.
(Reproduced with permission from Riordan-Eva, P, Augsburger JJ: *Vaughan & Asbury's General Ophthalmology*, 19th ed. New York, NY: McGraw Hill; 2018.)

into position. Additional laser treatment may be used to help secure the retina to the wall of the eye. Postoperatively, the patient is often positioned face down, allowing the gas to retain pressure on the retina.

The retina and choroid are highly vascularized structures and are susceptible to a variety of vascular pathologies. **Diabetic retinopathy** is a leading cause of blindness in the United States. It is estimated that >80% to 98% of patients with type 1 diabetes and approximately 60% to 90% of patients with type 2 diabetes will develop at least some diabetic retinopathy within 20 years of diagnosis. Early diabetic retinopathy is characterized by the selective loss of pericytes adjacent to capillary endothelial cells and microaneurysm formation. In addition, hard (white) exudates, cotton-wool spots (retinal nerve fiber layer infarcts), and venous beading can be seen (Figure 37–21). As the disease progresses, capillaries continue to close and drop out, creating larger areas of ischemia. With development of ischemia, multiple proangiogenic factors are made by the retina, and eventually new blood vessels begin to grow on the optic disk and retina. Thus, we separate diabetic retinopathy into nonproliferative diabetic retinopathy and the more advanced proliferative diabetic retinopathy based on the presence of new blood vessel growth. Vision loss caused by diabetic retinopathy is typically related to the development of macular edema in nonproliferative diabetic retinopathy and tractional retinal detachment and vitreous hemorrhage in proliferative disease. In addition, new blood vessels can also

develop on the iris and in the drainage angle of the eye, resulting in neovascular glaucoma. Patients with diabetes should be seen 12 months after their initial diagnosis of diabetes and should be seen at least every year after that for a dilated funduscopic examination. Treatment for diabetic retinopathy involves developing and maintaining control of the patient's blood sugars. In addition, focal laser and injection of anti–vascular endothelial growth factor (VEGF) medications can be used to control retinal edema. Proliferative disease often requires the use of panretinal photocoagulation, in which laser spots are placed in the peripheral retina in an attempt to ablate the unhealthy retina that is creating proangiogenic factors signaling neovascularization. The trade-off is development of scotomas at the sites where laser is applied.

Although **hypertensive retinopathy** is known to worsen diabetic retinopathy, hypertension can cause significant retinal pathology and vision loss itself. Hypertension can cause vasoconstriction of retinal arterioles as well as breakdown of the blood–retina barrier. Patients will present with arteriovenous nicking, copper or silver wiring of the arteries, microaneurysms, hemorrhages, exudates, and cotton-wool spots. In addition, the optic nerve can also show pathology with disk

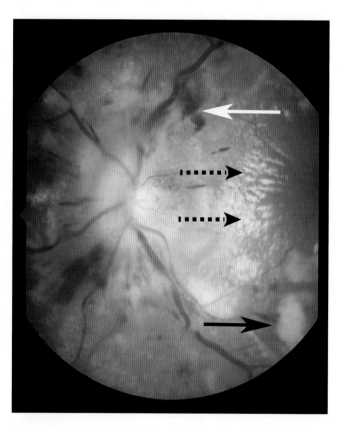

FIGURE 37–22 Malignant hypertensive retinopathy with optic nerve head edema (papilledema), flame hemorrhages (white arrow), cotton-wool spots (black arrow), and macular edema with exudates (dashed arrows). The patient was admitted to the hospital to treat malignant hypertension aggressively. (Reproduced with permission from Usatine RP, Smith MA, Mayeaux EJ, Chumley HS: *The Color Atlas and Synopsis of Family Medicine*, 3rd ed. New York, NY: McGraw Hill; 2019. Photo contributor: Paul D. Comeau.)

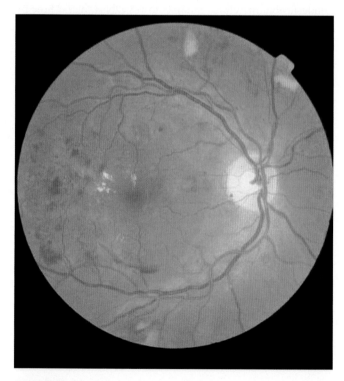

FIGURE 37–21 Moderate nonproliferative diabetic retinopathy with multiple microaneurysms and hemorrhages, mild macular hard exudates, and 2 cotton-wool spots in the superior retina. (Reproduced with permission from Riordan-Eva, P, Augsburger JJ: *Vaughan & Asbury's General Ophthalmology*, 19th ed. New York, NY: McGraw Hill; 2018.)

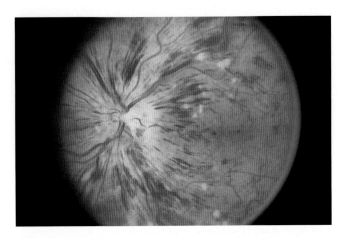

FIGURE 37–23 The amount of hemorrhage ("blood and thunder") is the most striking feature in this patient with a central retinal vein occlusion. Also note the blurred disk margin, the dilation and tortuosity of the venules, and the cotton-wool spots. In addition, retinal edema is suggested by blurring of the retinal details. (Reproduced with permission from Knoop KJ, Stack LB, Storrow AB, et al: *The Atlas of Emergency Medicine*, 4th ed. New York, NY: McGraw Hill; 2016. Photo contributor: Department of Ophthalmology, Naval Medical Center, Portsmouth, VA.)

edema and flame hemorrhages. Macular exudates may also be present (Figure 37–22). Patients may experience retinal ischemia and vision loss. Thus, any patient presenting with these signs and symptoms should have their blood pressure taken immediately while still in the office. Treatment is focused on the controlled lowering and maintenance of blood pressure because patients are at higher risk of multiple vision-threatening conditions (eg, retinal vein occlusion, ischemic optic neuropathies, worsening diabetic retinopathy) and life-threatening conditions (eg, stroke, heart attack, aneurysm).

A **central retinal vein occlusion** (CRVO) is typically caused by a thrombotic event within the central retinal vein posterior to the lamina cribrosa. This is the location where the retinal nerve fiber layer exits the eye and becomes the myelinated optic nerve. Patients will present with a sudden change in vision, and examination will reveal dilation and tortuosity of the retinal veins, extensive retinal hemorrhages in all 4 quadrants, disk edema, and/or macular edema. The retinal hemorrhages are often pathognomonic and are described as "blood-and-thunder" hemorrhages (Figure 37–23). Approximately two-thirds of patients avoid chronic widespread ischemia (nonischemic CRVO) and will typically have vision better than 20/200. The other one-third of patients will have extensive retinal ischemia (ischemic CRVO), which often carries a very poor visual prognosis. In addition, they are at high risk of neovascularization. Workup involves testing for hypertension, diabetes, glaucoma, hyperviscosity, and hypercoagulability, as well as other less common etiologies.

It is not uncommon for patients to present with temporary vision loss (typically <30 minutes) in 1 eye. This is known as **amaurosis fugax** or a *transient visual obscuration*. It is the ocular equivalent of a transient ischemic attack of the brain. Because the retina is a neurosensory organ, temporary loss of blood flow can cause loss of function, but as long as blood flow is restored in a reasonable time frame, vision loss is not

permanent. Although amaurosis fugax can be due to a variety of etiologies, the most common is embolic occlusion of the central retinal artery or 1 of its branches. Emboli are commonly from the carotid artery but may originate in the heart, heart valves, or aorta. The most common types of emboli are cholesterol (Hollenhorst) plaques, platelet fibrin, and calcium. In IV drug users, the differential should include talc emboli as well. Dilated examination should be focused on looking for an embolus, typically at an arterial bifurcation point. If giant cell arteritis is suspected, sedimentation rate and C-reactive protein values should be determined. Otherwise, initial workup should include carotid Doppler and cardiac echocardiography to look for an embolic source. Other risk factors include vascular insufficiency and hypercoagulable states.

If the acute, painless vision loss lasts longer than 30 minutes, there is a higher likelihood that the patient has experienced a **central retinal artery occlusion** (CRAO). In these patients, the embolic event does not self-resolve or the occlusion may be from another cause, such as thrombosis, giant cell arteritis, hypercoagulable states (eg, use of oral contraceptives, antiphospholipid syndrome, polycythemia), or other rarer etiologies such as lupus, migraine, syphilis, sickle cell disease, or polyarteritis nodosa. Patients with a CRAO will often present with global hypoperfusion and ischemia of the retina, giving it an edematous, opaque appearance. Because the fovea is thinner, the retina maintains a reddish transparency centrally; thus, a classic "cherry red spot" appearance can be seen (Figure 37–24). Vision loss is thought to become permanent after approximately 90 to 120 minutes of nonperfusion; therefore, attempts to reestablish blood flow by reducing the intraocular pressure are critical. This can be done by creating a paracentesis to release some aqueous fluid from

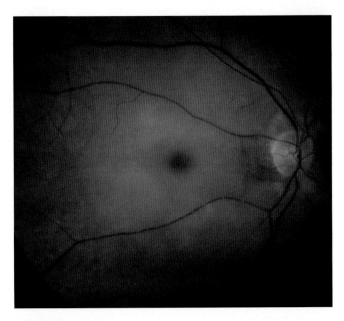

FIGURE 37–24 This central cherry red spot and peripheral cloudy swelling of the macula in a patient with central retinal artery occlusion was due to an embolus originating from a carotid artery atheromatous plaque. (Reproduced with permission from Kasper D, Fauci A, Hauser S, et al: *Harrison's Principles of Internal Medicine*, 19th ed. New York, NY: McGraw Hill; 2015.)

the eye, instilling intraocular pressure-lowering medications, administering oral intraocular pressure-lowering medications, performing ocular massage, and/or administering carbon dioxide inhalation.

In addition to causing embolic events, severe carotid artery stenosis can also cause global hypoperfusion of the entire eye. This is known as **ocular ischemic syndrome**. Patients may have a history of amaurosis fugax but often present with decreased vision and associated orbital or ocular pain. On dilated examination, these patients can have conjunctivitis, anterior cell uveitis, cataracts, optic nerve pallor, mid-peripheral retinal hemorrhages, and potentially neovascularization of the iris, angle, or posterior structures due to the global ischemia. Patients can have low intraocular pressure due to decreased ciliary body perfusion, but they may also have elevated pressure if there is evidence of angle neovascularization (ie, neovascular glaucoma). The physical exam should include carotid artery auscultation to evaluate for presence of a bruit. Treatment often requires a coordinated team effort, with the eye care specialist treating the neovascularization and glaucoma, if present, while the primary care team controls the systemic risk factors (hypertension, diabetes, and cholesterol). If occlusion of the carotid artery is significant, carotid endarterectomy is often considered.

In addition to vascular retinopathies, there are additional retinal pathologies that pose serious threats to vision. **Age-related macular degeneration** (AMD) is another leading cause of blindness in the United States. The primary risk factors for AMD are family history, age, female gender, white race, lightly colored irises, smoking, hypertension, ultraviolet exposure, and hyperopia. There are 2 forms of the disease. Approximately 90% of patients have the "dry" nonexudative form. In its early stages, dry AMD consists of pigmentation changes at the level of the RPE and presence of drusen. Drusen are excrescences of fatty lipid between the RPE and the Bruch membrane. On ophthalmic examination, drusen appear as small whitish-yellow deposits within the macula. As dry AMD progresses, the drusen become larger and more numerous. In addition, the RPE continues to change, and overlying photoreceptors begin to die off, creating geographic atrophy. Once photoreceptors have become damaged, they can no longer function properly, and the resulting scotomas are typically permanent. Once drusen reach a certain size, the use of a vitamin formulation containing vitamin C, vitamin E, β-carotene, zinc, and copper (ie, an Age-Related Eye Disease Study formula) has been shown to slow the progression of the dry form of the disease.

The other 10% of AMD patients have the "wet" exudative form of the disease. Wet AMD is characterized by the development of choroidal neovascularization that breaks through the Bruch membrane. The new blood vessels can cause detachment of the RPE from the Bruch membrane. In addition, the blood vessels can become leaky or bleed. The leaky blood vessels can cause folding or elevation of the retina. Thus, straight objects may look bent or distorted. If the blood vessels bleed, patients are at risk of developing scar tissue with large central scotomas. Patients can watch for AMD progression at home by using an Amsler grid to detect any early distortions in

vision. In addition, regular dilated funduscopic examinations and occasional fluorescein angiography and optical coherence tomography testing may be used to detect abnormal blood vessels and leakage as well as retinal morphologic changes. Although there are few available treatments for the dry form of AMD, the discovery of anti-VEGF therapy has revolutionized the treatment of wet AMD. The anti-VEGF medications are given via monthly intraocular injection. These medications work by shrinking choroidal neovascularization. For the first time, instead of a slow decline in vision, some patients with wet AMD are now able to maintain or even improve vision.

Retinitis pigmentosa (RP) is not a single disease, but instead a family of genetic disorders that cause a progressive rod-cone dystrophy. The inheritance pattern can be autosomal recessive (most common), autosomal dominant (least severe), X linked (rarest but most severe), or sporadic. The disease primarily affects the production of proteins within the photoreceptors, eventually causing them to die. The disease can eventually cause loss of the photoreceptor layer and the outer nuclear layer of the retina as well. The RPE migrates inward and will surround some of the retinal vascular structures in the area of pathology. This leads to the classic "bone spicule" pattern seen in the peripheral retina (Figure 37–25). In addition, patients are noted to have a waxy pallor of the optic nerve and increased choroidal visibility due to RPE migration and outer retinal thinning. The initial symptoms noted by patients are difficulty seeing at night (ie, night blindness) and peripheral vision loss. Patients eventually progress to having color vision deficits as well as decreases in central visual acuity. Electroretinography testing classically shows decreased scotopic a- and b-wave amplitudes early in the disease. In later stages,

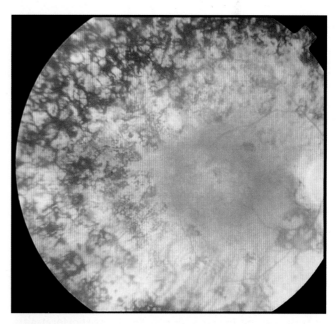

FIGURE 37–25 This patient with retinitis pigmentosa demonstrates arteriolar narrowing and peripheral retinal pigment clumping ("bone spicules"). (Reproduced with permission from Riordan-Eva, P, Augsburger JJ: *Vaughan & Asbury's General Ophthalmology*, 19th ed. New York, NY: McGraw Hill; 2018.)

electroretinography is flat with no response. RP can be seen in isolation or as part of a syndrome with associated systemic findings. Usher syndrome has an autosomal recessive inheritance and is associated with RP and deafness. Refsum disease is also autosomal recessive, and patients have a combination of RP symptoms and defects in fatty acid metabolism due to a deficiency of phytanic acid oxidase. Patients are instructed to avoid foods high in phytanic acid such as milk, animal fat, and leafy green vegetables. Bassen-Kornzweig syndrome is a combination of RP plus abetalipoproteinemia that is inherited in an autosomal recessive fashion. These patients can benefit from vitamin A and E treatment. Other conditions include chronic progressive external ophthalmoplegia and olivopontocerebellar atrophy.

Choroid

The choroid, located between the retina and sclera, has a primary role of providing the outer retinal layers with oxygen and nutrients. It is comprised of a highly vascular plexus of interconnected vessels and is thought to have one of the highest blood flow rates of any tissue in the body. Typically, the vascular choroid, in conjunction with the RPE, provide the reddish-orange reflection seen when examining the eye. Although the posterior pole is typically a relatively uniform color and texture, benign choroidal nevi can occasionally be seen.

Choroidal nevi are a normal occurrence in the general population and are thought to have a prevalence of anywhere from 2% to 8%. Choroidal nevi are composed of melanocytes and typically have clearly defined borders. They are typically roundish and flat or minimally elevated. Although their size remains stable over time, development of overlying drusen or RPE changes may be seen (**Figure 37–26**). They should be documented by fundus photography and observed regularly for any evidence of change.

The primary differential diagnosis for a choroidal nevus is choroidal melanoma. **Choroidal melanoma** is the most common primary intraocular malignancy in the white population and is composed of malignant uveal melanocytes. Typically, on examination, the melanoma will have a brown/black dome or mushroom shape. There may be associated drusen, but more worrisome is the presence of orange pigmentation, subretinal fluid, or contiguous exudative retinal detachment (see Figure 37–26). B-scan ultrasound can be helpful in distinguishing nevi from melanomas. Worrisome features include thickness >2 mm, diameter >7 mm, and low to medium internal reflectivity. Ocular melanomas are treated by local plaque radiation, excision, or enucleation of the eye depending on the clinical and diagnostic findings.

Certain pathologies can affect both the retina and the underlying choroid simultaneously. Concurrent inflammation of both layers at the same time is known as **chorioretinitis**. There are many causes; however, probably the most common cause is toxoplasmosis infection. Typically, *Toxoplasma gondii* is a congenital infection that is passed from the mother to

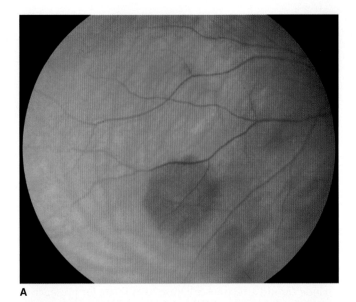

A

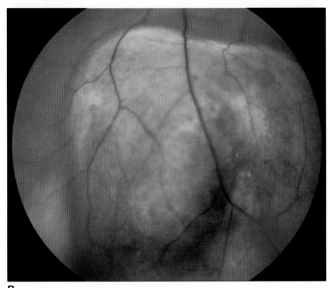

B

FIGURE 37–26 **A.** A typical melanocytic choroidal nevus is seen underlying the retinal blood vessels and is only about 0.25 mm thick by ultrasonography. **B.** This primary non–uniformly colored melanotic choroidal melanoma has a dome-shaped configuration. Note the central orangish pigment. On B-scan ultrasound, the lesion would have a low to medium internal reflectivity. (Reproduced with permission from Riordan-Eva, P, Augsburger JJ: *Vaughan & Asbury's General Ophthalmology*, 19th ed. New York, NY: McGraw Hill; 2018.)

the baby during pregnancy. It is the most common cause of both pediatric uveitis and posterior uveitis. The life cycle of *Toxoplasma* includes oocysts, tachyzoites, and cyst bradyzoites. In humans, only the tachyzoites and cysts are seen. The tachyzoite is responsible for the inflammation and can be treated with antibiotics. However, the treatment does not affect the cysts; thus, infections may recur throughout the patient's life. Steroids are used to target the inflammatory response. On examination, a pigmented chorioretinal scar can often be found in the macular region (**Figure 37–27**). Presence of an

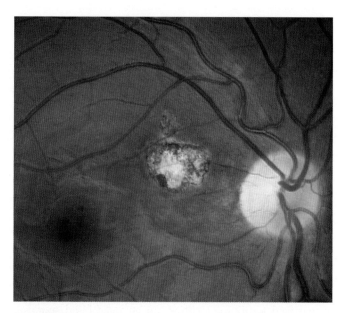

FIGURE 37–27 This chorioretinal scarring is due to old *Toxoplasma* chorioretinitis. The lesion is flat and pigmented. Areas of hypopigmentation are also present. (Reproduced with permission from Kasper D, Fauci A, Hauser S, et al: *Harrison's Principles of Internal Medicine*, 19th ed. New York, NY: McGraw Hill; 2015.)

active vitreous cell with a white fuzzy border adjacent to the scar may indicate reactivation.

The Optic Nerve

The optic nerve is composed of approximately 1.0 to 1.2 million retinal ganglion cell axons. The retinal ganglion cells are located in the inner retina (the ganglion cell layer), and their axons travel together in a coordinated fashion across the retina in the innermost retinal layer, the retinal nerve fiber layer. Once the axons reach the optic disk, they turn 90 degrees, pass through the lamina cribrosa, and exit the eye. Posterior to the lamina cribrosa, the axons become myelinated by oligodendrocytes and are packaged into bundles surrounded by astrocytes and microglia. The majority of axons terminate in the lateral geniculate nucleus. The optic nerve is composed of 4 major parts: the intraocular portion (1.0 to 1.5 mm), the intraorbital portion (30 to 40 mm), intracanalicular portion (5 to 8 mm), and the intracranial portion (10 mm). Damage at any of these locations can cause a profound impact on vision.

Glaucoma

Glaucoma, a leading cause of blindness in the United States, comprises a group of diseases characterized by a chronic, progressive optic neuropathy (optic nerve atrophy) with corresponding visual field defects. Depending on whether or not gonioscopic examination reveals an open anterior chamber drainage angle with visible trabecular meshwork structures, the disease is classified as either open-angle or angle-closure glaucoma, respectively. Primary open-angle glaucoma is

typically a bilateral but asymmetric disease, with individuals of African, Hispanic, and Asian descent appearing to be at a higher risk than whites. In addition, elevated intraocular pressure, advanced age, a first-degree family history of glaucoma, and a thin central cornea are some of the most commonly recognized risk factors. It should be noted that although a majority of patients with open-angle glaucoma have elevated intraocular pressure, approximately 30% of patients can have glaucomatous optic neuropathy and visual field defects while the intraocular pressure is within the normal range. For those with elevated intraocular pressure and an open drainage angle, the disease is thought to be related to an increased resistance to outflow of aqueous humor through the trabecular meshwork. There is some evidence of a genetic basis for the disease, with changes in the myocilin (*MYOC*) gene being some of the first genetic findings associated with the clinical diagnosis of glaucoma. However, the inheritance pattern appears to be quite complex, with a combination of genetic and possibly environmental factors.

Only during an acute angle closure attack, where intraocular pressure increases rapidly, do patients note a red, painful eye. Angle closure is typically caused by the iris pupillary margin making contact with the lens, causing pupillary block. This blockage of aqueous flow into the anterior chamber results in anterior bowing of the iris and acute obstruction of the outflow pathway with rapid elevation of intraocular pressure. Often in these cases, the patient may note "rainbow-colored halos" around lights due to the increased pressure causing corneal edema. Examination may reveal a mid-dilated pupil.

In open-angle glaucoma, the diagnosis is often made during a routine examination, and the patient will not have any visual complaints because the vision loss typically starts peripherally and slowly moves centrally. Not until late in the disease process is visual acuity lost. This is due to the pathophysiology of the disease. It is believed that axons are damaged as they pass through the lamina cribrosa. The axons at the superior and inferior poles appear to be at most risk. Due to the anatomic location of the retinal ganglion cells and axons, damage in these areas typically creates arcuate scotomas or nasal steps that respect the horizontal midline on visual field analysis. Optical coherence tomography of the retinal nerve fiber layer shows thinning. Examination of the nerve reveals an enlarged "cup-to-disk" ratio (Figure 37–28). This is a comparison of the diameters of the optic disk to the physiologic cup. The cup is the portion of the optic disk not occupied by axons. Thus, as the glaucomatous optic neuropathy progresses and the nerve becomes more atrophic, a smaller portion of the optic disk is occupied by axons and the cup-to-disk ratio increases. The only known treatment for glaucoma is the reduction of intraocular pressure, regardless of the type of disease. This is typically accomplished in 3 ways: use of topical or oral intraocular pressure-lowering medications (prostaglandin analogs, β-blockers, α-agonists, and carbonic anhydrase inhibitors), laser treatment of the trabecular meshwork, or conventional glaucoma surgery (typically a trabeculectomy or glaucoma shunt tube).

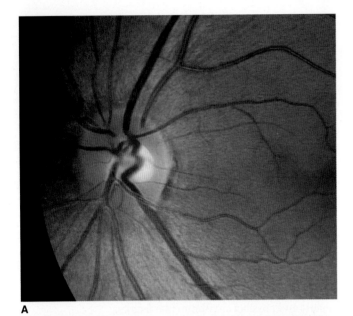

A

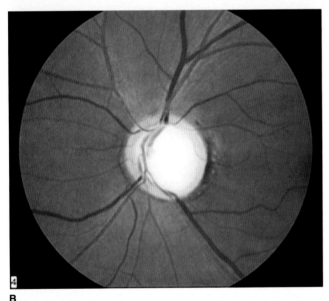

B

FIGURE 37–28 Glaucoma. **A.** An eye with a normal optic cup-to-disk ratio of 0.4 is seen. **B.** A patient with glaucoma has an increased optic cup-to-disk ratio of 0.8. (Part A, reproduced with permission from Usatine RP, Smith MA, Mayeaux EJ, Chumley HS: *The Color Atlas and Synopsis of Family Medicine*, 3rd ed. New York, NY: McGraw Hill; 2019. Photo contributor: Paul D. Comeau. B, reproduced with permission from Papadakis MA, McPhee SJ, Rabow MW: *Current Medical Diagnosis & Treatment 2020*. 59th ed. New York, NY: McGraw Hill; 2020.)

Papilledema

Just as increased intraocular pressure can cause damage to the optic nerve, so can increased intracranial pressure. Although the optic disk can become edematous as a result of other pathologies (eg, hypertensive emergency, inflammation, or infection), only edema caused by increased intracranial pressure is termed *papilledema*. The primary differential diagnosis for papilledema includes intracranial tumor, meningitis, and idiopathic intracranial hypertension (IIH; or pseudotumor cerebri). The first steps in narrowing down the diagnosis are to check the patient's blood pressure and then obtain a magnetic resonance imaging (MRI) or CT scan of the brain to rule out malignancy. Once malignancies have been ruled out, a lumbar puncture with opening pressure should be obtained. IIH is much more common in females than males and is often first diagnosed in the fourth decade of life. Patients are typically overweight and present with headache, possible nausea and vomiting, and possible pulsatile tinnitus. On ophthalmic examination, the severity of the disk edema can be quite variable. Thus, the Frisen Papilledema Scale (grades 0 to 5) is used for grading the severity (Figure 37–29). Initially, the nasal aspect of the optic disk margin becomes blurred. The edema then spreads superior and inferior. Eventually as papilledema progresses, the entire disk margin becomes involved. Flame hemorrhages at the disk margin often present in advanced stages, and dilation and tortuosity of the vasculature are seen. Visual field testing often shows an enlarged blind spot, but arcuate defects similar to those seen in glaucoma patients can also be present. In addition, patients may have an inability to abduct the eye due to a cranial nerve VI palsy. This is due to a shift in the brainstem position at higher intracranial pressure, which causes tension on the sixth cranial nerve. The nerve can be damaged near the clivus as it enters the Dorello canal. Although a definitive cause for IIH is often difficult to identify, it is associated with several medications (tetracycline, nalidixic acid, isotretinoin, vitamin A, steroids, and oral contraceptive pills), dural sinus thrombosis, and pregnancy. Treatment is centered on reducing intracranial pressure through the use of oral medications (acetazolamide and furosemide) and reduction of weight (approximately 10% of body weight) when appropriate. If vision loss is severe, surgical intervention is often required. Optic nerve sheath fenestration and ventriculoperitoneal shunt are 2 of the most common surgeries used in the treatment of refractory IIH cases. Failure to relieve the intracranial pressure can lead to permanent vision loss and blindness.

Optic Neuritis

Inflammation of the optic nerve, termed *optic neuritis*, is 1 of the most common optic neuropathies of early adulthood. Optic neuritis can be idiopathic, but it is often associated with multiple sclerosis, lupus, Lyme disease, sarcoidosis, syphilis, and other systemic diseases. Patients often present with a painful, unilateral loss of vision. Pain is typically exacerbated by eye movements. In addition, patients will likely have a relative afferent pupillary defect, decreased color vision (especially red desaturation), and visual field defects. Disk pallor may develop later in the disease process. Treatment for optic neuritis should include a consideration of IV steroids; however, oral steroids are contraindicated. The Optic Neuritis Treatment Trial has shown that approximately one-third of patients presenting with optic neuritis will go on to develop multiple sclerosis within 4 years. If the patient has had previous neurologic symptoms, the likelihood of multiple sclerosis is even higher.

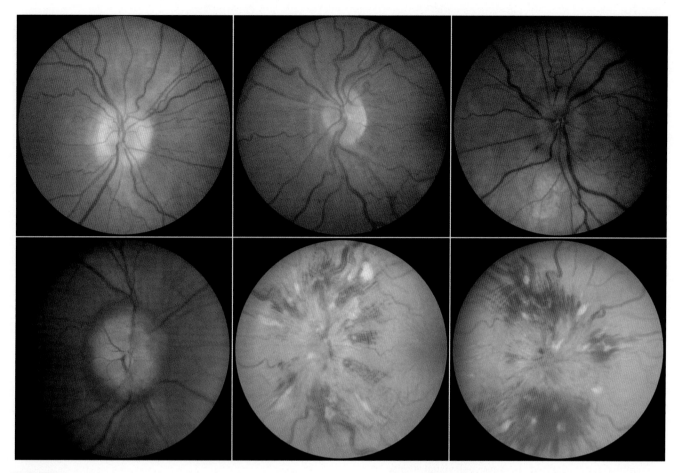

FIGURE 37–29 The 6 images represent optic nerves with progressively worse papilledema based on the Frisen Papilledema Scale (grades 0 to 5). (Reproduced with permission from McKean SC, Ross JJ, Dressler DD, et al: *Principles and Practice of Hospital Medicine*, 2nd ed. New York, NY: McGraw Hill; 2017.)

Optic Gliomas

The optic nerve and surrounding tissues are susceptible to tumor development as well. Optic nerve gliomas are common in children and have a high association with neurofibromatosis. Half of optic nerve gliomas remain intraorbital; however, half can also involve the intracranial portion of the optic nerve. When the intracranial portion is involved, there is always concern regarding extension to the hypothalamus due to the increased risk of mortality. Children often present with vision loss, strabismus, and optic disk edema and/or pallor. MRI is typically diagnostic. Optic nerve sheath meningiomas are also a concern. Typically, patients will present with decreased vision, an afferent pupillary defect, optic atrophy, and possibly retinochoroidal collateral shunt vessels coming off the optic nerve (Figure 37–30). Again, imaging is diagnostic, with calcification of the meninges showing up as a classic "railroad sign" along the length of the optic nerve.

Optic Nerve Trauma

Although trauma can affect the eyelids and globe, it can also affect the optic nerve proper. Traumatic optic neuropathy can be caused by compression due to a retrobulbar hemorrhage. However, the intracanalicular portion can also be damaged if

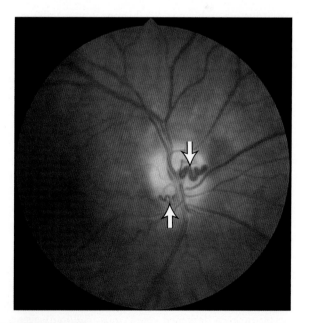

FIGURE 37–30 This optic disk shows secondary optic atrophy with retinochoroidal collateral shunt vessels (*arrows*) due to an optic nerve sheath meningioma. (Reproduced with permission from Riordan-Eva, P, Augsburger JJ: *Vaughan & Asbury's General Ophthalmology*, 19th ed. New York, NY: McGraw Hill; 2018.)

the canal is fractured. Patients typically present with decreased vision, visual field defects, and a relative afferent pupillary defect. CT of the head and orbits will show evidence of a fracture as well as hemorrhage. If hemorrhage is thought to be causing a significant problem, an urgent lateral canthotomy and cantholysis should be considered to decompress the orbit. For suspected traumatic optic neuropathy associated with optic canal fracture, use of high-dose steroids is common, although somewhat controversial.

PEDIATRIC CONDITIONS

Although a full discussion of pediatric eye problems is beyond the scope of this chapter, a few conditions deserve special mention.

Amblyopia

The development of good visual acuity relies on the proper development of the central nervous system's visual pathways and higher order visual processing centers after birth. Babies are actually born with poor visual acuity. Humans require the ability to obtain focused images on each retina for the final development of the central visual pathways, which allows perception of normal acuity. In addition, fixation with both eyes on the same target is required early in life for the development of stereoscopic vision (ie, depth perception). Without these early stimuli, children can develop amblyopia. If this is not recognized in time, it can lead to permanent visual loss.

Amblyopia is defined as abnormal visual acuity in an otherwise normal, healthy eye that cannot be corrected with glasses or contact lenses. There are multiple causes of amblyopia, including strabismic amblyopia, refractive amblyopia, and form deprivation amblyopia. **Strabismus** is an inability to fixate on a single object with both eyes at the same time due to a misalignment (Figure 37–31). If a preference develops for fixation out of 1 eye only, strabismic amblyopia can develop. The brain will ignore image information from the nonfixated eye in order to avoid diplopia. Refractive amblyopia is most commonly caused by a difference in refraction between the 2 eyes. One eye often has clearer vision; thus, it develops normally while information from the eye with the poorer image is ignored by the brain. Thus, the central pathways required for development of normal acuity do not fully develop. Finally, if the visual axis is blocked, preventing clear fixation on an object, form depravation amblyopia can develop. This can be caused by an eyelid covering the axis due to ptosis, corneal scaring, or cataract formation, to name a few.

Screening for congenital cataracts is critical in all children. As part of the newborn screening and well-child checkups, primary care physicians should examine the eyes of every child for lens opacification at every visit. This can be done quickly in the office. In a darkened room, most children's eyes will dilate sufficiently without need of pharmacologic assistance. A light source such as a Finnoff transilluminator or penlight can be used to directly examine the lens. However, the best method is to use a direct ophthalmoscope at arm's distance to

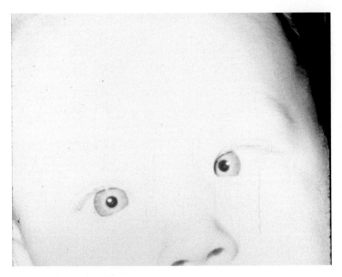

FIGURE 37–31 This baby has congenital esotropia (strabismus). The corneal light reflex of the left eye appears more temporal than that of the right eye. Therefore, the left eye is deviated inward. (Reproduced with permission from Wilbur JK, Graber MA, Ray BE. *Graber and Wilbur's Family Medicine Examination & Board Review*, 4th ed. New York, NY: McGraw Hill; 2017.)

evaluate the red reflex (Figure 37–32). The red reflex should be uniform without opacification. Any concern for congenital cataract should be referred to an ophthalmologist immediately because removal of amblyogenic cataracts is typically required by 3 months of age to avoid development of nystagmus and amblyopia.

Fortunately, if caught early in childhood, amblyopia is treatable. Typically, treatment for amblyopia must occur before the age of 10 years. In many cases, after the age of 10 years, the central visual processing pathways are no longer plastic enough to develop the appropriate connections to obtain normal visual acuity. Treatment for amblyopia should

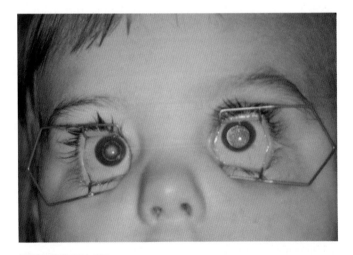

FIGURE 37–32 A congenital cataract is seen in the right eye of this patient with dilated pupils. Note the normal, uniform red reflex in the left eye compared to the opacification of the red reflex in the right eye. (Reproduced with permission from Riordan-Eva, P, Augsburger JJ: *Vaughan & Asbury's General Ophthalmology*, 19th ed. New York, NY: McGraw Hill; 2018.)

only be done by qualified eye care specialists. Treatment involves first eliminating any barriers in the visual axis that might cause form deprivation, and then any refractive errors must be corrected. Next, treatments focus on forced use of the poorer seeing eye by patching, atropinizing (instilling atropine), or blurring the corrective lens of the good seeing eye for a portion of the day. This in turn forces the development of the central nervous system pathways from the poorer seeing eye. Strabismus realignment surgery is the final step once visual acuity has been maximized.

Nasolacrimal Duct Disorders

One of the first things parents often note and become concerned about is epiphora, or watery eyes. Children can be born with a congenital nasolacrimal duct obstruction that results in excessive tearing. Often the tear duct will open spontaneously but gentle massage over the nasolacrimal system is recommended as a method that can assist in opening the system. In a small percentage of cases, the tear duct will need to be probed manually to develop patency.

In addition to congenital obstruction of the nasolacrimal system, it can also be the site of infection. The nasolacrimal sac is an ideal location for bacterial growth in both the pediatric and adult population. Infection of the nasolacrimal sac, or **dacrocystitis**, is often caused by *Staphylococcus, Streptococcus, Pseudomonas, and Haemophilus Influenza*. Dacryocystitis often presents with conjunctival injection and an erythematous swelling just below the medial canthal tendon (**Figure 37-33**). Gentle pressure often causes reflux of purulent material from the punctum. Systemic antibiotics are required while warm compresses can promote drainage. The goal is to avoid chronic conjunctivitis and/or extension to orbital cellulitis due to a prolonged course. If spontaneous drainage does not occur, surgical incision and drainage may be necessary, however probing of the nasolacrimal system should not be undertaken during an acute infection.

Retinoblastoma

The most common primary ocular tumor in children is retinoblastoma. It is critical that these tumors are diagnosed early as they are often fatal within 2 to 5 years of diagnosis if not treated. Retinoblastoma is a tumor developed from retinal progenitor cells within the eye during development. It is caused most often by a defect in the retinoblastoma tumor suppressor gene *RB1*. The congenital or hereditary form of retinoblastoma is a germline mutation that either occurs in utero or is passed down from the mother or father. These account for approximately one-third of the cases. Often in the congenital form of the disease, multiple tumors are seen within the eye and there is a higher chance of having bilateral involvement. "Trilateral" involvement is also possible with development of a pineoblastoma in the pineal gland. As these children grow into their late teens and early adulthood, they are also at a greater risk of developing other cancers, such as osteosarcoma (often the femur), soft tissue sarcomas, lymphoma, leukemia, melanoma, and others. Nonhereditary or sporadic retinoblastoma occurs in about two-thirds of the cases. These children do not have a germline mutation of the *RB1* gene, and instead have acquired 2 mutations sporadically. Typically the sporadic variety is more likely to be in 1 eye only. More than half of all retinoblastoma tumors are diagnosed based on the finding of leukocoria either by the parents when taking a photograph or during routine examination (**Figure 37-34**). Another one-fourth are diagnosed due to the patient having developed strabismus. On dilated fundus examination, a whitish retinal mass will be seen. Patients may also have uveitis, neovascularization

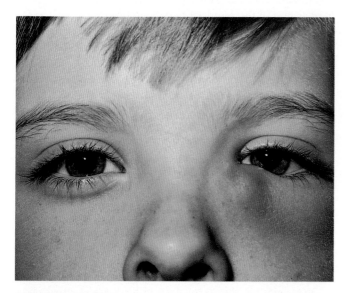

FIGURE 37-33 This 10-year-old patient with streptococcal pharyngitis developed swelling and erythema over the medial lower lid and lacrimal sac, indicative of dacryocystitis. (Reproduced with permission from Knoop KJ, Stack LB, Storrow AB, et al: *The Atlas of Emergency Medicine*, 4th ed. New York, NY: McGraw Hill; 2016. Photo contributor: Kevin J. Knoop, MD, MS.)

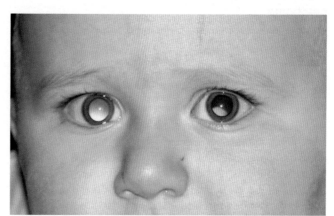

FIGURE 37-34 This patient with bilateral retinoblastomas has a white pupillary reflection (leukocoria) is seen in each eye. It is more pronounced in the right eye. Compare these reflexes to the normal red reflex seen in the left eye in Figure 37-32. (Reproduced with permission from Riordan-Eva, P, Augsburger JJ: *Vaughan & Asbury's General Ophthalmology*, 19th ed. New York, NY: McGraw Hill; 2018.)

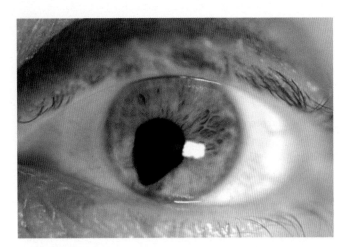

FIGURE 37–35 Iris Coloboma. Iris coloboma is a congenital finding resulting from incomplete closure of the fetal ocular cleft. It appears as a teardrop pupil and may be mistaken for a sign of scleral rupture. (Reproduced with permission from Knoop KJ, Stack LB, Storrow AB, et al: *The Atlas of Emergency Medicine*, 4th ed. New York, NY: McGraw Hill; 2016. Photo contributor: R. Jason Thurman, MD.)

of the iris, hyphema, or angle closure glaucoma. An ultrasound of the eye will show a solid tumor with high internal reflectivity. CT or MRI scan of the head should be completed to rule out optic nerve and pineal gland involvement. On CT, calcification of the tumor may be seen as hyperintensities. Treatment depends on the size, number, and location of the tumors and can range from local photocoagulation or cryotherapy, to plaque radiation, to external beam radiation, to enucleation. For those in which tissue samples can be taken, the severity of pathology is determined by the level of differentiation. Rosettes are the hallmark pathology seen in the disease with Homer-Write rosettes, Flexner-Wintersteiner rosettes, and Fleurettes being seen at different levels of tumor differentiation. With proper treatment and follow-up, survival rate is now nearly 90% to 95%.

Coloboma

During fetal development, if the optic fissure does not close appropriately during the 6th-7th week of life, an ocular coloboma may develop. A coloboma is a hole or dysgenesis in part of the eye. Typically the optic fissure begins closing at the inferior portion of the eye near the equator and the closure then moves anterior and posterior. A coloboma most often involves the iris, ciliary body, choroid, retina, and/or optic nerve. An iris coloboma (anterior segment) will commonly present as a "keyhole" pupil extending inferiorly (Figure 37–35). Chorioretinal colobomas (posterior segment) often present with an inferonasal defect. Retinal detachment is a common complication that can be addressed with prophylactic laser cerclage.

ADVERSE DRUG EFFECTS

Several medications can have adverse ophthalmic side effects. Chief among those is the use of hydroxychloroquine for the treatment of chronic conditions such as lupus and rheumatoid arthritis. While the most common side effects are associated with nausea and mild gastroenteritis, the most concerning are the retinal toxicity effects. Patients at highest risk are those taking >6.5 mg/kg/day (typically >400 mg/day), patients with a cumulative lifetime dose of 1000 g, a duration of treatment longer than 5 years, those 60 years and older, individuals with concurrent retinal/macular disease, and patients with renal or hepatic dysfunction. The mechanism causing toxicity is not fully understood but hydroxychloroquine is known to bind to the retinal pigmented epithelial cells and thought to affect metabolism in other retinal cells. Most patients are asymptomatic early; however, a central or paracentral scotoma can be elicited by visual field and objective changes seen with fundus autofluorescence, retinal optical coherence tomography or multifocal electroretinogram. The classic "bullseye" maculopathy is typically seen later in the disease process. Patients should have annual visual fields and at least 1 objective test (usually OCT). If toxicity is observed, the prescribing physician should be informed and discontinuation discussed. Because of the accumulation in the RPE melanin cells, toxicity can progress for some time even after stopping the medication.

Ethambutol is another medication that can cause significant ophthalmic side effects. Ethambutol is a drug commonly used for the treatment of tuberculosis. The drug can cause a bilateral toxic optic neuropathy that is thought to be related to alterations in the cytosolic and mitochondrial calcium levels in retinal ganglion cells. It is thought that patients on 25 mg/kg/day are at the greatest risk, in addition to those with renal impairment which can cause accumulation of the drug. Most people recommend that patients with intact renal function be placed on doses in the 15 mg/kg/day range if possible to minimize the risk of complications.

Corticosteroids, primarily prednisolone, are drugs that is used as part of the standard post-operative care as well as for treatment of chronic inflammatory pathologies such as uveitis. The key adverse effects are the potential for increased intraocular pressure (steroid response glaucoma) and the development of cataracts (primarily posterior subcapsular cataracts). Some of these risks can be minimized by aggressive initial treatment followed by a tapering to a lower maintenance dosage. In addition, less potent corticosteroids can sometimes have less severe elevations of pressure. Therefore switching to fluoromethalone or loteprednol may be helpful.

SELF-ASSESSMENT QUESTIONS

1. A 55-year-old woman presents to the emergency department with a headache, nausea, vomiting, and a red, painful eye. She describes the episode as starting after coming out of a movie theatre. She noticed halos around the lights in the parking lot. On examination, she has conjunctival injection and a fixed, mid-dilated pupil. You are concerned that the patient is

    A. having an aneurysm. An urgent computed tomography (CT) scan without contrast is needed to confirm presence of an aneurysm.

    B. experiencing a migraine with visual aura. Treatment would include use of an ergotamine and pain control until it resolves.

C. likely in pupillary block and is having an episode of acute angle closure glaucoma. The intraocular pressure should be checked, and ophthalmology consult should be obtained immediately.

D. having an acute attack of anterior uveitis. You should start topical steroids and have the patient follow up with an ophthalmologist.

2. A 17-year-old girl presents to your clinic with a painful right eye. She is otherwise healthy except for a lingering chronic sinusitis that she has been fighting. She is febrile (temperature 102°F) and has a best corrected visual acuity of 20/200. There is an afferent pupillary defect on the right side. Her right upper and lower eyelids are swollen and erythematous; however, there is no evidence of trauma. She has restricted eye movements. The conjunctiva is injected, the cornea is clear, the anterior chamber is quiet, and the lens is clear. The posterior segment does not appear to be involved. You plan to send the patient for a CT scan of the orbits with contrast because you suspect which of the following?

A. Preseptal cellulitis

B. Orbital cellulitis and possible periosteal abscess

C. Blunt force trauma and a retrobulbar hemorrhage

D. Type I hypersensitivity reaction

3. A 73-year-old man presents with transient visual obscuration (amaurosis fugax). On examination, you find a Hollenhorst plaque at an arterial bifurcation in the inferotemporal retina. Which of the following is the most likely source of the emboli?

A. Carotid artery

B. Aorta

C. Bicuspid aortic valve

D. Left ventricle of the heart.

SECTION VII Psychiatric Disorders

Thought Disorders

Nina Kraguljac

- Define the term *psychosis*.
- Understand the symptoms of schizophrenia and related disorders.
- Describe common pathophysiologic abnormalities associated with schizophrenia.
- Outline current available treatments for schizophrenia and related disorders.

PREVALENCE & BURDEN

Schizophrenia, the most common primary psychotic disorder, has a lifetime prevalence of approximately 1% worldwide, is equally common in males and females, and affects individuals from all racial and ethnic groups. The typical age of onset is in late adolescence to early adulthood, with females having an illness onset of approximately 5 to 10 years later. Prepubescent onset is rare, but those who present with early-onset schizophrenia have a more severe illness course. Late-onset schizophrenia after the age of 45 years is more common in females. The prevalence of schizophrenia is higher in densely populated areas and in developed nations. Life expectancy in patients is 10 to 20 years lower relative to the general population, which is attributed to increased rates of suicide (6% completed suicide rate), accidents, smoking, and poor physical health. Direct and indirect costs in the United States are estimated at about $100 billion annually, with productivity losses being the largest component of the overall societal cost.

MAJOR THOUGHT DISORDERS

Schizophrenia

Schizophrenia is a complex, heterogeneous syndrome believed to be multifactorial, with genetic and environmental components. Patients vary widely in their symptomatology, course of illness, and treatment response, to the point that the diagnosis may identify individuals who share few or no symptoms in common. The validity of traditional clinical subtypes (eg, paranoid schizophrenia, catatonic schizophrenia) as nosologic entities has been questioned, and their prognostic value is limited.

Dimensional models of psychosis suggest that symptoms and disease course are better explained in terms of continuous distributions. The psychopathology can be described along the following symptom domains: (1) positive symptoms, which include delusions, hallucinations, and disorganization of thought and speech; (2) negative symptoms, which include apathy, alogia, poor attention, flat affect, and anhedonia; and (3) cognitive deficits, which include working memory and episodic memory deficits, impairment in executive function, and decreased attention span. Negative symptoms can be divided into primary and secondary negative symptoms. Primary symptoms are regarded as part of the illness, whereas secondary negative symptoms have other causes, such as preoccupation with hallucinations or delusions, suspicious withdrawal, depression, medication side effects, or social isolation. Approximately 25% to 30% of patients suffer from persistent primary negative symptoms, also known as the deficit syndrome (see later discussion). Patients with significant negative symptoms may have poor awareness of their symptoms. Cognitive deficits are present in approximately 75% to 85% of all patients; the extent is variable, but patients typically score about a standard deviation lower on standardized assessments than would be expected for the general population. Memory is the cognitive domain showing the most pronounced deficits, with working memory and episodic memory appearing to be primarily affected. Cognitive dysfunction often predates emergence of positive symptoms and also is reported in high-risk individuals and unaffected family members of patients with schizophrenia, suggesting significant genetic contribution. The extent of these deficits is most predictive of long-term outcome and social functioning. Positive symptoms have a tendency to relapse and remit, but negative and cognitive symptoms tend to be chronic, even when patients receive antipsychotic treatment.

Affective flattening: Lack of range and intensity of emotional expression.

Akathisia: Extreme restlessness. May include pacing, rocking back and forth, or an inability to sit still.

Alogia: Synonym for poverty of speech.

Catalepsy: Passive induction of a posture held against gravity.

Catatonia: Unusual motor behavior, typically with lack of reactivity to the environment.

Delusion: A belief that is firmly maintained despite being contradicted by reality.

Dyskinesia: Abnormal, involuntary movement.

Dystonia: Abnormal muscle tone resulting in muscular spasm and abnormal posture.

Echolalia: Mimicking another's speech.

Echopraxia: Mimicking another's movement.

Extrapyramidal: Referring to the motor systems involving the basal ganglia, as opposed to the corticospinal tracts that pass through the medullary pyramids. Often used in the context of parkinsonian side effects of antipsychotic medications.

Formal thought disorder: A disturbance in the organization and expression of thoughts.

Hallucination: A sensory experience of something that is not present.

Ideas of reference: An unfounded belief that objects, events, or people are of personal significance.

Mannerisms: Odd caricature of normal actions.

Mutism: No or very little verbal response.

Negative symptoms: Normal behaviors or thought patterns lost as a feature of disease, such as apathy or social withdrawal.

Negativism: Opposing or not responding to instructions or external stimuli.

Positive symptoms: Abnormal behaviors or thought patterns that emerge as a feature of disease, such as delusions or hallucinations.

Posturing: Spontaneous and active maintenance of a posture against gravity.

Poverty of speech: Inability to start or take part in a conversation, mostly "small talk."

Stereotypy: Repetitive, abnormally frequent, non–goal-directed movements.

Stupor: A condition in which a person is immobile, mute, and unresponsive, but appears to be fully conscious.

Tardive: Appearance late in the treatment of a disease.

Thought broadcasting: The belief that one's thoughts are being made known to others.

Thought insertion: The belief that thoughts are put into one's mind.

Waxy flexibility: Slight and even resistance to positioning by examiner.

The diagnosis of schizophrenia is made clinically; no diagnostic tests or biomarkers are available. The patient must have 2 of the following 5 symptoms: (1) delusions, (2) hallucinations, (3) disorganized speech, (4) disorganized or catatonic behaviors, and (5) negative symptoms. To make a diagnosis, symptoms must have been present for 6 months (including prodromal and residual phase) with at least 1 month of active symptoms. A detailed personal and family history, physical examination, laboratory testing, and neuroimaging can help differentiate primary psychotic disorders from psychosis due to general medical conditions, delirium, and substance-induced psychosis.

The Deficit Syndrome

The deficit syndrome is a subtype of schizophrenia characterized by primary and enduring negative symptoms. These are present during and between episodes of positive symptom exacerbation and can be observed regardless of the patient's medication status. The deficit syndrome is associated with worse premorbid adjustment, more global impairment, lower quality of life, and poorer long-term outcome. Symptoms are evident at initial presentation and progress in severity in the first 5 years following the onset of the illness, with high temporal stability thereafter. Prevalence is estimated at 6% to 15% in first-episode patients and 25% to 30% in chronic schizophrenia. It is still unknown which neurodevelopmental or neurodegenerative processes manifest as negative symptoms in schizophrenia. Conventional antipsychotics, with the exception of clozapine, and psychosocial therapies have no clear effects on reducing primary negative symptoms.

Schizophreniform Disorder

Schizophreniform disorder is a type of psychosis that presents the same as schizophrenia, but the patient does not yet meet the time criterion for schizophrenia (ie, symptoms have been present for <6 months but >1 month). Treatment is the same as that for schizophrenia.

Brief Psychotic Disorder

This disorder is characterized by a sudden onset of 1 or more psychotic symptoms that last at least 1 day but <1 month. Negative symptoms are not part of the diagnostic criteria. The typical illness onset is 30 to 50 years of age, and the average brief psychotic episode lasts approximately 2 weeks. Brief psychotic disorders often occur in context of significant stressors. A higher incidence is also found among immigrants to developed countries and within 4 weeks postpartum. Short-term hospitalization and antipsychotic treatment may be required; cognitive-behavioral therapy can be used to help patients learn to cope with stress. Most people only have 1 episode, after which they return to their premorbid level of functioning; however, some will eventually develop a chronic psychotic condition.

Catatonia

Historically, catatonia has been conceptualized as a subtype of schizophrenia, but it frequently occurs in patients with a primary mood disorder and in association with neurologic diseases and other general medical conditions. Epidemiologic studies suggest that catatonia is associated with schizophrenia in approximately 20% of cases, with mood disorders in 45% of cases, and with somatic causes including epilepsy, systemic lupus erythematosus, intermittent porphyria, dementia, and encephalopathies in approximately 25% of cases.

Catatonia should be considered in any patient exhibiting marked deterioration in psychomotor function and overall responsiveness. Catatonia is defined as ≥3 of the following symptoms: (1) catalepsy; (2) waxy flexibility; (3) stupor; (4) agitation, not influenced by external stimuli; (5) mutism; (6) negativism; (7) posturing; (8) mannerisms; (9) stereotypies; (10) grimacing; (11) echolalia; and (12) echopraxia. The Bush-Francis catatonia rating scale is one of the most commonly used instruments to aid in the diagnosis. The prognosis of catatonia is good, especially with early and aggressive treatment, but longer duration of an episode is linked to a less favorable prognosis. Several recognized subtypes of catatonia are based on the predominant signs and symptoms. Retarded catatonia, the most common subtype is characterized by mutism, posturing, rigidity, and repetitive actions. Excited catatonia is marked by excessive and purposeless movements, agitation, restlessness, and talkativeness. Malignant catatonia is associated with hyperthermia and autonomic instability (diaphoresis, tachycardia, blood pressure instability, and varying degrees of cyanosis); the severe levels of metabolic decompensation can be lethal and warrant emergent treatment. Putative neurobiological mechanisms underlying catatonia include glutamatergic and γ-aminobutyric acid (GABA)-ergic neurotransmitter system abnormalities.

Schizoaffective Disorder

Schizoaffective disorder has features of both schizophrenia and a mood disorder. It is defined by intervals of significant mood disturbances and the presence of psychotic symptoms for >2 weeks in the absence of mania or depression. The mood episode must be present for the majority of the illness. Subtypes are defined as bipolar type (if manic episodes are part of the presentation) and depressive type (if only major depressive episodes occur). Schizoaffective disorder appears to occupy an intermediate position between schizophrenia and bipolar disorder in terms of symptomatology, neuroimaging findings, response to treatment, and prognosis.

Delusional Disorder

This disorder typically develops in middle to late adult life and is characterized by persistent delusional beliefs with minimal impairment of daily functioning and absence of negative or cognitive symptoms. Hallucinations are usually not present. Delusions cannot be due to effects of prescription or illicit drugs or a general medical condition. Delusional disorder cannot be diagnosed in patients with a prior diagnosis of schizophrenia. Six types of delusional disorder are described: (1) erotomanic, the belief that someone is in love with the patient, often someone who is famous; (2) grandiose, the belief that the patient is superior or unique; (3) persecutory, the belief that someone is wanting to harm the patient; (4) jealous, the belief that the partner is cheating on the patient; (5) somatic, the belief that someone has a medical condition; and (6) mixed, having features of >1 subtype of delusion. Personal beliefs should be evaluated with great respect to cultural and religious differences to avoid a false diagnosis of delusional disorder when the belief is widely accepted in the patient's culture.

Substance-Induced Psychosis

Intoxication or withdrawal from a number of substances is associated with acute onset of psychotic symptoms. Cocaine, amphetamines, phencyclidine, ketamine, cannabis, and alcohol have long been recognized to precipitate psychotic symptoms. More recently developed designer drugs including cathinones (bath salts) and synthetic cannabinoids have toxicity syndromes that often manifest with psychosis, agitation, and tachycardia. The main diagnostic feature is prominent delusions or hallucinations that are determined to be caused by effects of a psychoactive substance. If patients are aware that hallucinations are not real or psychotic symptoms occur only during delirium, a diagnosis of substance-induced psychosis cannot be made. Substance-induced psychoses manifest shortly after drug consumption and resolve quickly after cessation, often without the need for treatment. However, with continuing use, stimulants, cannabis, newer designer drugs, and alcohol seem to cause prolonged psychosis. Supportive therapy and drug counseling may be helpful after psychotic symptoms have resolved to prevent recurrence. If psychotic symptoms persist, antipsychotic medications should be considered.

Although illicit drug use is the most common cause of substance-induced psychosis, a number of prescription medications can also cause these symptoms. These include amphetamines, angiotensin-converting enzyme inhibitors, antihistamines, anticholinergics, β-blockers, cephalosporins, fluoroquinolone antibiotics, procaine derivatives, nonsteroidal anti-inflammatory drugs, salicylates, and dopamine receptor agonists, among others. Corticosteroid-induced psychosis often includes agitation, anxiety, insomnia, irritability, and restlessness. Symptoms often develop after a few days of corticosteroid treatment, but they can also occur late in the treatment. The risk for steroid-induced psychosis increases with greater corticosteroid doses, with an incidence of approximately 2%. Management includes tapering of corticosteroids or decreasing to the lowest possible dose. If a taper is not possible or symptoms are severe, low-dose antipsychotic medications can be prescribed. A history of psychiatric disorders or previous corticosteroid-induced psychosis is not predictive of future episodes, but steroids need to be used with caution in patients with psychotic disorders.

Psychosis Due to General Medical Conditions

Medical conditions associated with psychosis include autoimmune, endocrine, neurologic, and nutritional disorders. Endocrine conditions include thyroid and parathyroid dysfunction. Neurologic conditions include temporal lobe epilepsy, Parkinson disease, and Lewy body disease. A subacute onset of psychosis that is not primary should raise suspicion for an oncologic cause, such as a hormone-secreting tumor, space-occupying brain lesion, or paraneoplastic syndrome. Genetic or heritable diseases, such as Huntington disease, should also be considered. The temporal relationship and course of psychotic symptoms, as well as the patient's age, background, and general medical conditions, may provide diagnostic clues. A physical and neurologic exam with laboratory testing and neuroimaging may be necessary.

There has been a substantial increase in interest in autoimmune encephalitis that is characterized by brain inflammation and circulating autoantibodies, often in context of a paraneoplastic process. *N*-Methyl-D-aspartate (NMDA) receptors, α-amino-3-hydroxy-5-methylisoxazole-4-propionic acid (AMPA) receptors, and GABA receptors seem to be the main targets. Psychiatric symptoms generally occur early in the illness but may appear at any time during the course of the disease. Bizarre behaviors, confabulations, agitation, hallucinations and delusions, and confusion and disorientation are common. Neurologic symptoms may or may not be present. Magnetic resonance imaging can aid in the diagnosis. Nonspecific abnormalities on fluid-attenuated inversion recovery sequences are commonly found in the medial temporal lobes, basal ganglia, cerebellum, and cerebral cortex (Figure 38–1). Antipsychotics, benzodiazepines, and mood stabilizers have very limited effectiveness in the treatment of these symptoms. Steroid treatment, removal of antibodies by plasma exchange, or intravenous immunoglobulin therapy generally results in clinical improvement.

NATURAL HISTORY

Clinical staging is a useful tool in medicine. It assumes that pathologic indices are progressing in subsequent stages, that patients in individual stages present with similar pathologic changes, and that treatment should be most effective in earlier stages. Several stages are defined to characterize the clinical course of schizophrenia: the prodromal phase, the active phase (first psychotic episode followed by chronic phase), and the residual phase (Figure 38–2).

The term *prodrome* is derived from the Greek word *prodromos*, meaning the forerunner of an event. The prodromal phase typically predates the first psychotic break and is characterized by gradually increasing social withdrawal, poor

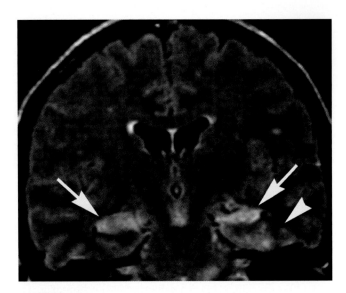

FIGURE 38–1 Magnetic resonance imaging (MRI) in a patient with limbic encephalitis. Coronal axial fluid-attenuated inversion recovery (FLAIR) images demonstrate abnormal hyperintensities involving the mesial temporal lobes (*arrowhead*) including the hippocampi (*arrows*) without significant mass effect. (Reproduced with permission from Jameson JL, Fauci AS, Kasper DL, et al: *Harrison's Principles of Internal Medicine*, 20th ed. New York, NY: McGraw Hill; 2018.)

motivation, restricted affective range, and cognitive deficits. Symptoms can also include brief self-limited intermittent psychotic symptoms (BLIPS; presence of psychotic symptoms of up to 7 days followed by remission with no hospitalization or treatment) and attenuated psychotic symptoms (APS; symptoms are present in attenuated form and duration and warrant clinical attention). It is important to note that only approximately 15% to 30% of patients with prodromal symptoms later develop a psychotic illness; therefore, a "watch and wait" approach with frequent clinical contact and regular assessment rather than antipsychotic medication is recommended in this population.

Active-phase symptoms emerge following the prodrome, often in context of significant life stress or substance use. There is considerable evidence that longer duration of untreated psychosis (ie, the time between symptom onset and first treatment) is related to poorer long-term outcomes. The average duration of untreated psychosis in the United States is estimated to be approximately 18 months. Clinicians are often concerned that an initial first episode schizophrenia diagnosis, if incorrect, may impede clinical care and lead to stigmatization, despite the high diagnostic stability of schizophrenia spectrum disorders. This may have profound effects, not only on pharmacotherapy and specific forms of psychotherapy used, but also on the prognosis provided to newly diagnosed patients and their families as to what lies ahead. Approximately one-third of patients with a first psychotic episode will have a favorable illness course, recovering with minimal or no long-term impairment. The remainder of patients have either an intermediate or poor outcome.

Stages of illness

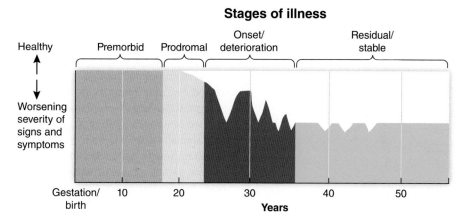

FIGURE 38-2   The illness trajectory of schizophrenia. The premorbid stage represents the stage of risk or genetic vulnerability, with no clinical signs or symptoms of the illness. The prodromal stage ushers in mild symptoms such as social isolation, functional decline, unusual thoughts, and suspicion. The stage of onset/deterioration is the stage of the manifest disease and usually involves multiple hospitalizations and gradual decline. The residual/stable stage is marked by deficit and cognitive symptoms, typically without full-blown psychotic episodes.

The residual phase is characterized by a stable course of persisting negative and/or cognitive symptoms, with only few positive symptoms. Frank psychotic behaviors may subside, but the patient may continue to hold strange beliefs. The residual phase is established after positive symptom severity is minimal for at least 1 year, in the absence of a neurodegenerative disease. It is recommended that antipsychotic medication be continued.

PATHOPHYSIOLOGY

Genetic & Environmental Factors

Epidemiologic studies suggest a greater concordance of schizophrenia in monozygotic than in dizygotic twins, supporting a genetic basis.

The heritable component is estimated to be approximately 70% to 80%. Genome-wide association studies have identified >100 distinct genetic loci containing fairly common alleles with small effects, suggesting that a range of single-nucleotide polymorphisms contribute to the risk. Eleven copy number variants that confer a relatively high risk have also been identified. Thus, genetic risk of schizophrenia is generally due either to the presence of a very rare, large-effect copy number variant or to the coincident inheritance of many alleles with small effect size. The genetic risk is also highly pleiotropic and does not map onto the existing disease definitions. For example, many risk alleles are shared between schizophrenia and bipolar disorder. Some of the risk variants identified encode glutamate receptors, voltage-dependent calcium channels, and the dopamine D_2 receptor. Others regulate neuronal plasticity, maturation, modulation, and regeneration. It is important to note that most genetic markers are considered to be associated with schizophrenia but do not serve as biomarkers per se.

The dominant paradigm for understanding the environmental contributions to schizophrenia has been the neurodevelopmental hypothesis, which posits risk factors that affect early neurodevelopment during pregnancy, including maternal stress, nutritional deficiencies, maternal infections, and birth complications. Other environmental risk factors include socioeconomic factors, childhood adversity, immigration, and being raised in cities. The use of cannabis is estimated to carry up to a 40% greater risk for development of psychosis, with a dose–effect relationship between cannabis use and schizophrenia risk. It is also thought that cannabis use in adolescence results in an earlier onset of psychosis than in those without a history of cannabis use.

Neurotransmitter Abnormalities

Dopamine has been a focus in investigating schizophrenia pathophysiology, based on the observations that drugs that cause psychosis increase dopaminergic neurotransmission and that antipsychotic medications act as dopamine receptor blockers. Research on mechanisms underlying schizophrenia indicates the following: (1) striatal dopamine synthesis and release capacity are increased; (2) dopamine release capacity in prefrontal cortical and other extrastriatal regions may be decreased; and (3) postsynaptic dopamine receptors and transporters are not consistently altered in the striatum or extrastriatal regions of the brain. However, dopaminergic alterations do not explain the full range of clinical symptoms, specifically negative symptoms and cognitive deficits.

The dissociative anesthetics phencyclidine (PCP) and ketamine act as noncompetitive NMDA receptor blockers. They have psychotomimetic effects in healthy humans that mimic symptoms of schizophrenia including some of the cognitive deficits. Ketamine also exacerbates psychotic symptoms in patients with schizophrenia. Alterations in NMDA receptors on parvalbumin-positive interneurons are thought to lead to disinhibition of excitatory pyramidal cells and result in a shift of the excitation/inhibition balance (Figure 38–3). This could interfere with brain synchronicity and cause some of

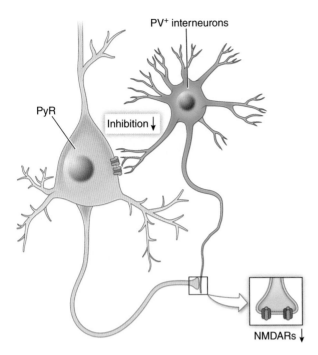

FIGURE 38–3 The *N*-methyl-D-aspartate receptor (NMDAR) hypofunction hypothesis of schizophrenia. Reduced NMDAR activation leads to reduced output from inhibitory γ-aminobutyric acid (GABA)-ergic interneurons, especially those that contain parvalbumin (PV⁺ interneurons). This then results in disinhibition of excitatory pyramidal neurons (PyR). (Reproduced with permission from Paoletti P, Bellone C, Zhou Q: NMDA receptor subunit diversity: impact on receptor properties, synaptic plasticity and disease, *Nat Rev Neurosci*. 2013 Jun;14(6):383-400.)

the symptom complexes observed in the illness. Evidence of GABAergic abnormalities comes predominantly from postmortem studies that find decreased interneuron numbers (predominantly fast-spiking interneurons) and decreased activity of glutamate decarboxylase, the enzyme that synthesizes GABA. Although glutamatergic and GABAergic alterations may be more proximal to the root causes of schizophrenia, this does not contradict the dopamine hypothesis. On the contrary, circuit-based models that integrate findings suggest that glutamate-related disinhibition in the hippocampus may result in malfunction of the feedback loop to the ventral tegmental area and result in a hyperdopaminergic state.

Structural & Functional Brain Abnormalities

Neuroimaging and postmortem studies have attempted to identify altered structure or function of particular brain regions and, more recently, brain circuits. The first evidence of structural brain abnormalities in schizophrenia was published in 1976, reporting enlarged ventricle size in patients compared to controls. The finding that is perhaps most replicated in volumetric studies in schizophrenia is hippocampal volume loss. In addition, reductions in cortical gray matter volume appear widespread, particularly in the medial temporal, superior temporal, and prefrontal areas, and may in part be associated with

exposure to antipsychotic medications. Interestingly, this volume loss does not appear to reflect a gross loss of cell bodies, but rather decreased neuropil (ie, reduced dendritic complexity and synaptic density).

Contemporary models postulate that schizophrenia is caused by faulty interactions between brain regions that lead to symptoms across domains, rather than abnormalities in isolated brain areas. White matter tracts that structurally connect spatially disparate brain regions have decreased integrity, which is thought to be related to dysmyelination and oligodendrocyte pathology. Abnormal interactions between networks of brain regions during cognitive tasks and at rest in patients with schizophrenia also support the dysconnectivity hypothesis.

MANAGEMENT & OUTCOMES

A Brief History of Antipsychotic Medications

Antipsychotic medications are the cornerstone of acute and maintenance treatment of schizophrenia and are effective in treating hallucinations, delusions, and thought disorders, regardless of etiology. The discovery of antipsychotic medications was serendipitous. More than half a century ago, the observation was made, quite accidentally, that the antihistamine chlorpromazine also relieves psychotic symptoms. Between 1954 and 1975, approximately 15 first-generation, or "typical," antipsychotic medications were introduced in the US market. All typical antipsychotics were found to have comparable efficacy but had significant neurologic side effects, such as neuroleptic malignant syndrome. In the late 1950s, a group of tricyclic compounds was synthesized based on the antidepressant imipramine. One of these compounds, clozapine, showed antipsychotic properties without causing disabling extrapyramidal side effects in trials in animals and humans. In 1975, soon after clozapine had slowly gained acceptance as a promising antipsychotic, a study reported severe blood dyscrasias in 18 patients with 9 fatalities, and clozapine was pulled off the market. In 1988, a seminal 6-week double-blind study comparing clozapine and chlorpromazine showed definitive superiority of clozapine for positive and negative symptoms. Because of the lack of extrapyramidal symptoms, the drug was considered "atypical." Based on these findings, clozapine was reintroduced and continues to be the drug of choice for treatment-refractory schizophrenia. In the 1990s, several other atypical (second-generation) antipsychotics were developed. They are considered as effective as the typical antipsychotics with lower propensity to develop extrapyramidal side effects, but with higher metabolic liability.

Mechanism of Action of First- & Second-Generation Antipsychotic Agents

All antipsychotic medications act as full or partial dopamine D_2 receptor antagonists in nigrostriatal, mesocortical, and tuberoinfundibular pathways (**Figure 38–4**). Oral

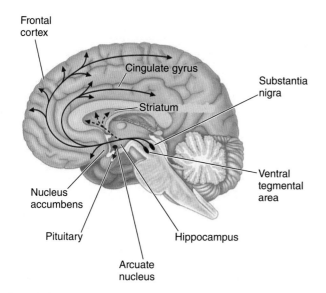

Frontal cortex

Cingulate gyrus

Substantia nigra

Striatum

Nucleus accumbens

Ventral tegmental area

Pituitary

Hippocampus

Arcuate nucleus

FIGURE 38–4 The 3 major dopaminergic projections in the central nervous system. *1.* The nigrostriatal pathway. Neurons in the substantia nigra pars compacta (SNc) project to the dorsal striatum (*upward dashed blue arrows*). *2.* Neurons in the ventral tegmental area project to the ventral striatum (nucleus accumbens), olfactory bulb, amygdala, hippocampus, orbital and medial prefrontal cortex, and cingulate gyrus (*solid blue arrows*). *3.* Neurons in the arcuate nucleus of the hypothalamus project by the tuberoinfundibular pathway in the hypothalamus, from which dopamine is delivered to the anterior pituitary (*red arrow*). (Reproduced with permission from Brunton LL, Hilal-Dandan R, Knollmann BC: *Goodman & Gilman's: The Pharmacological Basis of Therapeutics*, 13th ed. McGraw Hill; 2018.)

antipsychotics undergo extensive first-pass metabolism by the liver and are subject to extensive metabolism via the cytochrome P450 system, with 1 exception, paliperidone, which is predominantly excreted unchanged via the kidneys. Smoking may significantly affect drug levels through induction of the cytochrome system. Patients who are stabilized on antipsychotics in a nonsmoking environment such as a hospital may experience a decrease in serum levels upon resuming smoking, which may necessitate a dose increase.

Positron emission tomography studies have established that about 65% to 70% occupancy of the dopamine D_2 receptor is required to achieve therapeutic benefits. Exceptions are quetiapine and clozapine, which require substantially lower receptor occupancy to have therapeutic efficacy. Receptor occupancy of approximately 80% or higher leads to gross motor side effects.

Adverse Effects

Because of the widespread localization of dopamine binding throughout the central nervous system, dopaminergic antagonists can cause a variety of side effects, particularly extrapyramidal side effects. The immediate cause of acute and subacute extrapyramidal symptoms is considered to be the blockade of dopaminergic inhibition of striatal cholinergic neurons, leading to increased cholinergic activity in the basal ganglia. Several antipsychotic-induced extrapyramidal syndromes are

known. Acute dystonic reactions, such as torticollis, oculogyric crisis, or laryngospasm, are observed within a few hours of administration of a single dose of antipsychotic medications, especially after parenteral administration, and typically resolve within 24 to 48 hours. These can be painful and distressing and can erode patient trust and medication adherence. Risk factors include male gender, younger age, black race, previous dystonic reactions, family history of dystonia, cocaine use, hypercalcemia, hyperthyroidism, and dehydration. The risk of acute dystonic reactions is greater with high-potency, first-generation antipsychotics but can be mitigated by using prophylactic anticholinergics. Drug-induced parkinsonism is a subacute syndrome that mimics Parkinson disease; bilateral rigidity of the neck, trunk, and extremities, which can be "cogwheel," is a core finding. The risk of drug-induced parkinsonism is greater with older age, female gender, brain structural abnormalities, and preexisting extrapyramidal disease. Close monitoring for parkinsonian symptoms and antipsychotic dose adjustments are recommended in these cases, and evidence for use of anticholinergic drugs is limited. Akathisia is characterized by inner tension, restlessness, anxiety, an urge to move, and drawing sensations to the legs and has been associated with violence and suicide. Risk factors include older age, female gender, negative symptoms, iron deficiency, and concomitant parkinsonism. Benzodiazepines can be useful due to their anxiolytic and sedative properties, and β-blockers have been shown to be effective in some studies.

Neuroleptic malignant syndrome is a rare but potentially lethal form of extrapyramidal side effects. Classic signs are hyperthermia, tremor, altered consciousness, and "lead pipe" rigidity. In its severe form, patients develop elevated serum creatine kinase, myoglobinuria, leukocytosis, and hypoxia. Neuroleptic malignant syndrome may develop within hours but usually evolves over days, and many cases occur within 1 to 2 weeks of drug initiation. If not recognized, it can be fatal due to renal failure, cardiorespiratory arrest, disseminated intravascular coagulation, pulmonary emboli, or aspiration pneumonia. Risk factors include dehydration, agitation, catatonia, high doses of high-potency antipsychotics given parenterally at a rapid rate, use of multiple antipsychotics, and coincident treatment with lithium, selective serotonin reuptake inhibitors (SSRIs), or serotonin-norepinephrine reuptake inhibitors.

Tardive dyskinesia is a movement disorder that most commonly presents as choreiform movements often affecting orofacial and lingual musculature. It has an insidious onset after prolonged antipsychotic treatment and is often masked by ongoing treatment. Tardive dyskinesia is usually mild but often irreversible, and it can become socially stigmatizing and compromise eating, speaking, breathing, or ambulation. The cumulative incidence of tardive dyskinesia is estimated at 2% to 5% annually. The incidence of tardive dyskinesia with second-generation antipsychotics is 6- to 12-fold lower compared to haloperidol. Clozapine generally does not cause tardive dyskinesia. Risk factors include longer duration of antipsychotic treatment, higher cumulative drug doses, greater negative symptoms, substance abuse, and diabetes.

Atypical or second-generation antipsychotics potently block 5-hydroxytryptamine (5-HT) 2A serotonin receptors in addition to dopamine D_2 receptors, which is suggested to be the basis for lower overall risk of extrapyramidal side effects with second-generation antipsychotics. Common side effects associated with second-generation antipsychotics include weight gain and metabolic syndrome, hypotension, hyperprolactinemia, anticholinergic symptoms, extrapyramidal symptoms, and sexual dysfunction. Rare side effects include neuroleptic malignant syndrome, seizures, and agranulocytosis. There is increased risk of mortality from all causes, especially in older adults with dementia-related psychosis, for which the US Food and Drug Administration has issued a black box warning that should be weighed before prescribing these drugs in elderly patients. Metabolic monitoring is recommended for all patients chronically treated with second-generation antipsychotic medications. This include a baseline assessment of personal/family history of metabolic risk factors, quarterly assessments of the body mass index and waist circumference, and blood pressure, fasting glucose, and fasting lipids 12 weeks after antipsychotic initiation and annually thereafter.

The Clinical Antipsychotic Trials for Intervention Effectiveness (CATIE), a multicenter, double-blind, randomized controlled trial, compared the relative effectiveness of second-generation antipsychotic medications to the first-generation antipsychotic perphenazine. Surprisingly, efficacy measures did not differ between any of the antipsychotic medications included in the trial. Approximately three-quarters of patients discontinued the antipsychotic before the end of the 18-month trial; olanzapine had the lowest discontinuation rates but had the highest side effect burden overall. The Cost Utility of the Latest Antipsychotic Drugs in Schizophrenia Study (CUtLASS) from the United Kingdom similarly reported no advantage of second-generation antipsychotics in terms of quality of life or symptom burden over 1 year.

General Management Strategies

Acutely psychotic patients often require hospitalization for their safety. Oral second-generation antipsychotic agents are considered first-line treatment. For patients who are acutely agitated or likely to harm themselves or others, short-acting injectable antipsychotics, alone or in combination with benzodiazepines, are available. Electroconvulsive therapy (ECT) can be used as a last resort in acutely agitated patients or those with catatonia (see later discussion of ECT).

Most patients with chronic schizophrenia achieve a full response to a medication within 2 to 6 weeks. The goal of maintenance treatment is to prevent relapse and optimize functioning. The same medication dosage that resulted in control of acute symptoms is appropriate to use for maintenance treatment. In some cases, to minimize side effects or maximize clinical response, dosing can be further adjusted in clinically stable patients. In patients with multiepisode schizophrenia, treatment with antipsychotic medications will be indefinite. There is little evidence to support augmentation of nonclozapine atypical antipsychotic medications in non–treatment-resistant patients. Rather, a strategy of serial trials of antipsychotic monotherapy is preferred (Figure 38–5). When switching antipsychotic medications, cross-tapering of

---

CASE 38–1

D.J. is a 19-year-old man with no psychiatric history who presents to the emergency department with his parents. He reports that he is visiting home for his winter break from college and his parents have urged him to seek help. The patient denies any complaints and appears quite puzzled about his parents' concerns. He questions the psychiatry resident if his parents have paid the resident off in order to "fabricate something, and lock me up." The parents report an uncomplicated birth history, unremarkable upbringing, and no major medical problems in the past. D.J. had done well in high school and was excited to move out of state to pursue a degree in engineering. He had been in only sporadic phone contact with his parents, citing that he was busy with class work and was somewhat depressed because his grades were lower than expected. Upon his return home, D.J.'s parents noticed a number of odd behaviors. The patient would often close the curtains and peek out the window, wondering if they were being observed. He was suspicious about the new alarm system the parents had installed in his absence, believing that the equipment could be used as a surveillance tool by the National Security Agency. When

he was observed talking to himself, spending hours at a time documenting observations of meaningless events in his notebook, and hiding a knife under his pillow "for protection," the parents decided to have D.J. evaluated. His mother notes that her brother had displayed similar behaviors as a teenager and was later diagnosed with schizophrenia. A physical exam and basic lab workup including a urine drug screen are unremarkable, and a head computed tomography scan reveals no intracranial abnormalities. The patient is admitted to the inpatient psychiatric unit and started on 1 mg of risperidone, which is titrated to a total dose of 3 mg during the hospitalization. Within 2 weeks, delusions markedly improve, and the patient is able to be discharged home with close outpatient care. During his initial appointment, the patient reports only limited memory of the past few months, stating, "I feel as if everything was in a fog." After D.J. and his family receive psychoeducation, they gain better insight into his illness and are able to implement effective strategies in its management. Two months after the initial presentation, D.J. is able to return to school to continue his education.

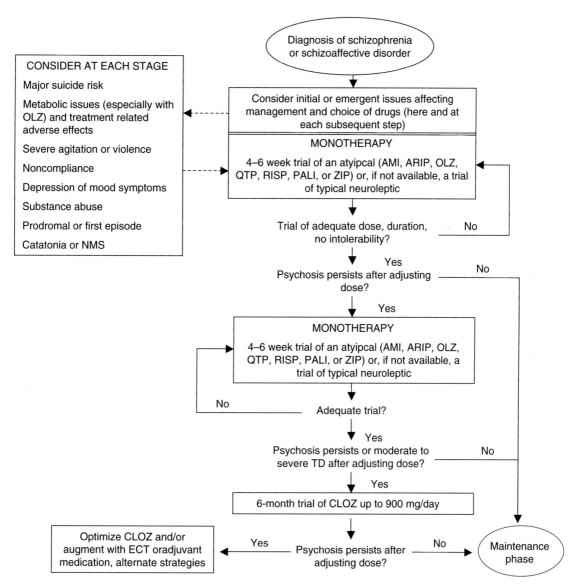

FIGURE 38–5 Algorithm for the pharmacologic treatment of patients with schizophrenia or schizoaffective disorder. First-line options include amisulpride (AMI; not available in the United States), aripiprazole (ARIP), olanzapine (OLZ), quetiapine (QTP), risperidone (RISP), paliperidone (PALI), or ziprasidone (ZIP). Clozapine (CLOZ) should be considered if a patient does not respond to 2 or more adequate medication trials. ECT, electroconvulsive therapy; NMS, neuroleptic malignant syndrome; TD, tardive dyskinesia. Adapted from the International Psychopharmacology Algorithm Project (IPAP) schizophrenia treatment algorithm, available online at www.ipap.org. (Adapted with permission from the International Psychopharmacology Algorithm Project (IPAP) algorithm for the treatment of schizophrenia, available at www.ipap.org.)

medications is advised, unless the patient has acute, severe adverse effects.

The United Kingdom National Institute for Health and Care excellence guidelines recommend that cognitive-behavioral therapy and family intervention should be offered to all patients with schizophrenia.

Management in First-Episode Schizophrenia

Evidence-based treatment guidelines in first-episode psychosis support the value of early intervention following a first episode of psychosis including low doses of antipsychotic medications, cognitive behavioral-psychotherapy, family education and support, and educational and vocational rehabilitation. Recovery-oriented first-episode clinics offer specialized services over a 2- to 5-year period after psychosis onset, with the goal to improve long-term clinical and functional outcomes. Initial results from the Recovery After an Initial Schizophrenia Episode (RAISE) research initiative indicates that mental health providers across multiple disciplines can implement the principles of coordinated specialty care for first-episode psychosis patients, which emphasizes shared decision making, addressing unique recovery goals of individuals, and engaging family members. Doses for most antipsychotics required for first-psychosis treatment are lower than those needed for multiepisode patients. The proper duration for trying a particular antipsychotic before switching due to lack of efficacy is considered 8 weeks at minimum, but approximately 25% of first-episode patients respond to longer treatments of up to 16 weeks. The recommended initial antipsychotic treatment should be risperidone, aripiprazole, quetiapine, or ziprasidone. If positive symptoms persist, a switch to another first-line medication is recommended. If risperidone was not the initial medication, it should be considered as the second. In addition, nonadherence as reason for lack of clinical response needs to be considered. If this is suspected, switching to a long-acting injectable formulation of risperidone is recommended as second trial. Clozapine can be considered for first-episode patients with persistent positive symptoms after trials of 2 antipsychotics, unless contraindicated or refused by the patient.

Management in Patients with Nonadherence to Oral Medications

Patients cite poor medication efficacy, difficult to tolerate side effects, personal beliefs that medication is unnecessary, stigma of taking antipsychotic agents, and cost as the most common reason for nonadherence with antipsychotic medications. For a significant subset of patients, nonadherence leads to relapse and hospitalization. Long-acting injectable antipsychotics were developed with the primary aim of addressing both hidden and overt nonadherence and are administered every 2 to 12 weeks. They offer several advantages, including more consistent bioavailability and reduced peak/trough plasma levels, transparency of adherence, and the possibility of early interventions if patients fail to take their medication. However, meta-analyses find no robust evidence of better tolerability or efficacy of long-acting injectables, with the possible exception of aripiprazole (this is likely at least in part explained by a selection bias, as those who would almost certainly benefit from a treatment are typically not recruited in clinical trials where they might not receive that medicine). It is recommended that the choice of formulation should be based on a shared decision-making process, taking into consideration patients' preference and pragmatic considerations on treatment adherence and potential risks of incorrect drug administration.

Management in Treatment-Resistant Schizophrenia

Patients with treatment-resistant schizophrenia are defined as patients who have experienced treatment failure with 2 different antipsychotic medications at adequate dose and duration (at least 6 weeks in duration at therapeutic doses in multiepisode schizophrenia). Clozapine is the only currently available antipsychotic medication with superior efficacy; it is estimated that approximately 30% to 50% of patients who fail to respond to other agents will respond to clozapine. Clozapine has a complex pharmacologic profile. It binds loosely and transiently to dopamine D_2 receptors. It has a high affinity for serotonergic, adrenergic, muscarinergic, and histaminic receptors. Receptor occupancy is approximately 40%, which is significantly lower than is needed for therapeutic effects of other antipsychotics. It is extensively metabolized by the cytochrome P450 system, and the elimination half-life averages about 14 hours. Clozapine is different from other antipsychotics in several ways, including its (1) absence of tardive dyskinesia; (2) lack of serum prolactin elevations; (3) ability to treat positive symptoms without exacerbating motor symptoms in patients with Parkinson disease who become psychotic due to exogenous dopaminergic agents; (4) ability to improve primary and secondary negative symptoms; (5) ability to improve some domains of cognition in schizophrenia; and (6) indication for persistent suicidality or self-injurious behavior. Pretreatment assessments include evaluation of the patient's cardiovascular health, complete blood count, electrocardiogram, abnormal involuntary movement scale, and pregnancy test in women of childbearing age. A slow titration with divided doses is recommended to minimize side effects such as orthostatic hypotension. The target dose of clozapine ranges between 200 and 900 mg/d (in divided doses) for most patients. Therapeutic plasma range is 250 to 350 ng/mL. Once an effective maintenance does is reached, most of the daily dose may be given at bedtime, which will aid in patients getting sleep while avoiding daytime sedation. If clozapine treatment is interrupted for >2 days, clozapine titration must be restarted at low doses, but titration can be done more quickly if tolerated by the patient.

Clozapine is associated with a number of severe adverse effects. Agranulocytosis occurs in approximately 0.8% of treated patients, and leukopenia occurs in 3%. These most commonly occur within the first 6 weeks of treatment. All patients, prescribers, and dispensing pharmacies have to be registered in the Clozapine Risk Evaluation and Mitigation Strategy (REMS) program, which provides guidelines for monitoring of leukopenia and agranulocytosis. It also documents routine neutrophil monitoring (weekly during the first 6 months, every other week during the second 6 months, and monthly thereafter for the duration of treatment). Myocarditis, likely an immunoglobulin E–mediated acute hypersensitivity reaction, can present with malaise, chest pain, shortness of breath, and elevated peripheral eosinophil counts, sedimentation rates, or troponin levels. Incidence is estimated to be between 0.001% and 0.2%. Clozapine needs to be discontinued promptly, and patients should not be rechallenged after myocarditis has resolved. The seizure risk associated with clozapine increases substantially in doses >600 mg/d; myoclonus can precede full-blown tonic-clonic seizures and can be valuable in determining when antiepileptic drugs are indicated. Gastrointestinal hypomotility is another potentially life-threatening side effect that can manifest in paralytic ileus, bowel obstruction, or acute megacolon. If patients do not respond to treatment with adequate doses of clozapine monotherapy for 6 months, the regimen may be augmented with another antipsychotic medication or a trial of ECT.

Management of Catatonia

A broad range of medical complications can occur in patients with catatonia. Some patients require a high level of nursing care, intravenous fluids and/or tube feeds, and anticoagulation therapies in order to reduce the risk of morbidity and mortality caused by immobility and poor nutrition. Antipsychotic agents should be discontinued because they may aggravate the catatonic state and can increase the risk of developing neuroleptic malignant syndrome. Benzodiazepines are the mainstay of treatment for catatonia, regardless of the underlying condition, and can also be helpful as a diagnostic probe. A positive lorazepam challenge validates the diagnosis of catatonia. After the patient is examined for signs of catatonia, 1 to 2 mg of lorazepam is administered intravenously. After 5 minutes, the patient is reexamined. If there is no change, a second dose of lorazepam is given, and the patient is assessed again 5 minutes later. The challenge is considered positive if marked improvement of symptoms is observed. However, a negative lorazepam challenge does not rule out a diagnosis of catatonia. With an adequate dose, response is usually seen within 3 to 7 days, but occasionally, response can be more incremental. A commonly suggested starting dose is 1 to 2 mg of lorazepam every 4 to 12 hours, with dose adjustments based on the patient's clinical response. Doses of 8 to 24 mg of lorazepam per day are common and tolerated without ensuing sedation. There is no consensus as to how long benzodiazepines are to be continued, but they are generally gradually tapered after the illness has remitted. If symptoms do reemerge during a taper, it is suggested that benzodiazepines be continued to be used for an extended period of time. Bilateral ECT should be started in patients who do not respond to benzodiazepines or in severe cases with life-threatening conditions such as malignant catatonia. Benzodiazepines need to be discontinued before initiation of ECT. Response rates with ECT are estimated at approximately 85%. The number of treatments needed to improve symptoms is variable. Often a rapid response is seen after only a few sessions. However, en block daily treatments for 3 to 5 days may be necessary for malignant catatonia. Maintenance ECT can be considered for sustained symptom remission. A few case reports suggest that zolpidem, a positive allosteric modulator of $GABA_A$ receptors, may be a treatment alternative in patients who have failed treatment with benzodiazepines and ECT. Treatment in children and adolescents should follow the same principles as in adults.

Management Strategies in Schizoaffective Disorder

Patients often receive a combination of antipsychotic medications and mood stabilizers or antidepressants. Antipsychotic treatment recommendations mirror those in schizophrenia, and management of mood symptoms is equivalent to that in bipolar disorder or major depressive disorder.

Management Strategies in Delusional Disorder

A major challenge in the management of delusional disorder is the lack of insight in many patients, which results in high rates of noncompliance with treatment recommendations. Antipsychotic medications typically do not work well. A small number of case reports suggest that pimozide may have superior efficacy in the somatic subtype of delusional disorder, but data from controlled trials are lacking. Pimozide acts as an antagonist of the dopamine D_2, D_3, and D_4 receptors as well as the $5\text{-}HT_7$ receptor. It is contraindicated in patients with acquired, congenital, or a family history of QT interval prolongation and is not advised in patients with a personal or family history of arrhythmias. It is also contraindicated in patients receiving SSRIs and those who receive CYP3A4, CYP1A2, and CYP2D6 inhibitors. Given these considerations, pimozide should be considered as a last resort. Psychotherapy can include cognitive-behavioral therapy or supportive therapy, with the goal to reduce the strength of conviction of the belief and improve social inclusion. Insight-oriented therapy is rarely indicated. ECT is not indicated in delusional disorder.

Management of Neuroleptic Malignant Syndrome

Initial management consists of early diagnosis and removal of the causative agent along with other potential contributing psychotropic agents (eg, lithium, anticholinergic medications, serotonergic agents). Supportive medical care includes maintenance of cardiorespiratory stability and an euvolemic state, use of cooling blankets for fevers, and use of benzodiazepines to control agitation if necessary. In addition, use of dopamine agonists and dantrolene has been reported to reduce mortality rates in retrospective studies, but a small prospective study suggests a more prolonged course and higher incidence of sequelae in those receiving dantrolene or bromocriptine compared to those receiving supportive care alone. ECT may decrease mortality rates and hasten recovery, but cardiovascular complications have been reported. ECT is generally only recommended for patients not responding to other treatments. Patients restarted on antipsychotic medications may or may not have a recurrent episode of neuroleptic malignant syndrome. To minimize the risk of recurrence, it is recommended to wait at least 2 weeks before resuming therapy, use lower potency agents, start low doses and slowly titrate, avoid concomitant lithium treatment, and prevent dehydration.

Management of Tardive Dyskinesia

Tardive dyskinesia usually appears after prolonged use of antipsychotic drugs. Prevention and early detection and treatment of potentially reversible cases of tardive dyskinesia are paramount, because symptoms are often irreversible despite cessation of the offending drug. Long-term use of antipsychotics in nonpsychotic illnesses should be discouraged, and patients with psychotic disorders should be maintained at the lowest effective antipsychotic dose. Withdrawal of antipsychotics may initially lead to worsening of tardive dyskinesia, but approximately 30% to 50% of patients will eventually have symptom reduction. However, a complete and permanent reversibility may be uncommon. Because of the risk of psychotic relapse, cessation of antipsychotic medication is generally not recommended. As a first step, a decision should be made about whether continuation of concomitant anticholinergic drugs is necessary, because these can probably worsen tardive dyskinesia. For patients who develop tardive dyskinesia on a first-generation antipsychotic, a switch to a second-generation antipsychotic can be considered, and the CATIE trial has shown reductions in severity of tardive symptoms when switching. Clozapine has been recommended for suppressing tardive movement disorders, especially the tardive dystonia variant. Vitamin E and its antioxidant properties have been thought to reverse possible toxic effects of free radicals produced during chronic antipsychotic treatment, but results from clinical trials were conflicting. A meta-analysis of 6 small, placebo-controlled trials suggests vitamin E does not improve tardive dyskinesia. Gingko biloba was found to be effective in a small randomized controlled trial, in which a 12-week treatment significantly reduced involuntary movements. Recently, the US Food and Drug administration has approved two dopamine depleting medications, valbenazine and deutetrabenazine, as treatments for tardive dyskinesia. Deep brain stimulation of the globus pallidus has been shown to improve symptoms in a small number of patients with severe tardive dyskinesia resistant to pharmacologic treatments.

Management of Antipsychotic-Induced Hyperprolactinemia

Prolactin level measurements prior to initiating antipsychotic medications and routine monitoring during antipsychotic therapy are not universally recommended. The strongest predictors of hyperprolactinemia are the type and dose of the antipsychotic prescribed, with increased levels observed at higher doses. Haloperidol and risperidone are among the most common antipsychotics that elevate prolactin level, whereas clozapine and aripiprazole rarely elevate prolactin. If a temporal relationship between prolactin level elevation and initiation of antipsychotic treatment cannot clearly be established, laboratory testing, including assessment of liver, renal, and thyroid function, as well as magnetic resonance imaging of the pituitary gland (especially if patient reports headaches and visual field defects), should be considered. Discontinuation of antipsychotic drugs is not recommended in asymptomatic patients or in female patients with only mild galactorrhea. However, known risks such as osteoporosis and elevated risk of pituitary adenomas may present a justifiable reason to reevaluate established antipsychotic therapy despite a lack of symptoms. If patients are significantly symptomatic, a switch to olanzapine, quetiapine, ziprasidone, or clozapine can be considered. Alternatively, aripiprazole as an adjunct medication, particularly in those who are psychiatrically stable, has been shown to result in normalization of prolactin levels in approximately 79% of patients. This may be because of its dual agonism/antagonism properties on the dopamine D_2 receptor, which may mitigate effects of other antipsychotic medications on the pituitary gland. Because the addition of a dopamine receptor agonist such as amantadine or bromocriptine may cause a psychotic relapse, this is typically not recommended in patients with primary psychotic disorders.

SELF-ASSESSMENT QUESTIONS

1. There is an association between the risk of schizophrenia and the use of which of the following?
   A. Alcohol
   B. Cannabis
   C. Ketamine
   D. None of the above

2. The worst functional outcome in schizophrenia is associated with the presence of which of the following?
   A. Hallucinations and delusions
   B. Disorganized thinking
   C. Blunted affect, social withdrawal
   D. Cognitive dysfunction

3. Which of the following statements is correct?
   A. Antipsychotic medications improve hallucinations and delusions.
   B. Antipsychotic medications improve blunted affect.
   C. Antipsychotic medications improve cognitive dysfunction.
   D. All of the above

Mood Disorders

Li Li

OBJECTIVES

After studying this chapter, the student should be able to:

- Understand the epidemiology, neurobiology, and psychopathology associated with mood disorders.
- Outline the *Diagnostic and Statistical Manual of Mental Disorders*, Fifth Edition, criteria for mood disorders, with a focus on major depressive disorder and bipolar disorders.
- List the psychopharmacologic agents for the treatment of mood disorders, especially major depressive disorder and bipolar disorders.
- Describe the social, medical, and psychological needs of patients with mood disorders.

PREVALENCE & BURDEN

Mood disorders are a major and common public health problem, with a 12-month prevalence of 9.5%. They consist of major depressive disorder and bipolar disorders. Both are serious medical illnesses with mood, cognitive, and physical symptoms. Major depression is relatively common, with a 12-month prevalence of 7% in the United States. It is more common in females, occurring 1.5 to 3 times more often than in males. The rate of major depression varies with age: 5.7% among youth aged 12 to 17 years, 20% among adults aged 20 and 30 years, and approximately 10% among adults aged 40 to 59 years. Adults age 60 years and older have a significantly lower rate of depression (5.4%).

In bipolar disorder, the individual experiences manic or hypomanic episodes alternating with depressive episodes, with periods of normal mood between episodes. The 12-month prevalence in the United States is between 0.6% and 0.8%. In contrast to major depression, bipolar disorder affects women and men at almost the same rate. The mean age at onset for bipolar disorder is approximately 25 years, and men have an earlier age of onset than women.

Mood disorders are associated with increased healthcare utilization, decreased qualify of life, and impairment in social and occupational functioning that significantly affects patients' lives. Studies have shown that major depression is a leading cause of disability. The economic burden of depression, including both direct and indirect costs, was estimated to be $210.5 billion in 2010 in the United States. Although bipolar illness is less common, on a per-case basis, it is the most expensive behavioral healthcare diagnosis because it costs more than twice as much as depression per affected individual due to medical care expenses and lost productivity.

ETIOLOGY

The cause of mood disorders remains unknown, but a combination of genetics, epigenetics, and environment is believed to contribute. Emerging evidence has shown the presence of neurochemical, structural, and functional brain abnormalities in patients with major depression and bipolar disorders.

Genetics

Both major depression and bipolar disorder clearly have inheritable risk factors. Increased risk for mood disorders in the first-degree relatives of patients with either major depression or bipolar disorder is well documented. For example, children of a parent with a mood disorder have a roughly 25% chance of developing a mood disorder themselves, and when both parents are affected, the risk is greater than 50%. First-degree relatives of patients with bipolar disorder have an estimated 12% lifetime prevalence of bipolar disorder, which is about 10 times higher than the general population. Despite this strong

VOCABULARY

Affect: Outward expression of emotions and mood that is observable.

Blunted affect: Diminution or absence of associated feeling.

Emotion: Subjectively experienced feelings that are related to affect and mood.

Episode: A certain number of symptoms for a certain period of time.

Flight of ideas: Shifts in frame of reference, but with meaning within the frame.

Grandiosity: Belief that one's ideas, capacities, or actions are superior to those of others.

Inappropriate affect: Incongruous association of idea and feeling.

Mood: Internal state of feeling at a particular time.

Poverty of speech: Reduced conversational output.

Pressured speech: Speech produced at an abnormally fast or rapid rate.

Racing thoughts: Thoughts or images experienced as occurring at an excessive rate.

evidence for a role of genetics, few individual genes for mood disorders have been identified, and at present, genetic testing for risk of mood disorders is not available.

Epigenetics

Epigenetic changes are modifications of chromatin, such as methylation of DNA or post-translational modifications of histone proteins, that can have long-lasting effects on gene expression. Work on epigenetic effects in mood disorders is just beginning, but initial findings seem quite promising. Alterations in DNA methylation of the glucocorticoid receptor gene are associated with stress vulnerability, altered histone modification is associated with use of antidepressants, and altered methylation status of DNA in the brains of patients with bipolar disorders has emerged as a potential factor in the pathogenesis of mood disorders. In addition, small noncoding RNA molecules known as microRNAs also appear to play a role in psychiatric disorders, including major depression and bipolar disorders. Together, these epigenetic changes emphasize the complex genetic and genomic factors that contribute to mood disorders.

Environment

Environmental factors also appear to contribute to mood disorders. Factors such as childhood maltreatment (ie, early life stress) may predispose to later development of mood

disorders. Mood disorders may also be caused or exacerbated by ongoing psychosocial stress. Although there are few hard data on gene–environment interactions, understanding these effects is likely to be critical to a full understanding of the etiology of mood disorders.

Chemical Abnormalities

Research in humans and animal models has revealed that there are abnormalities in multiple neurotransmitters and neuroendocrine systems in major depression and bipolar disorders (Figure 39–1). Common chemical pathways for bipolar disorders or major depression are believed to include the following: (1) deficiencies in serotonin, norepinephrine, dopamine, γ-aminobutyric acid, or the serotonin transporters; (2) regulators of intracellular signaling pathways, including phosphodiesterase 11A and brain-derived neurotrohic factor (BDNF); (3) components of the hypothalamic-pituitary-adrenal axis, including the glucocorticoid receptors; and (4) inflammatory factors.

Among these chemical pathways, the function of serotonin transmission and serotonin signaling has been well studied. Serotonergic abnormalities are believed to be central to depressive symptoms. The primary origins of serotonergic innervation of the brain are neurons located in the midline raphe nuclei in the brainstem. Serotonergic dysfunction is the basis for the most commonly used treatment of depressive disorders, selective serotonin reuptake inhibitors (SSRIs), which work by blocking serotonin transporters (SERTs) and increasing synaptic serotonin.

There are also structural changes in the brain in mood disorders. Reduced numbers of neurons are found in the anterior cingulate, hippocampus, and prefrontal cortex in bipolar disorders or major depression. Stress is a well-known risk factor or precipitator of depressive symptoms; stress can reduce both neuron number in the dentate gyrus as well as neural process length. Changes in neurotrophic factors have been proposed as an underlying mechanism (Figure 39–2). These changes in neuron structure and function may also, at least in part, be related to changes in serotonin because both effects can be prevented or reversed by SSRIs. In addition, serotonin has an effect on neurogenesis from neural stem cells in the brain. Studies of postmortem human brain samples show greater neurogenesis in the dentate gyrus in patients with major depression treated with SSRIs compared with patients with untreated major depression (see Figure 39–2).

Immune dysregulation in mood disorders has attracted growing attention, and a large number of studies have reported increased levels of inflammatory molecules, such as tumor necrosis factor-α, interleukin-6, and C-reactive protein, in the serum or postmortem brain samples of patients with major depression. Concentrations of proinflammatory cytokines are also reportedly elevated during mania or hypomania. Although most studies have focused on cytokines,

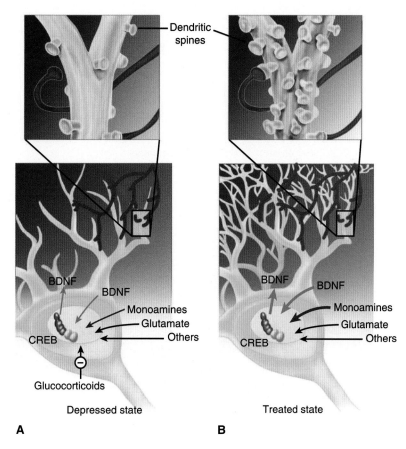

FIGURE 39-1 The neurotrophic hypothesis of major depression. **A.** Changes in trophic factors (especially brain-derived neurotrophic factor [BDNF]) and hormones appear to play a major role in the development of major depression. **B.** Successful treatment results in changes in these factors. CREB, cAMP response element-binding protein. (Reproduced with permission from Nestler EJ, Barrot M, DiLeone RJ: Neurobiology of depression, *Neuron.* 2002 Mar 28;34(1):13-25.)

additional support for the role of inflammation in mood disorders is derived from gene expression studies of peripheral blood mononuclear cells that have demonstrated the existence of increased messenger RNA expression for pro-inflammatory factors. However, most of these studies are observational; interventional studies will be required to establish a definite cause–effect relationship between inflammation and mood disorders.

Structural & Functional Changes in Brain

The recent widespread use of the structural and functional magnetic resonance imaging (MRI) has provided new information on the brain networks involved in mood disorders and how changes in these networks may affect mood regulation and cognition. The areas of the prefrontal cortex, anterior cingulate cortex, and amygdala are specifically implicated to be associated with mood symptoms. Reduced activity in the ventral and orbitofrontal cortices appears to be related to remission, whereas amygdala activity is persistently increased during remission. Taken together, all of these findings

indicate that causes of mood disorders are multifactorial and heterogeneous.

CLINICAL FEATURES OF MOOD DISORDERS

The core feature of any mood disorder is a distinct period of abnormally and persistently altered mood, during which patients suffer from impaired function at work, at school, or in the community. Although many patients with mood disorders have only 1 episode during their lives, most have multiple episodes, alternating with periods of remission or normal moods. However, some individuals may never experience remission. Therefore, another feature of any mood disorder is a tendency toward cycles of episodes, from response or remission to recurrence, which follows a longitudinal course. Besides altered mood, patients with mood disorders can also experience behavioral, cognitive, and psychomotor changes. Both depressive disorders and bipolar disorders have several subtypes, and each of them has very specific presentations, causes, and durations (Figure 39-3).

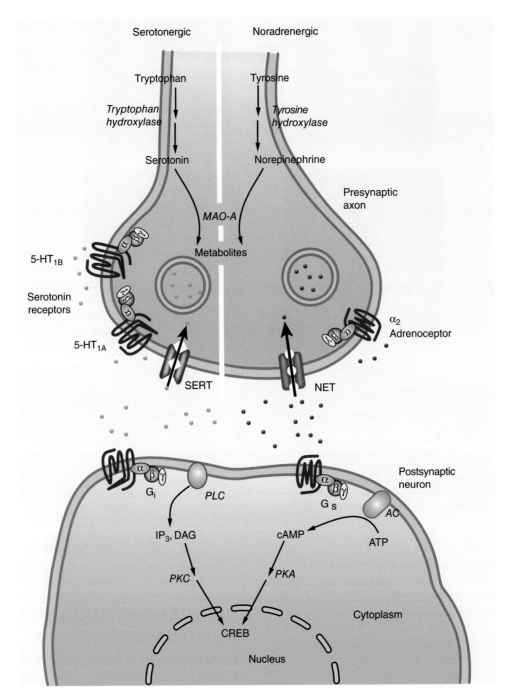

FIGURE 39–2 The amine hypothesis of major depression. Depression appears to be associated with changes in serotonin or norepinephrine signaling in the brain (or both) with significant downstream effects. Most antidepressants cause changes in amine signaling. AC, adenylyl cyclase; CREB, cAMP response element-binding protein; DAG, diacyl glycerol; 5-HT, serotonin; IP3, inositol trisphosphate; MAO, monoamine oxidase; NET, norepinephrine transporter; PKC, protein kinase C; PLC, phospholipase C; SERT, serotonin transporter. (Reproduced with permission from Belmaker RH, Agam G: Major depressive disorder, *N Engl J Med.* 2008 Jan 3;358(1):55-68.)

DEPRESSIVE DISORDERS

Major Depressive Disorder

Depression as a term in popular use is mostly considered to be synonymous with low mood or feeling down or blue. Major depressive disorder as a mental disorder, however, is characterized by a variety of psychological, behavioral, cognitive, and psychomotor symptoms. Major depression is also referred to as unipolar depression, which is differentiated from bipolar disorders. Different depressive symptoms are classified within diagnostic systems, such as the *Diagnostic and Statistical Manual of Mental Disorders*, Fifth Edition (DSM-V).

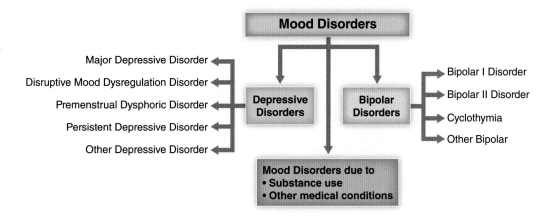

FIGURE 39-3 Classification of mood disorders.

According to the DSM-V, a person must experience 5 or more symptoms from the list below for a continuous period of at least 2 weeks to be diagnosed with an episode of major depressive disorder. Most symptoms must be present every day or nearly every day and must cause significant distress or problems in daily life function.

- Feelings of sadness, hopelessness, and depressed mood
- Loss of interest or pleasure in activities that used to be enjoyable (anhedonia)
- Change in weight or appetite (either increase or decrease)
- Change in activity: psychomotor agitation (being more active than usual) or psychomotor retardation (being less active than usual)
- Insomnia (difficulty sleeping) or sleeping too much
- Feeling tired or not having any energy
- Feelings of guilt or worthlessness
- Difficulties concentrating and paying attention
- Thoughts of death or suicide

Psychological Symptoms

Major depressive disorder is characterized by a pervasive and persistent depressed mood that is accompanied by low self-esteem or sense of inadequacy for at least 2 weeks. When describing their depressed mood, patients express it as "sad," "low," "down," or "blue" feelings. It may also be expressed as a feeling of emptiness or the need to cry. In addition, some patients may feel anxious, irritable, or even hostile, which is often seen in children or adolescents. Another psychological core symptom is anhedonia, the loss of interest or pleasure in normally enjoyable things, people, and activities. Patients state that they are not interested in things or activities they normally enjoy, such as food, sports, or sex, or that they just do not care anymore. They seem to have a flat or blunt affect and feel apathetic and unenthusiastic. Their anhedonia can be accompanied by fatigue or loss of energy, for which they feel guilty and worthless. Depressed patients also have intense pessimism and hopelessness. They feel that their future has

been destroyed and they will never feel "normal" or well again, triggering their anxious feelings. Fears of being alone and lack of support from others are common as well. A triad of worthlessness, hopelessness, and helplessness often leads to suicidal thoughts and suicidal behavior.

Suicide

Suicide is the act of intentionally causing one's own death. Since 2010, suicide has been the 10th leading cause of death in the general population in the United States. Approximately two-thirds of people who commit suicide suffered from depression. Depressed patients tend to feel extremely hopeless and pessimistic when their attempts to solve problems fail again, especially when they lack social support or feel their existence is a burden on family and friends. They frequently become angry, self-punishing, and self-critical. They often describe themselves as "miserable" and have distorted thoughts such as, "I will be better off dead" or "I deserve to die." Some depressed patients have constant suicidal thoughts but do not have the intent or wish to die (passive suicidal thoughts). In contrast, other patients with suicidal thoughts have an intense wish to die and then act on their thoughts and commit suicide. Another subset of depressed patients can present with deliberate nonsuicidal self-injurious behavior but without the wish to die (eg, multiple superficial cuttings). Many patients who engage in nonsuicidal self-injury state that they feel a sense of "relief" or even "euphoria" when they injure themselves.

Behavioral Symptoms

Depressed patients can have behavioral changes in sleep pattern, energy level, appetite, and libido. These symptoms are also referred as "vegetative" symptoms because they affect essential survival skills. Sleep disturbance can be divided into insomnia, hypersomnia, or daytime sleepiness. Insomnia is the most common complaint and includes difficulty falling asleep (sleep-onset insomnia), difficulty staying asleep (sleep-maintenance insomnia), and early morning awakening. Depressed patients may have 1 type of insomnia or a combination of the 3 types of insomnia. Up to 20% of depressed

CASE 39–1

Mr. A is a 32-year-old man with no history of psychiatric illness who presents accompanied by his wife with the following symptoms that have worsened over the past 2 months: severely depressed mood and anhedonia, insomnia with early morning awakening, diurnal variation with worse mood in the morning, and loss of appetite with a 10-pound weight loss. In the office, he is rocking in his chair with his arms wrapped around his body, saying, "Please help me!" His wife reports that he has been pacing around the house at night for the past 2 weeks.

patients report hypersomnia, especially patients with atypical features. Patients usually state they have no appetite to eat or do not feel hungry, leading to a significant weight loss during the depressive episode. Insomnia and poor appetite are the classic symptoms of depression. In contrast, some depressed patients present with hypersomnia and increased appetite, referred to as atypical depression. Physical fatigue or loss of energy occurs independently of sleep disturbance and appetite changes. Although it can be very frustrating to patients and their partners, a common symptom that patients may be reluctant or embarrassed to report is the loss of sex drive.

Cognitive Symptoms

Patients with major depression often report difficulty concentrating or completing tasks. For example, patients frequently report that they do not know where their mind is when they are reading. They have to read the same page over and over again but still do not comprehend the page. Another common frustration reported by depressed patients is the loss of memory, especially immediate or recent memories. They feel they are unable to remember anything. This cognitive dysfunction is usually not a simple matter of having distracting thoughts. Some patients exhibit frank confusion, are disoriented as to the time and place, and do not recognize people they know. This phenomenon is also referred as "pseudodementia" because it is transient in nature and secondary to the untreated depression. Pseudodementia occurs more often in aging patients and usually resolves when the depression is treated and improved.

Psychomotor Symptoms

Psychomotor activity is usually reduced in depressed patients, which is known as psychomotor retardation. Psychomotor retardation involves a slowing down of thoughts and speech, as well as a reduction of physical movements in patients. Patients with psychomotor retardation have difficulty performing activities that normally require little effort, such as getting out of bed. If psychomotor retardation is severe and combined with poor oral intake, severe apathy, and overall self-neglect, a medical emergency can result, and admission to an inpatient service is indicated. In contrast, some depressed patients may

exhibit psychomotor agitation, especially depressed patients with anxious features or children and adolescents. Psychomotor agitation can also be seen in patients who have just started taking antidepressants. However, it should subside in these patients over a few weeks, when they are more tolerant to the medication.

Severity of Major Depression

Depression can be categorized as mild, moderate, or severe. Besides clinical judgment, depression severity can be evaluated using standardized depression rating scales such as the Beck Depression Inventory (self-report) or the Hamilton Depression Rating Scale or the Montgomery-Asberg Depression Rating Scale (both administered by the physician). The assessment of depression severity is of clinical importance because it can guide the physician to select a treatment plan. Mild depression can be treated with psychotherapy alone. However, in moderate or severe depression, antidepressants are often part of the first-line treatment in adults, alone or in combination with psychotherapy, in order to stabilize patients rapidly to prevent or avoid adverse outcomes such as suicide.

Persistent Depressive Disorder

Persistent depressive disorder was previously called *dysthymia* before DSM-V. It is a mild but long-term form of depression that lasts at least 2 years. Its core symptom is a low, gloomy, or sad mood on most days for at least 2 years. In children or adolescents, the mood can be irritable instead of depressed and lasts for at least 1 year. In addition, 2 or more of the following symptoms are present almost all of the time: lost interest in normal activities, hopelessness, low self-esteem, low appetite, low energy, sleep disturbance, and poor concentration. Early morning awakening or worsening of mood in the morning, which are typical for major depression, are usually not present in patients with persistent depressive disorder unless patients also have an episode of major depressive disorder at some point in their lives. This coexistence of persistent depressive disorder and major depression is referred as *double depression*. Persistent depressive disorder tends to run in families and appear more frequently in women. Individuals with persistent depressive disorder often take a negative or discouraging view of themselves, their future, other people, and life events.

Premenstrual Dysphoric Disorder

Premenstrual dysphoric disorder is a mood disorder characterized by severe depressive symptoms, including irritability, extreme sadness, hopelessness, or anger, plus common premenstrual symptoms (breast tenderness, headache, and bloating) before menstruation. This specific condition causes extreme mood shifts that can disrupt work and damage relationships. Premenstrual dysphoric disorder follows a predictable and cyclic pattern. Symptoms begin in the late luteal phase of the menstrual cycle, remit within a few days of the follicular phase, and end in the week after menses.

Disruptive Mood Dysregulation Disorder

This is a fairly new diagnosis and was included for the first time in DSM-V. The diagnosis is only given to children between 6 and 18 years old. It is a childhood condition of extreme irritability, anger, and frequent outbursts that goes far beyond being a "moody" child. Patients often exhibit psychomotor agitation and suffer from severe functional impairments that warrant clinical attention. To be diagnosed with disruptive mood dysregulation disorder, patients must have the symptoms for at least 12 months in at least 2 settings with impaired quality of life and school performance and disrupted relationships with family and peers. Children with this diagnosis usually develop depressive disorders or anxiety disorders, rather than bipolar disorders, as they mature into adulthood.

BIPOLAR DISORDERS

Bipolar disorder is a mental disorder that causes unusual shifts in mood, energy, and activity levels and impairments in daily tasks. Patients with bipolar disorders have discrete periods of altered feeling, thought, and behavior. Most patients with bipolar disorders have manic or hypomanic (less severe form of mania) episodes as well as major depressive episodes. Depressive episodes in bipolar disorders are indistinguishable from those in major depression. The main types of bipolar disorders are presented in Figure 39–3, and all of them involve clear changes in mood, energy, and activity levels. Those who experience at least 1 manic episode are diagnosed with **bipolar I disorder**; however, an episode of major depression is not necessary to make a diagnosis of bipolar I disorder. Patients with episodes of both major depression and hypomania are diagnosed with **bipolar II disorder**. In the DSM-V, a diagnosis of bipolar disorder can be established if a full episode of mania or hypomania emerges during antidepressant treatment and persists at a fully symptomatic level beyond the immediate effects of the treatment.

Mania

A manic episode is defined by a distinct period of at least 1 week of abnormally elevated, expansive, or irritable mood accompanied by impairments in judgment and social and occupational function. Besides abnormal mood, at least 3 of the following symptoms should be present. If the person is only irritable, he or she must experience at least 4 of the following symptoms:

- Inflated self-esteem or grandiosity (ranges from uncritical self-confidence to a delusional sense of expertise)
- Decreased need for sleep

- More talkative than usual or pressure to keep talking
- Flight of ideas or subjective experience that thoughts are racing
- Distractibility (attention easily pulled away by irrelevant/ unimportant things)
- Increase in goal-directed activity (either socially, at work or school, or sexually) or psychomotor agitation (eg, pacing and hand-wringing)
- Excessive involvement in pleasurable activities that have a high potential for painful consequences.

Psychological Symptoms

Patients with manic episode describe their mood as euphoric; they feel they are "on top of the world" and are able to do or accomplish anything and that nothing can stop them (grandiosity). However, sometimes the mood can be irritable and even angry rather than elevated, especially if patients' wishes are curtailed or denied. Along with euphoric mood and unrealistic grandiosity, patients usually engage in significant goal-directed activities that frequently contain high potential for negative consequences.

Behavioral Symptoms

During the manic episode, mood abnormality is often accompanied by the decreased need for sleep. Patients usually sleep <3 hours at night but still feel rested and have excess energy for all kinds of tasks. Sometimes patients describe themselves as "a motor that is going too fast." Although patients may engage in multiple projects at the same time, often none of the projects are completed due to poor or no planning, resulting in frustrations. Their busy pace may also become unpleasant when patients have insomnia for several nights in a row. Mania can also manifest as increased sexual drive and indiscrete sexual behavior. Patients tend to have multiple partners and are more vulnerable to substance use, which may later result in feelings of shame and embarrassment.

CASE 39–2

Mr. B, a 40-year old man, was brought to the emergency department for a behavior evaluation. Mr. B describes similar severe episodes previously, where he becomes involved in impulsive and excessive behaviors such as spending large sums of money or traveling to other countries. He also describes a thought pattern characterized by an influx of ideas that he feels he must act upon. Mr. B describes the episodes as "amazingly intoxicating" and as giving him "lots and lots of pleasure and lots of energy even with decreased need for sleep." This energy and abundance of ideas are transferred into Mr. B's work, which in turn provides the wealth that supports his travels and money-spending pattern.

Cognitive Symptoms

Many manic patients have significant changes in their speech, thoughts, and attention. Patients may experience pressured speech, racing thoughts, and distractibility, which is often noticed by their family and friends. When mania is severe enough, racing thoughts can progress to *flight of ideas*, which is characterized by a series of tenuously connected thoughts. Irritable mood combined with other cognitive symptoms can result in psychomotor agitation. The extreme form of psychomotor agitation is manic delirium, in which patients are disoriented, act chaotically, and have incoherent speech. Patients with manic delirium warrant immediate medical intervention.

Suicide

In addition to the adverse psychosocial and vocational impacts of bipolar disorders, patients with bipolar disorders are also at increased risk for suicide. The lifetime risk of suicide in individuals with bipolar disorders is estimated to be 15 times higher than that of the general population. Suicide rate is higher in bipolar disorders than in major depressive disorder. The highest risk of suicide is seen in patients with bipolar disorders during depressed or mixed states. Indeed, bipolar disorders account for approximately one-quarter of all completed suicides.

Hypomania

Hypomanic and manic symptoms are similar, but a hypomanic episode is less severe than mania. Because hypomanic symptoms are less severe, patients with hypomania may not suffer from significant impairment in the social and occupational functions and are able to have a relatively normal quality of life. If patients stay in the hypomanic stage, they may not need to be hospitalized. Instead, some patients may be more productive at work or at school and may even state, "I've never felt so good before in my life." However, hypomanic patients can be "promoted" from hypomania to mania by the presence of 1 of the following 3 features: psychotic symptoms during the episode, severe symptoms warranting hospitalization, or marked social and occupational impairments. Of the 3 characteristics by which a patient is "promoted" from hypomania to mania, the presence of psychosis firmly indicates that the episode is mania rather than hypomania. Sometimes, hypomania may last for months, or it may occur for a few days before a full-blown manic episode develops.

Cyclothymia

As its name suggests, cyclothymia is a milder disorder or subsyndromal bipolar I or II disorder with cycling between depression and hypomania that lasts over several weeks to months. Patients experience emotional highs and lows alternating with normal or stable moods, but the highs and lows are much less extreme than those in bipolar I or II disorders. Due to its mild form, cyclothymic patients seek medical attention less frequently than those with full-blown bipolar I or II disorder. Although mood abnormalities in cyclothymia are less extreme, it is still critical to seek help managing these symptoms because they can interfere with patients' daily function and increase the risk for full-blown bipolar I or II disorder.

COURSE OF MOOD DISORDERS

Major Depressive Disorder

Episodes of major depression usually start gradually, and they can be self-limited and last approximately 6 to 9 months from time of onset to full recovery if untreated. However, a number of studies have shown the potential for recovery to take much longer or to not occur at all (never asymptomatic). It appears that for each episode of depression, approximately 10% of individuals remain ill for at least 5 years. Risk factors for prolonged time to recovery or chronic depression include a longer duration of the current episode before treatment is started, a family history of major depression, lower economic status, and comorbidity with other psychiatric illness, including alcohol and substance abuse. Only 25% of patients have only 1 episode of major depression. Thus, the majority of depressed patients will have >1 episode in their lives.

Approximately 20% of patients relapse within 1 year of follow-up evaluation. Factors predicting relapse include multiple episodes of major depression and a history of other psychiatric illness. Although none of these risk factors can significantly predict the likelihood of recurrence, the rate and timing of recurrence seem to depend on the type of recovery. Patients with full recovery (ie, asymptomatic on follow-up evaluation) have a much lower rate of recurrence than those with some residual symptoms. The time to recurrence is also much longer in the asymptomatic group compared with the group with residual symptoms. Therefore, it is important for depressed patients to reach recovery in each episode to reduce the risk for recurrence.

Bipolar Disorders

The degree of recovery between bipolar episodes varies. Episodes of mania and depression typically recur across the life span. Between episodes, most people with bipolar disorders are free of symptoms, but as many as one-third of people have some residual symptoms. Besides episodes of full-blown mania and major depression, patients can have episodes of milder depression, hypomania, or mixed states characterized by simultaneous occurrence of both depressive and manic symptoms. The natural course of bipolar disorders is for episode frequency to gradually increase and for a high percentage of episodes to be characterized by depressive symptoms rather than mania or hypomania. Although many patients are able to resume their normal activities within several weeks to months, a small percentage of patients may experience chronic unremitting symptoms despite treatment and have significant social and professional dysfunction for up to 2 years. The median duration of bipolar I episodes is approximately 3 months, and >75% of patients recover from their episodes within 1 year of onset. Factors that reduce the probability of recovery from a mood episode include severe onset of the mood episode, rapid cycling from one pole to the other, and greater cumulative morbidity. Patients with bipolar disorders tend to deteriorate without appropriate treatment, but proper treatment can help reduce the frequency and severity of episodes. Thus, patients with bipolar disorders can lead normal and productive lives when their illness is well managed.

Bipolar Disorders with Rapid Cycling

An important clinical phenomenon in bipolar disorders is rapid cycling, which is defined as having 4 (any combination of manic, hypomanic, mixed, or depressed episodes) or more episodes of bipolar disorder within a 12-month period in a patient. Episodes are demarcated by either partial or full remission for at least 2 months or a switch from one pole to the other with no intervening period of recovery (eg, major depressive episode to manic episode without a normal period). The prevalence of rapid cycling is estimated at 12% to 24% of patients with bipolar disorder and is more common in females than in males. Some patients experience multiple episodes very briefly or even in a single day, which is called *ultra-rapid cycling*.

Rapid cycling is an important marker of outcome in bipolar disorders because it predicts a relatively poorer outcome and worse response to mood stabilizers including lithium. Rapid cycling may occur at any time during the disorder; however, it tends to develop later in the course of illness. Several specific risk factors may be associated with rapid cycling, including earlier age at onset, comorbid substance use, greater severity of depressive episodes, antidepressant use, and prior or current thyroid dysfunction.

DIAGNOSIS & DIFFERENTIAL DIAGNOSIS

According to the DSM-V, identification of individual mood episodes is the basis for the diagnosis of major depression and bipolar disorders. A careful interview is essential to establish an accurate diagnosis. Due to the illness itself, some patients may not be able to engage in a meaningful and informative interview. In this case, it is useful to obtain collateral information from the patient's family and friends to understand patient's illness and baseline function. Sometimes it is difficult to determine what diagnosis a patient may have from a single interview. Considering the course of symptoms over time, including the timing, duration, and recurrence of episodes, is critical to avoid diagnostic errors. In addition, individuals with recurrent major depression often do not recognize or report prior hypomanic or even manic episodes, so these must be asked about specifically. The same holds true for evaluating manic episodes in bipolar disorder because patients may not be able to recognize their altered mood and abnormal behavior.

Similar to other psychiatric disorders, underlying medical causes and adverse effects of medications must be ruled out. Medical conditions and medications have been associated with both major depression and bipolar disorders. Common medical illnesses that induce mood disorders include endocrine disorders (eg, hypothyroidism, hyperthyroidism, Cushing disease), neurologic disorders (eg, cardiovascular diseases, dementia, temporal lobe epilepsy), and some cancers. Medication history should include both prescribed and over-the-counter medications.

Substance use is another major cause of mood disorders, and approximately half of patients with either major depression or bipolar disorders are affected by legal or illegal drugs. Most patients tend to self-medicate their mood disorders using substances such as alcohol, cocaine, and amphetamines. However, self-medication with these drugs usually causes or exacerbates their mood symptoms. Acute intoxication with stimulants such as cocaine or amphetamines may produce the same symptoms as mania or hypomania, although they last only a few hours to a few days. In contrast, withdrawal symptoms from these stimulants can mimic depression. Chronic alcohol use may cause depressive symptoms, but alcohol may also cause disinhibition that resembles hypomania, such as irritability. Substance use may likely contribute to diagnostic uncertainty. Thus, reassessment after a few months of abstinence is indicated.

Other psychiatric disorders may also have mood symptoms, such as schizoaffective disorder and delusional disorder (see Chapter 38). Persistent psychosis during periods of normal mood would be characteristic of schizoaffective disorder. Although sometimes patients may have comorbid psychotic disorders, mood symptoms should be the most prominent features in patients with mood disorders. Another common differential diagnosis is between mood disorders and anxiety disorders. Predominance of either anxiety or mood symptoms usually helps establish the correct diagnosis. Differential diagnosis is simplified if discrete episodes (depression, mania, or hypomania) are noted. However, mood disorders have a high rate of comorbidity with different anxiety disorders.

Similarly, personality disorders, including borderline, histrionic, and narcissistic personality disorders, can have some of the same symptoms as mood disorders. For example, borderline personality disorder frequently involves mood lability, instability of interpersonal relationships, periodic feelings of emptiness, and episodes of self-harm. All of these symptoms can be present in bipolar disorders. Although psychodynamic formulation can frequently differentiate the former from the latter, temporal course and relationship features are able to clarify the diagnosis. Thus, it is critical to ask what the patient's personality was like before the onset of mood symptoms. However, many patients may have comorbid mood disorders and personality disorders, both of which require treatment.

Medical Evaluation

Although the diagnosis of mood disorders is established primarily based on interview and collateral information, it is recommended that a thorough medical history, a physical examination, and laboratory tests be included to evaluate patients with mood disorders. There are several reasons to include this in routine evaluation. First, some medical conditions and substances can induce mood disorders. The management of these situations may lead to the resolution of the mood episodes. Second, medical evaluation is necessary to start some medications and to track medication-related adverse effects. Finally, for many patients with psychiatric illnesses, particularly chronic or severe illnesses, their first contact with a medical professional may be due to their psychiatric disorders. Thus, a thorough medical history and physical examination are necessary to provide appropriate and safe care for patients with mood disorders.

Routine laboratory tests include a complete blood count, basic metabolic profile, thyroid function panel, hepatic function panel, lipid profile, urine drug screening test, and urinalysis. An electrocardiogram may be ordered because of the cardiovascular effects of some medications, particularly QT_c prolongation with antipsychotic use. If it is the first onset of symptoms, brain imaging such as computed tomography or even MRI may be considered. Electroencephalography is considered in some patients with sedative abuse or suspected sedative abuse. Some workup results may indicate a need for consultation with other specialties.

TREATMENT

Major Depressive Disorder

What therapy to start first is determined by the severity of the depression. With mild or moderate major depression, especially mild depression, psychotherapy is usually the first option. If major depression is moderate or severe, the first-line therapy is to start and optimize an antidepressant, such as an SSRI or serotonin-norepinephrine reuptake inhibitor (SNRI; eg, bupropion and mirtazapine; Table 39–1). Most antidepressants act by increasing the amount of serotonin and/or norepinephrine (see Figure 39–2). Antidepressants are not rapidly effective medications, and it often takes 2 to 4 weeks to see an initial response (Figure 39–4). Patients may also experience adverse effects in the beginning before they see the benefits, so it is important to encourage patients to be compliant with antidepressants. However, if patients do not feel better by 4 to 6 weeks, it is probably better to switch antidepressants rather than maintain the current antidepressant. If there is a

TABLE 39–1 Different types of antidepressants.

Class	Medication	Usual Daily Dose (mg)	Mechanisms	Common Adverse Effects
SSRIs	Citalopram	20-40	Inhibit serotonin reuptake	Nausea, headache, insomnia, somnolence, nervousness, sweating, sexual dysfunction weight gain
	Escitalopram	10-20		
	Fluoxetine	20-80		
	Paroxetine	20-60		
	Fluvoxamine	100-300		
	Sertraline	50-200		
	Vilazodone	10-40		
SNRIs	Venlafaxine	150-375	Inhibit serotonin and norepinephrine reuptake	Nausea, sexual dysfunction, dry mouth, hypertension (at higher dosage)
	Desvenlafaxine	50		
	Duloxetine	60-120		
Newer SNRIs	Bupropion	300-450	Remains unknown, but may inhibit norepinephrine and dopamine reuptake	Overstimulation, lower seizure threshold, insomnia, dry mouth
	Mirtazapine	15-45	Inhibit α and several 5-HT receptors	Sedation, weight gain
	Trazodone	300-600	5-HT1$_A$ inhibitor	Very sedating (thus usually used as a hypnotic rather than as an antidepressant), priapism, nightmare
	Nefazodone	300-600	Serotonin reuptake inhibitor, 5-HT2$_A$ inhibitor	Sedation, hepatotoxicity
MAOIs	Phenelzine	45-90	Irreversibly inhibit monoamine oxidase, so increase the availability of norepinephrine, dopamine, and 5-HT	Orthostatic hypotension, insomnia, sexual dysfunction, dietary restrictions apply (at higher dosage)
	Selegiline (patch)	6-12 per 24 h		
	Tranylcypromine	30-60		
TCAs	Amitriptyline	100-250	Inhibit serotonin and norepinephrine reuptake; also block histaminic, cholinergic, and α₁ receptors	Dry mouth, sedation, urinary retention, weight gain, constipation, lower seizure threshold, fatal in overdose
	Doxepin	150-300		
	Imipramine	150-300		
	Clomipramine	150-250		

5-HT, serotonin; MAOIs, monoamine oxidase inhibitors; SNRIs, serotonin-norepinephrine reuptake inhibitors; SSRIs, selective serotonin reuptake inhibitors; TCAs, tricyclic antidepressants.

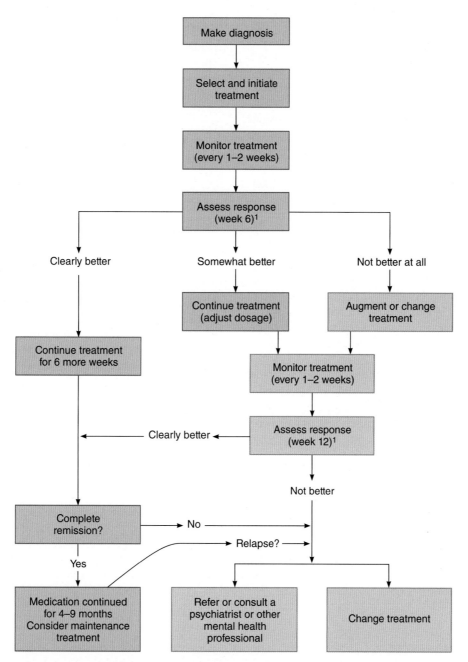

FIGURE 39-4 Overview of treatment for depression. (Reproduced with permission from the Agency for Health Care Policy and Research. *Depression in Primary Care. Vol. 2: Treatment of Major Depression.* Washington, DC: United States Department of Health and Human Services; 1993.)

partial response at 4 to 6 weeks at the full therapeutic dosage, adding another antidepressant from a different class or considering an augmenting strategy is indicated. Augmenting strategies include psychotherapy, thyroid hormone, lithium, or an approved atypical antipsychotic. Due to unpleasant and potentially lethal adverse effects, the tricyclic antidepressants (TCAs) and monoamine oxidase inhibitors (MAOIs) are usually not the first-line therapy except when treating atypical depression or treatment-resistant depression.

Several well-controlled studies, including the National Institutes of Health–funded STAR-D study, have shown that approximately one-third of patients with major depression do not respond to 2 trials with adequate treatments (adequate treatment duration and adequate dosage). There are a few other options available. Both repetitive transcranial magnetic stimulation and electroconvulsive therapy (ECT) have been demonstrated to be effective (efficacy as high as 80%) as treatments for major depression. The American Psychiatric

Association recommends ECT for patients who have had previous positive response to ECT or who are nonresponsive to antidepressants, as well as for patients who experience severe, psychotic, or acute suicidal depression. Although the mechanism for ECT remains unclear, ECT works rapidly and is relatively safe, even during pregnancy. In general, many patients feel better regarding their depression after 6 to 12 ECT sessions over a few weeks. After initial treatment, patients may still require maintenance ECT treatment (ie, weekly to monthly) and/or antidepressants to prevent relapse or reoccurrence. Another potential and promising therapy is ketamine; ketamine is experimental at present but may be a consideration in the future.

Another issue involves how long patients need to take antidepressants. If they have a single episode of major depression, continuation of treatment at the full dosage should be maintained for at least 6 months after the acute phase to prevent relapse. However, if patients have had >2 recurrent episodes of major depression with a family history of depression, treatment may need to be indefinite. If relapse occurs, the same medication is usually, but not always, effective.

For persistent depressive disorder and premenstrual dysphoric disorder, psychotherapy and antidepressants are usually effective treatments, and cognitive-behavioral therapy (CBT) may attenuate the functional impairments in patients.

Bipolar Disorders

Treating bipolar disorder is very different from treating major depression. Antidepressants appear to be much less effective for bipolar depression than major depression. The first step is starting mood stabilizers or optimizing current mood stabilizers. Medications commonly used in bipolar depression include olanzapine, olanzapine-fluoxetine combination (more effective than olanzapine alone), lamotrigine, quetiapine, and the recently approved drug lurasidone. Lithium and lamotrigine have antidepressant efficacy as well (Table 39–2). ECT should be considered in severe cases if it is available. As with major depression (see Figure 39–3), switching to a new drug is indicated if current mood stabilizers do not work in a few weeks.

It is often debated whether antidepressant therapy in bipolar depression has a risk of triggering mania. Recent studies have yielded inconsistent results, ranging from as high as 30% to 40% with the tricyclics to as low as placebo rates with SSRIs and other newer antidepressants. The natural switch rate from depression to mania in the absence of treatment may be as high as 40%, adding more variables to this discussion. On the whole, the benefit of antidepressant treatment appears to be low in patients with bipolar depression, and maximizing mood stabilizers appears to be the best intervention.

Lithium and anticonvulsants are the mood stabilizers that have generally been effective for acute mania (see Table 39–2). Lithium is widely used, with a 60% to 70% remission rate in patients with bipolar disorder, especially in patients with euphoric

TABLE 39–2 Mood stabilizers.

Medication	Usual Daily Dose (mg)	Therapeutic Blood Levels	Indications	Mechanisms	Adverse Effects and Comments
Lithium	Start at 600-900 mg, daily, and titrate up as indicated and tolerated	0.7-1.0 mEq/L	Acute and maintenance treatment of mania, aggression, suicidality; augment of antidepressants	Unknown but may be related to intracellular signaling pathways	Nausea, diarrhea, tremor, acne, excessive urination, affect thyroid function; avoid dehydration; narrow therapeutic window
Divalproex	Start at 250-500 mg, daily, and titrate up as indicated and tolerated	50-125 µg/mL	Refractory mania, rapid cycling, severe mood instability, intermittent explosive disorder	Remains poorly understood. Postulated mechanisms include to stabilize the cell membrane by interfering sodium and calcium channels and to enhance the inhibitory effects of γ–aminobutyric acid (GABA).	Nausea, weight gain, incoordination, confusion, affect liver function and platelet function, teratogenicity
Carbamazepine	Start at 200 mg daily, and titrate up as indicated and tolerated	6-12 µg/mL	Refractory mania, rapid cycling, severe mood instability, intermittent explosive disorder		Dry mouth, constipation, ataxia, diplopia, agranulocytosis (need to check white blood cell count), hepatitis
Lamotrigine	Start at 25 mg daily, with weekly 25 mg/d dose increment until 100 mg daily; then could increase by 50-100 mg/d as indicated and tolerated	n/a	Bipolar depression		Skin rash in about 10% patients, headache, nausea, dizziness, ataxia, somnolence, diplopia. The most serious side effect is Stevens-Johnsons syndrome.

mania or few or infrequent episodes, but it does not work well for rapid cyclers. Lithium has a narrow therapeutic window and lithium toxicity is an important complication. Symptoms include tremor, ataxia, confusion, lethargy, and nausea or diarrhea. When severe, lithium toxicity requires hemodialysis to correct.

Anticonvulsants, divalproex in particular, are more effective for bipolar disorder with rapid cycling than lithium (see Table 39–2). Sometimes patients may need to take both lithium and anticonvulsants to achieve an acceptable effect. In addition, atypical antipsychotics are also approved by the US Food and Drug Administration for mood stabilization in patients with acute mania and for long-term prevention.

It can take a week or more for mood stabilizers to act, and mood stabilizers do not have much sedative effect. Therefore, in the first few weeks of treating mania, antipsychotics and/or benzodiazepines may be used in combination with mood stabilizers to stabilize patients to ensure their safety and that of others. Improvements in psychomotor activation, insomnia, grandiosity, and psychotic symptoms are usually seen in a few days. Antipsychotics can be very helpful in treating hallucinations and delusions in patients with acute mania.

Suicide

Dealing with suicidality is probably the greatest challenge in the treatment of psychiatric illness, particularly in major depression and bipolar disorders. Suicidality needs to be assessed at every contact with patients. Predictors of an elevated suicide risk include depression severity, history of suicide attempts, active suicidal ideation/intent, hopelessness, unemployment, comorbid psychotic disorders (eg, substance use and personality disorder), a family history of completed suicide, male gender, and living single due to being widowed or divorced. Suicide events are most common right before initiating treatment and during the interval before treatment becomes effective, as well as within 1 to 3 months when patients are discharged from the hospital. Thus, frequent follow-up visits should be planned during these periods. In addition, it is important to involve family, friends, and caregivers in patients' treatment and recovery.

Psychotherapy in Managing Mood Disorders

In addition to the medication, psychotherapy is helpful in both major depression and bipolar disorders. CBT is well established, particularly in mild to moderate major depression.

Evidence suggests that CBT is as good as any antidepressant and, in some cases, may even be more effective at preventing relapse. Interpersonal therapy also has strong evidence to support its efficacy. This therapy focuses on interpersonal interactions and how to improve those interactions, which leads to improvement in depression.

In bipolar disorders, CBT possesses a good evidence base. Interpersonal therapy, social rhythm therapy, and family-focused therapies have been shown to decrease relapse, improve function, and help with treatment compliance. They are all used in conjunction with mood stabilizers to manage patients with bipolar disorders.

SELF-ASSESSMENT QUESTIONS

1. What is the treatment of choice for a patient with lithium intoxication who manifests with impaired consciousness, neuromuscular irritability, and seizures?
   A. Hemodialysis
   B. Sodium loading
   C. Osmotic diuresis
   D. Hyperbaric oxygen
   E. Transition to valproate

2. Venlafaxine acts primarily by inhibiting which neurotransmitter transporters?
   A. Serotonin
   B. Dopamine
   C. Norepinephrine
   D. A and C

3. A 47-year-old woman presents to her primary care physician with a chief complaint of fatigue. The patient reports that for the past 7 weeks, she has been waking up at 3 am every night and has been unable to go back to sleep. She dreads the day and the stresses of the workplace. She finds herself to be less motivated to complete her tasks at work and has been calling in sick sometimes. She has no interest and energy to pursue recreational activities. In addition, she does not feel hungry and has dropped 10% of her body weight in the past 3 to 4 months. She describes herself as feeling low and worried all the time. Her medical history is unremarkable. This patient's symptoms are most consistent with which of the following?
   A. Major depressive disorder
   B. Depression with atypical features
   C. Depression with melancholic features
   D. Adjustment disorder with depressive symptoms

Anxiety Disorders

Jesse Tobias C. Martinez, Jr.

OBJECTIVES

After studying this chapter, the student should be able to:

- Understand the basic biological mechanisms involved in the pathogenesis of anxiety disorders.
- Review the prevalence and severity of anxiety disorders.
- Understand the basic biological, psychological, and social factors that may render a person vulnerable to an anxiety disorder.
- State the various basic treatments of anxiety disorders.

Although anxiety is a normal emotion experienced by essentially everyone at some point in their lives, patients with anxiety disorders experience prolonged or abnormally intense feelings of anxiety that cause significant distress or impairment. In the fifth edition of the *Diagnostic and Statistical Manual of Mental Disorders* (DSM-V), these disorders are grouped into 3 categories. The first category, anxiety disorders, includes panic disorders, generalized anxiety disorder (GAD), and several disorders with anxiety caused by specific stimuli (including separation anxiety disorder, a childhood condition discussed in Chapter 44). The obsessive-compulsive disorders category includes obsessive-compulsive disorder, hoarding, and body dysmorphic disorder (the latter is discussed in Chapter 41 because it is considered a somatic disorder in the 10th revision of the International Statistical Classification of Diseases and Related Health Problems, ICD-10). The third category, trauma- and stressor-related disorders, includes posttraumatic stress disorder (PTSD).

PREVALENCE & BURDEN

Anxiety is a common feeling or emotion experienced by most people. In general, anxiety disorders have the highest prevalence of all psychiatric conditions, with a lifetime prevalence of approximately 25%. Phobias (specific phobia and social anxiety disorder/phobia) are the most common mental disorders in the United States. At least 5% to 10% of the population and possibly as much as 25% of the population may suffer from some type of a phobic disorder (eg, fear of needles, animals, heights). Prevalence estimates of anxiety disorders are generally higher in developed countries than in developing countries. Many anxiety disorders are more prevalent in women than in men, with a ratio of 2:1, except obsessive-compulsive disorder and social anxiety disorder, in which the female-to-male ratio is closer to 1:1. Most anxiety disorders start in childhood.

Studies have estimated the annual cost of anxiety disorders in the United States to be approximately $42.3 billion in the 1990s, a majority of which was due to nonpsychiatric medical treatment costs, per the Centers for Disease Control and Prevention. This estimate focused on short-term effects and did not include the effect of outcomes such as the increased risk of other disorders. Anxiety can be severely debilitating and can cause significant suffering and social isolation.

ANXIETY DISORDERS

Social Anxiety Disorder (Social Phobia)

Social anxiety disorder, also known as social phobia, is a marked fear or anxiety about 1 or more social situations in which the individual is exposed to possible scrutiny by others. The fear, anxiety, or avoidance is persistent and typically present for ≥6 months. Examples include fear of social interactions (eg, having a conversation, meeting unfamiliar people), fear of being observed (eg, eating or drinking), and fear of performing in front of others (eg, giving a speech). Of note, in children, the anxiety must occur in peer settings and not just during interactions with adults. Patients with social

VOCABULARY

Anxiety: Anticipation of a future concern, more often associated with muscle tension and avoidance behavior.

Anxiety disorder: Inappropriate experience of fear or worry and its physical manifestations (anxiety) that is incongruent with the magnitude of the perceived stressor.

Compulsion: Uncontrollable urge to engage in certain, often repetitive, behavior.

Fear: An emotional response to an immediate threat, usually associated with a fight or flight reaction, either staying to fight or leaving to escape danger.

Obsession: Recurrent, intrusive thought or impulse.

Panic attack: Abrupt onset of intense fear with somatic symptoms such as shortness of breath.

Phobia: Intense or irrational fear of something.

Worry: Continued apprehension despite identification of the threat.

phobia fear displaying anxiety symptoms that will be seen by others in a negative way. Patients are preoccupied with the fear of being humiliated or embarrassed, and this fear leads to a worry that they will be rejected by or offend others. Social situations almost always provoke fear or anxiety. In children, the fear or anxiety may be expressed by crying, tantrums, freezing, clinging, shrinking, or failing to speak in social situations. Social situations are avoided or endured with intense fear or anxiety. Fear or anxiety is out of proportion to the actual threat posed by the social situation and to the sociocultural context. Patients suffer clinically significant distress or impairment in social, occupational, or other important areas of functioning. For occasional anxiety-inducing situations such as public speaking, β-blockers or benzodiazepines may be treatment options. Cognitive-behavior therapy (CBT) and selective serotonin reuptake inhibitors (SSRIs) are the treatments of choice for most cases of social anxiety disorder.

CASE 40-1

A 19-year-old female college student presents with symptoms of depression and intense fear and avoidance of nearly all social functions at school. She is starting her second semester and has tried to register for as many online classes as possible. Her advisor informed her that all science labs have to be attended in-person and she must work in groups during labs. She is considering dropping out of college because of the requirement to attend labs and work in groups. This patient most likely has social anxiety disorder.

Phobic Disorders

Phobias are common disorders that cause a marked fear or anxiety about specific objects or situations (eg, flying, heights, animals, receiving an injection, seeing blood). In children, the fear or anxiety may be expressed by crying, tantrums, freezing, or clinging. The phobic object or situation almost always provokes immediate fear or anxiety. The phobic object or situation is actively avoided or endured with intense fear or anxiety. Fear or anxiety is out of proportion to the actual danger posed by the specific object or situation and to the sociocultural context. The fear, anxiety, or avoidance is persistent, typically lasting for ≥6 months, and causes clinically significant distress or impairment in social, occupational, or other important areas of functioning. When discussing phobias, it is important to describe the phobic stimulus. Systematic desensitization or graded exposure is considered first-line treatment for phobias. A short course of benzodiazepines or β-blockers may be helpful initially during desensitization to blunt autonomic hyperarousal.

Panic Disorder

Panic disorder consists of recurrent unexpected panic attacks with an average age of onset between 20 and 24 years old; it affects 2% to 3% of the population. A panic attack is an abrupt surge of intense fear or intense discomfort that reaches a peak within minutes and during which time ≥4 of the following symptoms occur (Table 40–1): palpitations, pounding heart, or accelerated heart rate; sweating; trembling or shaking; sensations of shortness of breath or smothering; feelings of choking; chest pain or discomfort; nausea or abdominal distress; feeling dizzy, unsteady, light-headed, or faint; chills or heat sensations; paresthesias (numbness or tingling sensations); derealization (feelings of unreality) or depersonalization (being detached from oneself); fear of losing control or "going crazy"; and fear of dying. Of note, the abrupt surge of

TABLE 40–1 Symptoms of panic attack.

Somatic symptoms
Racing heart or palpitations
Shortness of breath
Chest pain or discomfort
Diaphoresis
Nausea or gastrointestinal upset
Dizziness or lightheadedness
Choking sensation
Paresthesia
Psychological symptoms
Derealization or depersonalization
Fear of losing control or losing one's mind
Fear of dying

Data from American Psychiatric Association: *Diagnostic and Statistical Manual of Mental Disorders*, 5th ed. Arlington, VA, American Psychiatric Association, 2013.

these symptoms during a panic attack can occur from a calm state or an anxious state. At least 1 of the attacks must be followed by 1 month (or more) of 1 or both of the following: persistent concern or worry about additional panic attacks or their consequences (eg, losing control, having a heart attack, "going crazy"), and significant maladaptive change in behavior related to the attacks (eg, behaviors designed to avoid having panic attacks, such as avoidance of exercise or unfamiliar situations). Panic attacks may occur with other mental disorders such as depression or PTSD.

Agoraphobia

Agoraphobia is a condition of intense fear or anxiety related to anticipating or actually being in a situation where escape would be unlikely or help unavailable if panic or embarrassing or incapacitating symptoms were to occur. Patients report marked fear or anxiety about ≥2 of the following 5 situations: using public transportation (eg, automobiles, buses, trains, ships, planes); being in open spaces (eg, parking lots, marketplaces, bridges); being in enclosed places (eg, shops, theaters, cinemas); standing in line or being in a crowd; or being outside of the home alone. Patients fear or avoid these situations because of thoughts that escape might be difficult or help might not be available if they develop panic-like symptoms or other incapacitating or embarrassing symptoms (eg, fear of falling in the elderly; fear of incontinence).

Agoraphobic situations almost always provoke fear or anxiety, and patients will actively avoid agoraphobic situations and/or require the presence of a companion unless they choose to endure the situation with intense fear or anxiety. The level of fear or anxiety is out of proportion to the actual danger posed by the agoraphobic situations and to the sociocultural context. The anxiety associated with the situations must occur over the course of ≥6 months. If another medical condition (eg, inflammatory bowel disease, Parkinson disease) is present, the fear, anxiety, or avoidance is noticeably excessive.

It is important to be aware of the following medical conditions that are known to cause symptoms of panic disorders: hyperthyroidism, hyperparathyroidism, pheochromocytomatous, vestibular dysfunctions, seizure disorders, cardiopulmonary conditions (eg, arrhythmias, mitral valve prolapse), chronic obstructive pulmonary disease, asthma, and hypoglycemia.

Generalized Anxiety Disorder

Generalized anxiety disorder is a condition of uncontrollable worry, fear, or preoccupation about everyday situations and possibilities. Prevalence of GAD is 3% in adults, with an average age of onset at 30 years old; it effects females more than males at a rate of 2:1. Parental overprotection and childhood adversities play a role in the future development of GAD. Patients may report excessive anxiety and worry (apprehensive expectation), occurring more days than not for at least 6 months, about a number of events or activities (eg, work or school performance). Patients report great difficulty with

TABLE 40-2 Symptoms of generalized anxiety disorder.

Somatic symptoms
Poor sleep
Fatigue
Muscle tension
Restlessness or inability to relax
Cognitive symptoms
Impaired concentration
Mind going blank
Psychological symptoms
Irritability

Data from American Psychiatric Association: *Diagnostic and Statistical Manual of Mental Disorders*, 5th ed. Arlington, VA, American Psychiatric Association, 2013.

trying to control the worry. In GAD, the anxiety and worry are associated with ≥3 of the following 6 symptoms (Table 40–2), with at least some symptoms being present more days than not over the past 6 months: restlessness or feeling keyed up or on edge; being easily fatigued; difficulty concentrating or mind going blank; irritability; muscle tension; and sleep disturbance (difficulty falling or staying asleep or restless, unsatisfying sleep). Of note, in children, only 1 item is required to make the diagnosis. First-line treatment includes CBT, SSRIs, or a serotonin-norepinephrine reuptake inhibitor (SNRI) such as venlafaxine.

Substance-Induced Anxiety Disorder

In patients who suffer from a substance-induced anxiety disorder, panic attacks or anxiety is predominant in the clinical picture along with evidence from the history, physical examination, or laboratory findings of symptoms developing during or soon after substance intoxication or withdrawal or after exposure to a medication and evidence that the involved substance or medication is capable of producing the panic or anxiety symptoms. The disturbance described by the patient is not better explained by an anxiety disorder that is not substance or medication induced. Evidence of an independent anxiety disorder may include the following: the symptoms precede the onset of substance or medication use; the symptoms persist for a substantial period of time (eg, about 1 month) after the cessation of acute withdrawal or severe intoxication; or there is other evidence suggesting the existence of an independent non–substance or non–medication-induced anxiety disorder (eg, a history of recurrent episodes not related to substance or medication use). The patient's symptoms do not occur exclusively during the course of a delirium. The disturbance caused by reported substance-induced anxiety or panic attacks leads to clinically significant distress or impairment in the patient's social, occupational, or other important areas of functioning. Agents that may induce a clinical picture of substance-induced anxiety include, but are not limited to, the following:

anesthetics and analgesics, sympathomimetics or other bronchodilators, anticholinergics, insulin, thyroid preparations, oral contraceptives, antihistamines, antiparkinsonian medications, corticosteroids, antihypertensive and cardiovascular medications, anticonvulsants, lithium carbonate, antipsychotics, antidepressants, and heavy metals and toxins (eg, organophosphate insecticide, nerve gases, carbon monoxide, carbon dioxide, volatile substances such as gasoline and paint). Identifying and avoiding exposure to the substance should lead to improvement in symptoms.

Anxiety Disorder Due to Another Medical Condition

The critical feature of anxiety disorder due to another medical condition is clinically significant anxiety that is best attributed to be a physiologic effect of another medical condition. The presence of panic attacks or anxiety is predominant in the clinical picture. There is evidence from the history, physical examination, or laboratory findings that the disturbance is the direct pathophysiologic consequence of another medical condition. The disturbance cannot occur exclusively during the course of a delirium. The patient's disturbance causes clinically significant distress or impairment in social, occupational, or other important areas of daily functioning. In determining whether the anxiety symptoms are attributable to another medical condition, it is important to first establish the presence of the medical condition that may be causing the physiologic symptoms described by the patient. A number of medical conditions are known to include anxiety as a symptomatic manifestation (Table 40–3). Examples include endocrine disease (eg, hyperthyroidism, pheochromocytoma, hypoglycemia, hyperadrenocorticism), cardiovascular disorders (eg, congestive heart failure, pulmonary embolism, atrial fibrillation), respiratory illness (eg, chronic obstructive pulmonary disease, asthma, pneumonia), metabolic disturbances (eg, vitamin B_{12} deficiency, porphyria), and neurologic illness

TABLE 40–3   Selected medical conditions that can simulate an anxiety disorder.

- Cardiac
  Ischemic heart disease, mitral valve prolapse, arrhythmias
- Endocrine/metabolic
  Hyperthyroidism, hypoglycemia, pheochromocytoma, carcinoid
- Gynecologic
  Menopause, premenstrual syndrome
- Neurologic
  Transient ischemic attacks, seizure disorders
- Pharmacological
  Caffeine, alcohol, sympathomimetic agents, amphetamines, corticosteroids, theophylline, illicit drugs
- Respiratory
  Asthma, chronic obstructive pulmonary disease

Reproduced with permission from Feldman MD, Christensen JF, Satterfield JM, et al: *Behavioral Medicine: A Guide for Clinical Practice.* 5th ed. New York, NY: McGraw Hill; 2020.

(eg, neoplasms, vestibular dysfunction, encephalitis, seizure disorders).

OBSESSIVE-COMPULSIVE DISORDERS

Obsessive-Compulsive Disorder

Obsessive-compulsive disorder (OCD) includes the presence of either obsessions or compulsions that cause significant impairment in daily functioning or that are time consuming and interfere with routines, work, and interpersonal relationships. Obsessions are recurrent, intrusive thoughts or impulses that increase anxiety and are not simply excessive worries about real problems. Patients try to suppress the thoughts but are overpowered by them. Patients are able to realize that the thoughts are products of their own mind (patients have insight). Compulsions are repetitive behaviors that the patient feels compelled to perform to decrease anxiety. The compulsive behavior is intended to decrease distress, but there is no realistic link between the behavior and the distress. The person is aware that the obsessions and compulsions are unreasonable and excessive. Patients may have contamination obsessions followed by compulsive washing or avoidance; obsessional doubt, such as wondering if the doors are locked with compulsive checking to avoid potential danger; or intrusive thoughts (often violent or sexual in nature) without compulsions.

Hoarding was previously considered a form of OCD but is now a separate DSM-V diagnosis. A diagnosis of OCD requires the presence of obsessions and/or compulsions occurring for >1 hour a day that cause major distress and

---

CASE 40–2

A 22-year-old man presents to his family physician for evaluation of dry skin around his fingers and knuckles. He is home from college for the holidays, and his mother called to make the appointment. As you enter the exam room, you notice he is by the exam room sink washing his hands. He asks you about your hand hygiene and what procedures are in place to clean exam rooms between patients. On physical exam, his hands have severe chafing. He informs you that while in high school he would wash his hands up to 25 times a day, but since starting college his routine has increased to 40 times a day and he has started to add a small amount of bleach to ensure complete sanitation of germs from his hands.

This patient most likely has obsessive-compulsive disorder and may benefit from treatment with a selective serotonin reuptake inhibitor and/or cognitive-behavioral therapy.

impair work, social, or other important function. Approximately 1.2% of Americans have OCD, and among adults, slightly more women than men are affected. OCD often begins in childhood, adolescence, or early adulthood; the average age of onset is 19 years old. There is increased risk in patients with first-degree relatives who have Tourette syndrome.

TRAUMA- & STRESSOR-RELATED DISORDERS

Posttraumatic Stress Disorder

The essential feature of posttraumatic stress disorder (PTSD) is the development of characteristic symptoms following exposure to 1 or more traumatic events. Additional criteria focus on the presence of intrusion symptoms, avoidance behavior, negative effects on cognition or mood, and altered arousal (Table 40–4).

PTSD may develop after exposure to life-threatening events, serious injury, or sexual violence that is directly experienced, is witnessed in person, or affects a close friend or relative. The stressor (criterion A) can be repeated firsthand exposure to the aftermath of trauma (eg, by first responders); however, exposure through media does not qualify. Intrusion symptoms (criterion B) include recurrent, unwanted memories or thoughts related to the trauma, nightmares or distressing dreams, brief reliving of events (flashbacks), and

TABLE 40–4 Posttraumatic stress disorder.

Core symptoms
Flashbacks to the traumatic events
Intrusive memories of traumatic events
Nightmares related to traumatic events
Severe distress at reminders of traumatic events
Somatic symptoms
Poor sleep
Hypervigilance
Excessive startle response
Cognitive symptoms
Inability to recall parts of the traumatic events
Impaired concentration
Other psychological symptoms
Irritability or anger
Loss of interest in significant activities
Self-destructive or reckless behavior
Feeling of detachment from others
Excessive self-blame related to traumatic events
Negative emotions or beliefs

Data from American Psychiatric Association: *Diagnostic and Statistical Manual of Mental Disorders*, 5th ed. Arlington, VA, American Psychiatric Association, 2013.

psychological distress in response to cues. In children, this can manifest as repetitive play with traumatic themes. Avoidance (criterion C) includes efforts to avoid memories or cues related to the trauma or behavioral avoidance of trauma-related places, people, or objects. Persistent negative alterations in cognition or mood (criterion D) include inability to remember parts of the trauma (dissociative amnesia), exaggerated negative beliefs about self or others, distorted cognitions about causes of the trauma (self-blame), loss of interest in activities, feeling of detachment or estrangement from others, or inability to experience positive emotions. Alterations in arousal and reactivity (criterion E) include angry outbursts, reckless or self-destructive behavior, sleep problems, exaggerated startling, vigilance toward possible threats or repetition of the trauma, or impaired concentration. The PTSD symptoms must cause clinically significant distress or impairment in social, occupational, or other important areas of functioning for >1 month.

In the United States, the projected lifetime risk for PTSD is 8%. Rates of PTSD are higher among veterans and others whose vocation increases the risk of traumatic exposure (eg, police, firefighters, emergency medical personnel). Highest rates (ranging from one-third to more than one-half of those exposed) are found among survivors of rape, military combat and captivity, and ethnically or politically motivated internment and genocide. Symptoms usually begin within the first 3 months after the trauma, although there may be a delay of months, or even years, before criteria for the diagnosis are met. Often, an individual's reaction to a trauma initially meets criteria for acute stress disorder in the immediate aftermath of the trauma. Although the severity of a trauma is predictive of PTSD, the lasting impression of the stressor depends of the survivor's appraisal of its meaning. First-line treatment for PTSD includes trauma-focused CBT, SSRIs, or venlafaxine (SNRI). Studies have shown that prazosin may aid in reducing nightmares.

Acute Stress Disorder

Acute stress disorder describes symptoms exhibited in the early period following traumatic exposures. As such, the primary distinction between acute stress disorder and PTSD is the duration of symptoms, with acute stress disorder being limited to between 3 days and 1 month. Acute stress disorder is diagnosed when ≥9 symptoms emerge from the following 5 categories: intrusion, negative mood, dissociation, avoidance, and arousal.

Acute stress disorder is a strong predictor of PTSD. Prospective studies have found that 72% to 83% of individuals with acute stress disorder go on to develop PTSD 6 months after trauma and that 63% to 80% of those with acute stress disorder meet criteria for PTSD 2 years after trauma. CBT is considered first-line treatment for acute stress disorder, and in the majority of cases, psychopharmacologic treatment is not indicated.

TREATMENT OF ANXIETY DISORDERS

For most anxiety disorders, first-line treatment includes therapy or psychotropic medications or a combination of both. Medication options can be divided between those that are fast acting, including benzodiazepines and β-blockers, and those that are anxiolytic only with chronic treatment, including SSRIs, SNRIs, and buspirone.

At serotonergic synapses, signaling is terminated by reuptake of serotonin into the presynaptic terminal by the serotonin transporter (SERT). SSRIs inhibit SERT, reducing presynaptic reuptake and enhancing serotonergic neurotransmission. SSRIs are effective for the treatment of GAD, OCD, panic disorder, PTSD, and social anxiety disorder. They may also be helpful for select cases of specific phobias. They are also fairly easy to dose and inexpensive. In most cases, treatment of OCD requires higher doses of SSRIs. SSRIs are generally very well tolerated, with the most common side effects including mild gastrointestinal upset or decreased libido. Severe side effects may include serotonin syndrome, usually when multiple serotonergic drugs are combined. Serotonin syndrome manifests with hyperthermia, agitation, sweating, diarrhea, and miosis. There is a US Food and Drug Administration black box warning against using SSRIs or SNRIs for patients under the age of 18 years due to suicidal thoughts and behavior.

SNRIs, such as venlafaxine and duloxetine, are similar to SSRIs but also act at noradrenergic synapses, inhibiting the norepinephrine transporter that mediates reuptake of norepinephrine. Thus, SNRIs enhance both serotonergic and noradrenergic neurotransmission. They have similar indications and side effects to SSRIs.

Buspirone is a serotonin partial agonist that acts at serotonin 1A (5-HT$_{1A}$) receptors. It is primarily used in patients with GAD. It is well tolerated and does not cause sedation, addiction, or tolerance. Buspirone generally takes 1 to 2 weeks to take effect and does not interact with alcohol.

Tricyclic antidepressants include amitriptyline, nortriptyline, imipramine, desipramine, clomipramine, doxepin, and amoxapine. Their mechanism of action involves blockade reuptake of norepinephrine and 5-hydroxytryptophan. They are used in the treatment of major depressive disorder, OCD (clomipramine), and anxiety.

Benzodiazepines (alprazolam, lorazepam, clonazepam, and diazepam) are generally considered second-line medications for anxiety due to the potential side effects and their great potential for abuse, but they have the advantage of more rapid action. Benzodiazepines may serve as a bridge while patients wait the 4 to 6 weeks for SSRIs to reach therapeutic efficacy. Generally, they are most effective for panic disorder and can also be used with social anxiety disorder related to performance stressors. In most cases, benzodiazepines are not indicated for other anxiety disorders. There is evidence to indicate relative contraindication in PTSD due to potential for abuse. After taking benzodiazepines daily for 2 weeks, patients become physiologically dependent, leading to withdrawal symptoms in the absence of medication. Withdrawal from benzodiazepines may include severe anxiety, tremor, hypertension, tachycardia, diaphoresis, seizures, and hallucinations. Overdose from benzodiazepines may lead to respiratory depression and death.

β-Blockers, most commonly propranolol, are often used in the treatment of panic disorder and social anxiety disorder. Their mechanism of action aids in preventing the autonomic hyperarousal associated with symptoms of anxiety.

Psychological treatments used for anxiety disorder include various therapies. CBT is best suited to address symptoms of anxiety disorder and depressive disorders. CBT assists the patient in identifying and modifying cognitive distortions. Patients identify and examine cognitive distortions and replace anxious thoughts with more realistic helpful and positive thoughts. Cognitive interventions can be very helpful in the treatment of GAD. Other behavioral interventions include exposure response prevention for the treatment of OCD and graded exposure or systemic desensitization for the treatment of specific phobias, panic disorder, or PTSD. Other therapies include trauma processing therapy and prolonged exposure therapy for the treatment of PTSD and flooding for the treatment of specific phobias.

SELF-ASSESSMENT QUESTIONS

1. A 36-year-old nurse anesthetist states that he constantly wonders if he is capable of doing his job and feels as if he is not good enough. For the past year, he reports constant worry about making mortgage payments, paying telephone bills, making medication and billing code errors, and affording his children's education. His coworkers and wife have commented on his irritability, and he reports increased muscle tension and difficulty sleeping. The anesthesiologist he works with has requested a meeting with him due to increased errors he has made at work. The patient most likely has which of the following disorders?

   A. Social phobia
   B. Obsessive-compulsive disorder (OCD)
   C. Generalized anxiety disorder (GAD)
   D. Panic disorder
   E. Substance-induced anxiety disorder

2. During his first day on the emergency medicine clerkship rotation, a medical student is asked to assist his attending physician with repairing a laceration on a 35-year-old man who presented to the emergency department after a bar fight. The student has done his best to avoid situations involving human blood throughout his training until now. As he is preparing the patient for laceration repair, he starts to examine the wound and faints. The student would most likely benefit from which of the following?

   A. Eating a snack before starting his shift
   B. Systematic desensitization
   C. Dialectal behavioral therapy
   D. Starting a selective serotonin reuptake inhibitor (SSRI)
   E. Changing professions

3. A 59-year-old veteran presents to your office with complaints of ongoing troubling nightmares related to experiences he endured while in combat. He is currently prescribed an SSRI (sertraline) and reports improvement in his symptoms overall; however, his nightmares have not changed. He is worried because his wife has informed him that her sleep is also being affected by his nightmare experiences. Which of the following medications would be indicated in the treatment of this veteran's nightmares?

A. Alprazolam
B. Prazosin
C. Risperidone
D. Switching from sertraline to fluoxetine
E. Propranolol

Somatic Symptom Disorder & Related Disorders

Aaron D. Fobian & Lindsey Elliott

OBJECTIVES

After studying this chapter, the student should be able to:

- Identify and describe somatic symptom disorder and related conditions.
- Identify the etiology and diagnostic criteria for these disorders.
- Describe pharmacologic and nonpharmacologic evidence-based treatments for these disorders.

PREVALENCE & BURDEN

Somatic symptom disorder and related conditions such as conversion disorder present with physical symptoms that cause significant distress or impairment. A summary of somatic symptom disorder and related disorders is provided in Table 41–1. Individuals with these disorders commonly seek care in medical settings, such as primary care or emergency department settings, as opposed to psychiatric settings. Many patients with these disorders experience a chronic course, and they are often high utilizers of the medical system. Although these disorders are not often discussed, the prevalence is significant. Somatic symptom disorder occurs in 5% to 7% of the adult population, and conversion disorder is the second most common diagnosis in neurology clinics. In addition, previous estimates of hypochondriasis were as high as 10% of the population. These patients frequently seek medical care for their symptoms and are often significantly limited by their condition. Symptoms significantly interfere with many patients' ability to complete activities of daily living such as maintaining employment or living independently.

MIND–BODY CONNECTION

The *Diagnostic and Statistical Manual of Mental Disorders* (DSM), Fourth Edition, Text Revision (DSM-IV-TR, 2000), focused on medically unexplained symptoms in the diagnosis of somatic symptom and related disorders, which emphasizes mind–body dualism, or the idea that the mind and body are separable. However, our thoughts, feelings, and beliefs have been found to positively and negatively affect biological functioning, suggesting a significant mind–body connection. Over the past decade, it has become clear that the mind and body are not separate from each other but instead are closely connected. The placebo effect, which is when symptoms are improved or worsened (nocebo effect) by a patient's expectations about symptoms, has been found to significantly impact physical symptoms. Functional neuroimaging studies have demonstrated that the placebo effect and unexplained medical occurrences involve similar cerebral mechanisms. Studies using positron emission tomography found increased activation in the right orbitofrontal and anterior cingulate cortices, as well as an absence of activity in the right primary motor cortex, in both a case of unexplained (functional) paralysis of the leg and a case of hypnotic left leg paralysis. This indicates that suggested paralysis and conversion paralysis may both involve the inhibition of primary motor activity in the prefrontal cortex, emphasizing that these symptoms are not "fake" and are being experienced by the patient.

Having a medical diagnosis does not exclude the presence of a mental health disorder, including a diagnosis of somatic symptom and related disorders, and it is not appropriate to diagnosis a mental health disorder based solely on the absence of a medical explanation. The emphasis on the absence of a medical diagnosis has historically been understood by patients to mean that doctors believe their symptoms are fake or "in their head," often angering and alienating patients and resulting in the patient searching for a different doctor to diagnose their symptoms. These diagnostic criteria were also difficult for doctors in primary care settings to use, which is where most patients with somatic symptom disorders initially present. Therefore, the fifth edition of the DSM (DSM-V, 2013) revised this section of disorders to make the diagnostic criteria clearer and more practical for use in medical settings. The current criteria no longer emphasize the presence of medically unexplained symptoms and instead focus on positive

627

VOCABULARY

Body-focused attention: Attention to physical symptoms and frequent scanning of the body to monitor symptoms.

Functional: A term used to describe symptoms that affect physiologic or psychological functions but not organic structure. Functional symptoms suggest there is a functional problem, such as a miscommunication between the brain and nerves, that is not detected by diagnostic tests.

Mind–body connection: The idea that the mind and body are inseparable and that a person's thoughts, feelings, and beliefs can positively or negatively affect biological functioning.

Somatic symptoms: Symptoms experienced in the body such as physical sensations or movements.

CASE 41–1

J is a 7-year-old girl diagnosed with juvenile rheumatoid arthritis at the age of 5. Her parents withdrew her from kindergarten and began homeschooling her due to pain. J frequently refused to walk due to pain and would scream and cry if she had to walk. Her mother carried her around the house, and she almost always used a wheelchair to get around outside of the home. She saw her rheumatologist, who, after examination, laboratory work, and scans, determined that her pain was greater than expected given her disease state. She was diagnosed with somatic symptom disorder.

symptoms, such as distress and abnormal thoughts, feelings, and behaviors about symptoms, and/or the incompatibility of symptoms with recognized medical disorders.

As demonstrated in Figure 41–1, all physical symptoms, regardless of etiology, have many factors that may contribute to or exacerbate physical symptoms. These include biological, psychological, social, and behavioral factors and activities of daily living. In addition, physical symptoms may also affect these factors. For example, a patient with arthritis may experience increased joint pain during a time of increased stress, such as after an argument with his or her spouse. At the same time, joint pain associated with arthritis may increase a patient's stress level. This bidirectional explanation may increase patients' acceptance of their somatic symptom disorder diagnosis. To effectively treat these symptoms, each of these factors should be addressed in treatment, and using Figure 41–1 to explain the diagnosis may help patients understand why they are being referred to a psychologist and/or physical therapist for treatment.

SOMATIC SYMPTOM DISORDER

Somatic symptom disorder, previously called somatization disorder (in 10th revision of the *International Statistical Classification of Diseases and Related Health Problems* [ICD-10]), is characterized by 1 or more physical symptoms that are distressing to the individual and/or disrupt the patient's daily life and are present for at least 6 months. Commonly reported somatic symptoms include general pain, headaches, fatigue, chest pain, stomachaches, dizziness, and insomnia. In the previous version of the DSM, a diagnosis of somatization disorder required that the physical symptoms could not be explained by a medical diagnosis. Under current criteria, somatic symptom disorder can occur with or without a medical explanation for the somatic symptoms, but patients must exhibit inappropriate thoughts, feelings, or behaviors in response to the somatic

symptoms. This change was due in part to the understanding that the disorder is characterized not by the somatic symptoms, but instead by an individual's expectation and interpretation of symptoms and the individual's response to the symptoms. This can include thoughts about the symptoms that are disproportionate to the severity of the symptom (eg, interpreting normal bodily sensations as a sign of serious illness), excessive anxiety related to one's health or symptoms (eg, increased attention to physical symptoms, worry about becoming ill, fear of physical activity causing harm to one's body), or spending excessive time or energy on one's symptoms or health concerns (eg, body-focused attention, seeking frequent medical care, or avoiding physical activity). Brief somatic symptom disorder may be diagnosed when a patient exhibits symptoms that meet the criteria for somatic symptom disorder but that have been present for <6 months.

Given the recent shift in diagnostic criteria, the prevalence of somatic symptom disorder is unknown. Its predecessor, somatization disorder, had a prevalence of <1%, but it is suggested that the prevalence of somatic symptom disorder is higher, at an estimated 5% to 7% of the adult population. Typically, individuals with somatic symptom disorder are more likely to present for treatment in a medical setting than a mental health setting. In general, females report more somatic symptoms than males; therefore, it follows that the prevalence of somatic symptom disorder is also likely to be higher in females than males.

CONVERSION DISORDER (FUNCTIONAL NEUROLOGIC SYMPTOM DISORDER)

Conversion disorder, also called functional neurologic symptom disorder, is a disorder in which a person experiences neurologic symptoms that are not due to a neurologic condition, as confirmed by a medical professional. Conversion disorder is found in approximately 5% of referrals to neurology clinics, making it the second most common diagnosis in these clinics. Onset of conversion disorder is found throughout the life span, and symptoms

TABLE 41-1 Diagnostic criteria, epidemiology, and comorbidity of somatic symptom disorder and related disorders.

Disorder	Diagnostic Criteria	Epidemiology	Comorbidity
Somatic symptom disorder	≥1 somatic symptom that is distressing or disrupts daily life Excessive thoughts, feelings, or behaviors related to symptoms Symptoms are persistent (>6 months)	5%-7% of adult population Likely higher in females than males	Medical disorders Anxiety and depressive disorders
Brief somatic symptom disorder	Same criteria as somatic symptom disorder, but lasting <6 months		
Conversion disorder (functional neurologic symptom disorder)	≥1 symptom of altered voluntary motor or sensory function Incompatibility between symptoms and neurologic or medical conditions	5% of referrals to neurology clinics	Anxiety disorders; in particular, panic disorder Depressive disorders Somatic symptom disorder Personality disorders Neurologic or other medical conditions
Illness anxiety disorder	Preoccupation with having or acquiring serious illness (if medical illness present, preoccupation excessive) Mild or no somatic symptoms Anxiety related to health Excessive health-related behaviors or maladaptive avoidance Preoccupation present ≥6 months	Unavailable based on new criteria, but hypochondriasis prevalence was between 1.3% and 10% Similar prevalence in males and females	Anxiety disorders (eg, generalized anxiety disorder, panic disorder, and obsessive-compulsive disorder) Depressive disorders Elevated risk for somatic symptom disorder and personality disorder
Brief illness anxiety disorder	Same criteria as illness anxiety disorder, but lasting <6 months		
Illness anxiety disorder without excessive health-related behaviors	Same criteria as illness anxiety disorder, but without excessive health-related behaviors or maladaptive avoidance		
Body dysmorphic disorder	Preoccupation with perceived flaws in physical appearance not apparent to others Repetitive behaviors in relation to perceived flaw	Estimated prevalence of 2.4% in US adults	Major depressive disorder Social anxiety disorder Obsessive-compulsive disorder Substance-related disorders
Psychological factors affecting other medical conditions	Medical symptom or condition Psychological or behavioral factors that adversely affect medical condition	Prevalence unclear	
Factitious disorder	Falsification of physical or psychological symptoms or induction of injury or disease in self (or another) Presents self (or another) as ill, impaired, or injured No evidence of external incentive	Estimated prevalence of 1% in hospital settings	
Malingering	Intentional production of symptoms External incentive for symptoms		

may present in various ways and can change over time. Short duration of symptoms, childhood onset, and acceptance of the diagnosis are positive prognostic factors. Conversion disorder is 2 to 3 times more common in females than males. If they do not obtain timely diagnosis and treatment, these patients can experience significant disability, often similar to those with medical disorders.

Symptoms can include physical weakness, abnormal gait, paralysis, dystonic movements, tingling, dizziness, syncope, or episodes of seizures or tremors. Other symptoms may include impaired hearing or vision, diplopia, dysarthria, dysphonia, and aphonia, and it must be determined that the presenting symptoms are not associated with a neurologic disorder. However, confirming this may be difficult. Although psychogenic nonepileptic seizures (PNES) can be confirmed through electroencephalography (EEG), other symptoms, such as paralysis or syncope, do not have a gold standard test to definitively rule out a neurologic disorder. Therefore, absence of positive test

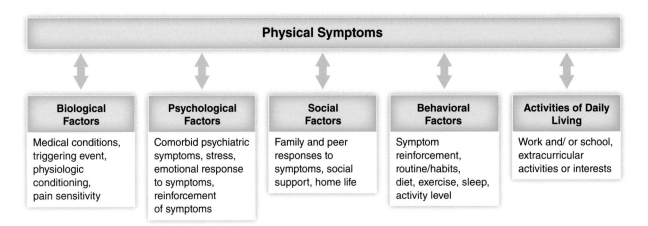

FIGURE 41-1 Factors that affect physical symptoms.

results does not automatically indicate a diagnosis of conversion disorder.

Instead of relying on the absence of a medical diagnosis alone, the DSM-V diagnostic criteria now focus on the incompatibility between the patient's symptoms and a recognized neurologic or medical disorder. There are several ways to examine patients' symptoms and determine if they are consistent with a medical disorder (Table 41–2). For example, patients with PNES often present with closed eyelids and pelvic thrusting during episodes, which are both rare in epilepsy. Although physicians are sometimes hesitant to make this diagnosis, research has demonstrated that neurologists' impression of conversion disorder based on clinical presentation is commonly confirmed with further medical examination, such as EEG. Although physicians should not rely solely on the incompatibility of symptoms, when paired with reasonable medical tests, an accurate diagnosis can be made.

Traditionally, conversion disorder was believed to be the direct result of trauma or stress. However, it is important to note that although conversion disorder is more common in people who have a history of trauma or stress, trauma or stress is not the direct cause of conversion disorder, and not all of those with conversion disorder have a history of trauma or stress. Due to recent research demonstrating this, the DSM-V removed the requirement that psychological factors need to be associated with the symptoms to make the diagnosis. Instead, trauma and stress are considered risk factors for, but not required contributors to, the development of conversion disorder. In addition, the presence of a neurologic disease with similar symptom presentation in either the patient or the patient's family members is also a risk factor. For example, patients with epilepsy or a family history

TABLE 41-2 Signs of incompatibility between common symptoms of conversion disorder and neurologic disorders.

Hoover sign	Hip extension is weak when directly tested but normal when opposite hip is flexed
Tremor entrainment	Tremor changes or stops when individual is distracted from tremor; typically done by asking patient to copy rhythmical movements
Tubular visual fields	Tunnel vision is the same width when tested at different distances
Ankle plantar flexion	Patient has no ankle plantar flexion while lying down but is able to stand on tiptoes

Psychogenic nonepileptic seizure signs (inconsistent with epileptic seizures)
- Closed eyes, resistant to opening
- Duration >2 minutes
- Gradual onset
- Asynchronous movements
- Side-to-side head shaking

CASE 41-2

Ms. M is a 23-year-old woman with a medical history significant for sinus node dysfunction with syncopal spells from documented sinus arrest. She has been unable to work due to her medical condition. To treat her syncopal episodes, Ms. M had a pacemaker implanted. With the pacemaker, Ms. M continued to have episodes with a slightly different presentation. The symptoms were similar to those she had experienced prior to the implantation of the pacemaker but without accompanying loss of consciousness. She reported that she felt "foggy" and was unable to move or speak, but she could hear what was happening around her. These fainting episodes occurred at the same time of day and in the same location as the syncopal episodes she had prior to receiving her pacemaker. Ms. M presented to a neurology clinic where her episodes were monitored, and results showed normal sinus rhythms and normal electroencephalogram during the events. She was diagnosed with psychogenic nonepileptic seizures, a form of conversion disorder.

of epilepsy are at greater risk of developing PNES. Previous exposure to neurologic disorders may have created symptom expectations for these patients, consistent with the idea that the placebo effect may be a causal mechanism for conversion disorder.

Neurobiological evidence has demonstrated abnormal brain activity during conversion movements despite employing voluntary motor pathways. One study compared brain activity in conversion patients during their functional tremors and while mimicking their tremor. Results showed hypoactivity in the right temporoparietal junction during functional tremors, which is associated with discerning between self-generated and externally generated sensations, suggesting symptoms are perceived to be involuntary despite the use of voluntary motor pathways.

ILLNESS ANXIETY DISORDER

Illness anxiety disorder, previously called hypochondriasis, is characterized by excessive concern surrounding currently having or developing a serious illness. Notably, to be diagnosed with illness anxiety disorder, patients cannot have any somatic symptoms or their somatic symptoms must be mild in intensity. Often, the somatic symptoms that are present are normal physiologic sensations (eg, dizziness upon standing) or symptoms not typically indicative of a medical condition (eg, belching). If the individual has a current medical condition or is at high risk for a medical condition, the worry must be excessive or disproportionate to the severity. In illness anxiety disorder, an individual's distress stems not from the somatic symptom, if present, but instead from what that symptom might mean (eg, serious illness). In addition, individuals with illness anxiety disorder either perform excessive health-related behaviors (eg, body-focused attention) or display avoidance (eg, avoiding hospitals or individuals who are ill). Individuals with illness anxiety disorder typically do not experience relief from their health-related anxiety as a result of negative test results or reassurance from physicians about their health. The preoccupation with health must last for at least 6 months to merit a diagnosis of illness anxiety disorder. Individuals who have symptoms for <6 months are diagnosed with brief illness anxiety disorder. Similarly, individuals who meet criteria for most symptoms but do not engage in excessive health-related behaviors are diagnosed with illness anxiety disorder without excessive health-related behaviors.

The primary change between the fourth edition DSM (DSM-IV) and DSM-V definitions is that a DSM-IV diagnosis of hypochondriasis also involved significant somatic symptoms, whereas the DSM-V definition specifies that individuals with illness anxiety disorder cannot have somatic symptoms or the symptoms must be mild in nature. With the changes in diagnostic criteria between DSM-IV and DSM-V, approximately 75% of individuals who would have previously been diagnosed with hypochondriasis now meet criteria for somatic symptom disorder instead. Estimates of the prevalence of illness anxiety disorder are not available because the diagnostic criteria have changed significantly. However, previous estimates of hypochondriasis ranged from 1.3% to 10%.

FACTITIOUS DISORDER & MALINGERING

Factitious disorder is a disorder in which an individual falsely reports physical or psychological symptoms or purposefully induces injury or disease. Individuals with factitious disorder may lie about medical history, falsify medical records, or induce symptoms in themselves. The individuals present themselves as ill or injured to others and often seek medical treatment. Deception is the key element of factitious disorder, and the deception must occur without any obvious external rewards (eg, disability income). Individuals with factitious disorder may have an existing medical condition, but to merit a diagnosis of factitious disorder, the individuals must present themselves in such a way that makes them appear more ill or impaired to others.

An individual may also receive the diagnosis of factitious disorder imposed on another (factitious disorder by proxy in DSM-IV). This diagnosis would be merited if an individual falsely presents another person as ill or disabled or induces illness or injury in another person. Notably, the individual who is falsifying information receives this diagnosis, not the individual who is presented as ill.

Malingering is similar to factitious disorder but differs in that there is an external motivation for the falsification of symptoms. This could include monetary gain, avoiding school or work, avoiding criminal prosecution, or obtaining drugs.

The prevalence of factitious disorder is particularly hard to determine due to the element of deception. However, within the hospital setting, it is estimated that 1% of individuals meet criteria for diagnosis. Factitious disorder often develops after a hospitalization for a medical or mental disorder or, in the case of factitious disorder imposed on another, the hospitalization of a family member.

BODY DYSMORPHIC DISORDER

DSM-V moved body dysmorphic disorder from under the category of somatic symptom disorders and into the category of obsessive-compulsive and related disorders. However, the ICD-10 currently classifies it under somatoform disorders, and therefore, it has been included in this chapter.

Body dysmorphic disorder involves individuals having an irrational preoccupation with what they believe to be a defect or a flaw in their physical appearance. Common areas of preoccupation include the skin (eg, acne, scars, wrinkles), hair (eg, thinning hair or unwanted body or facial hair), and nose. However, the preoccupation can focus on any part of the body. These preoccupations are unwanted, difficult for the individual to control, and often very time consuming. On average, individuals with body dysmorphic disorder spend 3 to 8 hours per day thinking about their perceived flaw or defect. Notably, these flaws or defects are not noticed by others, or the individual's concerns about a flaw are disproportionate to what others perceive. Individuals with body dysmorphic disorder also engage in repetitive behaviors or thoughts at some point during their disorder. Examples of these thoughts and behaviors include excessive mirror checking, excessive grooming, repeatedly applying makeup, seeking reassurance from peers, or comparing him- or herself to others. These repetitive behaviors are the basis for moving body dysmorphic disorder from the somatoform disorders classification into the obsessive-compulsive and related disorders classification in the DSM-V. Individuals with body dysmorphic disorder often receive cosmetic treatment such as dermatologic treatment or cosmetic surgery to try to fix their perceived flaws. However, cosmetic treatment rarely relieves the symptoms of body dysmorphic disorder and may instead worsen the severity of the preoccupation.

Body dysmorphic disorder with muscle dysmorphia is a specific form of body dysmorphic disorder that occurs primarily in males. This form of body dysmorphic disorder involves the preoccupation with the idea that their body is not muscular enough, despite being normal looking or very muscular. Individuals with muscle dysmorphia often diet and exercise excessively and may use steroids or other substances to compensate for their perceived flaws.

The prevalence of body dysmorphic disorder in the United States is 2.4% overall, 2.5% in females, and 2.2% in males. The prevalence in dermatology and cosmetic surgery patients is higher, with a prevalence of 9% to 15% and 7% to 8% in those settings, respectively. The majority of individuals with body dysmorphic disorder have an onset in adolescence, with two-thirds of individuals with the disorder having onset prior to the age of 18 years.

PSYCHOLOGICAL FACTORS AFFECTING OTHER MEDICAL CONDITIONS

The defining characteristic of psychological factors affecting other medical conditions is the existence of psychological or behavioral factors that have a negative effect on an existing medical condition. Psychological factors may include psychological distress (eg, depression or anxiety), poor coping skills, current life stressors, and interpersonal relationships. Behavioral factors include poor health behaviors such as symptom denial or difficulty with adherence to medical recommendations. These factors may exacerbate symptoms, resulting in nonadherence to or avoidance of treatment, or may be a well-established health risk. To receive a diagnosis of psychological factors affecting other medical conditions, the individual's psychological or behavioral factors must significantly affect either the course or outcome of the medical condition. In addition,

the factors must exist prior to diagnosis of the medical condition. If an individual develops psychological or behavioral symptoms following the diagnosis of a medical condition, a diagnosis of adjustment disorder is likely more appropriate.

The prevalence of psychological factors affecting other medical conditions is unknown. However, based on insurance billing within the United States, it is more commonly diagnosed than somatic symptom disorder.

OTHER SPECIFIED & UNSPECIFIED SOMATIC SYMPTOM & RELATED DISORDERS

A diagnosis of other specified somatic symptom and related disorder is appropriate when an individual exhibits symptoms of a somatic symptom and related disorder but does not meet all diagnostic criteria for a diagnosis. These diagnoses include brief somatic symptom disorder, brief illness anxiety disorder, and illness anxiety disorder without excessive health-related behaviors, all of which have been discussed previously in this chapter. Pseudocyesis is also encompassed in the other specified category. Pseudocyesis is the incorrect belief that one is pregnant without any objective signs or symptoms of pregnancy. Similarly, unspecified somatic symptom and related disorder is an appropriate diagnosis when an individual does not meet full criteria for a diagnosis of a somatic symptom and related disorder. However, this diagnosis should only be given when information is lacking for a more specific diagnosis.

DIAGNOSIS & TREATMENT

Providing an accurate diagnosis and explanation of the diagnosis to the patient is the first step to providing appropriate treatment for these patients. Physicians often avoid officially diagnosing somatic symptom disorder or conversion disorder, and instead opt to diagnose the symptoms, such as "tremor" or "pain." However, providing an accurate diagnosis is important for patients. This prevents them from continuing to search for a medical explanation and reduces their risk for obtaining improper medical treatment and iatrogenic illness.

After making the diagnosis, providing a clear explanation is crucial to helping the patient understand the diagnosis and treatment. It is important to emphasize that the symptoms are real and not "in their head" or "fake." Most patients do not respond well to psychiatric explanations for their symptoms, such as "stress-related" or "depression-related," and as discussed earlier, stress and depression are usually exacerbating factors or risk factors, not causal factors. Instead, patients have been found to prefer the word "functional" to describe the symptoms, meaning affecting physiologic or psychological functions but not organic structure. This suggests that although medical tests were negative, there is a functional issue, such as a miscommunication between the brain and nerves, that is not detected by diagnostic tests. In addition, use of Figure 41–1 can be helpful in explaining how symptoms can be exacerbated by many factors and can aid in patients' understanding as to why they are being referred to a psychologist, psychiatrist, or physical therapist.

Pharmacologic Treatment

A number of pharmacologic treatments (eg, antidepressants, antiepileptic drugs, and antipsychotics) have been proposed for somatic symptom disorders. However, research indicates they generally are not effective. Antidepressants have several proposed underlying mechanisms of action for the treatment of somatic symptom disorders. Individuals with somatic symptom disorders have been found to have abnormal brain activity in areas of the brain associated with serotonin and norepinephrine, and some have postulated that serotonin and norepinephrine may suppress somatic symptoms. Antidepressants may also directly affect organ systems. For example, they may slow the gastrointestinal tract, providing symptom relief for individuals with irritable bowel syndrome. Furthermore, antidepressants have immunoregulatory effects that are speculated to decrease symptoms of fatigue, sleep disturbance, and psychomotor retardation. Finally, antidepressants may reduce comorbid psychiatric conditions, including anxiety and depressive disorders, possibly resulting in a decrease in functional symptoms. Antiepileptic drugs are thought to treat somatic symptom disorders through their analgesic, anxiolytic, and sedative effects. Similarly, antipsychotics have been used in the treatment of somatic symptom disorders for their analgesic effects.

Randomized controlled trials of pharmacologic treatment for somatic symptom disorders have demonstrated very little support for pharmacology as an effective treatment. There is limited evidence for new-generation antidepressants, with some studies showing a reduction in depressive symptoms and functional disability. However, this evidence is inconsistent across studies.

Nonpharmacologic Treatment

Systematic reviews of randomized controlled trials for the treatment of somatic symptom and related disorders show cognitive-behavioral therapy (CBT) to be the most effective treatment. CBT has been found to be consistently effective in treating the range of somatic symptom and related disorders, including somatic symptom disorder, conversion disorder, illness anxiety disorder, and body dysmorphic disorder.

CBT treatment may focus on a number of aspects of somatic symptom disorders, including reducing attention to symptoms, cognitive reframing of catastrophic thinking related to symptoms (eg, "I'm going to die!"), behavioral modifications (eg, reduction in seeking medical help for somatic symptom disorder and reduction in mirror checking for body dysmorphic disorder), and reducing functional disability (eg, returning to work or school). Secondary to direct reduction in symptoms, CBT is also effective at treating comorbid anxiety or depression, which may exacerbate or be related to symptoms.

Most somatic symptom and related disorders respond to general CBT techniques, but some require specific treatments. Specifically, illness anxiety disorder is effectively treated with exposure and response prevention techniques used in CBT. Typically, this includes imaginal exposure and in vivo exposure (eg, visiting a hospital), as well as relaxation techniques and cognitive reframing of thoughts related to illness. Conversion disorder often requires an interdisciplinary approach to CBT, including physicians, psychologists, and physical therapists. Physical therapists are involved with the rehabilitation process for functional gait disorders, tremors, and paralysis, using techniques similar to those used for organic neurologic conditions, and research has found this approach to improve symptoms in both inpatient and outpatient settings. Similarly, physical therapists treat pain symptoms with techniques that increase functionality and mobility and desensitization techniques for relief of pain.

SELF-ASSESSMENT QUESTIONS

1. A patient presents with complaints of a left-handed tremor that results in tapping of her right hand. She also complains of frequent headaches and abdominal pain. After full examination, there is no evidence that suggests the symptoms are due to a medical or psychiatric condition. What would be the best diagnosis for her symptoms?

   A. Conversion disorder
   B. Illness anxiety disorder
   C. Somatic symptom disorder
   D. Body dysmorphic disorder

2. Appropriate treatment for the patient described in Question 1 would include which of the following?

   A. Physical therapy
   B. Cognitive-behavioral therapy (CBT)
   C. Antidepressants
   D. CBT and antidepressants
   E. Continued medical tests to rule out an organic cause

3. Mrs. H presents to her primary care physician with concerns that she may have a brain tumor. She indicates that she has a headache about once every 2 months, which she rates as a 2 out of 10 on the pain scale, and it subsides immediately when she takes ibuprofen. She has no other symptoms. She extensively tracks all of her headaches and brings the logs to each appointment. Her primary care physician runs several tests, all of which come back negative. She is referred to a neurologist who agrees with her doctor that she does not have a medical condition and that the occasional headaches are normal. However, Mrs. H returns to the doctor because she has been researching brain tumors on the Internet and is convinced her doctors have missed something. Mrs. H should be diagnosed with which of the following disorders?

   A. Factitious disorder
   B. Body dysmorphic disorder
   C. Illness anxiety disorder
   D. Somatic symptom disorder

4. Appropriate treatment for Mrs. H from Question 3 would include which of the following?

   A. Referral to another neurologist to rule out a brain tumor
   B. Prescription for an anxiolytic
   C. Refusal to treat Mrs. H on the grounds that she is malingering
   D. CBT with focus on exposure and response prevention

Personality Disorders

Merida Grant

OBJECTIVES

After studying this chapter, the student should be able to:

- Understand what distinguishes personality disorders from other psychiatric disorders.
- Recognize the clinical presentation and prevalence of the 10 recognized personality disorders.
- Describe the potential interventions for personality disorders.

Personality disorders are characterized by trait-like, inflexible, and unhealthy patterns of thought and behavior that deviate from cultural norms and are associated with significant distress or impaired social or occupational function. A key feature is that they are enduring, with typical onset in adolescence or early adulthood and persistence over a long duration and across a variety of contexts.

The *Diagnostic and Statistical Manual of Mental Disorders*, Fifth Edition (DSM-V) classifies personality disorders into 3 categories. Cluster A is the odd or eccentric group, and includes paranoid, schizoid, and schizotypal personality disorders. Cluster B is the dramatic, emotional, or erratic group, and includes antisocial, borderline, histrionic, and narcissistic personality disorders. Cluster C is the anxious or fearful group, and includes avoidant, dependent, and obsessive-compulsive personality disorders. In practice, patients do not usually present with a single, clearly defined personality disorder, and the lines between these syndromes are not precise. In fact, the majority of personality disorders probably go undiagnosed, often until some predisposing event or other medical or psychiatric issue brings them into the healthcare system.

Prior editions of the DSM classified personality disorders as Axis II disorders, in contrast to Axis I disorders such as major depressive disorder or schizophrenia. Although DSM-5 does not use this axis categorization, personality disorders are still sometimes referred to as Axis II disorders.

PREVALENCE & BURDEN

Personality disorders are common, affecting a little under 10% of the adult population. On the whole, they are equally common in men and women, although certain personality disorders are more common in one sex or the other. The most common personality disorder varies by country. In the United States, the most common personality disorders are obsessive-compulsive, narcissistic, and borderline personality disorder.

By definition, personality disorders are associated with impaired functioning in work, relationships, and society. Personality disorders are often comorbid with other psychiatric diagnoses. Anxiety disorders are particularly common (over half of patients with personality disorders), and substance use disorders occur in approximately 25% of patients with personality disorders. The suicide rate in borderline personality disorder, in particular, is much higher than that of the general population.

CLUSTER A: ODD OR ECCENTRIC PERSONALITY DISORDERS

Paranoid personality disorder is characterized by a pervasive and enduring distrust and cynical view of the world. Furthermore, the disorder is also characterized by hypervigilance to physical, verbal, or interpersonal threats. As a result, individuals with paranoid personality tend to have few if any close or intimate connections. Their interpersonal style is

VOCABULARY

Cluster A: The odd or eccentric personality disorders.

Cluster B: The dramatic, emotional, or erratic personality disorders.

Cluster C: The anxious or fearful personality disorders.

Histrionic: Overly dramatic or theatrical.

Narcissism: Egocentric self-absorption; excessive self-interest or admiration of one's own appearance.

Personality disorder: Trait-like inflexible and unhealthy patterns of thought and behavior that deviate from cultural norms and are associated with significant distress or impaired social or occupational function.

best described as detached and distrustful. They often appear guarded and secretive, as well as inflexible. Moreover, any perceived criticism typically elicits a response of hostility and defensiveness.

Paranoid personality disorder is a nonpsychotic disorder involving dysfunctional and maladaptive personality characteristics, rather than a thought or mood disorder. Individuals with paranoid personality disorder may develop brief psychotic reactions under stress, but these episodes do not endure. However, paranoid personality disorder is characterized by genuine belief that others have hidden motives or are out to harm them. Similarly, depressive disorders may present with paranoid ideation, often with an underlying focus on persecution. However, a detailed longitudinal history of illness will differentiate between paranoid personality disorder and ideation that only occurs in the presence of a concurrent mood disorder.

Schizoid personality disorder is characterized by a lack of close personal relationships or even a desire for such relationships. People with this personality disorder are described as cold, aloof, detached, or withdrawn. They display a restricted range of emotions and affect. They do not seek or enjoy close relationships with family or friends, and instead prefer solitary activities and are often seen as loners. People with this disorder are able to function in everyday life but may prefer solitary jobs that involve little interaction with others. This disorder generally appears by early adulthood and is more common in males than females.

The "schiz" in the term *schizoid personality disorder* comes from "schizophrenia," with the suffix "-oid" meaning schizophrenia-like, based on symptoms such as the detachment from others and flat affect. However, unlike people with schizophrenia, people with schizoid personality disorder do not have active psychotic symptoms such as paranoia or hallucinations, nor do they have disorganized speech (ie, they generally make sense in conversation). Schizoid personality disorder is often associated with depression but generally is not a precursor to schizophrenia.

Schizotypal personality disorder, like schizoid personality disorder, is characterized by difficulty forming relationships. The key difference is that those with schizotypal personality disorder, unlike those with schizoid personality disorder, may desire and seek personal relationships. However, their odd beliefs, eccentric appearance, peculiar behavior, and discomfort with other people make forming such relationships difficult. In other words, someone with schizotypal personality disorder may try and fail to form relationships and has anxiety and discomfort around others, whereas someone with schizoid personality disorder is indifferent and does not even desire to form relationships.

Strange beliefs are an important aspect of schizotypal personality disorder. Those affected often believe in special powers such as clairvoyance or telepathy or in aliens or witchcraft. Patients are likely to misperceive social cues or take offense at inoffensive things. The word *schizotypal* comes from *schizophrenic phenotype* because, like schizoid personality disorder, there are some similarities to schizophrenia. One way to think about the difference between schizoid and schizotypal personality disorders is that those with schizoid personality disorder exhibit some *negative* symptoms of schizophrenia (flat affect, restricted emotional range, indifference to others), whereas those with schizotypal personality disorder exhibit some positive symptoms of schizophrenia (magical thinking, delusions, odd speech, paranoia). (Mnemonic hint: Associate the "p" in schizoty**p**al with **p**ositive symptoms.) Both of these personality disorders may share some of the same genetic predispositions as schizophrenia and be part of a schizophrenia spectrum.

CLUSTER B: DRAMATIC, EMOTIONAL, OR ERRATIC PERSONALITY DISORDERS

Narcissistic personality disorder is characterized by a pervasive pattern of grandiosity, lack of empathy for others, and a need for admiration (narcissism is defined as excessive interest in oneself). Individuals with narcissistic personality disorder are often described as arrogant, self-absorbed, and manipulative, with fantasies of success and attractiveness. Moreover, these individuals perceive themselves as deserving of special treatment. People with narcissistic personality disorder believe they are superior and often try to associate with other people who they believe are unique or gifted in some way. This association enhances their self-esteem, which is typically quite delicate. Individuals with narcissistic personality disorder have difficulty tolerating criticism or defeat and may feel humiliated or empty following criticism or rejection. Narcissistic personality disorder may present as either a grandiose, attention-seeking, entitled, or arrogant subtype or a hypersensitive, inhibited, chronically envious, and anxious subtype. Individuals with narcissistic personality disorder can also fluctuate between grandiose and vulnerable states.

The differential diagnosis for narcissistic personality disorder includes bipolar illness and other mood disorders, substance abuse, and anxiety disorders.

Histrionic personality disorder is characterized by excessive emotionality and attention seeking. People with this disorder need to be the center of attention and, as a result, may be overly dramatic, theatrical, flirtatious, or seductive. They tend to focus on their physical appearance as a way to draw attention to themselves (eg, dressing provocatively) and are uncomfortable when they are not the focus. They are usually very social and vivacious and often seen as the "life of the party." Their emotional states can shift rapidly.

Histrionic personality disorder shares some features with narcissistic personality disorder, particularly the fact that people with both conditions seek the admiration and attention of others. However, what lies behind these traits is quite different: Whereas narcissists are convinced of their own superiority and do not need the approval of others to be convinced of their special qualities, histrionics are often very suggestible, easily influenced, and sensitive to criticism; histrionics lack a sense of self-worth and seek reassurance and others' approval through their dramatic appearance or behavior. Narcissistic personality disorder is diagnosed more commonly in males, whereas histrionic personality disorder is more commonly found in females.

Borderline personality disorder is characterized by instability in interpersonal relationships and impulsive behavior. People with this condition tend toward emotional extremes and can swing suddenly between them. For example, they may quickly develop a close, intimate relationship, which tends to be intense but stormy, and then may suddenly turn on the partner, considering them an enemy and cutting off the relationship. They have intense bouts of anger, depression, or anxiety that can last hours to days. They tend to act impulsively and without considering the consequences, and given the tendency toward bouts of depression, they are at risk of self-injurious behavior and suicidal thoughts or threats. Many of these behaviors can be seen as efforts to avoid abandonment, whether real or imagined.

Borderline personality disorder is one of the more common personality disorders in both women and men. Those affected have a high rate of hospitalization, accounting for about 20% of psychiatric admissions. The term *borderline* dates back to when neurosis and psychosis were considered the 2 main types of mental disorders; people with this disorder had features of both and thus were considered as occupying the "border" between the 2 types.

Borderline personality disorder has similarities to histrionic personality disorder in the tendency to display provocative or intensely emotional behavior, and these 2 disorders overlap to some extent, but the driving force is different. The key feature of borderline personality disorder is extreme difficulty with emotional regulation and erratic behavior, lacking the goal-directed nature in histrionic personality disorder, which is driven by a desire to temporarily enhance self-esteem.

Antisocial personality disorder is characterized by disregard for moral or ethical standards and the rights of others. Those with the disorder often violate rules or laws and have no guilt or remorse for doing so. They may be superficially charming but are manipulative and aggressive and tend to exploit others for their own purposes. Affected individuals are often hostile, callous, disrespectful, and/or deceitful. Their behavior is impulsive, reckless, and without concern for others.

Antisocial personality disorder is much more common in males than females and is prevalent among those in prison.

CLUSTER C: ANXIOUS OR FEARFUL PERSONALITY DISORDERS

Obsessive-compulsive personality disorder is characterized by preoccupation with rules, orderliness, and a need for control. People with this disorder tend toward perfectionism, even to the point of interfering with task completion due to rigid adherence to an unrealistically high standard. This can be exacerbated by unwillingness to delegate, because of the associated loss of control and fear that things will be done incorrectly. They can be workaholics, with a fixation on their vocation at the expense of relationships. People with obsessive-compulsive personality disorder are often overly adherent to rules and inflexible about moral or ethical standards. They can be miserly, with tight control over spending, and they can be

CASE 42-1

A 40-year-old man and his wife present for marital counseling. He graduated from both high school and college with honors, although he had few close friends because he devoted himself to studying. Although his wife was initially attracted by his strong sense of morality and attention to detail, she has since found that his rigid adherence to a schedule and workaholic nature have left no time for his family. He now runs a small business that by all accounts is doing well, and he is perceived as the key to its success. He does not take vacation and expects everyone around him to adhere to his sense of values. His employees view him as a micromanager and are frustrated by his inability to delegate. They feel that the company would be much more successful if he allowed others to do their jobs and focused on the big picture. He recently fired a valuable coworker who had made what most people thought was a trivial violation of office policy, but he felt that adhering to the rules was more important. His wife is now seeking counseling because his behavior, such as missing important children's events due to rigid adherence to his work schedule and disciplining his children for seemingly minor infractions, has resulted in family stress.

This history is consistent with obsessive-compulsive personality disorder, given the long-term pattern of inflexible and perfectionistic behavior with an overly rigid adherence to rules and the impaired function in his interpersonal relationships.

reluctant to part with old items and thus have a tendency to hoard.

Obsessive-compulsive personality disorder is one of the most common personality disorders, with a prevalence between 2% and 8%, and it is more common in males. There are obvious similarities to obsessive-compulsive disorder (OCD), but there are several differences that distinguish the 2 conditions. First, obsessive-compulsive personality disorder lacks true obsessions (uncontrollable intrusive thoughts) or compulsions (irresistible urges to repeatedly perform purposeless behaviors). Second, and perhaps more importantly, whereas people with OCD are distressed by their condition and aware of its negative effects on them and those around them and thus usually seek treatment, people with obsessive-compulsive personality disorder tend to think that their inflexible behaviors are adaptive and appropriate and see no need to change or seek treatment.

Avoidant personality disorder is characterized by social anxiety and isolation, with feelings of inadequacy. People with this disorder fear embarrassment or rejection, are easily hurt by any criticism, and feel socially inept. They tend to be preoccupied with their own weaknesses and suspect that they are unappealing to others. As a result, those affected cope with these feelings of inferiority by isolating themselves socially and avoiding intimate relationships. People with avoidant personality disorder may be perceived as shy and risk averse, with low self-esteem.

Although both avoidant and schizoid personality disorders have social isolation as a defining feature, the key difference is that those with avoidant personality disorder have a great deal of anxiety and distress about what might happen in a relationship, whereas those with schizoid personality disorder simply have no interest in forming relationships.

Dependent personality disorder is characterized by a pervasive and abnormal need for the approval and assistance of others. People with this disorder find it difficult to make even simple decisions like what to wear, let alone major choices such as where to live or work, without input from others. They require constant reassurance. They do not trust their own instincts and put themselves in need of caregiving from others. They may be viewed as passive, clingy, naïve, oversensitive to criticism, and submissive, with low self-confidence. People with dependent personality disorder fear abandonment and do not like to be alone; they often place their own needs below those of others and even tolerate mistreatment.

Borderline personality disorder is also associated with a fear of abandonment, but the difference with dependent personality disorder lies in how the individual responds: A person with borderline personality disorder is likely to lash out, rage, and be highly demanding, whereas someone with dependent personality disorder tends toward submissiveness and appeasement to maintain the relationship. The similarity between patients with dependent personality disorder and those with histrionic personality disorder is that both seek approval from others; however, those with histrionic personality disorder do so in a highly outgoing, flamboyant, or seductive way, whereas those with dependent personality disorder do so in a meek, childlike way. Finally, although both avoidant and dependent personality disorders feature feelings of inadequacy, the response is quite different, with the former avoiding social relationships and the latter strongly seeking them, even to the point of sacrificing their own autonomy.

CAUSES & RISK FACTORS

The factors that influence the development of personality disorders are not well understood, but both genetic vulnerability and childhood experiences are thought to underlie the risk for personality disorders. They are more common when there is a family history of personality disorders or other psychiatric disorders, which could be due to either genetic or environmental influences. Twin studies indicate fairly high genetic heritability, estimated at 30% to 60%, which is consistent with growing evidence for genetic determinants of personality traits in general, apart from personality disorders. Approaches such as genome-wide association studies are beginning to identify some candidate genes, including several involved in neuronal development and differentiation or neurotransmitter pathways. In many cases, the genetic risk factors for personality disorders are related to those for related psychiatric disorders. For example, there are shared factors between schizophrenia and Cluster A personality disorders and between bipolar disorder and Cluster B borderline personality disorder.

Environmental factors in childhood also likely contribute to many personality disorders. Abuse (eg, sexual, physical, verbal, or psychological abuse or neglect) is associated with higher rates of personality disorders in all 3 clusters. Childhood abuse is particularly associated with borderline personality disorder, but it is also associated with most other personality disorders.

Given evidence that both genetics and experience substantially contribute to the development of personality disorders, there is increasing interest in gene–environment interactions. That is, adverse childhood experiences may have a particularly detrimental effect on those with certain genetic backgrounds, whereas others with a less vulnerable genetic susceptibility may have more resilience after abuse.

TREATMENT OF PERSONALITY DISORDERS

Because by definition personality disorders reflect a long-standing pattern of behavior, often since young adulthood, they can be difficult to treat or modify. Because of their enduring nature, the prognosis for spontaneous remission is rather low. Furthermore, given the symptoms of many personality disorders, particularly the ones associated with social isolation, those affected may not even seek treatment because they may not believe there is anything wrong them. Because it is among the most common personality disorders and because it engenders behavior such as suicidal gestures that may drive hospitalization, borderline personality disorder has the most literature on treatment.

The mainstay of treatment is psychotherapy. Cognitive-behavioral therapy (CBT) addresses ingrained thought patterns (rather than life events) that may drive problematic behaviors. A type of CBT that has been well-studied for borderline personality disorder is dialectical behavioral therapy. *Dialectical* refers to integrating opposite ideas, such as accepting patients as they are while simultaneously emphasizing the need for change. Randomized controlled trials indicate that these approaches can reduce some of the frequency of self-injurious behavior or other symptoms, although they probably do not reduce the number of patients meeting diagnostic criteria for the disorder. Psychodynamic therapy, which focuses on discussing past experiences and increasing insight, is another evidence-based approach for borderline personality.

Pharmacotherapy is viewed as an adjunct treatment for personality disorders, particularly during periods of decompensation or acute behavior changes. Guidelines recommend treatment aimed at 3 symptom clusters: neuroleptics for cognitive/perceptual symptoms, selective serotonin reuptake inhibitors (SSRIs) for affective symptoms, and SSRIs or low-dose neuroleptics for impulsivity and irritability.

SELF-ASSESSMENT QUESTIONS

1. A 50-year-old man is scheduled for a routine colonoscopy. As plans are made for postprocedure care, he says he has no close friends who can help. He is estranged from his family, who no longer invite him to gatherings because he does not seem to enjoy them and prefers to play video games. He lives alone and has never married or even had a significant dating relationship, going back to high school. He works as a truck driver, spending weeks on the road by himself. He has been through several jobs and had difficulty maintaining any that involved working closely with others. In conversation, he is somewhat cold and detached but otherwise seems appropriate. When asked why he has few friends, he says he just "doesn't see the point." Which of the following is the most likely diagnosis?

   A. Avoidant personality disorder
   B. Schizoid personality disorder
   C. Schizotypal personality disorder
   D. Paranoid personality disorder
   E. Antisocial personality disorder

2. A 32-year-old woman presents to the emergency department after a sleeping pill overdose. She says her boyfriend recently broke up with her. Apparently the relationship had formed a couple months before and become serious shortly after they had met, and ended because the boyfriend found her too volatile after several episodes when she became enraged about seemingly minor issues. The patient acknowledges a feeling of emptiness and says she has a difficult time controlling her temper. She has several prior hospitalizations for self-injurious behavior including cutting herself, dating back to college. Which of the following is the most appropriate diagnosis?

   A. Narcissistic personality disorder
   B. Histrionic personality disorder
   C. Dependent personality disorder
   D. Borderline personality disorder
   E. Schizotypal personality disorder

3. What is most likely to be an effective approach to treating the patient in Question 2?

   A. Dialectical behavioral therapy
   B. Haloperidol
   C. A combination of citalopram and olanzapine
   D. Psychodynamic psychotherapy
   E. Either A or D

Substance Use Disorders

CHAPTER

43

Stephen Brackett, Samantha Schiavon,
Michelle Sisson, & Karen Cropsey

OBJECTIVES

After studying this chapter, the student should be able to:

- Recognize common drugs of abuse, associated symptoms of substance use disorders, and physiologic pathways associated with addiction.
- Understand the prevalence and common medical comorbidities associated with substance use disorders.
- Identify treatment approaches for each class of substance use disorders.

PREVALENCE & BURDEN

Approximately 20.2 million adults (8.4%) had a substance use disorder in the past year, making substance use disorders one of the most prevalent mental health disorders in the United States. Nicotine use disorder is the most prevalent, with an estimated lifetime prevalence of 27%. Alcohol use disorder is also common, with an estimated 8% of adults meeting criteria during their lifetime. Lifetime prevalence of an illicit drug use disorder is approximately 2% to 3%. The National Institute on Drug Abuse estimates the total cost of substance use to our country to be $740 billion annually. This includes not only associated healthcare cost, but also lost productivity and crime-related costs.

SUBSTANCE USE DISORDERS & THE REWARD PATHWAY

It is important to understand the role of the reward pathway and the effects of drugs on this part of the brain. The reward pathway of the brain increases pleasurable behaviors that enhance our survival. For example, on a more basic level, drinking a bottle of water after a run or eating meal when hungry activates the reward pathway to create the feeling of satiation. The reward pathway also plays a role in more complex behaviors such as forming relationships, sexual intercourse, and child rearing.

The reward pathway is also known as the mesolimbic pathway. It originates in a portion of the midbrain called the ventral tegmental area (VTA). From the VTA, dopaminergic neurons project into an area of the ventral striatum called the nucleus accumbens (NAcc) (Figure 43–1). When dopamine is released at the NAcc, it causes pleasure, partially through the release of endorphins. Generally, the more dopamine a given

stimulus releases at the NAcc, the more pleasurable is the experience. The NAcc is able to assign various stimuli differing amounts of salience. This stimulus–reward phenomenon plays a vital role in both classical and operant conditioning (Figure 43–2).

In some individuals, the reward pathway is able to be "highjacked" through a variety of substances. The very nature of the reward system itself can lead to substantial changes in behavior through the salience phenomena. In some circumstances, this system, which developed as a means to ensure survival, can lead to destructive behaviors that all too frequently increase morbidity and mortality.

Individuals develop what is known as a substance use disorder, when through repeated use of a given substance, physiologic and psychologic changes occur, leading to maladaptive behaviors. The *Diagnostic and Statistical Manual of Mental Disorders*, Fifth Edition (DSM-V) lists 11 criteria for substance use disorder, with the severity of the disorder determined by the number of criteria met as follows: 2 to 3 for mild, 4 to 5 for moderate, and ≥6 for severe substance use disorder. These criteria can be thought of as occurring in 1 of 4 domains, as shown in Table 43–1.

SUBSTANCE USE DISORDERS

This section reviews common drugs of abuse (Table 43–2), including the associated neurotransmitters and neural pathways, symptoms of intoxication and withdrawal, and common treatment modalities, including pharmacotherapies. Although this chapter is focused specifically on substance use disorders, it is important to realize that these disorders often have many other substance, psychiatric, and medical comorbidities. For example, it is common to see patients who meet criteria for multiple substance use disorders with comorbid psychiatric

VOCABULARY

Addiction: A condition characterized by compulsive engagement in rewarding stimuli, despite adverse consequences.

Dependence: An adaptive state that occurs from continued administration of a given substance.

Intoxication: A substance-specific syndrome occurring after a substance has been administered at a sufficient dose.

Salience: A want or strong desire assigned to a rewarding stimulus.

Tolerance: A decreasing effect of a substance due to continued administration of a given dose.

Withdrawal: A substance-specific syndrome occurring after administration of a given substance has been discontinued.

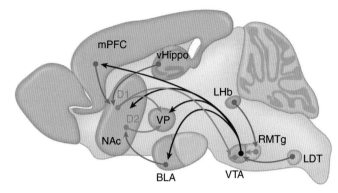

FIGURE 43-2 Major connections of the mesolimbic dopamine system in the brain. Schematic diagram of the brain illustrating that the dopamine projections (red) originate in the ventral tegmental area (VTA) and target the nucleus accumbens (NAc), prefrontal cortex (mPFC), basolateral amygdala (BLA), and ventral pallidum (VP). Neurons in the NAc fall into 2 classes, one expressing type 1 dopamine receptors (D1s) and the other expressing type 2 receptors (D2s). Both classes contain GABAergic projection neurons (green); the D1 receptor neurons send their axons to both the VP and the VTA (where they target primarily the γ-aminobutyric acid [GABA] interneurons), whereas the D2 receptor neurons send their axons selectively to the VP. The NAc is also a site of convergence of excitatory projections from the mPFC, the ventral hippocampus (vHippo), and the BLA. The midbrain dopamine neurons receive a direct excitatory input (blue) from the lateral dorsal tegmentum (LDT), while the GABA neurons of the rostromedial tegmentum (RMTg) at the tail of the VTA are excited by neurons from the lateral habenula (LHb), typically when an aversive stimulus occurs. (Reproduced with permission from Lüthi A, Lüscher C: Pathological circuit function underlying addiction and anxiety disorders, *Nat Neurosci*. 2014 Dec;17(12):1635-1643.)

disorders. Many patients will have comorbid medical problems directly due to their use of substances.

Alcohol

Humans have consumed alcohol for thousands of years, beginning somewhere between 3000 and 2000 B.C. Alcohol is produced during the process of fermentation in which yeast breaks down sugar into alcohol and carbon dioxide. The antiseptic properties of alcohol allowed for potable beverages prior to modern water sanitation systems.

Unlike the other substances of abuse, there is no "alcohol receptor" in the human brain. Alcohol exerts its effect primarily due to the molecule's interactions at the amino

acids level. The net result leads to a general decrease in the amount of glutamate transmission and general increase in the amount of γ-aminobutyric acid (GABA). In addition, alcohol has been shown to cause the release of endorphins

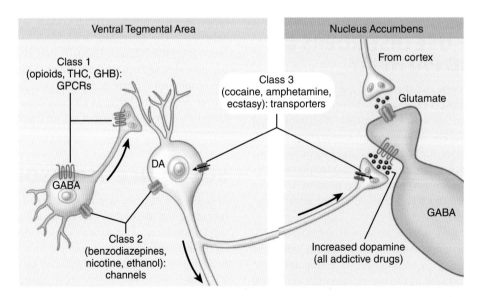

FIGURE 43-1 Neuropharmacologic classification of addictive drugs by primary target. DA, dopamine; GABA, γ-aminobutyric acid; GHB, γ-hydroxybutyric acid; GPCRs, G-protein–coupled receptors; THC, Δ9-tetrahydrocannabinol. (Reproduced with permission from Katzung BG: *Basic and Clinical Pharmacology*, 14th ed. New York, NY: McGraw Hill; 2018.)

TABLE 43–1 *Diagnostic and statistical manual of mental disorders,* **fifth edition substance use criteria.**

Impairment of control
- Using a larger amount of a substance than one intended to or using for a longer period of time than intended
- A continual desire to stop using or unsuccessful efforts to cut down on use
- Spending large amounts of time finding, using, or recovering from having used a substance
- Cravings (both positive and negative)

Impairment of social functioning
- Role obligation failure (home, school, or work)
- Continued use in the context of worsening social problems caused by the substance
- Reducing (or eliminating) previously pleasurable activities

Use with increased risk
- Hazardous situations (driving, heavy machinery, guns)
- Continued use despite knowledge of worsening physical or psychological problems caused by the substance

Physiologic
- Tolerance
- Withdrawal

Mild substance use disorder, 2–3 symptoms; moderate substance use disorder, 4–5 symptoms; severe substance use disorder, ≥6 symptoms.

Data from American Psychiatric Association: Diagnostic and Statistical Manual of Mental Disorders, 5th ed. Arlington, VA, American Psychiatric Association, 2013.

at the NAcc, leading to the phenomenon of alcohol-induced cravings.

Alcohol is primarily metabolized in the body by 2 enzymes: alcohol dehydrogenase (ADH) and aldehyde dehydrogenase (ALDH). ADH breaks alcohol down into acetaldehyde, which ALDH further degrades into acetate. Acetaldehyde is a known carcinogen, and higher concentration of this chemical are known to cause flushing and nausea. A mutation in the gene for ADH (*ADH1B*2*) is commonly found in people of East Asian descent and is thought to be protective against developing alcohol use disorder.

At low levels of consumption, alcohol reduces anxiety. As the amount of alcohol consumed increases, intoxication occurs, leading to symptoms of ataxia, slurred speech, and cognitive impairment. As the concentration of alcohol increases in the blood, a transient anterograde amnesia (blackout) can occur. Coma and respiratory depression are signs of alcohol poisoning.

Alcohol withdrawal occurs in individuals who have become physiologically dependent on alcohol. Its symptoms commonly include anxiety, nausea, tremor, sweating, hypertension, and tachycardia. Withdrawal symptoms may begin as early as 6 hours after consumption, but generally, they begin within 24 hours and, in most people, subside within 2 days. Individuals who consume large amounts of alcohol for long periods of time may experience withdrawal symptoms before the blood alcohol concentration reaches zero. Life-threatening complications of alcohol withdrawal include seizures and delirium tremens (DT). DT is the most severe form of alcohol withdrawal and is a medical emergency. It occurs in the context of the previously mentioned alcohol withdrawal symptoms, but also includes confusion, disorientation, fever, agitation, and hallucinations (visual, auditory, and tactile). Generally, DT begins within 3 to 4 days after the last alcohol consumption and typical resolves after 3 days. If untreated, the DT mortality rate may reach 40%.

Benzodiazepines are commonly used to treat alcohol withdrawal symptoms. Longer acting forms such as chlordiazepoxide, clonazepam, and diazepam allow for less frequent dosing in addition to a smoother detoxification course and are especially useful in the outpatient setting. For patients who are hospitalized, lorazepam is a common choice to treat withdrawal symptoms. Lorazepam is available in a variety of formulations (oral, intramuscular, and intravenous) and does not require oxidation, but only glucuronide, to be excreted. This may be of use in patients whose alcohol use has led to liver disease, and its shorter half-life reduces the chance of accumulation in the plasma.

Several pharmacotherapies have US Food and Drug Administration (FDA) approval for the treatment of alcohol use disorders. These medications include disulfiram, acamprosate, and naltrexone. Disulfiram produces sensitivity to alcohol by inhibiting the enzyme acetaldehyde dehydrogenase, such that ingestion of even a small amount of alcohol causes flushing, throbbing in the head and neck, headache, respiratory difficulty, nausea, vomiting, sweating, thirst, chest pain, dyspnea, tachycardia, hypotension, syncope, weakness, blurred vision, and confusion. These unpleasant effects generally prevent individuals from drinking alcohol. However, disulfiram is not widely used because adherence to the medication is generally poor. Acamprosate is believed to be an *N*-methyl-D-aspartate (NMDA) receptor antagonist and modulator of $GABA_A$ receptors that helps regulate chemical signaling in the brain. However, the efficacy of acamprosate is limited, and the pill burden (2 pills taken 3 times daily) often makes adherence to the medication problematic. However, acamprosate is metabolized through the kidneys and may be the best option for alcohol treatment among patients with severe liver disease. Naltrexone, an opioid antagonist, is available in both oral and monthly intramuscular injectable formulations. Naltrexone is believed to reduce the rewarding effects of alcohol and reduce cravings. Naltrexone cannot be used for patients who are prescribed chronic opioids because it will precipitate withdrawal. Although these medications are all FDA approved for alcohol use disorders, none has shown strong efficacy or is widely used in practice.

Caffeine

Caffeine is a legal and unregulated central nervous system stimulant that belongs to the methylxanthine class. It is an antagonist for adenosine receptors and therefore blocks the lethargic effects of adenosine. Caffeine is found in several South American and East Asian native plants and is typically sourced from *Coffea* plants. It is most typically consumed through drinking beverages such as coffee, tea, and carbonated

TABLE 43–2 Categories of substance use disorders, prevalence, and medical sequelae.

Substance Type	Common Examples	Street Names	Route of Administration	12-Month Prevalence of a Substance Use Disorder	Medical Sequelae
Alcohol	Beer, wine, liquor (eg, vodka, gin)	"Hooch," "juice," "sauce," "moonshine"	Oral	8.5% of adults	Liver disease, pancreatitis, ulcers and gastrointestinal problems, cancer, malnourishment, brain damage, heart disease. Accidents, injury, and death, particularly when combined with other central nervous system depressants such as opioids, sedatives, hypnotics, or anxiolytics.
Caffeine	Coffee, tea, soda, energy drinks	"Java," "Joe," "go juice"	Oral	7% of adults	Anxiety, gastrointestinal distress. Very high doses (>400 mg) can result in grand mal seizures and respiratory failure.
Cannabis/marijuana	Sativa, indica, ruderalis	"Weed," "pot," "reefer," "Mary Jane"	Oral, inhalation (smoked)	3.4% of children age 12-17 years 1.5% of adults	Respiratory symptoms of bronchitis, sputum production, shortness of breath, wheezing.
Hallucinogens/ other hallucinogens	Lysergic acid diethylamide (LSD), phencyclidine (PCP), psilocybin, ketamine, 3,4-methylenedioxy-methamphetamine (MDMA)	"Acid," "blotter," "angel dust," "doses," "dots," "shrooms," "magic mushrooms," "special K"	Oral, inhalation	Unknown; 2.5% of population has ever used hallucinogens	Cardiovascular and neurologic toxicities may result from intoxication. Memory problems with chronic use.
Inhalants	Nitrous oxide, paint thinners, gasoline, glue, felt-tip markers	"Poppers," "snotballs," "spray," "snappers"	Inhalation	0.4% of children age 12-17 years 0.02% of adults	Arrhythmias, respiratory illnesses and respiratory depression, asphyxiation, aspiration, accident, injury, death
Opioids	Heroin, codeine, fentanyl, hydrocodone, oxycodone, methadone, buprenorphine	"Dope," "smack," "black tar," "China white," "K9," "OC"	Oral, intravenous, rectal, inhalation (snorted or smoked)	0.37% of adults	Viral infections (HIV, hepatitis C virus), bacterial infections (cellulitis, endocarditis, tuberculosis), sexually transmitted infections, and death (1.5%-2% per year). Overdose is more likely when combined with other central nervous system depressants such as sedatives, hypnotics, or anxiolytics or alcohol.
Sedatives/ hypnotics/ anxiolytics	Barbiturates, zolpidem, eszopiclone, alprazolam, clonazepam, diazepam, lorazepam	"Yellows," "barbs," "downers," "tranks," "ludes," "sleepers," "benzos," "roofies"	Oral, intravenous	0.3% of children age 12-17 years 0.2% of adults	Accident, injury, or death, particularly when mixed with other central nervous system depressants such as alcohol or opioids. Cognitive problems and falls among elderly.
Stimulants	Amphetamines, methamphetamine, cocaine, crack cocaine	"Speed," "uppers," "coke," "powder"	Oral, inhalation (snorted or smoked), intravenous	Amphetamines: 0.2% of adults and children age 12-17 years Cocaine: 0.2% of children age 12-17 years and 0.3% of adults	HIV and sexually transmitted infections, cardiovascular (myocardial infarction, chest pain, palpitations) and respiratory problems, seizures, death (respiratory or cardiac arrest).
Tobacco	Cigarettes, cigars, cigarillos, pipe tobacco, hookah, smokeless tobacco	"Smokes," "ciggies," "cigs"	Inhalation (smoked), buccal (smokeless)	13% of adults	Cardiovascular illnesses, chronic obstructive pulmonary disease, and cancers.

drinks. Although >85% of adults and children consume caffeine, only about 7% of caffeine users experience ≥5 symptoms and functional impairment indicating caffeine intoxication.

Caffeine use disorder is included in the Conditions for Further Study section of the DSM-V, because additional research is needed to determine a consistent manner of identifying cases with adequate severity to warrant the diagnosis of a disorder. A strict diagnostic threshold needs to be determined due to the high rate of nonproblematic daily use in the general population. Current research has provided enough evidence supporting the establishment of a proposed disorder, and the World Health Organization recognized caffeine dependence in the 10th revision of the International Statistical Classification of Diseases and Related Health Problems.

Caffeine intoxication usually occurs with doses >250 mg and is characterized by restlessness, nervousness, excitement, insomnia, flushed face, diuresis, gastrointestinal disturbance, muscle twitch, rambling thought and speech, tachycardia or arrhythmia, and psychomotor agitation. Given the short half-life of caffeine (4 to 6 hours), caffeine intoxication usually ends within a day and generally does not produce any long-term negative effects. Abrupt cessation of caffeine used regularly usually results in withdrawal symptoms of headache, fatigue or drowsiness, difficulty with concentration, and the flulike symptoms of nausea, vomiting, and muscle aches or stiffness. Onset of withdrawal is usually within 12 to 24 hours of last caffeine use; withdrawal peaks after 1 to 2 days and can last between 2 and 9 days, although the caffeine headache can persist up to 21 days after discontinuation of caffeine.

Cannabis

Cannabis is a genus of flowering plant that has been used by humans for thousands of years (Figure 43–3). The plant can be used to form hemp fibers used in rope and textiles. The plant also contains a variety of chemicals known as cannabinoids. These chemicals have been shown to interact with the endocannabinoid system in various ways. Tetrahydrocannabinol (THC) is the most psychoactive of these substances, at least in terms of addiction. Marijuana is the dried leaves and flowers from the plant and is typically smoked. More concentrated amounts of THC can be found in hashish (a dried resin), with an even greater concentration found in hash oil.

THC has endogenous receptors in the brain, the CB1 and CB2 endocannabinoid receptors. Through its binding action, it is able to cause a variety of effects throughout the body, including appetite stimulation, suppression of nausea, and analgesia. It is also known to cause euphoria, in addition to impairing both motor function and memory. Cannabis use, particularly during adolescence, is associated with a higher risk of schizophrenia and may also worsens its symptoms.

Cannabis intoxication is associated with dry mouth, tachycardia, euphoria, hunger, and relaxation in lower amounts. In some individuals, cannabis may cause lightheadedness and paranoia; in higher amounts, it may heighten anxiety or cause panic. Chronic, heavy use has been shown to induce tolerance. Upon cessation, prominent withdrawal symptoms include anorexia, nausea, insomnia, irritability, and anxiety.

Although the use, possession, and sale of cannabis remain illegal under federal law, approximately half of the states in the United States have passed laws allowing for some medical use of marijuana, whereas 8 states allow medical as well as recreational use of marijuana. Two FDA-approved medications available in oral form, dronabinol and nabilone, contain cannabinoids and are prescribed for nausea and to increase appetite. Cannabidiol (CBD) oil, which does not contain THC or produce psychoactive effects, has also shown promise for seizure disorders that do not respond to conventional medications. CBD oil does not have FDA approval for any medical condition.

Hallucinogens

Hallucinogens or psychedelics represent a classification of drugs that produce changes in perceptual experiences. These changes may be associated with short-term alterations in cognition and mood that may produce lasting changes in cognitive beliefs. Hallucinogens span a wide range of drugs including phencyclidine (PCP), ketamine, psilocybin (mushrooms), lysergic acid diethylamide (LSD), and 3,4-methylenedioxymethamphetamine (MDMA). Serotonergic psychedelics such as LSD and psilocybin cause more hallucinogenic and less stimulatory effects. Serotonergic hallucinogens alter thinking and produce illusions and visual hallucinations. Glutamatergic NMDA receptor antagonists, such as PCP and ketamine, were first developed as anesthetic drugs for humans or large animals and produce a dissociative state of being. Interestingly, MDMA (catecholamine-like psychedelic) is chemically similar to both stimulants and hallucinogens, which causes this drug to produce mixed subjective effects including increased energy, pleasure, and emotional warmth as well as distorted sensory and time perception.

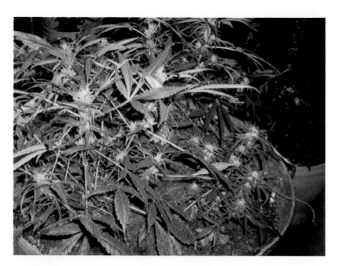

FIGURE 43–3 Home-grown marijuana plant. (Reproduced with permission from US Drug Enforcement Administration.)

Although hallucinogens may produce varied subjective effects and act on several different receptors, all hallucinogen-related disorders are classified as either PCP use or other hallucinogen use. PCP intoxication is characterized by vertical or horizontal nystagmus, hypertension or tachycardia, numbness or diminished responsiveness to pain, ataxia, dysarthria, muscle rigidity, seizures or coma, and hyperacusis. These symptoms are typically present within 1 hour of use. Repetitive, uncontrolled movements of the eyes coupled with bizarre and violent behavior may help distinguish individuals suffering from PCP intoxication versus intoxication with other substances. Symptoms of other hallucinogen intoxication occur shortly after ingestion and include pupillary dilation, tachycardia, sweating, palpitations, blurring of vision, tremors, and incoordination. Although suicide is rare among hallucinogen users, hallucinogen intoxication may lead to increased suicide risk or death due to secondary effects (eg, increased severity of visual hallucinations may cause individuals to place themselves in dangerous situations).

Although some hallucinogens produce tolerance, not all hallucinogens have been associated with physical withdrawal symptoms, and most withdrawal symptoms are likely experienced psychologically rather than physically. One notable exception is with repeated use of PCP, which often produces cravings, headaches, and sweating withdrawal symptoms upon abrupt cessation.

On rare occasions, the use of hallucinogens has been associated with long-term effects. *Hallucinogen persisting perception disorder* is the reexperiencing of perceptual distortions (eg, hallucinations, false perceptions of movement, flashes of color, images of moving objects, positive afterimages, halos around objects, macropsia, and micropsia) after the cessation of hallucinogen use. Similarly, there are anecdotal accounts of flashbacks from hallucinogen users. A flashback is the reexperience of a hallucinogen's subjective effects that can happen a few day or years after drug use and often occurs without warning.

Although hallucinogens are commonly considered drugs of abuse, some hallucinogens have been studied as pharmacotherapeutic agents. For example, recent research has investigated the use of ketamine to treat severe depression. Some studies have shown that a single dose of ketamine can decrease depression for up to 2 weeks, and therapeutic benefits begin immediately. This is especially important considering that it takes approximately 2 weeks before individuals begin to experience any benefit from most antidepressant medications. Similarly, a recent pilot study among individuals with terminal cancer demonstrated that a single-dose session of psilocybin significantly reduced patients' end-of-life anxiety and improved their depressed mood, which was maintained for up to 3 and 6 months, respectively.

Inhalants

Inhalant use (also known as *huffing, sniffing,* or *bagging*) is the intentional inhalation of chemical vapors to achieve a short-acting altered mental state. Inhalants include commonly found household products, such as solvents (paint thinners or removers, gasoline, lighter fluid), aerosols (spray paints, hair or deodorant sprays, aerosol computer cleaning products), gases (butane lighters, propane tanks, whipped cream aerosols), adhesives (glue), and nitrates (room odorizer, leather cleaner, liquid aroma). Inhalants affect the central nervous systems to produce short-term effects that are similar to the effects of alcohol, including slurred or distorted speech, lack of coordination, euphoria, and dizziness. Inhalants are predominately used by youths, with 2017 trends revealing that >8% of adolescents age 12 to 17 years reported having used an inhalant. In particular, nitrates are primarily used among older adolescents as sexual enhancers. Nitrates produce vasodilatation, which is thought to increase sexual satisfaction.

Inhalant intoxication is characterized by the experience of the following symptoms shortly after inhalant use: dizziness, nystagmus, incoordination, slurred speech, unsteady gait, lethargy, depressed reflexes, psychomotor retardation, tremor, generalized muscle weakness, blurred vision or diplopia, stupor or coma, and euphoria. Abusers of inhalants may be particularly susceptible to overdose because solvents and aerosol sprays may be highly concentrated. Inhaling the high volume of chemicals can cause *sudden sniffing death syndrome.* Butane and propane are particularly associated with sudden sniffing death syndrome due to rapid-onset, potentially fatal cardiac arrhythmias.

Although inhalants do not have significant withdrawal symptoms, chronic abuse of inhalants is associated with serious damage to the heart, lungs, liver, and kidneys. Other serious complications include peripheral and central nervous system damage, dementia, loss of cognitive functioning, gait disturbances, and loss of coordination. Due to these possible cognitive impairments, psychotherapies and other standard approaches to substance abuse treatment must be adapted to accommodate the short attention span and poor impulse control associated with chronic inhalant abuse.

Opioids

The opium poppy, *Papaver somniferum* (Figure 43–4), is native to the eastern Mediterranean, and its uses were known to ancient civilizations. The term *opiate* is reserved for naturally occurring alkaloids found in the latex of the poppy plant (eg, codeine, morphine, and thebaine). Originally, the term *opioid* was used to describe the semisynthetic (eg, buprenorphine, hydrocodone, oxycodone) and fully synthetic (eg, methadone, fentanyl) chemicals with similar clinical effects, but now, it is commonly used to describe any chemical in this class.

Although multiple opioid receptors and subtypes have been discovered, this chapter will primarily focus on the effects of the mu (μ) opioid receptor, because it is the most relevant to substance use disorders. The μ receptors are present in the NAcc, cortex, and thalamus, in addition to others areas of the central nervous system and body. Its endogenous ligands are endorphins and enkephalins. Depending on the area in

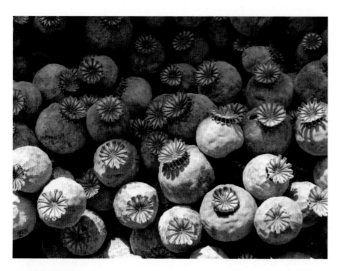

FIGURE 43–4 Harvested poppy capsules from Afghanistan. (Photograph by Wikipedia contributor Zyance, distributed under a CC-BY 2.5 license. https://en.wikipedia.org/wiki/Poppy_straw#/media/File:Mohn_z06.jpg. Accessed January 23, 2020.)

the brain in which the receptor is found, activation may cause euphoria, analgesia, or respiratory depression. The μ receptors are also found in the gastrointestinal tract, where activation causes a decrease in motility, leading to constipation.

Opioid intoxication is characterized by a decrease in heart rate, respirations, and blood pressure, in addition to pupillary constriction and euphoria. As serum levels increase, respiratory suppression occurs and leads to death. Opioid overdose can be reversed by naloxone, a μ-receptor antagonist that can be given by nasal spray or by injection, either intramuscular or intravenous.

Opioid withdrawal is often described as a flulike syndrome. Common symptoms include alternating hot and cold sweats, body aches, diarrhea, nasal congestion, rhinorrhea, sweating, restless legs, and pupillary dilation. It is important to note that withdrawal symptoms can occur in some individuals after as little as a 2-week course of pain medication. As a result, symptoms of tolerance and withdrawal cannot be counted as criteria used to make the diagnosis of opioid use disorder in individuals who have been taking medications as prescribed by their physician. Opioid withdrawal is generally not life threatening; however, these are cases where extreme caution should be used due to the vasoconstrictive effects of opioid withdrawal. Individuals with severe coronary artery disease should be closely monitored during withdrawal to avoid myocardial infarction. In addition, uterine artery constriction can cause fetal distress in pregnant females, and current practice is to maintain these women on opioids such as buprenorphine or methadone throughout the duration of the pregnancy.

Treatment of Opioid Use Disorder

Unlike other substances discussed so far in this chapter, pharmacotherapy treatment for opioid use disorder is to maintain individuals on long-acting opioids while under the supervision of a physician, following federal guidelines. Patients with opioid use disorder who meet certain criteria may be able to participate in methadone treatment programs. Methadone is a long-acting μ-receptor agonist that can be titrated to a dose sufficient to alleviate not only cravings, but also withdrawal symptoms. Initially, methadone is dispensed daily from the treatment program in liquid form under direct observation to prevent diversion and ensure adherence. The titration schedule is set by federal regulation. Individuals are also required to meet with an individual counselor and establish a treatment plan and are monitored with urine drugs screens. Over time, individuals who adhere to their treatment plan may earn "take-home" doses of up to 1 month of medication. Methadone can prolong the QTc interval, and electrocardiograms should be obtained periodically to reduce the chance of torsades de pointes.

Another maintenance treatment option for opioid use disorder is buprenorphine. Unlike methadone, buprenorphine is a partial agonist for the μ receptor. This characteristic causes a ceiling effect, such that dosages >24 mg show little to no effect in regard to respiratory suppression, analgesia, or cravings when taken sublingually. In addition, buprenorphine has a very high affinity for the μ receptor, and thus, it can prevent the euphoria caused by full μ agonists if a full μ agonist is taken after buprenorphine (eg, heroin). Conversely, individuals must be in moderate to severe opioid withdrawal (12 hours since last use of an opioid) prior to being induced on buprenorphine, because its displacement of lower affinity, full μ agonists (eg, heroin) would cause a precipitated withdrawal. An additional benefit of buprenorphine is that federal law allows for its use in an office-based practice as opposed to an opioid treatment center. This allows for a physician who has been trained and has a waiver on their Drug Enforcement Administration license to see patients in their regular practice. The physician can determine the amount of medication prescribed and the interval indicated for follow-up for an individual patient, as opposed to following a strict federally mandated schedule for dosing adjustments and visits. Buprenorphine is typically prescribed in a form that includes a coating of naloxone in a 4:1 ratio of buprenorphine to naloxone. Naloxone, a μ-receptor antagonist, was added to the formulation to prevent dissolving buprenorphine in saline and injecting it intravenously. When taken as directed in sublingual form, very little naloxone is absorbed into the bloodstream, and there is no clinically relevant effect.

Patients who are abstinent from opioids for at least 7 to 10 days but who are at high risk for opioid relapse could be prescribed naltrexone. Naltrexone is an opioid antagonist and blocks opioid effects if opioids are administered after naltrexone. Naltrexone requires detoxification from all opioids prior to administration to avoid precipitating withdrawal. This medication may be a particularly good choice for individuals at high risk for opioid relapse who are leaving a controlled environment such as a drug treatment program, inpatient treatment program, or a correctional facility. Naltrexone comes in both oral and monthly intramuscular formulations, which can increase adherence.

Withdrawal can occur after the discontinuation of opioids that are being abused or taken as prescribed for analgesia or maintenance. Although withdrawal symptoms can be reduced by tapering the opioid over time, it is virtually impossible to eliminate them completely through tapering. Withdrawal is managed symptomatically, that is, by giving medications targeted at relieving the individual symptoms, such as loperamide for diarrhea and ibuprofen for muscle aches. The α_2-adrenergic agonist clonidine is useful for symptoms related to sympathetic outflow from the central nervous system, such as sweating and tachycardia.

Sedatives, Hypnotics, & Anxiolytics

For the purpose of this chapter, sedatives refer to medications commonly used for their sedating effects, namely benzodiazepines and barbiturates. In clinical practice, these medications are often used to treat panic disorder, anxiety, insomnia, and seizures. These medications typically act as agonists at the GABA receptor, although they have different binding sites.

Barbiturates were first used clinically in 1904. They can be divided into short-, intermediate-, and long-acting groups. They act by binding to the $GABA_A$ receptor at locations between the individual subunits. Barbiturates tend to increase the duration of chloride channel opening. Tolerance develops with regular use; however, the lethal dose varies greatly between individuals. There is no antidote to barbiturate overdose. As such, barbiturates began to fall out of favor clinically after the development of benzodiazepines in the 1960s, although phenobarbital, due to its very long half-life, is sometimes used as treatment for alcohol withdrawal and for some cases of epilepsy.

Benzodiazepines were first marketed in the 1960s for the treatment of anxiety. Like barbiturates, they can be divided into short-, intermediate-, and long-acting forms. They act by binding to $GABA_A$ receptors at the benzodiazepine site. Benzodiazepines tend to increase the frequency of chloride channel opening.

Sedative use initially causes relaxation and a reduction in anxiety. As serum concentrations rise, slurred speech, ataxia, and nystagmus can be seen. At still higher levels, coma and respiratory depression occur. An important point is that although tolerance may develop to the therapeutic effects of sedatives, there is no increase in the levels required to cause coma or respiratory depression. Flumazenil is a GABA/benzodiazepine receptor antagonist that can be used to reverse the effects of benzodiazepine overdose, but it must be used with caution because use can precipitate a seizure. No maintenance pharmacotherapy exists to treat sedative, hypnotic, or anxiolytic use disorder.

Sedative withdrawal symptoms may occur after as little as 2 months of continuous use. Anxiety, tremor, tachycardia, hypertension, irritability, and insomnia are common when withdrawing from lower dosages. When higher dosages are abruptly discontinued, seizures and delirium can occur. Thus,

alcohol and sedative intoxication and withdrawal syndromes have similarities due to these substances acting in similar ways at the $GABA_A$ receptor.

Detoxification from sedatives typically requires a prolonged taper over weeks to months, depending on the substance that had been abused. Generally speaking, higher dosages or shorter acting agents cause more severe withdrawal symptoms. As with alcohol, longer acting benzodiazepines are typically used because they are able to better control withdrawal symptoms and require less frequent dosing.

Stimulants (Cocaine & Amphetamines)

Cocaine is a stimulant derived from the leaves of the coca plant, *Erythroxylum coca*. It is native to South America, where the leaves have been chewed by the local population as a mild stimulant for perhaps 8000 years. Cocaine is clinically useful due to its anesthetic and vasoconstrictive properties. This makes it especially useful for surgeries involving the face and nasopharynx. It is not uncommon to find perforations of the nasal septum in individuals who chronically insufflate cocaine due to these vasoconstrictive properties. Illicit cocaine is found in 2 forms: a salt that is nasally insufflated or intravenously injected and a base (crack cocaine) that is typically smoked. When consumed in the presence of alcohol, the chemical cocaethylene is formed, which has significant cardiotoxic effects.

Cocaine affects the brain by increasing the amount of neurotransmitters in the synaptic cleft (Figure 43–5). Primarily, it blocks presynaptic reuptake of dopamine by binding to the dopamine reuptake transporter. It also affects norepinephrine and serotonin reuptake.

Cocaine use initially causes feeling of euphoria, increased energy, and pupillary dilation. As serum levels increase, symptoms of tachycardia, hypertension, anorexia, and agitation become apparent. Paranoia and hallucinations may also occur; however, it should be noted these are typically of the nonbizarre type. Death may occur through the sequelae of seizures, strokes, or arrhythmias.

Cocaine withdrawal is noted to cause fatigue, hypersomnia, increased appetite, psychomotor retardation, and dysphoria. Withdrawal is not life threatening. Unfortunately, there are no proven pharmacotherapeutic agents effective for the treatment of stimulant disorders. Behavioral treatment approaches, such as cognitive-behavioral therapy and contingency management, are the most effective for stimulant disorders.

Amphetamines were first discovered in the late 19th century. Current medicinal uses include the treatment of attention-deficit/hyperactivity disorder (ADHD), narcolepsy, and obesity. Amphetamine and the more potent methamphetamine are structurally related to bupropion and MDMA (ecstasy). Amphetamine is taken orally when used for approved purposes, but it is often crushed into a powder and nasally insufflated when abused. Although methamphetamine does come in an oral preparation for treatment of ADHD, its

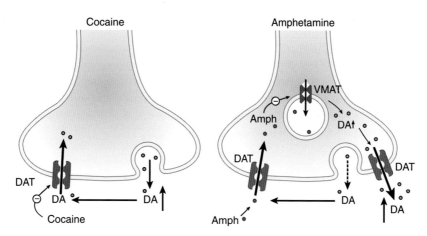

FIGURE 43–5 Mechanism of action of cocaine and amphetamine on synaptic terminal of dopamine (DA) neurons. *Left:* Cocaine inhibits the dopamine transporter (DAT), decreasing DA clearance from the synaptic cleft and causing an increase in extracellular DA concentration. *Right:* Because amphetamine (Amph) is a substrate of the DAT, it competitively inhibits DA transport. In addition, once in the cell, amphetamine interferes with the vesicular monoamine transporter (VMAT) and impedes the filling of synaptic vesicles. As a consequence, vesicles are depleted and cytoplasmic DA increases. This leads to a reversal of DAT direction, strongly increasing nonvesicular release of DA and further increasing extracellular DA concentrations. (Reproduced with permission from Katzung BG: *Basic and Clinical Pharmacology*, 14th ed. New York, NY: McGraw Hill; 2018.)

use is uncommon. The vast majority of methamphetamine that is abused is manufactured outside of the pharmaceutical industry, either by drug cartels or by individuals, using various household chemicals.

Like cocaine, amphetamines also cause an increase of neurotransmitters in the synaptic cleft, but via different mechanisms (see Figure 43–5). Although amphetamines block reuptake of synaptic dopamine via the dopamine transporter, they are able to cause the dopamine transporter to work in reverse, effectively pumping cytoplasmic dopamine into the synaptic cleft. This effect is compounded by the intracellular effects of amphetamines, which result in dopamine release from intracellular storage vesicles through its effects on the vesicular monoamine transporter.

Due to the similar mechanisms of action, the intoxication and withdrawal syndromes for amphetamines are similar to those of cocaine. Feelings of euphoria and a state of alertness progress to anxiety, agitation, and paranoia as serum levels rise. Insomnia is another side effect especially prominent with methamphetamine, causing binge users to remain awake for days at a time, exacerbating hallucinations and paranoia. Skin picking also may occur. This may be evident as sores or scabs, typically on the face or arms. Unlike amphetamine, methamphetamine is a neurotoxin.

Tobacco (Nicotine)

Nicotiana tabacum is a plant native to Central and South America from which the stimulant nicotine is derived. Commonly known as the tobacco plant, it has been smoked by indigenous people for thousands of years for a variety of purposes. It was introduced to Europe in the 1500s. Nicotine can be inhaled in cigarettes, cigars, or pipes or can be chewed by placing it between the gums and oral mucosa.

Nicotine is active at the nicotinic acetylcholine receptor. The receptors are found throughout the brain and not surprisingly affect dopamine in the reward pathway. When consumed via smoking, additional chemicals are inhaled, many of which are carcinogenic. Interestingly, some of these inhaled chemicals are also monoamine oxidase inhibitors (MAOIs). These MAOIs are the reason many people report that smoking has an antidepressant effect. Although there is no nicotine intoxication syndrome, nicotine is known to cause relaxation and to have anxiolytic properties despite being a mild stimulant.

Nicotine replacement therapy (NRT) is often the first pharmacologic method used for smoking cessation. The FDA has approved gum, lozenges, and patches as over-the-counter medications, whereas an inhaler and nasal spray are available with a prescription. The patch is long acting and applied daily. The patch can be worn for 24 hours, and common side effects include irritation at the patch site and vivid dreams. The patch can be removed before bed if the patient finds the vivid dreams unpleasant or has insomnia. The other shorter acting forms or NRT are used to substitute for cigarettes when cravings occur. The patch and a short-acting form of NRT can be used together for optimal effectiveness.

Bupropion is a norepinephrine-dopamine reuptake inhibitor that is most commonly used as an antidepressant, although it now has a second indication for smoking cessation treatment under the trade name of Zyban. It also has nicotine receptor antagonist properties that have been shown to decrease both nicotine withdrawal symptoms and cravings. Patients are allowed to continue smoking after starting the medication and commonly report "losing the taste" or experiencing a "bad taste" for cigarettes between 1 and 2 weeks of therapy. Bupropion has been shown to be effective alone or in combination with NRT to improve cessation outcomes.

CASE 43-1

Mrs. Jones is a divorced, 35-year-old white woman seen in the emergency department for an opioid overdose. She has been using heroin daily but is interested in treatment because local agencies recently removed her children from her home. She has a history of sexual abuse as a child (by her uncle) and has been sexually assaulted during the course of her drug use. She describes multiple incidents of being in life-threatening situations, including 2 sexual assaults, domestic violence from her ex-husband, and having a gun waved in her face. She reports using heroin daily for the past 12 months, and her longest period of abstinence was for 1 month during a 30-day inpatient treatment program 6 months ago. She had previously been prescribed hydrocodone 3 years earlier due to a fractured wrist from domestic violence. She reports that her physician prescribed this medication for about 3 months, and then she bought "pills" off the street until she progressed to heroin. When asked about her heroin use, she endorses using larger amounts than she initially intended, a desire to stop but being unable to quit using, spending most of her time trying to get heroin or being affected by use, cravings, inability to care for her children, needing more heroin to get the same effect (tolerance), and withdrawal symptoms. She meets criteria for

a severe opioid use disorder. In addition, she reports smoking cannabis daily for the past 10 years for her anxiety and admits to cravings for cannabis but denies any other symptoms or functional impairment due to her cannabis use. She reports regular use of alcohol and experimentation with cocaine and methamphetamine in her 20s but denies any regular use of these substances now. She also reports difficulties with sleep due to nightmares. When queried, she endorses symptoms consistent with posttraumatic stress disorder (PTSD), including intrusive and distressing memories of the sexual abuse, nightmares, increased arousal (hypervigilance, exaggerated startle response), avoidance of people and places that remind her of the abuse, feelings of shame and guilt, and distrust of others, particularly men. She notes that these symptoms have been present since her abuse as a child and cause impairment in her ability to form and maintain relationships. Treatment recommendations include medication-assisted therapy (buprenorphine or methadone), referral for outpatient substance abuse treatment for her opioid and cannabis use, referral to psychiatry for medication to help with her PTSD symptoms, and referral to a clinical psychologist for therapy focusing on prolonged exposure treatment for PTSD.

Varenicline functions as both a partial agonist and antagonist at the nicotine receptor. As such, it is able to prevent nicotine from binding to the receptors, while activating the receptor itself, but at lower levels of activity. Because varenicline is cleared through the kidneys, this medication may be preferred for patients with severe liver disease. Studies have shown varenicline to be the most effective single-medication treatment, and its effectiveness is comparable to that of combination NRT for smoking cessation.

SELF-ASSESSMENT QUESTIONS

1. Which of the following is not classified as a stimulant?
   A. Amphetamines
   B. Cocaine
   C. Methamphetamine
   D. Cannabis

2. Prolonged and heavy use of which substance generally requires medical detoxification?
   A. Alcohol
   B. Cocaine
   C. Cannabis
   D. Opioids

3. Which medication is used to reverse opioid overdoses?
   A. Methadone
   B. Buprenorphine
   C. Naltrexone
   D. Naloxone

4. Which substance is associated with the highest number of users?
   A. Alcohol
   B. Tobacco
   C. Caffeine
   D. Cannabis

Child & Adolescent Psychiatry

Yesie Yoon

PREVALENCE & BURDEN

Almost 1 in 5 children either currently or at some point during their life will have a severe mental disorder. Mental and substance use disorders are the leading cause of disability in children and youth worldwide, and depression is the number 1 cause of loss of disability-adjusted life-years. These conditions can affect children's development, educational attainment, and potential to live fulfilling and productive lives.

DISORDERS

In this chapter, psychiatric disorders prevalent in child and adolescent years are discussed. Some disorders will gradually improve with maturation, some will persist through adulthood, and some will worsen without adequate intervention. We will also note the different presentations of some common psychiatric disorders in children and adolescents. Eating disorders are also included in this chapter because their onset often occurs in adolescence.

Neurodevelopmental Disorders

Neurodevelopmental disorders are characterized by developmental deficits of the central nervous system, which can have prominent effects on personal, social, academic, or occupational functioning. These can vary from very specific impairments (eg, communication disorder) to global impairments (eg, intellectual disability). It is common for these disorders co-occur (eg, intellectual disability with autism spectrum disorder, or attention-deficit/hyperactive disorder [ADHD] with

a specific learning disorder). Because the etiology of these conditions varies, their presentation is also heterogeneous. There are few pharmacologic treatments indicated specifically for neurodevelopmental disorders, other than stimulants for ADHD. However, nonpharmacologic interventions such as speech therapy, occupational therapy, educational support, and psychotherapy can improve overall prognosis and daily functioning.

Intellectual disabilities are the result of a variety of prenatal, perinatal, and postnatal etiologies. Congenital causes include fetal alcohol syndrome (FAS), genetic conditions such as trisomy 21 and fragile X syndrome, and infections during pregnancy such as toxoplasmosis. In some cases, intellectual disability may result from severe head injury, infection, or other acquired factors after birth. Intellectual disability is characterized by deficits in general mental abilities and impairment in everyday adaptive functioning, compared with an individual's age-, gender-, and socioculturally matched peers. Examples of areas of impaired functioning may include reasoning, problem solving, planning, abstract thinking, judgment, academic learning, and learning from experience. With severe intellectual disability, delay in major milestones in the motor, language, and social aspects can be identified within 2 years of life, but mild cases may not be diagnosed until school age. Approximately 1% of the general population is affected by intellectual disabilities, and severe intellectual disability is estimated to be present in approximately 6 per 1000 population. Males are more likely than females to be diagnosed with intellectual disabilities. After childhood, the disorder is lifelong. When a delay in development is suspected either from caregiver's report or during routine screening, a child can be assessed for the possibility

VOCABULARY

Binge eating: Eating much more rapidly than normal, until feeling uncomfortably full; consuming large amounts of food when not hungry; eating alone because of feeling embarrassed about how much one is eating; or feeling disgusted with oneself, depressed, or guilty after overeating.

Encopresis: Repeated passage of feces in inappropriate places.

Enuresis: Repeated voiding of urine in inappropriate places.

Hyperactivity: Excessive motor activity or excessive fidgeting, tapping, or talkativeness.

Impulsivity: Hasty actions that occur in the moment without forethought and that have a high potential for harm to the individual.

Inattention: Wandering off task, lacking persistence, having difficulty sustaining focus, and being disorganized; not due to defiance or lack of comprehension.

of intellectual disability through comprehensive evaluation of intellectual capacity and adaptive functioning. Further workup to identify genetic and nongenetic etiologies should be considered. Given their various etiologies, there is no single pharmacologic treatment identified to treat intellectual disabilities. Early and ongoing nonpharmacologic treatment and intervention may improve adaptive functioning.

Speech sound disorder, a communication disorder, is defined as persistent difficulty with speech sound production that interferes with speech intelligibility. The disturbance causes limitation in effective communication. The onset of symptoms occurs in the early developmental period. Most children master mostly intelligible speech by 3 years of age, and other misarticulation should be corrected by 8 years of age. However, children with speech sound disorder continue to use immature misarticulation past community norm. When the diagnosis is suspected, regional, social, or cultural/ethnic variations of speech should be considered. Most children respond well to speech therapy, and speech difficulties improve over time.

In the United States, approximately 1 in 68 children has been diagnosed with **autism spectrum disorder** (ASD). It is reported to occur in all racial, ethnic, and socioeconomic groups. ASD is about 4.5 times more common among boys (1 in 42) than among girls (1 in 189). Worldwide prevalence is estimated to be between 1% and 2%. Heritability is estimated to be between 37% and 90% based on twin studies. Symptoms are typically recognized during the second year of life (12 to 24 months of age). Patients often initially present with delayed language development with lack of interest in social interaction, odd play patterns, and unusual communication patterns. Its key features include persistent impairment in reciprocal social communication and social interaction and restricted,

repetitive patterns of behavior, interests, or activities. These symptoms are present from early childhood, and the impairments limit everyday functioning. ASD is not a degenerative disorder, and learning and compensation continue throughout life. It is a spectrum disorder, which means the severity of symptoms and level of functioning vary greatly, and early detection and intervention are thought to be the key to a better prognosis. The Modified Checklist for Autism in Toddlers (M-CHAT) is applied to screen for ASD during pediatric check-ups between 16 and 30 months of age. The final diagnosis is made clinically based on the *Diagnostic and Statistical Manual of Mental Disorders*, Fifth Edition (DSM-V) criteria that emphasize clinical features; there is no biomarker or imaging study that is diagnostic. Standardized behavioral diagnostic instruments (eg, Autism Diagnostic Observation Schedule) are also available to improve the reliability of diagnosis. After a diagnosis is made, structured educational and behavioral interventions including Picture Exchange Communication System, pragmatic language skills training, applied behavioral analysis, and structured educational approaches have been shown to be effective and are associated with better outcomes.

ADHD has been reported in approximately 5% of children and 2.5% of adults in population surveys, but recent data show a higher prevalence in the United States. Its key features include a persistent pattern of inattention and hyperactivity-impulsivity that interferes with functioning or development. The dysfunction of brain areas for executive function and inhibitory control (frontal-striatal regions), catecholaminergic dysregulation, and delays in cortical maturation are all associated with ADHD. Before the age of 4 years, the symptoms of ADHD are difficult to distinguish from highly variable normative behaviors. In preschool, the main symptom is hyperactivity, which becomes less obvious in adolescence and adulthood. Restlessness, inattention, poor planning, and impulsivity may remain problematic. Some symptoms improve over time. Diagnosis can be made based on DSM-V criteria if there is consistent information from at least 2 separate contexts. Rating scales can be helpful to obtain an objective report from informants other than the primary caregiver. Prior to making the diagnosis, other causes of inattention, hyperactivity, or impulsivity such as ASD, anxiety disorder, depressive disorder, and substance use disorder should be evaluated.

The first-line pharmacologic treatments for ADHD are *methylphenidate* and *amphetamine.* These are stimulants medications and have been proven to be effective in the treatment of core symptoms. Both increase norepinephrine and dopamine in the synaptic cleft by inhibiting reuptake and increasing release from presynaptic neurons. Prior to treatment with these drugs, a physical exam and careful family history should be obtained because they may have serious adverse effects on the cardiovascular system. Insomnia and decreased appetite are common and problematic side effects. Other possible side effects include hypertension, tachycardia, psychosis, anxiety, nausea, and headache. Other nonstimulant pharmacologic treatments such as *clonidine* and *guanfacine* can also be considered. Clonidine is a nonselective α_2-adrenergic agonist, and guanfacine is a selective α_{2A}-adrenergic agonist. They both decrease activity of the locus coeruleus, which may have increased basal activity in individuals with ADHD. Side effects of an α_2 agonist include rebound hypertension and tachycardia, sedation, dizziness, constipation, headache, and fatigue. *Atomoxetine* can be used for ADHD patients with comorbid anxiety disorder who report worsening anxiety with stimulants. Atomoxetine is a norepinephrine reuptake inhibitor that can cause decreased appetite, dizziness, dyspepsia, and sedation as side effects.

Specific learning disorder is defined as persistent difficulties learning keystone academic skills including the reading of single words, reading comprehension, written expression and spelling, arithmetic calculation, and mathematical reasoning. The individual with a specific learning disorder has well-below-average skill for age, that is not due to lack of opportunity of learning or inadequate instruction. The disorder is apparent in the early school years in most individuals, and the prevalence is estimated to be 5% to 15% of school-age children. Diagnosis of a specific learning disorder usually occurs when children are required to learn to read, spell, write, and learn mathematics. Psychological testing, neuropsychological testing, and projective testing can be applied to support the diagnosis. Symptoms typically persist into adulthood, but the course is variable. Educational support using accommodation modification such as an individualized education plan is important.

Tic disorders are characterized by a sudden, rapid, recurrent, nonrhythmic motor movement or vocalization. Simple motor tics include eye blinking, shoulder shrugging, and extension of the extremities. Simple vocal tics include throat clearing, sniffing, and grunting. Complex motor tics are a stereotyped combination of movements. Examples of complex vocal tics are repeating sounds or words, repeating the last heard word of the phrase, or uttering socially unacceptable words. Patients report a premonitory urge before a tic and a feeling of tension reduction after the expression of the tic. Tics are often suppressible for a period of time. The diagnosis of a tic disorder can be made when there are motor and vocal tics and the symptoms are present for >1 year. If the symptoms are present for <1 year, *provisional tic disorder* is an appropriate diagnosis. **Tourette syndrome** is diagnosed when both multiple motor tics and 1 or more vocal tics have been present at some time during the illness, although not necessarily concurrently. Tics are common in childhood but transient in most cases. The estimated prevalence of Tourette syndrome is 3 to 8 per 1000 school-age children. Males are 2 to 4 times more likely to be diagnosed with tic disorder than females. Onset is typically between ages 4 and 6 years, and peak onset occurs between ages 10 and 12 years; severity then declines during adolescence. Many adults with tic disorders experience diminished symptoms, but a small number of patients will have persistent or worsening symptoms in adulthood. Tics wax and wane in severity and change in affected muscle groups and vocalizations over time. ADHD, obsessive-compulsive disorder, and anxiety disorders are common comorbidities with tic disorders (Figure 44–1).

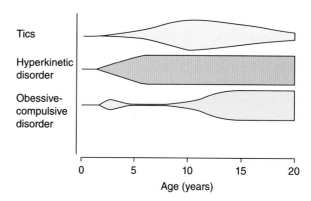

FIGURE 44–1 Age at which tics and coexisting disorders affect patients. Width of bars shows schematically the amount the disorder affects a patient at a particular age. (Reproduced with permission from Leckman JF: Tourette's syndrome, *Lancet*. 2002 Nov 16;360(9345):1577-1586.)

Effective nonpharmacologic treatment options include habit reversal training, where individuals are trained to replace a tic with a competing response that is a more comfortable or acceptable movement or sound. Pharmacologic treatment is recommended only when tics result in significant subjective discomfort, pain, or ongoing social problems. α_2-Adrenergic agonists such as *clonidine* and *guanfacine* reduce symptoms by decreasing sympathetic nerve impulses. Atypical antipsychotic agents, such as risperidone, and high-potency, first-generation antipsychotics such as *haloperidol* can also be considered if the benefit outweighs the risk. Significant and possibly life-threatening side effects can occur with antipsychotics, including neuroleptic malignant syndrome, extrapyramidal symptoms including tardive dyskinesia, sedation, increased appetite, and weight gain.

Mood Disorders in Children & Adolescents

Mood disorders are common in childhood and adolescence. **Major depressive disorder** (MDD) is estimated to be present in approximately 2% of children and 4% to 8% of adolescents. There is no significant difference in prevalence between males and females during childhood, but in adolescence, females have a higher prevalence compared to males. The cumulative prevalence of MDD is 20% by age 18 years. Children and adolescents with MDD often report irritability rather than depressed mood. They also exhibit poor concentration that affects academic performance. Depression in children is associated with childhood neglect, parental mental illness (eg, depression, substance use disorder), domestic violence, marital conflict, or persistent parental conflict following separation, divorce, or child abuse. Some children and adolescents who experience a major depressive episode may eventually develop **bipolar disorder**. Children with bipolar disorder are more likely to have a family history of this illness. In individuals with bipolar disorder, mood usually alternates between high mood (mania) and low mood (depression) more rapidly than in adults. This rapid and severe cycling between moods may produce a type of chronic irritability with few clear periods of peace between episodes. Patients may also experience symptoms of mania and depression at the same time, which is defined as a mixed episode. See Chapter 39 for further information on mood disorders.

Anxiety Disorders in Children & Adolescents

Anxiety can be normal for children and adolescents when faced with an unfamiliar or especially stressful situation. It becomes pathologic or problematic when it is excessive or persists beyond developmentally appropriate periods.

Separation anxiety disorder is the most prevalent anxiety disorder in children younger than age 12 years. The 6- to 12-month prevalence is estimated to be approximately 4% in children and 1.6% in adolescents. Increased anxiety related to separation from attachment figures is normal in early development. However, the anxiety can be viewed as problematic if it is excessive for the child's age or cultural norm. Children who are diagnosed with separation anxiety disorder have exacerbations and remissions, although in some cases, symptoms may persist through adulthood. The disorder is characterized by excessive fear or anxiety concerning separation from home or attachment figures. Younger children are more reluctant to go to school or may avoid school altogether. As children age, they often worry about specific dangers (eg, accidents, kidnapping, or death) or not being reunited with attachment figures. Repeated nightmares about separation or physical symptoms may occur when separation is anticipated. To meet the diagnostic criteria, fear, anxiety, or avoidance needs to be persistent, lasting at least 4 weeks in children and adolescents and 6 months or more in adults. See Chapter 40 for further information on anxiety disorders.

Trauma- & Stress-Related Disorders

Traumatic events such as neglect, physical or sexual abuse, natural or manmade disasters, violent crimes such as kidnapping or school shooting, and motor vehicle accidents can lead to the development of **posttraumatic stress disorder** (PTSD). It is estimated that approximately 5% of adolescents will meet criteria for PTSD in their lifetime, whereas the number of children exposed to traumatic events is much higher. Children and adolescents experience symptoms of PTSD that are similar to those of adults, including intrusion symptoms, negative alterations in cognition and mood, avoidance and numbing, and hyperarousal symptoms. Some school-age children may experience visual flashbacks or amnesia, but others will have *time skew* and *omen formation*, symptoms that are not typically seen in adults. Time skew refers to a child missequencing trauma-related events when recalling the memory. Omen formation is a belief that there were warning signs that predicted the trauma. The child's trauma is often exhibited in play, drawings, or verbalization. Adolescents tend to engage in traumatic reenactment, in which they incorporate aspects of the trauma into their daily lives. Adolescents are also more likely to exhibit impulsive and aggressive behaviors compared to children and adults with PTSD. Due to these distinctive features of PTSD in children, play therapy can help children process the traumatic memories. Other therapies and pharmacologic treatment that are effective in adults with PTSD can also be applied in children and adolescents.

Reactive attachment disorder is seen in children who have absent or underdeveloped attachment with putative caregiving adults. When distressed, they show no consistent effort to obtain comfort, support, nurturance, or protection from caregivers. It often co-occurs with delays in cognition and language. The clinical features include absent to minimal attachment behaviors in children between the ages of 9 months and 5 years. There is also a consistent pattern of inhibited, emotionally withdrawn behavior toward adult caregivers, which causes persistent social and emotional disturbance. Without a normative caregiving environment to remediate, symptoms may persist for several years.

Feeding & Eating Disorders

Feeding and eating disorders are characterized by a persistent disturbance of eating or eating-related behavior that results in the altered consumption or absorption of food. These behaviors significantly impair physical and psychological health and functioning. Abnormal eating behaviors seem to develop as a way of handling stress and anxieties. Although many disorders under this category share some features, there are substantial differences in clinical course, outcome, and treatment needs. In brief, anorexia is a form of self-starvation, bulimia nervosa is related to repetitive cycles of binge eating alternating with self-induced vomiting or starvation, and binge-eating disorder is when an individual has binge-eating behaviors without compensatory behaviors. Some individuals with these disorders report symptoms such as craving and compulsion, which are typical symptoms of substance use disorders.

Anorexia nervosa (AN) commonly begins during adolescence and young adulthood. The onset is often associated with a stressful life event, and the course is variable. The 12-month prevalence among young females is approximately 0.4%, and lifetime prevalence is 0.5% to 1%. It is 10 times more prevalent in females compared to males. After the onset of symptoms, many patients exhibit a fluctuating pattern, and some experience a chronic course over many years. Long-term follow-up shows a mortality rate of 7% at 10-year follow-up and 18% to 30% at 30-year follow-up, which is higher than any other mental illness. Individuals with AN report fear of gaining weight or of becoming fat and exhibit persistent behavior that interferes with weight gain. These behaviors include restriction of energy intake relative to requirements, leading to a significantly low body weight in the context of age, sex, developmental trajectory, and physical health. Body mass index (BMI) for adults or BMI percentile for children and adolescents can be used to determine a healthy weight for each patient. In the *restricting type* of AN, weight loss is accomplished primarily through dieting, fasting, and excessive exercise. The *binge-eating/ purging type* of AN involves recurrent episodes of binge eating or purging behavior during the past 3 months. Binge eating is defined as eating an amount of food that is greater than what most individuals would consume. It is also accompanied by a sense of lack of control. Examples of purging behavior include self-induced vomiting; misuse of laxatives, diuretics, or other medications; fasting; or excessive exercise. Treatment consists of nutritional rehabilitation to restore weight, normalizing eating patterns, reestablishing normal perception of hunger, and correction of malnutrition. With severe malnutrition, hospitalization with close monitoring for refeeding syndrome is recommended. Psychotherapy has shown utility in adults, especially family-based therapy. However, medications are not generally effective for AN.

Bulimia nervosa is characterized by recurrent episodes of binge eating without abnormally low body weight. The 12-month prevalence among young females is 1% to 1.5%. After binge-eating behavior, recurrent inappropriate compensatory behaviors follow to prevent weight gain. Patients are often ashamed of their eating problems and attempt to conceal their symptoms. There is also excessive emphasis on body shape or weight, which affects self-esteem. The course may be chronic or intermittent, with periods of remission. The crude mortality rate for bulimia nervosa is nearly 2% per decade. The pharmacologic treatment *fluoxetine* is effective in decreasing binge and purge episodes. Because it is an antidepressant that works by selectively inhibiting reuptake of serotonin, it also treats comorbidities such as depression and obsessive-compulsive disorder. The most effective treatment strategy is combining antidepressant medication and cognitive-behavioral therapy. Other forms of therapy such as family-based therapy and dialectical behavioral therapy can also be helpful.

In contrast to bulimia nervosa, **binge-eating disorder** is not accompanied by compensatory behaviors. This disorder typically begins in adolescence or young adulthood but can also begin in later adulthood. Like bulimia, recurrent episodes of binge eating occur, but they are not associated with the recurrent compensatory behavior such as purging after binge eating. It can occur in normal-weight or overweight/obese individuals, and the remission rates are higher for binge-eating disorder than for bulimia or AN. For pharmacologic treatment, antidepressants (eg, selective serotonin reuptake inhibitors) have been shown to improve symptoms of binge-eating behavior. Antiepileptic drugs (eg, topiramate) can decrease appetite and overall improve binge-eating behavior. However, topiramate has side effects such as cognitive impairment, paresthesia, and somnolence. Stimulants (eg, lisdexamfetamine) also decrease appetite and weight, but there are side effects including anorexia, gastrointestinal distress, headaches, insomnia, and sympathetic nervous system arousal. Nonpharmacologic treatment, including cognitive-behavioral therapy, interpersonal therapy, dialectical behavioral therapy, and family therapy, can also be considered to improve symptoms.

Pica is defined as eating 1 or more nonnutritive, nonfood substances on a persistent basis over a period of at least 1 month. This abnormal eating must be developmentally, culturally, and socially inappropriate. It is important to recognize that pica may be caused by vitamin or mineral deficiencies, particularly iron and zinc. Pica can cause medical complications such as intestinal obstruction, intestinal perforation, toxoplasmosis, toxocariasis, and lead poisoning.

Elimination Disorders

Elimination disorders involve the inappropriate elimination of urine or feces. In infancy and toddler years, lack of continence is developmentally appropriate. Therefore, these diagnoses have minimal age requirements based on the level of development, not chronologic age. Both enuresis and encopresis can be voluntary or involuntary.

Enuresis is defined as repeated voiding of urine in inappropriate places. *Primary enuresis* is when urinary continence was never established and the developmental level is at least 5 years, and *secondary enuresis* is when the disturbance develops after a period of established urinary continence. In the United States, 30% of children achieve continence by age 2, and both primary and secondary enuresis have a spontaneous remission rate of 5% to 10% per year. Most children become continent by adolescence, but 1% of cases continue into adulthood. The *nocturnal-only subtype* is the most common, with the incontinence occurring only during nighttime sleep. *Diurnal-only subtype* is the absence of nocturnal enuresis and may be referred as to as urinary incontinence. Workup should rule out a physical cause of incontinence, especially if a child presents with repeated urinary tract infections. Ultrasounds and voiding cystourethrograms can help reveal underlying physical abnormalities such as detrusor hypertrophy and overactive bladder. Other evaluations including electroencephalogram or sleep study can be considered if there are other symptoms concerning for seizure or obstructive sleep apnea, which also can cause incontinence. Education for the family and patient and watchful waiting should be tried prior to considering interventions. *Bell-and-pad therapy* is a nonpharmacologic treatment that relies upon classical and operant conditioning. A child sleeps on the pad, which triggers an alarm when the child begins to urinate. It takes a few months to work and the success rate is 80% to 90%, but the relapse rate can be up to 40%. Other interventions such as bladder volume alarm, timed night awakening, and bladder training exercises can be considered. In terms of pharmacologic treatment, *desmopressin* is a long-acting arginine vasopressin (antidiuretic hormone [ADH]) that increases water reabsorption at the renal collecting duct, which results in reduced urine output. The success rate is between 10% and 65%, with a relapse rate as high as 80%. When desmopressin is used, sodium should be monitored due to risk for hyponatremia. *Imipramine* is a tricyclic antidepressant, and its anticholinergic properties cause relaxation of the bladder detrusor muscle and increase sphincter tone. It also increases the release of ADH, which results in free water retention and suppresses rapid eye movement sleep, which helps the child to wake up. The partial success rate is around 50%, but complete remission occurs in only about 25% of patients. Imipramine also has significant side effects including lethality in overdose, suicidal ideation, cardiac dysrhythmias, convulsions, and coma. In addition, 10% of patients report more common side effects related to its anticholinergic properties including drowsiness, dry mouth, dizziness, constipation, blurred vision, difficulty starting urine stream, and palpitation.

Encopresis is defined as repeated passage of feces in inappropriate places, which can be involuntary or intentional. When the passage of feces is involuntary, it is often related to constipation, impaction, or retention with subsequent overflow. Its prevalence is approximately 1% of 5-year-old children, and it occurs more often in males than females. Inadequate, inconsistent toilet training and psychosocial stress may be predisposing factors. *Primary encopresis* is when a child has never established fecal continence, and *secondary encopresis* is when the disturbance develops after a period of established fecal continence. When the diagnosis is suspected, physical exam and gastrointestinal imaging may be informative to assess stool burden. Other medical conditions, such as Hirschsprung disease, should be ruled out by barium enema and anorectal manography. Education for the family and patient including encouraging high-fiber food, increased fluid intake, and regular bathroom times should be provided. If encopresis is the retentive type, laxatives and stool softeners can be given to assist in emptying of the bowel.

Disruptive, Impulse-Control, & Conduct Disorders

Disruptive, impulse-control, and conduct disorders include conditions involving problems in the self-control of emotions and behaviors. These disorders are unique in that these behaviors violate the rights of others and bring the individual into significant conflict with societal norms and authority figures. They all tend to be more common in males than in females, although the relative degree of male predominance may differ. Although there is a developmental relationship between **oppositional defiant disorder** (ODD) and conduct disorder, not every child with ODD develops conduct disorder later in life.

Usually, ODD first appears during the preschool years and rarely after early adolescence. Angry or irritable mood, argumentative or defiant behavior, and vindictiveness characterize this disorder. Patients often justify their behavior as a response to unreasonable demands or circumstances. Children with defiant, argumentative, and vindictive symptoms develop a conduct disorder. Those with angry, irritable mood symptoms carry the risk of developing anxiety disorder or depression. Parent–child interaction therapy is a useful nonpharmacologic treatment option. There is no medication indicated for ODD, but it is important to identify and treat comorbidities such as ADHD, depression, PTSD, and bipolar disorder.

Diagnosis of **conduct disorder** can be made when there are symptoms of aggression to people and animals, destruction of property, deceitfulness or theft, and serious violations of rules. The onset may occur as early as the preschool years, but it occurs mostly in childhood and adolescence and rarely after the age of 16 years. The early-onset type has a poor prognosis and has more risk for criminal behavior and substance-related disorders. The 12-month prevalence is anywhere from 2% to >10%, and it is higher among males. Multisystemic therapy involving the individual, family, peers, school, and neighborhood can be effective and helpful.

Other Conditions

Fetal alcohol syndrome is a consequence of prenatal alcohol exposure, but not all exposure leads to FAS. Individuals affected by FAS can have facial anomalies including short palpebral features, flat or indistinct philtrum, and a thin vermillion border of the upper lip (Figure 44–2). There is also growth retardation that affects height more than weight. Central nervous system dysfunction is also significant. Microcephaly, structural brain abnormalities, and other neurologic

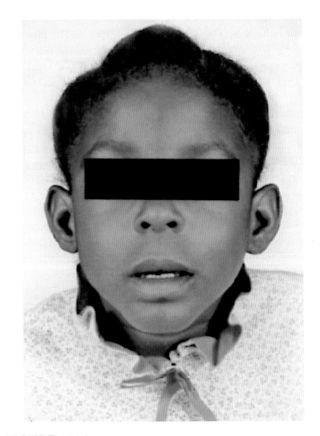

FIGURE 44–2 Fetal alcohol syndrome: midface hypoplasia, absent philtrum, and microcephaly. (Reproduced with permission from Fuster V, Walsh RA, Harrington RA: *Hurst's the Heart*. 13th ed. New York, NY: McGraw Hill; 2011.)

CASE 44–1

A mother brings her 20-month-old boy, Adam, to the pediatrician's office for a well-child check. The mother had no complications during pregnancy and delivery, and Adam was examined at birth by a pediatrician who discharged him from newborn nursery with no concerns. The mother tells the pediatrician that Adam has always been a fussy infant and an extremely picky eater but otherwise has been healthy. The mother was concerned that he has not been able to produce any meaningful words yet. Adam has an older brother who has developmental delay and is in a special education class. She says that Adam expresses his frustrations by throwing extreme temper tantrums, is aggressive to his newborn sister and mother, and has no interest in playing with other children. He rocks himself back and forth when stressed, does not adapt well to changes in routine, and focuses on lining up his toy cars for hours at a time. The family struggles with going to new places, traveling, and visiting relatives due to his behavior. As a part of routine screening, the Modified Checklist for Autism in Toddlers (M-CHAT) is applied, which shows an abnormal result. After examining him in the office and reviewing the M-CHAT, the pediatrician orders hearing testing and measurement of lead level, which are both normal. The pediatrician then refers Adam to a neurodevelopmental specialist who diagnoses him with autism spectrum disorder after obtaining the history, observing the child, and administering the Autism Diagnostic Observation Schedule.

problems occur. In terms of psychiatric symptoms, cognitive impairments, developmental delay, executive functioning deficits, learning disabilities, poor academic achievement, language problems, visual-spatial impairment, and memory impairment are all observed.

Rett syndrome is a postnatal neurologic disorder that is caused by mutations on the X chromosome in a gene called *MECP2*. It occurs worldwide in 1 in 10,000 female births and

only rarely in males because the mutation in Rett syndrome is almost exclusively on the paternally derived X chromosome. Symptoms appear after an early period of apparently normal or nearly normal development until 6 to 18 months of life. After this period, there is stagnation following regression of development. The course and severity of Rett syndrome are determined by the location, type, and severity of the mutation as well as X-inactivation. The main symptoms include stereotypic hand movements, gait disturbances, and slowing of head growth. Psychiatric symptoms include inconsolable cries, irritability, lack of social/emotional reciprocity, impaired use of nonverbal communication, sensory problems, extreme tantrums, and language impairments.

SELF-ASSESSMENT QUESTIONS

1. Which of the following is the most effective treatment for attention-deficit/hyperactivity disorder (ADHD)?
    A. Fluoxetine
    B. Clonidine
    C. Valproate
    D. Methylphenidate
    E. Atomoxetine

2. Which of the following is a true statement about tic disorder?
    A. The onset of tic disorder is rarely before the age of 12 years.
    B. Prevalence of tic disorder is higher in females.
    C. Tourette syndrome is diagnosed when both multiple motor tics and 1 or more vocal tics have been present at some time during the illness, although not necessarily concurrently.
    D. Tic disorder continues to worsen throughout adolescence, and most people live with severe symptoms throughout adulthood.
    E. Medication should be started as soon as the first symptom occurs.

3. Which of following symptoms of major depressive disorder (MDD) is more prominent in child and adolescents compared to adults?
    A. Insomnia
    B. Irritable mood
    C. Loss of energy
    D. Loss of interest
    E. Feeling worthless

Answers

Chapter 1

1. **D.** The vast majority of axonal proteins are synthesized in the cell soma. Axonal transport includes fast and slow axonal transport from the cell soma along the axon to the presynaptic terminus. Fast axonal transport is for transport of large organelles and vesicles and depends on microtubules and microtubule motors (kinesins for anterograde transport and dyneins for retrograde transport). Slow axonal transport is for cytosolic and cytoskeletal proteins. (Recent studies suggest that slow transport may also involve microtubules, but the cytosolic and cytoskeletal cargoes may stop more along the way.)

2. **B.** White matter is found in only the CNS (not the PNS) and contains myelinated axons, white matter astrocytes, and the myelinating oligodendrocytes. Pericytes line the brain capillaries (and white matter does have capillaries), but ependymal cells are located only in the ventricles.

3. **C.** Brain capillaries are formed by vascular endothelial cells surrounded by pericytes. Astrocytes form end feet on these capillaries; transport a variety of nutrients, including energy substrates; and release substances that can regulate blood flow. Microglia are the immune cells of the CNS, and neuronal processes such as dendrites or dendritic spines form the postsynaptic component of the synapse. Astrocytes can surround the synapse, forming the tripartite synapse.

4. **A.** No matter its function, be it a sensory neuron, motor neuron, or interneuron, all neurons form synapses or contacts with target cells and signal or communicate with their targets. Depending on their function, different neurons can have very different types of morphologies, and not all have an axon or branched dendrites. Neuronal cell bodies can be present in the PNS (dorsal root ganglia and autonomic ganglia); not all axons are myelinated (about half are not) or branched; and not all dendrites are spiny.

5. **E.** The BBB does not prevent entry of hydrophobic molecules, only hydrophilic molecules. The BBB prevents the entry of the majority of pathogenic and immune cells. The majority of neurons do not contact the brain capillaries and hence depend on astrocytes for essential nutrients and energy substrates. The BBB forms late in development after neurogenesis and gliogenesis. As described earlier, the BBB is formed by vascular endothelial cells, which are surrounded by pericytes.

Chapter 2

1. **A.** Neural induction occurs after gastrulation, when the notochord at the midline (and surrounding paraxial mesoderm) releases morphogens to the overlying ectoderm. These morphogens inhibit the BMP signaling pathway in the ectoderm and instruct the ectoderm to form the neural plate (neuroectoderm). Once the plate is formed, it undergoes neurulation followed by segmentation and flexure.

2. **D.** Errors in neurogenesis and gliogenesis cause microcephaly. Errors in neuronal migration cause cortical malformations such as heterotopias. Neural tube defects result from errors in closing of the neural tube. The neural tube forms from the neural plate via the process of neurulation. The neural tube gives rise to almost all the neurons and glia of the CNS (a small number of neurons that end up in the CNS arise from placodes or neural crest). The lumen of the neural tube forms the brain ventricles and central canal.

3. **B.** The myelencephalon gives rise to the medulla oblongata. The mesencephalon gives rise to the midbrain. The telencephalon gives rise to the cerebral hemispheres and several subcortical structures. The diencephalon gives rise to the thalamus and hypothalamus. The metencephalon gives rise to the pons and cerebellum.

4. **C.** For most cortical regions, neurons develop before glia. The vast majority of CNS neurons and glia develop from the neural tube, whereas all the PNS neurons and glia develop from neural crest cells. Neural stem cells and neural progenitor cells are the precursors of both neurons and glia during neurogenesis and gliogenesis. Both neurogenesis and gliogenesis occur both prenatally and postnatally. Neurogenesis and gliogenesis occur after neurulation.

5. **E.** Synapses form between presynaptic axons and their targets, which can be other neurons (on dendrites, the cell soma and other axons) or muscles or glands. Apoptosis refers to cell death, and although some are lost, not all synapses are eliminated during critical periods. Synapses are dynamic structures that are formed both prenatally and postnatally and in the adult CNS. Radial glial cells guide axons during migration before synapses form. Synapses are dynamic structures that undergo synaptic plasticity and can form or be eliminated, weakened, or strengthened.

Chapter 3

1. **E.** The left and right cerebral hemispheres are separated by the longitudinal fissure (also known as the deep sagittal fissure). Only the parietal, occipital, and temporal lobes contain substantial cortical areas dedicated to sensory processing, and only the frontal lobe has substantial cortical areas dedicated to motor function. However, because they are all well connected, all the lobes do contribute to sensory processing and motor function. The locations of the primary gyri and sulci are very similar among humans, but the

secondary and tertiary gyri and sulci can be located differentially among individuals. The right and left hemispheres are not functionally identical because some functions such as language are lateralized and/or more prominent on 1 side of the brain. The insular lobe and limbic lobe are considered the fifth and sixth "functional" lobes but are not visible from the exterior view of the brain.

2. **C.** The human brain contains both neocortex (6 layers) and allocortex (3 to 4 layers); for example, the hippocampus is allocortex. Association cortices are mainly involved in processing either sensory or motor information, but not both. The cortical column is considered the smallest functional unit, and columns have been identified in both visual and somatosensory cortex. The human neocortex is large and represents about 75% of cerebral gray matter. The cortical gray matter lies on top of the cerebral white matter and underneath the meninges.

3. **D.** The amygdala processes many emotions, including pleasant and negative emotions such as fear. Although the hippocampus and associated structures are required for encoding declarative and spatial memories, most explicit memories are thought to be stored in many other areas of the cerebral cortex. Olfactory sensory information is not relayed by way of the thalamus. The primary and secondary auditory cortices are located in the temporal lobe. The ventral regions of the temporal lobe form the ventral stream, or "what" pathway involved in visual processing that aids in object and facial recognition.

4. **B.** As the "gateway" to the cerebral cortex, the thalamus transmits sensory, motor, and cognitive information between the cerebral cortex and the spinal cord, basal ganglia, brainstem, and cerebellum. The thalamus contains at least 60 individual nuclei that form specific connections. The basic life functions listed are the job of the hypothalamus. As mentioned earlier, the thalamus does not relay information from the olfactory nerve.

5. **A.** The BG control voluntary movements including motor initiation and motivation-based movements and procedural (a type of implicit) learning and is involved in cognition of motivation and reward. Anatomically, the BG do not include the thalamus. The BG communicate with the cerebral cortex by way of the thalamus; they do not have direct input to the cerebral cortex. The BG are not required for declarative memory, only for nondeclarative/procedural memory. Loss of neurons in the substantia nigra, a component of the BG, is associated with only Parkinson disease and Huntington disease.

Chapter 4

1. **C.** The brainstem includes the midbrain, pons, and medulla but not the basal ganglia (although some anatomists may include the diencephalon). Voluntary motor information that controls body movement and sensory information from the body are transmitted via white matter tracts that travel through the brainstem but do not require relay there. The brainstem is required for life-sustaining control of breathing, sleep, and other functions. Damage to the brainstem often lead to loss of consciousness and is often life threatening, especially because of the loss of breathing control. The brainstem houses sensory and motor tracts and the majority (10 of 12) of cranial nerve nuclei.

2. **E.** The cerebellum receives inputs from the cerebral cortices via the pons through the cerebellar peduncles. The main functions of the cerebellum are in control and coordination of movement, posture and balance, motor learning, and some cognitive functions. The cerebellum contains only 3 functional regions, as there is no bulbar cerebellum. Damage to the cerebellum leads to loss of coordination of movement, abnormal gait, and inability to judge distances.

3. **D.** Answer choice D is not true because motor axons exit the SC via the ventral roots, whereas axons enter the SC via the dorsal roots.

4. **B.** The ventricles contain the choroid plexus and are lined with ependymal cells, which both synthesize CSF. Only the cerebral aqueduct and fourth ventricle lie within the brainstem since the third ventricle is surrounded by the thalamus. The ventricles and CC are formed from the lumen of the neural tube. CSF flows from the lateral ventricles to the third ventricle to the fourth ventricle and then via the cisterna magna to the subarachnoid space.

5. **A.** The blood supply to the brain and spinal cord depends on 2 paired branches of the dorsal aorta (the internal carotid arteries arise from bifurcation of the left and right common carotid arteries, and the vertebral arteries are branches of the left and right subclavian arteries). The vertebral arteries supply the posterior part of the brain. The internal carotid arteries supply the anterior part of the brain. In addition to arteries, arterioles, veins, and venules, there are many capillaries that supply the brain. The main outflow from the brain is the jugular vein.

Chapter 5

1. **C.** The negative potential inside neurons causes exiting of chloride ions through leakage channels.

2. **A.** The Na+/K+ ATP pump is necessary for the ionic concentration differences underlying the action potential.

3. **B.** Amino acids and neurotransmitters are transported across neural membranes by active pumps.

4. **D.** The K+ ion channel causes the relative refractory period.

5. **E.** *Ligand-gated* means opened by binding a neurotransmitter.

Chapter 6

1. **A.** The potential difference across the membrane is a result of the separation charge and is called the resting membrane potential. The potential difference across the membrane

is a direct function the numbers of positive and negative charges on either side of the membrane. As the separation of charge (ie, the differences between the charges) across the membrane is reduced, the membrane is said to be depolarized. Conversely, as the difference between the charges is increased, the membrane becomes hyperpolarized. In the latter case, the inside of the cell is made more negative with respect to the outside. If a cell has only a single channel in its membrane (eg, for K^+), the gradients for the other become irrelevant and the membrane will approach the equilibrium potential for the single ion (K^+ in this example). There is a tendency for ions to leak down their electrochemical gradients from one side of the membrane to the other. For there to be a steady resting membrane potential, the gradients across the membrane must be held constant. Changes in ionic gradients are avoided, despite the leak, by the presence of an active Na^+/K^+ pump (a membrane protein) that moves Na^+ out of the cell and at the same time brings K^+ into the cell. Such pumping mechanism requires energy because it is working against the electrochemical gradients of the 2 ions. This energy is derived from hydrolysis of ATP.

2. **A.** In the late phase of the action potential, potassium channels become opened and potassium efflux produces a hyperpolarization of the membrane. During the repolarization of the membrane, sodium channels are closed (sodium inactivation). Recall that activation of sodium channels is associated with the generation of the action potential. Calcium has a strong electrochemical gradient that drives it into the cell; this coincides with the upstroke of the action potential. A number of different types of calcium-gated potassium channels have been described that are activated during the action potential. Thus, it would appear that calcium influx during the action potential could generate opposing effects. On the one hand, calcium influx carries a positive charge into the cell, which contributes to the depolarization of the membrane. On the other hand, calcium influx may help to open up more potassium channels, which contributes to an outward ionic flow of potassium that causes repolarization of the membrane.

3. **D.** The trigger zone for the initiation of impulses from a neuron includes a specialized region of the cell body—the axon hillock—together with the section of the axon that adjoins this region—the initial segment. Other components of the neuron, such as the dendrites and cell body, receive inputs from afferent sources but are not capable of initiating impulses at these sites. The same is true about more distal aspects of the axon over which the impulse is conducted.

4. **A.** Because the membrane is a leaky one, the sodium-potassium pump assists in actively transporting ions from one side of the membrane to the other. The membrane is permeable to ions other than potassium, such as sodium and chloride. This fact is taken into consideration in the Goldman equation. This equation includes the distribution of all of these other ions in its formula for determining the value of membrane potential. Accordingly, the resting membrane potential is dependent upon the concentration of these other ions as well as potassium. Although it is true that the Nernst equation considers the relative distribution of potassium ions across the membrane, this statement in itself does not explain why the equilibrium potential for potassium differs from the resting potential of the neuron. The statement that the Nernst equation does not take into account differences in temperature is false. But, again, even if that statement were true, it would not account for the differences between the equilibrium potential for potassium and the resting potential of the neuron.

5. **E.** The action potential is characterized by an all-or-none response in which the overshoot may reach an amplitude of up to 100 mV. The mechanism involves separate ion channels for sodium and potassium. The resting potential is characterized by a relatively steady potential, usually in the region of 270 mV, but that may range from 235 to 270 mV. This potential is mainly dependent on potassium and chloride channels.

Chapter 7

1. **D.** Electrical synapses do not involve neurotransmitter and thus do not require synaptic vesicles. A typical postsynaptic neuron receives thousands of inputs, with synaptic inputs from excitatory, inhibitory, and modulatory neurons. Because there is no neurotransmitter release or receptors, synaptic delay is much shorter at electrical synapses. Ionotropic receptors are neurotransmitter gated ion channels, whereas metabotropic receptors can regulate ion channels indirectly. Indirect gating of ion channels involves G proteins, which can interact with ion channels, or G proteins that produce second messengers, which control protein kinases that phosphorylate and regulate ions channels.

2. **E.** Although voltage-gated Na^+ and K^+ channels are involved in the generation and conduction of the action potential (with Na^+ influx and K^+ efflux), which is necessary to depolarize the presynaptic membrane potential, it is the influx of Ca^{2+} through the activation of voltage-gated Ca^{2+} channels that directly activates the fusion of synaptic vesicles and neurotransmitter release by the presynaptic axon.

3. **B.** The action potential has a fairly consistent (stereotypical) magnitude and duration, which does not change. Voltage-gated Na^+ channels inactivate, but voltage-gated K^+ and Ca^{2+} channels do not typically inactivate. The frequency and pattern of presynaptic action potentials determine how long the voltage-gated Ca^{2+} channels will be open and thus how much presynaptic Ca^{2+} influx there is and how much neurotransmitter is released and for how long. The synaptic delay does not affect the level or extent of neurotransmitter release.

4. **C.** Astrocytic end feet would not have access to neurotransmitters at the synapse. There are no neurotransmitter

channels. Neurotransmitter transporters transport glutamate, GABA, glycine, and monoamines and biogenic amines, whereas acetylcholine is degraded by acetylcholine esterase. Most neurotransmitters are not oxidized at the cleft (monoamine oxidases were previously thought to be present in the synapse but have now been shown to be mainly intracellular).

5. **A.** After synaptic vesicles fuse with the presynaptic membrane, they undergo endocytosis and are either refilled or traffic to the early/synaptic endosome. Vesicles are not released into the cleft; only their content, the neurotransmitter, is released. The endocytosed vesicles do not traffic to the secretory pathway. Most endocytic vesicles are not degraded by lysosomes. Endocytic vesicles do not traffic back to the cell body where the TGN (Golgi) is located.

Chapter 8

1. **E.** Cholinergic neurons are located in the brainstem and spinal cord (lower somatic motor neurons and preganglionic autonomic neurons), interneurons in the brain (basal forebrain, striatum, and brainstem), and autonomic ganglia (majority of postganglionic parasympathetic neurons).

2. **B.** GABA has predominantly inhibitory actions in the adult CNS (it has some excitatory actions in the developing brain). The GABA receptor is a ligand-gated Cl⁻ channel, which when open, usually leads to Cl⁻ influx and hyperpolarization of the membrane potential and inhibition. GABA is formed from glutamate. Decreased GABA function is associated with seizures. GABA is present in both the brain and spinal cord, whereas glycine is found mainly in the spinal cord.

3. **A.** The NMDA receptor is a ligand (glutamate)-gated channel, but at the resting membrane potential, it is blocked by Mg^{2+} binding inside the channel pore. The NMDA receptor is a nonselective cation channel permeable to Na^+, K^+, and Ca^{2+}. NMDA is selective for 1 subtype of glutamate ionotropic receptor. Excess glutamate acting through NMDA receptors is thought to cause excitotoxic cell death. Glutamate opens the channels if the membrane is depolarized to remove the Mg^{2+} block, leading to Na^+ and Ca^{2+} influx (because of the larger driving forces for Na^+ and Ca^{2+} than for K^+), which leads to depolarization of the postsynaptic cell.

4. **D.** Although they can receive inputs from all types of neurons in the brain, the only types of neurons in the cerebral cortex are glutamatergic and GABAergic neurons. Cortical local circuit neurons are GABAergic or glutamatergic. Cortical projection neurons are mainly glutamatergic. Cortical neurons receive inputs from other cortical regions as well as the thalamus and brainstem. The majority of glutamatergic neurons are projection neurons.

5. **C.** Summation refers to the summation of all the responses from synaptic inputs, which are the postsynaptic excitatory (EPSPs) and inhibitory (IPSPs) responses in neurons. Summation occurs everywhere in the neuron, but it

is important at the axon hillock initial segment since that is the place where, if the summed depolarization is above threshold, the action potential is triggered.

Chapter 9

1. **C.** All the monoamine/biogenic amine cell bodies are located in the brainstem or hypothalamus.

2. **D.** The monoamine/biogenic amine neurons project throughout the brain and spinal cord to many areas of the cerebral cortex, to key subcortical regions such as the basal ganglia and hippocampus, and to the spinal cord.

3. **B.** Second messengers often lead to desensitization of receptors. Second messengers regulate protein kinases, which can control transcription and translation and hence affect gene expression. Second messengers can directly gate ion channels and also regulate protein kinases, which can also control opening or closing of ion channels. Activation of metabotropic glutamate receptors is typically excitatory. NMDA receptors are gated by glutamate binding (although they can be indirectly affected by second messengers and protein kinases).

4. **E.** NPs are typically released far away from the active zone. NPs activate only metabotropic receptors. NPs are packaged into larger secretory granule or dense core vesicles, not transported into synaptic vesicles. NPs typically require high-frequency action potential trains to be released because they are located further away from the active zones where the voltage-gated Ca^{2+} channels are located. NPs are synthesized as larger precursor peptides and undergo cleavage inside vesicles and maturation; they are trafficked by fast axonal transport along microtubules to the axon terminus.

5. **A.** Classical neurotransmitters are small organic molecules or peptides. Nitric oxide (NO) is a free radical gas. NO is usually modulatory in its function and does not directly cause inhibitory postsynaptic potentials or excitatory postsynaptic potentials. NO is typically released by classical neurotransmitter action in neurons. NO is released by neurons in the central nervous system. As a free radical gas, NO is hydrophobic and is not packed into vesicles because it can diffuse across the lipid bilayer.

Chapter 10

1. **D.** Neuroplasticity occurs in both the developing and adult brain. Neuroplasticity is the mechanism that allows the brain to become rewired after injury and disorders. Neuroplasticity is what leads to a change in neurotransmission and circuit activity. Neuroplasticity is thought to underlie all types of learning and memory. Neuroplasticity likely involves modification of individual synapses, overall neuronal activity, neuronal circuits, and even formation of new neurons (neurogenesis).

2. **E.** Synapses form (synaptogenesis) prenatally, postnatally, and in the adult brain. Synapses can occur between a

presynaptic neuron and another neuron (on the dendrite, axon, or cell body), a muscle, or a gland. Synaptogenesis occurs both prenatally and postnatally, and the critical period is when a significant amount of activity-dependent synaptic refinement occurs. Some synapses are not completely stable in adulthood. A typical interneuron receives thousands of synapses. Synapses are modified by postnatal experience and activity.

3. **B.** Synaptogenesis is the formation of new synapses. Synaptic plasticity refers to changes (increase or decreases) in synapse number and strength (response). Synaptic transmission usually refers to the electrical or other response at the postsynaptic target. Synaptic integration can refer to summation of excitatory postsynaptic potentials and inhibitory postsynaptic potentials. Adult neurogenesis is the formation of new neurons in the adult.

4. **C.** LTP has been shown to occur in many regions of the brain (hippocampus, cerebellum, and striatum) and with several types of neuronal circuits. LTP in the SC is generally a postsynaptic effect with increased AMPA receptors, although a presynaptic increase in glutamate is observed. LTP at the SC requires Ca^{2+}-dependent protein kinases, transcription of new mRNA, and translation of new proteins. LTP in the SC involves regulation of gene expression that involves transcription factors and epigenetic mechanisms. LTP at the SC involves the unsilencing of previously silent synapses.

5. **A.** One of the main functions for hippocampal LTD may be to reverse LTP after information has been transferred to cortical circuits via consolidation so that the hippocampus can be used to encode new information. Plasticity molecules are synthesized de novo and probably do not need to be recycled. Encoded information is most likely not transferred within the hippocampus and LTD is probably not required for synaptic or systems consolidation. Once induced, LTP is fairly stable, and although activity is increased at some synapses, the potentiation is not high enough to cause excitotoxicity. LTP is stable for hours to days, and the idea is that only relevant information association produces LTP.

Chapter 11

1. **E.** In 1 form of retinitis pigmentosa, there is a genetic defect with respect to rhodopsin. The result of this defect is the production of defective opsin. As a consequence, rod cells are affected, leading to a reduced response to light. Consequently, there is degeneration of photoreceptors, which die by apoptosis. At a later time, cone cells also appear to degenerate. Other components of the retina (eg, retina/ganglion cells) and central nervous system neurons (eg, those located in area 17) are not directly affected, and vision is not totally lost.

2. **D.** The only cell in the retina that is capable of producing an action potential is the ganglion cell. As indicated earlier,

the ganglion cell gives rise to optic nerve fibers, which terminate as optic tract fibers in the lateral geniculate nucleus. As a result of action potentials generated in the ganglion cells, volleys of impulses are transmitted over these fibers, resulting in the appropriate responses in the neurons of the lateral geniculate nucleus. Therefore, the patient became blind due to damage to the ganglion cells, whose axons form the optic nerve and optic tract, thus depriving the lateral geniculate nucleus and visual cortex from receiving visual inputs.

3. **C.** To correct for farsightedness, a person is prescribed a convex lens because objects focus behind the retina. The convex lens helps to refocus the object onto the retina. The reason that the focus of the object is behind the retina is because the eyeball is too short.

4. **B.** Low-contrast, achromatic vision is mediated primarily by the magnocellular pathway. Parvocellular ganglion cells operate at higher contrast and mediate color and detail vision. Loss of horizontal or amacrine cells tends to produce blur, whereas dopaminergic amacrine cell loss affects dark and light adaptation.

5. **C.** Open-angle glaucoma has a slow painless progression, but that of closed-angle glaucoma is rapid and often associated with pain and headaches. Retinitis pigmentosa presents first as night blindness due to rod death. Macular degeneration is slow, with loss mainly in the central retina. Diabetic retinopathy also has a slow, symptomless onset.

Chapter 12

1. **C.** Disruption of optic tract fibers destined for the lateral geniculate nucleus will cause a homonymous hemianopsia because it affects fibers arising from the temporal retina of the ipsilateral side and from the nasal retina of the contralateral side. Because the damage occurred in the left optic tract, the loss of vision is reflected on the right visual field (ie, the left temporal retina is associated with the nasal or right visual field of the left eye, and the right nasal retina is associated with the temporal or right visual field of the right eye). Therefore, such a lesion would result in a right homonymous hemianopsia.

2. **D.** Face identification is particularly dependent on a right temporal lobe area called the fusiform face area. Damage to the parietal lobe would result in visual apraxia, whereas occipital lobe damage would tend to compromise multiple visual functions.

3. **B.** The patient is exhibiting left-sided hemineglect, which is caused by a parietal lobe lesion on the right side. Right-sided hemineglect, due to lesions on the left side of the parietal lobe, is much rarer. Temporal lobe damage compromises pattern recognition, whereas occipital lobe damage usually results in compromise of multiple visual functions.

4. **A.** Damage to the superior colliculus causes loss of orienting to peripheral stimuli and inability to make head movements and eye movements toward those stimuli.

5. B. The retinal loss progression in glaucoma starts with ganglion cells. A particular type of ganglion cell that has its own photopigment (intrinsically photoreceptive) mediates circadian rhythms via its projection to the suprachiasmatic nucleus. Patients with glaucoma typically also lose circadian rhythm synchronicity to sunrise and sunset, whereas patients with photoreceptor loss often retain normal circadian rhythms. A tumor or stroke involving the suprachiasmatic nucleus would not, by itself, cause blindness.

Chapter 13

1. D. Several tests can be conducted to distinguish between conduction deafness and sensorineural deafness. These include the Weber test and Rinne test, which were presented in this case. In the Weber test, the sound was localized in the left ear, suggesting that if the loss were conduction deafness, the affected ear would be the left ear. If it were sensorineural loss, the sound would appear stronger on the left side. The convincing feature here is that Rinne test showed that when the sound from the tuning fork was placed near the right ear, it sounded louder, whereas the sound did not appear louder when the tuning fork was placed on the mastoid process of the right side, which would have signified conduction loss on the right side (and likewise for the test when conducted for the left side). Therefore, it is reasonable to conclude that the patient suffers from sensorineural loss on the right side, which quite often may involve an acoustic neuroma affecting Schwann cell sheaths associated with cranial nerve VIII. This argument excludes all other choices except the last choice (E). A tumor of the cerebellar vermis could produce different symptoms, which include principally a wide-based gait ataxia and nystagmus, with no effect on hearing.

2. B. A lesion of the vestibular labyrinth could result in the symptoms described for this patient because the receptors in this complex mediate vestibular sensation and impulses and its disruption would induce these sensory aberrations. Damage to the cochlea or middle ear would produce hearing deficits. A lesion of the dorsolateral medulla may affect vestibular function, but would also affect a number of other functions, such as eye movements, and would induce nystagmus as well as produce a Wallenberg syndrome. A lesion of the medial longitudinal fasciculus would also result in nystagmus and/or other eye movement disorders.

3. A. Along the auditory pathway from the periphery to the cerebral cortex, there are multiple sites in this circuit where auditory discrimination of tone can take place. The first site is actually in the periphery along the basilar membrane. Different parts of the basilar membrane respond most effectively to different frequencies of sound (ie, the base of the basilar membrane responds most effectively to high frequencies, whereas the apex responds to low frequencies). The tympanic membrane, located at the end of the auditory canal, receives sound waves, causing it to vibrate, but it lacks properties of tonotopic discrimination. The otolithic membrane is related to the vestibular component of the eighth nerve, not the auditory component. The superior olivary nucleus is part of a feedback system, where its axons are believed to provide feedback to the auditory receptors. Its function, in part, is to localize sound in space by discriminating the time of arrival of sounds or by differentiation of sound intensity. The middle temporal gyrus is associated with perception of moving objects and not with sound.

4. D. Aging, particularly in men, is associated with high-frequency hearing loss, called presbycusis. Young adults typically hear well to frequencies up to 20 kHz, but this limit drops to 15 kHz or less in older adults.

5. E. Auditory hair cells in the organ of Corti are contacted by the processes of spiral ganglion cells, whose cell bodies are located near the tympanic membrane in the bony part of the cochlea. These are pseudo-unipolar cells that extend 1 input process to the auditory hair cells and another output process to the cochlear nucleus where conventional synapses are made on cells. Cells in the cochlear nucleus project to the superior olive.

Chapter 14

1. C. The olfactory receptor and its primary afferent fiber terminate upon dendrites of mitral cells. This relationship is important because it is the axon of the mitral cell that projects out of the olfactory bulb (forming the major component of the lateral olfactory stria). The granule cell processes make synaptic contact with dendrites of mitral cells, forming dendrodendritic synapses, but are not known to make synaptic contact with primary afferent terminals. Cells arising in the olfactory tubercle are not known to project to the olfactory bulb. Instead, projections of cells situated in the olfactory tubercle contribute fibers to the medial forebrain bundle and stria medullaris.

2. D. Experimental evidence indicates the prefrontal cortex is a key region for the conscious perception of smell. This conclusion is based on 2 observations. First, the prefrontal cortex receives major inputs from the olfactory bulb by the following routes: olfactory bulb to pyriform cortex to prefrontal cortex, or olfactory bulb to pyriform cortex (and olfactory tubercle) to mediodorsal thalamic nucleus to prefrontal cortex. Second, lesions of the prefrontal cortex result in a failure to discriminate odors. Olfactory functions are not known to be associated with any of the other choices. Instead, the primary auditory receiving area is located in the auditory cortex, the posterior parietal lobule is concerned with such processes as the programming mechanisms associated with complex motor tasks, the cingulate gyrus has been associated with such functions as spatial learning and the modulation of autonomic and emotional processes, and the precentral gyrus contains the primary motor area.

3. **E.** The olfactory cilia are extensions of the receptor cell, and it is this part of the cell that initially responds to an olfactory stimulus. The cilia contain protein membranes that bind with different odorants, which constitutes a necessary condition for excitation of the olfactory cell. Mitral and granule cells are situated in the olfactory bulb and, consequently, are not part of the receptor mechanism. Sustentacular cells are supporting cells and are not part of the receptor mechanism. Basal cells are the precursors for receptor cells and, thus, are also not directly part of the receptor mechanism.

4. **B.** A number of recent studies have indicated that different olfactory glomeruli respond to different kinds of olfactory stimuli. In a sense, this represents a type of organization of the olfactory bulb that bears a functional similarity to the spatial organization that exists for other sensory systems and that is now disrupted by the continuous exposure to the strong odorant. There is no evidence that such a spatial arrangement exists for other components of the olfactory system, nor is there any evidence that temporal summation plays any role in the process of olfactory discrimination.

5. **B.** Mitral cell axons enter the lateral olfactory stria and project caudally through this bundle to supply the medial amygdala and pyriform cortex. Olfactory projections to other nuclei, such as the hippocampal formation, prefrontal cortex, medial thalamus, and septal area, require at least 1 additional synaptic connection, such as in the pyriform cortex, amygdala, or olfactory tubercle.

Chapter 15

1. **D.** To generate an excitatory focus with an inhibitory surround, 3 types of inhibition are present in the dorsal column nuclei. First-order neurons ascending in the dorsal columns make synaptic contact with different cells in the dorsal column nuclei and excite those cells. One such cell may be an inhibitory interneuron that makes synaptic contact with a neighboring dorsal column nuclear cell, thus inhibiting that cell (ie, feedforward inhibition). In addition, the dorsal column cell that is excited by the first-order neuron may make synaptic contact with another inhibitory interneuron (in addition to its classical ascending projection to the ventral posterolateral nucleus of the thalamus). This inhibitory interneuron makes synaptic contact with an adjacent dorsal column cell and inhibits that cell (ie, feedback inhibition). Finally, a descending fiber from the postcentral gyrus can make synaptic contact with inhibitory interneurons that inhibit dorsal column cells (descending inhibition).

2. **E.** As a general rule, neurons that are situated in the cortex in association with any of the sensory systems take on a much higher level of complexity than neurons that are situated at lower levels of the relay network. In the case of the somatosensory system, direction-sensitive cells in the somatosensory cortex will respond to 1 direction of movement of a stimulus along the receptive field and not to another direction. Orientation-sensitive neurons respond best to movement along 1 axis of the receptive field. This is not true of neurons that are situated in lower levels of the somatosensory pathway. Thus, a tumor or lesion of this region of cortex is likely to disrupt the neuronal process essential for such discriminations to be made.

3. **C.** Referred pain is a phenomenon in which pain impulses, arising from primary afferent fibers from 1 part of the body (eg, from deep visceral structures), terminate on dorsal horn projection neurons that normally receive cutaneous afferents from a different part of the body (eg, the arm). In this situation, a person who is suffering a heart attack experiences pain that appears to be coming from the arm. It is the convergence of these distinctly different inputs onto the same projection neurons that provides the basis for this phenomenon. None of the other possible mechanisms listed in this question have an anatomic or physiologic basis.

4. **D.** Primary nociceptive afferent fibers would have to release an excitatory transmitter in order for normal transmission to take place. Two excitatory transmitters have been identified in association with different classes of primary nociceptive afferents: (1) substance P and (2) excitatory amino acids. The best candidate as an excitatory amino acid is glutamate. Because enkephalins have been shown to be inhibitory transmitters in the pain system, they are not likely to be released from the primary afferents. Instead, other CNS neurons impinge upon the primary afferents, and enkephalins are released from those neurons.

5. **B.** Perhaps one of the most important discoveries in pain research made over the past 25 years is that of a descending pathway that originates in the midbrain periaqueductal gray and makes synaptic contacts in the medulla. From the medulla, this pathway descends to the dorsal horn, where these fibers provide the anatomic substrate for suppression of pain inputs that enter the spinal cord from the periphery. There are no known inputs to the cortex that directly produce analgesia. The mechanism governing analgesia appears to operate at lower brainstem and spinal cord levels. The ascending fibers for transmission of pain impulses reach thalamic nuclei directly, and thus, local interneurons within the midbrain would not be able to interfere with such transmission. The pathway to the ventral posterolateral nucleus of the thalamus is an excitatory one and is not known to have any inhibitory properties. Cholinergic neurons in the basal forebrain have been implicated in memory functions and are not known to have any role in the regulation of pain sensation.

Chapter 16

1. **C.** The premotor areas play an important role in the programming or sequencing of responses that compose complex, learned movements. They receive significant inputs for this process from the posterior parietal lobule

and, in turn, signal appropriate neurons in the brainstem and spinal cord (both flexors and extensors). Lesions of the postcentral gyrus produce a somatosensory loss. Lesions of the precentral gyrus produce paralysis. Neither lesions of the prefrontal cortex nor those of the cingulate gyrus have been reported to produce apraxia.

2. **D.** Although the postcentral gyrus is referred to as "somatosensory" cortex, it contributes many fibers to the corticospinal tract and plays an important role in motor behavior. In essence, it is the sensory feedback that is essential for motor behavior to occur. Without such sensory information, the sequences of motor responses necessary for simple tasks such as playing the piano or swinging a baseball bat would lose their smoothness and sequential characteristics; or on a simpler level, the motor behavior described in this question requires sensory feedback, and without it, motor behavior breaks down. The other choices presented as alternate answers represent regions where lesions produce entirely different kinds of deficits unrelated to those described in the stem of this question. These include pseudobulbar palsy that would be associated with lesions of the far lateral precentral gyrus, inability to detect movement of objects after lesions of the middle temporal gyrus, a hemianopsia following damage to the primary visual cortex, or intellectual and emotional changes associated with lesions of the prefrontal cortex.

3. **C.** This patient is suffering from the disorder of apraxia, which is defined as a state where an attentive patient has lost the ability to carry out a previously learned task in the absence of motor deficits such as ataxia, muscle weakness, loss of sensory functions, or disorders associated with the basal ganglia. Apraxia occurs most commonly when there is a lesion of the posterior parietal cortex (areas 5 and 7) or premotor cortex. The region of the posterior parietal cortex serves as a kind of integrating mechanism of various sensory modalities for the transmission of signals to the premotor region that serve as a sequencing mechanism for the expression of complex acts of movement such as the completion of tasks described in the question stem. When the sequencing mechanism is disrupted, apraxia occurs. The other choices represent regions that are not associated with this disorder. Lesions of the precentral gyrus result in paralysis; the superior temporal gyrus is associated with complex discrimination and the interpretation of sounds, and the lateral prefrontal cortex relates to higher intellectual and emotional forms of behavior.

4. **A.** Medial aspects of the right primary motor cortex control voluntary movements of the left leg, from the hip down. Lesions of the supplementary or premotor areas would have more complex coordination effects.

Chapter 17

1. **C.** The basic principle governing how the basal ganglia control motor activity is that they do so by modulating neurons of the motor cortex and premotor areas (of the ipsilateral side) via synaptic connections in the ventrolateral (VL) and ventral anterior (VA) nuclei of the thalamus. One can see from the following circuits that damage to the basal ganglia on 1 side of the brain will affect cortical neurons on the same side:

Globus pallidus (medial segment) → VL nucleus → area 4 of cortex

Globus pallidus (medial segment) → VA nucleus → area 6 of cortex

This will result in dyskinesia expressed on the contralateral side of the body because the corticospinal tract is crossed. The other possibilities listed in the question are not viable. Projections of the basal ganglia to the brainstem nuclei are minimal. The basal ganglia do not project fibers down to the spinal cord, nor do they project to the cerebellum.

2. **C.** In Huntington disease, the essential neurochemical change is in the basal ganglia, where there is a significant reduction in the 2 transmitters ACh and GABA. In particular, there are reduced levels of enzymes associated with the synthesis of ACh and GABA (ie, choline acetyltransferase and glutamic acid decarboxylase, respectively) and GABA directly.

3. **C.** MPTP was discovered by accident when drug abusers who were using a synthetic heroin derivative developed signs of Parkinson disease. It was discovered that their drug included the contaminant MPTP. As a consequence, MPTP has been applied systemically in a number of experimental animals, resulting in significant decreases in dopamine content of the brain due to the loss of dopaminergic neurons in the substantia nigra. These animals also developed symptoms similar to those seen in Parkinson patients. For these reasons, this drug is currently being used for research purposes in order to develop a better understanding of this disease and to establish possible drug therapies for its treatment and eventual cure.

4. **A.** One of the most important features of the anterior lobe of the cerebellum is that it receives major inputs from structures that mediate information concerning muscle spindle and Golgi tendon organ activity (sometimes referred to as unconscious proprioception). The pathways that mediate unconscious proprioception include the dorsal and ventral spinocerebellar tracts and the cuneocerebellar tract. Accordingly, the cerebellar anterior lobe is sometimes referred to as the spinocerebellum. The fastigial and dentate nuclei receive their principal inputs from the cerebellar cortex, and their axons project out of the cerebellum. The posterior lobe receives few, if any, inputs from pathways that mediate unconscious proprioception information.

5. **B.** Purkinje cells are inhibitory neurons whose axons supply the deep cerebellar nuclei. The Purkinje cells of the lateral aspects of the hemispheres supply the dentate nucleus; those in the intermediate region supply the interposed

nuclei; and those situated in the vermal region supply the fastigial nucleus. The outputs of the cerebellum to the other regions (with the exception of spinal cord) listed in this question receive their direct inputs from deep cerebellar nuclei. The spinal cord receives its inputs from cerebellum only indirectly via cerebellar projections to such regions as the red nucleus, cerebral cortex, vestibular nuclei, and reticular formation.

Chapter 18

1. **A.** The transmitter released from preganglionic endings of both sympathetic and parasympathetic fibers is acetylcholine (ACh). The other transmitters listed are not involved at this synapse. Evidence in support of this view is derived, in part, from studies that demonstrated that drugs that block nicotinic receptors (eg, hexamethonium chloride, curare) also block the output of these systems.

2. **C.** The solitary nucleus of the medulla plays a significant role in the neural control of autonomic functions because it receives input from several different regions of the brain that regulate such functions. These inputs include fibers that arise from the hypothalamus, central nucleus of the amygdala, midbrain periaqueductal gray, and sensory processes (ie, visceral afferents) of the glossopharyngeal and vagus nerves. The last signal reflects changes in blood pressure and levels of oxygen and carbon dioxide in the blood. The ventrolateral nucleus of the thalamus, red nucleus of the midbrain, and ventral horn cells of the spinal cord are associated with somatomotor rather than autonomic function. The nucleus accumbens is believed to be associated with motivational processes.

3. **C.** A tumor of the posterior fossa would interfere with descending (and possibly ascending) autonomic pathways from the medulla and thus account for the impairment of blood pressure. The lateral thalamus is associated with ascending somatosensory information (eg, ventroposterolateral nucleus) and motor signals (eg, ventrolateral thalamic nucleus), and therefore, a tumor in this area would not likely impair blood pressure. A tumor of the premotor cortex would likely result in an apraxia of movement. A tumor in the midline region of the basilar pons would likely affect movements associated with the cerebellar hemispheres because the transverse pontine pathways passing through that region supply the cerebellar hemispheres. A tumor of the midline region of the dorsal midbrain affecting the superior colliculus could affect tracking movements of the eyes but would not likely affect autonomic functions such as blood pressure.

4. **D.** One of the principal causes of orthostatic hypotension relates to lesions of postganglionic sympathetic neurons. All of the other choices involve either central or peripheral components of the parasympathetic system, none of which are involved in this disorder.

Chapter 19

1. **B.** The lateral region of the thalamus and the posterior limb of the internal capsule are supplied by choroidal branches of the internal carotid artery. Infarct of this artery most frequently results in contralateral hemiparesis and dysarthria. Although lesions associated with this artery may affect only motor functions, they may also cause loss of pain, touch, and sometimes visual functions. The other choices given in this question are not associated with this constellation of deficits.

2. **C.** Studies conducted on fear conditioning in rats have demonstrated that the amygdala plays a very important role in this process. Rare evidence obtained from patients has shown that individuals suffering from a rare autosomal recessive condition called Urbach-Wiethe disease, in which there is bilateral atrophy of the portion of the temporal lobe that includes the amygdala, have no sense of the emotion of fear. They are unable to recognize it and are not capable of depicting it in a drawing. Other regions listed in this question have not been linked to the emotion of fear.

3. **D.** Failure to recognize complex sounds such as those of animals, individuals, bells, or whistles can occur with a lesion of the superior temporal cortex, while the ability to discriminate tones and hear sounds is preserved. A lesion of the inferior parietal cortex would result in other forms of agnosia such as finger agnosia (Gerstmann syndrome); a lesion of the superior parietal cortex results in a syndrome called sensory neglect; a lesion of the inferior temporal cortex typically results in a failure to recognize faces called prosopagnosia; and a lesion of the medial geniculate nucleus is rare in man, but if it were to occur, the effect would presumably be to affect hearing directly, especially discrimination of tones. There is no evidence that such a lesion would produce an auditory agnosia.

4. **C.** Damage to the prefrontal cortex results in social disinhibition and impairment of judgment, insight, and foresight. The patient may retain basic cognitive functions; however, the patient may display behaviors that are inappropriate without feeling any regret or guilt about such responses. Other regions presented as alternative choices in this question do not display these forms of dysfunctional responses. For example, lesions of the superior parietal and premotor cortices are more closely associated with apraxia, lesions of the hippocampal formation with short-term memory disorders, and lesions of the amygdala with the loss of fear responses and changes in aggressive behavior.

Chapter 20

1. **D.** A combination of human functional imaging studies and research in rodents has demonstrated that short-term working memory involves specific regions in the prefrontal cortex, posterior parietal cortex, and temporal cortex.

2. **A.** Human studies (eg, patient H.M. and others) have demonstrated that the hippocampus is required for semantic

and episodic (together with declarative or explicit) and spatial memory. Encoding of implicit/nondeclarative and short-term memory involves other brain regions.

3. **E.** Although encoding and formation of new declarative/explicit memories require the hippocampus, studies in rodents suggest that memories are transferred from the hippocampus to the cerebral cortex following encoding and learning over a period of days to weeks to months. Human studies also suggest that some episodic memories, especially autobiographical memories, are either stored in the hippocampus or require the hippocampus for retrieval.

4. **C.** Sensory memory involves very short-lived enhancement of synaptic transmission, whereas short-term working memory involves increased circuit activity, most likely via reverberating circuits in the prefrontal cortex. Neither sensory nor short-term working memory involves long-term synaptic changes, including biochemical changes. So only hippocampal-dependent memory (declarative and spatial memory) is thought to require LTP. That said, it is anticipated that other types of long-term memory such as nondeclarative, procedural, and motor memory will likely involve similar LTP and/or long-term depression mechanisms.

5. **B.** Although all of these ideas have been proposed, are plausible, and are not mutually exclusive, the theory that many neuroscientists are most keen on at the moment is that during sleep there is reduced incoming sensory activity to the hippocampus, and thus synaptic and systems consolidation can proceed without interference.

Chapter 21

1. **B.** A lesion of the operculum and convexity of the frontal lobe (which lies rostral to the precentral gyrus of the left side of the cortex and is called the Broca area) results in aphasia. This form of aphasia is characterized by nonfluency in speech, as well as difficulty in word naming and repetition of words, while comprehension of speech is preserved. Frequently, such lesions extend beyond this region and include wide parts of the precentral gyrus, thus resulting in hemiparesis of the right side of the body. A lesion of the medial convexity of the premotor cortex would result in loss of motor functions mainly of the lower limb; lesions of the supramarginal gyrus or angular gyrus produce forms of aphasia in which fluency is preserved; and a lesion of the inferior parietal lobule might also produce a form of aphasia where fluency is preserved or a Gerstmann syndrome.

2. **D.** A lesion of the posterior aspect of the superior temporal cortex, known as Wernicke area, results in a reduction in fluency in speech, and this form of aphasia is sometimes referred to as receptive aphasia. A lesion of the medial convexity of the premotor cortex would produce apraxic movement disorders; a lesion of the lateral convexity of the precentral gyrus would produce a limb paralysis; a lesion

of the medial aspect of the occipital cortex would produce visual deficits; and a lesion of the superior parietal lobule could produce a form of apraxia.

3. **C.** The language problem is an example of Broca aphasia, a deficit seen with lesions of the Broca area and manifested by defects in the motor aspect of speech, leaving the patient's speech halting and nonfluent. People with Broca aphasia tend to repeat certain phrases, as well as leave out pronouns. Because the language centers are usually located on the dominant side of the brain (the left side for a right-handed person), this lesion must be on the left side of the patient's brain. Wernicke aphasia is a problem with the sensory aspect of speech, where the patient can speak fluently, but the speech sounds like gibberish. The area of disruption in this type of aphasia is usually in Wernicke area, a region of the posterior superior temporal lobe. Dysarthria is slurred speech that makes grammatical sense. Alexia is the inability to read. Pure word deafness is a type of sensory aphasia whereby language, reading, and writing are only mildly disturbed, but auditory comprehension of words is very abnormal. This arises from lesions of the posterior temporal lobe.

Chapter 22

1. **B.** The amygdala is specifically involved with memories of fearful items associated with dangerous or punishing contexts from the past. Damage to the hippocampus would interfere with the acquisition of all new memories. Damage to the insula does not eliminate emotional learning but interferes with visceral consciousness and empathy. Prefrontal damage interferes with all emotional judgement, not just emotional learning.

2. **D.** Damage to ventromedial prefrontal cortex, as in the case of Phineas Gage, results in poor social judgement, risk taking, and utilization behavior. Damage to the hippocampus interferes with the acquisition of new memories. Thalamic damage results in deficits in sensory processing, motor control, and attention. Damage to the dorsolateral prefrontal cortex would interfere with working memory tasks.

3. **B.** The left prefrontal cortex, ventromedial prefrontal cortex more than dorsolateral, is biased to approach, while the right is biased toward withdrawal. Damage to the left side biases activity toward right side–mediated withdrawal, whereas damage to the right biases toward left-mediated approach and manic activity. Amygdala damage compromises fear learning.

Chapter 23

1. **A.** Soon after the origin of life is the correct answer.

2. **C.** Entrainment allows continuity in clock phase to be robust with respect to temporary changes in light levels, such as from cloud cover or volcanoes.

3. **B.** The suprachiasmatic nucleus of the hypothalamus is the central pacemaker brain area in mammals.

4. **D.** Intrinsically photoreceptive retinal ganglion cells compose the retinal output to the suprachiasmatic nucleus.

5. **A.** *Per2* is the gene involved in circadian clocks.

6. **D.** Sleep problems are the most common circadian rhythm disorder.

7. **D.** The retinal contains a class of ganglion cells called intrinsically photosensitive that contain their own photopigment and react directly to light (although they may also be driven by photoreceptors through bipolar cells, like other ganglion cells). These project to the suprachiasmatic nucleus via the retino-hypothalanic tract. Neither photoreceptors, amacrine cells, or other ganglion cell classes are involved in this projection.

Chapter 24

1. **C.** This patient has a right visual field cut. Although some of these fibers traverse the left middle cerebral artery territory, other neurologic deficits would be expected to be present. An isolated visual field cut is typical of a posterior cerebral artery territory infarction.

2. **B.** An irregularly irregular heart rhythm is suggestive of atrial fibrillation, a common stroke mechanism. In these patients, the stroke is thought to originate from an embolism from the appendage of the left atrium.

3. **A.** This is a typical location for a hypertensive hemorrhage. Cerebral amyloid angiopathy typically affects older patients and causes lobar hemorrhage. Although a venous sinus thrombosis can cause hemorrhage, they are more often cortical, and thrombosis of the superior sagittal sinus would not affect the deep nuclei. Herpes simplex virus preferentially affects the temporal lobe rather than the deep nuclei.

4. **B.** This patient is having a cerebral venous sinus thrombosis. The treatment of choice is therapeutic anticoagulation, typically heparin or low-molecular-weight heparin, followed by transitioning to oral anticoagulation for 3 to 12 months.

Chapter 25

1. **B.** Glioblastomas are the most common malignant brain tumors in adults.

2. **B.** Pilocytic astrocytomas are low-grade (World Health Organization grade I) astrocytomas that are found predominately in the pediatric age group, most commonly occurring around 9 to 10 years of age, and they are most often found in the posterior fossa, specifically in the cerebellum. Patients often present with signs of increased intracranial pressure, such as headache. Histologically, they are sparsely cellular without anaplasia or mitoses. These tumors often contain Rosenthal fibers, which are corkscrew-shaped, eosinophilic

intracytoplasmic inclusions, and eosinophilic granular bodies, which are globular aggregates within astrocytic processes.

3. **C.** GBM is a World Health Organization grade IV astrocytoma. Histologically, GBMs have anaplasia and increased mitotic activity and *either* microvascular proliferation *or* necrosis.

4. **E.** Schwannomas consist of alternating highly cellular regions (Antoni A regions) that have areas of nuclear palisading (Verocay bodies) and loosely arranged hypocellular regions (Antoni B regions). Most schwannomas strongly express the S100 protein.

Chapter 26

1. **A.** The patient has episodic migraine without aura. Given her obesity and no history of renal calculi or glaucoma, topiramate would be the treatment of choice. Propranolol is contraindicated in patients with asthma. Acetazolamide is used for idiopathic intracranial hypertension. Sumatriptan is a migraine abortive treatment.

2. **C.** This patient has episodic migraine with aura and should be treated with migraine-specific therapy in the setting of no contraindications. Triptans work via agonism of 5-HT 1B/1D receptors. The 5-HT 1B subreceptor is thought to decrease nociception via vasoconstriction of vessels that mediate pain. The 5-HT 1D subreceptor inhibits trigeminal neuromediator release and activation of the trigeminal vascular system. This leads to decreased neurogenic inflammation, peripheral and central sensitization, and headache.

3. **E.** This patient's presentation is typical of cluster headaches. Cluster headache is a diagnosis of exclusion, and this patient needs neuroimaging as the next best step. Increasing verapamil might help with his cluster bout if his blood pressure can tolerate it, but secondary causes of cluster symptoms need to be ruled out. Sumatriptan injection is the treatment of choice for symptomatic relief of a cluster attack, but imaging is the next best step. Scheduled caffeine is used for hypnic headache, which does present as a headache causing nocturnal awakenings in older individuals but does not have associated autonomic features or restlessness. A sleep study is not likely to contribute to this clinical pictures, as there is no clinical suspicion of sleep apnea based on history.

Chapter 27

1. **D.** The boy is having episodes of daydreaming while in class and not always following directions while at home. Both of these are likely related to absence seizures, which typically occur between the ages of 3 and 8 years. In typical absence seizures, we would expect to see only staring with minimal additional movements, and there would be a minimal, if any, postictal period. The EEG performed

is abnormal with generalized discharges at 3 Hz, which is classic for typical absence epilepsy. Typical absence epilepsy usually remits by early adulthood, and the need for lifelong medication is rare. Although staring could be a manifestation of ADD, the EEG should be normal in that case. Abnormal EEG epileptiform discharges would alter this boy's behavior, and he is unable to "try harder" and make his events go away.

2. **C.** This woman has signs of phenytoin toxicity with ataxia, nystagmus, and confusion. The phenytoin dose was increased in the emergency room due to a breakthrough seizure. Due to the zero-order kinetics of phenytoin, a small increase in the dose can lead to large increases in serum concentrations. Complex partial seizures are unlikely to cause constant symptoms of ataxia, nystagmus, and confusion. Cerebellar ataxia generally has a more chronic and insidious onset. Opioid intoxication can cause confusion but does not typically cause ataxia or nystagmus.

3. **B.** The patient has not had a complete workup yet and has not obtained a definitive diagnosis of epilepsy. Although it is possible that she has intractable epilepsy, it is also possible that she has PNES. Further EEG evaluation is necessary. A sleep-deprived EEG could be performed since sleep obtained on EEG will increase the probability of noting interictal epileptiform discharges. Likewise, evaluation in an epilepsy monitoring unit would also be appropriate in a patient with frequent events and normal routine EEG who is not responding to medication trials. Further increasing medications without a clear diagnosis is not ideal since this patient could have PNES. You should not assume the patient has PNES just because she has had a negative initial workup and has not responded to medication. Lastly, referring for epilepsy surgery is not appropriate without a definitive diagnosis.

Chapter 28

1. **E.** Parkinsonism plus apraxia or other asymmetric cortical signs is classic for corticobasal syndrome (CBS). The patient does not have the classic features of any of the other disorders. This vignette describes the classic alien limb phenomenon. Disproportionate lateralized atrophy on brain imaging can also be seen in CBS.

2. **B.** This is drug-induced parkinsonism from metoclopramide, which potently antagonizes central dopamine. Even without knowledge of the offending medication, parkinsonism that was symmetric at onset should be a clue because idiopathic Parkinson disease is nearly always unilateral at onset. There are no atypical features to suggest a Parkinson-plus disorder.

3. **D.** The patient has dopamine dysregulation syndrome, resulting in an impulse-control disorder. This phenomenon is a problematic side effect of the dopamine agonists, which include pramipexole, ropinirole, and rotigotine.

4. **A.** Young-onset dystonia with parkinsonism should prompt consideration of dopa-responsive dystonia, even with no family history. Because autosomal recessive mutations causing dopa-responsive dystonia are common, a positive family history may not be present. Huntington disease presenting at this young age would almost certainly have a positive family history and impairment of eye movements. If dopa-responsive dystonia is a consideration, the patient should undergo a trial of carbidopa/levodopa.

Chapter 29

1. **E.** Depression commonly presents with cognitive symptoms, especially in older people. Hypothyroidism and vitamin B_{12} deficiency are both reversible causes of cognitive impairment, and screening for these abnormalities is standard of care for a dementia evaluation.

2. **E.** Anticholinergics such as diphenhydramine are the drugs most commonly associated with adverse cognitive effects.

3. **D.** First-line treatment for Alzheimer disease is a centrally acting cholinesterase inhibitor. Memantine is indicated in later stages of the disease. Selective serotonin reuptake inhibitors can be used as adjuncts. There is no evidence for the effectiveness of *Ginkgo biloba*. Peripherally acting cholinesterase inhibitors would have no effect on cerebral function.

4. **D.** The ε4 polymorphism in *APOE* is the strongest genetic risk factor for late-onset Alzheimer disease (AD). Mutations in presenilin or amyloid precursor protein (*APP*) cause early-onset AD. *LRRK2* mutations cause Parkinson disease, and progranulin mutations cause frontotemporal dementia .

Chapter 30

1. **A.** Longitudinally extensive transverse myelitis is a hallmark of neuromyelitis optica and idiopathic transverse myelitis (TM). Multiple sclerosis–related TM is almost always shorter than 2 vertebral body heights in length.

2. **C.** A diagnosis of progressive MS according to the 2010 revised McDonald Criteria must include a history of 1 year of progressive myelopathy plus 2 of the following 3 findings: (1) brain MRI with 1 or more lesions typical of demyelination; (2) spinal MRI with 2 or more lesions typical of demyelination; and (3) spinal fluid with elevated IgG index or oligoclonal bands unique to the cerebrospinal fluid. Abnormal somatosensory evoked potentials would be further confirmation of spinal dysfunction but would not be sufficient to support a diagnosis of MS.

3. **C.** Postsynaptic acetylcholine receptors are bound by antagonist proteins, which results over time in the downregulation of the density of postsynaptic receptors for acetylcholine. This leads to rapid fatigue with muscle use.

Chapter 31

1. **A.** This patient has ocular myasthenia gravis. The underlying mechanism is antibody-mediated attack on the postsynaptic acetylcholine receptors. This is different from Lambert-Eaton syndrome, where the specific antibodies bind to the presynaptic voltage-gated calcium channels, as in choice B. The answer in choice C represents the case in botulism, where the botulinum toxin targets the synaptobrevin protein in the acetylcholine-containing vesicle membrane. In chronic inflammatory demyelinating polyradiculoneuropathy, the proposed mechanism is CD8 cytotoxic lymphocytes and monocytes attacking the myelinated nerve fibers (choice D). In polymyositis, major histocompatibility antigen complex-1 (MHC-1) is upregulated on the surface of muscle membrane, leading to activation of the CD8 cytotoxic lymphocytes (choice E).

2. **A.** This is a case of Guillain-Barré syndrome where the primary pathology is immune attack on myelinated peripheral nerves. Choice B represents the pathophysiology in diphtheria, where the specific toxin penetrates through the blood–nerve barrier. In vasculitic neuropathy, immune complex disposition occurs in the walls of epineurial arterioles and venules (choice C). Choice D represents the case in Charcot-Marie-Tooth disease, likely type 1A.

3. **D.** A common peroneal nerve injury is common at the level of the fibular neck, where the nerve is superficial and overlying the bone. It can happen in patients who have the habit of crossing their legs, especially in the setting of weight loss. The classic picture is weakness in ankle dorsiflexion (tibialis anterior) and eversion (peroneus longus and brevis) with loss of sensation over the dorsum of the foot. The ankle jerk is still preserved as it is mediated through the tibial nerve. With L5 radiculopathy, we expect weakness of the ankle inverters (tibialis posterior muscle) too. In cases of lumbosacral plexopathy, more patchy muscle weakness involving multiple proximal and distal lower limb muscles is expected with more diffuse sensory loss. Sciatic neuropathy could cause weakness of knee flexion and loss of all muscle movements below the knee. Tibial nerve injury is rare on its own and theoretically leads to weakness in ankle planter flexion (gastrocnemius and soleus) and inversion with loss of ankle jerk.

Chapter 32

1. **A.** Tabes dorsalis is a late complication of syphilis due to degeneration of posterior columns in the spinal cord. Symptoms include sensory disturbance as well as gait ataxia.

2. **E.** Arboviruses include West Nile virus, Japanese encephalitis, and St. Louis encephalitis. These require an insect vector for transmission. JC virus is not an arbovirus.

3. **B.** Multiple small calcified brain lesions are characteristic of neurocysticercosis and represent an inactive form of the parasite. Strokes in the basal ganglia are a common finding in CNS tuberculosis, or other infections causing vasculitis.

4. **C.** In North America, Lyme disease is transmitted by the deer tick, *Ixodes scapularis*.

Chapter 33

1. **B.** The patient described in the vignette would score a 3 for eye opening to voice and a 5 on the motor response subscale for localizing to pain. The description of his verbal response is consistent with a score of 3, for inappropriate words. Therefore, the total GCS score would be 11.

2. **A.** The patient's cerebral perfusion pressure is equal to her mean arterial pressure (58 mm Hg) minus her intracranial pressure (19 mm Hg), or 39 mm Hg.

3. **C.** To maintain adequate cerebral blood flow, it is important to maintain a cerebral perfusion pressure (CPP) >50 mm Hg. However, there is no evidence that raising the CPP >70 mm Hg is beneficial, and there is some concern that doing so may predispose patients to intracranial hypertension and/or worsening cerebral edema. Removing cerebrospinal fluid is unlikely to have any lasting effect on perfusion pressure. Steroids increase mortality in traumatic brain injury patients and therefore should not be used in this setting; hyperventilation causes cerebral vasoconstriction, as opposed to vasodilation, and would not be indicated in this scenario. Therefore, choice C is the most appropriate choice.

4. **A.** Central cord syndrome classically occurs in the setting of hyperextension injuries to the cervical spine, which is the scenario described in the vignette. It is typified by motor impairment that is disproportionately greater in the upper extremities than in the lower extremities. The exam is inconsistent with Brown-Sequard syndrome, which causes unilateral weakness, or with cauda equina syndrome, which affects only the lower extremities. Pseudotumor cerebri does not typically involve motor weakness, nor does it typically present following trauma.

Chapter 34

1. **B.** The symptoms this patient describes are excessive daytime sleepiness, hypnopompic hallucinations, sleep paralysis, and cataplexy. These are the 4 cardinal features of narcolepsy with cataplexy. The neurotransmitter that is deficient in the brains of these patients is orexin, which is normally localized in the lateral hypothalamus.

2. **D.** The patient describes episodes that are most consistent with rapid eye movement (REM) sleep behavior disorder. This is a condition that is characterized by the loss of normal atonia-producing mechanisms, leading to dream enactment behavior. Longitudinal studies following patients with this disorder demonstrate the later development of Parkinson disease and other α-synucleinopathies years after their sleep disorder manifests.

3. B. This patient describes symptoms that are very consistent with restless legs syndrome, or Willis-Ekbom disease. There are several conditions that can be associated with the emergence of this disorder, including iron deficiency, pregnancy, chronic kidney disease, and neuropathy.

4. C. K complexes and spindles are the 2 features on the EEG that define stage N2 sleep. Posterior occipital sharp transients can be seen during drowsiness and sleep onset. Delta activity dominates the EEG of stage N3 sleep, whereas the alpha rhythm is the pattern that characterizes wakefulness. Sawtooth waves are an EEG pattern occasionally seen in REM sleep but are not a defining characteristic.

Chapter 35

1. D. Proximal leg weakness, delayed walking, and toe walking in the context of normal cognitive development are indicative of a muscular dystrophy, most likely Duchenne muscular dystrophy. The first test to order in this scenario is a CK level, which is generally 10 to 30 times above average. After an elevated CK level has been verified, the diagnosis can be made with genetic testing.

2. C. A generalized seizure lasting <15 minutes in a neurologically normal child between the ages of 6 months and 6 years without symptoms concerning for meningitis is considered a simple febrile seizure and does not require further workup or management. Parental reassurance and seizure education are most important and appropriate.

3. B. The description of stagnation of verbal, language, and social skills; decelerated head growth; irritability; and stereotyped hand movements is typical of children with Rett syndrome, which is associated with a mutation in the *MECP2* gene. *FMR1* gene mutations cause Fragile X Syndrome, which is more common in males. *FXN* mutations cause Friedreich ataxia, a multisystem disorder without noteworthy cognitive impairment. Uniparental disomy on chromosome 15 causes Prader-Willi syndrome when both chromosomes are inherited from the mother or Angelman syndrome when both chromosomes are inherited from the father.

Chapter 36

1. A. The patient exhibits the classic phenomenon of head motion–triggered spells of vertigo that are typical of BPPV. Age is the major risk factor for BPPV. Spells are brief and are triggered by vertical head movements because they are due to the movement of otoliths that have fallen into the semicircular canal that migrate as the head is moved in relation to gravity.

2. B. This patient has eustachian tube dysfunction, with her major risk factor being recurrent childhood ear infections. She likely has patulous eustachian tubes (ie, tubes that stay persistently open). Thus, the sound and pressure from the nasopharynx are transmitted into the middle ear.

The patient may sniff or perform the Valsalva maneuver repeatedly in order to clear her ears.

3. D. This patient has otitis externa, inflammation of the external auditory canal. Although this is colloquially referred to as *swimmer's ear*, it can be seen in any condition where moisture gets trapped in the external auditory canal. Hearing aids and impacted cerumen are additional risk factors. Acute inflammation is associated with pain, redness, swelling, and fever. Chronic inflammation can lead to progressive stenosis of the canal.

Chapter 37

1. C. Time in a dark environment has likely caused the pupil to dilate slightly, which increases the chance for pupillary block. Once the pupillary block occurs, the aqueous humor is trapped in the posterior chamber and cannot pass to the anterior chamber. As additional aqueous humor is created, the iris will bulge forward (iris bombe), and appositional blockage of the trabecular meshwork will occur. This results in a sudden increase in intraocular pressure, which is painful and often causes nausea and emesis. In addition, the elevated pressure will cause fluid within the anterior chamber to be forced into the cornea, with resultant corneal edema. Lights will appear to have halos around them (often described as "rainbow colored") due to the prismatic effect that occurs. The pupil will often be stuck in a mid-dilated position. Treatment includes topical and oral intraocular pressure–lowering drops and possibly a laser peripheral iridotomy, which will create a hole in the iris and break the episode. If laser treatment is impossible, a surgical peripheral iridotomy may be necessary.

2. B. In the setting of a chronic sinus infection, a febrile patient with decreased vision, relative afferent pupillary defect, a red painful eye with eyelid involvement, restricted eye movement, and the absence of eyelid trauma or abrasion should prompt the suspicion of orbital cellulitis. This patient should be admitted for intravenous antibiotics and drainage of any periosteal abscess if found. Further, serial eye examinations should be completed to ensure that the patient is getting better.

3. A. Amaurosis fugax with visualization of a calcific Hollenhorst plaque should prompt concern for carotid occlusive disease because this is the most likely source of the emboli. Although the heart, heart valves, and aorta can also be sources of emboli, they are less common. You should order a carotid Doppler to determine whether atherosclerosis is present and to what degree.

Chapter 38

1. B. Use of cannabis, particularly during adolescence and in those with genetic susceptibility or family history of psychosis, is associated with a higher risk of schizophrenia.

2. **D.** Cognitive deficits are present in approximately 75% to 85% of schizophrenia patients and tend to emerge before positive symptoms. The extent of these deficits is most predictive of long-term outcome and social functioning.

3. **A.** Antipsychotic medications are most effective against the positive symptoms of schizophrenia, such as hallucinations and delusions, and less effective against the negative symptoms, such as blunted affect or the cognitive symptoms.

Chapter 39

1. **A.** When a patient presents with these toxicity symptoms, the level of lithium is likely >1.8 to 2.0 mEq/L; thus, hemodialysis is needed to save the patient's life.

2. **D.** Venlafaxine is a serotonin-norepinephrine reuptake inhibitor (SNRI). Although it may weakly affect dopamine at high doses, this is not generally considered its likely mechanism of action.

3. **A.** This patient meets the diagnostic criteria of major depressive disorder.

Chapter 40

1. **C.** The patient's symptoms are most consistent with generalized anxiety disorder. They have been ongoing for several years and include anxiety and worry associated with increased irritability (at home and work), difficulty concentrating, muscle tension, and difficulty sleeping. Substance-induced anxiety disorder would be a consideration given his access to drugs, but there is no mention of substance abuse or drug testing to confirm.

2. **B.** This medical student most likely suffers from a specific phobia—fear of blood (hemophobia). Treatment of choice for phobia is systematic desensitization. There is no evidence to support that the student has diabetes or hypoglycemia. Dialectal behavioral therapy is the treatment of choice for borderline personality disorder. SSRI pharmacotherapy would not be indicated for these symptoms. Phobias are treatable with therapy, and it would be best to encourage the student to seek treatment before entertaining ideas of changing professions.

3. **B.** Of the medications listed, prazosin is the treatment of choice to help with the patient's nightmares. There is no indication to change the SSRI from sertraline to fluoxetine as the patient reports improvement in symptoms with sertraline. Propranolol is indicated in the treatment of performance anxiety. No psychotic symptoms were described, and there is no indication to initiate an antipsychotic such as risperidone. Benzodiazepines such as alprazolam are not indicated in the treatment of posttraumatic stress disorder.

Chapter 41

1. **C.** This patient has neurologic symptoms and other somatic complaints, such as abdominal pain, so the best choice would be somatic symptom disorder. If tremor were the only symptom and the nonneurologic symptoms were absent, conversion disorder would be the better answer.

2. **B.** CBT has been shown to be most effective in treating somatic symptom and related disorders. The patient has no psychiatric symptoms, so antidepressants would not be the best choice for first-line treatment.

3. **C.** Mrs. H is exhibiting significant preoccupation with having an illness, despite relevant symptoms being mild. She is engaging in maladaptive behaviors related to this worry (eg, continued medical help seeking and excessive tracking of her symptoms). Mrs. H should be diagnosed with illness anxiety disorder.

4. **D.** Illness anxiety disorder is best treated using cognitive-behavioral therapy with exposure and response prevention. This can include imaginal exposure or in vivo exposure.

Chapter 42

1. **B.** The patient has no significant interest in developing long-term relationships, which is a long-term pattern of behavior for him and results in impaired social and occupational performance. The difference from schizotypal personality disorder, another Cluster A disorder, is that this patient has no desire for relationships and does not appear particularly unusual in terms of his demeanor and beliefs; those with schizotypal personality disorder may seek relationships, but their odd and eccentric behavior impairs their ability to form them. His impaired relationships are not due to suspicion or perceived threats from others, as in the other Cluster A disorder, paranoid personality disorder. The history is not consistent with antisocial personality disorder (Cluster B), which is characterized by a disregard for rules and unethical behavior; this patient does not seem to disregard the rights of others, but he just is not interested in having relationships with them. The history is also not consistent with avoidant personality disorder (Cluster C) because the patient is not avoiding relationships due to a fear of rejection or sense of inferiority.

2. **D.** The patient has a history of volatile emotional states, unstable relationships, episodes of intense anger and rage, and self-injurious behavior, all of which are typical of borderline personality disorder. She does not have the arrogance and grandiosity associated with narcissistic personality disorder or the history of attention-seeking provocative behavior and seductive appearance associated with histrionic personality disorder, other Cluster B diagnoses. She does not have the bizarre beliefs and peculiar

behavior and speech patterns typical of schizotypal personality disorder (Cluster A) or the passive, submissive nature or difficulty making decisions typical of dependent personality disorder (Cluster C).

3. **E.** Both dialectical behavioral therapy and psychodynamic psychotherapy have shown benefit for borderline personality disorder in randomized trials. Although pharmacotherapy can be used as an adjunct to therapy, neither first-generation neuroleptics nor polypharmacy would be an ideal choice.

Chapter 43

1. **D.** Cannabis is not a stimulant.

2. **A.** Alcohol use is associated with the strongest withdrawal symptoms, including delirium tremens, which requires medical treatment. Opioid use often requires long-term medical treatment with methadone or buprenorphine, but this involves medical treatment to treat the use disorder with a less problematic opioid, not for detoxification.

3. **D.** Naloxone and naltrexone are both opioid antagonists, but naltrexone is longer acting with a slower onset and thus is not suitable for treatment of acute intoxication, for which the more rapidly acting naloxone is the agent of choice.

4. **C.** Of the choices listed, caffeine has the most users. If the question had asked about use disorders instead of simply users, tobacco/nicotine would have the highest number, followed by alcohol. This highlights the different rates of developing use disorders; for example, those who experiment with cigarettes develop nicotine use disorder at about twice the rate that those who experiment with alcohol develop alcohol use disorder.

Chapter 44

1. **D.** The most effective treatment for ADHD is a stimulant such as methylphenidate or amphetamine. Fluoxetine is a selective serotonin reuptake inhibitor and is used for a variety of depressive and anxiety disorders. Clonidine is an α agonist that can be used to treat ADHD, but it is not the first-line treatment. Valproate is an antiepileptic drug that can be used to treat seizures or bipolar disorder in adolescents. Atomoxetine is a selective norepinephrine reuptake inhibitor that can also be used in ADHD but is not as effective as stimulants in most patients.

2. **C.** The onset of tic disorder is typically between age 4 and 6 years, and peak onset occurs between ages 10 and 12 years. Prevalence of tic disorder is higher in males. Symptoms of tic disorder wax and wane in severity and change in affected muscle groups and vocalizations over time. Many adults with tic disorders experience diminished symptoms in adulthood. Medication is recommended when tics result in significant subjective discomfort, pain, or ongoing social problems.

3. **B.** In children and adolescent, depression often presents as irritability rather than depressed mood.

Index

Note: Page numbers followed by *f* and *t* indicate figures and tables.